AF516653

3rd Edition

Compendium of Dermatology for Examinations

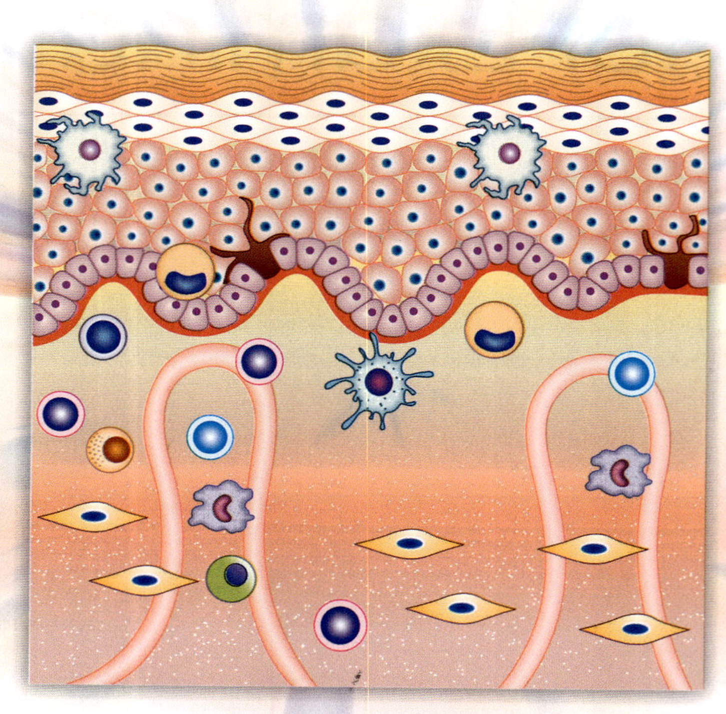

3rd Edition

Compendium of Dermatology for Examinations

Editors

Kabir Sardana MD DNB MNAMS
Director Professor and Head
Department of Dermatology and STD
Atal Bihari Vajpayee Institute of Medical Sciences and
Dr Ram Manohar Lohia Hospital, New Delhi
Former Professor
Department of Dermatology
Maulana Azad Medical College, New Delhi

Surabhi Sinha MD DNB MNAMS
Assistant Professor
Department of Dermatology and STD
Lady Hardinge Medical College and
Associated Hospitals
New Delhi

Seema Rani MD
Professor
Department of Dermatology and STD
Lady Hardinge Medical College and
Associated Hospitals
New Delhi

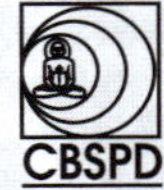

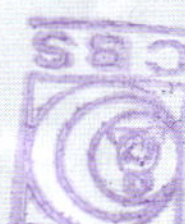

CBS Publishers & Distributors Pvt Ltd
New Delhi • Bengaluru • Chennai • Kochi • Kolkata • Lucknow • Mumbai
Hyderabad • Jharkhand • Nagpur • Patna • Pune • Uttarakhand

Disclaimer

Science and technology are constantly changing fields. New research and experience broaden the scope of information and knowledge. The editors have tried their best in giving information available to them while preparing the material for this book. Although all efforts have been made to ensure optimum accuracy of the material, yet it is quite possible some errors might have been left uncorrected. The publisher, the printer and the editors will not be held responsible for any inadvertent errors or inaccuracies.

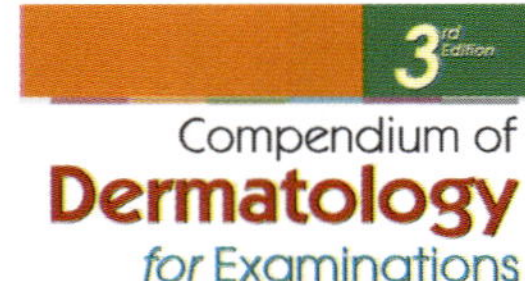

ISBN: 978-93-5466-689-6

Third Edition: 2024
First Edition: 2020
Second Edition: 2021

Published by Satish Kumar Jain and produced by Varun Jain for

CBS Publishers & Distributors Pvt Ltd
4819/XI Prahlad Street, 24 Ansari Road, Daryaganj, New Delhi 110 002, India
Ph: 011-23289259, 23266861 Website: www.cbspd.com
e-mail: delhi@cbspd.com

Corporate Office: 204 FIE, Industrial Area, Patparganj, Delhi 110 092, India
Ph: 011-4934 4934 Fax: 011-4934 4935 e-mail: publishing@cbspd.com; publicity@cbspd.com

Branches

- **Bengaluru:** Seema House 2975, 17th Cross, K.R. Road, Banasankari 2nd Stage, Bengaluru 560 070, Karnataka, India
  Ph: +91-80-26771678/79 Fax: +91-80-26771680 e-mail: bangalore@cbspd.com
- **Chennai:** 7, Subbaraya Street, Shenoy Nagar, Chennai 600 030, Tamil Nadu, India
  Ph: +91-44-26680620, 26681266 Fax: +91-44-42032115 e-mail: chennai@cbspd.com
- **Kochi:** 42/1325, 1326, Power House Road, Opp KSEB, Power House, Ernakulam, Kochi, 682 018, Kerala, India
  Ph: +91-484-4059061-65,67 Fax: +91-484-4059065 e-mail: kochi@cbspd.com
- **Kolkata:** 147, Hind Ceramics Compound, 1st Floor, Nilgunj Road, Belghoria, Kolkata 700 056, West Bengal, India
  Ph: +91-33-25633055/56 e-mail: kolkata@cbspd.com
- **Lucknow:** Basement, Khushnuma Complex, 7-Meerabai Marg (behind Jawahar Bhawan), Lucknow 226 001, UP, India
  Ph: +91-522-4000032 e-mail: tiwari.lucknow@cbspd.com
- **Mumbai:** PWD Shed, Gala no. 25/26, Ramchandra Bhatt Marg, Next to JJ Hospital Gate no. 2, Opp. Union Bank of India, Noorbaug, Mumbai 400 009, Maharashtra, India
  Ph: +91-22-66661880/89 e-mail: mumbai@cbspd.com

Representatives

- **Hyderabad** 0-9885175004 • **Jharkhand** 0-9811541605 • **Nagpur** 0-9421945513
- **Patna** 0-9334159340 • **Pune** 0-9923910676 • **Uttarakhand** 0-9716462459

Printed at: Magic International Pvt. Ltd. Greater Noida, UP, India

to

All the Doctors, Residents and HCW
who laid down their lives in the COVID Epidemic
and
Those who continue to Serve Humanity
God
My Parents, My Family
My Students, friends, Colleagues and Critics
To the trio who left no stone unturned to
destroy a career but forgot that destiny is
not made by mortals and life usually comes back full circle!

—Kabir Sardana

My Parents, whose prayers have given me all I have.
My husband, Dr Tarun Bhatnagar, for wholeheartedly partnering everything I choose to do.
My son, Rishit Bhatnagar, the most positive little being I know.
My teachers, past and present, for their sincere guidance.
Dermatology postgraduates everywhere.

—Surabhi Sinha

God—the Almighty
The important people in my life for their constant encouragement
during my professional career—my loving husband—Dr Kumar Ardhendu Shekhar,
my two wonderful sons Ishaan and Inesh
and
my Parents Mr Satish Prasad and
Mrs Meena Prasad for their enormous love and blessing.
All senior and junior colleagues of my department.

—Seema Rani

"Live Everything as it were"

"Don't search for the answers which could not be given to you now, because you would not be able to live them

And the point is to live everything. Live the questions now. Perhaps then, someday far into the future, you will gradually, without even noticing it, live your way into the answer."

—Rainer Maria Rilke, Letters to a Young Poet

Preface to the Third Edition

"There are only two mistakes one can make along the road to truth: not going all the way and not starting."

—Buddha

Dear readers

Thanks for the stupendous response to the first two editions which encouraged us to take out this edition. This book is not just aimed at postgraduates; it will be helpful for anyone interested in core dermatology, as we have retained the basic premise of gleaning data from books and journals by sitting and sifting through libraries—yes physically sitting in them! This book is a distillate of the top ranking books and journals in Dermatology.

What's new?

We have divided each topic into sections for easy readability and added numerous diagrams of pathogenesis and flowcharts of treatment. We have added chapters on acne, adverse drug reactions, atopic dermatitis and structure and function of skin. Also there is a chapter on Immunodermatology, which is essential for any student of dermatology. The existing chapters have been made more comprehensive with the addition of certain disorders that we felt were important for postgraduates. The chapter on dermatopathology has been made more exhaustive with addition of the basics of dermatopathology and numerous images with detailed descriptions have been added at the end of the book. Also an index of short and long cases has been given in the beginning. The layout is single column which will make it easy to read!

What we have not done?

No e-book or no PDF access, as of course it is a copyright issue when it is put in various online sites, but, more importantly, a good book is worth holding! Save your eyes, use the tablet for seeing movies, read this book as a physical copy!

What's even more exhaustive!

Special emphasis has been laid on STDs, leprosy and the latest updated data and recommendations have been incorporated. We daresay it is a great, quick and exhaustive text for these two topics and you may not need to see any other books for these topics. And yes, we have some new contributors to make it more complete and comprehensive.

Many topics are essential for theory exams and have been added throughout the book.

And now what can the PG hope for?

Well, if you have an examiner who wants to know what you know—We assure you the book will help you across all examinations: State, national or board levels. Of course, if you have an examiner who wants to know what you do not know, well, then this is not the book to read! And do not ask us which book to read in that scenario, as there is none actually! Luckily such examiners are rare nowadays!

We are thankful to Mr SK Jain CMD, Mr Varun Jain Director, Mr YN Arjuna Senior Vice President—Publishing, Editorial and Publicity, Mrs Ritu Chawla GM—Production and Mr SK Verma Vice President—Marketing and Operations. Here we must acknowledge the effort of the great team of CBS, with a special thanks to the diligence and perseverance of the dedicated reformatting by Mr Vikrant Sharma (DTP Operator), Mr Neeraj Prasad (Cover Artist), Mrs Baljeet Kaur (Graphic Designer) and Mr Dinesh Chandra Gupta (Senior Editor).

To all readers, postgraduates, board examinees, institutional faculty and practitioners, we assure that there may be more topics beyond this book in dermatology, but what is in it, is rigorously sourced and scientifically vetted from the best literature available!

A video is given in the QR code below that gives an overview of the MD dermatology examination.

Happy reading!

Editors

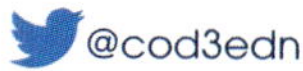

Approach the MD Dermatology Examination

Preface to the First Edition

Intelligence is the ability to adapt to change. **—Stephen Hawking**

Many years back when I was a PG, my Guide and Head Dr RC Sharma, used to say that for every case you see in the OPD go back and read the case and the differentials and in one year you would have learned dermatology! With 4 volumes of Rook's that seemed impossible! It was many years later that I realized that in the days when my Head passed dermatology Rook's had only 2 volumes! Rook's gave way to Fitzpatrick and then Bolognia and the volumes have been replaced by iPads which I find impossible to comprehend, as nothing beats the good old book and the feeling of marking them—though our PGs would disagree!

Nevertheless the focus nowadays unfortunately is on cosmetology—for which an MD degree is probably becoming a stepping stone—and the PG is just keen to pass the examinations. For this kind of audience there are two kinds of books: The first is based on questions and answers where the questions are probably dictated by the examiner and writers of the book and are the individual's personal views and not necessarily always asked in examinations. I feel such books are a waste and are of a little use as "your answer may not be my answer"! And also the knowledge is "person" based and not "text" based. The second is the textbooks, great but impossible to finish in 3 years time, especially in the rapidly changing dermatology world with conferences and workshops constantly bombarding us with more cosmetology information!

Postgraduate dermatology examinations are a test of not only just theoretical knowledge but also of practical skills and updated information. Most dermatology textbooks provide elaborate and extensive knowledge, but are not very exam-friendly! Nor are they "carrier friendly" and can easily cause a sprain or dislocation!

Thus this book is based on two premises—one to cover the topics covered in the practical dermatology examinations and two a book that is not based on our views—but a summary of the data from the standard textbooks—hence each line is from a textbook. Plus, we have added, data from published review articles as and when required. Prolific diagrams hand-drawn by an artist have been added for full body representations of uncommon disorders—classically genodermatoses. Spotters (short cases) and long cases are presented in a reader-friendly manner, with numerous flowcharts and pictures to aid quick grasp and retention of the matter. Special emphasis has been laid on STDs and leprosy and the latest updated data and recommendations have been incorporated. Tables have been added wherever possible for a quick look before the examinations.

The book is an effort of some amazingly talented contributors and the great team of CBS, which includes the data entry Mr Tarun Rajput and artist Mr Ram Murti, Readers Mr Prasenjit Paul and Mohanty, Mrs Ritu Chawla, Mr YN Arjuna, Mr SK Verma, Mr Varun Jain and Mr SK Jain.

I hope this book serves as a useful ready reckoner for postgraduates and I am confident that this book will serve them well beyond their resident years!

Kabir Sardana

https://www.facebook.com/2019TheCompendium-334891597202026

Life's Philosophy in Three Paragraphs

"You can't skip chapters, that's not how life works. You have to read every line, meet every character. You won't enjoy all of it. Hell, some chapters will make you cry for weeks. You will read things you don't want to read, you will have moments when you don't want the pages to end. But you have to keep going. Stories keep the world revolving. Live yours, don't miss out."

—Pillow Thoughts II

At the end the understated truth determines most things in life and is learnt sooner or later—

We get that which we are meant to get
Even the Gods cannot change that
And so I do not despair
Nor am I Surprised at loss or gain
That which is mine will be mine
No Other can take it away

—Panchatantra

Honor and disgrace both surprise us.
Great esteem brings trouble
because one is bound to
their own sense of self-importance.
This is why honor and disgrace surprise us.
Gaining praise makes one fall–
To receive it feels like fear.
This is why honor and disgrace surprise us.
Trouble is caused
by a strong sense of self.
Without a sense of self,
what can trouble you?
Therefore, if one treasures themselves
by servicing others,
One is able to hold the world in her hands.

—Tao Te Chung

List of Contributors

Aastha Agarwal
MBBS MD (Dermatology) DNB MRCP SCE
Senior Resident
Deen Dayal Upadhyay Hospital, New Delhi

Ananta Khurana MD DNB MNAMS FRCP (London)
Professor, Department of Dermatology
ABVIMS and Dr RML Hospital
New Delhi

Bhavya Sangal MD DNB MNAMS
Assistant Professor, Department of Dermatology
Government Doon Medical College
Dehradun

Bhawuk Dhir MD DNB MNAMS MRCP (SCE)
Senior Resident, Department of Dermatology
ABVIMS and Dr RML Hospital
New Delhi

Geeti Khullar MD DNB MNAMS
Assistant Professor
Department of Dermatology
LHMC and Associated Hospitals, New Delhi

Kabir Sardana MD DNB MNAMS
Director Professor and Head
Department of Dermatology
ABVIMS and Dr RML Hospital, New Delhi

Kumari Ritu
Postgraduate Resident
Department of Dermatology
ABVIMS and Dr RML Hospital, New Delhi

Pooja Arora Mrig MD DNB MNAMS
Professor, Department of Dermatology
ABVIMS and Dr RML Hospital, New Delhi

Purnima Paliwal MD
Specialist, Department of Pathology
ABVIMS and Dr RML Hospital, New Delhi

Rahul Mahajan MD MNAMS FRCP (Edinburgh)
Associate Professor
PGIMER, Chandigarh

Seema Rani MD
Professor
Department of Dermatology
LHMC and Associated Hospitals, New Delhi

Sinu Rose Mathachan MD DNB MNAMS
Senior Resident
Department of Dermatology
ABVIMS and Dr RML Hospital, New Delhi

Snigdha Saxena MD MRCP (SCE)
Consultant Dermatologist
Nav Imperial Hospital, Jaipur, Rajasthan

Sumitra Meena
Postgraduate Resident
Department of Dermatology
ABVIMS and Dr RML Hospital
New Delhi

Surabhi Sinha MD DNB MNAMS
Assistant Professor
Department of Dermatology
LHMC and Associated Hospitals, New Delhi

Sweta Singh MD DNB MNAMS
Consultant Dermatologist
Max Smart Super Speciality Hospital
Saket, New Delhi

Image Contributors

Dr Aditi Gupta
Dr Ananta Khurana
Dr Balachandra Ankad
Dr Chanchal Singh
Dr Deepak Jakhar
Dr Mala Bhalla
Dr Prashant Jakhmola
Dr Rakhi Ghodge
Dr R Madhu
Dr Roberto Arenas

Contents

Long and Short Cases

Long Cases

Short Cases

Fundamentals of Dermatology

Kabir Sardana

STRUCTURE AND FUNCTION OF SKIN

The skin is the interface between humans and their environment. It weighs an average of 4 kg and covers an area of 2 m^2. It acts as a barrier, protecting the body from harsh external conditions and preventing the loss of important body constituents, especially water.

The aim of this section is to dwell on the salient aspects of the skin and its applied functions.

Embryology

- Skin is composed of cells from different lineages:
  - Ectodermal: Keratinocytes, melanocytes, Merkel cells, neurons
  - Mesodermal: Fibroblasts, Langerhans cells, endothelial cells
- Epidermis
  - Development milestones
    - 5 weeks: Outer periderm and inner basal epidermal layer
    - 8 weeks: Stratification of embryonic epidermis
    - 12 weeks: Terminal differentiation of keratinizing epidermal cells
    - 12–16 weeks: Epidermal melanin production
    - 15 weeks: Early cornification within hair canal
    - 20 weeks: Melanosome transfer to keratinocytes
    - 22–24 weeks: Cornification in interfollicular epidermis (head → palms, soles)
    - 24–26 weeks: Cornified cell layer formation
    - 30–34 weeks: Epidermis similar to adult skin
    - Full skin barrier function at 3 weeks postpartum
  - Epidermal cells
    - 9–12 weeks: Melanocytes, Langerhans cells and Merkel cells migrate into epidermis.
- Adnexal structures
  - Hair follicle
    - 12–14 weeks: Hair peg is formed
    - 14–20 weeks: Concentric layers of hair follicles undergo maturation

- 18–21 weeks: Hair canal fully formed
- 24–28 weeks: Hairs continue to grow

– Nail
  - 8–10 weeks: Fingernail development begins
  - 11 weeks: Nail bed keratinizes
  - 13 weeks: Proximal nail fold develops
  - 20 weeks: Development complete

– Sebaceous glands—development parallels follicular development
  - 13–16 weeks: Develop as superficial bulge on developing hair follicle.

EPIDERMIS

The epidermis is composed of multiple layers of cells known as Keratinocytes **(Fig. 1)**.

Keratinocytes

- Ectodermal is derived during the first few weeks of embryonic development
- Composed of intermediate filaments (IF), the predominant IF being keratin. There are 54 functional keratins (37 epithelial and 17 hair keratins): 40–70 kDa.

Types of Keratins

a. **Acidic keratins:** Keratin 9 (K9)-K20, chromosome 17
b. **Basic keratins:** K1–K8, chromosome 12

Keratinocytes also have other Intermediate filaments as listed in the **Table 1**.

The acidic and basic keratin are paired together. Important keratins and their defects are listed below in **Table 2**. A schematic diagram of the main pairs is depicted in **Fig. 2**.

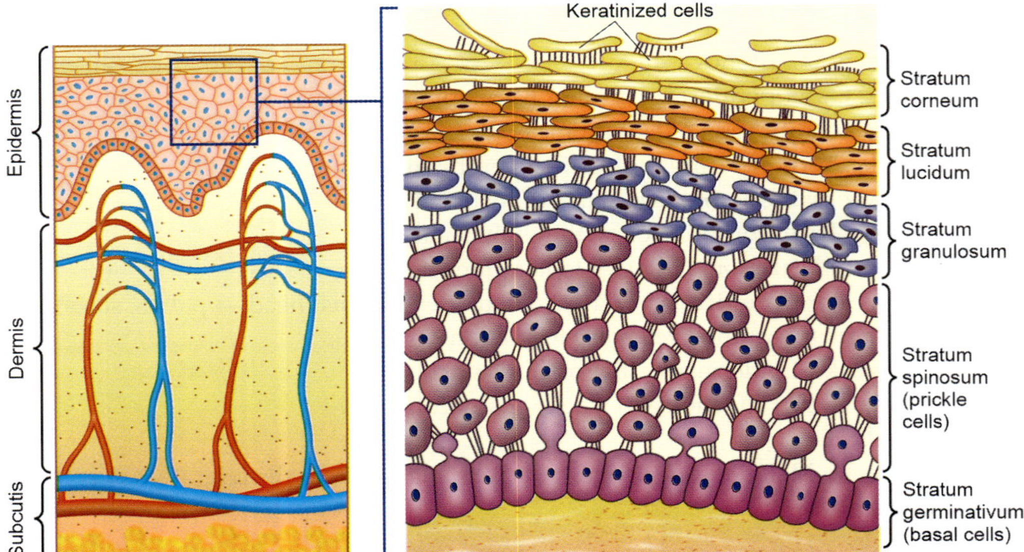

Fig. 1: A depiction of the layers of the skin with the various layers of the epidermis depicted on the right

TABLE 1: Types of intermediate filaments in epidermis

Type I	Type II	Type III	Type IV	Type V	Type VI	Others (Unclassified)
Keratins 9–20	Keratins 1–8	Vimentin	NF-L, NF-H	Lamin A/C	Nestin	Filensin
20 (acidic)	8 (basic)	Desmin	NF-M	Lamin B1		Phakinin
		GFAP	α-Intermexin	Lamin B2		
		Peripherin	Syncoilin			
			Synemin			

TABLE 2: Keratin expression patterns and disease associations

Type II	Type I	Location	Hereditary disease association
K1	—	Suprabasal keratinocytes	Ichthyosis hystrix of Curth-Macklin Diffuse nonepidermolytic PPK (Unna-Thost)
K1	K10	Suprabasal keratinocytes	Bullous congenital ichthyosiform erythroderma, EHK (corrugated scale)
K1	K9	Palmoplantar suprabasilar keratinocytes	Epidermolytic PPK, diffuse nonepidermolytic PPK
K2e	K10	Upper spinous and granular layers	Ichthyosis bullosa of Siemens (milder EHK)
K3	K12	Cornea	Meesmann's corneal dystrophy
K4	K13	Mucosal epithelium	White sponge nevus (Cannon): Buccal
K5	K14	Basal keratinocytes	Epidermolysis bullosa simplex 1. Dowlin–Meara (head or tail of central rod domain) 2. Koebner (segment 1a or 2b of rod domain) 3. Weber–Cockayne (nonhelical parts)
K5	K15	Mucosal basal layer	
K6a	K16	Outer root sheath, hyperproliferative keratinocytes	Pachyonchia congenita type I (Jadassohn–Lewandowsky), focal nonepidermolytic PPK
K6b	K17	Nail bed	Pachyonychia congenita type II, steatocystoma multiplex (Jackson–Lawler)
K8	K18	Simple epithelium	Cryptogenic cirrhosis
hHb1	—	Hair follicle	Monilethrix
hHb6	—		
—	K19	Bulge cells and simple epithelium	Paget's: CK7, KC20 are other markers
—	K20	Basal layer of epidermis	Merkel cell carcinoma
K1	K16		Nonepidermolytic PPK
—	K17		Steatocystoma multiplex
K5	—		EBS mottled pigmentation (nonhelical V_1 domain)
—	K14		EBS (autosomal recessive)
—	K14		Naegeli–Franceschetti–Jadassohn syndrome/ dermatopathia pigmentosa reticularis

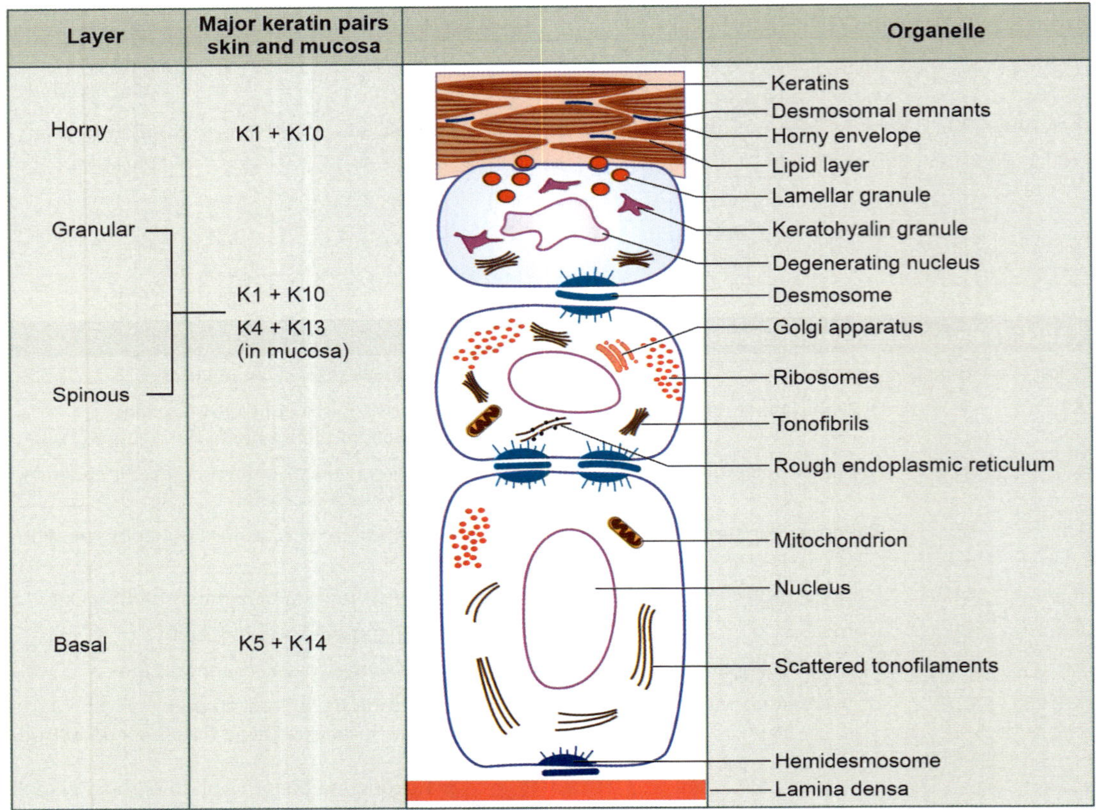

Fig. 2: A depiction of the salient Keratin pairs in the layers of the epidermis

Stratum Corneum (SC)

- Provides mechanical protection, barrier to water loss, and to permeation of environmental soluble substances.
- Consists of keratin in **filaggrin-rich** matrix.
- Normal SC cells have no nuclei; nuclei may persist in incompletely keratinized cells (parakeratosis).
- "Bricks and mortar" model: Corneocytes (bricks) and extacellular lipid matrix (from loricrin)/lamellar lipid barrier (mortar).

Stratum Granulosum

- The keratohyalin granules contain **profilaggrin** and **loricrin**, which form the cornified cell envelope.
- **Cornified cell envelope (CE):** Composed of proteins synthesized in spinous/granular layers and have various components including envoplakin, involucrin and loricrin.
- **Filaggrin:** This is a histidine rich; filament-aggregating component of keratohyalin granules and it is defective in ichthyosis vulgaris and AD. Profilaggrin is converted to monomeric

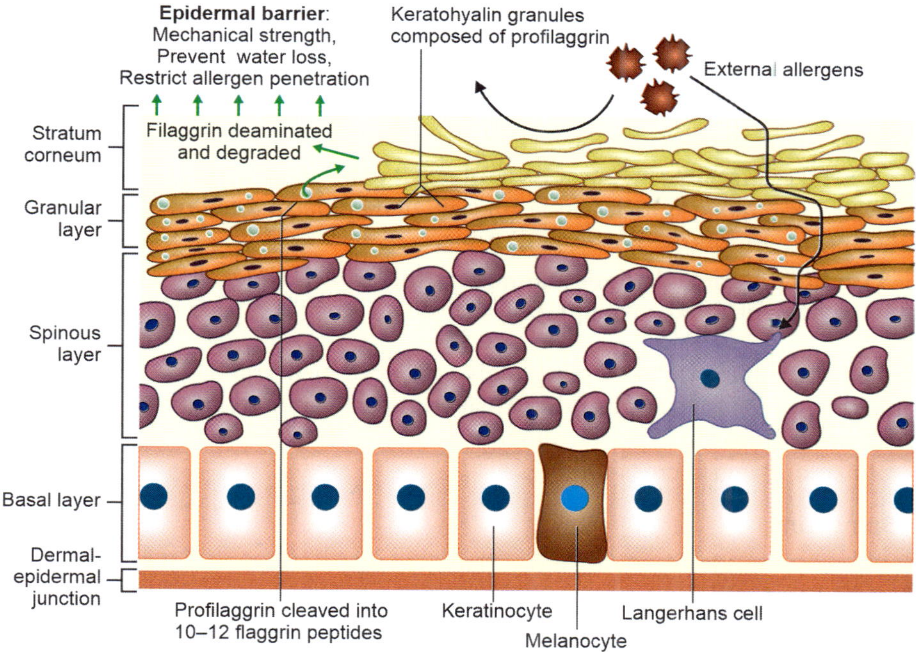

Fig. 3: Role of filaggrin in formation of cornified envelope (CE). In the granular layer, profilaggrin is cleaved into filaggrin peptides and its subsequent deamination and degradation products provides the skin with mechanical strength and restricts transepidermal water loss as it produces natural moisturizing factors. Filaggrin also prevents allergen penetration

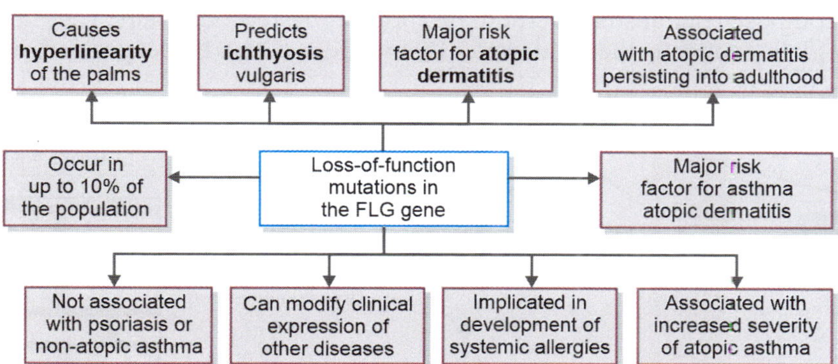

Fig. 4: Various disorders that arise from mutation in the *FLG* gene

filaggrin subunits when granular layer is transformed to cornified layer and this is a calcium-dependent process. This is believed to promote aggregation and disulfide bonding of keratin filaments in cornified cells (like a glue). It is degraded into urocanic acid and pyrrolidone carboxylic acid which form natural moisturizing factor (NMF) and hydrate stratum corneum and block UV radiation **(Fig. 3)**. The various disorders caused by loss of function of filaggrin are depicted in **Fig. 4**.

- **Transglutaminase (TG):** This helps in cross-linking the cornified envelope (calcium-dependent process). Three types:
  a. **TG-1:** Keratinocyte transglutaminase, membrane associated, defect causes lamellar ichthyosis type I (TGM1 gene) and nonbullous congenital ichthyosiform erythroderma (TGM1 +ALOX12B + ALOXE3)
  b. **TG-2:** Fetal epidermis and basal layer of adult epidermis
  c. **TG-3:** Present in hair follicles and differentiated epidermal cells. In sublamina densa, it is the antigen for dermatitis herpetiformis.

The process of **Epidermal differentiation/keratinization** is triggered by calcium and results in formation of the cornified envelope, and the salient steps are listed below and depicted in **Fig. 5**.

a. Cross-linking of envoplakin, periplakin, along cell membrane
b. Lamellar granule formation and extrusion into extracellular space
c. Loricrin cross-linking of the envelope
d. Keratin and filaggrin cross-linking.

Stratum Spinosum

- The cells have rounder nucleus, more flattened appearance and they contain lamellar granules (Odland bodies).
- Lamellar granules contain ceramides.
- They express K5/K14 and this changes to K1/K10 which is indicative of keratinization.
- Hyperproliferative markers are: K6, K16, Ki–67.
- In **psoriasis**, **actinic keratoses**, and **wound healing**, suprabasilar keratinocytes downregulate K1/K10 and there is ↑ K6/K16.
- This layer has **desmosomes** which are complex structures and hold cells together **(Fig. 6)**. They are composed of transmembranous desmoglein-desmocollin pairs. There are four types of desmoglein found in the epidermis. Desmoglein (Dsg) 1 is expressed in the upper

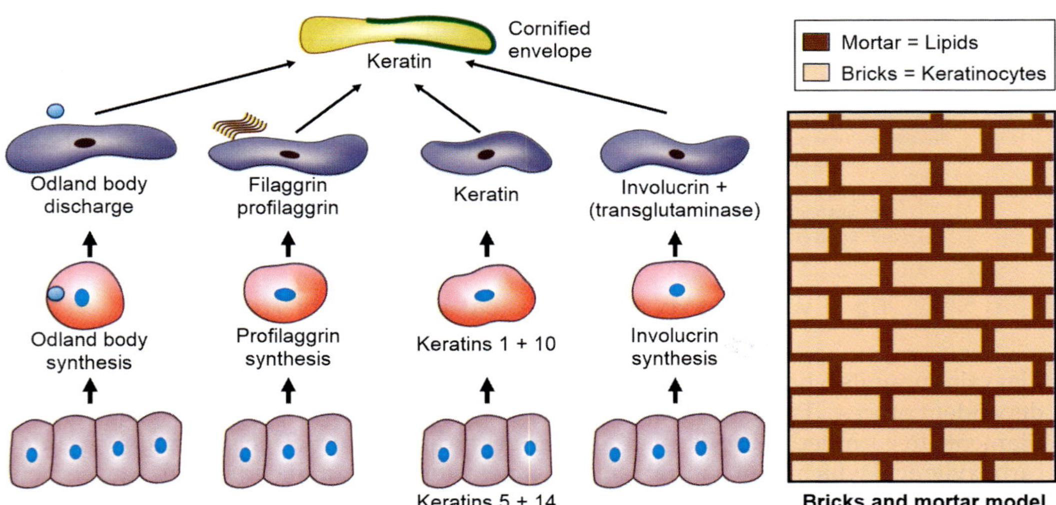

Fig. 5: A depiction of the various steps of keratinization

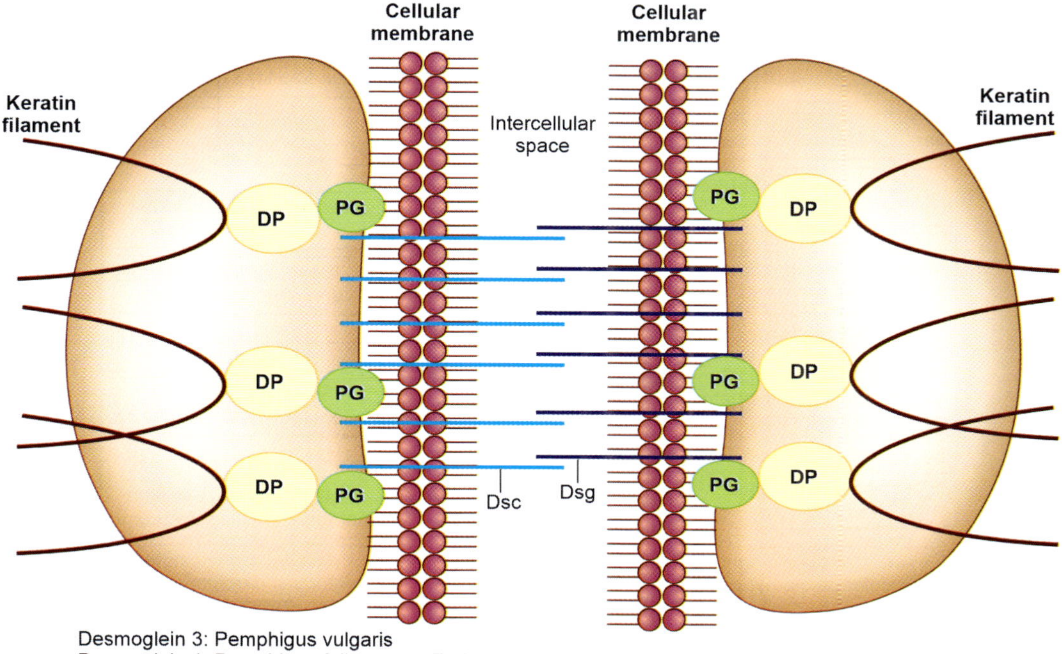

Fig. 6: Structure of desmosomes. They are composed of desmoplakin (DP) and plakoglobins (PG), and the former binds to keratin filaments in the keratinocytes adding to the epidermal integrity. The desmosomal cadherins desmocollin (Dsc) and desmoglein (Dsg) anchor two neighboring cells

epidermis while Dsg 3 is mostly expressed in the basal epidermis. A depiction of the various disorders affecting the components of desmosomes is depicted in **Fig. 7**.

- **Gap junctions** are more abundant in stratum spinosum compared with stratum basale. The common disorders in which these are involved are listed in **Table 3**.
- **Lamellar granules "Odland bodies"**: They are membrane-bound intracellular structures, 0.2–0.3 µm in diameter and are responsible for forming ceramide which is the major lipid for barrier function of the skin. They are seen in upper stratum spinosum and stratum granulosum, but their primary activity is in the stratum corneum. They discharge their contents into the extracellular space at the junction of the granular and horny layers, establishing a barrier to water loss, and alongwith filaggrin, mediate stratum corneum adhesion. They secrete glycoproteins, glycolipids, phospholipids, free sterols, and glucosylceramides (predominant lipid of stratum corneum).

TABLE 3: List of disorders affecting gap junctions

Connexin 26	Vohwinkel's syndrome, keratitis-ichthyosis-deafness (KID) syndrome, palmoplantar keratoderma (PPK) with deafness
Connexins 30.3 and 31	Erythrokeratodermia variabilis
Connexin 30	Hidrotic ectodermal dysplasia

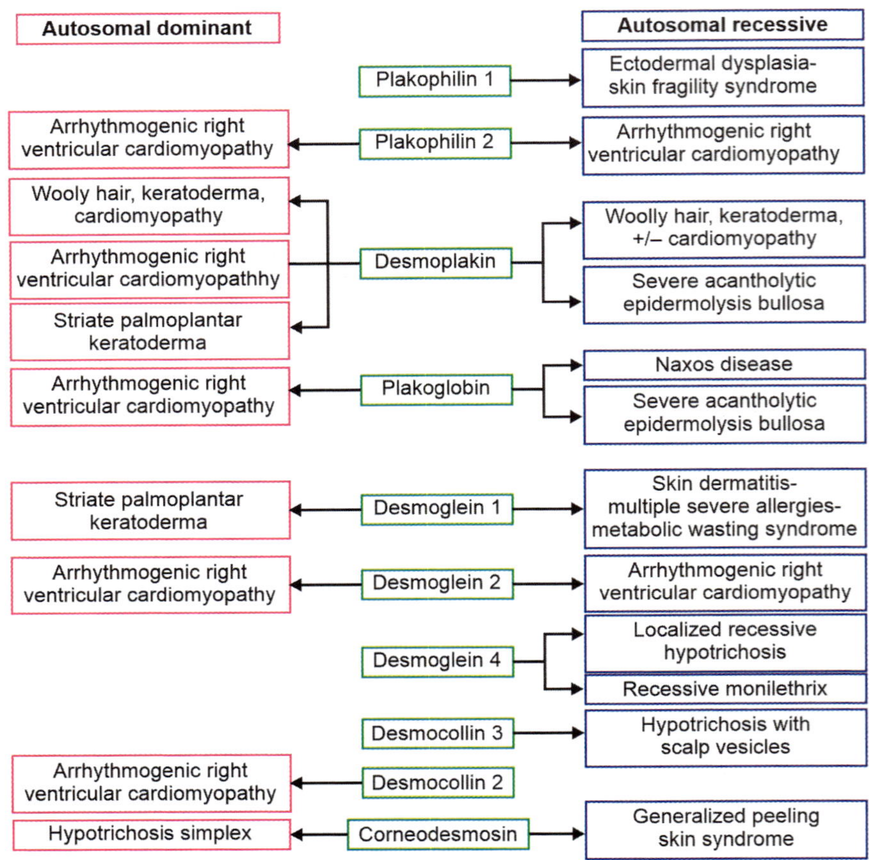

Fig. 7: An overview of disorders caused by defects in the components of desmososmes

Affected in

a. Flegel's disease: Decreased lamellar granules.
b. Harlequin ichthyosis: Lamellar granules uniformly abnormal or absent. Defect in ABCA12 at 2q34 (also defective in lamellar ichthyosis type II).
c. X-linked ichthyosis: Steroid sulfatase missing in lamellar granules.

Stratum Germinativum (Basale)

- The basal cells contain ornithine decarboxylase (marker of proliferative activity); **stimulated** by trauma, UV, epidermal growth factor (EGF), estrogens, β-agonists, tumor promoters; **Inhibited** by retinoids.
- It expresses **K5** and **K14**
- Microfilaments (actin, myosin, and α-actinin) assist in upward movement of cells as they differentiate.

The term "**Malpighian layer**" includes both stratum basale and stratum spinosum.

BASEMENT MEMBRANE ZONE

This is composed of the hemidesmosome-anchoring filament-anchoring fibril complex at the dermal-epidermal junction **(Fig. 8)**. It serves as an important structure for attachment of cells, template for tissue repair, influences differentiation, morphogenesis, and apoptosis of epithelial cells.

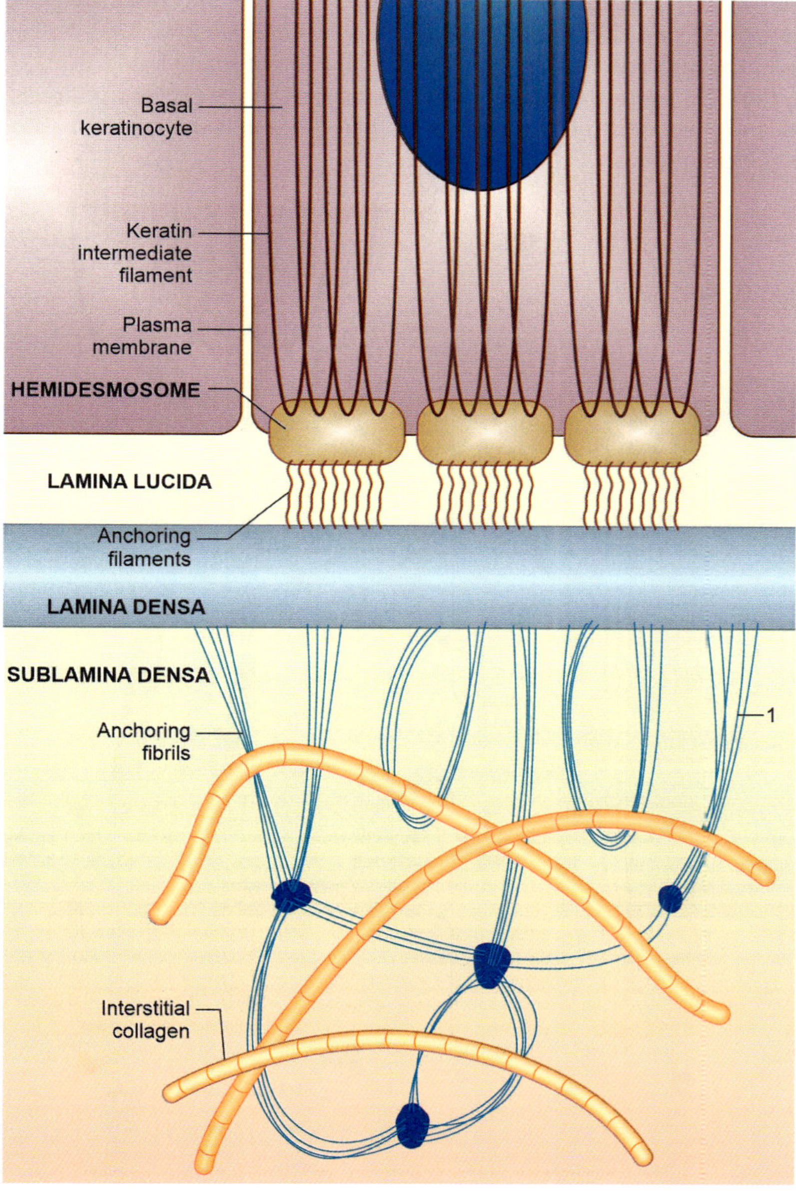

Fig. 8: A depiction of the various components of the BMZ

Four major ultrastructural subregions: basal keratinocyte, lamina lucida, lamina densa, and sublamina densa **(Fig. 8)**.

a. **Basal keratinocyte:** Hemidesmosome is the adhesion complex that attaches basal keratinocyte to extracellular matrix. The inner plaque attaches to the keratin filaments while the outer plaque is attached to anchoring filaments that traverse the lamina lucida **(Fig. 9)** to attach to the lamina densa.

   Hemidesmosome plaque consists of plectin, BP230, BP180, and integrins.

   - **BPAg1: 230-kDa protein** (desmoplakin), Intracellular, at attachment plaque, Attaches intermediate filaments (keratins) to hemidesmosomal plaque.
   - **BPAg2: 180-kDa protein (collagen XVII)** Transmembrane protein, interacts with BPAg1, integrin, and plectin intracellularly; Its NC16A domain is the target of autoantibodies in bullous pemphigoid.

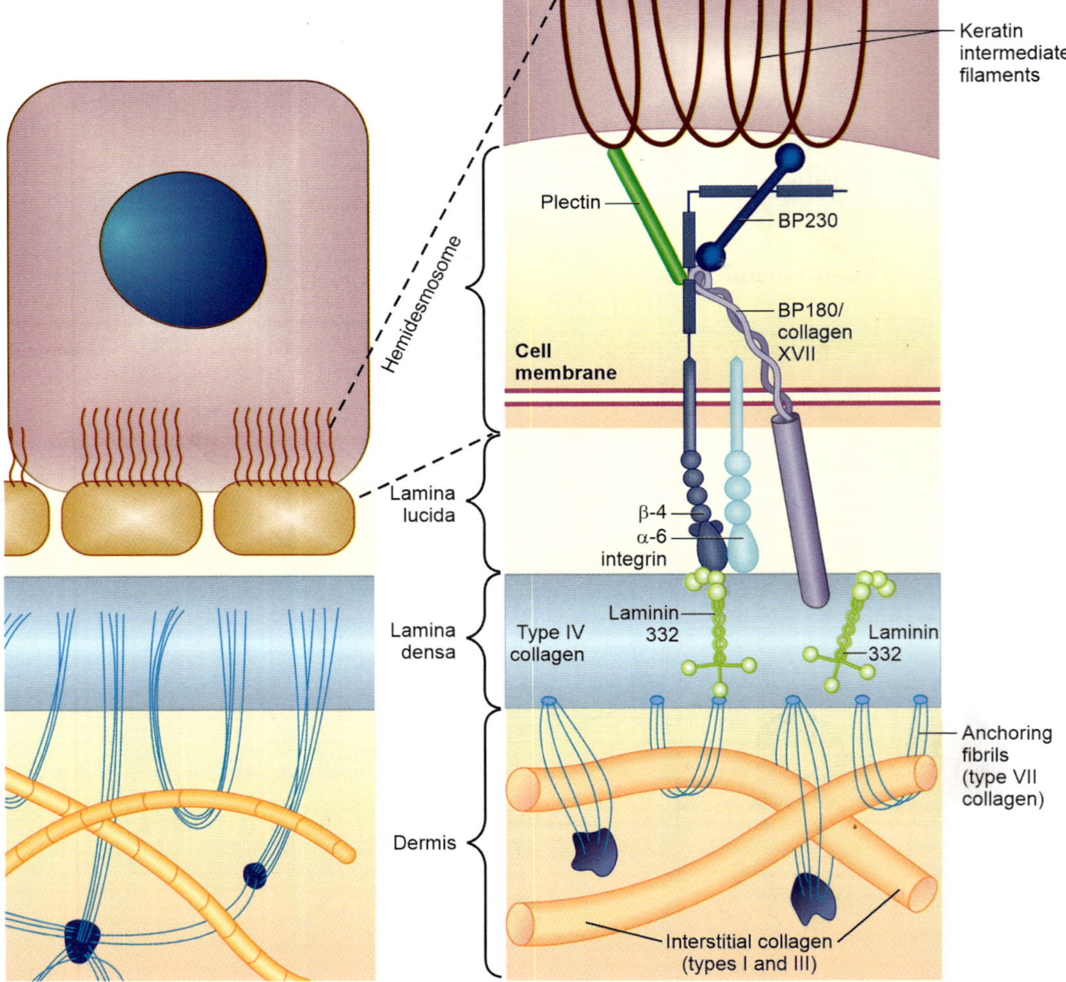

Fig. 9: Molecular structure of the components of the BMZ

TABLE 4: Disease associations of molecular structures of BMZ

BPAg1/BPAg2-NC16A BPAg2	Bullous pemphigoid Generalized atrophic benign EB
Plectin	EBS with muscular dystrophy, PNP
K5, K14	EBS Dowling-Meara
α6β4-Integrin	• JEB with pyloric atresia • α4-integrin ocular CP
Laminin 332	JEB, CP with increased risk of cancer (anti-Lam332 autoantibodies, previously termed anti-laminin 5 or anti-epiligrin MMP)
Type VII collagen	Epidermolysis bullosa acquisita and bullous lupus erythematosus, dominant and recessive DEB

b. **Lamina lucida:** Electron lucent region. It has the anchoring **filaments** that consist of laminins, BP180, and nidogen (connects hemidesmosomal plaque to lamina densa) and integrins. The major laminin is the laminin 332 **(Fig. 9)**.

c. **Lamina densa:** Contains laminins, type **IV collagen** (triple helical structure Gly-X-Y), nidogen, and heparin sulfate proteoglycans (perlacan is prototype) **(Fig. 9)**.

d. **Sublamina densa:** Anchoring fibrils consist of **collagen VII**, which binds types I and IV collagen, laminin 332, microfibrils (composed of desmosine, isodesmosine) and microthread like fibers **(Fig. 9)**.

The clinical relevance of various parts of BMZ is listed in **Table 4** and is also depicted in **Fig. 9**.

CELLS

Melanocytes

- Derived from neural crest cells. The progenitor cells are derived from 2 sources—formed along the dorsal neural tube and migrate via dorsolateral then ventral pathway AND from Schwann cell/melanocyte precursor cells that migrate along nerves to skin via ventral pathway.
- KIT receptor activation is required for melanocyte development/migration.
  - KIT ligand (aka steel factor or stem cell growth factor)
  - KIT mutation responsible for piebaldism
- Located in basal layer: Interface via cadherins in 1:10 ratio with keratinocytes in basal layer, 1 melanocyte distributes melanin to 30–40 surrounding keratinocytes, forming the **epidermal melanin unit**.
- Melanosomes (lysosomal organelles) produce melanin, which is in turn transported to neighboring keratinocytes via dendritic processes.
  - Tyrosine → DOPA → DOPAquinone → pheomelanin/eumelanin
  - First two steps require tyrosinase (Cu-dependent enzyme)

  Two types of pigment are formed:
  - Pheomelanin: yellow/red, made by round melanosomes
  - Eumelanin: black/brown, made by elliptical melanosomes.

  Major determinant of skin color is activity of melanocytes and not their density.

- Melanin production is induced by MSH and ACTH activity on melanocortin 1 receptor (MC1-R) on the melanocytes. Eumelanin is synthesized at the expense of pheomelanin following activation of the MC1R.
  - MC1-R mutation is responsible for red hair/fair skin phenotype, ↑ risk of melanoma, ↑ pheomelanin: eumelanin ratio.

Langerhans Cells

Dendritic cells responsible for immune surveillance (APC of skin) found in stratum spinosum, constitute 3–5% cells

- Express langerin (CD207), CD45, CD1a, S100, CD34, vimentin, actin.
- After processing antigen, they migrate to lymph nodes to activate T cells.
- Contain reniform nuclei with characteristic Birbeck granules (tennis racket-shaped) seen on electron microscopy.

Merkel Cells

- Epidermal lineage neuroendocrine cells involved in mechanoreception.
- Express CK20 in perinuclear dot pattern, S100, synaptophysin, chromogranin, neuron-specific enolase.
- Found in fingertips, lips, oral cavity, hair follicle ORS.

Epithelial Stem Cells

- Lineage-specific cells that can multiply and differentiate to mediate epidermal renewal/turnover. They are found within the interfollicular epidermis, base of sebaceous glands and bulge area of hair follicles.
- Keratinocyte stem cells: Express markers such as delta 1, MCSP, α6-and β1-integrins, LRIG1; low levels of CD71.
- Melanocyte stem cells: Express markers such as ax3, TYRP1, TYRP2; negative for KIT, tyrosinase.
- Hair follicle stem cells: Express markers such as SOX9, keratin 15, α6-and β1-integrins, CD200, PHLDA1, follistatin, frizzled homolog 1, LGR5; low levels of CD24, CD34, CD71, CD146.
- Merkel cell stem cells: Express markers such as α6-integrin, keratin 17, ATOH1, CD200, GLI1, SOX2.

Mononuclear Phagocytic Cells

- Monocytes, macrophages, and dermal dendrocytes from bone marrow.
- All phagocytic skin macrophages express integrins that play a role in phagocytosis, cell adherence and migration-CD6; CR4 (CD11c).

Mast Cells

- Greatest density in the papillary dermis, in sheaths of the appendages, and around blood vessels and nerves of the subpapillary plexus.
- Diseases: Mastocytosis, solitary mastocytoma, diffuse erythrodermic mastocytosis, telangiectasia macularis eruptiva perstans (TMEP), urticaria pigmentosa.
- Derived from bone marrow CD34 + stem cells.

- Proliferation depends on the c-Kit receptor and its ligand stem-cell factor (SCF). Mutations in c-Kit (CD117) may result in mastocytosis or piebaldism.
- Stain cells for CD34, c-Kit, SCF or with Giemsa, Teledyne, Leder stain (naphthol chloroacetate esterase.

HAIR

Embryogenesis

- Hair follicle development happens only once during skin development.
- 100,000 scalp hair follicles.
- Hair bulb resides in subcutis in terminal follicles, situated at oblique angle to epidermal surface.
- **Follicular unit:** 2–4 terminal and 1–2 vellus hair follicles that share arrector pili muscle (12–14 follicular units in 4 mm punch biopsy).
- **Infants:** Lanugo hair formed first, shed, and second coat formed and shed.
- **Pre-pubertal:** Vellus hair on face, trunk, extremities; terminal hair on scalp, eyelashes, eyebrows.
- **Puberty:** Vellus hairs terminally differentiate due to androgens.

Anatomy

Outer root sheath (trichilemmal keratin): Most peripheral of cellular components **(Fig. 10)**.

Inner root sheath: Three compartments, stains red because of citrulline:

1. Henle's layer: Keratinizes first
2. Huxley's layer
3. Cuticle

Hair shaft: Three compartments:

1. Cuticle
2. Cortex: Forms bulk of hair; no keratohyalin granules
3. Medulla: Central

Critical line of Auber: Widest diameter of the bulb; bulk of mitotic activity that gives rise to the hair and the inner root sheath occurs below this level.

Hair Cycle (Fig. 11)

1. **Anagen:** 84%, 3–4 years
    - Follicle traverses entire epidermis, the matrix keratinocytes in the bulb region proliferate rapidly; these cells are pluripotent cells and are capable of differentiating into cuticle, cortex, and medulla of hair shaft.
    - Divided into six substages (I to VI): The first five are collectively called proanagen—defined by progressively higher levels of new hair tip position within the follicle; the 6th stage, meta-anagen, is defined by emergence of hair shaft above the skin surface.
    - End of anagen: Apoptosis.
    - Duration of anagen phase by hair location
        - Scalp: Lasts 2–6 years
        - Leg: 19–26 weeks

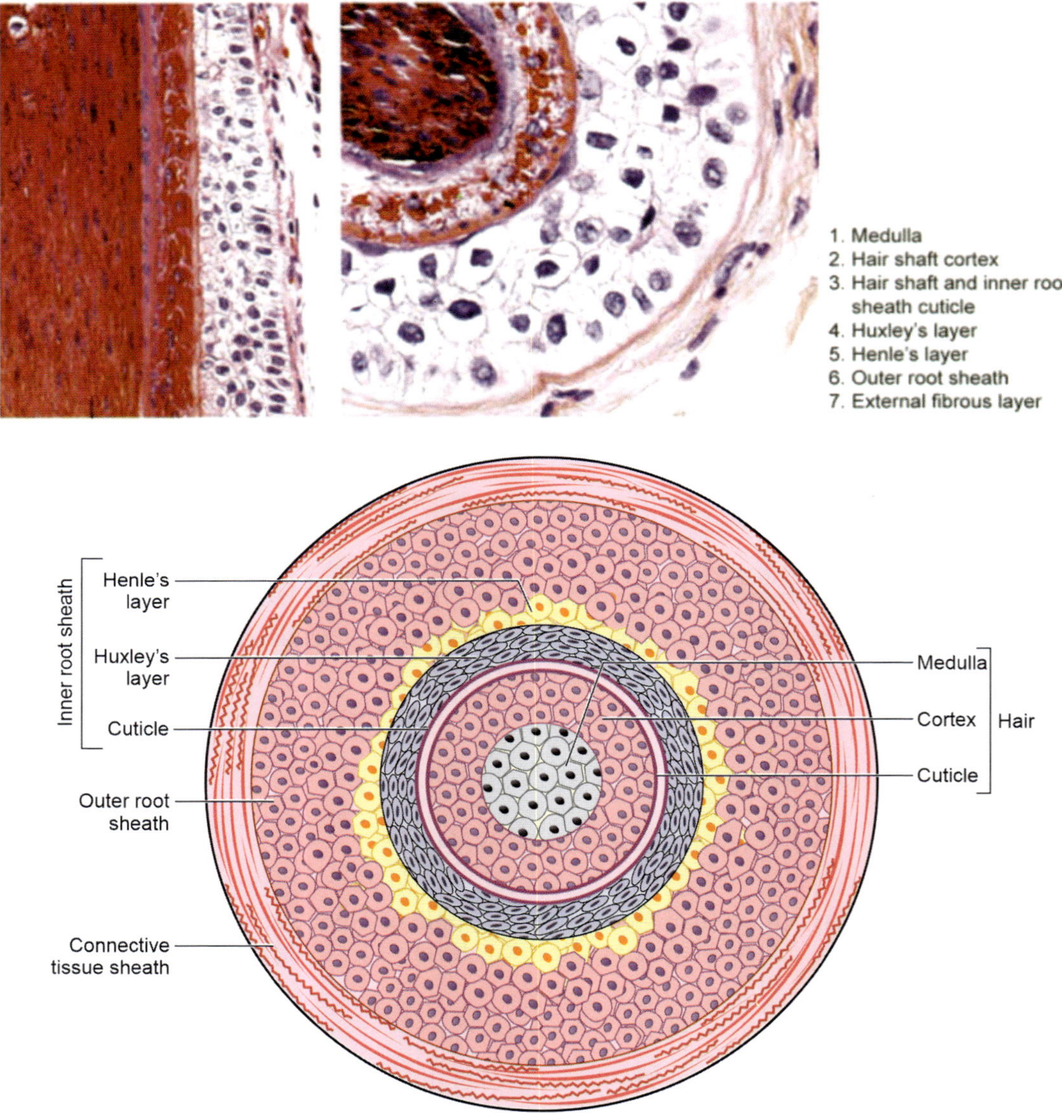

Fig. 10: Histological and schematic depiction of the various layers of a terminal hair

- Arm: 6–12 weeks
- Moustache: 4–14 weeks.

2. **Catagen**
   - 2%, club ends, lasts 3 weeks
   - Scalp hairs show gradual thinning and lightening of the pigment at the base of the hair shaft and the melanocytes in the matrix cease producing melanin and undergo apoptosis.

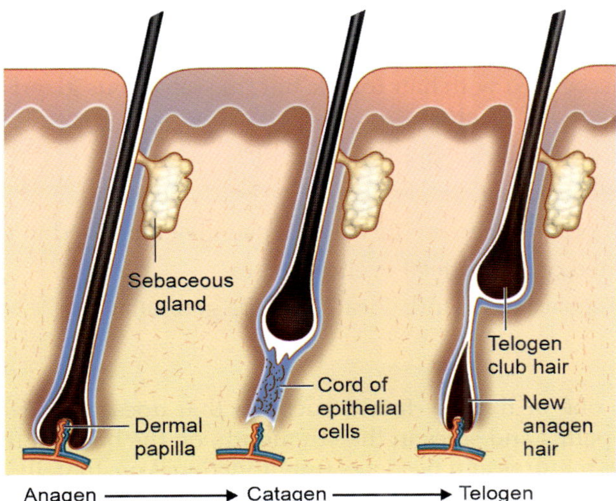

Fig. 11: A depiction of the phases of hair cycle

TABLE 5: Major determinants of the hair cycle	
Transition from anagen to telogen	• FGF5, Hairless and vitamin D receptor • Defects lead to "angora hair" and atrichia
Transition of telogen to anagen	• Sonic hedgehog (SHH) • Patched (receptor for SHH) • β-Catenin
Size of the follicle	• SHH, β-catenin, noggin, bone morphogenetic protein (BMP), FGFs, TGF-β, laminin 10

Thus there is involution of lower two-thirds of hair follicle by keratinocyte apoptosis. The matrix keratinocytes abruptly cease proliferating and undergo terminal differentiation. At end of catagen, the follicular papilla comes to rest at the bottom of the permanent portion of the hair follicle.

3. **Telogen**
   - 14%, duration is 3 months.
   - Hair has club-shaped proximal end, and is typically shed from the follicle. The inner root sheath is totally absent from the telogen follicle. Hair growth occurs in a "wave pattern" in humans *in utero*, with the first telogen phase entered near the time of birth with shedding 2–3 months later.

The important mediators of the various phases are listed in **Table 5**.

The various glands and nerve fibers are discussed in brief below.

SEBACEOUS GLANDS

- They enlarge at puberty in response to increased androgens and are important in the pathogenesis of acne.
- They are found everywhere on the skin except the palms, soles and prepuce.

- They consists of several lobules that empty into a sebaceous duct and the secretion is known as Holocrine secretion.
- They are usually associated with hair follicle but free sebaceous glands not associated with hairs are found in specific locations.

Montgomery's areolar tubercles: Nipple and areola.

Fordyce's spots: Free sebaceous glands on vermillion border of the lips and on the buccal mucosa.

Meibomian glands: Located deep on the eyelids, usually embedded in tarsal plate.

Glands of Zeis: Located on superficial eyelid margin.

Tyson's glands: Free sebaceous glands located on the genitalia.

ECCRINE GLANDS

- **Embryology:** It is one of the few fetal structures that does not develop craniocaudally (develops first on palms and soles in the 4th month, on the body in the 5th month). Fully formed at birth but matures and becomes fully functional postnatally.
- **Structure:** They are characterised by a long thin duct that open to skin and have a thermoregulatory function. They are supplied by postganglionic sympathetic fibers. Composed of three segments: The intraepidermal duct (acrosyringium), the intradermal duct, and the secretory portion. The basal coil exists either in the lower portion of the dermis or at the border of the dermis and the subcutaneous fat.
- **Site:** They are present everywhere on the skin, but absent in modified skin that lacks cutaneous appendages: Vermillion border of the lips, nail beds, labia minora, glans penis, clitoris, external auditory canal. They have the highest density on palms and soles.
- **Sweat formed in two steps:** Secretion of primary fluid, isotonic NaCl; then reabsorption of NaCl by the duct. Other components of sweat include lactate, urea, ammonia, amino acids, proteins, and proteases.
- **Markers:** S100, carcinoembryonic antigen (CEA), keratin positive.

APOCRINE GLANDS

- **Embryology:** They develop from mantle of hair follicle. First seen week 24 on scalp.
- **Structure and function:** They are innervated by sympathetic fibers. Tubular glands that demonstrate decapitation secretion; part of cell pinched off during secretory process. Like eccrine glands, composed of three segments: Intraepidermal duct, intradermal duct, and secretory portion. Duct of apocrine gland usually leads to a pilosebaceous follicle above entrance of the sebaceous duct.

  They begin functioning at puberty and they have a unclear functional role and possibly serve as a tool for olfactory communication. The secretion is in response to emotive stimuli mediated by the limbic system-through action of epinephrine/norepinephrine. Denervation does not abolish this response, though apocrine sweating requires intact nerve supply. During sleep, the glands are inactive, which supports the idea of emotional control.

  Initial secretion is odorless. The odor is derived from C6–C11 acids; the most abundant is 3-methyl-2-hexenoic acid.
- **Site:** Apocrine glands found in axillae, anogenital region, external ear canal (ceruminous glands), in the eyelids (Moll's glands), in the breast (mammary glands), and periumbilical region.
- **Stain:** Glands stain positive for keratin, S100, CEA, lysozyme.

- **Diseases:**
  - Fox-Fordyce disease: Occlusion of apocrine ducts
  - Chromhidrosis: Pigmented sweat due to lipofuscin context
  - Bromhidrosis: Abnormal body odor by apocrine gland secretion.

NERVES AND RECEPTORS OF THE SKIN

Sensory nerve fibers may exist alone (free nerve endings) or in conjunction with specialized receptors of touch, pain, temperature, itch, and mechanical stimuli and are more often seen in hairless areas.

Function

- They innervate the sweat glands (cholinergic for eccrine; adrenergic for apocrine), vascular smooth muscle (adrenergic → vasoconstriction) and hair follicles (adrenergic → contracting). Innervation of the skin is derived from the musculocutaneous branches of the spinal nerves.
- Itch is transmitted via afferent fibers of the Aδ and C-polymodal nociceptor class.
- Adrenergic innervation controls vasoconstriction, apocrine secretion, and contraction of arrector pili muscles.
- Eccrine sweating is under the control of cholinergic nerves.
- Sebaceous glands are not under neuronal control, and only respond to chemical stimuli such as hormones.
- Sympathetic nerve fibers innervate various glands (eccrine gland [acetylcholine]), vascular smooth muscle, arrector pili, apocrine and sebaceous glands (respond to chemical stimuli [hormones]).
- Adrenergic receptors in the sympathetic nervous system play a key role in modulating the cutaneous vasculature, and individual receptor subtypes vary in tissue distribution and function.
- Activation of α1-and α2-adrenergic postsynaptic receptors results in vasoconstriction that may improve persistent erythema associated with rosacea.

Free Nerve Endings

- They are widespread.
- Penicillate fibers found subepidermally in hair-bearing skin: Detect touch, pain, temperature, and itch; function in fine discrimination in the nonhairy, ridged areas of skin.
- Papillary nerve endings are found at the orifice of the hair follicle and are particularly sensitive to cold.
- Free nerve endings also penetrate the epidermis to contact Merkel cells.

Corpuscular Receptors

- Contain a capsule and inner core, and contain both neural and nonneural constituents
  Meissner's corpuscle: Ovoid, elongated mechanoreceptor located in the dermal papillae of digital skin; detect touch and light pressure.
  Pacinian (Vater–Pacini) corpuscle: Exists in deep dermis and within subcutis in weight-bearing sites of the body; functions as an adapting mechanoreceptor that responds to vibrational stimuli.
  Krause end bulbs: Mucocutaneous receptors found on glans penis, clitoris, labia minora, perianal area, and vermillion border of the lips.

IMMUNODERMATOLOGY

It is important for any student of dermatology to know the basic and advanced aspects of immunology as this defines most disorders and their therapy. In fact the basis of almost all the biological therapies and the JAKib drugs is firmly entrenched in the basic principles of immunology.

Adult human skin is home to abundant populations of memory αβ T cells, dendritic cells (DCs) and macrophages, as well as lesser numbers of natural killer (NK) cells, γδ T cells and innate lymphoid cells (ILCs) **(Fig. 12)**.

INNATE RESPONSE

This is the initial response to a foreign antigen and is characterized by **(Fig. 13)**:

- Rapid response-"first line of defence"
- Low specificity

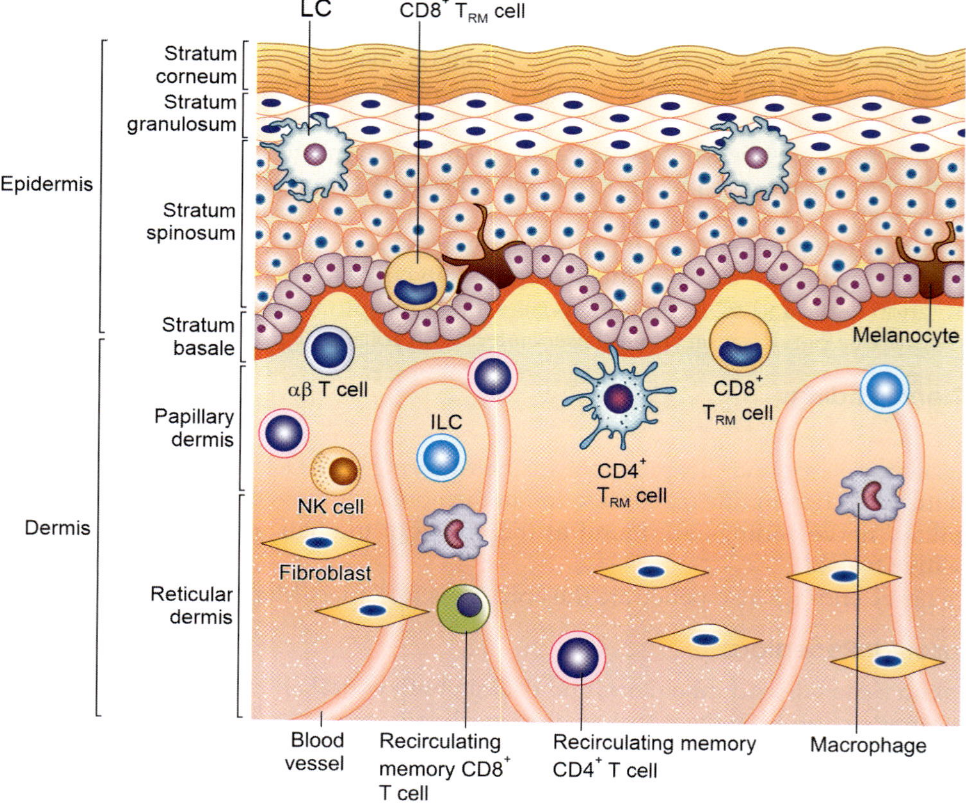

Fig. 12: A depiction of the major immune cells in the epidermis. The most prevalent immune cell types in the human epidermis are Langerhans cells (LCs) and CD8+ tissue-resident memory T (T_{RM}) cells. Other cells include dendritic cells (DCs), macrophages, innate lymphoid cells (ILCs), natural killer (NK) cells and CD8+ T_{RM} cells

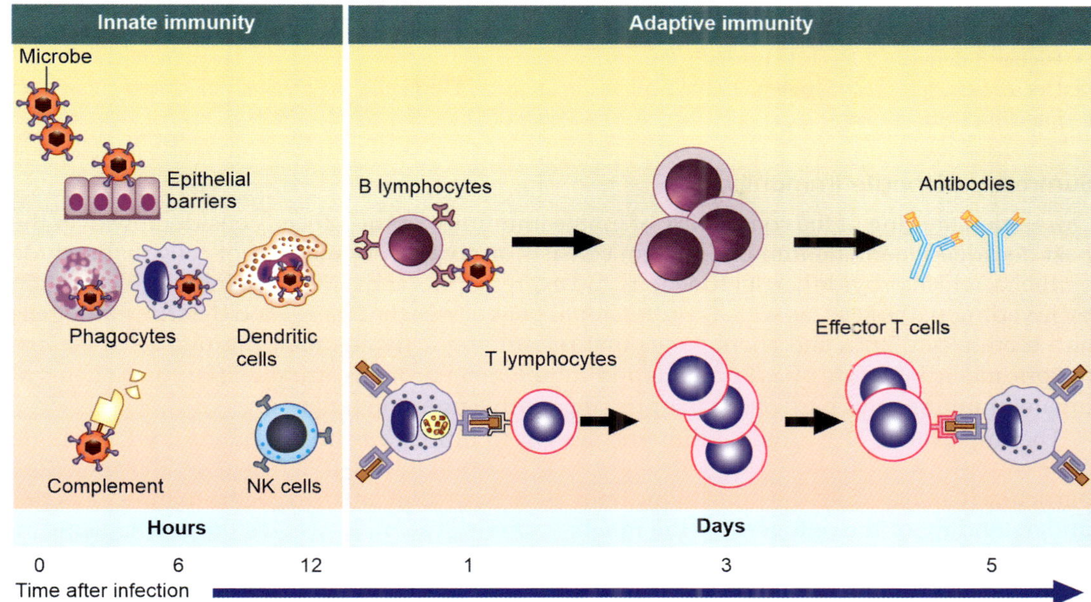

Fig. 13: Overview of the immune response with the initial (innate) and late (adaptive) responses

- Lack of memory cells
- Provides initial inflammatory signals that recruit lymphocytes (adaptive immunity)
- Lack of innate inflammatory signal may induce tolerance by adaptive immunity
- It is mediated by cells, cytokines, complement, PRRs and AMPs
- The main cells that play a role include macrophages, neutrophils, natural killer cells, mast cells, eosinophils.

  The main mediators are:

  i. **Pattern recognition receptors (PRRs)** that include toll-like receptors (TLRs) and nucleotide oligomerization domain (NOD) receptors; these receptors recognize PAMPs (pathogen-associated molecular patterns). These are instrumental in recognizing the foreign antigen and play an important role in the initial defence mechanisms. Out of these the TLRs are important.

- **TLR7 binds imiquimod,** activates **antigen-presenting cell (APC) and cytokine production (IL-12, interferon [IFN]-γ, TNF-α)**
- **TLR2** may be activated in **inflammatory acne**
- **TLR2** and **TLR9** polymorphisms are associated with **atopic dermatitis.**

  ii. **Innate immunity cytokines**

  Particularly TNF-α, IL-1, IL-10, IL-12, IFN-α, IFN-γ

  iii. **AMPs**

  Antimicrobial peptides: Defensins and cathelicidins are produced by phagocytes and keratinocytes and directly kill bacteria, fungi and viruses.

- Defects in **HBD-2** and **LL 37** are seen in lesions of **atopic dermatitis**.
- **Higher β-defensin 2 levels** in **psoriatic** lesions are associated with more severe disease activity.
- Decreased expression of antimicrobial peptides in atopics *vs* psoriatics may explain increased cutaneous infection in the former.

Summary of Innate Immunity

Our understanding of the complexity of innate immunity has advanced considerably over the past decade. The innate immune system consists of diverse populations of cells that include epithelia, which provide barrier functions and express PRRs and AMPs that inhibit colonization by invading pathogens, as well as professional phagocytes that ingest and destroy pathogens and secrete cytokines and chemokines that recruit and activate other immune cells. Plasma factors, including acute phase proteins and complement proteins, are essential components of innate immunity and participate in optimal adaptive immune function.

The importance of the innate immune system to human health is underscored by single gene mutations, such as *IRAK4* deficiency, that result in immune deficiencies and infection, particularly in early life. As innate immunity is expressed in an age-specific manner, a better understanding of the ontogeny of the innate immune system, as well as the mechanisms by which innate and adaptive immunity interact, will guide development of more effective vaccines and tumour immunotherapy. The innate immune response does not depend on immune recognition by lymphocytes, but has co-evolved with and is functionally integrated with the adaptive immune system **(Fig. 13)**.

ADAPTIVE IMMUNITY

It has a delayed response (initially), high specificity with a memory response (stronger elicitation responses on re-exposure). There is increasing focus on the tissue resident memory **(Trm)** cells which are now known to be the cause of relapse in varied autoimmune disorders. The adaptive immune response is of two types: humoral and cell mediated, and is depicted in **Fig. 14**.

The various mediators include the cells, cytokines, antibodies and complement activation.

A. Cells in Adaptive Immune Response

- **Lymphocytes:** They are triggered by a specific antigen to produce antibodies (B cells) or cytokines (CD4+ T cells), or cause direct cytotoxicity (CD8+ T cells)

  Cytokines: Particularly **IL-2, IL-4, IL-5, IFN-γ, TGF-β**
- **Natural killer cells**
  - **CD56** cell surface markers identify virally infected or transformed (tumor) host cells due to downregulation of self-MHC I on these cells
  - Destroy target cells via **perforins and granzymes** (same as T-effector cells)
  - Are activated by **IL-12** and **IL-15**, secrete **IFN-γ**
  - Mediate **antibody-dependent cellular cytotoxicity**
- **B cells**
  - **CD19/20** cell surface marker
  - Progenitors in the bone marrow develop into immature B lymphocytes that express an antigen-specific receptor

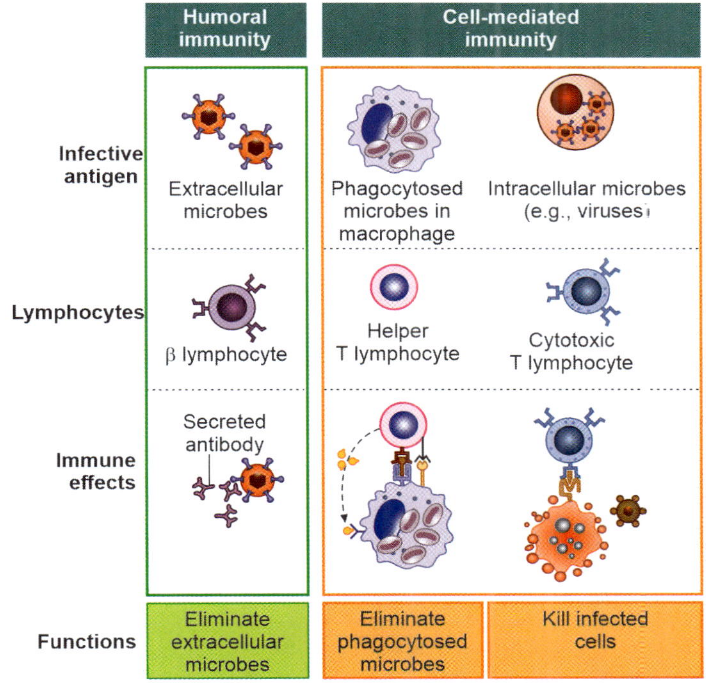

Fig. 14: The interaction of the two major classes of T lymphocytes, CD4 and CD8 via MHC leads to humoral and cell-mediated immune responses

- Express **MHC II molecules**, receptors for complement, and Fc receptor
- They undergo isotype switching of antibodies

- **T cells**
  - Progenitors arise in the bone marrow, but migrate to thymus for maturation
  - There are distinct populations of helper (CD4+) and cytotoxic (CD8+) T cells
  - Respond to stimulation by production of cytokines (CD4+) or causing cell lysis (CD8+)

Role of the CD4 and CD8 Coreceptors In T Cell Activation

The host immune response is initiated by the CD4 and CD8 cells that interact with MHC molecules and facilitate signaling by the TCR complex during T cell activation ***(see* Fig. 4)**. CD8 and CD4 interact with class I and class II MHC molecules, respectively, and are responsible for the class I or class II MHC restriction of these classes of T cells.

The activation of T cells require **two signals** (costimulation):

- **Signal 1** involves T cell receptor (TCR) binding to MHC molecule on APC
- **Signal 2** involves CD28 on T cell interacting with B7 molecule on APC

(CTLA-4 binding to B7 causes inhibition of response (checkpoint inhibition), this is blocked by ipilimumab (enhances immune response to cancer).

A detailed overview of the coreceptors is detailed in the **Fig. 15** and the consequences of MHC-APC interaction are detailed in the **Fig. 16**.

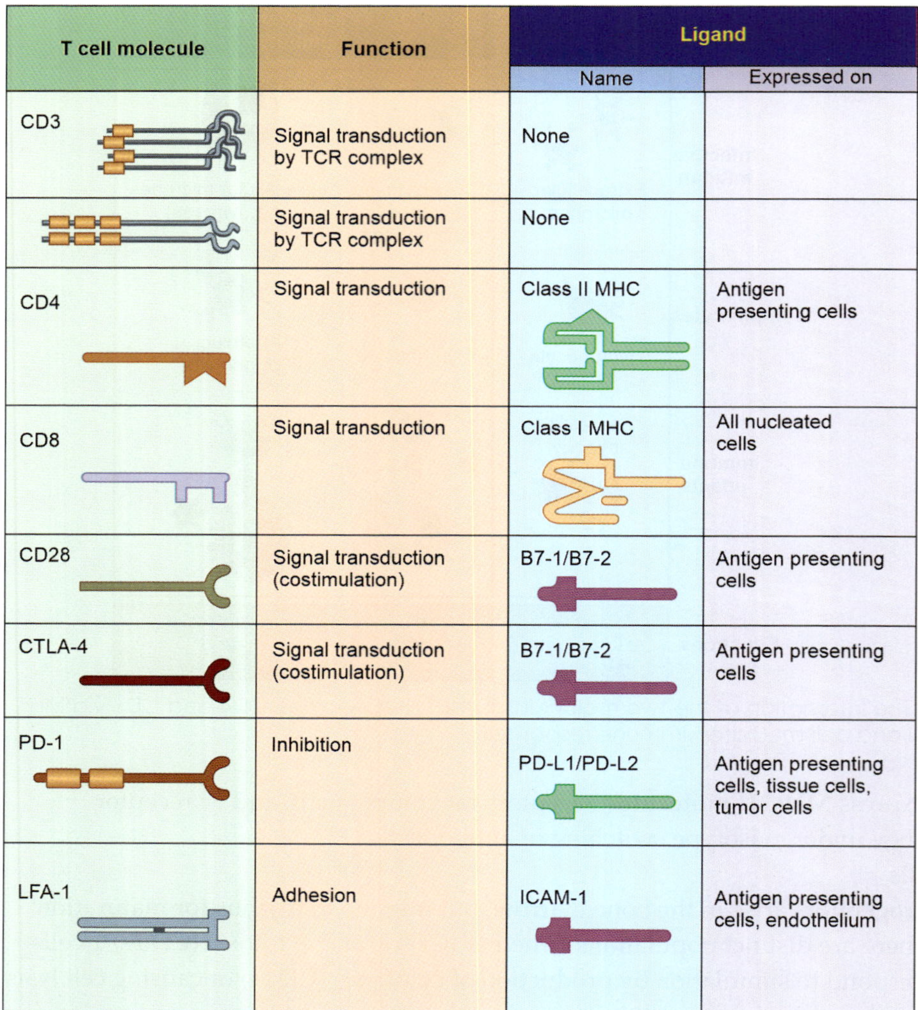

T cell molecule	Function	Ligand	
		Name	Expressed on
CD3	Signal transduction by TCR complex	None	
	Signal transduction by TCR complex	None	
CD4	Signal transduction	Class II MHC	Antigen presenting cells
CD8	Signal transduction	Class I MHC	All nucleated cells
CD28	Signal transduction (costimulation)	B7-1/B7-2	Antigen presenting cells
CTLA-4	Signal transduction (costimulation)	B7-1/B7-2	Antigen presenting cells
PD-1	Inhibition	PD-L1/PD-L2	Antigen presenting cells, tissue cells, tumor cells
LFA-1	Adhesion	ICAM-1	Antigen presenting cells, endothelium

Fig. 15: Interaction between major surface molecules of T cells and their ligands on APCs

Types of T Cells

The T cells have the following subtypes:

1. CD4+ T cells

- CD4+ T cells (helper T cells) are divided into four main subtypes: Th1, Th2, Th17, T reg, and a few more-Tfh, Th22, Th9!
- CD4+ cells [Th] interact with MHC class II (HLA-DR and HLA-DQ) molecules, which primarily present exogenous antigens (such as allergens or haptens) to T cells.
- **Differentiation and functions of CD4+ effector T cells**

  The sequence of events in the responses of CD4+ T cells involves the initial activation of these cells in lymphoid organs to generate effector and memory cells, migration of many of

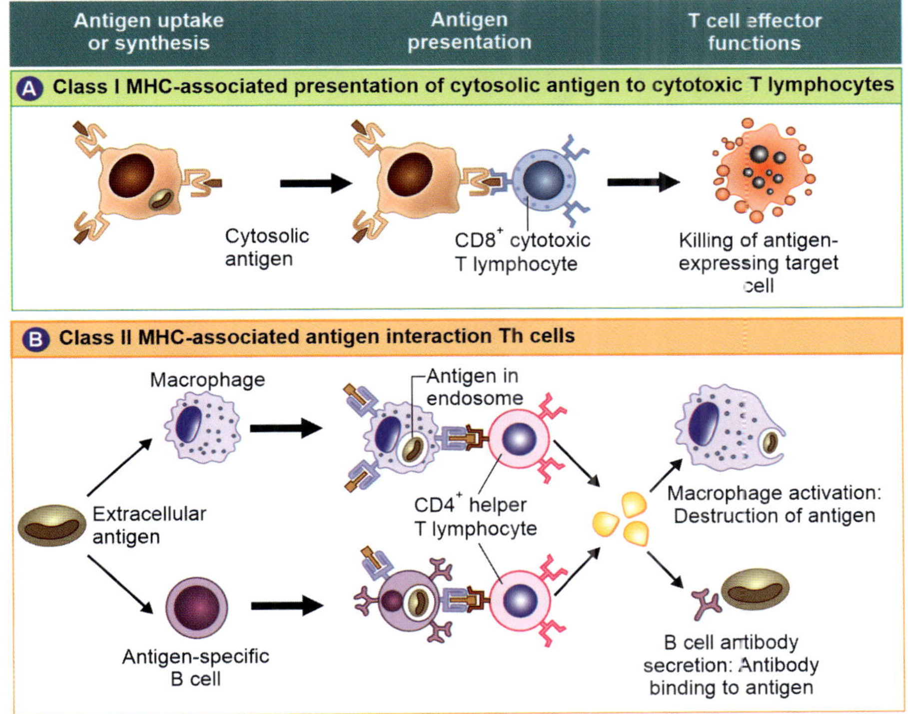

Fig. 16: Role of MHC and APC interaction in the host immune response

these effector cells to sites of infection, and elimination of infectious pathogens at these sites **(Figs 16 and 17)**.

While there are many CD4+ effector T cells, Th1, Th2, and Th17 secrete different sets of cytokines, and help in host defense against distinct types of infectious pathogens, and are involved in different types of tissue injury in immunologic diseases **(Fig. 18)**. In essence, Th1 cells are associated with cell-mediated inflammatory reactions and Th2 cells are associated with strong antibody and allergic responses. Th17 cells are important for defense against certain infections, involving the mucosal surfaces. An overview of the subtypes of CD4 T cells is given in **Fig. 18** and the salient functions are given in **Table 6**.

2. Regulatory T Cells

CD4+ Tregs

These cells are a distinct population of CD4+ T cells and their function is to control immune reactions to self and foreign antigens. Thus these cells are important as they have a dominant suppressive effect. Several **types** of T cells with regulatory activity have been described, including subpopulations of γδ T cells, NKT cells, CD8+ and CD4+ T cells. Some of these Tregs are naturally produced in the immune system, while others are induced from naïve T cells as a product of a particular mode of antigen stimulation in a particular cytokine milieu.

The CD4 Tregs can be divided into two categories: Naturally occurring and induced. The naturally occurring Foxp3+ Tregs, also referred to as CD25+ Tregs because of their constitutive expression of CD25, are primarily generated in the thymus in a functionally mature form,

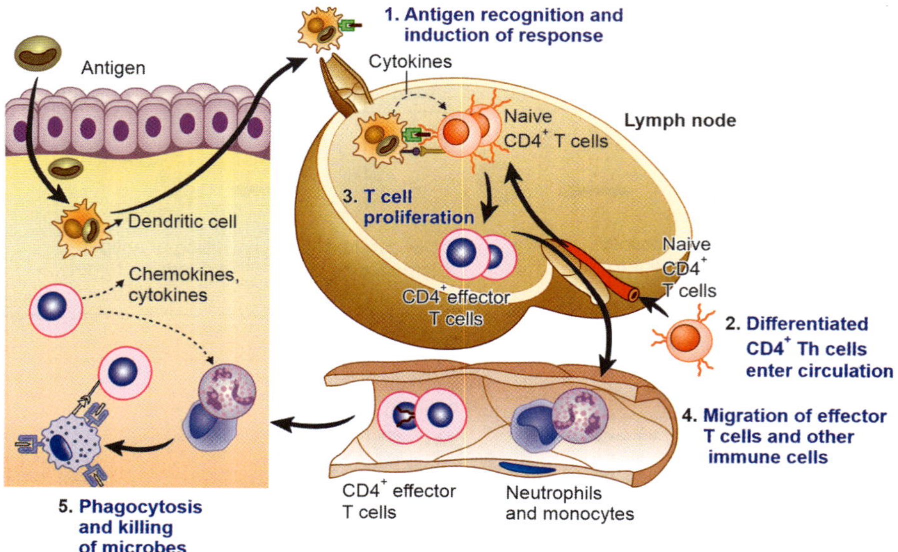

Fig. 17: A depiction of the host immune response following antigen presentation and recognition by the naïve CD4 cells which differentiate into the effector CD4 Th cells and lead to destruction of the antigen

TABLE 6: Overview of the salient Th cell subtypes and their functions	
Th1	• Augment **T cell-mediated immunity**, activate **macrophages**, and downregulate Th2 responses via IFN-γ • Release IFN-γ, IL-2, TNF-α and TNF-β (LT-α) • Promote phagocytosis • **Play a role in**–Psoriasis, tuberculoid leprosy (high immune), Leishmaniasis (cutaneous-self resolving), CTCL (non-Sezary), DLE, allergic contact dermatitis, sarcoidosis.
Th2	• Suppress macrophage activity, **activate eosinophils**, induce isotype switching to **IgE and IgG4**, and **downregulate Th1 responses** via IL-10 • Produce IL-4, IL-5, IL-6 and IL-10 • Increase degranulation through FcεRI cross-linking and IL-5-mediated eosinophil activation • **Play a role in:** Atopic dermatitis, lepromatous leprosy (low immune), leishmaniasis (chronic indolent), Sezary syndrome, scleroderma, systemic lupus, helminth infections, pemphigus.
Th17	• Proinflammatory; implicated in the pathogenesis of **psoriasis** • Activate local endothelium, induce cytokine and chemokine production, increase infiltration by neutrophils, activate cell-mediated inflammation • Secrete IL-17A, IL-17F, IL-21, IL-22, IL-23, and TNF-α • Differentiation induced by IL-6 and TGF-β. • Proliferation and survival mediated by IL-23
Treg	• Downregulation of the immune response • Express high levels of **CD25** (IL-2 receptor α chain) and are characterized by expression of transcription factor **FOXP3** • Suppress immune response through direct contact inhibition or the secretion of IL-10, TGF-β, or CTLA-4 • Important role in leprosy reactions

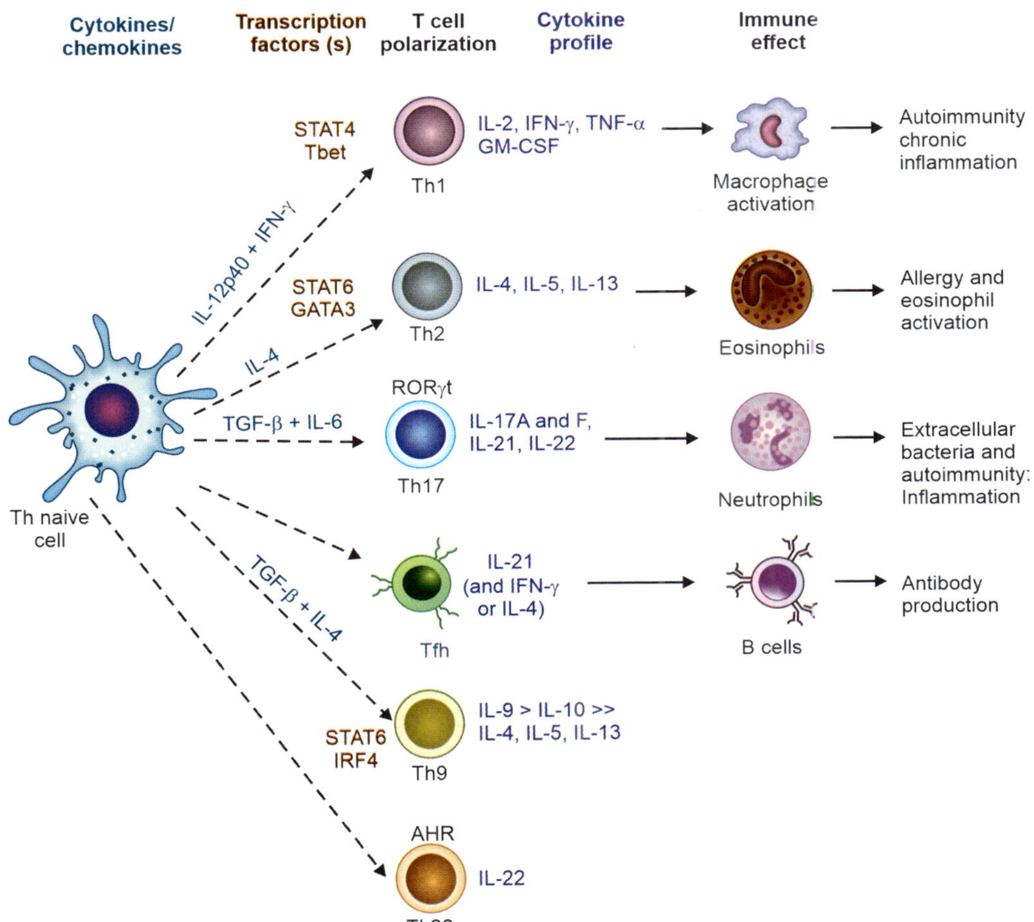

Fig. 18: The Th naïve cell on stimulation by an appropriate antigenic stimulation via defined transcription factors and cytokines can differentiate into varied T cell subtypes which via predetermined cytokines mediate immune effects.

though they can also arise *de novo* in the periphery from naïve CD4 T cells **(Fig. 19)**. Peripheral (extra-thymic) development of CD4+ Tregs and CD8+ Tregs is due to high concentrations of TGF-β, IL-10, or antigen priming. The importance of **Foxp3** in the development of **CD4+CD25+ Tregs** is that it helps in increased expression of CD25 and induces **suppressor function**. The generation, survival, and functional competence of Tregs is dependent on the cytokine **IL-2**.

Induced CD4 Tregs, are of two types, the IL-10-secreting type 1 regulatory T cells (Tr1) and TGF-β-secreting T helper 3 cells **(Th3) (Fig. 20)**. These two sublineage cells have a difference in expression of Foxp3. Hence the **adaptive/induced Treg cells are** similar to natural Tregs and are capable of suppressing CD4 and CD8 T-cell responses *in vitro* and *in vivo*.

The Foxp3+ Tregs suppress aberrant immune response by multiple mechanisms secreting soluble and cell surface-bound mediators **(Fig. 21)**. Unlike natural Tregs, which function in a cell-contact-dependent manner, adaptive Tregs appear to function at least in part through

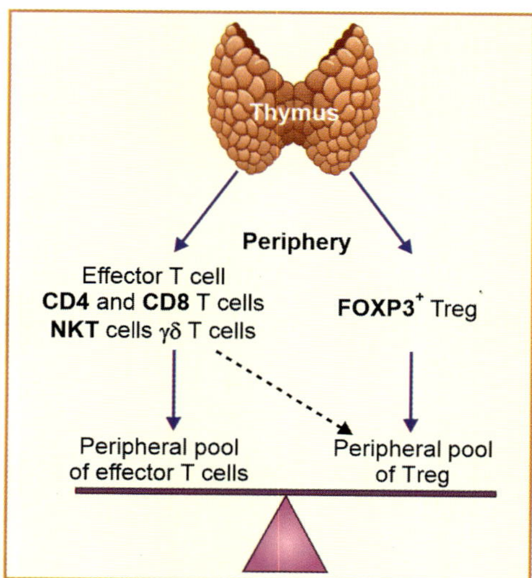

Fig. 19: Treg cells can develop either in the thymus or the periphery and are vital for maintaining tolerance as a counter-balance to effector T cells. The signals that control differentiation of γδ T cells and NKT cells to cells with regulatory properties are less well defined

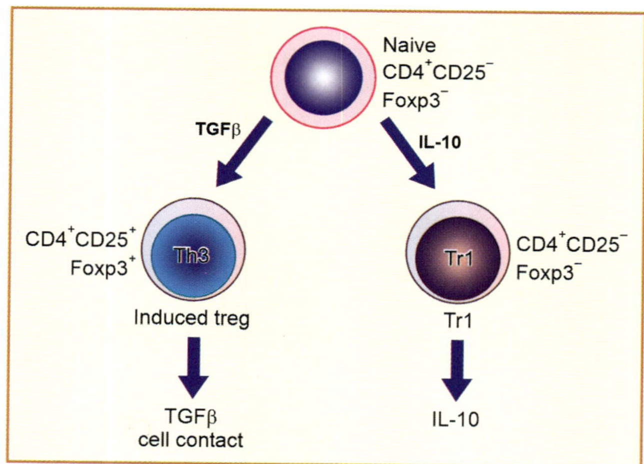

Fig. 20: The fate of naive CD4+CD25—cells in the periphery depend on the cytokine milieu. If TGFβ is present, cells upregulate Foxp3 and CD25 expression. In the presence of IL-10, these cells can become suppressive, but do not express Foxp3 or CD25 (RA, retinoic acid)

the secretion of IL-10 and TGF-β. These cytokines may directly regulate effector T cells or may inhibit dendritic cell activity.

The suppression effected by Tregs is at multiple steps-at the level of naive T cell activation in lymphoid organs as well as the effector phase of these responses in tissues. They control cell responses mainly by inhibiting the stimulatory ability of dendritic cells (DCs), and also by suppressing T cell activation. Tregs may also suppress B cell activation and inhibit the

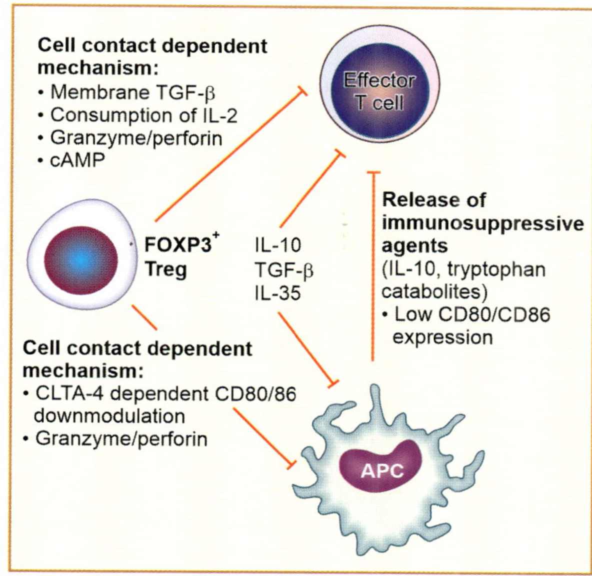

Fig. 21: Foxp3+CD25+ Tregs can inhibit many different types of effector cells by multiple mechanisms as depicted

proliferation and differentiation of natural killer (NK) cells. The main mechanisms of action are:

a. CTLA-4-mediated inhibition of costimulation.
b. Production of the immunosuppressive cytokines IL-10 and TGF-β.
c. Consumption of IL-2.

CD8+ Tregs

They need to be primed by CD4+ cells during a primary response; they then suppress secondary immune responses. They can target activated effector T cell, kill by direct lysis of target cells and suppress immune responses through the secretion of cytokines such as IL-10.

The clinical importance of Treg cells is listed in **Box 1**.

BOX 1: Clinical importance of Treg cells

Reduction of FOXP3$^+$ Treg suppression or reducing Treg numbers

- Enhanced tumor immunity, clearance of infections, improved response to vaccine.

Boost of FOXP3+ Treg function or increasing Treg numbers

- Treatment of autoimmunity, allergic response, induction of transplantation tolerance.

Role in infections

- CD4$^+$ Tregs have a protective role against immune-mediated pathology and they are also important in reducing inflammation.
- CD4$^+$ Tregs can also suppress virus-specific responses. Many pathogens induce high levels of IL-10 and TGFβ, which promote the induction of CD4+CD25+ Tregs. In chronic viral infections, including HIV, cytomegalovirus (CMV), and herpes simplex virus (HSV) infections, increased numbers of Tregs are responsible for decreased antigen-specific responses by CD4+ and CD8+ T cells. This can lead to disease development.

How can the same CD4+ cells elicit such different responses?

The answer lies in the fact that CD4+ T cells consist of subsets of effector cells that produce distinct sets of cytokines, elicit different reactions, and are involved in host defense against different microbes, as well as in distinct types of immunologic diseases. The first two subsets that were discovered were called types 1 and 2 helper T cells, or Th1 and Th2. The Th17 subset, so named because its characteristic cytokine is interleukin-17 (IL-17), was identified many years later.

Notably these subtypes are defined by **(Fig. 18)**:

a. The cytokines they produce
b. The transcription factors they express.

The signature cytokines produced by the major CD4+T cell subsets are

- **Interferon (IFN)-γ** for Th1 cells
- **IL-4, IL-5, and IL-13** for Th2 cells and
- **IL-17 and IL-22** for Th17 cells **(Fig. 22)**

IFN-γ released by Th1 inhibits **Th2 and Th17, IL-10** released by Th2 inhibits **Th1 cells, while IL 17A** release by Th 17 cells inhibits **Th1 cells;** thus there is an intrinsic counterbalancing of cytokines and T cells.

Different inflammatory diseases are caused by excessive reactions of different helper T cell subsets. In general, Th1 and Th17 cells play prominent roles in autoimmune diseases associated with inflammation, whereas allergic reactions are dominated by Th2 cells.

What is T cell Plasticity?

It has been shown that Th cells have considerable developmental plasticity. In particular, TH17 cells can be induced to produce IFNγ (a TH1 cytokine) and shut down production of IL-17A if they are stimulated in the presence of IL-12 **(Fig. 11)**. Similarly, at least *in vitro*, TH2 cells can be driven to a mixed TH2/1 phenotype by culture with type one IFNs and IL-12, where cells coexpress IL-4 and IFNγ. The reasons for this flexibility in cytokine production remains to be further explored, but it is thought that such plasticity may enable rapid site-specific immune responses to infections to occur.

There is also a reciprocal link between Treg cells and Th17 cells **(Fig. 23)**. Thus both induced Treg and TH17 cells are dependent on **TGFβ** for their development. In the presence of TGFβ,

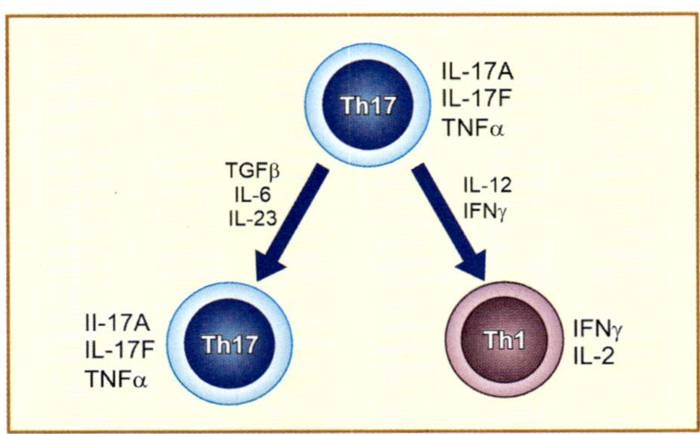

Fig. 22: Cytokines are released by Th17 cell and its interaction with Th1 cell

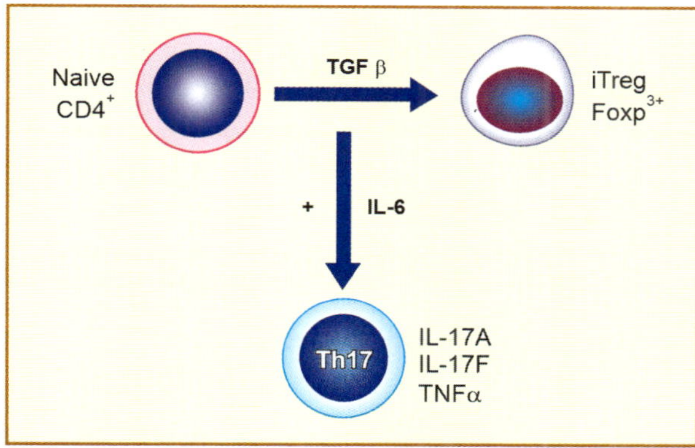

Fig. 23: Differentiation of Th17 cells and Tregs from naïve CD4+ cells is regulatec by cytokines. TGFb is common to both cell lineages; in additional presence of IL 6, Th17 cells are formed

naive $CD4^+$ T cells upregulate Foxp3 and develop into induced Tregs. In the presence of inflammatory cytokines such as **IL-6 or IL-1β**, naive T cells develop into inflammatory TH17 cells that secrete cytokines such as IL-17A, IL-17F, and TNFα. This dichotomous relationship shows the important role for cytokines derived from the innate immune system in determining the outcome of an adaptive immune response.

3. CD8 cells

- Cytotoxic CD8+ cells (Tc) interact with MHC class I (HLA-A and HLA-B) molecules; primarily endogenous antigens such as viral and tumor peptides **(*see* Fig. 16)**.
- They act by releasing granules containing perforin and granzymes, which induce apoptosis.
- Also induce apoptosis by presenting Fas ligand (FasL) to Fas receptor on target cells.

4. γδ T cells

- These are T cells that possess a γδ TCR as opposed to the more common αβ TCR (as seen in CD4+ and CD8+ T cells).
- Primarily found in epithelia and appear to play a role in immunoregulation and immuno-surveillance.
- Suppress Th1 cells through release of IL-10.
- May play important roles in cancer surveillance and resistance to graft-*vs*-host disease.

B. Cytokines

These are classified on the basis of the type of the receptor they bind: Type I (hematopoietin family) and type II (interferon family) cytokine receptors, tumor necrosis factor (TNF) family receptors, interleukin (IL)-1 receptor and the related Toll-like receptors (TLRs), IL-17 receptors, receptor tyrosine kinases, and the transforming growth factor-β (TGF-β) family **(Fig. 24)**. Cytokines are a large group of proteins that function as mediators of immunity and inflammation. We have already discussed cytokines in innate immune responses, which are produced mainly by dendritic cells and macrophages. In adaptive immunity, cytokines are secreted by T cells, mainly CD4+ cells The first **cytokine** to be produced by **CD4+ T cells**, within 1–2 hours after activation, is **interleukin-2 (IL-2)**. Activation also rapidly enhances the ability of T cells to bind and respond to IL-2, by increasing the expression of the high-affinity

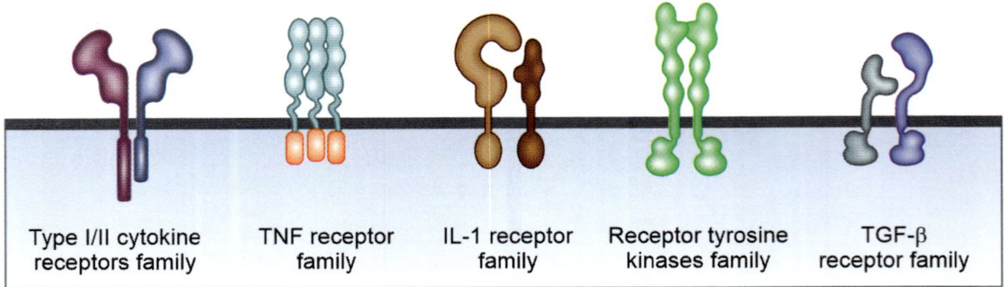

Fig. 24: Schematic representation of prototypical receptors from five of the major cytokine receptor superfamilies

TABLE 7: Overview of the salient cytokines

Th1 cytokines	**IFN-γ:** Differentiation toward Th1 cells; ↑ MHC I and II on APCs; ↑ macrophage activity and ↓ of Th2 **IL-2:** Proliferation and activation of T cells (clonal expansion), B cells (antibody production), and NK cells **IL-12:** Heterodimer of p40 and p35 subunits. ↑ cytolytic activity and IFN-γ production by T cells and NK cells. **Ustekinumab** binds to the p40 subunit of both IL-12 and IL-23.
Th2 cytokines	**IL-4:** Differentiation toward TH2 cells; isotype switching to IgE and IgG4, inhibition of macrophage activation. **IL-5:** Activates eosinophils and B-cell differentiation, ↑ IgA secretion. **IL-6:** Proliferation and differentiation of B cells, induces acute-phase reactants. **IL-10:** ↓expression of MHC II and costimulatory molecules on APCs; decreases IL-12. **IL-13:** Related to IL-4; implicated in allergic inflammation. **Dupilumab** is a monoclonal antibody against IL4Rα (blocks IL-4 and IL-13) designed for treatment of atopic dermatitis and asthma.
Th17 cytokines	**IL-17:** Family of cytokines that are proinflammatory, resulting in production of many cytokines including IL-6 and TNF-α. IL-17 members include IL-17A and IL-17F, which are implicated in allergic and autoimmune inflammation as seen in asthma, SLE, and RA. **IL-22:** Member of IL-10 family that mediates inflammation through STAT transcriptional activation pathway; stimulates keratinocyte proliferation. **IL-23:** Heterodimer of p40 (as in IL-12) and p19 subunits. Required for survival and proliferation of Th17; may be key cytokine in development of psoriasis. IL-23A encodes p19.

*JAK it can inhibit multiple cytokines and CD4/CD8 cell lines.

IL-2 receptor. T lymphocytes activated by antigen and costimulation begin to proliferate within 1 or 2 days, resulting in expansion of antigen-specific clones. The salient actions of the cytokines with drugs that inhibit the cytokines are detailed **Table 7**.

C. Signaling Pathway

There are certain signalling pathways that mediate the action of cytokines in the immune system and the salient ones are JAK-STAT, NF-κB, PI3K-AKT-mTOR, MAPK and Keap1-Nrf2-ARE, and for each specific pathway, there are immunosuppressive drugs and therein lies the importance of these pathways in dermatology.

JAK STAT

Cytokine receptors of the type I and type II receptor families mediate the signal transduction pathways that involve non-receptor tyrosine kinases called Janus kinases (JAKs) and transcription factors called signal transducers and activators of transcription (STATs). There are four known JAKs (JAKs1 to 3 and TYK2) and **seven** STATs (STATs 1 to 4, 5a, 5b, and 6).

The sequence of events in the JAK-STAT signaling pathways are depicted in **Fig. 25**.

a. Inactive JAK enzymes are noncovalently attached to the cytoplasmic domains of type I and type II cytokine receptors.
b. When two receptor molecules are brought together by binding of a cytokine molecule, the receptor-associated JAKs are activated and phosphorylate tyrosine residues in the cytoplasmic portions of the clustered receptors. Some of these phosphotyrosine moieties of the receptors are then recognized by and bind SH2 domains of monomeric cytosolic STAT proteins. The STAT proteins are thus brought close to JAKs and are phosphorylated by these receptor-associated kinases.
c. The STAT dimers that are generated migrate to the nucleus, where they bind to speci?c DNA sequences in the promoter regions of cytokine-responsive genes and activate gene transcription.

Expression of JAK and Action of Cytokines

The effect of various cytokines is mediated by the JAK STAT pathway and thus JAKib drugs blocking these cytokines may lead to side effects **(Fig. 26)**.

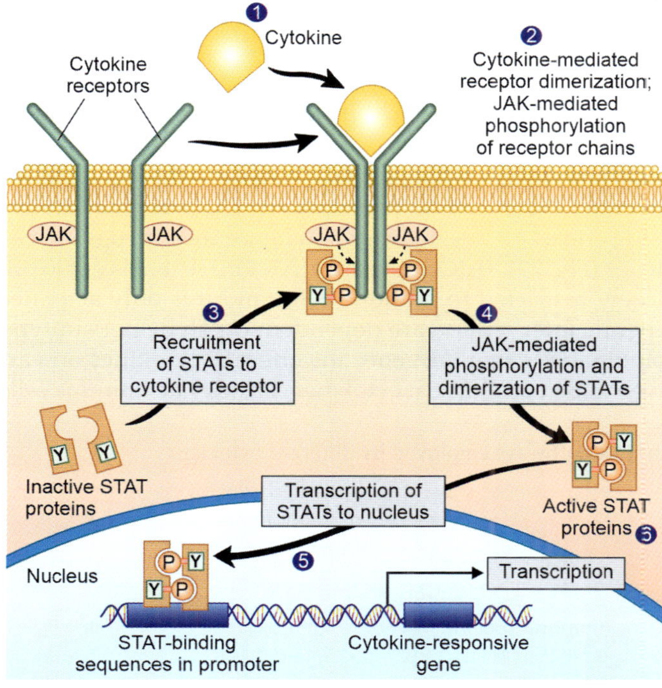

Fig. 25: Sequence of events in the JAK-STAT signaling pathways

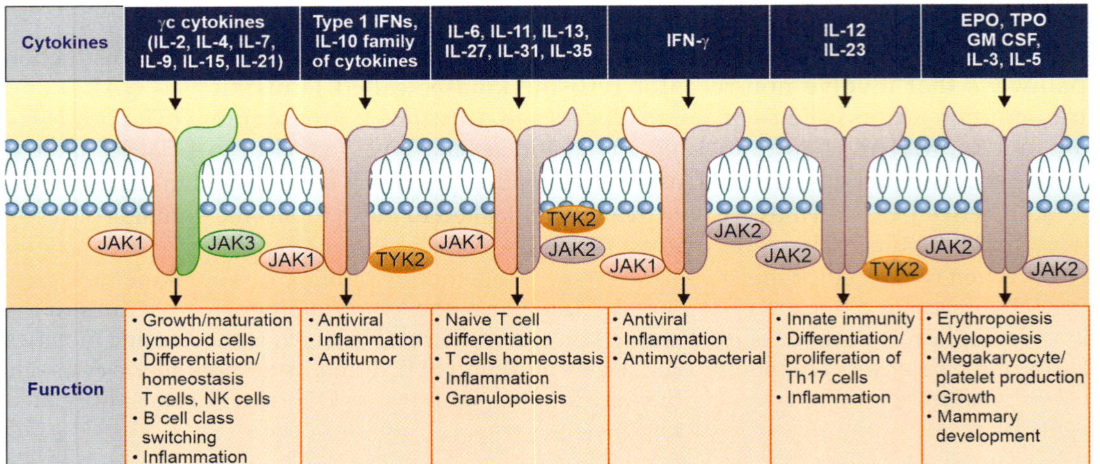

Fig. 26: Schematic diagram of the JAK signaling pathway employed by certain cytokine families and their respective functions

JAK3 is primarily expressed in hematopoietic cells and is critical for signal transduction of IL-2, IL-4, IL-7, IL-9, IL-15, and IL-21. JAK3 only signals in combination with JAK1. These cytokines are integral to lymphocyte activation, function, and proliferation. Hormone-like cytokines erythropoietin, thrombopoietin, growth hormone, granulocyte-macrophage colony-stimulating factor (GM-CSF), IL-3, and IL-5 signal through **JAK2**. IL-6, IL-10, IL-11, IL-19, IL-20, IL-22, and IFN-α, IFN-β, and IFN-γ signal through **JAK1**. **TYK2** facilitates signaling for IL-12, IL-23, and type 1 IFNs. TYK2 pairs with either JAK1 or JAK2 to facilitate signaling. TYK2 inhibitors are under development as oral therapies for psoriasis due to inhibition of IL12/23 activity, as well as for systemic lupus erythematosus (SLE), due to inhibition of IFN-α and other inflammatory cytokines **(Box 2)**.

There is a significant amount of combinatorial diversity in the signaling that can be generated from a limited number of JAK and STAT proteins. The JAK subtypes are present on most cells accounting for the side effects of JAK ib drugs and hence these drugs are classified as selective and non-selective drugs **(Fig. 27)**. **JAK3** is the only JAK kinase that is not expressed ubiquitously. Its expression is largely restricted to immune cells, and it is only activated by γc-containing receptors. As therapeutic intervention are dependent on Th helper subtypes, a list of the JAK STAT signalling combinations that influence the effect of cytokines on varied cells including T lymphocytes is given in **Box 2**. Different cytokines can activate immune cells via a combination

BOX 2: Predominant JAK pathways employed by different cytokines

JAK1	Many cytokines • IL-6, IL-10, IL-11, IL-19, IL-20, IL-22, and IFN-α, IFN-β, and IFN-γ
JAK 2	Hematopoiesis • EPO, TPO, G-CSF, IL-3, IL-5
JAK 3	Immune specific JAK • IL-2, IL-4, IL-7, IL-9, IL-15, and IL-21
TYK2	IL-12, IL-23, and type 1 IFNs

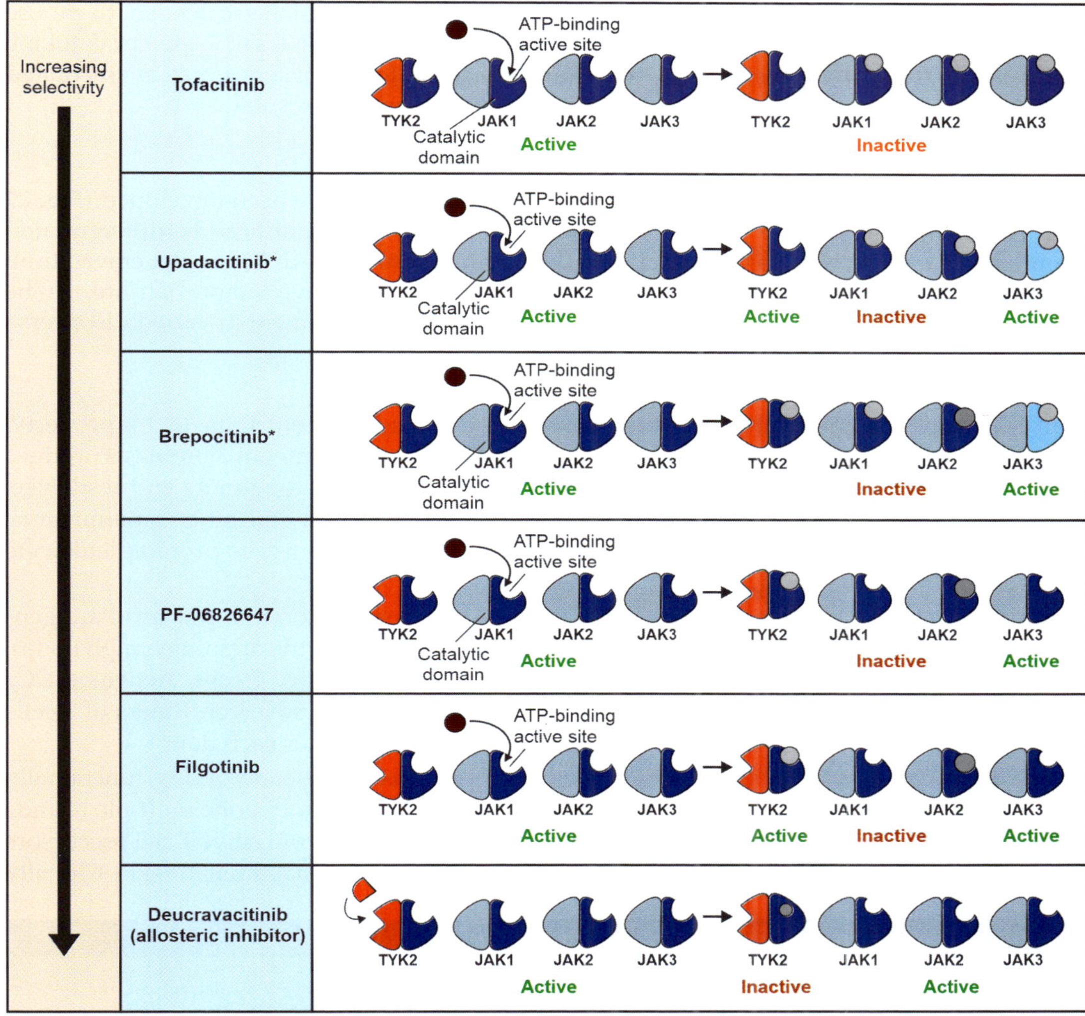

Fig. 27: Activity of nonselective and selective JAK inhibitor (JAKib) drugs

of JAK STAT receptors thus a knowledge of the JAK combinations on various cells can be useful. JAK1, 2 are seen on **Th1** cells and JAK 1, 3 on **Th2** and **Th17** cells, hence AD and Prurigo that are mediated by Th2 cells can be managed by a JAK 1, 3 inhibitor which would preferentially inhibit the Th2 cells. The most important advantage of these drugs is that they can inhibit multiple key cytokines and immune responses:

i. Type 1 (Th1) immunity: IL-2, IFN-γ, IL-15 (JAK1, 2)
ii. Type 2 (Th2) immunity: IL-4, IL-15, IL-13 (JAK1, 3)
iii. Type 3 (e.g. Th17) immunity: IL-12, IL-23 (JAK1, 3)

Thus the cytokines that mediate Th1 (Type 1), Th2 (Type 2) and Th17 (Type 3) can be inhibited if an appropriate JAKib drug is given depending on their action on JAK/TYK2 receptors.

While ideally gene expression data of cytokines and JAK expression are needed, to choose an ideal JAKib drug, a knowledge of the predominant cell (Th1, Th2, Th17, etc.) or cytokine can also help in choosing the ideal JAKib. Thus Th12 mediated disorders which are mediated by JAK1 and 3 have been treated by Tofacitinib with encouraging results.

Classification of Janus Kinase Inhibitors

In recent years, various JAKi with different isotype specificity have been developed **(Fig. 27 and Table 8)**. Less selective JAKi (for example, tofacitinib, peficitinib) can be differentiated from selective JAKi, such as upadacitinib (JAK1i), abrocitinib (JAK1i), or deucravacitinib (TYK2i) In contrast to biologics, JAKi are small molecules. They have a short half-life, can be applied orally or topically, and offer effective steroid-sparing treatment in varied disorders.

GENERATION OF EFFECTOR T CELL RESPONSES IN SKIN

Skin is a formidable physical barrier, and many of its intrinsic cells contribute to this property, like keratinocytes differentiate and form the impermeable stratum corneum, fibroblasts produce collagens, elastin and other glycoproteins that give the dermis its toughness and resilience. Most cells can, upon stimulation, produce chemokines, cytokines and other inflammatory mediators that activate cells of the innate and adaptive immune systems and promote leukocyte recruitment from blood **(Fig. 28)**.

Innate immune activation of dermal DCs leads to their maturation into powerful antigen-presenting cells. Mature DCs migrate through afferent lymphatics to the draining lymph nodes, where they can activate naive T cells or recirculating central memory T cells. Activated DCs can also activate recruited or tissue-resident T cells in the skin. Episodic recruitment of T cells and other leukoytes into inflamed or injured skin occurs many times each day.

Adult skin contains large populations of **memory T cells** that are phenotypically, functionally and clonally diverse and are derived from naive T cells that have undergone multiple rounds of clonal expansion. Skin-tropic effector T cell clones are generated from naive T cell precursors that have been activated by antigen-presenting DCs in lymph nodes that drain the skin. Clonally

TABLE 8: Less selective and selective JAKi

Less selective JAKi		
Tofacitinib	**JAK1/2/3**	**RA, PsA, UC**
Baricitinib	**JAK1/2**	**RA, AD, AA**
Peficitinib Delgocitinib	**Pan JAK**	AD (Topical delgocitinib)
Ifidancitinib	**JAK1/3**	
Selective JAKi		
Upadacitinib Abrocitinib	**JAK1**	**RA/AD, PsA** **AD**
Deucravacitinib	**TYK2**	**Psoriasis**
Brepocitinib PF-06826647 Ritlecitinib	**JAK3**	**AA**

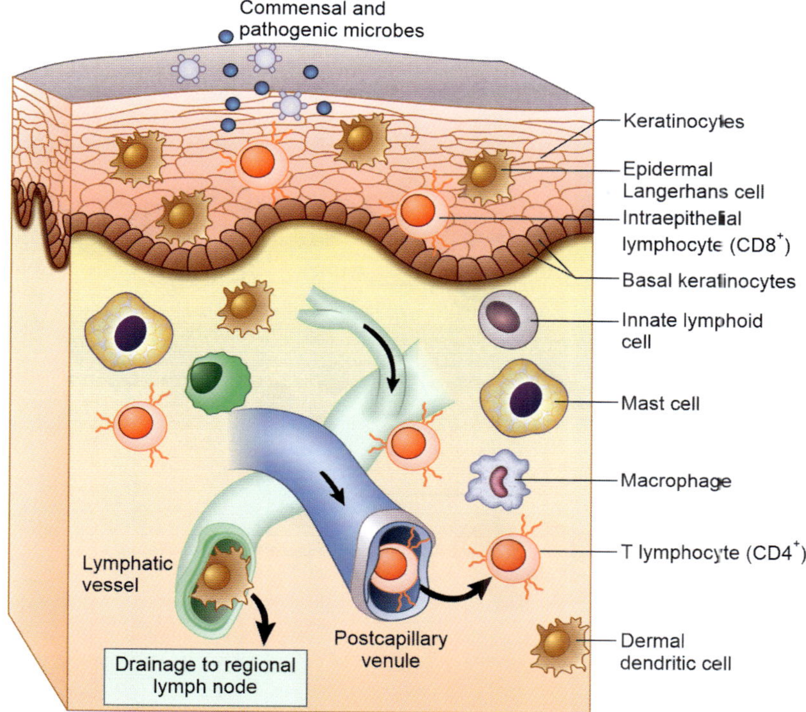

Fig. 28: Leukocyte recruitment from blood by stimulated cells through secretion of chemokines, cytokines and other inflammatory mediators that in turn activate cells of the innate and adaptive immune systems.

expanded effector T cells generated under these conditions traffic to skin, accumulating in highest abundance at the site of initial antigen encounter **(Fig. 29)**.

The steps of immune response in skin are:

1. Following microbial invasion, antigen-presenting cells **(APCs)** migrate from the site of insult to the secondary lymphoid tissues via afferent lymphatic vessels **(Fig. 28)**.
2. T cell priming occurs within the secondary lymphoid tissue, resulting in the generation of effector T cells (T_{eff} cells, which include **memory T** (T_M) cell precursors) that travel to the site of inflammation. This pool of T effector cells eradicates the infection, concluding the effector phase of an immune response, which typically lasts **3–10 days (Fig. 29)**.
3. Following microbial clearance, the majority of T_{eff} cells die, while subsets of T cells become recirculating memory cells or are maintained in the tissue as **tissue-resident memory** T (T_{rm}) cells **(Fig. 29)**.
4. Recirculating memory T cells leave skin in response to gradients of sphingosine-1-phosphate and CC-chemokine ligand 21 (CCL21), which bind to sphingosine-1-phosphate receptor 1 (S1PR1) and CC-chemokine receptor 7 (CCR7), respectively. The generation of T_{rm} cells results from a specific transcriptional signature that has been characterized. T_{rm} cells are defined as cells that persist in the absence of inflammation or infection, usually >25 days after the original exposure **(Fig. 29)**.

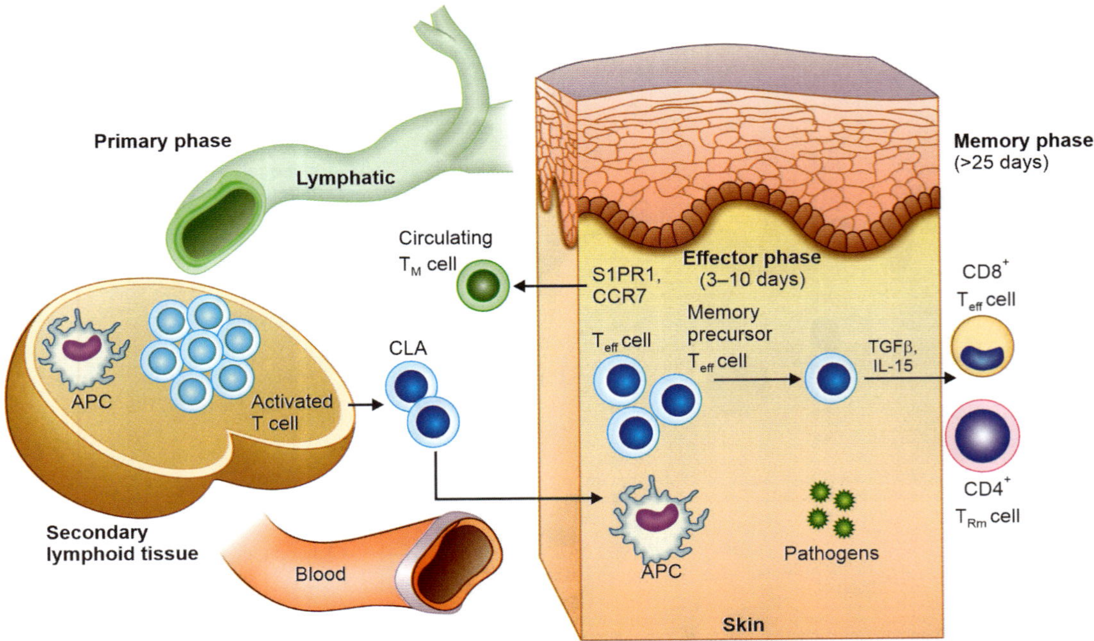

Fig. 29: T cell priming resulting in generation of effector T cells including a subset of tissue-resident memory T cells

Skin-resident T Cells

In 2001, it was demonstrated that, after the resolution of systemic viral infection **(Fig. 29)**, T cells are detected and persist for long periods of time in peripheral nonlymphoid tissues. These were referred to as skin-resident T cell and corresponded to the memory T cells that were found in lesions of fixed drug eruptions, which appear at the same location after repeated exposure to the same drug. In 2004, Boyman et al. reported that non-lesional skin from patients with psoriasis (but not normal control skin) developed a psoriatic phenotype when grafted onto immunocompromised mice, suggesting that pathogenic T cells reside in normal-appearing adult skin. In 2006, a seminal report by Clark et al. demonstrated that there were roughly four times as many memory T cells in adult human skin as there were in peripheral blood. These skin T cells were heterogeneous and retained potent effector functions, with different subsets producing IFNγ, IL-17 or IL-13 overexpressing a regulatory T (T reg) cell phenotype. More recently, the same group described **four** distinct populations of memory T cells in skin. A population of T_{CM} cells, a population of migratory memory T cells and two populations of T_{rm} cells.

Non-recirculating T_{rm} cells in human skin were mostly CD4+ and CD69 +. **CD8+ T_{rm}** cells were mainly epidermal, a more rapidly recirculating population of T cells that expressed CLA, CCR4, L-selectin and CCR7 were identified as skin **T_{CM}** cells, whereas a more slowly recirculating population of skin T cells that expressed CCR7 (but not L-selectin) were termed migratory memory T (T_{MM}) cells, and it was proposed that these cells may be the direct precursors of T_{rm} cells. As T_{MM} cells clearly recirculate, this may explain why multiple discrete skin lesions can develop in both benign and malignant T cell-mediated skin disorders.

TABLE 9: Role of T cells in common dermatoses with the therapeutic targets utilized in their management

Psoriasis	• IL-17 is a key cytokine in psoriasis • Th17 cells and IL-17-producing CD8+ T cells (Tc17) cells play an important role • IL-23 is critical for the expansion of IL-17-producing T cells • Recurrence is due to T_{rm} cells • **Rx** – Ixekizumab, Secukinumab (Neutralize IL-17A) – Ustekinumab (Neutralizes p40 subunit of IL-12 and IL-23) – Guselkumab (Neutralizes p19 subunit of IL-23)
Atopic dermatitis	• Two main defects-Skin barrier and immune dysregulation (IL-/4-IL-13 axis.) • Th2 cells, Th22 cells and Th17 cells • The role of these may be age related • Important role of TSLP-activated DCs that polarize naive CD4+ T cells to produce IL-4, IL-5, IL-13 and TNF while downregulating IL-10 and IFNγ • Thymic stromal lymphopoietin (TSLP) mediates its stimulation of Th2 via CCL17 • The Th2 cell-type cytokines such as IL-13 and IL-31, stimulate nerve fibres directly and upregulate the release of cellular pruritogens. • Also a role of IL-33 and IL-22 • **Rx** Dupilumab (IL-4 and IL-13), and now JAKi may prove to be the therapy for AD (moderate-severe)
Alopecia areata	• Loss of immune privilege results in a subsequent assault on the hair follicle at the level of the bulb by oligoclonal and autoreactive CD8+ T cell • Cytotoxic CD8+ NKG2D + T cells • Cytokines-IFNγ and IL-5 • **Rx** JAK inhibitors (tofacitinib, baricitinib)
Vitiligo	• CD8+ T cells • IFNγ and IFNγ-dependent genes, including those encoding CXCR3 and its ligands, CXCL9, CXCL10 and CXCL11 • Recurrence due to T_{rm} cells • Antibody blockade of CD122 (a component of the IL-15R) in a mouse model of vitiligo results in the depletion of pathogenic T_{rm} cells in lesional skin and reversal of disease.

The role of T cells in common dermatoses along with the therapeutic targets utilized in their management is given in **Table 9**.

BIBLIOGRAPHY

1. Immunology, 8th edn, https://www.inkling.com/read/immunology-male-brostoff-roth-roitt-8th/chapter-11/t-cell-regulation-of-the-immune-system.
2. Clinical Immunology: Principles and Practice Fourth Edition © 2013, Elsevier Limited All rights reserved.

Chapter

1

Acne Vulgaris

Kabir Sardana, Surabhi Sinha

Acne vulgaris (acne) is an inflammatory disease of the pilosebaceous gland. It presents as open and closed comedones that develop into inflammatory red papules or pustules. Atrophic or hypertrophic acne scars may ensue, as can post-inflammatory hyperpigmentation or post-acne erythema. Acne can develop into refractory cysts, nodules, and subcutaneous fistulas. Lesions appear on the sebaceous follicle–rich areas like face, neck, chest, and upper back.

ETIOPATHOGENESIS

The classical etiology of acne vulgaris is believed to involve increased sebum excretion rates, abnormal keratinization of the follicular infundibulum, bacterial proliferation, and subsequent inflammation.

1. Sebaceous Gland in Acne

Sebaceous follicles are located on the face, chest, and upper back. The part of the isthmus where the sebaceous gland attaches to the hair follicle is referred to as the Junctional zone. Cells of the junctional zone give rise to the infundibulum and sebaceous gland **(Fig. 1.1)** and play an important role in acne. Comedo-associated sebaceous glands are atrophic suggesting abnormal differentiation of progenitor cells that are responsible for generating the sebaceous gland and infundibulum-this is known as the 'comedo switch' theory (Saurat), whereby growth of the infundibulum is aberrantly promoted in lieu of that of the sebaceous gland. (Clayton et al., 2019). Undifferentiated sebocytes in acne differentiate into sebaceous duct cells and infundibular keratinocytes instead of mature sebocytes, resulting in the abnormal keratinization of follicular channels **(Fig. 1.2)**.

Among signaling pathways, Wingless (Wnt) and Hedgehog signals are important. Low levels of Wnt signaling favor sebaceous differentiation, while high levels promote differentiation of follicular lineages. Androgens promote sebocyte differentiation and inhibit Wnt signaling. Aryl hydrocarbon receptors (AHRs) are linked to chloracne. AHRs also inhibit sebaceous differentiation by promoting the differentiation of junctional zone stem cells into infundibular keratinocytes. Fibroblast growth factor (FGF) 2 stimulates proliferation of the pilosebaceous unit, and epidermal growth factor receptors (EGFRs) can enhance the hyperproliferation of sebaceous glands and increase sebum production.

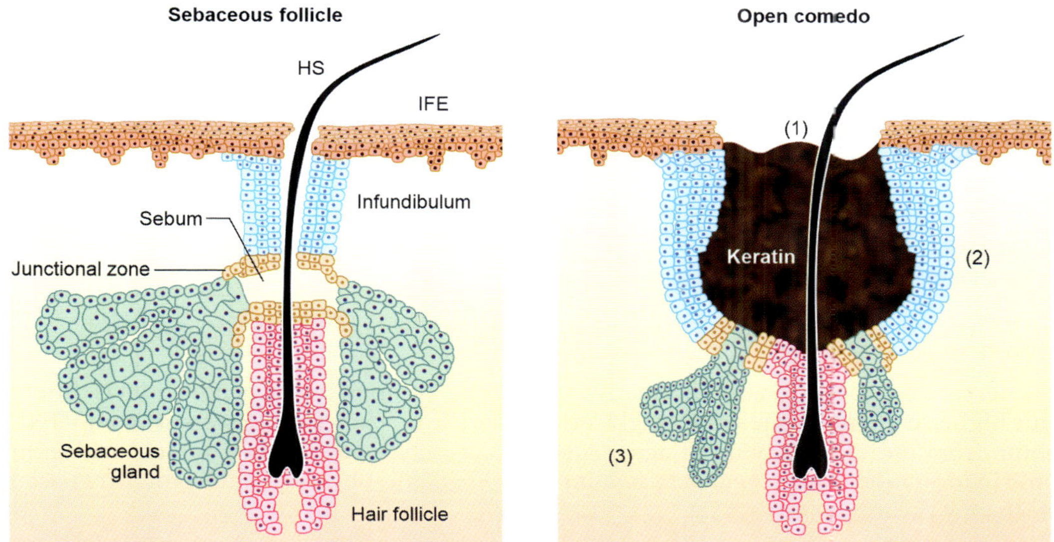

Fig. 1.1: Depiction of normal sebaceous follicle and acne pilosebaceous unit: (Left) Healthy human sebaceous follicle with multilobular sebaceous gland (SG) and normal infundibulum. Cells of the junctional zone (JZ) give rise to the infundibulum and SG. (Right) Comedo, composed of sebum and infundibular-derived keratin. Other aspects are (2) hyperplasia and abnormal keratinization of the infundibulum, and (3) atrophy of the associated SGs.

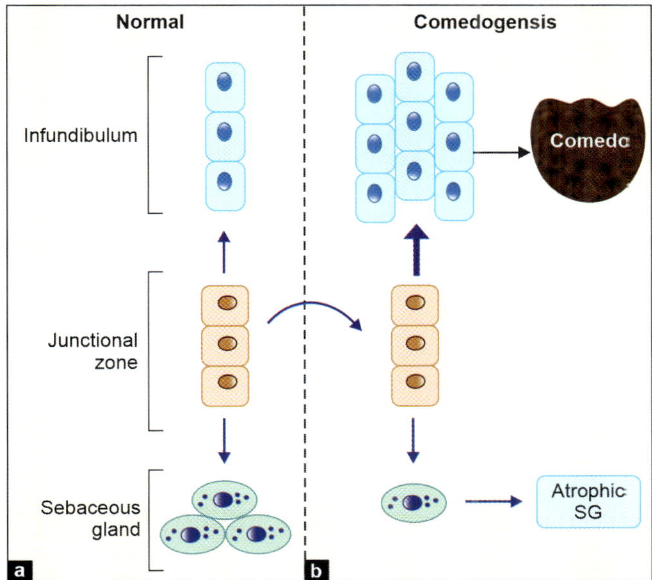

Fig. 1.2: The "comedo switch" hypothesis. (a) Progenitor cells within the junctional zone (JZ) contribute to infundibulum and the sebaceous gland (SG). (b) A comedogenic stimulus acts on cells in the JZ, causing a switch in lineage determination that favors the infundibulum, resulting in the atrophy of SG

An overview of the factors that determine activity of the SG are listed in **Box 1.1**.

BOX 1.1: Factors determining the activity of Sebaceous Glands

- Sex steroids: Androgens, testosterone, 5 alpha-reductase, estrogens, progesterone
- Peroxisome proliferator-activated receptor
- Wnt signaling: Androgens ↓Wnt signaling
- Aryl hydrocarbon receptor
- Fibroblast growth factor receptors
- ErbB family receptor signaling
- Insulin/insulin-like growth factor-1 signaling

Sebum

In acne, sebum production is abnormally high and the composition of acne sebum is different with higher content of squalene, triglycerides, and wax/cholesterol esters as compared to sebum from individuals without acne. Also, certain sebaceous lipids like oleic acid induce comedo formation in rabbit ear skin. Sebum also serves as a substrate for the growth of bacteria which may contribute to acne.

2. Keratinization in Acne

Abnormal keratinization is an important factor in acne pathogenesis. Expression of the hyperproliferative keratins **(K6, K16, and K17)** is increased in acne lesions. Significant filaggrin expression in the infundibulum is closely associated with the abnormal keratinization involved in acne. **IL-1α** is involved in abnormal keratinization, and inflammation is believed to precede abnormal keratinization.

3. Immunological Aspects and Inflammation

In acne, *Cutibacterium acnes* (*C. acnes*) in the follicular channel stimulates Langerhans cells in the infundibulum via TLR-2, resulting in the production of IL-12 and IL-8 by activating Th1 cells. *C. acnes* also stimulates follicular keratinocytes in the infundibulum via TLR-2, resulting in the production of IL-6 and IL-8, followed by the formation of inflammatory lesions. A Th1 shift occurs in acne lesions with the additional role of Th17. *C. acnes* is a potent inducer of Th17 and Th1. IL-1β and TNF-α are additionally involved in acne inflammation.

An overview is given in **Fig. 1.3** and a summary is detailed in **Box 1.2**.

4. The Cutaneous Microbiome

Under normal circumstances with a "balanced skin microbiome", *Staphylococcus epidermidis* limits overcolonization and the inflammatory response of the skin by the different *C. acnes* strains and suppresses *C. acnes*-induced IL-6 and TNF-α production by keratinocytes. Conversely, *C. acnes* limits the proliferation of *S. aureus* and *S. pyogenes* by maintaining an

BOX 1.2: Role of *C. acnes* in acne

- *C. acnes* activates TLR2 and stimulates release of proinflammatory mediators
- IL-1α, IL-8 (causes neutrophil recruitment), IL-12 (promotes Th1 response), TNF-α, MMP
- *C. acnes* increases keratinocyte expression of TLR2 and TLR4
- *C. acnes* activates NOD-like receptor protein 3 (NLRP3) of inflammasomes in cytoplasm of neutrophils and monocytes → release of proinflammatory IL-1β

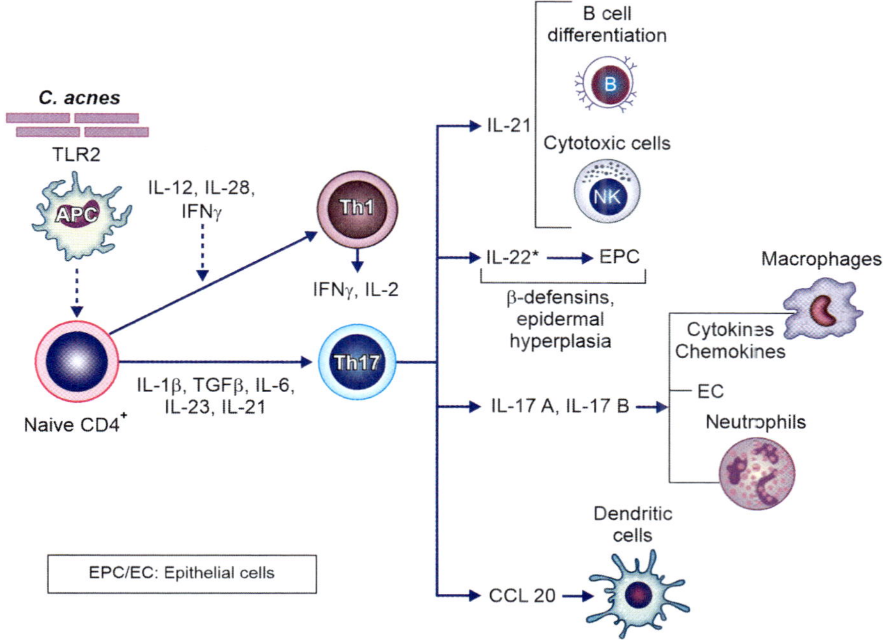

Fig. 1.3: Overview of the immunological mechanisms triggered by *C. acnes*

acidic pH of the pilosebaceous follicle due to hydrolysis of sebum triglycerides and by secreting propionic acid (Ramasamy et al., 2019).

Multiple studies have incriminated *C. acnes* in the causation of acne but phylogenetic, biochemical and microscopic *C. acnes* analyses reveal distinct evolutionary lineages, known as **types I, II and III** with recA analysis dividing type I into subclades IA and IB. Moreover, 16S rRNA analysis reveals that certain *C. acnes* strains are highly acne-associated while others are associated with healthy skin. It has been shown that phylotypes **IA-1** are strongly associated with inflammatory acne and acne fulminans.

Therefore, any modification of the natural microbiome composition may lead to a disturbed skin barrier, an effect called "dysbiosis" which triggers the activation of the innate immunity leading to inflammation. In acne, dysbiosis may be paralleled by a qualitative and quantitative change of the sebum, called "dys-seborrhea" and a modified profile of *C. acnes*.

Genetic Findings

The following genes are postulated to pay a role:

- 21-hydroxylase (*CYP21A2*),
- Steroid 5α-reductase type I (*SRD5A1*),
- Androgen receptor (*AR*),
- Growth hormone axis-*GH1*, *GHR*, *IGF1*, *IGFBP3*, and *IGF1R*,
- Peroxisome proliferator-activated receptor (*PPARA*, *PPARB*, *PPARG*, *PPARD*),
- FGF-2 (*FGF2*),
- Melanocortin receptor (*MC5R*, *MC1R*),

- Matrix metalloprotease (*MMP1, MMP2, MMP3, MMP9, MMP13*),
- TNF-α (*TNF*),
- IL-1α (*IL1A*),
- Toll-like receptors (*TLR2* and *TLR4*).

Diet and Acne

A diet rich in dairy protein and high glycemic index carbohydrates may induce acne by various mechanisms as depicted in **Boxes 1.3** and **1.4**.

BOX 1.3: Interplay between FoxO1 and mTORC1 in acne

- The cell's nutritional status is primarily sensed by the forkhead box transcription factor O1 (FoxO1) and the serine/threonine kinase mammalian target of rapamycin complex 1 (mTORC1).
- High glycemic load and dairy protein consumption both increase insulin/insulin-like growth factor-1 (IGF-1) signaling.
- FoxO1 reduces IGF-1 secretion by liver, sebaceous gland lipogenesis, androgen signaling, oxidative stress and enhances antimicrobial peptide (AMP) synthesis.
- Conversely, mTORC1 stimulates gene transcription and translation, protein synthesis, cell growth, cell proliferation and lipid synthesis. An abundance of dairy and meat protein overactivates mTORC1, leading to increased proliferation of acroinfundibular keratinocytes, sebaceous gland hyperplasia and lipogenesis.
- FoxO1 acts as a rheostat regulating mTORC1 under normal conditions. Insulinotropic diets impair gene regulation by FoxO1 and lead to unchecked activity of mTORC1.

BOX 1.4: Mechanisms of diet-induced acne

Dietary agent	***Mechanism***
Milk, whey protein	• Promotes anabolic mTORC1 signaling • Promotes IGF-1 synthesis • Stimulates sebaceous gland lipogenesis • Inhibits mRNA expression of PTEN, which downregulates nuclear FoxO1
Chocolate	• Increases cytokine production
High glycemic index carbohydrates	• Increase IGF-1 level
Fish, curcumin, silymarin, resveratrol	• Decrease inflammation • Suppress sebaceous gland lipogenesis • Inhibit SREBP-1
Omega-3 fatty acids	• Suppress production of inflammatory cytokines • Decrease IGF-1 level • Inhibits TLR-1 and TLR-2 signaling • Inhibits mTORC1 signaling • Downregulates SREBP-1c pathway

FoxO1-forkhead box transcription factor O1, mTORC1-serine/threonine kinase mammalian target of rapamycin complex 1.

LESIONS OF ACNE

Comedones—the earliest lesion to develop. Can be open ("blackheads") or closed ("whiteheads") **(Fig. 1.4)**. Open comedones allow oxidation of the debris within the follicle leading to the black color. Types of comedones are as follows:

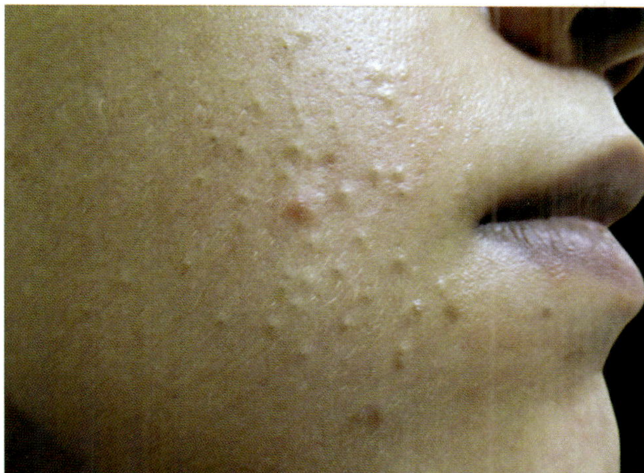

Fig. 1.4: Multiple comedones in a case of mild acne

- Sandpaper comedones—multiple, very small whiteheads usually on the forehead. Give a gritty feel to the skin and respond poorly to treatment.
- Macrocomedones—large whiteheads >1 mm in diameter. Respond poorly to treatment.
- Submarine comedones—large comedones >0.5 cm in diameter. Reside deep within the skin and associated with recurrent nodules.

Inflammatory Lesions

Papules, pustules (<5 mm), nodules (>5 mm) which often heal with pigmentation **(Figs 1.5 and 1.6)**.

Sinus tracts may form between deep-seated nodules leading to scarring.

Inflammatory macules may persist for many weeks.

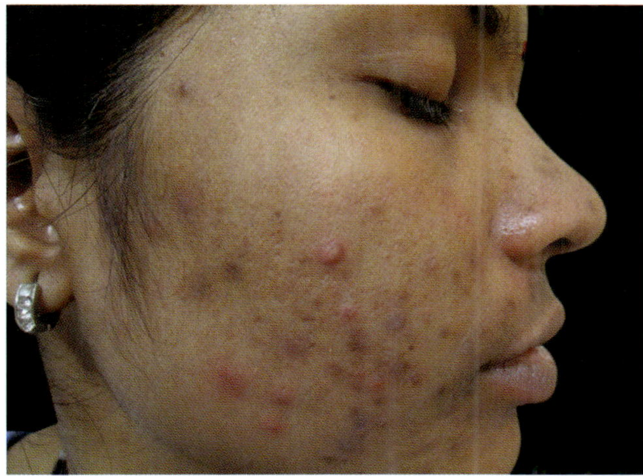

Fig. 1.5: Multiple papules, pustules and associated PIH in a case of acne

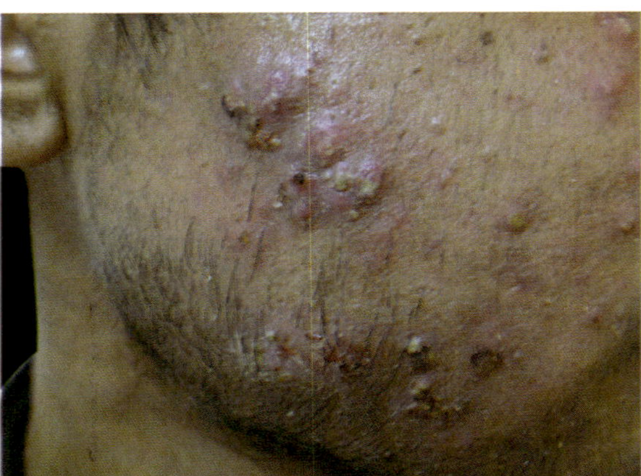

Fig. 1.6: Nodules and pustules in a case of acne

CLINICAL VARIANTS OF ACNE

- **Adult female acne/post-adolescent acne (Fig. 1.7)**
  - *Androgen source in females*: Androgen excess disorders manifest by an interaction between circulating androgen levels and the sensitivity of hair follicles to androgen stimulation **(Fig. 1.8)**. In women, the major circulating androgens (in descending order of serum concentration) are dehydroepiandrosterone sulfate (DHEA-S), dehydroepiandrosterone (DHEA), androstenedione, testosterone, and DHT. DHEA-S, DHEA, and androstenedione can be considered prehormones because they have little or no intrinsic androgenic activity and require conversion to testosterone to exert androgenic effects. DHEA-S is produced almost exclusively by the adrenal glands, DHEA is produced by both the adrenals (50%) and the ovaries (20%) and by peripheral conversion of DHEA-S (30%). Androstenedione production is divided equally between the ovaries and the adrenals and testosterone

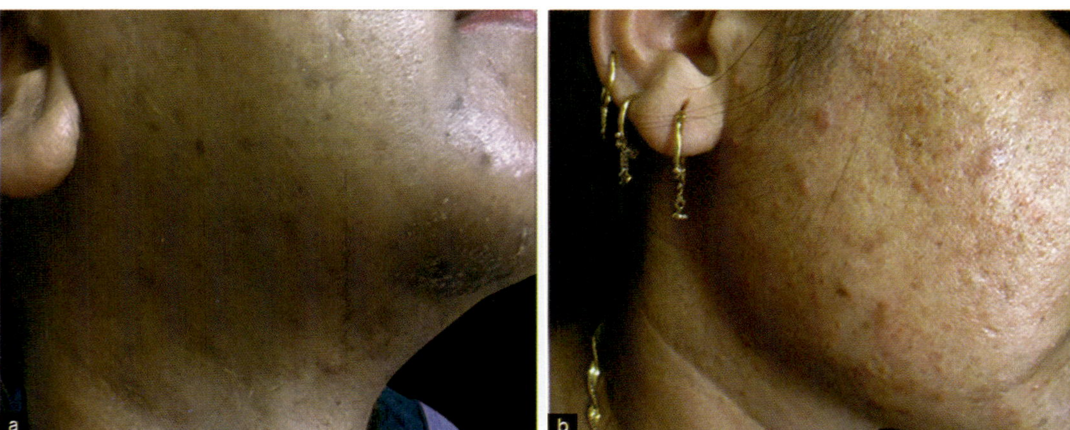

Fig. 1.7: Hormonal or adult female acne has usually jawline acne with hirsutism with signs and symptoms of hyperandrogenism including ovulatory dysfunction (manifesting as irregular menstrual cycles)

production derives from the adrenals (25%), the ovaries (25%), and from peripheral conversion of androstenedione (50%) **(Fig. 1.8)**. In normal women, about 80% of circulating testosterone is bound to a beta globulin known as sex hormone-binding globulin (SHBG), another 19% is loosely bound to albumin, leaving only about 1% unbound or free. 3α-androstanediol is the peripheral tissue metabolite of DHT, and its glucuronide conjugate, 3α-androstanediol glucuronide (3α-AG), can be used as a marker of peripheral androgen metabolism specially in those with normal testosterone levels. The common etiology of androgen excess is listed in **Table 1.1**.

- Clinical manifestations of hyperandrogenism include hirsutism, acne, androgenic alopecia, and virilization. Hirsutism, defined as excessive growth of terminal hair in women in a male-like pattern, is the most commonly used clinical diagnostic criterion of

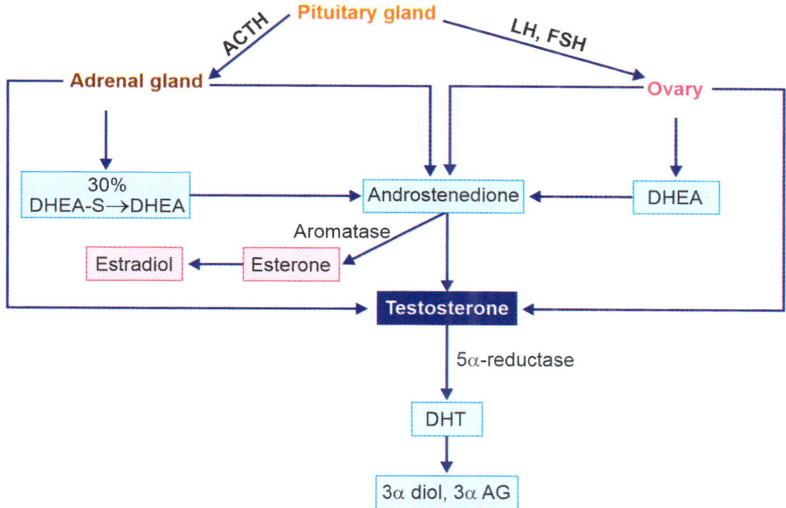

Fig. 1.8: Pathway showing the production and distribution of preandrogens and testosterone and its end organ metabolites which determine hormonal acne

TABLE 1.1: Androgen excess disorders among women (Azziz et al., 2004)

Diagnosis	Number	Prevalence (%)
Specific disorders		
Androgen-secreting neoplasm	2	0.23
Classical congenital adrenal hyperplasia	6	0.69
Nonclassical congenital adrenal hyperplasia	18	2.06
Hair-AN syndrome	33	3.78
Disorders of exclusion		
Polycystic ovary syndrome	716	82.02
Idiopathic hirsutism	39	4.47
Hyperandrogenemia, hisutism, and normal ovulation	59	6.75
Total	873	100.00

hyperandrogenism. The presence of hirsutism is usually determined by using a standardized scoring system of hair growth and may be seen in up to 80% of patients with hyperandrogenism. Acne and androgenic alopecia are other common androgenic skin changes, and might be observed without hirsutism in some hyperandrogenic women. However, isolated presence of any of these manifestations is not usually considered as a diagnostic criterion for hyperandrogenism. Virilization is a relatively uncommon feature of hyperandrogenism, and its presence often suggests an androgen-producing tumor. A thorough history and a focused clinical examination are extremely helpful in diagnostic evaluation of patients with suspected hyperandrogenism (Yildiz BO, 2006).

- Adult female acne (AFA) is acne that is seen beyond 25 years of age and can present either as "isolated" acne or with hyperandrogenic signs. While acne per se can be a feature of HA routine hormonal tests may not reveal an underlying abnormality except PCOS. End-organ hypersensitivity is the most plausible explanation and thus justifies the use of antiandrogens in its management (Bansal et al., 2021).
- A recent study found that of the AFA subtypes, the late onset subtype was more common in adult acne patients (56.6%) but the persistent acne subgroup (43.33%) had a younger age at onset, a past history of adolescent acne (51.92%), truncal predilection (44.23%), polycystic ovary syndrome (PCOS) (44.23%), significant presence of irregular menses (40.38%) and hirsutism (57.69%), and increased TT (13.46%), 17-OHP (76.92%), AMH (44.23%), and increased LH/FSH (15.38%) ratio. PCOS was seen more in the persistent acne patients with clinical HA and increased 17-OHP levels (Sardana K et al., 2012)

- **Acne fulminans:** This is a rare severe variant predominantly occurring in adolescent males. Sudden onset of febrile ulcerative necrotic acne covered with hemorrhagic crusts, with fever, arthralgia and other systemic symptoms are seen and they fail to respond to antibiotics. Rx-prednisone monotherapy for 2–4 weeks followed by low-dose isotretinoin for 4 weeks, then slowly increase isotretinoin (to avoid paradoxical flare during the acute inflammatory phase).
  Others: Topical/intralesional corticosteroids, oral antibiotics, TNF-α inhibitors, IL-1 antagonists, azathioprine, cyclosporine, dapsone.
- **Acne conglobata:** This is a severe acne variant with multiple grouped (polyporous) comedones, interspersed with papules, tender inflammatory nodules which may be suppurative and coalesce to form sinus tracts with extensive scarring as usual outcome.
  Part of **follicular occlusion tetrad:** Dissecting cellulitis of scalp, hidradenitis suppurativa, pilonidal cyst, acne conglobata.
  Other syndromes associated:
  - PAPA-sterile pyogenic arthritis, pyoderma gangrenosum, acne conglobata (PSTPIP1 mutation)
  - PAPASH-pyogenic arthritis, pyoderma gangrenosum, acne, suppurative hidradenitis
- Acne associated with **psychiatric disease:**
  - Acne excoriee
  - Body dysmorphic disorder
  - Eating disorders
- **Granulomatous acne**
- **Neonatal acne/Neonatal cephalic pustulosis:** Seen in >20% healthy newborns around 2 weeks of age, resolves within 3 months, papules and pustules on cheeks, foreheads, eyelids, chin, upper trunk.

TABLE 1.2: Variants of acne/Acneiform eruptions
• **Drug-induced acne:** Anabolic steroids, bromides, corticosteroids, EGFR inhibitors, iodides, isoniazid, lithium, MEK inhibitors (trametinib), phenytoin, progestins
• **Occupational acne:** Comedones with papules, pustules, cystic lesions due to exposure to insoluble, follicle-occluding substances such as cutting oils, petroleum-based products, chlorinated aromatic hydrocarbons, coal tar derivatives
• **Acne cosmetica:** Comedonal acne (mostly closed comedones) due to chronic exposure to follicle-occluding cosmetics
• **Pomade acne:** Comedonal facial acne at the forehead and temples due to follicle-occlusion by hair products
• **Chloracne:** Occurs several weeks after systemic exposure to halogenated aromatic hydrocarbons (percutaneous absorption, inhalation, ingestion)—found in insecticides, insulators, fungicides, herbicides, wood preservatives
• **Acne mechanica:** Comedo formation due to repeated mechanical and frictional obstruction of pilosebaceous unit
• **Tropical acne:** Acneiform eruption after exposure to extreme heat
• **Radiation acne:** Comedo-like papules at sites of previous exposure to therapeutic ionizing radiation
• **Pseudoacne of the nasal crease:** Transverse nasal crease with milia, cysts, and comedones lining up along the fold
• **Idiopathic facial aseptic granuloma:** Affects young children, usually single painless nodule on cheek, resolve spontaenous after 1 year
• **Childhood flexural comedones:** Discrete, double-orifice comedones localized to axillae > groin, usually single lesion, with no association with hidradenitis suppurativa, acne vulgaris, or precocious puberty

- **Mid-childhood acne:** Seen in children between 1 and 7 years, possibility of underlying hyperandrogenic condition should be considered.
- **Preadolescent acne:** Presents between 7 and 12 years of age with prominent comedo formation, pitted scarring, occasional deep suppurative nodules.
  Resolves within 6–18 months but associated with ↑ severe acne during adolescence.

A list of acneiform eruptions is listed in **Table 1.2**.

INVESTIGATIONS AND WORK UP FOR ACNE

Microbiologic and Endocrinological

Routine microbiologic testing is not recommended in the evaluation and management of patients with acne though some scenarios are detailed below.

- Those who exhibit acne-like lesions suggestive of gram-negative folliculitis may benefit from microbiologic testing.
- Routine endocrinologic evaluation (e.g. for androgen excess) is not recommended for most patients with acne except in cases of adult female acne and when there are signs of androgen excess.

An overview of the investigations is detailed in **Table 1.3**.

A significant number of female patients have hormonal acne and this should be suspected especially in adult female acne. Indications for testing for hormonal acne and the suggested tests are listed in **Table 1.4**.

TABLE 1.3: List of investigations in acne

Test for organisms	• Pyogenic bacterial folliculitis due to *Staphylococcus aureus* which may mimic acne • Gram negative folliculitis • Malassezia folliculitis • Tinea faciei due to a dermatophyte fungus such as *Trichophyton rubrum* or *Microsporum canis* • In suspected cases of resistance culture and 16-S-RNA verification of *C. acnes*
Hormonal tests	• Possibility of pregnancy, which would influence what treatment was appropriate • Signs suggesting hyperandrogenism including PCOS and NCCAH • Signs suggesting excessive prolactin • Signs suggesting Cushing syndrome
Imaging	• USG, CT, MRI whenever indicated
Tests for monitoring Rx	• LFT, Lipids and UPT

TABLE 1.4: Work up in a suspected case of hormonal acne

When to evaluate for a hormonal cause?	• Postadolescent acne/acne tarda • A male patient who has cystic acne and has failed therapy • Prepubertal children with acne, early-onset body odor, axillary or pubic hair, accelerated growth, advanced bone age, and genital maturation • A female patient who has failed multiple courses of recommended therapy • Signs of hyperandrogenism • In women, polycystic ovary syndrome (PCOS) • Rapid appearance of acne in conjunction with virilization suggestive of an underlying adrenal or ovarian tumor • Patients with Cushing's disease or syndrome and late-onset congenital adrenal hyperplasia
Which tests to perform	• Total testosterone and free androgen index • DHEA-S • Prolactin • TSH • Anti-Mullerian hormone (AMH) (a sensitive tool to diagnose PCOM: polycystic ovarian morphology and PCOS) • 17-hydroxyprogesterone (to diagnose nonclassic congenital adrenal hyperplasia [NCCAH]) • USG, CT, MRI whenever indicated

Endocrinological Investigations

The aim of investigations are **twofold:**

a. To elicit the source of androgens
b. To eliminate the common causes and differentials including PCOS.

Testosterone levels are usually the best way to start the investigative profile and its levels can predict the possible causes. As free testosterone levels are erratic and inconsistent due to lack of sensitive tools and its miniscule levels in the blood, various calculated indices are used, one of which is free androgen index **(FAI)**. While PCOS is a common cause, in AFA the conventional tool to diagnose it, **USG**, has a notable drawback. Polycystic ovarian syndrome (PCOS) diagnosis in adult female acne (AFA) using a TV USG can be an issue, specially in the population that is commonly seen by dermatologists, as most patients are unmarried and may not consent for a TV USG which is the gold old standard for sonographic diagnosis of PCOS. Also transabdominal USG is not sensitive in obese females (Bell et al., 2021). Also the criterion of PCOM is restricted to the Rotterdam criterion and is not universally accepted as the presence of PCOM is neither necessary nor sufficient for diagnosis of PCOS. There is no evidence that the presence of PCOM has any implications with regard to the endocrine or metabolic features of PCOS. There is also no evidence to support the addition of assessment of PCOM to the diagnosis of NIH PCOS. Thus a large body of evidence suggests that assessment of PCOM is not needed for the endocrine management of PCOS or hirsutism; use of accurate ovarian sonography is limited to reproductive endocrinology.

A recent study (Bansal et al., 2020) found that AFA with PCOS had significant clinical hyperandrogenism, truncal and adolescent acne, and raised hormones (AMH, TT, FAI, LH, and LH/FSH). The **AMH levels** were significantly higher in the PCOS group (6.91 ± 3.85 ng/mL) and positively correlated with TT, FAI, 17OHP, LH, and LH/FSH ratio. AMH at >5.1 ng/mL (sensitivity-70.97% and specificity-82.02%) predicted PCOS and correlated with PCOM. Thus AMH (>5.1 ng/mL) is a sensitive tool to diagnose PCOS (Bansal et al., 2020). Here it is important to understand that this test can have a variation due to the assay used, but as a general rule higher the value "beyond 5", more the chances of PCOS (Rudnicka et al., 2021) and this is a more sensitive tool than a USG for diagnosis of PCOM.

While some feel that NCCAH is common in AFA, this is not true in most cases, and we do not think 17OHP is needed in the majority of cases of AFA.

The values of various tests depend a lot on the reference values which do vary between laboratories. It is accepted that tests should be performed on the 5th day of the cycle with a proviso of avoidance of any hormonal medicine for 3 months. A few **cut off values** that can be used to diagnose hyperandrogenism and include: normal levels of total testosterone should not exceed 1.1 ng/mL (54.5 ng/dL), normal levels of DHEA should not exceed 430 µg/dL, FAI should not exceed 5 and AMH beyond 5 ng/mL indicates PCOM. The interpretation of tests depends on the experience of the clinician and an important adage is to minimize unnecessary tests.

TREATMENT OF ACNE

The therapeutic agents can be classified according to the major pathogenic steps they modify in acne **(Fig. 1.9)**, though some would work on more than one of the major factors.

Many treatment guidelines have been published by various bodies of dermatological experts worldwide. Select recommendations from the American Academy of Dermatology's acne clinical guidelines (2016) are listed in **Table 1.5**.

An overview of the current treatment guidelines are depicted in the **Figs 1.10 and 1.11** and the details will in the text below.

Certain general measures that can be advised include use of noncomedogenic products and avoiding use of excessive hair oil which is a common cause of acne localized to the forehead.

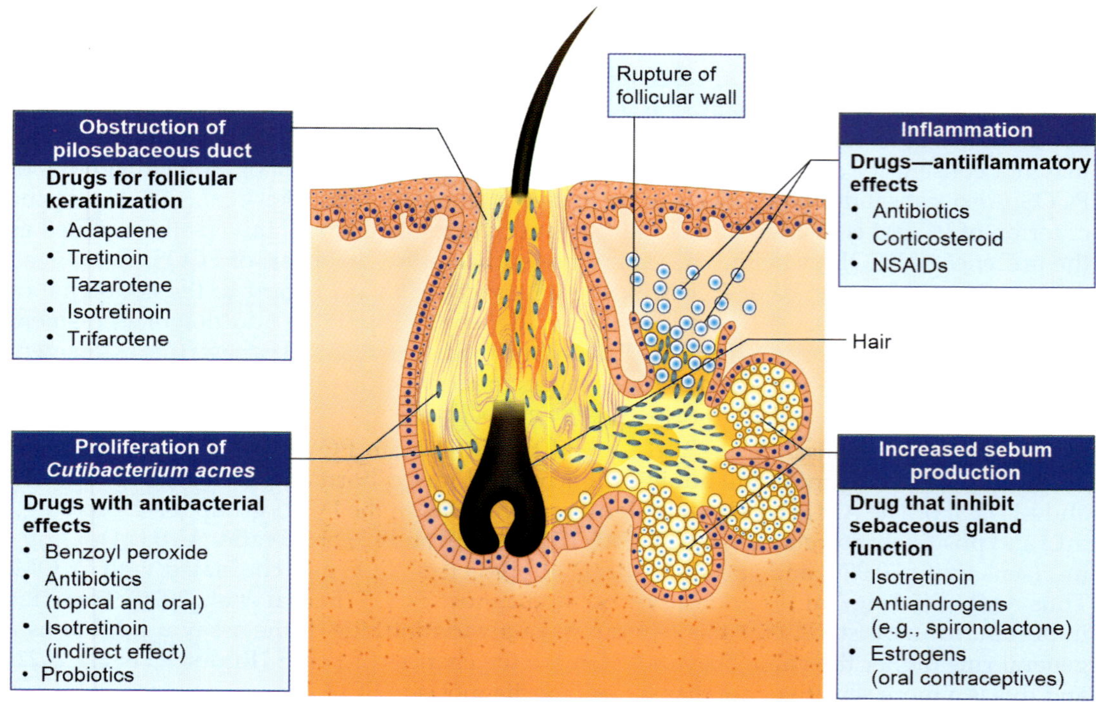

Fig. 1.9: Overview of the major targets of therapeutic agents in acne vulgaris

TABLE 1.5: Recommendations from the American Academy of Dermatology's acne clinical guidelines (Zaenglein AL, 2016)

AAD recommendation	Topical therapy
Recommendation 1	Benzoyl peroxide is recommended for all patients using a topical or systemic antibiotic to prevent antibiotic resistance
Recommendation 2	Topical antibiotics are not recommended as monotherapy because of the risk of bacterial resistance
Recommendation 3	Combination therapy with multiple topical agents that target different aspects of acne pathogenesis (i.e. topical retinoid + topical antibiotic) is recommended for most patients with acne
	Systemic therapy
Recommendation 4	Systemic antibiotic monotherapy is not recommended because of the risk of antibiotic resistance
Recommendation 5	Topical benzoyl peroxide or topical retinoids should be used concurrently with systemic antibiotic therapy

1. Topical Agents

A list of common agents is listed in **Table 1.6**.

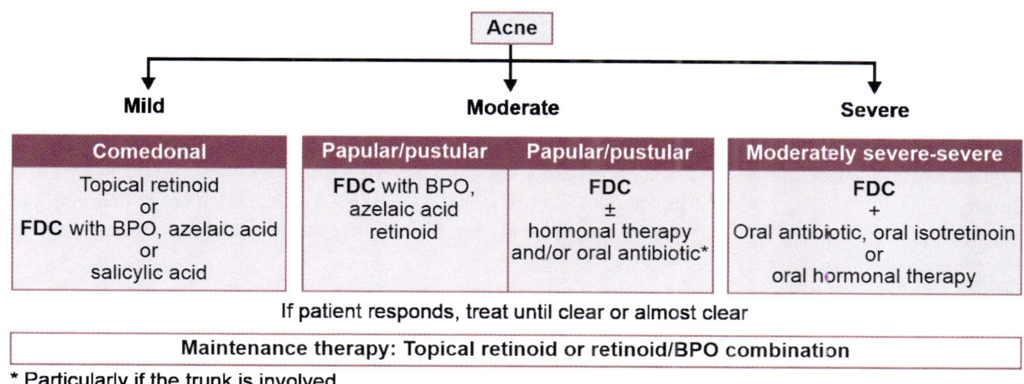

Fig. 1.10: Overview of standard treatment for various grades of acne

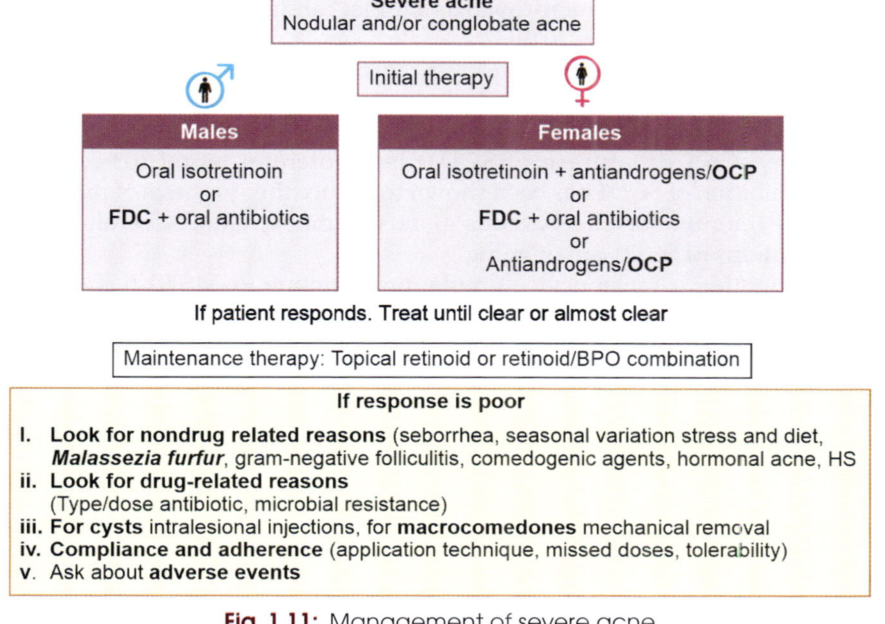

Fig. 1.11: Management of severe acne

A recent systematic review and network meta-analysis on topical treatment of mild-to-moderate acne concluded that adapalene plus benzoyl peroxide may be the most effective therapy but with a slightly higher incidence of withdrawal (Stuart et al., 2021).

TABLE 1.6: Overview of topical agents*	
Benzoyl peroxide (BPO)	If irritation is not a factor, BP or combination with clindamycin are effective treatments and are recommended as monotherapy for mild acne, or in conjunction with a topical retinoid, or systemic antibiotic therapy for moderate to severe acne.
Topical antibiotics	Avoid as monotherapy
Retinoids	Ideal initial agents and can be used alone for comedonal acne, or in combination with topical or oral antimicrobials in patients with mixed or primarily inflammatory acne lesions.
Azelaic acid	Aside from retinoids, azelaic acid is a useful adjunctive acne treatment and is recommended in the treatment of postinflammatory dyspigmentation
Topical dapsone 5% gel	In adult female acne
Combination agents	Stable, fixed-combination agents are available with erythromycin 3%/BPO 5%, clindamycin 1%/BPO 5%, and clindamycin 1%/BPO 3.75%., Adapalene 0.3%/ benzoyl peroxide 2.5%.

*Sardana K, Narang I; IADVL Textbook of Dermatology 5th edn 2022

Novel Topical Agents

- **Trifarotene**, a novel fourth-generation retinoid, selective for gamma-RAR, has demonstrated improved tolerability compared with existing topical retinoids.
- **Clascoterone** is a novel first-in-class antiandrogen that topically addresses the hormonal etiology of acne. It was US FDA approved as a topical androgen receptor inhibitor for acne in patients 12 years and older in 2020.
- **SB204**. This agent contains a nitric oxide-releasing macromolecule formulated in an alcoholic gel.
- Topical **minocycline 4% foam**. This formulation is not yet launched in India.
- Agents that inhibit sebum production is a novel approach and is based on the fact that the enzyme stearoyl-CoA desaturase 1 **(SCD1)** is a potential target for reducing sebum production. Inhibition of SCD1 has been shown to reduce the synthesis of monounsaturated fatty acids and the number of sebaceous glands in mouse skin. Several clinical trials of topical formulations of SCD1 are ongoing.
- Melanocortin peptide α-melanocyte-stimulating hormone **(α-MSH)** has demonstrated a sebotrophic effect in mice and an α-MSH mimetic compound is being tested in subjects with acne in a phase 2 study.
- **Nitiricoxide (NO)** releasing particles are under investigation due to their potential to suppress the release of multiple cytokines from human monocytes and keratinocytes and to prevent *C. acnes* induced inflammation.
- N-acetyl-GED-0507-34-LEVO **(NAC-GED)** gel 5% which acts as a selective peroxisome proliferator-activated receptor-c (PPARγ) modulator, has been recently tried (Br J Dermatol 2022; 187:507–14).

2. Systemic Agents

Systemic antibiotics have been the mainstay of acne treatment for years and are probably the most misused drugs even though elaborate guidelines have been made to restrict their misuse. Notably acne is not an "infection" and thus suppressing *C. acnes* is not needed to treat it. Evidence supports the efficacy of erythromycin, azithromycin, amoxicillin, tetracycline, doxycycline, minocycline, trimethoprim, trimethoprim/sulfamethoxazole (TMP/SMX), and cephalexin. An overview of the general principles that dictate use of systemic agents is given in **Table 1.7**. A pilot study confirmed high resistance of *P. acnes* (identified by 16S RNA PCR) and the antibiotic sensitivity pattern to various antibiotics in India is depicted in **Figure 1.12** and gives data of the ideal antibiotic that can be prescribed which in India seems to be minocycline and **not** azithromycin (Sardana K, et al., 2021).

Sarecycline is a once-daily, oral, narrow-spectrum, tetracycline-derived antibiotic with anti-inflammatory properties. At 1.5 and 3.0 mg/kg, it significantly reduced inflammatory lesion counts from baseline compared with placebo (by 52.7%, 51.8%, and 38.3%, respectively), with no significant difference from placebo in noninflammatory lesion counts in a phase 2 trial of patients with moderate or severe acne. Sarecycline, being a narrow-spectrum tetracycline, is notable for being very effective against *Cutibacterium acnes* without affecting other bacteria and thus seems to preserve the natural microbiome. It has not yet been launched in India.

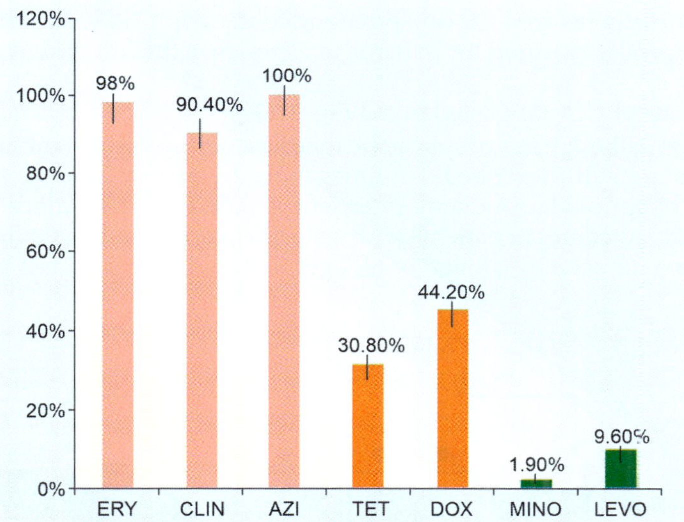

Fig. 1.12: Antibiotic sensitivity pattern in India in *C. acnes* isolates showing high rates of resistance to azithromycin and erythromycin (Sardana K, et al., 2021)

TABLE 1.7: Overview of the general principles that dictate use of systemic antibiotics in acne
Systemic antibiotics are recommended in the management of moderate and severe acne and forms of inflammatory acne that are resistant to topical treatments.
Doxycycline and minocycline are equally effective but Indian data show that minocycline has negligible resistance and is the preferred tetracycline.
Although oral erythromycin and azithromycin can be effective in treating acne, their use should be limited to those who cannot use the tetracyclines (i.e. pregnant women or children <8 years of age).
Response should be evaluated at 6–8 weeks and therapy should be given for a maximum of 3 months.
Benzoyl peroxide or a retinoid should be used concomitantly.
Subantimicrobial dose antibiotics are useful but trials are not yet confirmatory for their efficacy.
The minocycline ER (extended release) formulation is not subantimicrobial, thus it can potentially cause resistance. It is not superior to conventinal minocycline.

Recommendations for Hormonal Agents

While antiandrogens target obvious signs of hyperandrogenism, women with Idiopathic Hyperandrogenism relating to increased end-organ sensitivity to androgens can benefit from treatments that lower free/active androgen concentrations or block the androgen receptor. The clinical response correlates with circulating levels of 3α-androstanediol glucuronide (the peripheral metabolite of DHT), supporting increased peripheral 5α-reductase activity as the cause of IH.

- Estrogen-containing **combined oral contraceptives (COC)** are effective and recommended in the treatment of inflammatory acne in females.

  COC containing estrogen and progestin, address the hormonal pathogenesis of acne, decreasing free testosterone **by 40–50%** on an average. In addition, estrogen also reduces the conversion of testosterone to dihydrotestosterone in the pilosebaceous unit, further decreasing sebum production. Trials comparing drospirenone containing COCs to other COCs have generally favored the drospirenone containing COCs. A course of 3–6 months of therapy is typically required for patients to experience the full benefit of treatment with a COC.

  The major actions of COC are listed in the **Fig. 1.13**.
- **Spironolactone:** Although use of spironolactone has increased substantially in recent years, oral antibiotics are still prescribed 3–5 times more frequently among women with acne. Increased use of spironolactone may represent an opportunity to improve antimicrobial stewardship and outcomes in patients with acne. It is important to note that spironolactone may be effective for acne in women of <u>all ages</u> and its use should not be limited only to

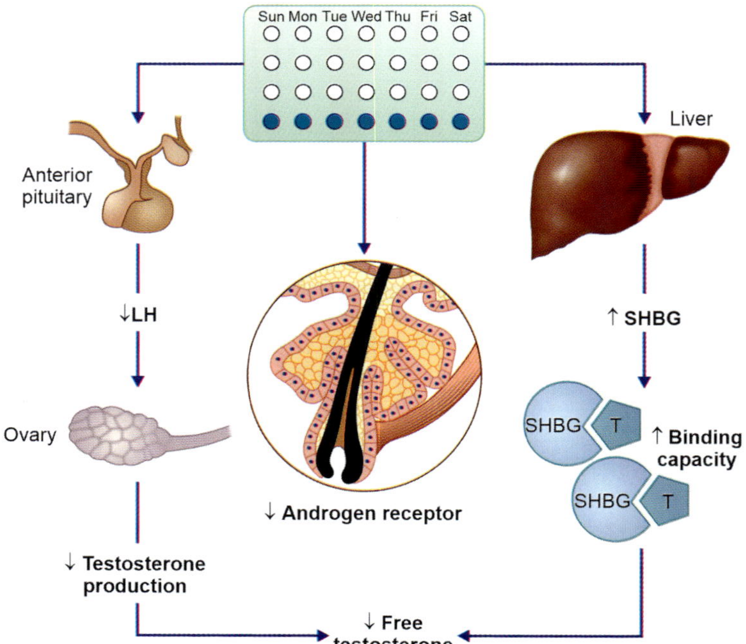

Fig. 1.13: A depiction of the major actions of combined oral contraceptives

adult women or women with prominent acne on the lower face or acne that flares with their menstrual cycle. (Krunic A, et al., 2008)

MOA: It competes with DHT for binding to the androgen receptor and, to a varying extent, also inhibits ovarian and adrenal androgen synthesis. Although serum androstenedione levels decrease, those of DHEA, DHEA-S, and cortisol do not significantly change during treatment with spironolactone.

Does: Starting dose is typically 100 mg/day in the evening with a maximum of 200 mg/d. The effects of spironolactone are dose dependent, and best results are achieved with doses of 50–100 mg twice daily. Ideally it should be combined with COC, preferably drospirenone containing COC.

- In classic congenital adrenal hyperplasia, glucocorticoids are effective in suppressing ACTH-stimulated adrenal androgen production. In **NCCAH**, glucocorticoids should **not be the first-line therapy** to treat symptoms/signs of hyperandrogenism other than for ovulation induction. In fact, oral contraceptives are more effective in improving hirsutism compared with dexamethasone (Frank-Raue K, et al., 1990).

Recommendations for Isotretinoin (Zaenglein AL, et al., 2016)

- Oral isotretinoin is recommended for the treatment of severe nodular acne.
- Oral isotretinoin is appropriate for the treatment of moderate acne that is treatment-resistant or for the management of acne that is producing physical scarring or psychosocial distress.
- Low-dose isotretinoin can be used to effectively treat acne and reduce the frequency and severity of medication-related side effects. Intermittent dosing of isotretinoin is not recommended.
- A recent Delphi consensus study evaluated laboratory monitoring for isotretinoin and arrived at the following consensus: alanine aminotransferase and triglycerides should be checked within a month prior to initiation and at peak dose (not monthly); complete blood cell count, basic metabolic panel parameters, gamma-glutamyl transferase, bilirubin, albumin, total protein, low-density lipoprotein, high-density lipoprotein, or C-reactive protein do not need to be checked at any point during isotretinoin treatment (Xia E, et al., 2022.)
- All patients treated with isotretinoin must adhere to the iPLEDGE risk management program.
- Females of child-bearing potential taking isotretinoin should be counseled regarding various contraceptive methods including user-independent forms.
- Prescribing physicians also should monitor their patients for any indication of inflammatory bowel disease and depressive symptoms and educate their patients about the potential risks with isotretinoin **(Table 1.8)**.

MANAGING ACNE DURING PREGNANCY AND LACTATION

The topical agents azelaic acid, BPO, and clindamycin (**"ABC"**) and the systemic medications amoxicillin, cephalexin, and erythromycin (mnemonic **"ACE"**) can be used during pregnancy **(Table 1.9)**.

OTHER THERAPEUTIC AGENTS

- Light therapy
  - Blue light (1–2 times per week for 4 weeks), Red + blue light (15 min daily for 12 weeks).
- PDT
  - ALA + red light or blue light

TABLE 1.8: Optimization of isotretinoin use in acne (Landis, Megan N 2020; Sardana K 2021)

Dose	• Low dose: <0.5 mg/kg/d (for mild to moderate acne) • High dose: >**220** mg/kg cumulative dose (for **severe acne only**!) (relapse rate at 1 year was 26.6% among those who received >220 mg/kg cumulative dose compared to 43.8% among those treated with lower doses.) • Post-treatment effect: Lasts for 5 months, hence second course can wait for this duration. • Duration of treatment: Continue till complete clearance and a further 2 months irrespective of cumulative dose.
Relapse	• Majority relapse within first 3 years of stopping therapy. • More in truncal acne or in those receiving a total cumulative dose of <120 mg/kg. • Relapse rates in those receiving a total cumulative dose of 120–150 mg/kg of isotretinoin range between 20% and 60%. • Younger age at initial treatment and male gender are associated with an increased risk of relapse, with those under 16 years of age having approximately a 25% increased rate of relapse.
Tests	• Baseline fasting lipid profile and liver function tests. • If these test results are normal and the dose of isotretinoin remains stable, discontinue laboratory monitoring. • Women of childbearing potential must have a monthly serum or urine pregnancy test throughout the duration of therapy. A pregnancy test also should be performed 1 month after the last dose of isotretinoin. • Those with serum triglyceride concentration increases to at least >89 mg/dL (1.0 mmol/L) during isotretinoin therapy (hyper-responders) are prone to future hyperlipidemia and metabolic syndrome.

- Chemical Peels (e.g. salicylic acid, glycolic acid)
- 1450 nm diode laser
  - Fluence 10–14 J/cm^2, 6 mm spot size, 250 ns pulse duration and cooling at 35 ms with 2 passes, treatments monthly for 3–6 months.

ACNE SCARRING

Acne scars can be divided into **three different types:** Atrophic, hypertrophic and red-pigmented macular acne scars. Strictly speaking, the macular acne scars are not "scars" as they are transient) **(Fig. 1.14)**.

Hypertrophic scars are divided into two types:

- Simple: Not exceeding the margins of the initial lesions, usually regress after 12–18 months.
- Keloid: Exceeding the margins, more frequent in the prethoracic region, the back, or the mandible.

Atrophic acne scars are related to particular inflammatory mediators and enzymatic degradation of collagen fibers and fat. **Atrophic acne scars** are the most common (80–90% of all acne scars patients), and they can be further divided into the following types: ice-pick scars, rolling scars, boxcar scars, perifollicular elastolysis, and complex scars **(Fig. 1.14)**.

For clinical types of acne scars the **depth** is important with respect to the procedures employed to treat them and thus a random robotic use of therapies is of little use. Lasers, especially fractional ablative, can achieve both depth and width and can correct most atrophic scars if a proper depth is achieved. (Sardana K, et al., 2012)

TABLE 1.9: Acne therapies: pregnancy categories

Acne severity	Medication	Pregnancy category	Comments
	Topical		
	Azelaic acid	B	About 4%–8% absorption; no known fetal effects
	Benzoyl peroxide	C	May be used on limited areas
	Clindomycin, erythromycin	B	Minimal data: no known fetal effects
	Dapsone	C	Limited data: use during pregnancy has not been associated with increased risk of fetal malformations
	Glycolic acid	N	No evidence of adverse effects during pregnancy
	Salicylic acid	C	Low risk if restricted to local areas for limited duration
Mild/ moderate/ severe	Topical retinoids	C-X	Not recommended during pregnancy
	Systemic		
	Amoxicillin	B	Short-term; avoid in first trimester—associated with oral clefts
	Cephalexin	B	No malformations in animal studies
	Macrolides (erythromycin is drug of choice)	B	Short-term use; avoid in first trimester; ***AVOID*** erythromycin estolate, as it is associated with hepatotoxicity in the second trimester
	Spironolactone	D	Feminization of male fetus
	Tetracyclines	D	Contraindicated after the 15th week of pregnancy
	Zinc	C	<75 mg/day; no increased risk of fetal abnormalities in animal and human studies
	Photodynamic therapy		
	Narrowband and broadband ultraviolet B light		Considered acceptable during pregnancy
Severe/acne fulminans	Isotretinoin	X	Teratogenic; contraindicated in females of childbearing potential unles patient is not pregnant or breasfeeding and agrees to comply with mandatory contraceptive measures (e.g. concurrent use of two forms of contraception) in accordance with the System to Manage Accutane Related Teratogenicity™ (SMART™)
	Oral glucocorticoids	C	Human studies showed an increased risk of oral cleft and a slight increase in miscarriage rates and preterm births; short-term use after first trimester Doses limited to <20 mg/day over a course of ≤1 month during the third trimester

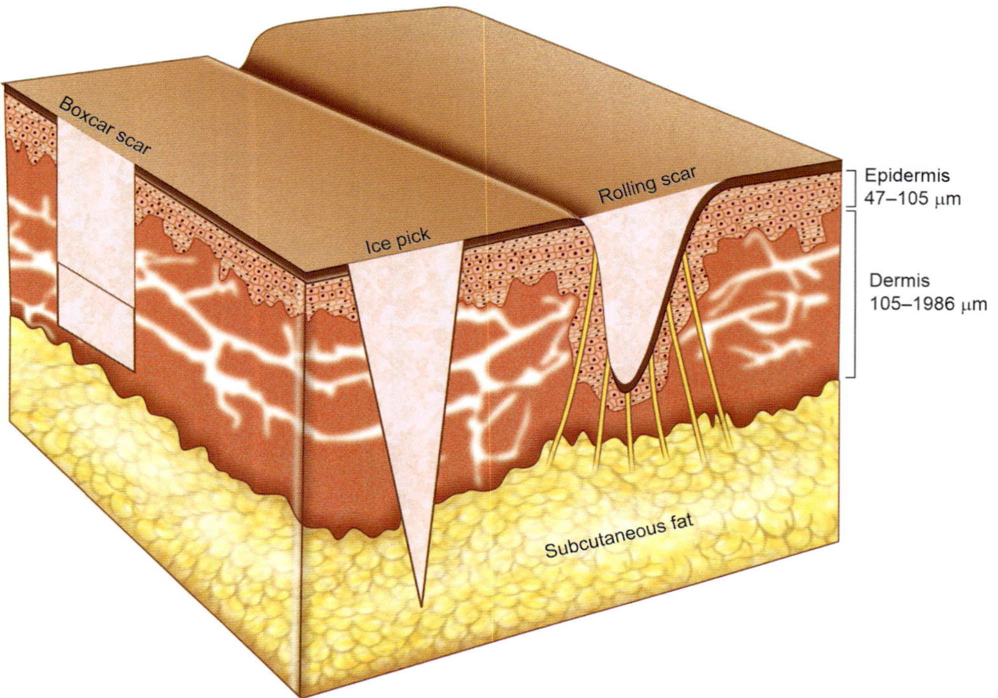

Fig. 1.14: A depiction of the various types of atrophic acne scars

1. Rolling Scars

Rolling or M-shaped scars have a rolling appearance on the overlying skin. They are superficial with an irregular surface, have a diameter >4 mm and are consequent to the destruction of the subcuticular fat, which leads to abnormal fibrous anchoring of the dermis to the subcutis **(Fig. 1.14)**. Abnormal fibrous anchoring of the dermis to the subcutis leads to superficial shadowing and a rolling or undulating appearance to the overlying skin **(Fig. 1.15)**. Although they tend to be shallow, the subdermal tether precludes treatment from the surface above. Correction of the subdermal component is essential for treatment success. Clinical experience suggests that they are amenable to lasers that penetrate up to the papillary dermis.

2. Ice Pick Scars

V-shaped, narrow **(<2 mm)**, deep, sharply marginated epithelial tracts that extend vertically to the deep dermis or subcutaneous tissue apex and it is believed that their depth is below the depth reached by conventional skin resurfacing options and they rarely respond to fractional lasers unless the whole length of the scar is ablated **(Figs 1.14 and 1.16)**.

3. Boxcar Scars

U-shaped scars that have sharply demarcated vertical edges and a diameter of **2–4 mm**. They may be **shallow (0.1–0.5 mm) or deep (≥0.5 mm)** and are most often **1.5–4.0 mm in diameter (Figs 1.14 and 1.17)**. Shallow boxcar scars and most deep boxcar scars are amenable to fractional lasers.

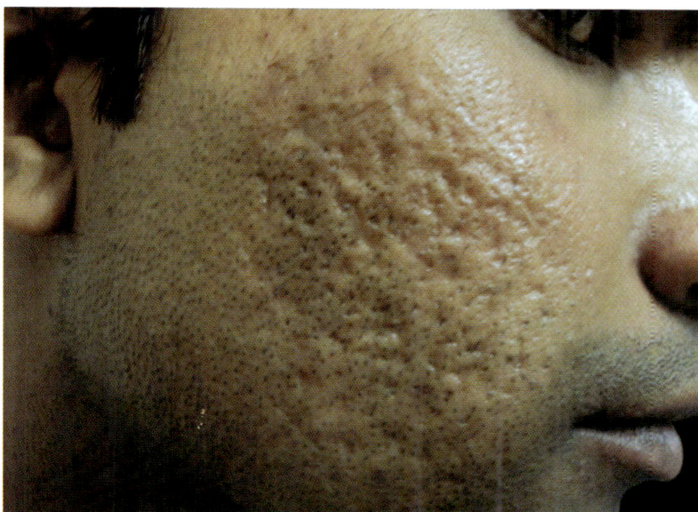

Fig. 1.15: Rolling scars in a male, amenable to fractional laser

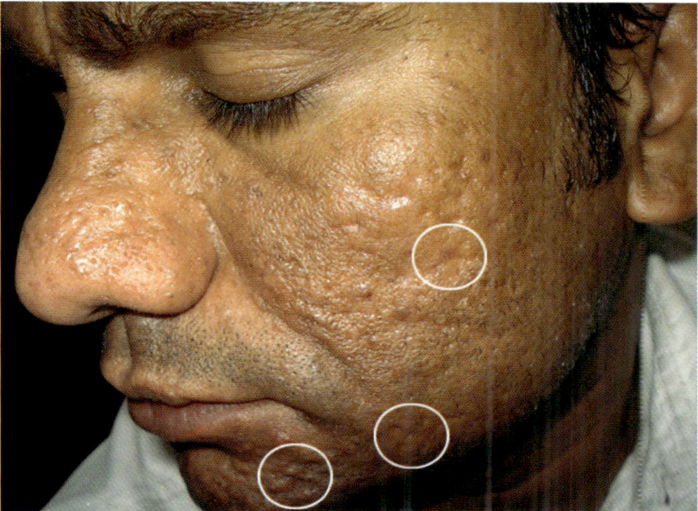

Fig. 1.16: Patient with variable scars-papular scars on the chin, ice pick scar on the jawline and rolling scars on the cheek

4. Perifollicular Elastolysis

Small, round, white spots with a follicle in the center with a soft texture, probably due to the presence of elastase secreting *Staphylococcus epidermidis* **(Fig. 1.18)**.

5. Complex Scars

Associating cords, bridges, intradermal epithelialized tunnels, multiporous comedones, and often a persistent inflammatory disease.

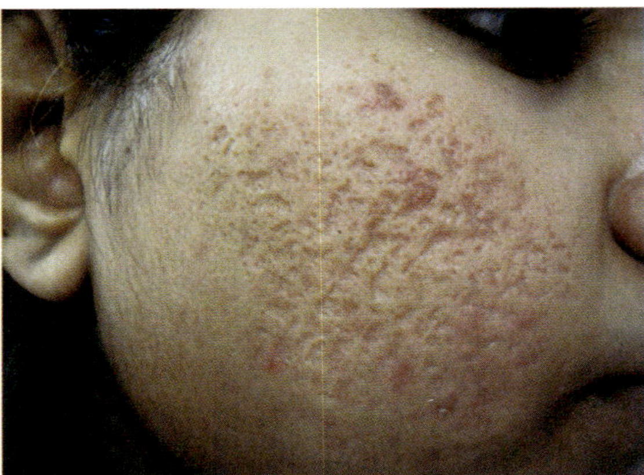

Fig. 1.17: Boxcar scars in a female

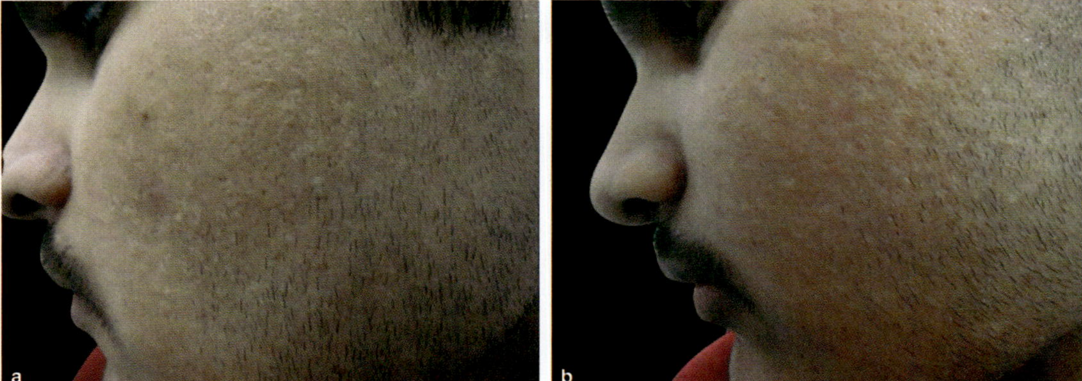

Fig. 1.18: Perifollicular elastolysis

In real world settings, most patients have more than one type of atrophic acne scar **(Figs 1.16 and 1.19)** and while a list of measures is given below it must be understood that scars can be treated primarily by either destroying the tethering-rolling-scars or by volumizing the atrophic scars.

Treatment of Acne Scars

There are comparatively few methods of treating an acne scar and often several selected methods will need to be combined in the patient to treat one difficult area of scarring and sometimes to treat different scars in the same patient (Goodman GJ, 2000). Simply put, one can:

1. **Alter the color:** Color may be the main visual clue to the presence of macular, atrophic or hypertrophic scarring. In Indian skin the major issue is post-inflammatory hyper-pigmentation which is often perceived as "scarring" by the patient and is responsive to medical therapy including in some cases light chemical skin peeling. Hypopigmented lesions are more problematic but uncommon.
2. **Induce (or reduce) collagen:** This is the most common method utilized in the treatment of post-acne atrophic scars. Inducing new collagen formation is a common pathway used by

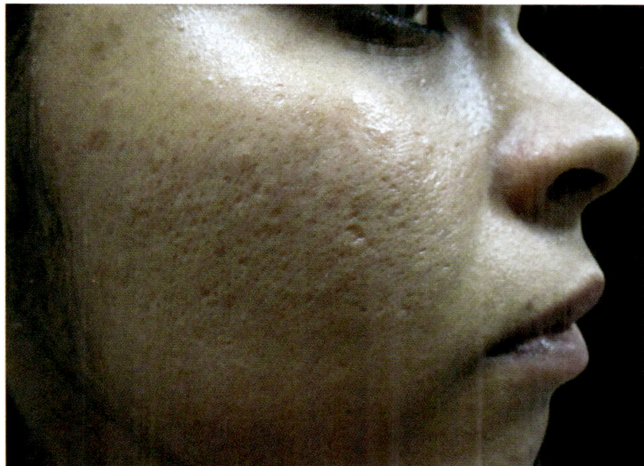

Fig. 1.19: Female with an admixture of boxcar and ice pick scars

all resurfacing techniques from the most minor home care to superficial treatments such as microdermabrasion, light chemical skin peeling through to the deeper resurfacing techniques represented by medium and deep chemical peeling including the "CROSS" technique, skin needling or rolling, dermabrasion, ablative laser skin resurfacing (CO_2, erbium), plasma skin resurfacing and fractional resurfacing.

When treating hypertrophic and keloid scars, multiple and often periodically repeated therapies are required to change the excessive collagen production by the fibroblasts.

3. **Fill the scar:** This includes autologous (autologous collagen, dermal and fat grafting) and non-autologous temporary, semipermanent and permanent augmentation techniques and agents.

   In essence:

   1. **Surface** treatment revolves around altering the color of the scar as well as inducing or reducing collagen in the underlying tissue.
   2. **Volume** requires augmentation or filling to decrease volume deficits or sometimes decrease the volume in terms of hypertrophic scarring.
   3. **Movement** involves neurotoxins to minimize the action of muscle on diseased, atrophic or sometimes hypertrophic scarring.
   4. **Surgical options** include punch techniques, excision or subcision.

An overview of techniques dependent on the type, mobility and distensibility of the scar is depicted in **Table 1.10** (Goodman GJ, 2000). We do not feel that LADD (laser-assisted drug delivery) has any advantage and may be a "fancy" treatment which may not be of any great value as the MTZ that are formed by Ablative Fractional lasers close within 3 hrs and thus the penetration of agents via the MTZ seems unlikely.

Fractional Lasers

While various techniques have been suggested, the fractional energy devices are useful and both lasers and RF devices have been used. The most important aspect is the depth of penetration of the laser beam or MTZ created by the energy device. This is more important than the density as that determines the response to various sub types of acne scars. As can be seen in the depictive **Fig. 1.20**, various simulation formulas have been used to determine the depth of the fractional

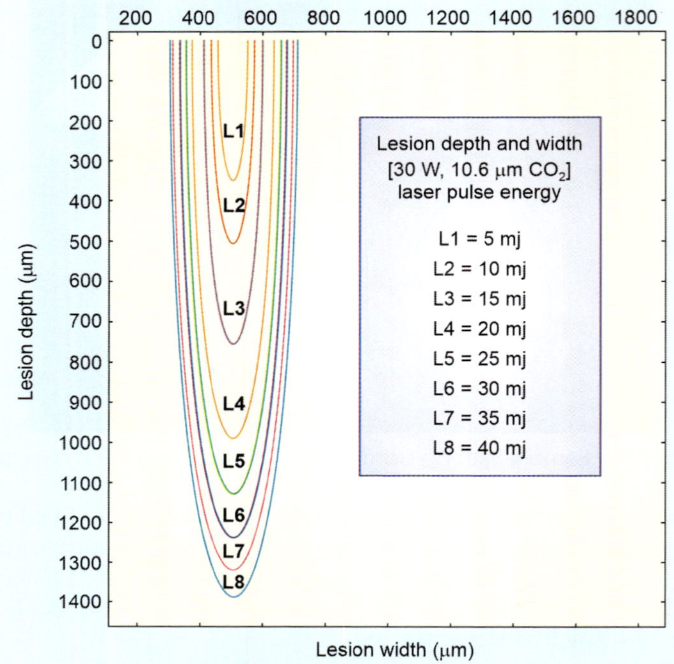

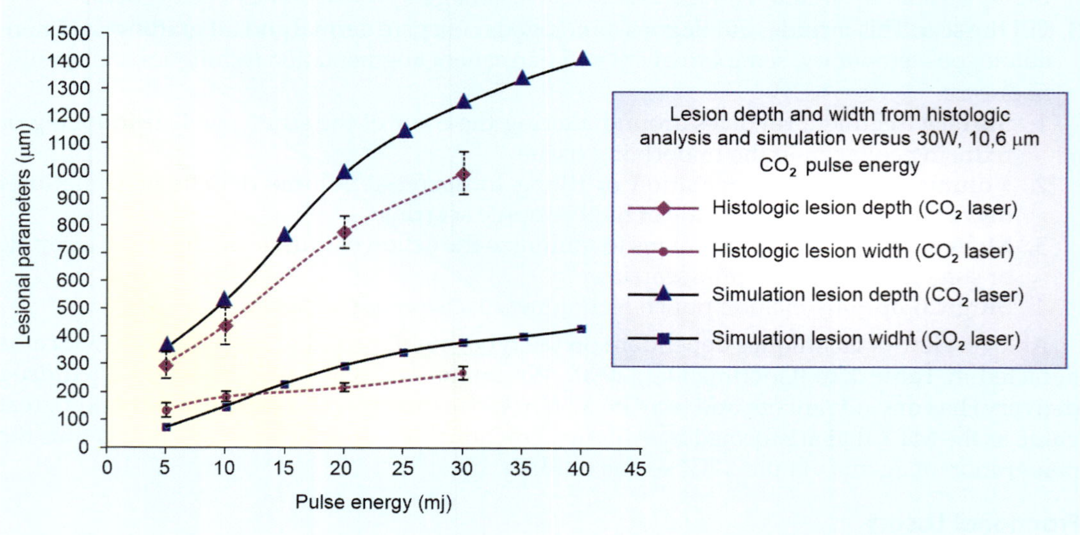

Fig. 1.20: Lesional depth achieved by a fractional CO_2 laser at various pulse energies and the lower image lower compares the simulated depth and width with histological depth and width. This depth, if correlated with the depth of the atrophic acne scar, can help in modulating the treatment settings. This concept is important, as excessive energy would have no additional effect and would also lead to PIH in skin of color

TABLE 1.10: An overview of the treatments for acne scars

		Ice-pick	Boxcar	Rolling	Papular	Keloid
Surgical modalites	Excision	++	++ [deep and nondistensible]			
	Punch elevation		++ [deep and nondistensible]			
	Subcision			+		
Laser and EBD	Ablative fractional	+	++ [superficial boxcar]	+++	+	++ [combination with ILC]
	Fractional RF	+	++ [superficial boxcar]	+++	+	++
Chemical agents	TCA	+	+	+		

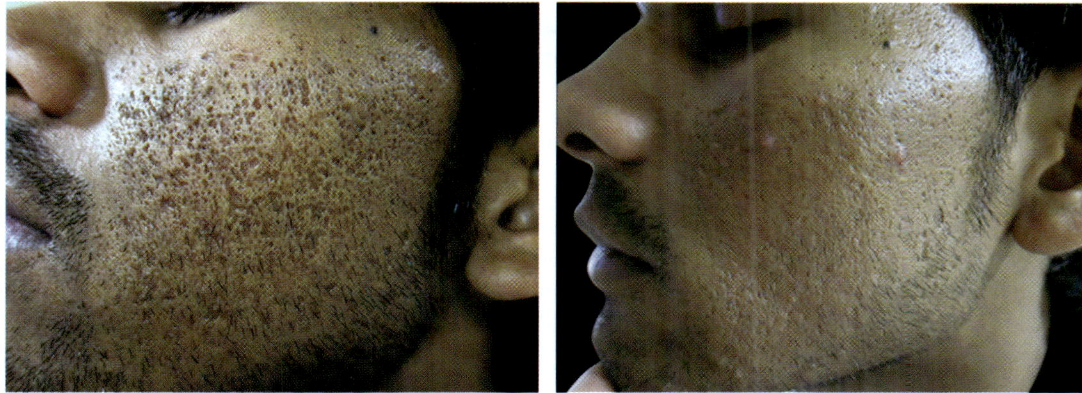

Fig. 1.21: A case of boxcar scars after 4 sessions of fractional Er:YAG

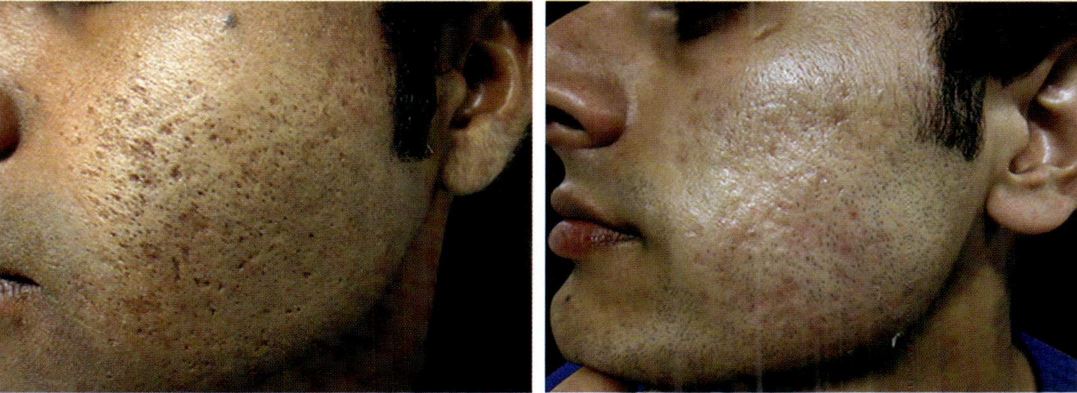

Fig. 1.22: A case of boxcar scars after 3 sessions of fractional Er:YAG

lasers, which may overestimate the depth achieved, but are important as they give a generic idea of the depth of the laser MTZ at various dose settings. Thus one would need pulse energies in excess of 35 mJ to achieve a depth to treat ice pick scars which can extend up to the subcutaneous fat, thus ice pick scars with deep bases are ideally treated with punch excision.

For almost all atrophic acne scars, except ice pick scars, ablative fractional lasers give an excellent improvement **(Figs 1.21 and 1.22)**. A combined approach may be needed in deep scars. There is a need for more tissue depth studies of the MTZ of fractional lasers, coupled with histology of acne scars to arrive at an ideal dose parameter for treatment of atrophic acne scars, which at present is based on "experience" and not "science".

BIBLIOGRAPHY

1. Lasers and Energy Devices in Aesthetic Dermatology Practice 1st edn. 2018. Jaypee.
2. Clinical Approach To Acne Vulgaris (Hb- 2015) 1st edn. CBS.
3. K. Shokrollahi (ed.), Laser Management of Scars.

Journals

1. Azziz R, Sanchez LA, Knochenhauer ES, et al., Androgen excess in women: experience with over 1000 consecutive patients, J Clin Endocrinol Metab 89(2):453, 2004.
2. B. Stuart;E. et al. Topical preparations for the treatment of mild?to?moderate acne vulgaris: systematic review and network meta?analysis*. Br J Dermatol 2021, doi:10.1111/bjd.20080
3. Bansal P, Sardana K, Arora P, Khurana A, Garga UC, Sharma L. A prospective study of anti-mullerian hormone and other ovarian and adrenal hormones in adult female acne. Dermatol Ther. 2020 Nov;33(6):e13974
4. Bansal P, Sardana K, Sharma L, Garga UC, Vats G. A prospective study examining isolated acne and acne with hyperandrogenic signs in adult females. J Dermatolog Treat. 2021 Nov;32(7):752–755.
5. Bell RJ, Islam RM, Skiba MA, Herbert D, Martinez Garcia A, Davis SR. Substituting serum anti-Müllerian hormone for polycystic ovary morphology increases the number of women diagnosed with polycystic ovary syndrome: a community-based cross-sectional study. Hum Reprod. 2021 Dec 27;37(1):109–118.
6. Clayton, R.W., Göbel, K., Niessen, C.M., Paus, R., van Steensel, M.A.M. and Lim, X. (2019), Homeostasis of the sebaceous gland and mechanisms of acne pathogenesis. Br J Dermatol, 181: 677-690. https://doi.org/10.1111/bjd.17981.
7. Dréno, B. (2017), What is new in the pathophysiology of acne, an overview. J Eur Acad Dermatol Venereol, 31: 8-12. https://doi.org/10.1111/jdv.14374
8. Frank-Raue K, Junga G, Raue F, et al. [Therapy of hirsutism in females with adrenal enzyme defects of steroid hormone biosynthesis: comparison of dexamethasone with cyproterone acetate]. Klin Wochenschr 1990;68(12):597–60.
9. Goodman GJ. Post-acne scarring: A review of its pathophysiology and treatment. Dermatol Surg 2000;26:857–71.
10. Krunic A, Ciurea A, Scheman A. Efficacy and tolerance of acne treatment using both spironolactone and a combined contraceptive containing drospirenone. J Am Acad Dermatol. 2008;58(1):60–62.
11. Landis, Megan N. (2020). Optimizing Isotretinoin Treatment of Acne: Update on Current Recommendations for Monitoring, Dosing, Safety, Adverse Effects, Compliance, and Outcomes. American Journal of Clinical Dermatology, (), -. doi:10.1007/s40257-020-00508-0
12. Mayslich C, Grange PA, Dupin N. Cutibacterium acnes as an Opportunistic Pathogen: An Update of Its Virulence-Associated Factors. Microorganisms. 2021 Feb 2;9(2):303. doi: 10.3390/microorganisms9020303. PMID: 33540667; PMCID: PMC7913060.
13. Ramasamy S, Barnard E, Dawson TL Jr, L, H. The role of the skin microbiota in acne pathophysiology. Br J Dermatol 2019; 181: 691–699. https://doi.org/10.1111/bjd.18230

14. Rudnicka E, Kunicki M, Calik-Ksepka A, Suchta K, Duszewska A, Smolarczyk K, Smolarczyk R. Anti-Müllerian Hormone in Pathogenesis, Diagnostic and Treatment of PCOS. Int J Mol Sci. 2021 Nov 19;22(22):12507
15. Sardana K, Bansal P, Sharma LK, Garga UC, Vats G. A study comparing the clinical and hormonal profile of late onset and persistent acne in adult females. Int J Dermatol. 2020 Apr;59(4):428–433.
16. Sardana K, Garg VK, Arora P, Khurana N. Histological validity and clinical evidence for use of fractional lasers for acne scars. J Cutan Aesthet Surg. 2012 Apr;5(2):75–90.
17. Sardana K, Narang I. Acne vulgaris. In: Sacchidanand S, Savitha AS, Shilpa K, Shashi Kumar BM, eds. IADVL Textbook of Dermatology. 5th ed. Mumbai: Bhalani Publishing House; 2022:1419–1448.
18. Sardana K, Mathachan SR, Gupta T. Antibiotic resistance in acne an emergent need to recognize resistance to azithromycin and restrict its unapproved use in acne vulgaris. J Eur Acad Dermatol Venereol. 2021 May;35(5):e347–e348.
19. Saurat JH: Strategic Targets in Acne: The Comedone Switch in Question. Dermatology. 2015;231(2):105–11. 10.1159/000382031
20. Xia E, et al. Isotretinoin Laboratory Monitoring in Acne Treatment: A Delphi Consensus Study. JAMA Dermatol. 2022 Aug 1;158(8):942-948. doi: 10.1001/jamadermatol.2022.2044. PMID: 35704293.
21. Yildiz BO. Diagnosis of hyperandrogenism: clinical criteria. Best Pract Res Clin Endocrinol Metab. 2006 Jun;20(2):167–176.
22. Zaenglein AL, et al. Guidelines of care for the management of acne vulgaris. JAAD 2016.
23. Zaenglein AL, et al. Guidelines of care for the management of acne vulgaris. J Am Acad Dermatol S0190962215026146-. doi:10.1016/j.jaad.2015.12.037.

Chapter

2

Acne Rosacea

Pooja Arora Mrig

INTRODUCTION

Rosacea is a centrofacial skin disease characterized by flushing, erythema, telangiectasias and papulopustular lesions on the cheeks and nose. The clinical spectrum varies from mild involvement with erythema to severe disfiguring variants.

Epidemiology

- It is more common in fair skin types.
- It usually affects the middle aged and elderly with an age of onset between 30 and 50 years.
- Rosacea can rarely occur in children. Children more commonly present with rosacea-like conditions like perioral dermatitis.
- Gender predilection varies between different populations.

Pathogenesis

Pathogenesis of rosacea is multifactorial with interplay of several factors.

Genetics: Association found with polymorphisms nearby the BPTK316 as well as signals in the MHC class II molecules.

Environmental factors: Temperature changes, caffeine, hot and spicy foods, alcohol, sunlight, exercise, psychological stress, menstruation, demodex mites and certain medications. Role of *H. pylori* is not clear.

Toll-like receptors, cytokines and antimicrobial peptides: Toll-like receptor 2 (TLR2) and Toll-like receptor 4 (TLR4) found to be over-expressed in rosacea skin. AMPs are also increased.

Immune cells: T cells (especially Th1/Th17 immune cells), macrophages, mast cells and neutrophils play an important role in pathogenesis. Reactive oxygen species (ROS) and other proteases are produced by inflammatory cells that lead to inflammation, angiogenesis, and telangiectases. Recently, an involvement of B cells in the pathogenesis of rosacea was shown as well.

Blood vessels: Papillary dermal vessels are dilated resulting in erythema.

Nerves: Sensory nerve endings are activated to release vasoactive peptides that cause flushing and erythema.

Clinical Features and Differential Diagnosis

In 2002, the American National Rosacea Society had classified rosacea into various types based on clinical features. There was overlap in the clinical manifestations and one patient could have more than one subtype. The various manifestations are depicted in **Fig. 2.1**. Recently, a schema based on encompassing the diversity of clinical presentations was proposed by the global **ROS**acea **CO**nsensus **(ROSCO)** panel in 2017 and endorsed by the National Rosacea Society. **Table 2.1** lists the diagnostic features of rosacea under this schema.

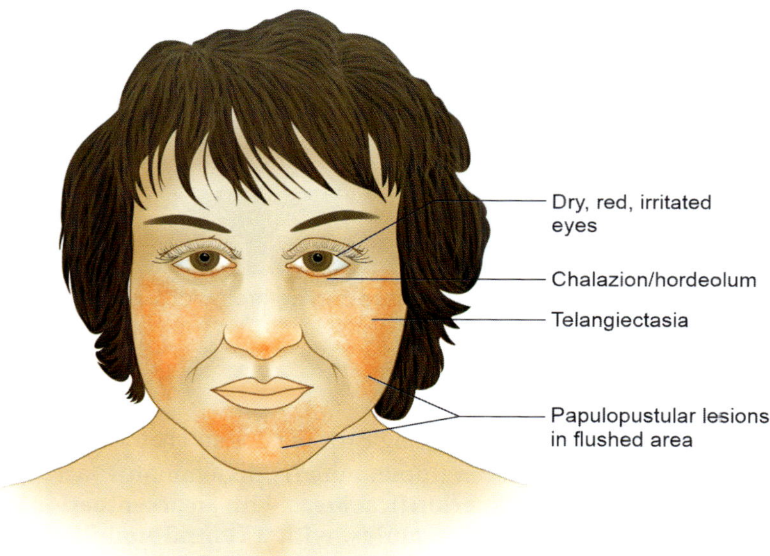

Fig. 2.1: Depiction of the various manifestations of rosacea

TABLE 2.1: Diagnostic, major and minor cutaneous features of rosacea (Tan J et al., 2017)

Diagnostic features	Major features	Minor features
• Persistent centrofacial erythema with periodic intensification by potential trigger factors • Phymatous changes Facial skin thickening due to fibrosis and/or sebaceous glandular hyperplasia. Most commonly on the nose.	• Flushing/transient centrofacial erythema **(Fig. 2.2)** • Inflammatory papules and pustules • Telangiectases (not only in the alar area)	• Burning sensation of skin • Stinging sensation of skin • Dry sensat on of skin • Edema

*Diagnostic features are independently diagnostic. Two or more major features are diagnostic. Ocular manifestations include lid margin telangiectases, blepharitis, keratitis, conjunctivitis and anterior uveitis and require a referral to an ophthalmologist for treatment.

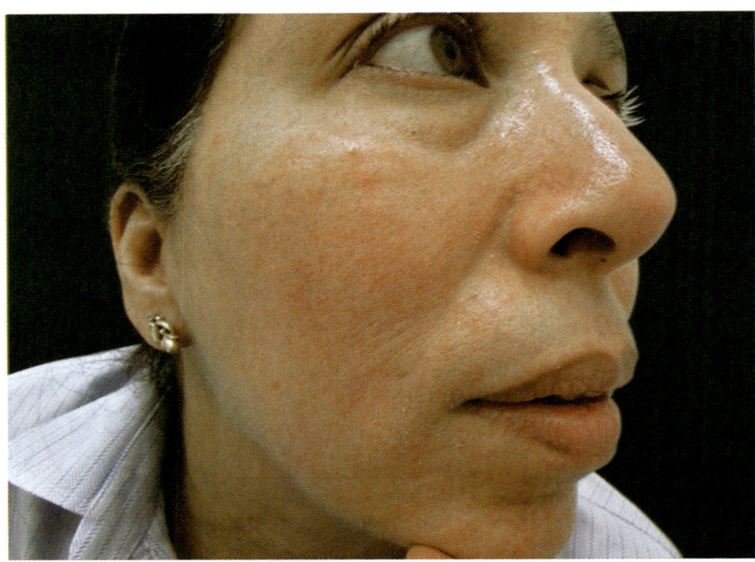

Fig. 2.2: A patient with flushing attacks on the nose and centrofacial aspect of the face (erythemato-telangiectatic rosacea) (subtype I)

Other Variants

- **Extrafacial rosacea:** Neck, presternal or epigastric regions and hairless area of the scalp in men.
- **Lupoid or granulomatous rosacea** (lupus miliaris disseminatus faciei): In this disorder, lesions occur on the **cheeks and periorifical areas with an accentuation periorbitally and are yellowish brown papules and nodules, with a central umbilication and heal with atrophic, punched-out scars**. The biopsy shows epithelioid granulomas with central caseous necrosis. It is believed to be a variant of either rosacea or sarcoidosis or an entity that has overlapping features of both.
- **Morbihan disease:** Solid, persistent facial edema, restricted to the upper part of the face, worsens progressively, impacts vision if eyelids are involved.
- **Rosacea fulminans** (pyoderma faciale): Previously called rosacea congloblata, presents as sudden eruption of erythema, sterile papulopustules, cystic nodules and draining sinuses in young females.
- **Rosacea aggravated or induced by medicines:** Examples—amiodarone, amineptine, EGFR inhibitors, phosphodiesterase type 5 inhibitors.
- **Rosacea induced by steroids or aggravated by corticosteroid treatment (iatrosacea):** This is common and is due to the use of steroids which lead to skin atrophy, telangiectases and then the appearance of papules, pustules and nodules, associated with localized discomfort **(Fig. 2.3)**.

Diagnosis

Clinical

Diagnosis of rosacea is mainly clinical. Extensive scaling, sharp demarcation of erythema, scarring, unilateral involvement, exclusive perioral or periorbital involvement are less compatible with a diagnosis of rosacea.

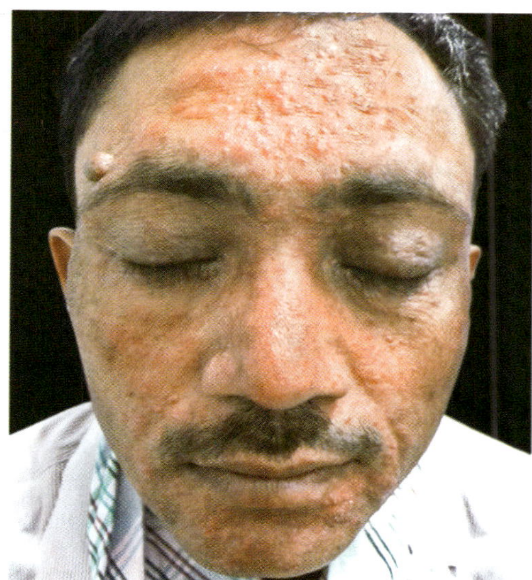

Fig. 2.3: Steroid abuse leading to erythema, papules, pustules and nodules—"iatrosacea"

HPE

- Usually not needed.
- Dilated blood and lymphatic vessels in upper and mid-dermis with superficial perivascular and perifollicular mononuclear lymphohistiocytic infiltrate. Edema and thickened elastic fibers can be seen.
- Granulomatous rosacea—noncaseating epithelioid cell granulomas in dermis.
- Demodex mites are seen in 10% of routine biopsies.

Treatment

Treatment of rosacea is outlined in **Tables 2.2** and **2.3**. Some general tips are given below:

- **Combination treatment**
  - Brimonidine in morning and ivermectin in evening are effective for treating erythema and papules/pustules.
- **Maintenance treatment**
  - Topical ivermectin 1%, metronidazole 0.75% and azelaic acid 15% are effective for maintenance.

A recent study has shown that paroxetine in a dose of 25 mg is useful for the flushing attacks of rosacea.

TABLE 2.2: Facial skin care recommendations in rosacea
• Educate regarding nature of disease • Advise to avoid triggers • Sun avoidance • Use sunscreen with SPF >30 with both UVA and UVB protection • Use soap-free gentle skin cleansers • Moisturizers to repair epidermal barrier • Avoid harsh products on face like astringents and exfoliators

TABLE 2.3: Medical and surgical therapies of rosacea (Zuuren et al., 2019)

Clinical subtype	Therapy	Comments
Erythematotelangiectatic	Topical **brimonidine tartrate** (0.33% gel)	Alpha-2 adrenergic receptor agonist, once daily, improves erythema
	Topical **oxymetazoline**	Alpha-2 adrenergic receptor agonist, improves erythema
	Topical azelaic acid, metronidazole	May reduce erythema
	Topical tacrolimus, Topical pimecrolimus	Tried in small studies with improvement
	Beta blockers	Propanolol, nadolol, carvedilol have been tried
	Lasers	(Nd:YAG), pulsed dye laser (PDL) or intense pulsed light (IPL) reduce erythema and telangiectases
Papulopustular	Topical **metronidazole** (0.75–1%)	
	Topical tacrolimus	Not recommended as it only reduces erythema
	Topical **azelaic acid** (15%/20%)	Anti-inflammatory
	Topical **ivermectin** (1% cream)	
	Topical retinoids (tretinoin 0.025% and adapalene)	
	Topical permethrin	
	Topical benzoyl peroxide	Anti-inflammatory
	Topical dapsone, topical erythromycin, Nd:YAG	Anti-inflammatory
	Topical minocycline foam (1.5%)	**USFDA approved in 2020**
	Oral **doxycycline** (**40 mg** daily for 4–8 weeks)	
	Oral **minocycline (100 mg)**	
	Oral metronidazole	Trial showed good efficacy
	Oral azithromycin (500 mg thrice a week then tapered)	
	Oral **isotretinoin (0.3 mg/kg)**	Better than doxycycline
	Oral ivermectin	Tried in case reports
	Oral rifaximin (400 mg TDS) × 10 days	**Inhibits small intestinal bacterial overgrowth**
Phymatous	**Isotretinoin** (0.3 mg/kg) Doxycycline—low dose	Off label
	Ablative lasers, surgery	
Ocular	Lid hygiene, lid massages, application of warm wet tissues, tear replacement	All therapies are off label
	Topical ciclosporin (0.05% ophthalmic emlusion)	
	Azithromycin, tetracyclines Omega-3 fatty acids	Omega-3 fatty acids improve symptoms of dry eyes and tear gland function
	Blepharoplasty	
Granulomatous	Minocycline, dapsone, isotretinoin, and intense pulsed light	Tried in case reports

The drugs in bold have maximum evidence

Prognosis

Rosacea is a chronic disease with likelihood of exacerbations with various aggravating factors. Patients need to be educated regarding the benign nature of disease, avoidance of triggers and need for compliance with treatment.

BIBLIOGRAPHY

1. Alexis AF, Callender VD, Baldwin HE, et al. Global epidemiology and clinical spectrum of rosacea, highlighting skin of colour: Review and clinical practice experience. J Am Acad Dermatol 2019 Jun;80(6):1722–29.e7.
2. Anzengruber F, Czernielewski J, Conrad C, et al. Swiss S1 guideline for the treatment of rosacea. J Eur Acad Dermatol Venereol 2017 Nov;31(11):1775–91.
3. Juliandri J, Wang X, Liu Z, et al. Global rosacea treatment guidelines and expert consensus points: The differences. J Cosmet Dermatol 2019 Aug;18(4):960–965.
4. van Zuuren EJ, Fedorowicz Z, Tan J, et al. Interventions for rosacea based on the phenotype approach: an updated systematic review including GRADE assessments. Br J Dermatol 2019 Jul;181(1):65–2.
5. van Zuuren EJ, Arents BWM, et al. Rosacea: New concepts in classification and treatment. Am J clin Dermatol 2021;22:457–65.
6. Tan J, Almeida LM, Bewley A, et al. Updating the diagnosis, classification and assessment of rosacea: recommendations from the global ROSCO panel. BJD 2017;176:431–8.
7. Schaller M, Almeida LMC, Bewley A et al. Recommendations for rosacea diagnosis, classification and management: Update from the global ROSacea COnsensus (ROSCO) 2019 panel. BJD 2020 May;182(5):1269-1276. doi:10.1111/bjd.18420

Chapter

3

Adverse Drug Reactions

Kabir Sardana, Kumari Ritu

INTRODUCTION

The cardinal features of a drug reaction are

- Symmetric rash
- Sudden onset
- Itchy
- Self-limiting, if drug is discontinued.

Classification

Drug reactions can be classified in many ways. One useful approach is to separate **predictable reactions** occurring in patients with no particular susceptibility from **unpredictable reactions** occurring in susceptible patients.

Predictable Adverse Reactions

- Overdosage (wrong dosage or defect in drug metabolism)
- Side effects (sleepiness from antihistamines)
- Indirect effects (antibiotics change normal flora)
- Drug interactions (alter metabolism of drugs; most commonly the cytochrome P-450 system).

Unpredictable Adverse Reactions

- Intolerance (known side effect occurs at low dose)
- Allergic reaction (drug allergy or hypersensitivity; immunologic reaction to drug; requires previous exposure or cross-reaction)
- Pseudoallergic reaction (nonimmunologic activation of mast cells)
- Idiosyncratic reaction (unexplained reaction, not related to mechanism of action, without known or suspected immunologic mechanism).

Pathogenesis

In some instances, a drug reaction can be clearly assigned to an immunologic reaction type, although more often the mechanisms are not understood. These are listed **Table 3.1**.

TABLE 3.1: Overview of the immunological sub-types of drug reactions		
Immune (allergic hypersensitivity)		
Type I (IgE antibody-mediated)	Varied types: Anaphylaxis, bronchospasm, cardiovascular collapse, urticaria, angioedema	Penicillins; cephalosporins; neuromuscular blockers; quinolones; pyrazolones; PPI; L-asparaginase; mAbs
Type II [antibody (IgG, IgM)-mediated cytotoxic reactions]	Drug-induced haemolytic anaemia, immune thrombocytopenia, immune form of agranulocytosis	Penicillins; cephalosporins; quinine; quinidine; sulphonamides; thiouracil; gold salts; oxaliplatin; fludarabine; irinotecan; suramin; mAbs
Type III (immune complex-mediated via IgG, IgM)	Serum sickness, drug-induced vasculitis	Penicillins; cephalosporins; sulfonamides; tetracycline; NSAIDs; carbamazepine; allopurinol; mAbs; oxaliplatin
Type IV (DTH)	Large number of reactions	NSAIDs; penicillins; other anti-microbials; anticonvulsants (carbamazepine); local anesthetics; sulfonamides; hydroxychloroquine; cytarabine; tamoxifen; imatinib; mAbs
Non-immune (non-allergic sensitivities)		
	Pseudoallergy (termed anaphylactoid)	Most reactions to NSAIDs. Direct mast cell degranulation (neuromuscular blockers; opioids; contrast media; vancomycin)
	Idiosyncratic reactions	Halothane hepatitis; malignant hypothermia; drug-induced anaemia in G6PD deficient individuals (antimalarials, sulfonamides, dapsone)
	Intolerance	Tinnitus induced by small doses of aspirin. Some reactions to contrast media and NSAIDs

The majority of allergic drug reactions are caused by **type IV cell-mediated immune reactions**, which can present in a number of forms, most commonly as maculopapular eruption or morbilliform erythema. Helper **CD4+ T cells** occur more frequently in the more common morbilliform eruptions, while cytotoxic **CD8+ T cells** predominate in blistering eruptions and FDE.

The International **CON**sensus **(ICON)** on Drug Allergies classifies drug hypersensitivity reactions into **immediate** and **non-immediate** types, according to the time of onset after drug exposure. The immediate type usually refers to the symptoms appearing within 1–6 hours after exposure to the suspected drugs. The common presentations of immediate-type drug hypersensitivity include angioedema, urticaria and anaphylaxis. Delayed-type drug hypersensitivity frequently involves skin reactions, ranging from mild reactions [e.g. maculopapular exanthema (MPE), and fixed drug eruption (FDE)] to severe cutaneous adverse

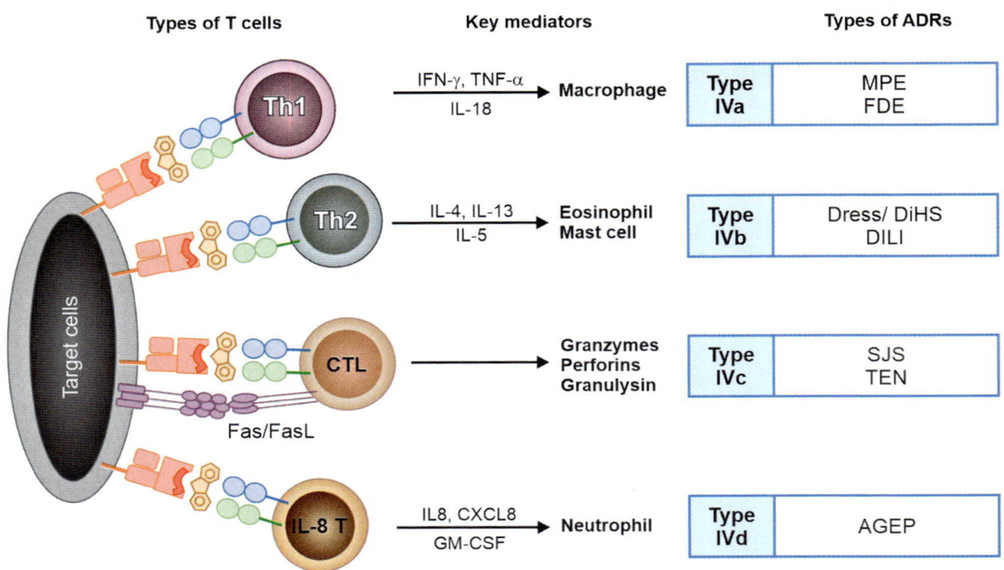

Fig. 3.1: Overview of subtypes of type IV hypersensitivity reaction and their morphological types. FDE, fixed drug eruption; MPE, maculopapular eruption; AGEP, acute generalized exanthematous pustulosis; DRESS, drug reaction with eosinophilia and systemic symptoms; DiHS, drug-induced hypersensitivity syndrome; DILI, drug-induced liver injury; SJS, Stevens–Johnson syndrome; TEN, toxic epidermal necrolysis.

reactions (SCARs) (e.g. drug reaction with eosinophilia and systemic symptoms (DRESS) (also called DiHS, drug-induced hypersensitivity syndrome), Stevens–Johnson syndrome (SJS), toxic epidermal necrolysis (TEN), and acute generalized exanthematous pustulosis (AGEP).

The **delayed-type hypersensitivity** reaction, also called a type IV reaction, is essentially mediated by T cell-antigen recognition, accompanied by the activation of other leukocytes. This has been further subclassified as IVa, IVb, IVc, and IVd **(Fig. 3.1)**. Type IVa, IVb, and IVd are mediated by Th1, Th2 and IL-8-producing Th cells, respectively, and involve other inflammatory cells, such as macrophages, eosinophils, and neutrophils. Thus the type IVa is classically involved in maculopapular exanthem and FDE. The type IVb reaction mainly involves Th2 cell activation and thus mediates DRESS/DiHS and DILI. The CXCL8/IL-8-producing Th cells mediate the type IVd reaction via producing CXCL8 and GM-CSF to activate neutrophils, which are predominately in drug-related AGEP. The last type IVc involves the cytotoxic T cells via the Fas/FasL pathway and is seen in SJS/TEN **(Fig. 3.1)**.

ERYTHEMA MULTIFORME

EM minor and major, determined by presence or absence of mucosal involvement and systemic symptoms.

Etiology

Infections (about 90% cases): HSV 1 > 2 (usually EM minor), *Mycoplasma* (usually EM major), histoplasmosis, hepatitis C, EBV, coxsackie virus.

TABLE 3.2: Etiology of EM

Virus	HSV type 1 causes **recurrent** EM **Non recurrent EM**-parvovirus B19, VZV, HCV, EBV, Orf virus, and SARS-CoV2
Vaccinations	Polyvalent measles mumps rubella vaccine, hepatitis B vaccination and vaccination with polyvalent HPV vaccine
Other infections	*Mycoplasma pneumoniae, syphilis, Trichophyton mentagrophytes, Histoplasma capsulatum, or Gardnerella vaginalis*
Hormones	EM rarely occurs parallel to menstruation; cases of progesterone-dependent EM have been described.
UV	EM-like polymorphic light eruption, EM-like photoallergic reaction after medication
Others	Malignancies, systemic diseases, ACD

Drugs (<10% cases): Allopurinol, phenobarbital, phenytoin, valproic acid, sulfonamide antibiotics, penicillins, erythromycin, nitrofurantoin, tetracyclines, acetylsalicylic acid, statins, TNF-α inhibitors.

In up to 60% of cases no trigger is identified.

A list of common causes is listed **Table 3.2**.

Clinical Features

Typical target lesion with 3 distinct zones **(Fig. 3.2)**

- Can have atypical target lesions—round, edematous, palpable but only 2 zones and/or poorly defined border
- Prefers face, upper extremities (dorsal hands, forearms, palms), neck, trunk
- Koebner phenomenon is seen
- Vesiculobullous mucosal lesions → progress into painful erosions on buccal mucosa and lips > ocular/genital mucosae
- Systemic features are suggestive of EM major → precede/accompany skin lesions: fever, asthenia, arthralgias + joint swelling, atypical pneumonia
- Rapid development of lesions within 24 hours, fixed for 7+ days, heals without sequelae (except rare ocular damage).

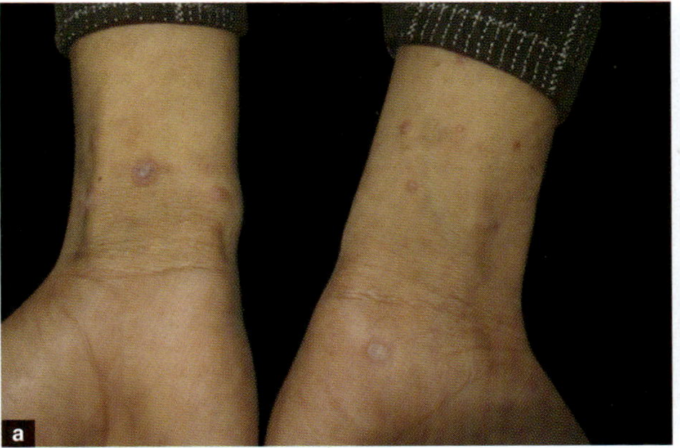

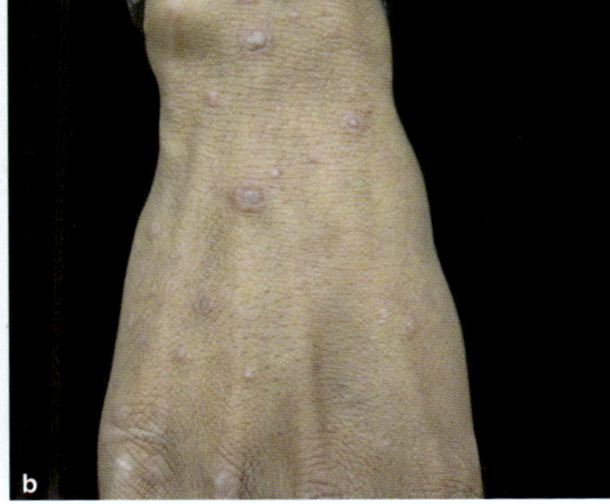

Fig. 3.2: Classical lesions of EM on the extremities

Histopathology

- Apoptosis of keratinocytes, mild spongiosis, focal vacuolar degeneration of basal keratinocytes, superficial dermal edema, perivascular lymphocytes.
- DIF nonspecific-granular IgM, C3 around blood vessels and at DEJ.

Treatment

- Oral antihistamines, systemic corticosteroids or pulse methylprednisolone
- Treatment for HSV and *Mycoplasma* as indicated
  - Prophylaxis × 6 months with acyclovir 400 mg BD, valacyclovir 500–1000 mg/day, famciclovir 250 mg BID. This is advised in case there is evidence of recurrent HSV associated EM.
- Antiviral-resistant cases of recurrent HSV-related EM
  Consider azathioprine, mycophenolate mofetil, dapsone, thalidomide.

What is New in Treatment?

A recent paper has shown that Tofacitinib can be a useful drug based on its inhibition of the key cytokines that are involved in EM. Thus JAKinibs (Murphy MJ, 2021) inhibit the IFN-γ (JAK1/2) and IL-15 (JAK1/3). As cytotoxic response against keratinocytes appears to be a hallmark of EM and IFN-γ and IL-15 have well-established roles in promoting cytotoxic response, JAKi can have an important role to play in EM.

SEVERE CUTANEOUS ADVERSE REACTIONS

STEVENS–JOHNSON SYNDROME/TOXIC EPIDERMAL NECROLYSIS

- Prodrome of upper respiratory tract symptoms, fever, painful skin
- Mortality 1–5% SJS, 25–35% TEN
- Almost always drug-related–due to extensive keratinocyte cell death resulting in separation of skin at DEJ **(Fig. 3.3)**.
- F > M

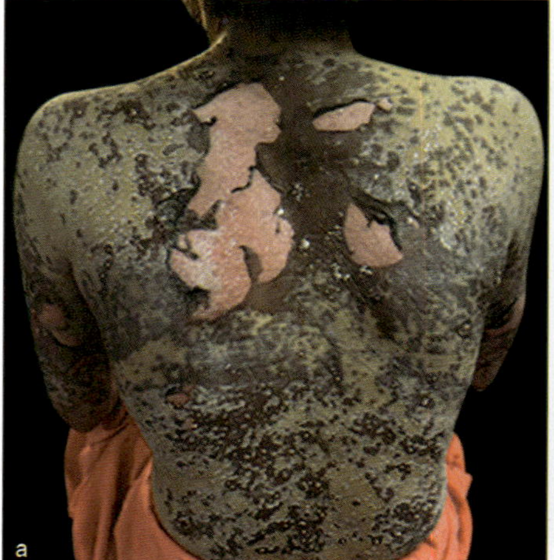

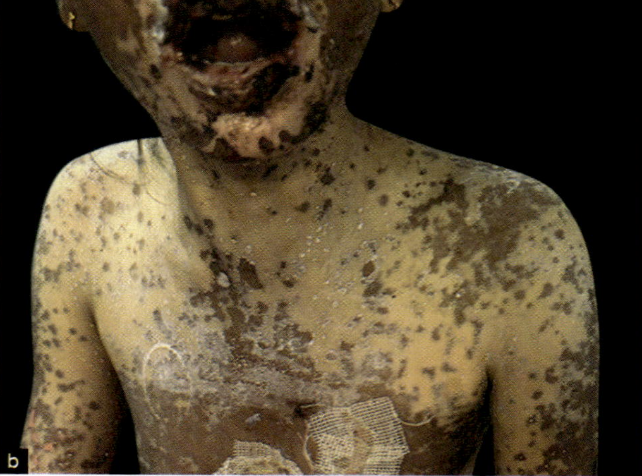

Fig. 3.3: A case of SJS TEN overlap secondary to oxcarbamazepine

- *Drugs*: Allopurinol, antibiotics, NSAIDs, aromatic anticonvulsants
  Sulfonamides most strongly associated > aminopenicillins, quinolones, cephalosporins, tetracyclines, antiretrovirals.
  A case-control study of patients hospitalized for SJS/TEN in selected hospitals in France, Germany, Italy, and Portugal between 1989 and 1993, reported by Roujeau et al., (1995) divided the drugs in two categories.
  a. Those that can induce SJS/TEN over a **short period of time** (trimethoprim-sulfamethoxazole and other sulfonamide antibiotics, aminopenicillins, cephalosporins, quinolones, and chlormezanone).
  b. Those that cause when used **over prolonged periods of time** (aromatic antiepileptics [carbamazepine, phenytoin, phenobarbital], valproic acid, NSAIDs of the oxicam type, allopurinol, and corticosteroids).
     Amongst the newer drugs common implicated drugs are nevirapine, lamotrigine, and sertraline.
- *Risk factors*: HIV infection, *Mycoplasma pneumoniae* infection, underlying autoimmune disease, underlying hematologic malignancy, HLA-B*15:02 or HLA-A*31:01 for carbamazepine in South Asians and Asians, HLA-B*58:01 for allopurinol.
- *Onset*: **7–28 days** after first exposure, <48 hours with reexposure; risk limited to 8 weeks after starting drug. Useful for etiological diagnosis.
- The extent of skin involvement is a major prognostic factor in SJS and TEN. It should be emphasized that only necrotic skin that is already detached (e.g. blisters, erosions) or detachable skin (Nikolsky positive) should be counted for evaluation of extent of the skin involvement. Bastuji-Garin et al., proposed to classify patients into 3 groups according to the degree of skin detachment. SJS, SJS-TEN overlap and TEN **(Table 3.3)**.

Pathogenesis

It is thought to involve exposure to drug, that leads to immune reaction to a drug or its metabolite, resulting in expression of cytolytic molecule FasL on keratinocytes and secretion of granulysin from CTLs, NK cells and NKT cells and annexin A1 from monocytes

- FasL-and granulysin-mediated apoptosis and/or annexin-dependent necroptosis of keratinocytes, epidermal necrosis and detachment.
- Based on our knowledge to date, **CD8 T cells** as well as the cytolytic molecules **FasL and granulysin** are key players in the pathogenesis of SJS/TEN **(Fig. 3.1)**.

Clinical Features

- **Initial features are—usually nonspecific** and include fever, stinging eyes, and discomfort on swallowing. The morphology of early skin lesions includes erythematous and livid macules, which may or may not be slightly infiltrated and which have a tendency to rapidly coalescence. The development to SJS or TEN from a harmless-looking macular eruption to bullous detachment can occur rapidly, within a few hours. In a second phase, large areas of epidermal detachment develop **(Fig. 3.3)**.
  A severity scoring is useful to prognosticate and help in planning aggressive or supportive treatment **(Table 3.4)**.
- Mucosal erosions in >90% patients
  i. Early ophthalmology consult for ocular symptoms (seen in ~80%) like severe conjunctivitis with purulent discharge, bulla formation, corneal ulceration, anterior uveitis, panophthalmitis **(Fig. 3.4)**.

TABLE 3.3: Clinical features that distinguish SJS, SJS–TEN overlap, and TEN

Clinical entity	SJS	SJS–TEN overlap	TEN
Primary lesions	Dusky red lesions Flat atypical targets	Dusky red lesions Flat atypical targets	Poorly delineated erythematous plaques Epidermal detachment—spontaneous or by friction Dusky red lesions Flat atypical targets
Distribution	Isolated lesions Confluence (+) on face and trunk	Isolated lesions Confluence (++) on face and trunk	Isolated lesions (rare) Confluence (+++) or face, trunk, and elsewhere
Mucosal involvement	Yes	Yes	Yes
Systemic symptoms	Usually	Always	Always
Detachment (% body surface area)	<10	10–30	>30

TABLE 3.4: SCORTEN severity-of-illness score

SCORTEN parameter	Individual score
Age >40 years	Yes = 1, No = 0
Malignancy	Yes = 1, No = 0
Tachycardia (>120/min)	Yes = 1, No = 0
Initial surface of epidermal detachment >10%	Yes = 1, No = 0
Serum urea >28 mg/dL	Yes = 1, No = 0
Serum glucose >252 mg/dL	Yes = 1, No = 0
Bicarbonate <20 mmol/L	Yes = 1, No = 0
SCORTEN (sum of individual scores)	**Predicted mortality (%)**
0–1	3.2
2	12.1
3	35.8
4	58.3
≥5	90

   ii. Late sequelae include pain, dryness, synechiae development.
   iii. Early obs and gyne or urology consult for urogenital symptoms (seen in ~66%): Urethritis, genital erosions/ulcerations, genital synechiae development.

- Photophobia, painful micturition
- SCORTEN: **Poor outcomes:** Age >40 years, HR > 120, malignancy, BSA >10% on day 1, urea ↑, bicarb ↓, glucose ↑.

  The average reported mortality rate of SJS is 1–5%, and that of TEN 25–35%; it can be even higher in elderly patients and those with a large surface area of epidermal detachment **(Table 3.4)**.

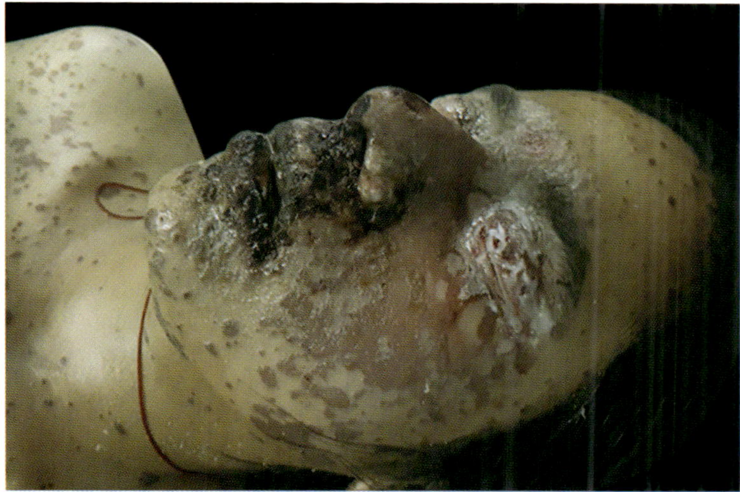

Fig. 3.4: Marked ocular involvement in TEN

- Death usually due to infection (*S. aureus*, *Pseudomonas aeruginosa*)
- Reepithelialization starts within days, complete within 3 weeks
  - Proliferation/migration of keratinocytes from "reservoir" sites (explains why skin grafting not required)
- Sequelae: Symblepharon, synechiae, entropion, ingrowth of eyelashes, scarring, irregular pigmentation, eruptive melanocytic nevi, persistent erosions of mucous membranes, urethral stenosis, phimosis, vaginal synechiae, nail dystrophy, diffuse hair loss, sicca syndrome.

Histopathology

Full thickness epidermal necrosis.

Differential Diagnosis

EM major, generalized FDE, autoimmune bullous disease, Kawasaki disease, SSSS, drug-induced linear IgA, DRESS, acute GVHD, lupus erythematosus (Rowell syndrome—usually resembles EM but can have TEN-like presentation).

Management

Prompt withdrawal of culprit drugs and supportive care. Garcia-Doval et al., (2000) have shown that the earlier the causative drug is withdrawn, the better the prognosis, and that patients exposed to causative drugs with long half-lives have an increased risk of dying.

Supportive Care

1. **Fluid resuscitation:** Lactated Ringer's solution to maintain urinary output of 0.5–1.0 cc/kg/h. (1.5–2 mL/kg/–1 affected area).
2. **Nutritional support:** Enteral therapy titrated according to prealbumin and C-reactive peptides every 3 days. Consider nasogastric tube placement and feedings if more than 20% TBSA epidermal loss or mucosal involvement.

3. **Wound care:** Debridement to remove sloughed epidermis, fibrinous exudate, and debris. Consider a silver-impregnated antimicrobial dressing (Acticoat/Excalt). Facial dressing with 2% mupirocin or plain petroleum gauze. Currently, nanocrystalline gauze materials containing silver are being used to replace the use of petrolatum-impregnated gauze for the coverage of denuded skin, although controlled trials have not been performed. Castillo et al. (2018) conducted a literature review to compare the efficacy of different dressing types in TEN/SJS and they looked at the time required for reepithelialization. They compared simple older style dressings such as ointment with bandages and more modern biosynthetic and silver impregnated dressings. While no significant difference was found in healing time, more modern dressings could be left in place for longer and thus facilitated improved patient comfort. This reinforces the benefits of the above mentioned use of nanocrystalline dressings. Thus dressings that can left for longer periods of time are preferred.
4. **Ophthalmic care:** Aggressive corneal lubrication. Frequent ocular exams utilizing fluorescein dye to assess for denudation and ulceration of the conjunctiva and cornea, along with early ophthalmology service consultation if indicated. An amniotic membrane graft may be necessary with severe ocular involvement.
5. **Pain control:** Multimodal therapy with opioid and nonopioid analgesics; consider adjunctive anxiolytics prior to wound care.
6. Catheters should be changed and cultured regularly, and bacterial sampling of the skin lesions must be performed at least every 48 hours.
7. Pulmonary care includes aerosols, bronchial aspiration, and physical therapy. Intubation and mechanical ventilation are nearly always necessary if the trachea and bronchi are involved.

An overview of the wound care is depicted in **Figs 3.5** and **3.6** and is the basis of SJS TEN management beyond systemic drugs.

Antibiotics

Prompt identification and management of secondary infection in this cohort are imperative. Sepsis and pneumonia are the most common complications in TEN/SJS. A recent Japanese study (Wang Q, et. al., 2018) compared the sensitivity of procalcitonin (PCT) and C-reactive protein (CRP) in detecting systemic infection. They demonstrated that PCT levels were significantly higher in patients with systemic bacterial infections, than in patients with only superficial cutaneous infection or no infection. The PCT and SCORTEN were also positively correlated. This was the first study to highlight PCT as a superior diagnostic tool and further prospective multicenter studies are required.

Disease Modifying Agents

To date, a disease modifying agent for SJS and TEN which has shown efficacy in controlled clinical trials, does not exist. Thus we are listing the varied therapeutic options but the overiding principle would be to avoid the use of steroids in all cases, a practice which is well entrenched in routine practice.

1. *High-dose Intravenous Immunoglobulins*

The majority of studies suggest that there may be a benefit of IVIG used at total doses greater than 2 g/kg over 3–4 days on the mortality associated, but it should be administered early in the disease. Only 1 cycle of IVIG treatment administered over a period of 3–5 days is usually required in this condition.

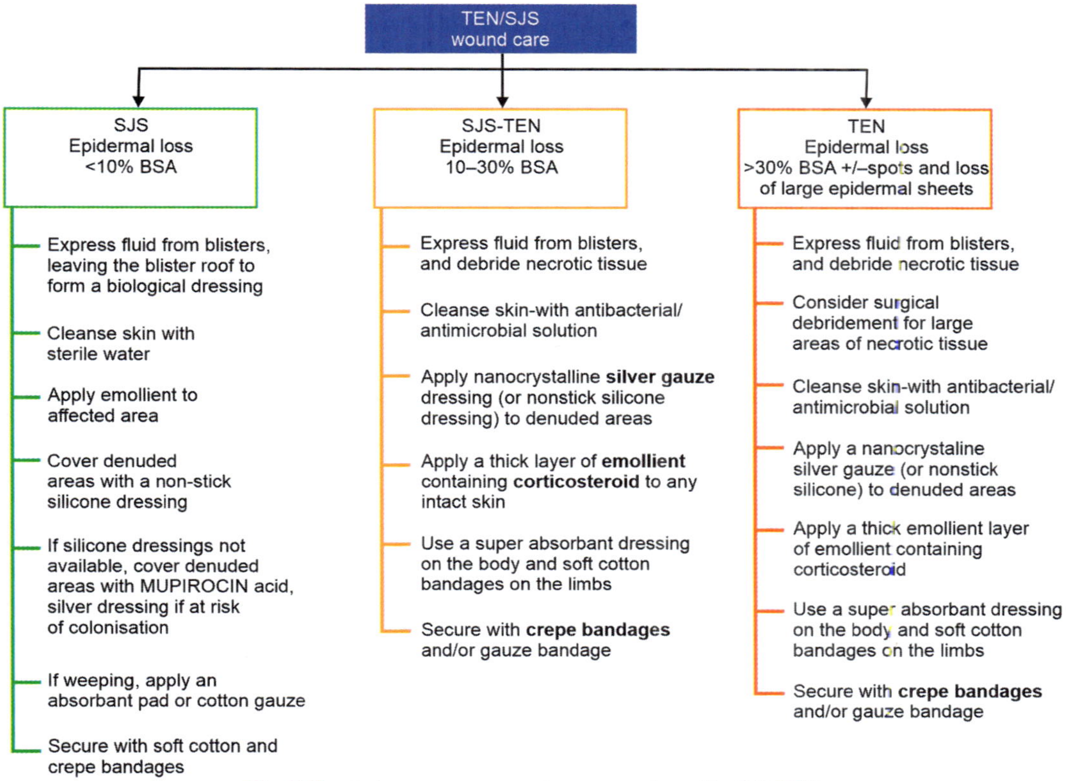

TEN/SJS wound care
SJS Epidermal loss <10% BSA
Express fluid from blisters, leaving the blister roof to form a biological dressing
Cleanse skin with sterile water
Apply emollient to affected area
Cover denuded areas with a non-stick silicone dressing
If silicone dressings not available, cover denuded areas with MUPIROCIN acid, silver dressing if at risk of colonisation
If weeping, apply an absorbant pad or cotton gauze
Secure with soft cotton and crepe bandages
SJS-TEN Epidermal loss 10–30% BSA
Express fluid from blisters, and debride necrotic tissue
Cleanse skin-with antibacterial/ antimicrobial solution
Apply nanocrystalline **silver gauze** dressing (or nonstick silicone dressing) to denuded areas
Apply a thick layer of **emollient** containing **corticosteroid** to any intact skin
Use a super absorbant dressing on the body and soft cotton bandages on the limbs
Secure with **crepe bandages** and/or gauze bandage
TEN Epidermal loss >30% BSA +/–spots and loss of large epidermal sheets
Express fluid from blisters, and debride necrotic tissue
Consider surgical debridement for large areas of necrotic tissue
Cleanse skin-with antibacterial/ antimicrobial solution
Apply a nanocrystaline silver gauze (or nonstick silicone) to denuded areas
Apply a thick emollient layer of emollient containing corticosteroid
Use a super absorbant dressing on the body and soft cotton bandages on the limbs
Secure with **crepe bandages** and/or gauze bandage

Fig. 3.5: Cutaneous wound care protocol in SJS/TEN

Eyes/mouth/urogenital wound care
Ocular involvement
Necrotic tissue not removed nowadays as per latest consensus. It acts as protective covering.
1–2 hourly application of lubricating eyedrops
Require corticosteroid drops and/ or antibiotic drops
Apply white paraffin to eyelids and surrounding skin
Mouth involvement
Apply white soft paraffin every 2 hours
Cleanse mouth and oral cavity with warm normal saline
Antiseptic, anti- inflammatory and anaesthetic mouthwash
Assessment of airway patency and need for intubation
Urogenital involvement
Full back foreskin and gently clean genitals with antimicrobial solution
Remove synechia
Apply white soft paraffin and replace foreskin
Silver sulfadiazine may also be used
Topical CS /Ab combinations
Gently clean vulva and vagina with antimicrobial solution
Remove synechia
Use a dilator (one can be made with a finger from a sterile glove packed with gauze and lubricant applied) or a tampon

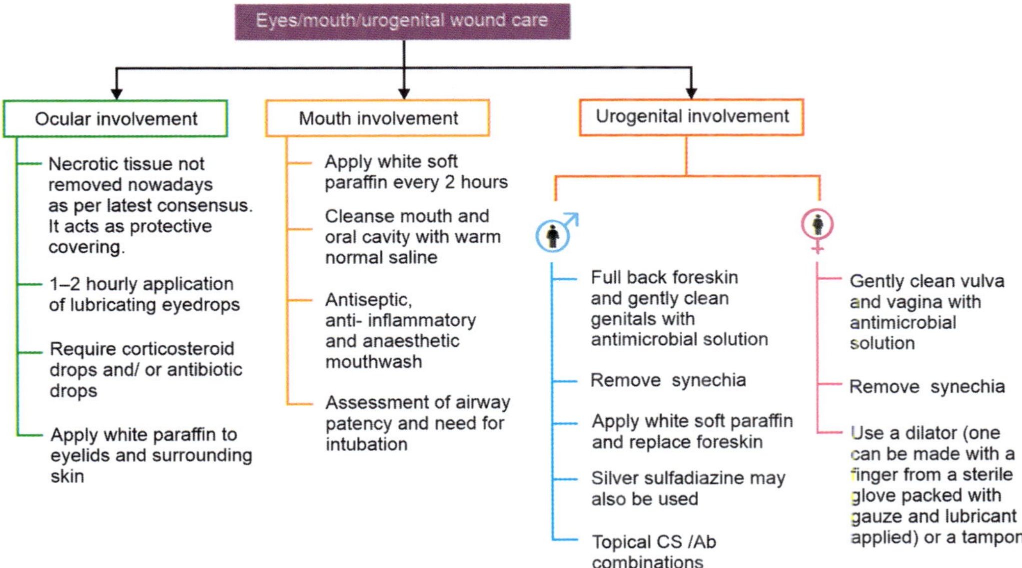

Fig. 3.6: Regionwise mucosal wound care protocol in SJS/TEN

2. *Cyclosporine*

Cyclosporine solution, administered orally through a nasogastric catheter at an initial dose of 1.5 mg/kg twice daily for 10 days, 1 mg/kg twice daily for the following 10 days, and finally 0.5 mg/kg twice daily for 10 days for a total treatment period of a 30 days is a useful measure with the caveat that this tends to work better in young patients.

The high rate of acute renal insufficiency in patients with SJS/TEN could limit or complicate the use of this medication and thus results are better in young patients with a normal kidney function.

3. *TNF-alpha Inhibitors*

They have been used to halt the disease, shorten disease duration, improve mortality, and decrease SJS/TEN related adverse events.
- Etanercept 50 mg subcutaneously once
- Infliximab 5 mg/kg infusion once.

4. *Systemic Corticosteroids*

Historically, high-dose corticosteroids have been used to treat SJS/TEN, despite lack of demonstrated efficacy. Dexamethasone 100 mg IV for 3 days and methylprednisolone 1000 mg IV for 3 days have decreased mortality in small case series, but the dearth of data supporting their use is notable and the most recent guidelines do not recommend corticosteroid therapy (Kardaun SH, et. al., 2007). Furthermore, some data suggests that lower doses of corticosteroids given 48 hours or more prior to admission can cause an increase in infections, length of stay, and mortality.

It must be noted that oustide of a trial, most centres adopt a combination of drugs to treat SJS/TEN, including, steroids, IVIg, and cyclosporine alone or in combination as the overiding aim is to save the patient (Papp A, et. al., 2018). But unless scrupulous nursing and wound care is effected, monotherapy with steroids is ill-advised and can lead to medico legal ramifications.

ACUTE GENERALIZED EXANTHEMATOUS PUSTULOSIS

Definition

AGEP is an acute febrile, generalized rash, with small uniform noninfective, nonfollicular pustules, with a tendency for accentuation in the intertriginous and flexural regions and a predilection for females.

Drugs

The EuroSCAR study has identified pristinamycin (macrolide), ampicillin/amoxicillin, quinolones, aromatic sulfonamides, (hydroxy-) chloroquine, terbinafine, and diltiazem as the leading culprits; notably, HAART drugs such as nevirapine do not seem to be associated with an elevated risk of inducing AGEP, contrary to the increased risk for SJS and TEN.

The interval between drug intake and the onset of AGEP can be generally divided into groups of 5 days or less of intake and 22 days or less of intake (Baker H, et al., 1968). Typically anti-infectious drugs (pristinamycin, aminopenicillins, quinolones, and anti-infective sulfonamides) lead to development of rash within 5 days, whereas chloroquine, diltiazem, terbinafine, and hydroxychloroquine tend to lead to delayed induction of rash **(Box 3.1)**.

BOX 3.1: Drugs commonly known to cause AGEP

- Ampicillin/amoxicillin
- Anti-infective sulfonamides
- Diltiazem
- Hydroxychloroquine
- Pristinamycin
- Quinolone
- Terbinafine

Clinical Features

- Characterized by small pustules that appear on face, intertriginous sites → become generalized within hours **(Fig. 3.7)**.
  Due to its marked flexural predilection some believe that AGEP is similar to symmetric drug-related intertriginous and flexural exanthema (SDRIFE).
- Associated with high fever, small sterile pustules on background of edema.
- Can present with purpuric or EM-like lesions, mucosal involvement, and edema of hands/face.
- Other features: ↑WBC, peripheral neutrophilia, hypocalcemia, eosinophilia, renal insufficiency.
- Patch test + in 50–60%.
- Histopathology: Subcorneal and intraepidermal pustules, dermal edema, eosinophils.

Differential Diagnoses

- Generalized pustular psoriasis (Zumbusch psoriasis) where pustules typically manifest on lesional skin, with polyarthritis and palmoplantar involvement. In addition, a positive family history for psoriasis usually exists, and relapses of generalized pustulation occur often.
- Subcorneal pustulosis (Sneddon-Wilkinson disease) and subcorneal IgA dermatosis often present with similar clinical features to the aforementioned disease, but sometimes mucosal

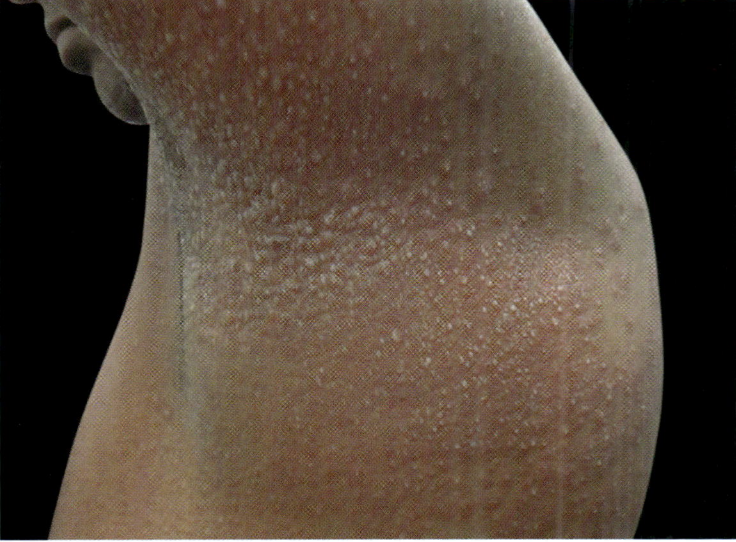

Fig. 3.7: A case of AGEP wih nonfollicular, monomorphic pustules

involvement is seen, and only diagnostic procedures such as a skin biopsy can distinguish the diseases.
- Infectious folliculitis is always a major differential diagnosis of AGEP although the typical manifestations are follicular-associated abscesses of bacterial, fungal, or viral pathogens.

Treatment: Systemic corticosteroids

DRUG REACTION WITH EOSINOPHILIA AND SYSTEMIC SYMPTOMS (DRESS) AND DRUG-INDUCED HYPERSENSITIVITY SYNDROME (DIHS)

- Multi-organ drug reaction.
- Pathogenesis not fully understood—can be linked to HHV-6, HHV-7, EBV–HLA-A*3101 (Northern Europeans—carbamazepine), HLA-B5801 (Han Chinese—allopurinol).
- **Drugs:** Aromatic anticonvulsants, lamotrigine, sulfonamides, minocycline, dapsone, allopurinol, abacavir, nevirapine.
- Develops **2–6 weeks** after drug initiation.

Clinical Features

- Fever, morbilliform punctuation eruption → edematous with follicular accentuation **(Fig. 3.8)**.
- Face, upper trunk extremities (**facial edema** is frequent and hallmark finding–up to 25% cases) **(Fig. 3.8)**. A recent sign reported is the ear lobe sign **(Fig. 3.9)**.
- Mucosal involvement mild, if present.

  The Registry of Severe Cutaneous Adverse Reactions (RegiSCAR), the Japanese Consensus Group (J-SCAR) and Boequet et al., are all scoring systems which use a set of defined criteria to make the determination of DRESS. The J-SCAR includes the detection of HHV-6 viral reactivation. If present, the Japanese refer to the condition as DIHS (Drug-induced hypersensitivity syndrome). It is important to note that while these tools are helpful, some of the scoring criteria are for symptoms that may occur later in the disease or may be transient

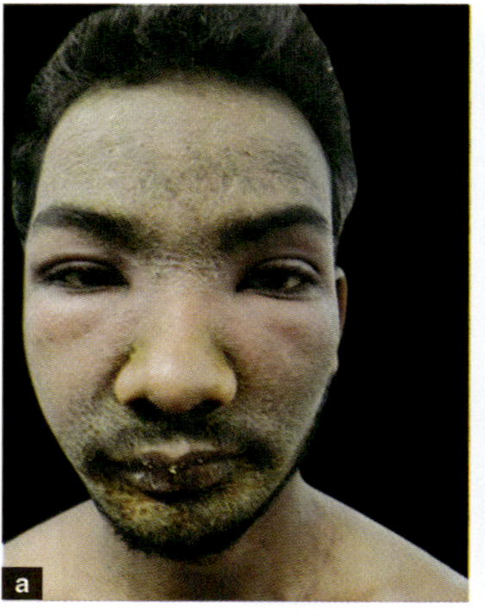

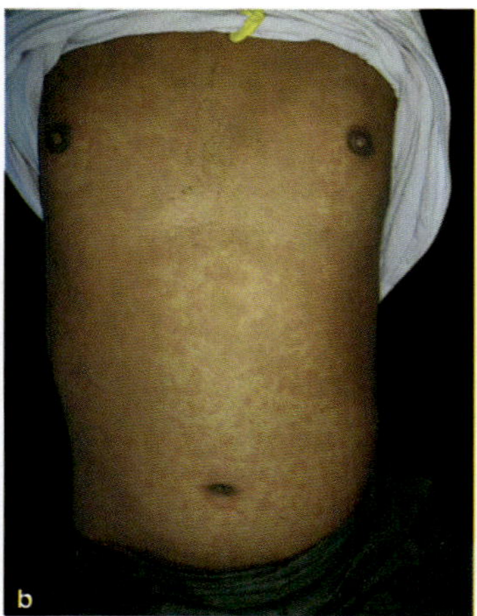

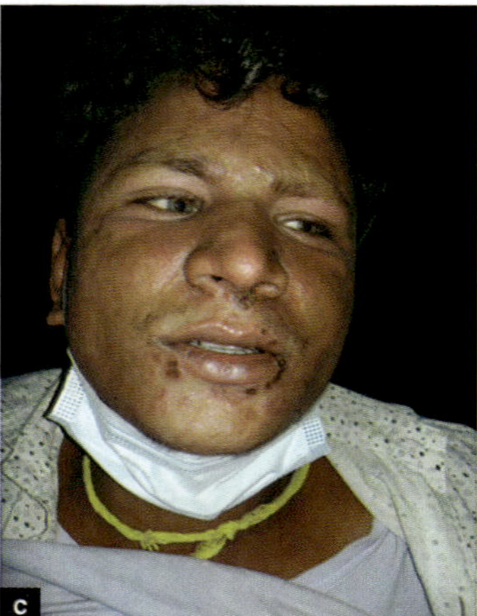

Fig. 3.8: DRESS manifests with a generalized rash, mild mucosal involvement and marked facial edema

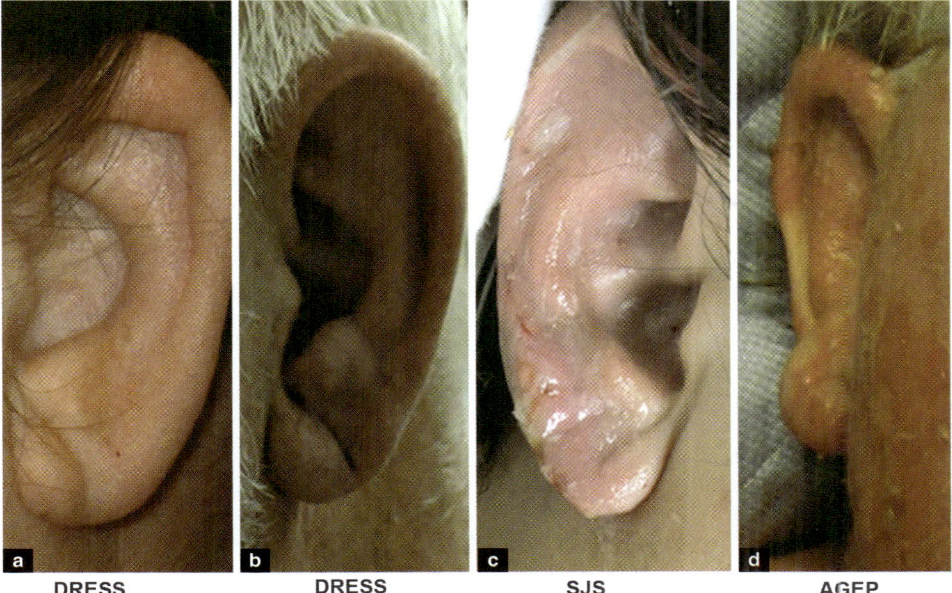

Fig. 3.9: Oblique earlobe crease in two patients diagnosed with DRESS syndrome; Ear lobes without an oblique earlobe crease in control patients diagnosed with Stevens-Johnson Syndrome (SJS) and acute generalized exanthematous pustulosis. https://doi.org/10.1111/jdv.18270

and not detectable at the time of diagnostic testing. The golden rule should be to assume DRESS in a patient who has taken medication and presents with: **fever, rash, facial edema/swelling and enlarged lymph nodes**.

There are many diagnostic criteria and are listed in **Table 3.5**.

- **Systemic features:** Lymphadenopathy, hepatic involvement, interstitial nephritis, myocarditis, pneumonitis, thyroiditis.
- Eruption and internal manifestations may persist for months even with treatment.
- They also have late involvement of visceral organs even after tapering steroid, hence, check thyroid profile for 2 years after DRESS.

An overview of some common myths and clinical pearls of DRESS are listed in the **Box 3.2**.

Investigations

A list of tests that can be ordered are listed in **Table 3.6**.

Treatment

The mainstay of treatment are systemic corticosteroids (oral prednisone). They are indicated when organs are affected and could decrease the chance of flare-ups and also autoimmune complications. Steroids are typically started as high dose and weaned very slowly to reduce the chance of disease recurrence. Patients who have a difficult time being weaned off steroids without a flare in symptoms may be put on additional, supportive medications like cyclosporine, intravenous immunoglobulin (IVIG), mycophenolate mofetil and rituximab.

TABLE 3.5: A comparsion of the major diagnostic criteria of DRESS

RegiSCAR study group	Japanese consensus group	Boequet et al.
More than 3 criteria are required for the diagnosis of DRESS: 1. Hospitalization 2. Reaction suspected to be drug related 3. Acute rash 4. Fever above 38°C 5. Enlarged lymph nodes involving at least two sites 6. Involvement of at least one internal organ 7. Blood count abnormalities: • Lymphocytes above or below laboratory limits • Eosinophils above laboratory limits (in percentage or absolute count) • Platelets below laboratory limits	Typical DRESS (presence of all 7 criteria); atypical DIHS (all criteria present except lymphadenopathy and HHV-6 reactivation): 1. HHV-6 reactivation 2. Prolonged clinical symptoms 2 weeks after discontinuation of causative drug 3. Maculopapular rash developing >3 weeks after starting drug 4. Fever above 38°C 5. Lymphadenopathy 6. ALT >100 U/L or other organ involvement 7. Leukocyte abnormalities (at least one) • Leukocytosis (>11 × 10^9/L) • Atypical lymphocytosis (>5%) • Eosinophilia (1.5 × 10^9/L)	DRESS is confirmed by presence of 1 and 2 and 3: 1. Cutaneous drug eruption 2. Adenopathies >2 cm in diameter or hepatitis (liver transaminases >2 times upper limit of normal) (or) interstitial nephritis (or) interstitial pneumonitis (or) carditis 3. Hematologic abnormalities • Eosinophilia >1.5 × 10^9/L (or) • Atypical lymphocytes

DRESS: Drug reaction with eosinophilia and systemic symptoms; ALT: Alanine aminotransferase; HHV-6: Human herpes virus-6; DIHS: Drug-induced hypersensitivity syndrome.

BOX 3.2: Common factoids on DRESS

Myths
- DRESS syndrome may only be diagnosed when the clinical criteria satisfy one of the established scoring systems.
- If the eruption is not morbiliform, then if is not DRESS syndrome.
- Patients who have had an allergic reaction to sulfonamide antibiotics will have a cross-reaction to nonantibiotic sulfonamides.
- Myocarditis secondary to DRESS syndrome will present with chest pain at the time of the cutaneous eruption.

Pearls
- The most commonly involved organ in DRESS syndrome is the liver.
- New-onset proteinuria, hematuria, and sterile pyuria indicate acute interstitial nephritis that may be associated with DRESS syndrome.
- Facial edema noted during physical examination is an important clue to DRESS syndrome.
- Vancomycin is an important cause of DRESS syndrome.
- Steroids are not the only treatment used to control DRESS syndrome.
- DRESS patients need to be monitored for long-term sequelae such as autoimmune disease.
- Small cases series suggest differences between adult and pediatric DRESS syndrome, but there are no large studies in children.

Cyclosporine has been found to be as effective as steroids and can be administered twice a day for a total of 2–3 mg/kg/day for 1 week, with a subsequent dose reduction to 1–1.5 mg/kg/day for extended treatment. Antiviral medications, like ganciclovir, may be indicated along with systemic steroids or IVIG in those patients who have viral reactivation.

TABLE 3.6: Investigations in a case of DRESS

Investigation	Findings
Complete blood count with differential counts and peripheral blood smear (CBC)	• Eosinophilia (>700/μL) • Lymphocytosis (absolute lymphocyte count >4500/μL), and/or • Atypical lymphocytes on peripheral smear
Liver function tests (LFT)	• Elevated enzymes 1.5–2 times the normal value
Serum creatinine and urinalysis	• Moderate elevation in creatinine level • Low grade proteinuria • Indications of kidney involvement: Abnormal urinary sediment with occasional eosinophils
Serology for viral hepatitis	• Hepatitis A IgM antibody • Hepatitis B surface antigen • Hepatitis B core IgM antibody • Hepatitis C viral RNA

MISCELLANEOUS DRUG ERUPTIONS

Some common patterns and their causes are listed below:

Acne-inducing Drugs

- Adrenocorticotropic hormone (ACTH)
- Phenytoin
- Isoniazid (INH)
- Lithium
- Oral steroids

Acute Generalized Exanthematous Pustulosis (AGEP)

- Calcium channel blockers
- Cephalosporins
- Macrolide antibiotics
- Mercury
- β-Lactam antibiotics

Fixed-drug Eruptions (FDEs)

- Barbiturates
- Erythromycin
- NSAIDs, naproxen
- Pseudoephedrine hydrochloride (nonpigmenting FDE)
- Sulfonamides
- Tetracyclines

Lichenoid Eruptions

- Antimalarials
- Captopril
- D-Penicillamine

- Gold
- Hydrochlorothiazide
- NSAIDs

Linear IgA Dermatosis

- Amiodarone
- Captopril
- Lithium
- Penicillin
- Vancomycin

Psoriasis-inducing Drugs

- Corticosteroid withdrawal
- Interferons
- Interleukin-2
- Lithium
- Propranolol (β-blockers)
- TNF alpha inhibitors (palmoplantar pustulosis)

Subacute Cutaneous Lupus Erythematosus (SCLE)-like Eruption

- Azathioprine
- Glyburide
- Griseofulvin
- Hydrochlorothiazide
- Penicillamine
- Penicillin
- Piroxicam
- Terbinafine

Drug-related Pigmentation

- **Amiodarone:** The drug is known to cause a slate-gray hyperpigmentation in photo-exposed areas. Histologically, periodic acid-Schiff (PAS)-positive yellow-brown granules are seen in macrophages in the dermis; on electron microscopy, membrane-bound structures resembling lysosomes are visualized.
- **Clofazimine:** Can cause a "drug-induced lipofuscinosis". The skin initially turns pink and then red-brown in lesions of patients with Hansen's disease **(Fig. 3.10)**. Granular pigment thought to be lipofuscin is seen in macrophages.
- **Chlorpromazine, thioridazine, imipramine, and clomipramine** cause a sun-exposed purple-gray hyperpigmentation, with corneal and lens opacities.
- **Gold, silver, and bismuth** can induce a slate-gray hyperpigmentation in sun-exposed areas
- **Bismuth** can cause pigmentation of the gingival margin.
- **Arsenical melanosis** causes truncal hyperpigmentation with depigmented raindrop-like macules.

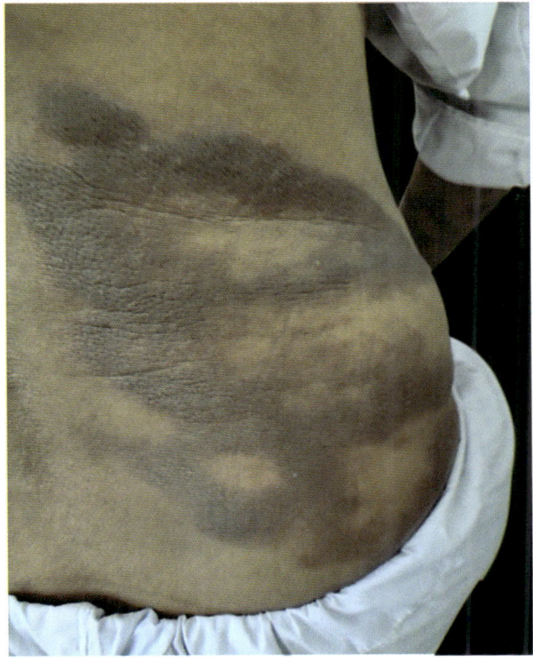

Fig. 3.10: Clofazimine induced pigmentation

COMMON CUTANEOUS SIDE EFFECTS OF ANTICANCER AGENTS

1. Cytotoxic Drugs

Hand Foot Syndrome

- Clinical presentation: Initial tingling sensation in palms/soles, then tender diffuse, symmetric erythema with or without scale on the palms and soles, may progress to blistering and desquamation **(Fig. 3.11)**.
- Common drugs: Cytarabine, pegylated liposomal doxorubicin, capecitabine, fluorouracil.
- There may be temporary loss of fingerprints with capecitabine.

Hair Pigmentary Changes

- "Flag sign" with methotrexate: Alternating bands of hyperpigmentation of hair on the scalp, eyebrows and eyelashes which corresponds to periods of treatment and no treatment.
- Cisplatin, cyclophosphamide, and combination regimens containing these drugs may abruptly change hair color.

Chemotherapy-induced Alopecia

- Primarily anagen punctuation effluvium with onset 7–10 days, most prominent 1–2 months after starting chemotherapy. Cyclophosphamide and busulfan can cause permanent alopecia.
- Docetaxel can cause prolonged and/or permanent alopecia.
- Scalp cooling may minimize the alopecia (Brunner C, 2022).

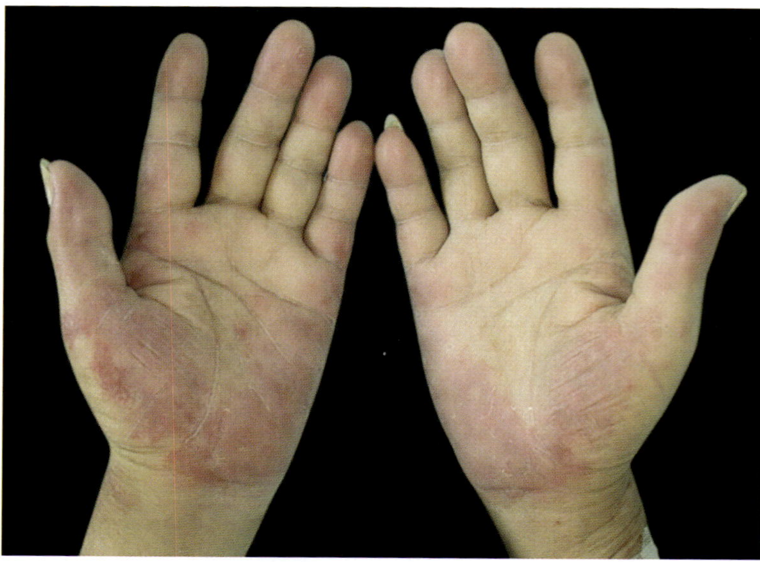

Fig. 3.11: Palmar–plantar erythrodysesthesia syndrome due to capecitabine

Scalp cooling: Use 30 minutes prior to infusion, throughout infusion and 90–120 min after infusion. Contraindicated in leukemias/lymphomas (systemic treatment required; discuss with primary team if a lymphoma); solid tumors with continuous-infusion chemotherapy >1 day; cranial irradiation; sensitivity to cold; cold agglutinins; cryoglobulinemia; post-traumatic cold dystrophy; caution with abnormal liver function.

Sclerodermoid-like Changes

- Clinical presentation: Trunk and extremities develop edema, tightening and indurated skin.
- Drugs: Bleomycin, gemcitabine, docetaxel.

Radiation Recall Dermatitis

- Clinical presentation: Previously irradiated skin with new onset acute inflammation with erythema after administration of chemotherapy; there can be vesiculation, desquamation, ulceration.
- Drugs: Dactinomycin, anthracyclines and anthracycline-like drugs.

Hyperpigmentation

Varied forms of pigmentation have been reported and are detailed in the **Table 3.7**.

2. Targeted Therapies (Solid Tumors)

Epidermal Growth Factor Receptor (EGFR) Inhibitors are usually given for nonsmall cell lung cancers.

These are of two broad categories:

- **Monoclonal antibodies:** Cetuximab, panitumumab, necitumumab
- **Small molecule EGFR inhibitors:** Gefitinib, erlotinib, lapatinib, afatinib, osimertinib.

TABLE 3.7: Cutaneous and mucosal hyperpigmentation with chemotherapeutic agents	
Generalized pattern	**Causative agents**
Diffuse	• Busulfan ("busulfan tan") • Methotrexate • Procarbazine
Diffuse and pressure induced	• Hydroxyurea • Cisplatin
Localized pattern	**Causative agents**
Flexural areas, palmar creases	• Bleomycin • Cyclophosphamide • Busulfan • Doxorubicin
Cutaneous and mucosal hyperpigmentation	• Busulfan • Cyclophosphamide (gingiva) • Tegafur (prodrug of 5-fluorouracil; lower lip, glans penis, also acral) • Doxorubicin (tongue, buccal mucosa) • Cisplatin • Fluorouracil
Specific pattern	**Causative agents**
Serpentine hyperpigmentation	• Fluorouracil • Taxanes • Cyclophosphamide, doxorubicin, vincristine, predn solone (CHOP)
Flagellate hyperpigmentation	• Bleomycin (often with preceding generalized pruritus) **(Fig. 3.12)**
Reticular hyperpigmentation	• Paclitaxel • Cytarabine • Fluorouracil • Idarubicin

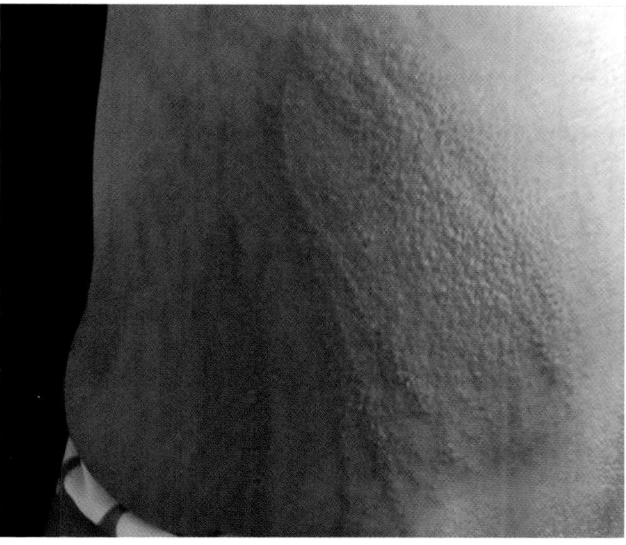

Fig. 3.12: Flagellate pigmentation with bleomycin

Papulopustular Rashes (Acneiform Eruptions)

Clinical presentation

- There is an acneiform eruption with folliculocentric erythematous papules and pustules with or without pruritus on the face, trunk, and extremities, sparing the palms and soles; no comedonal component
- Seen 1–2 weeks after EGFRi initiation and improves significantly around 8 weeks of treatment; if it persists after 8 weeks of treatment, there is a need to rule out superinfection.
- It is dose-dependent and correlates with the survival and is seen in majority of cases.

Treatment

Petroleum jelly for xerosis, strict photoprotection, low-mid potency topical steroid ointments for pruritus, topical antibiotics, systemic antibiotics if needed (doxycycline or minocycline, cautioning on photosensitivity).

The other reactions seen with this class of drugs are listed in **Table 3.8**.

3. Small Molecule Tyrosine Kinase Inhibitors

The drugs in this class are Sorafenib, sunitinib, pazopanib, regorafenib, axitinib, cabozantinib.

Hand-foot Skin Reaction

- Seen with sorafenib and sunitinib, ~40% of patients; different from hand foot syndrome induced by traditional chemotherapies.
- Clinical presentation: localized areas on the palms, soles, interdigital web spaces, and lateral aspect of the feet with focal hyperkeratotic callus-like lesions on an erythematous base with onset approximately 2–4 weeks after initiation of therapy **(Fig. 3.13)**.
- Associated with paresthesias, tingling, burning, soreness, decreased tolerance with hot objects.
- Associated with increased tumor response rate and overall survival.
- Manage with cushioned shoes, decrease friction, keratolytics +/– topical retinoids, topical steroids if erythema, topical lidocaine, acitretin, oral/topical gabapentin.

Other cutaneous rashes seen are listed in **Table 3.9**.

TABLE 3.8: Summary of EGFR inhibitor reactions

Site of reaction	Type of reaction
Cutaneous	• Papulopustular rashes (*see* above) • Exfoliative eruptions • Bullous eruptions • Hand-foot skin reaction (*see* MTKIs) • Pruritus • Telangiectasias • Urticaria • Xerosis and desquamation
Mucosa	• Aphthous ulceration of oral, nasal mucosa
Hair	• Abnormality or change in scalp hair, facial hair or eyelash growth
Nails	• Paronychia +/– pyogenic granuloma

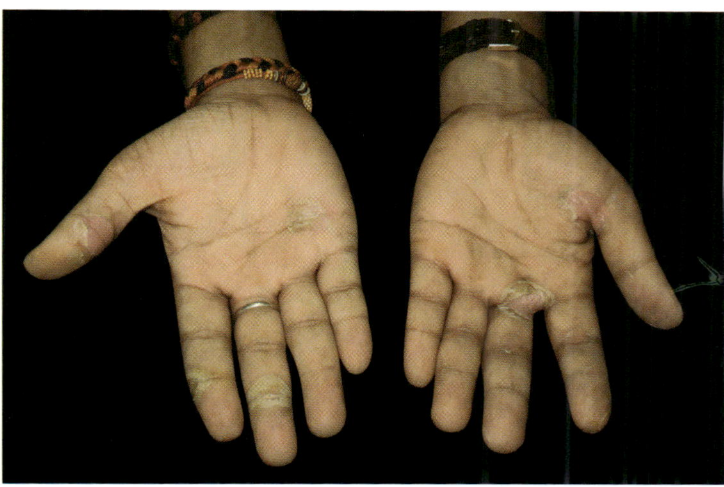

Fig. 3.13: Focal hyperkeratotic erythematous lesions on the palms due to Sorafenib

TABLE 3.9: Reactions to sorafenib and sunitinib

Site of reaction	Type of reaction
Cutaneous	• Acquired perforating dermatosis • Eruptive melanocytic lesions • Erythema multiforme and EM-like eruptions • Exanthematous rashes • Hand-foot skin reaction (*see* above) • Keratoacanthomas, squamous cell carcinoma* • Pyoderma gangrenosum** • Scalp dysesthesia • Seborrheic dermatitis-like reaction • SJS • Yellow discoloration of skin** • Xerosis
Mucosa	• Mucositis • Geographic tongue
Hair	• Alopecia-temporary • Hair depigmentaiton-reversible upon drug holiday or discontinuation
Nails	• Subungual splinter hemorrhages • Periungual erythema

*MC sorafenib
**MC sunitinib

4. BRAF Inhibitors

The common drugs in this class are vemurafenib, dabrafenib, and encorafenib, and they are commonly used for nonsmall cell lung cancers.

The skin rashes seen with this of drugs are listed in **Table 3.10**.

TABLE 3.10: Reactions to BRAF inhibitors

Site of reaction	Type of reaction
Cutaneous	• Eruptive nevi[v] • Grover disease[d] • Keratoacanthomas* • Melanoma—second primary[d] – Unclear if secondary to therapy or higher risk at baseline due to primary melanoma • Papulopustular eruption* • Photosensitivity[v] • Plantar hyperkeratosis[d] • Pyogenic granuloma[v] • Radiation enhancement[v] • SJS/TEN[v] • Benign and malignant squamous proliferative disorders* • Highest risk in patients >60 years, first 3 months of treatment; occur in sun-protected sites more commonly than sporadic SCCs; risk is decreased when combined with MEK inhibitors • Xerosis*
Hair	• Alopecia +/– structural hair changes*
Nails	• Acute paronychia* • Brittle nails[v] • Onycholysis[d]

*Vemurafenib and dabrafenib
[v]Vemurafenib
[d]Dabrafenib

5. MEK Inhibitors

- MEK inhibitors: Trametinib and cobimetinib. These are used for melanoma.
- Trametinib
  - Acneiform rash
  - Pruritus
  - Xerosis
- Cobimetinib
  - Acneiform eruption
  - Photosensitivity.

6. Targeted Therapies (Hematologic Malignancies)

Bruton Tyrosine Kinase (BTK) Inhibitors (Ibrutinib, Acalabrutinib)

They are approved for mantle cell lymphoma, CLL/SLL, chronic graft-versus-host disease (GVHD), WM, and marginal zone lymphoma as monotherapy or combined therapy. The cutaneous side effects are:

- Petechiae, ecchymoses, hematomas, bleeding diathesis
- Non-palpable petechial eruption
- Palpable purpuric rash (clinically resembling leukocytoclastic vasculitis)
- Neutrophilic panniculitis.

BCR-ABL Inhibitors (Imatinib, Dasatinib, Nilotinib, Bosutinib, Ponatinib)

They are approved for CML and the skin rashes seen are minor and include:

- Non-specific dermatitis with morbilliform papules on face > trunk > extremities
- Lichenoid dermatitis
- Pruritus: Common and can be severe
- Periorbital edema: Around 6 weeks after initiation
- Pigmentary changes: Blue-gray hyperpigmentation or hypopigmentation in darker skin or hypopigmentation.

Proteasome Inhibitors (Bortezomib, Carfilzomib, Ixazomib)

- Erythematous nodules and plaques.
- Morbilliform exanthem or maculopapular rash, with small vessel vasculitis on pathology but no associated systemic vasculitis.
- Sweet syndrome.

PI3Kδ inhibitors (Idelalisib, Duvelisib, and Copanlisib)

- Nonspecific maculopapular rash in 10–20% but severe in up to 2%.
- Desquamative/exfoliative erythroderma with islands of sparing and keratoderma, "EM-like" epidermal necrosis on pathology.
- May have delayed onset and protracted course.

7. Checkpoint Inhibitors

This class of drugs has numerous indications including nonsmall cell lung cancer; squamous cell carcinoma; renal cell carcinoma; triple negative breast cancer; hepatocellular carcinoma; gastric cancer; small cell lung cancer; squamous cell carcinoma of head and neck and melanoma.

There are varied class of drugs in this class.

Programmed Cell Death Receptor 1 (PD-1) Inhibitors

- Nivolumab, pembrolizumab, and cemiplimab
- PD-1 is on T cells.

Programmed Cell Death Receptor Ligand 1 (PD-L1) Inhibitors

- Atezolizumab, avelumab and durvalumab
- PD-L1 is on tumor cells
- PEARL: PD-1 and PD-L1: Can get delayed reactions, up to months and years.

Cytotoxic T-lymphocyte-associated Antigen 4 (CTLA-4)

- Ipilimumab and tremelimumab (in development)
- Side effects are due to immunologic enhancement and include dermatologic, rheumatologic, gastrointestinal, hepatic, endocrinological.

The varied side effects of these drugs are listed in **Table 3.11**.

TABLE 3.11: Reactions to checkpoint inhibitors

Site of reaction	Type of reaction
Cutaneous	• Bullous disorders including BP • Follicular eruption • Granulomas • Lichenoid dermatitis • Maculopapular eruption • Papulopustular eruption • Pruritus without dermatitis • Psoriasiform dermatitis • SJS/TEN • Sweet's syndrome • Urticarial eruption • Vitiligo
Mucosa	• Gingivitis • Lichenoid mucositis • Mucositis (PD-1 inhibitors >> CTLA-4 inhibitors) • Sicca syndrome
Hair	• Alopecia (alopecia areata)

BIBLIOGRAPHY

1. Baker H, Ryan TJ. Generalized pustular psoriasis. A clinical and epidemiological study of 104 cases. Br J Dermatol 1968;80:771.
2. Brunner C. Hair safe study: Effects of scalp cooling on hair preservation and hair regrowth in breast cancer patients receiving chemotherapy - A prospective interventional study. Breast. 2022 Aug;64:50–55.
3. Castillo B, Vera N, Ortega-Loayza AG, SeminarioVidal L. Wound care for Stevens-Johnson syndrome and toxic epidermal necrolysis. J Am Acad Dermatol 2018;79:764.e1–767.e1.
4. Garcia-Doval I, LeCleach L, Bocquet H, et al. Toxic epidermal necrolysis and Ste-vens-Johnson syndrome: does early withdrawal of causative drugs decrease the risk of death? Arch Dermatol 2000;136:323.
5. Kardaun SH, Jonkman MF. Dexamethasone pulse therapy for Stevens-Johnson syndrome/toxic epidermal necrolysis. Acta Derm Venereol. 2007;87(2):144–8.
6. Murphy MJ, Treatment of Persistent Erythema Multiforme With Janus Kinase Inhibition and the Role of Interferon Gamma and Interleukin 15 in Its Pathogenesis. JAMA Dermatol. 2021 Dec 1;157(12):1477–1482.
7. Papp A, Sikora S, Evans M, Song D, Kirchhof M, Miliszewski M, Dutz J. Treatment of toxic epidermal necrolysis by a multidisciplinary team. A review of literature and treatment results. Burns. 2018 Jun;44(4):807–815.
8. Pereira FA, Mudgil AV, Rosmarin DM. Toxic epidermal necrolysis. J Am Acad Dermatol. 2007;56(2):181–200.
9. Roujeau JC, Kelly JP, Naldi L, et al. Medication use and the risk of Stevens-John-son syndrome or toxic epidermal necrolysis. N Engl J Med 1995;333:1600.
10. Sidoroff A, Dunant A, Viboud C, et al. Risk factors for acute generalized exan-thematous pustulosis (AGEP)-results of a multinational case-control study (EuroSCAR). Br J Dermatol 2007;157:989.
11. Wang Q, Tian X, Liu W, Zhang L. Procalcitonin as a diagnostic indicator for systemic bacterial infections in patients with Stevens-Johnson syndrome/toxic epidermal necrolysis. J Dermatol 2018;45:989–993.

Chapter

4

Amyloidosis

Surabhi Sinha

Definition and Types

- *Amylum* (L)—starch-like (though it is a protein and not carbohydrate)
- Extracellular deposition of autologous proteins which show highly conserved **antiparallel β-sheet conformation** and nonbranching linear fibrils of variable lengths and diameter of 7.5–10 nm.
- **Functional versus disease-causing amyloid**
  a. Functional amyloid—in mammals, insects, fungi and bacteria
    – Involved in various structural and protective roles
  b. Disease-causing amyloid—toxic effects of deposition

Types of Cutaneous Amyloidosis

a. Acquired
b. Hereditary

Types of Acquired Amyloidosis

a. Primary localized cutaneous amyloidosis (PLCA)
b. Secondary localized cutaneous amyloidosis (SLCA)
c. Systemic amyloidosis with cutaneous involvement (e.g. plasma cell dyscrasias)
d. Secondary cutaneous amyloidosis originating from other systemic diseases (e.g. inflammatory disorders like rheumatoid arthritis, chronic infection).

We shall primarily discuss PLCA here.

Types of PLCA

a. Macular (35%) **(Fig. 4.1)**
b. Papular (35%) **(Fig. 4.2)**
c. Mixed/biphasic/allotropic/maculopapular (15%)
d. Nodular (1.5%)—rare, only 100 cases reported, may rarely develop systemic amyloidosis

Epidemiology

- More common in South-East Asia, China and South America. PLCA more frequent near equator.
- Asia—papular PLCA is the most common (75%), mixed/maculopapular (15%) and macular (10%)
- Female:male—2–3:1 (papular—more in M and macular—more in F)

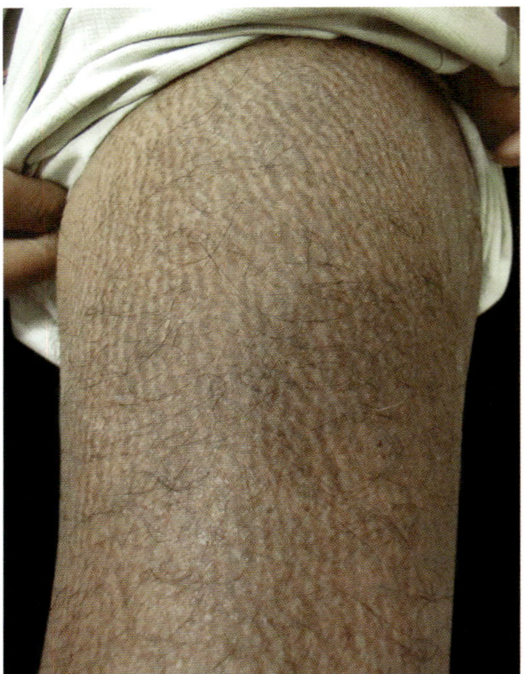

Fig. 4.1: Macular amyloidosis with characteristic rippled pigmentation

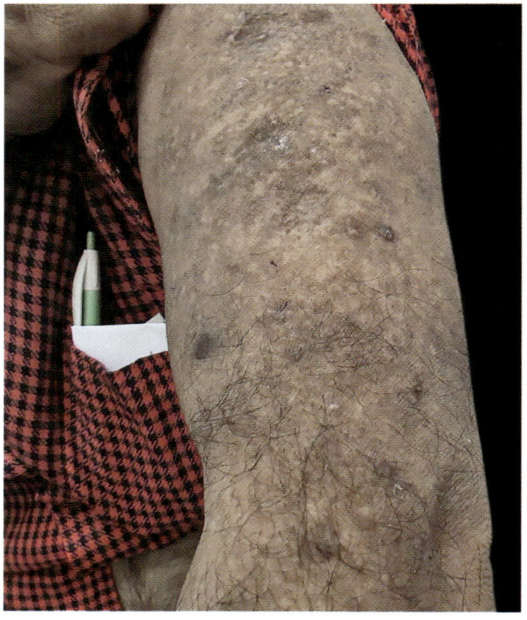

Fig. 4.2: Papular amyloidosis (raised papules on a background of macular amyloidosis)—biphasic amyloidosis

Predisposing Factors

- Prolonged friction
- Genetic predisposition
- Epstein-Barr virus
- Environmental factors.

Pathogenesis (Flowchart 4.1)

It must be noted that there is a well accepted "itch scratch" cycle that play a role in cutaneous amyloidosis like in other Th2 mediated disorders like prurigo nodularis and atopic dermatitis. It has also been shown that type 2 cytokines directly activate sensory neurons and the itch is dependent on on neuronal IL-4Rα and JAK1 signaling and would respond to JAK inhibitors. (Oetjen LK, 2017)

Flowchart 4.1: Pathogenesis of PLCA

Apoptotic basal keratinocytes (reason not known)

↓

Cytokeratins are released

↓

Get coated by autoantibodies

↓

Phagocytosed by macrophages and then enzymatically degraded to **amyloid K** (key feature)*

*Cytokeratin 5 (and 1, 10, 14) is the major constituent of AK amyloid

Clinical Features

See **Table 4.1**.

Differential Diagnosis

Tables 4.2 and **4.3** give a list of differential diagnosis for macular and papular amyloidosis, respectively.

Complications

1. Pruritus can be bothersome.
2. Esthetic issues

Diagnosis

Dermoscopy

- Macular amyloidosis—a central hub either white or brown in color, surrounded by various configurations of pigmentation.
- Papular/lichen amyloidosis—the central hub is replaced by scar-like morphology.

TABLE 4.1: Overview of amyloidosis

Type of amyloidosis	Clinical findings	Distribution	Variants	Associated disorders	Differential diagnosis	HPE
Macular (amyloid cytokeratin—mainly CK5)	Pruritic or asymptomatic hyperpigmented, vaguely demarcated or confluent plaques, characteristic rippled pattern (+/–)	Interscapular region, extremities, trunk	• Mixed/biphasic/allotropic (macular + papular) • Poikilodermatous (macules, blisters and poikilodermatous lesions) • Anosacral (Japan) Amyloidosis cutis dyschromica (hyper- and hypopigmented macules)	• MEN2a • Primary biliary cirrhosis	Atopic dermatitis, PIH, LSC, FDE, atrophoderma of Pasini-Pierini, morphea, anetoderma	Amyloid deposits in papillary dermis
Papular/lichenoid (amyloid cytokeratin—mainly CK5)	Discrete firm, scaly, skin-colored or hyperpigmented brownish lichenoid, papules, which later coalesce to form hyperkeratotic plaques	Lower leg, trunk, forearm	• Mixed (macular and papular) • Poikilodermatous (lichenoid papules, blisters, poikilodermatous lesions)	—	LSC, hypertrophic LP	Amyloid deposits in papillary dermis
Nodular PLCA (amyloid from Ig light chains κ, λ)	Solitary/multiple waxy nodules with atrophic telangiectatic surface, <100 cases	Feet, nose, genitals, trunk	—	• Diabetes • Sjögren syndrome • CREST syndrome	Nevus lipomatosus, cutaneous lymphomas	Amyloid deposits found in reticular dermis and subcutaneous fat (like systemic amyloidosis)
SLCA (amyloid cytokeratins—mainly CK5)	Similar to papular PLCA	Similar to papular PLCA		Skin tumors*, DLE, collagenoses	According to association	Amyloid deposits in papillary dermis
Hereditary—familial PLCA (AApo-E4—amyloid apolipoprotein E4, amyloid cytokeratin)	Similar to macular/papular PLCA	Similar to macular/papular PLCA		Lipid metabolism disorders	According to association dermis	Amyloid deposits in papillary

*Skin tumors—nevi, sweat gland tumors, pilomatricomas, actinic keratoses, seborrheic keratoses, porokeratosis of Mibelli, Bowen disease, basal cell carcinoma, trichoepithelioma.

TABLE 4.2: Important differential diagnosis of macular amyloidosis	
Disease	**Differentiating features**
Post-inflammatory hyperpigmentation	Rippled pigmentation like amyloid is absent No amyloid deposits on histopathology
Notalgia paraesthetica	Histopathology: Melanophages are seen but no amyloid deposits
Ashy dermatosis	• Macules with different shades of grey on the trunk mainly • Dermoscopy: Gray-bluish small dots over a bluish background corresponding to melanophages/melanin deposits in deeper dermis

TABLE 4.3: Important differential diagnosis of lichen amyloidosis	
Disease	**Differentiating features**
Hypertrophic lichen planus	Plaques have a violaceous hue No amyloid deposit on histopathology Dermoscopy: • Rippled surface • Comedo-like structures • Round corneal structures (corn pearls)
Lichen simplex chronicus	Lichenification is the more prominent feature No amyloid deposits seen on histopathology Dermoscopy: • Accentuated skin markings with mottled light brownish and white pigmentation • No characteristic central hubs or scar seen

Histopathological Examination (HPE) and Special Stains

- **Epidermis:** Acanthosis and compact orthohyperkeratosis
- **Dermis:** Amyloid deposits present as:
  - Homogeneous, hyaline, eosinophilic deposits on **H&E** stain **(Fig. 4.3)**
  - **Metachromasia** on crystal violet or methyl violet stain
  - Positive staining with alkaline **Congo red and thioflavin** T
  - **Dichroism:** Apple-green birefringence under **polarized light** after Congo red staining.
  - **On fluorescence microscopy:** Amyloid deposits are seen on staining with **Thioflavin T**.
- Blood vessels are not affected in macular and lichenoid amyloidosis (c.f. systemic amyloidosis).

Immunohistochemistry

- Antibodies against cytokeratins 5 > 1 > 14 > 10 in PLCA and cytokeratins 5 > 1 > 10 > 14 in SLCA. IHC studies have shown intense staining of the amyloid with cytokeratin 5 (CK5) antibody and high molecular weight keratin (HMWK)—which proved superior to Congo red staining (Sari Aslani F, et al., 2020).
- Pan-CK antibodies can also be used against all four basal keratinocyte CKs (1, 5, 10 and 14).
- Antibodies against Ig light chains in nodular PLCA and systemic amyloidosis.

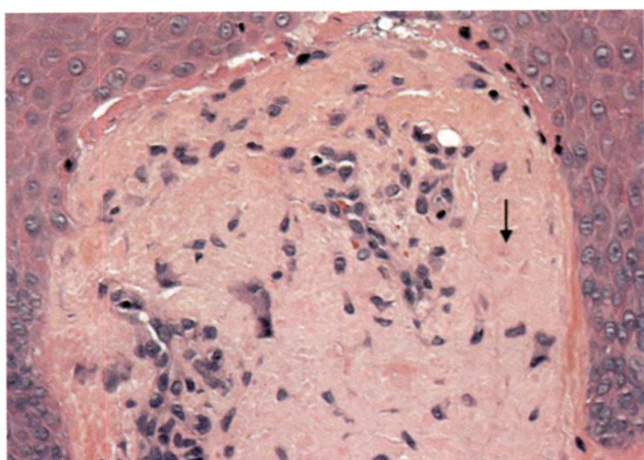

Fig. 4.3: Pink hyaline material deposited in the papillary dermis with dendritic melanophages on histopathology (H&E stain)

Electron Microscopy

Can definitively confirm amyloid in tissues—seen as fibrils 7.5–10 nm in diameter. Useful in differentiating nodular PLCA from systemic amyloidosis.

- For **nodular PLCA**—important to **rule out systemic amyloidosis**.
  Investigations:
  - Detailed history and physical examination
  - ECG
  - CBC, LFT with enzymes, KFT
  - Serum protein electrophoresis and urine protein electrophoresis
  - Skin biopsy
  - Abdominal fat pad biopsy to rule out systemic amyloidosis
  - Abdominal fat pad FNAC

Treatment

The main aim is cosmetic improvement and relief of pruritus. **Flowchart 4.2** gives an algorithm that can be used in a patient with PLCA.

A recent systematic treatment review analysed a variety of treatment options for PLCA including retinoids, corticosteroids, cyclophosphamide, cyclosporine, amitriptyline, colchicine, tacrolimus, dimethyl sulfoxide, vitamin D3 analogs, capsaicin, menthol, hydrocolloid dressings, surgical modalities, laser treatment, and phototherapy. However, it concluded that no definitive recommendation of preferable treatment procedures could be made based on the available literature (Weidner, et al., 2017).

Considering the importance of Th2 cytokines and the fact that amyloid deposition is thought to be driven by a chronic itch–scratch cycle, which is similar to other Th2 mediated disorders JAKi have been tried successfully in PLCA and include tofacitinib, baricitinib and recently upadicitinib. (Fakhraie S, 2023)

Flowchart 4.2: Treatment algorithm for PLCA

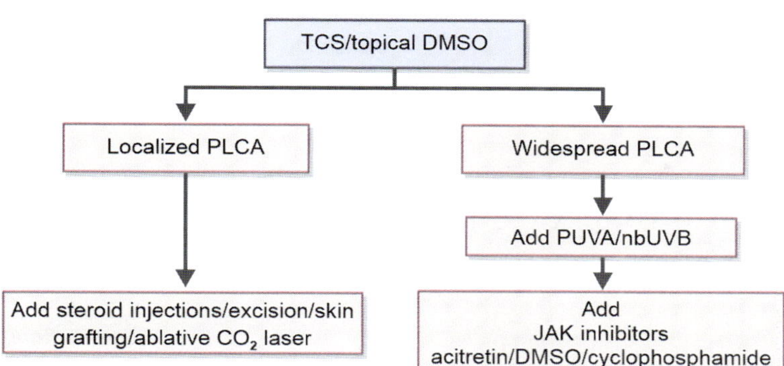

TCS, topical corticosteroid; DMSO, dimethyl sulfoxide

Recently, intralesional injection of tranexamic acid (TXA) was seen to be more effective than topical application of Kligman combination in macular amyloidosis in an RCT (Ghassemi et al., 2022).

Among lasers, in a recent study 4 areas of 1 sq cm diameter were treated simultaneously with PDL, Q-Switched Nd-YAG, CO_2 and combined CO_2 and Nd-YAG Lasers. The authors inferred that PDL was not effective, the Q-Switched Nd-YAG was effective in only 3/17 patients whereas all areas of the 17 patients treated with CO_2 laser were cleared, alone or in combination (Radmanesh, 2021).

BIBLIOGRAPHY

Books

1. Bolognia. Dermatology, 4th ed. Chapter 47, sec 8 metabolic and systemic diseases.
2. Rook's Textbook of Dermatology, 9th ed. Part 5 Chapter 58 "Cutaneous Amyloidoses". Pg 1579–91.

Journal

1. Fakhraie S, . Lichen amyloidosis: towards pathogenesis-driven targeted treatment. Clin Exp Dermatol. 2023 Mar 1;48(3):261–262.
2. Ghassemi M, Roohaninasab M, Kamani SA, Sadeghzadeh-Bazargan A, Goodarzi A. Comparison of the efficacy and safety of intralesional injection of tranexamic acid and the topical application of Kligman combination drug in the treatment of macular amyloidosis. Dermatol Ther. 2022 Jan 35(1):e15213. doi: 10.1111/dth.15213. Epub 2021 Nov 30. PMID: 34797597.
3. Oetjen LK, Sensory Neurons Co-opt Classical Immune Signaling Pathways to Mediate Chronic Itch. Cell. 2017 Sep 21;171(1):217–228.e13.
4. Radmanesh M, Ghanatir F, Radmanesh R. Comparing the efficacy of pulsed dye laser, Q-Switched Nd-YAG, CO2, and combined CO_2 and Q-Switched Nd-YAG lasers for the treatment of cutaneous macular amyloidosis. J Dermatolog Treat. 2021 Mar;32(2):258-260. doi: 10.1080/09546634.2019.1654071. Epub 2019 Aug 25. PMID: 31415215.
5. Sari Aslani F, Kargar H, Safaei A, Jowkar F, Hosseini M, Sepaskhah M. Comparison of Immunostaining with Hematoxylin-Eosin and Special Stains in the Diagnosis of Cutaneous Macular Amyloidosis. Cureus. 2020 Apr 9;12(4):e7606. doi: 10.7759/cureus.7606.
6. Weidner T, Illing T, Elsner P. Primary Localized Cutaneous Amyloidosis: A Systematic Treatment Review. Am J Clin Dermatol. 2017 Oct;18(5):629-642. doi: 10.1007/s40257-017-0278-9. PMID: 28342017.

Chapter

5

Annular (Figurate) Erythemas

Seema Rani, Bhavya Sangal

Annular Erythemas

- Lesions have an annular, arciform or polycyclic appearance.
- Self-limiting and without associated systemic symptoms.
- The eruptions may start in infancy or in teenage years.
- An autosomal dominant inherited form has been reported.
- **Four** classical types **(Table 5.1)**:
  - **Erythema annulare centrifugum (EAC)**
  - **Erythema marginatum (rheumaticum)**
  - **Erythema (chronicum) migrans (ECM)**
  - **Erythema gyratum repens (EGR)**

TABLE 5.1: Important differentiating features of annular erythemas (gyrate erythemas)

	Erythema annulare centrifugum (EAC)	Erythema marginatum (rheumaticum)	Erythema (chronicum) migrans	Erythema gyratum repens
Classic lesion	• Annular, polycyclic, erythematous plaques with scaling behind the advancing edge **(trailing scale) (Fig. 5.1)**	• Annular and sometimes polycyclic, serpiginous, erythematous eruption	• Erythema slowly migrates from site of tick bite • Due to the spirochete ***Borrelia burgdorferi*** (**Ixodes** tick bite)	• Mobile, concentric, often palpable, erythematous rings with **'woodgrain'** appearance of the skin
Epidemiology	• Occurs at any age • No sex predilection	• Most common in children, age group 5–15 years	• No sex predilection • Tick must be attached for >1 day, usually >48 hours • Bimodal age distribution (5–19 years and 55–69 years)	• Usually in seventh decade M:F = 2:1

(Contd.)

5

TABLE 5.1: Important differentiating features of annular erythemas (gyrate erythemas) *(Contd.)*

	Erythema annulare centrifugum (EAC)	Erythema marginatum (rheumaticum)	Erythema (chronicum) migrans	Erythema gyratum repens
Associated factors	• Concurrent infection (EBV, bacterial, parasitic, dermatophytes) • Thyroid and liver disorders • Pregnancy • Drugs • Malignancy	• Rheumatic fever • Psittacosis • Angioedema (C1 inhibitor deficiency—acquired or hereditary)	• Lyme disease	• Paraneoplastic dermatosis—carcinoma of the lung (47%) esophagus, breast, stomach, kidney, pharynx, urinary bladder, uterus and/or cervix, hematological cancers
HPE	• Perivascular **'sleeve-like'** lymphohistiocytic infiltrate in dermis—superficial, deep or mixed	• Perivascular polymorphous infiltrate of neutrophils and mononuclear cells in the papillary dermis and upper portion of the reticular dermis, leukocytoclasia is often present	• Inflammatory dermal infiltrates contain eosinophil and plasma cells, apoptotic cells seen in epidermis • *Borrelia* spp. + on silver stains	• Hyperkeratosis, parakeratosis, acanthosis and spongiosis • Superficial and occasionally deep perivascular lymphohistiocytic infiltrate in the papillary dermis
Clinical features	• Expanding polycyclic, annular, erythematous plaques with 'central clearing' • 'Trailing scale' (inner margin shows desquamation) is common in superficial lesions, but not in deep lesions	• Begin as erythematous macules or papules (urticarial) that spread peripherally and may merge to produce the typical serpiginous, polycyclic annular eruption • Non-scaly	• An erythematous, expanding annular plaque (rapid growth rate of up to 3 cm/day) with lighter colored central area or a **bull's eye** appearance • The advancing edge may be crusted or even vesicular • Sensations of warmth, pruritus and pain +/–	• Rings, swirls or waves appear within existing lesions to form a concentric pattern of sequential eruptions, resembling the *'grain of wood'* (rapid rate of up to 1 cm/day) • Pruritus + • Cutaneous lesions develop 1 year prior/after diagnosis of the neoplasm • May be associated with acquired ichthyosis and palmoplantar keratoderma
Sites	• May be localized or generalized, involve buttocks, thighs and trunk mostly, rarely involve palm, sole, scalp or mucous membranes	• Trunk, axillae and proximal extremities, with sparing of the face	• Favor the trunk, axillae, groin and popliteal fossa	• No specific site

(Contd.)

TABLE 5.1: Important differentiating features of annular erythemas (gyrate erythemas) *(Contd.)*

	Erythema annulare centrifugum (EAC)	Erythema marginatum (rheumaticum)	Erythema (chronicum) migrans	Erythema gyratum repens
Disease course and prognosis	• Chronic, with waxing and waning course • Variable duration, lasting from days to to decades (mean 2.8 years). May regress spontaneously or with t/t of associated conditions	• Resolving and reappearing skin lesions	• Untreated lesions usually last 4 to 6 weeks, 60% have mono- or oligoarticular arthritis, 10% neurological (facial nerve palsy) and 5% have cardiac complications	• Resolves once underlying malignancy is treated • Course parallels underlying malignancy
D/D	• Erythema chronicum migrans • Annular SCLE • Annular urticaria • Erythema multiforme • Tinea corporis • Annular psoriasis • Mycosis fungoides	• Other figurate erythemas • Annular urticaria • Annular erythema of infancy • Neutrophilic figurate erythema of infancy	• Cellulitis • Erysipelas • Fixed drug eruptions	• Figurate erythemas • Erythrokeratoderma variabilis • Psoriasis • Pityriasis rubra pilaris • Tinea corporis • Tinea imbricata • Mycosis fungoides
Investigations	• Culture from skin or nail to rule out fungal infections • Skin biopsy, DIF, ANA, ACE level, HIV serology, PET and CT scan, if suspected malignancy	• Throat swab C/S • ASO titres • CRP • ESR • All routine tests and ECG	• Skin biopsy with silver stain for pathogenic organism visualization • PCR in skin biopsy • Tissue culture • ELISA • Western blot for anti-*Borrelia* antibodies	• All routine tests, CT scan of chest, abdomen and pelvis (screen for a possible underlying malignancy)
Treatment	*First line* • Treatment of underlying cause • Topical steroids • Topical calcipotriol *Second line* • Topical tacrolimus • Phototherapy *Third line* • Chloroquine or hydroxychloroquine • Systemic steroids	• Aspirin or non-steroidal anti-inflammatory drugs • Penicillin or erythromycin	• Doxycycline 100 mg oral 12 hourly for 2–3 weeks (>8 years of age) • Amoxycillin 50 mg/kg 8 hourly for 2–3 weeks (<8 years of age)	• Identification and treatment of underlying cause

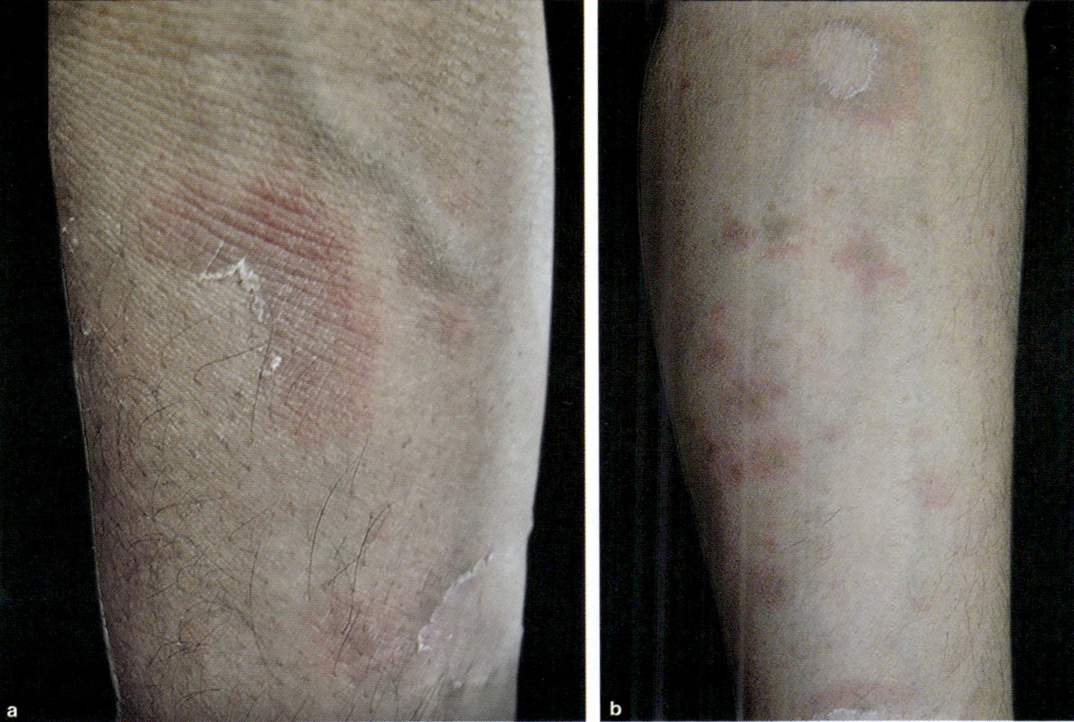

Fig. 5.1: Erythema annulare centrifugum. Note the annular plaques with a trailing scale

BIBLIOGRAPHY

1. Dermatology. Eds: Bolognia, Schaffer, Cerroni. Chapter 19: FigurateErythemas.
2. Fitzpatrick's Dermatology, 9th edition. Chapter 46: Erythema Annulare Centrifugum and Other Figurate Erythemas.
3. Rook's Textbook of Dermatology, 9th ed. Chapter 47: Reactive inflammatoryerythemas.

Chapter

6

Atopic Dermatitis

Kabir Sardana, Sumitra Meena

DEFINITION

The word atopic derives from Greek word *'a-topos'* which means "a strange disease without a precise place". "Eczema" is derived from the Greek word *"Ekzein"* which meaning to "boil out". Dermatitis means inflammation of skin. (Coca AF et al., 1923) Atopic dermatitis (AD) is a multifactorial, chronic, relapsing inflammatory skin condition that is commonly associated with other atopic conditions such as food allergy, allergic rhinitis, and asthma (Bieber T, et al., 2009).

EPIDEMIOLOGY

It affects approximately 15–20% of children and 1–3% of adults worldwide. Onset is most commonly seen by 5 years of age but it can be seen at any age.

AD commonly resolves by increasing age, and only about **10–30%** of patients will continue with symptoms of disease (Ellis CN, et al., 2012).

- Early onset: Within 2 years—most common, 50% develop allergen-specific IgE Ab by 2 years of age
- Late onset: After puberty
- Senile onset: After 60 years (unusual).

PATHOPHYSIOLOGY

It is a multifactorial heterogenous disorder in which various factors are implicated (genetic, epigenetic alteration, environmental, epidermal barrier dysfunction and immunological factors). (Bieber T, et al., 2009)

Three main factors mediate the disorder **(Fig. 6.1)**:

1. Genetics

It has been shown that mutation in filaggrin (*FLG*) gene located on chromosome 1q2, leads to a defect in the epidermal barrier and an increase in trans-epidermal water loss (TEWL) associated with a decrease in natural moisturizer factor (NMF). (Palmer CN, et al., 2006)

- Filaggrin deficiency-early onset AD, severe, ↑atopy, infections
- FLG mutations are only seen in 50% of AD

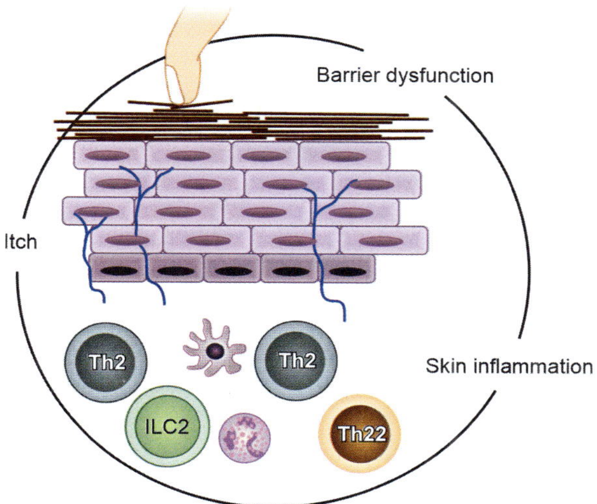

Fig. 6.1: Atopic dermatitis is characterized by an interplay of 3 factors: Barrier dysfunction, skin inflammation and itch. ILC2, group 2 innate lymphoid cells; Th, T-helper cell of the immunological cells Th2, Th22 play a dominant role

2. Epidermal Dysfunction

Th-2 cytokines, external antigens and systemic inflammatory responses downregulate the production of epidermal barrier proteins. (Kim J, et al., 2019)

3. Immune Dysregulation

Th2 cytokines, e.g. **IL-4** and **IL-13**, play roles in chemokine production, skin barrier dysfunction, suppression of antimicrobial peptides (AMP), and allergic inflammation. IL-31 enhances the release and production of brain-derived natriuretic peptide and coordinates cytokine and chemokine release from skin cells, thereby inducing itch in patients of AD. (Kim J, et al., 2019). Notably the IL-13 cytokine has a predominant role in AD. There is also a role of the Th17 cells and Th22 cells. A summary of the immunological process is depicted in **Fig. 6.2** and is given in the **Box 6.1**.

JAK Pathway

The JAK kinase family comprises **four** receptor-associated kinases: JAK1, JAK2, JAK3, and TYK2 (tyrosine kinase 2), and the STAT family comprises **seven** proteins: STAT1, STAT2, STAT3, STAT4, STAT5A, STAT5B, and STAT6. As most cytokines act via the JAK STAT pathway (Villarino AV, et al., 2017) they in turn modulate Th2, Th1 and Th 17 pathways involved in AD.

Depending on their dose-dependent selectivity for one or several JAKs, the JAK inhibitors (JAKi) exert a broad immunopharmacological impact because they block the signal transduction pathways of multiple type I (hematopoietic family) and type II (interferon) cytokine receptors. This also determines their side effects. With regard to their respective selectivity, JAKi approved for AD or in clinical development for this indication can be classified into three main categories:

a. Nonselective (pan-)JAKi (delgocitinib, cerdulatinib, jaktinib, CEE321)
b. Dual inhibitors (baricitinib, ruxolitinib, brepocitinib, ATI-1777)
c. Selective JAK1 inhibitors (upadacitinib, abrocitinib, SHR0302).

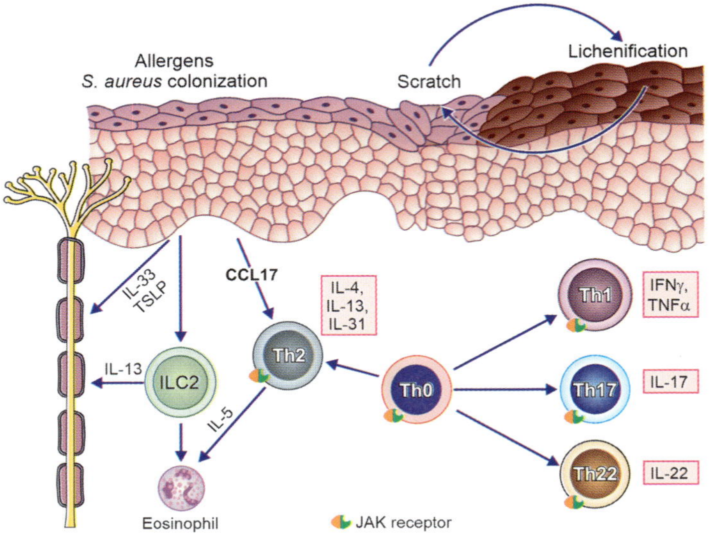

Fig. 6.2: There is interplay between the skin barrier dysfunction, inflammation and itch. Itching tends to lead to allergen ingress and the keratinocytes release immunoregulatory cytokines, like thymic stromal lymphopoietin (TSLP), interleukin (IL)-25 and IL-33. These cytokines induce a type 2 immune response which inhibit barrier function by downregulating fllaggrin (FLG) expression. The cytokines also mediate nerve stimulation and cause itch in addition to the induction of inflammation and barrier disruption. (IgE, immunoglobulin E; ILC2, group 2 innate lymphoid cells; Th, T-helper cell)

BOX 6.1: Role of various immune cells and cytokines in AD

- ↑ **Th2 and Th22** reduce the terminal differentiation of keratinocytes
- **Innate cytokines** ↑ TSLP, IL-25, IL-33
- Th2 → ↑ **IL-4 and IL-13**, act via type 1, type 2 and type 3 receptor via specific JAK receptors and lead to
  - ↑ Signaling of Th2 cytokines and chemokines
  - Inappropriate IgE class switching
  - Weakened epidermal barrier function
  - ↓ AMPs
  - ↓ Keratinocyte differentiation
  - ↓ Epidermal lipids
  - Via IL-5 attract basophils and eosinophils
- **TSLP** (thymic stromal lymphopoietin)—IL-7-like cytokine, known as "master-switch of allergic inflammation" → evokes Th2 response via dendritic cell activation
- **IL-33**-activates Th2 and also leads to itching
- **IgE**-production is increased by IL-4

  Two types—↑ IgE (extrinsic type) and non IgE (intrinsic type)
- **Itching**
  - Itch signals are transmitted to the spinal cord and brain
  - TRPA1 channels mediate histaminergic itch, TRPV1 other itch pathways
  - IL-4, IL-13 and IL-31 mediate the itch response pathway

Acute lesion: ↑↑ Th2 cytokines, IL-4 and IL-13, **and also Th22** cytokines (e.g. IL-22)

Chronic lesion: Th1, Th17 and Th22-related inflammation, ↑ IL-5, IL-13, IL-10, IL-31, CCL5, CCL13, and CCL18.

Notably most of the lymphoid cells express JAK3 and JAK2 has a widespread expression hence side effects are more in case of JAK2 inhibition. Also all JAKib drugs inhibit JAK1. A summary of the salient JAK receptors that mediate the action of cytokines is listed below.

IL-4 → JAK1/3 and STAT6
IL-5 → JAK2/1
IL-13 → JAK1 or JAK2/(TYK2), STAT6
IL-22 → JAK1 and TYK2, STAT 1, 3, 5
TSLP → JAK1/2 and STAT5
IL-31 → JAK1/2 and STAT 1, 3, 5
IL-22 → JAK1 and TYK2
IL-17 → SYK pathway

Thus IL-4 is mediated by JAK1 and JAK3, while IL-13 is mediated by JAK1, JAK3 and TYK2. It is obvious that JAKib drugs that can target the varied JAK would be useful. As all JAKib drugs block JAK1 equally, what matters is the JAK2 and JAK3 selectivity but at present with little comparative data on JAKib, varied drugs have been given approval (*see* page 118).

4. Environmental Factors

Allergens, microbiome, diesel exhaust, cigarette smoke, and chemical irritants increase TSLP production.

5. Factors Involved in Onset and Exacerbation

Exposure to environmental allergens, sweating, psychological stress, wool fibers, food, viral infections and alcohol are considered for induction and exacerbating factors of itch in AD. (Wahlgren CF, et al., 1991)

Summary

A background genetic predisposition and environment factors may induce skin barrier impairment along with the invasion of allergens and skin microbiota (mostly *Staphylococcus aureus*). TSLP, IL-25, and IL-33 released from keratinocytes and activated skin LCs and IDECs lead to the activation of Th2 axis immune response through ILC2 and Th2 cells. In the **acute phase** of atopic dermatitis, the production of various Th2 cytokines including IL-4, IL-5, IL-13, IL-31 results in barrier dysfunction. In the **chronic phase** of atopic dermatitis, Th17 and Th22 cytokines cooperatively modulate local inflammation through upregulation of proinflammatory cytokines stimulating epidermal hyperplasia. Th1 immune response also plays a role in the chronic phase of atopic dermatitis.

1. Skin barrier defects lead to allergen penetration and itching with activation of keratinocytes and immune activation.
2. There is release of chemokines like CCL17, IL-33, TSLP which activate itch and Th2 cells and ILC2 cells.
3. Th2 cells release cytokines, disrupt barrier, attract eosinophils and basophils.
4. Chronic stage has more of Th1, Th17 and Th22 activity.

CLINICAL FEATURES OF AD

AD is characterized by erythematous, itchy, papules or papulovesicular rashes which have typical distribution and morphology with predominant involvement of cheeks, scalp and extensors in infants and flexures in children and adults. (Odhiambo JA, et al., 2009)

Lesions of AD generally present in 3 clinical phases:

1. **Acute:** Vesicular, weeping and crusted lesion
2. **Subacute:** Erythematous, dry and scaly lesions
3. **Chronic:** Lichenification and thickening due to repeated scratching (Berke R, et al., 2017).

Diagnostic Criteria

Diagnostic criteria (as given by the Japanese Dermatological Association)

1. **Pruritus**
2. **Typical morphology and distribution**
   a. Diagnostic criteria for eczematous dermatitis
      - **Acute lesions:** Erythema, exudation, papules, vesiculopapules, scales, and crusts
      - **Chronic lesions:** Infiltrated erythema, lichenification, prurigo, scales, and crusts

   b. Symmetrical distribution
      - Predilection sites: Forehead, periorbital area, perioral area, lips, periauricular area, neck, joint areas of limbs, and trunk
      - Age-related characteristics
        Infantile phase: Starts on the scalp and face, often spreads to the trunk and extremities
        Childhood phase neck, flexural surfaces of the arms and legs
        Adolescent and adult phase face, neck, anterior chest, and back.
3. **Chronic or chronically relapsing course (usually coexistence of old and new lesions)**
   More than 2 months in infancy
   More than 6 months in childhood, adolescence, and adulthood

Definitive diagnosis of AD **needs all three** features without consideration of severity.

Differential Diagnosis and Associations

Contact dermatitis, seborrheic dermatitis, prurigo simplex, scabies, miliaria, ichthyosis, xerotic eczema, hand dermatitis (nonatopic).

Complications

Ocular complications (cataract and/or retinal detachment, especially in patients with severe facial lesions), infections such as molluscum contagiosum, Kaposi's varicelliform eruption and impetigo contagiosa.

Severity Assessment and Biomarkers (Table 6.1)

SCORAD index, EASI and IGA (Hanifin JM, et al., 2001)

The importance of assessing the severity of AD lies in its impact on treatment selection:

- **Assessment of eruption severity**. The selection of topical steroids, a key treatment, depends on "severity of individual eruption".
- **Assessment of pruritus—NRS** (numerical rating scale) and **VAS** (visual analog scale), **Behavioural rating scale** for evaluating the degree of scratching. These are subjective assessment methods.
- **IGA**—(Investigator's Global Assessment)-frequently used in clinical studies.

Serum TARC Level

TARC (CCL17) is a ligand of the chemokine receptor CCR4 and induces Th2 cell migration. Serum TARC level in patients with AD increases consistently with severity, and it reflects disease progression more strongly than serum IgE levels, LDH levels, or peripheral eosinophil counts. Moreover, patient education and treatment can be reviewed using serum TARC levels as an index. However, test values should be carefully interpreted because TARC levels are generally higher in younger children, especially in children aged <2 years.

TABLE 6.1: Useful biomarkers in AD for diagnosis and severity assessment		
Biomarkers	**Cause**	**Clinical implications**
Serum IgE level	• Immune state with excessive Th2 activity (high IL-4 levels) • A high level (500 IU or higher) is often observed in patients with AD	Indicates allergic diathesis and reflects disease progression of AD
Specific IgE levels	Allergen-specific antibody produced via the same mechanism as above	Sensitization is **not always related** to causes
Peripheral eosinophil count	• IL-5 is the cause • No definitive reference level is available (>300/mm^3)	Reflects disease progression of AD
Serum LDH level	Indicative of cell damage	Reflects disease progression of AD
Serum TARC level (CCL17)	It is produced by chemokines and induces Th2 cell migration	It is more relevant than eosinophil count or LDH level. It is covered by national health insurance as a marker for AD in Japan

MANAGEMENT APPROACHES

AD is a relapsing skin disease, and currently no curative treatment is available.

Treatment measures revolve around 3 aspects.

- Skin care
- Drug therapy
- Elimination of exacerbating factors.

An algorithm of treatment of AD is given in **Fig. 6.3**.

Skin Care

Topical Moisturizers

Helps to prevent allergen invasion, relapse, recovering and maintaining skin barrier function and suppress itching.

'Emollients' are defined as 'topical formulations with vehicle-type substances without active ingredients', whereas 'emollients plus' refers to 'topical formulations with vehicle-type substances plus additional active, nonmedicated substances'.

Emollients usually contain a humectant or moisturizer (promoting stratum corneum hydration) such as urea or glycerol and an occlusive agent (reducing evaporation such as lipids or petrolatum).

Bathing, Showering, and Washing

The water temperature during bathing or showering for skin barrier function recovery is 38–40°C.

The bath should be of short duration (approx. 5 minutes) and the use of bath oils (added for the last 2 min of bathing) are aimed at avoiding epidermal dehydration.

Bleach bath therapy—Bleach bath therapy is not currently recommended.

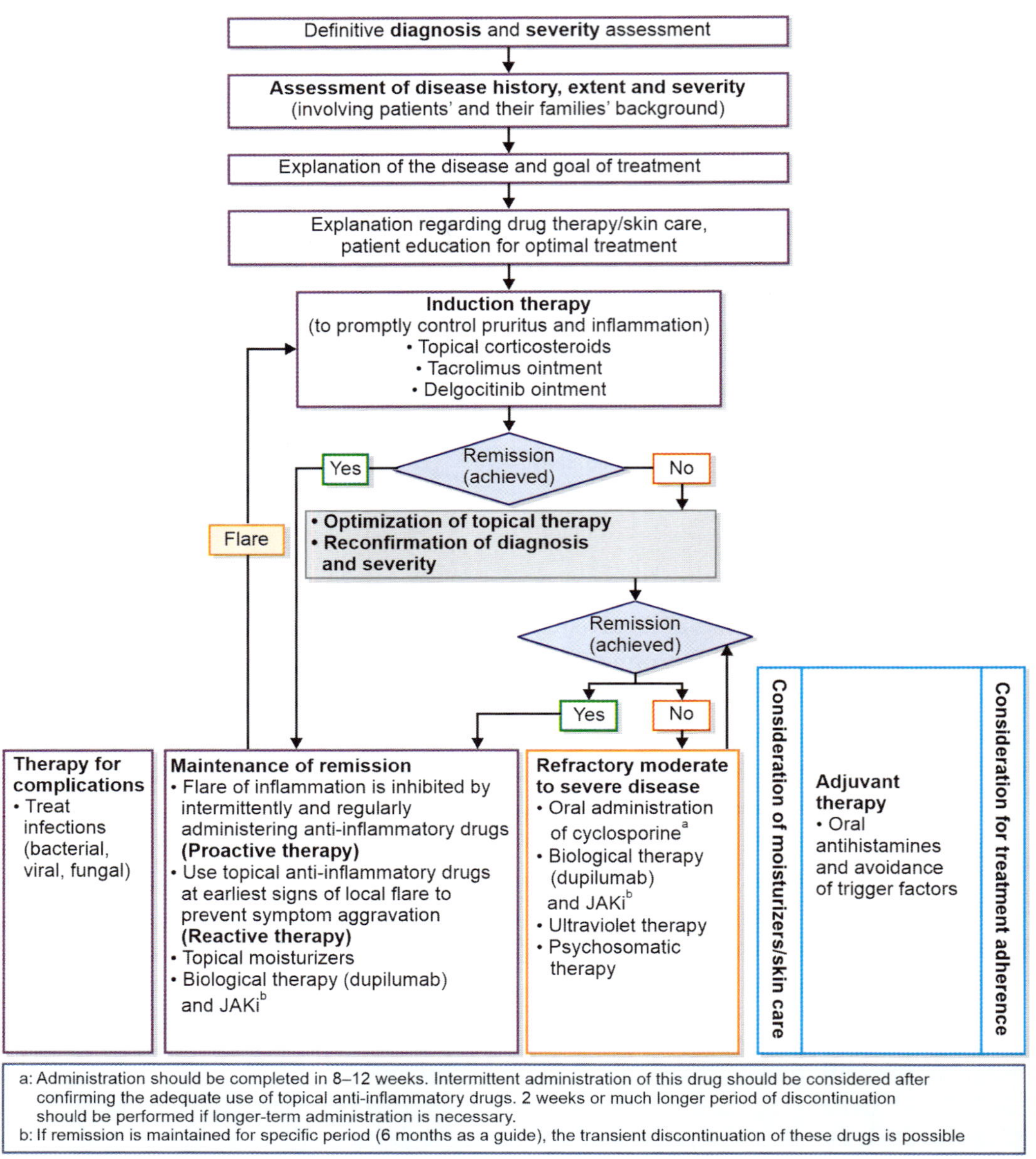

Fig. 6.3: An approach to management of AD (Saeki H, 2022)

Nonspecific Irritants

Nonspecific irritation present in daily life such as **contact with saliva, sweat, hair, and friction** against clothes may exacerbate AD. **Saliva or sweat** should be washed away or wiped off with soft wet gauze. In some cases even minor stimulation, including irritation from the **rough texture of clothes, such as from wool**, are a concern and using synthetic material like nylon towel, leads to a decline in the skin barrier function and progression of eczema.

Sweating: Patients with AD generally have a decreased sweat volume and the sweat reduction-related increase in the skin temperature or skin dryness leads to a deterioration of dermatitis.

Drug Therapy

Principles of Treatment

Apart from the conventional agents that include moisturizers, steroids and immunosuppressive agents many novel agents, have been used based on the predominant cytokines that have been implicated in AD. The ideal drug should be chosen to:

- Maximize the outcome of treatment.
- Lead to control of biomarkers
- Help in treatment adherence
- Cost effective.

Topical Anti-inflammatory Drugs

1. Topical corticosteroids (TCS)
2. Topical calcineurin inhibitor (TCI)
   a. Tacrolimus ointments (0.1% for adults and 0.03% for children), in patients ≤1 year of age, its safety has not yet been established
3. Topical Janus kinase inhibitor-Delgocitinib ointments for patients with AD aged ≥2 years.
4. Crisaborole 2%
   - PDE4-inhibitor
   - PDE4 degrades cAMP, leading to ↑ production of IL-4, IL-10.

The use of topical agents has been stratified into 3 steps and are detailed in **Fig. 6.4**.

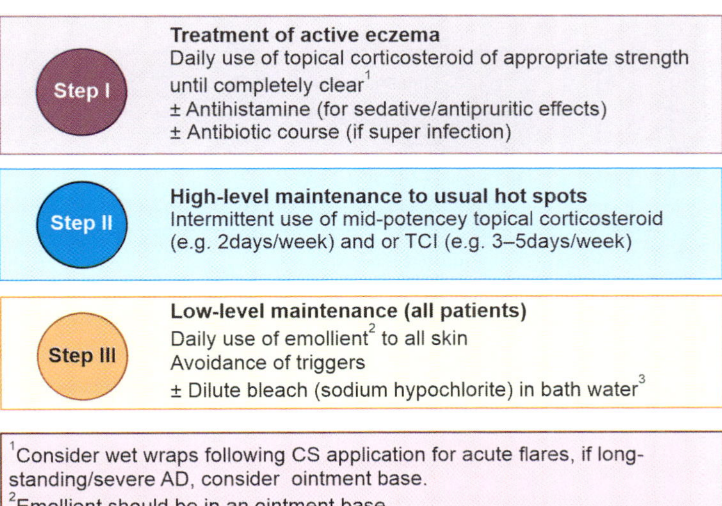

Fig. 6.4: Summary of the steps involved in the application of topical therapy in AD

Proactive and Reactive Therapy

The therapy of AD should combine an active arm and a maintenance arm where therapy is directed to the localized affected areas only **(Fig. 6.5)**.

TCS or tacrolimus (e.g. twice a week), are used to maintain remission of disease, in addition to skin care with moisturizing topical drugs. This concept is based on the fact that there is histological evidence of inflammatory cells in visibly normal-appearing skin following the resolution of inflammation. There can be a relapse because of external or internal factors. Intensive treatment **for 1–3 months** results in sufficient improvement for up to 1 year.

Systemic Drugs

- **Antihistamines**—2nd generation nonsedating are preferred
- **Ciclosporine**
  - Approved in Japan, for very severe AD patients
  - Dose-initial dose of this drug is 3 mg/kg per day, but should not exceed 5 mg/kg per day.
  - Duration-8–12 weeks
- **Newer cytokine based drugs**

While a list of agents is given below, it is now known that the expression levels of IL-13 in lesional skin strongly correlate with disease severity in other words, IL-13 may be a more important mediator for type 2 inflammatory responses in the skin lesions of AD and play a more crucial role in the pathophysiology of AD than IL-4. A list of the major agents that work on the important cytokines in AD is listed below and depicted in **Fig. 6.6**. It should be noted that in chronic AD the cytokine mileu changes and here lies the role of JAKib.

IL4: Dupilumab-IL-4Rα monoclonal antibody
IL13/IL 4: Tralokinumab, lebrikizumab
IL-31: Nemolizumab-Reduces pruritus
IL-22: Fezakinumab-useful in chronic stage

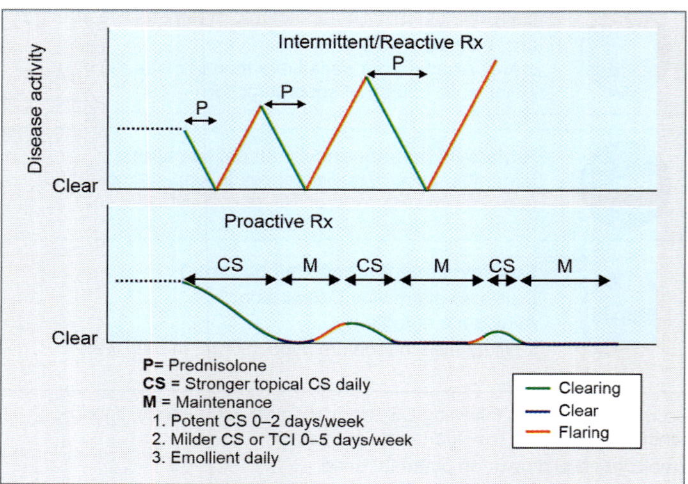

Fig. 6.5: A depiction of proactive therapy in AD which entails reduction in use of CS 2/weekly dose that helps to mantain the disease in remission than a reactive approach wherein the disease tends to flare.

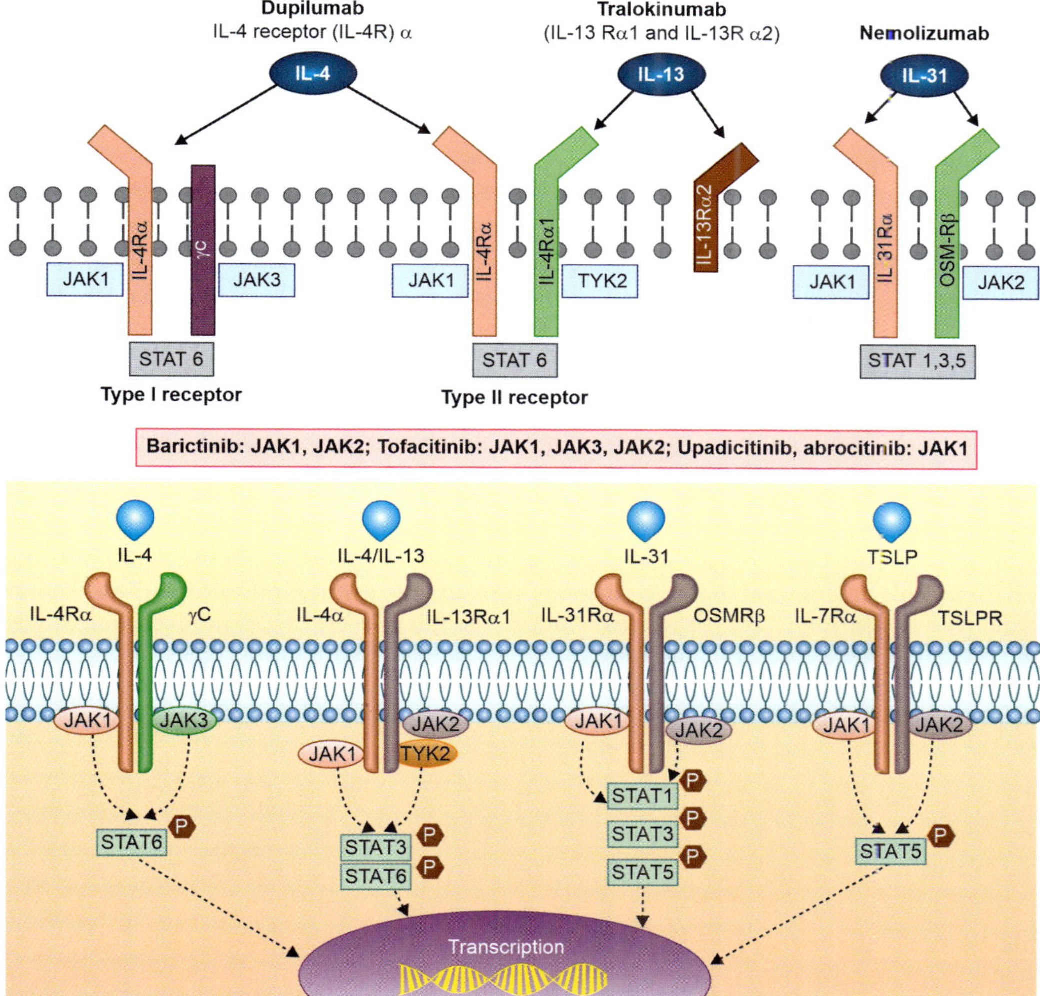

Fig. 6.6: (a) Structures of interleukin (IL)-4 and IL-13 receptors. IL-4 binds to type I receptor while IL-13 binds to type II receptors. These in turn act via Janus kinase (JAK)/signal transducer and activator of transcription (STAT). (b) Major cytokines and their mediation of action via JAK STAT pathway. It is obvious that JAKib can target multiple cytokines.

Dupilumab (Recommendation Grade 1, Evidence Level A)

- Recombinant human IgG4 monoclonal antibody, IL-4Rα antagonist
- The US FDA approved dupilumab for adults and children ≥6 months of age with moderate-to-severe atopic dermatitis whose disease is not adequately controlled with topical prescription therapies or when those therapies are not advisable.
- Most commonly reported side effect is conjunctivitis (up to 30% in some studies).
- Dose-initial dose of 600 mg f/b 300 mg (subcutaneous injection) every 2 weeks.
- Discontinued if there is no response in 16 weeks after initiation of therapy.

It must be noted that less than 50% of patients achieved clear or almost clear skin during a 16-week course of dupilumab monotherapy (Simpson EL, et al., 2016), leading to the search for more effective therapeutic options. Compared with the 50% success rate for dupilumab, patients treated with upadacitinib presented substantially better results, with ≥75% of patients achieving an improvement in EASI score from baseline (EASI75) (Blauvelt A et al., 2021). Recently there have been reports of JAKib being used as a rescue therapy in refractory cases uncontrolled by dupilumab.

JAKib Drugs

The major cytokines implicated in AD including IL-4, IL-13, IL 31 and TSLP play a role in both the inflammatory pathway and chronic itch through Janus kinase (JAK) pathway **(Figs 6.6 and 6.7)**. As the signal of IL-4 is mediated by JAK1 and JAK3, while that of IL-13 is mediated by JAK1, JAK3 and TYK2, appropriate JAK inhibitor drugs will be useful for AD. First-generation JAK inhibitors, such as baricitinib, target more than one JAK, while second-or next-generation JAK inhibitors, including upadacitinib and abrocitinib, target selective JAK. The findings of clinical trials on JAK inhibitors have shown their benefits in reducing the skin signs and symptoms of AD. Notably, they very rapidly control pruritus and also lead to a more rapid or faster resolution of inflammatory responses than classic biologics. Topical ruxolitinib, upadacitinib and abrocitinib are the 3 JAKib drugs which are **US FDA** approved for AD currently. Baricitinib has been approved by the EMA for adults with AD but US FDA has delayed its approval. Tofacitinib is not approved but is as effective and in chronic stage of AD better than selective JAKib as it can inhibit multiple cytokines and cells.

A list of drugs in this class used in AD is given below:

Pan-JAKi: Delgocitinib, CEE312, Jaktinib, Cerdulatinib, Tofacitine
JAK1/JAK2: Baricitinib, Ruxolitinib*
JAK1: Upadacitinib*, Abrocitinib*, SHR0302
JAK1/TYK2: Brepocitinib

*(US FDA)

Baricitinib

- Selective, reversible JAK1/JAK2 inhibitor
- MoA-suppresses inflammatory or immune responses by inhibiting the JAK1-JAK2 mediated intracellular signal transduction of cytokines
- Indicated for patients with AD in whom conventional treatment is ineffective
- Dose-adults at 4 mg once a day, decreased to 2 mg in patients with moderate renal dysfunction.
- The amelioration of itch is achieved as early as week 1 for 4 mg and week 2 for 2 mg.
- The most common adverse events in patients treated with baricitinib were nasopharyngitis and headache.

Upadacitinib

- Upadacitinib, is an oral reversible JAK inhibitor with greater inhibitory potency for JAK1 than JAK2, JAK3, and TYK2.
- US FDA has approved upadacitinib for the treatment of moderate to severe atopic dermatitis in adults and children ≥12 years of age whose disease did not respond to previous treatment

and is not well controlled with other drugs, including biologics, or when other drugs cannot be recommended.
- AD aged 12–64 years: Dose is initiated from 15 mg/day and titrated up to 30 mg/day if necessary.
- Upadacitinib has been found to be superior to dupilumab in terms of several secondary endpoints, including the percentage of patients achieving ≥90% and 100% improvement in EASI score (EASI90 and EASI100) and the percentage change of Pruritus NRS at week 16.
- Patients receiving upadacitinib presented higher rates of serious infection, eczema herpeticum, herpes zoster, and laboratory-related AEs than patients receiving dupilumab.
- The adverse events associated with JAK2 and JAK3, such as anemia and infections, may be minimized with a JAK1 inhibitor like upadacitinib.

Evidence of Comparative Effectiveness from Network Meta-analysis

Numerous novel small molecules and biologics have been developed. Choosing the most appropriate treatment for patients with AD recalcitrant to conventional treatment can be challenging. Among all steroid-sparing topical treatments for AD, twice-daily doses of tofacitinib 2%, delgocitinib 3%, and ruxolitinib 1.5% demonstrated superior efficacy when compared with other topical JAK and PDE4 inhibitors (Zhang L, et al., 2021). Regarding the choice of systemic therapy, Drucker et al. conducted a network meta-analysis to compare the efficacy among all systemic immunomodulatory therapies for AD (Drucker AM, et al., 2022). In the reported analysis, the 200-mg dose of abrocitinib and 30-mg dose of upadacitinib demonstrated greater improvements in EASI scores than dupilumab, whereas the 15-mg dose of upadacitinib demonstrated similar efficacy to dupilumab.

Phototherapy

- MoA-UV light has inhibitory effects on immune-related cells of the skin, which explains the improvement of eruption in AD.
- UVA1-wavelength of 340–400 nm, is more effective in acute phase of AD but has an increased risk of skin carcinogenesis.
- Narrowband UVB with a peak wavelength of 311 nm is useful in the chronic phase of AD
  - Safety of long-term treatment in children is limited.
  - Should be avoided in history of skin cancer, photosensitivity, with immunosuppressive drugs.

Prevention of Exacerbation of AD

- **Antibiotics**—to treat secondary infection
- **Sunscreen**—when spending extended time outdoors
- **Avoid contact with animals**
- **Allergen elimination diet**—eliminating a specific food is not recommended (except for cases in which AD progression due to a certain food is confirmed using an allergen elimination test).
- **Probiotics or prebiotics**—not recommended for the prevention of AD onset.

Management Algorithm for Atopic Dermatitis

Treatment of AD has been reviewed recently by a specialised group and they have given recommendations for adults and children **(Figs 6.7 and 6.8)**. Also therapeutic options of treatment differ in children and pregnant or lactating women and suggested drugs are given in **Fig. 6.9**.

A list of systemic drugs and their uses guidelines are is given in **Table 6.2**.

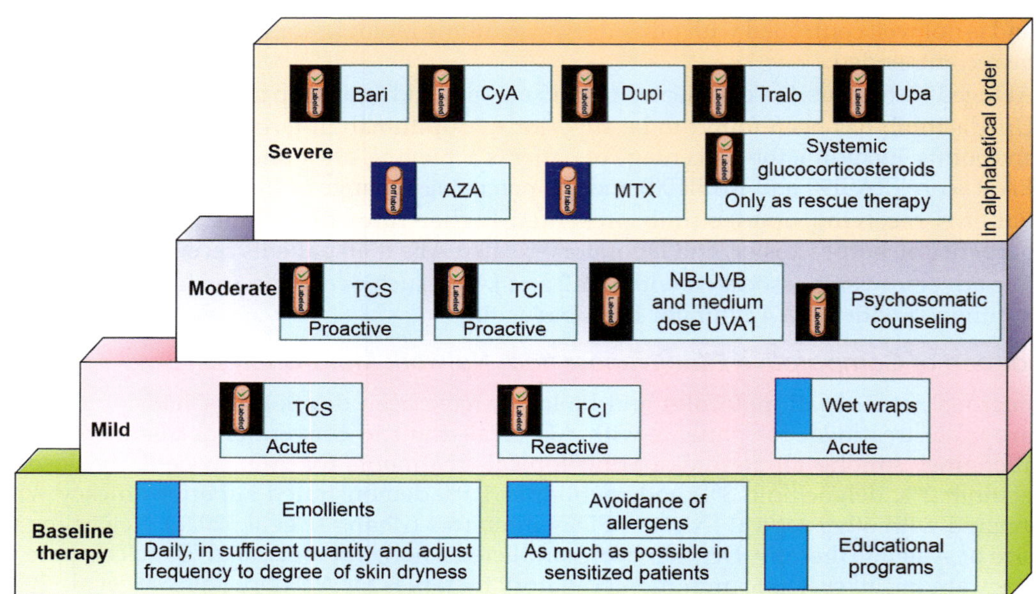

Fig. 6.7: Management protocol of AD in adults (Wollenberg A, et al., 2022)
Abro, Abrocitinib; AZA, azathioprine; Bari, baricitinib; CyA, ciclosporin; Dupi, dupilumab; MTX, methotrexate; TCI, topical clacineurin inhibitors; TCS, topical cotricosteroids; Tralo, tralokinumab; Upa, upadacitinib; UVA1, ultraviolet A1, NB-UVB, narrow-band ultraviolet B.

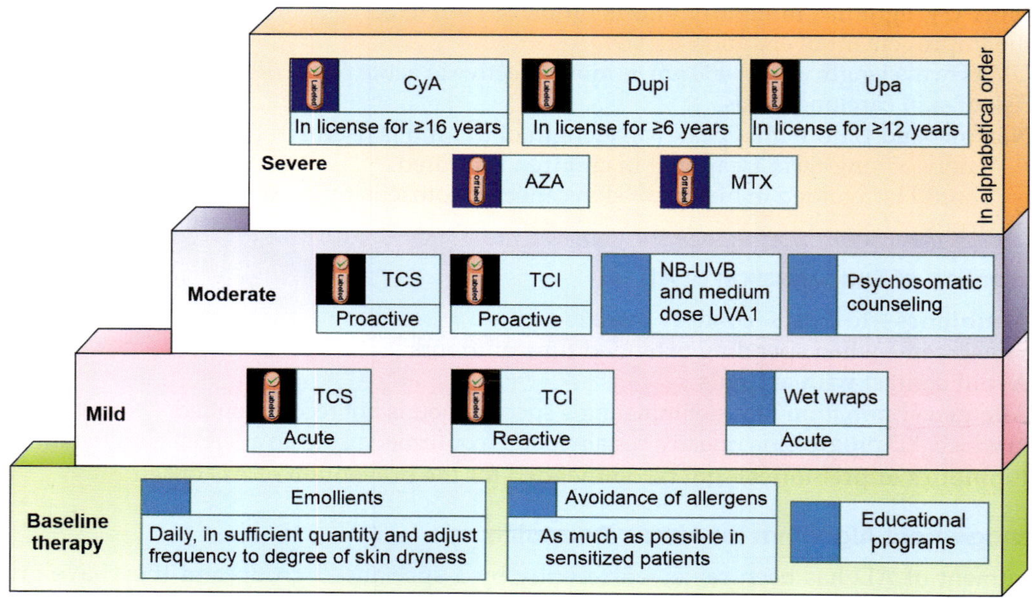

Fig. 6.8: Management protocol of AD in children (Wollenberg A, et al., 2022)
AZA, azathioprine; CyA, ciclosporin; Dupi, dupilumab; MTX, methotrexate; TCI, topical calcineurin inhibitors; TCS, topical corticosteroids; Upa, upadacitinib; UVA1, ultraviolet A1; NB-UVB, narrow-band ultraviolet B.

TABLE 6.2: General recommendations for systemic drugs in adults AE patients who are candidates for systemic treatment (for details see corresponding chapter)

	Conventional systemic treatments			Biologics		JAK-inhibitors		Rescue therapy
	Ciclosporin	**Methotrexate**	**Azathioprine**	**Dupilumab**	**Tralokinumab**	**Baricitinib**	**Upadacitinib**	**Systemic corticosteroids**
Recommendations	↑↑	↑	↑	↑↑	↑↑	↑↑	↑↑	↑
Dose for adults[1]	Licensed ≥16 years standard dosage adult: 2.5–5 mg/kg per day in two single doses	Off-label; commonly used dosage adults: Initial dose: 5–15 mg/per week; maximum dose: 25 mg/week	Off-label; commonly used dosage adults: 1–3 mg/kg per day	Licensed ≥6 years; adults: Initially 600 mg sc day 1 followed by 300 mg Q2W	Licensed for adults; initially 600 mg sc day 1 followed by 300 mg Q2W; consider Q4W dosing at week 16 in those achieving clear or almost clear skin	Licensed for adults; dosage adult: 4 mg per day, reduction to 2 mg per day possible, depending on treatment response	Licensed ≥12 years; dosage adult: 15 or 30 mg per day based on individual patient presentation; age ≥65: 15 mg per day; the lowest effective dose for maintenance should be considered 1–2	General licence for adults and children; dosage maximum: 1 mg/kg per day
Time to response (weeks)[2]	1–2	8–12	8–12	4–6	4–8	1–2	1–2	1–2
Time to relapse (weeks, based on expert experience)[2]	<2	>12	>12	>8	>8	<2	<2	<2
Monitoring	Complete blood count, renal and liver profile, blood pressure	Complete blood count, renal and liver profile, PIIINP if available, screen for chronic infections	Complete blood count, renal and liver profile, TPMT activity if available, screen for chronic infections	Not required	Not required	Complete blood count, lipid profile, liver profile	Complete blood count, lipid profile, liver profile	Not required for short-term treatment, consider blood glucose and testing for adrenal gland suppression with high doses/longer-term treatment

(*Contd.*)

TABLE 6.2: General recommendations for systemic drugs in adults AE patients who are candidates for systemic treatment (for details see corresponding chapter) *(Contd.)*

	Conventional systemic treatments			Biologics		JAK-inhibitors		Rescue therapy
	Ciclosporin	**Methotrexate**	**Azathioprine**	**Dupilumab**	**Tralokinumab**	**Baricitinib**	**Upadacitinib**	**Systemic corticosteroids**
Recommendations	↑↑	↑	↑	↑↑	↑↑	↑↑	↑↑	↑
Selection of most relevant adverse events	Serum creatinine ↑, blood pressure ↑	Nausea, fatigue, liver enzymes ↑, myelotoxicity	Gastrointestinal disturbances, idiosyncratic hypersensitivity reactions, hepatotoxicity, myelotoxicity	Conjunctivitis, upper respiratory tract infections, arthralgia	Upper respiratory tract infections; conjunctivitis	Upper respiratory tract infections, increase in LDL cholesterol; thrombocytosis, nausea and abdominal pain herpes virus infections, acne	Upper respiratory tract infections, acne; headache, anaemia and neutropenia, CK elevation, increase in LDL cholesterol, nausea and abdominal pain herpes virus infections	Skin atrophy, weight gain, sleep distrubance, mood changes, hyperglycemia or new onset diabetes, peptic ulcers/gastritis, osteoporosis

	Conventional systemic treatments			Biologics		JAK-inhibitors		Rescue
	Ciclosporin	Methotrexate	Azathioprine	Dupilumab	Tralokinumab	Baricitinib	Upadacitinib	Corticosteroids
Children and adolescents	↑↑ Licensed for ≥16 years **dose** children: **2.5–5** mg/kg per day in two doses	↑ off-label, commonly used dosage children: **0.3–0.4** mg/kg per week	↑ off-label, commonly used dose children: **1.3** mg/kg per day	↑↑ licensed for >=6 months of age *	off-label	off-label	↑↑ Licensed for ≥12 years: Age 12–17 (≥ 30kg bw): **15 mg** per day	Steroid responsive skin disease dosage maximum: **1mg/kg** per day
Pregnancy (in candidates for systemic treatment)	↑	↓↓	↑	0		↓↓	↓↓	Prednisolone ↑ (0.5mg/kg/d) only as rescue therapy for acute flares
Breastfeeding	↓	↓	↓	0		↓	↓	Prednisolone ↑ (0.5mg/kg/d) only as rescue therapy for acute flares

* **6 months–5 years:** Administer with a pre-filled syringe Q4W based on weight (200 mg for children ≥5 kg to <15 kg and 300 mg for children ≥15 kg to <30 kg)

* **Age 6–11:** 15 kg < 60 kg, 300 mg s.c. day 1 and 15 f/b 300 mg Q4W, ≥60 kg, 600 mg s.c. day 1 f/b 300 mg Q2W

* **Age 12–17:** <60 kg: 400 mg s.c. day 1 f/b 200 mg Q2W, ≥60 kg: 600 mg s.c. day 1 followed by 300 mg Q2W

Note: Up- arrows and down-arrows - Refer to the strength of recommendation of the drug where dark green is a strong recommendation FOR using the drug and dark red is a strong recommendation AGAINST using the drug.

Fig. 6.9: Therapy of AD in special scenarios

BIBLIOGRAPHY

1. Berke R, Singh A, Guralnick M. Atopic dermatitis: An overview. *Am Fam Physician*. Volume 23, Issue 8, 2017.
2. Bieber T, Novak N. Pathogenesis of atopic dermatitis: New developments. Current allergy and asthma reports. 2009 Jul;9(4):291–4.
3. Blauvelt A, Teixeira HD, Simpson EL, Costanzo A, De Bruin-Weller M, Barbarot S, et al. Efficacy and safety of upadacitinib vs dupilumab in adults with moderate-to-Severe atopic dermatitis: A randomized clinical trial. JAMA Dermatol (2021) 157(9):1047–5.
4. Coca AF, Cooke RA. On the classification of the phenomena of hypersensitiveness. J Immunol 1923 8:163–182.
5. Drucker AM, Morra DE, Prieto-Merino D, Ellis AG, Yiu ZZN, Rochwerg B, et al. Systemic immunomodulatory treatments for atopic dermatitis: Update of a living systematic review and network meta-analysis. JAMA Dermatol (2022) 158 (5):523–32.
6. Du D, Wang L, Guo L, Jiang X. Efficacy and safety of topical janus kinase and phosphodiesterase inhibitor-4 inhibitors for the treatment of atopic dermatitis: A network meta-analysis. J Dermatol (2021) 48(12):1877–83.
7. Ellis CN, Mancini AJ, Paller AS, Simpson EL, Eichenfield LF. Understanding and managing atopic dermatitis in adult patients. *Semin Cutan Med Surg*. 2012;31(suppl 3): S18-S22. doi: 10.1016/j.sder.2012.07.006.
8. Hanifin JM, Thurston M, Omoto M, Cherill R, Tofte SJ, Graeber M. The eczema area and severity index (EASI): assessment of reliability in atopic dermatitis. EASI Evaluator Group. Exp Dermatol. 2001; 10:11–8.
9. Kim J, Kim BE, Leung DYM. Pathophysiology of atopic dermatitis: Clinical implications. Allergy Asthma Proc. 2019 Mar 1;40(2):84–92. doi: 10.2500/aap.2019.40.4202. PMID: 30819278; PMCID: PMC6399565.
10. Odhiambo JA, Williams HC, Clayton TO, Robertson CF, Asher MI, Group IPTS.Global variations in prevalence of eczema symptoms in children from ISAAC Phase Three. J Allergy Clin Immunol 2009;124(6):1251–8. e23
11. Palmer CN, Irvine AD, Terron? Kwiatkowski A. Common loss? of? function variants of the epidermal barrier protein filaggrin are a major predisposing factor for atopic dermatitis. Nat Genet 2006;38:441–6.
12. Saeki H, Ohya Y, Furuta J, Arakawa H, Ichiyama S, Katsunuma T, et al. Executive summary: Japanese guidelines for atopic dermatits (ADGL) 2021. Allergol Int 2022;71(4):448–58. https://doi.org/10.1016/j.alit.2022.06.009
13. Severity scoring of atopic dermatitis: the SCORAD index. Consensus report of the European Task Force on atopic dermatitis. Dermatology. 1993; 186:23–31.
14. Simpson EL, Bieber T, Guttman-Yassky E, Beck LA, Blauvelt A, Cork MJ, et al. Two phase 3 trials of dupilumab versus placebo in atopic dermatitis. N Engl J Med (2016) 375(24):2335–48.
15. Villarino, A., Kanno, Y. & O'Shea, J. Mechanisms and consequences of Jak–STAT signaling in the immune system. Nat Immunol 18, 374–384 (2017). https://doi.org/10.1038/ni.3691
16. Wahlgren CF. Itch and atopic dermatitis: clinical and experimental studies. Acta Derm Venereo Suppl. 1991;165:1–53.
17. Wollenberg A, Kinberger M, Arents B, Aszodi N, Avila Valle G, Barbarot S, et al. European guideline (EuroGuiDerm) on atopic eczema: part I-systemic therapy. J Eur Acad Dermatol Venereol 2022;36(9):1409–31.
18. Zhang L, Du D, Wang L, Guo L, Jiang X. Efficacy and safety of topical Janus kinase and phosphodiesterase inhibitor-4 inhibitors for the treatment of atopic dermatitis: A network meta-analysis. J Dermatol 2021;48(12):1877–83. 10.1111/1346-8138.16126

Chapter

7

Autoimmune Bullous Diseases

Surabhi Sinha, Sinu Rose Mathachan, Kabir Sardana

INTRODUCTION

The autoimmune blistering diseases may be subdivided into intraepidermal (pemphigus group) and subepidermal (pemphigoid group) blistering disorders on the basis of the level at which blistering occurs **(Fig. 7.1)**.

PEMPHIGUS

The word 'pemphigus' was derived from the Greek word *'pemphix'* meaning blister or bubble. The incidence of pemphigus in India varies from 0.09 to 1.8% and occurs in a relatively younger age group (mean 40 years). Both males and females are equally affected, but some studies have suggested a slight female preponderance.

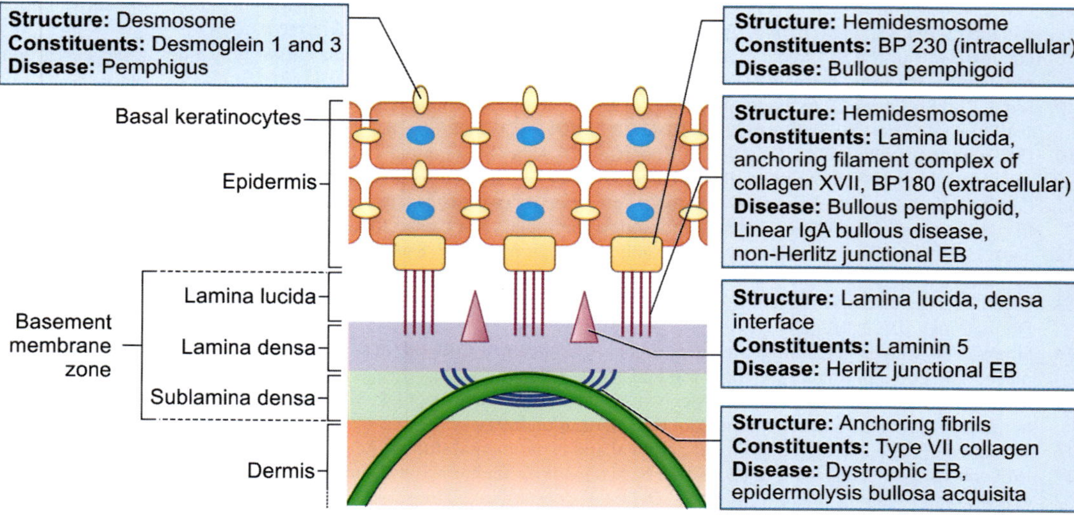

Fig. 7.1: A depiction of the intercellular-subepidermal structure relevant to autoimmune bullous disorders (EB, epidermolysis bullosa)

Classification

Table 7.1 gives a classification and **Table 7.2** lists the antigens and autoantibodies in pemphigus group of disorders.

Etiopathogenesis

The binding of autoantibodies to the target antigens leads to disruption of adhesions between the cells leading to intraepidermal blistering (acantholysis).

Physiological Intercellular Adhesions (Fig. 7.2a)

1. **Adherens junctions:** Classic cadherins (calcium-dependent adherens; E-, P-, and N-cadherins) are transmembrane proteins that bind to the armadillo family intracytoplasmic

TABLE 7.1: Classification of pemphigus
Pemphigus vulgaris Variant: Pemphigus vegetans • Neumann type • Hallopeau type (synonyms—pyodermite végétante, pyoderma vegetans)
Pemphigus foliaceus Variants: • Fogo selvagem: Endemic pemphigus • Pemphigus erythematosus (Senear-Usher syndrome) • Pemphigus herpetiformis
Induced pemphigus
Intercellular IgA pemphigus
Paraneoplastic pemphigus

TABLE 7.2: Antigens and antibodies in pemphigus group

Disease	Antigens	Autoantibodies
Pemphigus vulgaris • Mucosal-dominant type • Mucocutaneous type	 Desmoglein 3 (130 kDa) Desmoglein 1 and 3	 IgG IgG
Pemphigus foliaceus	Desmoglein 1 (160 kDa)	IgG
Drug-induced pemphigus	Desmoglein 1 and 3	IgG
Paraneoplastic pemphigus	• Envoplakin (210 kDa) and periplakin (190 kDa)—**most consistent*** • Desmoplakin I and II (250 and 210 kDa, respectively)* • BPAG1 (230 kDa) • Plectin (>500 kDa) • Plakoglobin • Unidentified 170 kDa antigen • Dsg3 and Dsg1	 IgG
IgA pemphigus	Desmocollin 1 (110/100 kDa)	IgA

Dsg, desmoglein
*Antibodies against plakin proteins are characteristic of PNP and are not found in other forms of pemphigus usually.

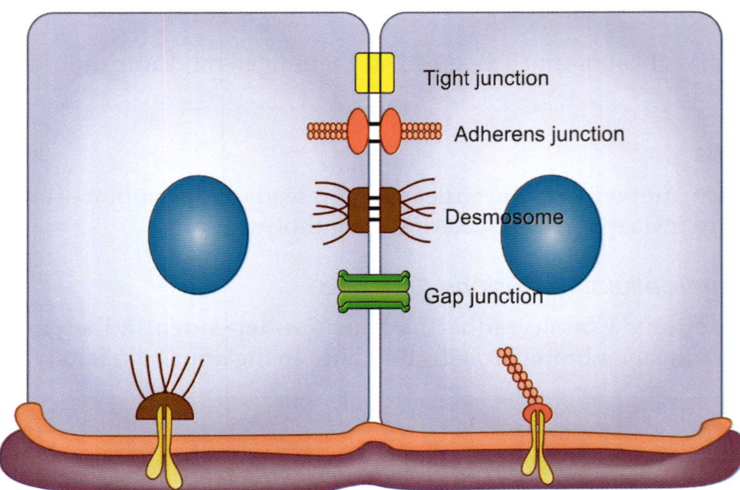

Fig. 7.2a: Types of intercellular junctions: Simple epithelial cells have multiple intercellular junctions polarized along their apical to basal axis. **Tight junctions** restrict the paracellular passage of ions and solutes. **Gap junctions** are channels made up of connexins that link the cytoplasm of two cells together for exchange of ions, second messengers, and small metabolites. The cadherin-based junctions, **adherens junctions** (comprising classic cadherins and their interacting proteins) and **desmosomes** (comprising desmosomal cadherins called desmogleins and desmocollins and interacting proteins), occupy the lateral membranes between neighboring cells where they anchor actin and intermediate filaments, respectively

plaque proteins (α/β/γ-catenin and plakoglobin → which bind to intracytoplasmic vinculin → in turn bind to bundles of α-actin microfilaments. Mediate quick but weak cellular adhesion.

2. **Desmosomes:** Desmosomal cadherins (calcium-dependent adherens—desmogleins and desmocollins) are transmembrane proteins that bind to the armadillo family intracytoplasmic plaque proteins (plakophilin and plakoglobin) → which bind to intracytoplasmic plakins (desmoplakin I and II, BPAG1, plectin, envoplakin, and periplakin) → which in turn anchor keratin intermediate filaments. Mediate slow but strong cellular adhesion **(Fig. 7.2b)**.

Desmoglein localization

i. **Desmoglein 1:** Expressed in all levels of the epidermis (**top > bottom**)—explains the level of split in pemphigus foliaceus
   - Dsg1 can compensate for Dsg 3 loss in skin → therefore, if only Dsg 3 is targeted (as in pemphigus vulgaris), the skin remains intact.
   - Dsg1 has no significant role in mucosal epithelial adhesion → cannot compensate for Dsg 3 loss in **mucosa** → if Dsg 3 function is lost (as in pemphigus vulgaris), mucosal blisters can form. Also neonatal skin is like oral mucosa; hence pemphigus foliaceous is rare in neonates.
   - Dsg1 is cleaved by ***S. aureus*** exfoliative toxin (bullous impetigo, SSSS)
   - Dsg1 mutation is also present in striate PPK 1 (desmoplakin is mutated in striate PPK 2, and keratin 1 in striate PPK 3; all are part of the desmosome complex.)

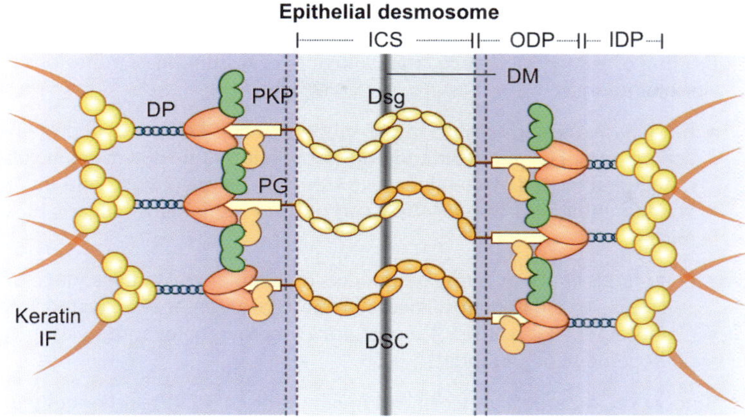

Fig. 7.2b: Structure of desmosome: Desmosomes anchor intermediate filaments to the desmosomal cadherins, desmogleins and desmocollins, through a series of adapter proteins, whereas adherens junction anchor microfilaments to cadherins (DM, Desmosome; ICS, Intercellular space; Dsg, desmoglein; DSC, desmocollin; DP, desmoplakin; IF, intermediate filaments; PKP, plakophilin; PG, plakoglobin; ODI, outer dense plaque; IDP, inner dense plaque)

ii. **Desmoglein 3:** Expressed mostly in lower portion of epidermis and throughout mucosal epithelium.
   - Dsg 3 cannot compensate for Dsg1 loss in superficial epidermis → if Dsg1 is targeted (as in P. foliaceus and mucocutaneous pemphigus vulgaris); the skin develops blisters.
   - Dsg 3 is the major desmoglein involved in mucosal epithelial adhesion.

iii. **Desmoglein 4:** Important role in hair follicles.
   - Dsg 4 is mutated in autosomal recessive localized hypotrichosis and also autosomal recessive monilethrix.

iv. **Desmoglein 2:** Important in cardiomyocyte adhesion and in simple epithelium.

Acantholysis

Acantholysis can be broadly classified into primary and secondary types.

Primary acantholysis occurs due to direct injury/hereditary defects in desmosomes causing dissociation and separation of keratinocytes while **secondary acantholysis** occurs due to alteration or damage to keratinocytes by various factors (keratinocytes are injured first followed by subsequent disintegration of desmosomes). **Box 7.1** lists some important causes of both types of acantholysis. The various postulated mechanisms of acantholysis are explained in **Table 7.3**.

BOX 7.1: Important causes of primary and secondary acantholysis

Primary acantholysis	Secondary acantholysis
Pemphigus vulgaris and its variants	Epidermolytic hyperkeratosis
Pemphigus foliaceus and its variants	Epidermolysis bullosa (EB)
	Acantholytic Dowling–Meara type of EB simplex
Hailey–Hailey disease	Herpes simplex and zoster
	Condyloma acuminatum
Darier disease	Tinea corporis
Transient acantholytic dermatosis (Grover disease)	Adenoid squamous cell carcinoma
Bullous impetigo	Basal cell carcinoma
Staphylococcal scalded skin syndrome (SSSS)	Keratoacanthoma

TABLE 7.3: Mechanisms of acantholysis	
Steric hindrance	Binding of autoantibodies to target antigens → disruption of adhesions between cells by steric hindrance
p38 mitogen-activated protein kinase (p38MAPK) pathway	• Binding of antibody results in phosphorylation of keratinocyte proteins, including activation of EGF receptor and phosphorylation of its downstream substrates p38 mitogen-activated protein kinase (p38MAPK) → apoptolysis and inflammation • Specific inhibition of p38MAPK can prevent pemphigus vulgaris blistering *in vivo* in mice
Complement pathway	• Pemphigus antibody fixes components of complement to the surface of epidermal cells → release of inflammatory mediators and recruitment of activated T cells • Complement activation, though not essential for acantholysis, may enhance the pathogenicity of antibodies
Cellular acetyl-choline receptor (AChR) pathway	Binding of antibodies to peripheral myelin protein (PERP) and/or cellular acetylcholine receptor (AChR) → dissociation of adhesion molecules
Apoptolysis hypothesis	Binding of pathogenic autoantibodies to keratinocyte via receptor–ligand interaction → activation of signaling pathways → elevation of intracellular Ca^{2+} → activation of caspases → initiates cell death enzymatic cascades (apoptotic cascade) → basal cell shrinkage → suprabasal acantholysis
Multiple hit hypothesis	Apart from anti-desmoglein 1 and 3 antibodies, patient may also develop antibodies against non-desmosomal proteins
Role of T cells	Unclear role, but autoreactive T cell responses to Dsg 3 may be critical in its pathogenesis. Most patients with PF have circulating T cells that specifically proliferate in response to Dsg1
Drug-induced	• Drugs and food items of the thiol or phenol groups can trigger pemphigus • The proposed mechanisms for thiol-induced acantholysis include direct biochemical effect by formation of thiol–cysteine bonds disturbing cell adhesion, protease activation, and immunological reaction with the formation of a neoantigen • Possible mechanisms of phenol-induced acantholysis include induction of IL-1α and TNF-α release from keratinocytes, which results in the dysregulation of proteases-like plasminogen activator

PEMPHIGUS VULGARIS (PV)

Potentially fatal autoimmune bullous disease of the skin and mucous membranes with a peak incidence between 4th and 6th decades but occurs at a younger age in India.

May be associated with other autoimmune diseases: Myasthenia gravis, thymoma, and autoimmune thyroiditis.

Pathogenesis

The interplay of the following leads to acantholysis:

- **Autoantigens:** Desmoglein 3 (mucosal), desmoglein 1 (mucocutaneous)
- Patient serum contains antibodies against non-conformational epitopes of Dsg 3.
- **Autoantibodies:** IgG **(IgG4 > IgG1)** and C3. IgG4 titers diminish during remission, whereas circulating IgG1 may continue to be present. Relapse is commonly preceded by rising IgG4 antibody titers. Active disease correlates with the presence of antibodies directed against the NH2-terminal aspect of Dsg 3, in particular ectodomains 2–4.

- Oral disease is particularly associated with reactivity to ectodomains 1–4, which is less in cutaneous pemphigus.
- **Genetic:** HLA-DRB1*04, HLA-DRw6, HLA-DRB1*14
- **T cells:** CD4+ memory T cells are predominantly involved and both T-helper 1 (Th1) and Th2 Dsg 3-specific subtypes are represented.
  - Th1 → IFN-γ inhibits IgG1 gene transcription.
  - Th2 → Interleukin (IL)-4 and IL-13 → B cell-derived IgG4, IgG1 increased.

  Tumor necrosis factor alpha (TNF-α), Fas- ligand and IL-1 are the key mediators. An overview of the salient aspects of the pathogenesis is depicted in **Fig. 7.3**.

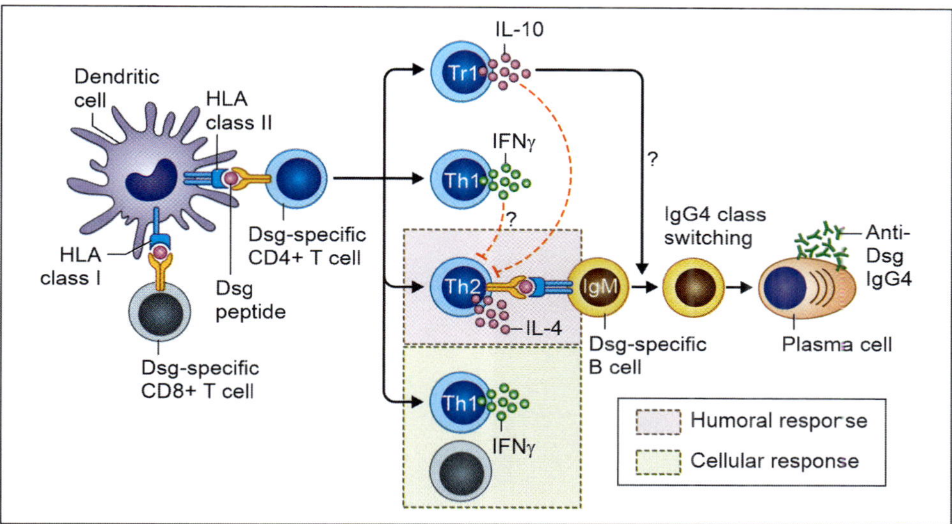

Fig. 7.3: Pathogenesis of pemphigus vulgaris: Dendritic cells presenting desmoglein (Dsg) antigens can activate CD4+ and CD8+ T cells. These autoreactive T cells can be identified even in healthy individuals and mainly produce IL-10 and interferon-γ (IFN-γ). IL-4-producing Th cells can be isolated from patients with pemphigus (but not healthy individuals) and presumably drive anti-Dsg antibody production by B cells. Acantholysis seen in pemphigus is induced by a humoral autoimmune response. Dsg-reactive (or reactive to other epidermal autoantigens) CD4+ and CD8+ T cells with cytotoxic activity are occasionally generated and mediate a cellular autoimmune response that causes interface dermatitis, which can be observed in paraneoplastic pemphigus (TCR, T cell receptor; Tr1, T regulatory type 1)

Box 7.2 lists some important facts about pemphigus vulgaris.

BOX 7.2: Factoids about pemphigus vulgaris[Q]

• Why do some patients have active pemphigus with intercellular antibodies detectable on direct or indirect IF but **do not** have Dsg antibodies?	There may be significant non-Dsg targets and antibodies against desmocollins, plakoglobin, E-cadherin and acetylcholine receptors (85%).
• What is the reason for predominant scalp involvement?	• Abundant antigen in the follicular outer root sheath and germinal matrix. • Hence, plucked hair follicles may serve as an adequate substrate for direct immunofluorescence analysis.

Clinical Features

- Flaccid blisters filled with clear fluid → the contents may become turbid or the blisters rupture → producing painful erosions which extend at the edges **(Fig. 7.4a** and **b)** → healing occurs without scarring but with pigmentary alteration. Pruritus is uncommon (unlike bullous pemphigoid).
- Lesions persist on the scalp **(Fig. 7.4c)** and in severe cases may involve the whole body **(Fig. 7.4d)**.
- Two subgroups:
  1. Mucosal-dominant type
  2. Mucocutaneous type
- Nikolsky sign—positive. Marginal Nikolsky sign—more sensitive and direct Nikolsky sign—more specific.

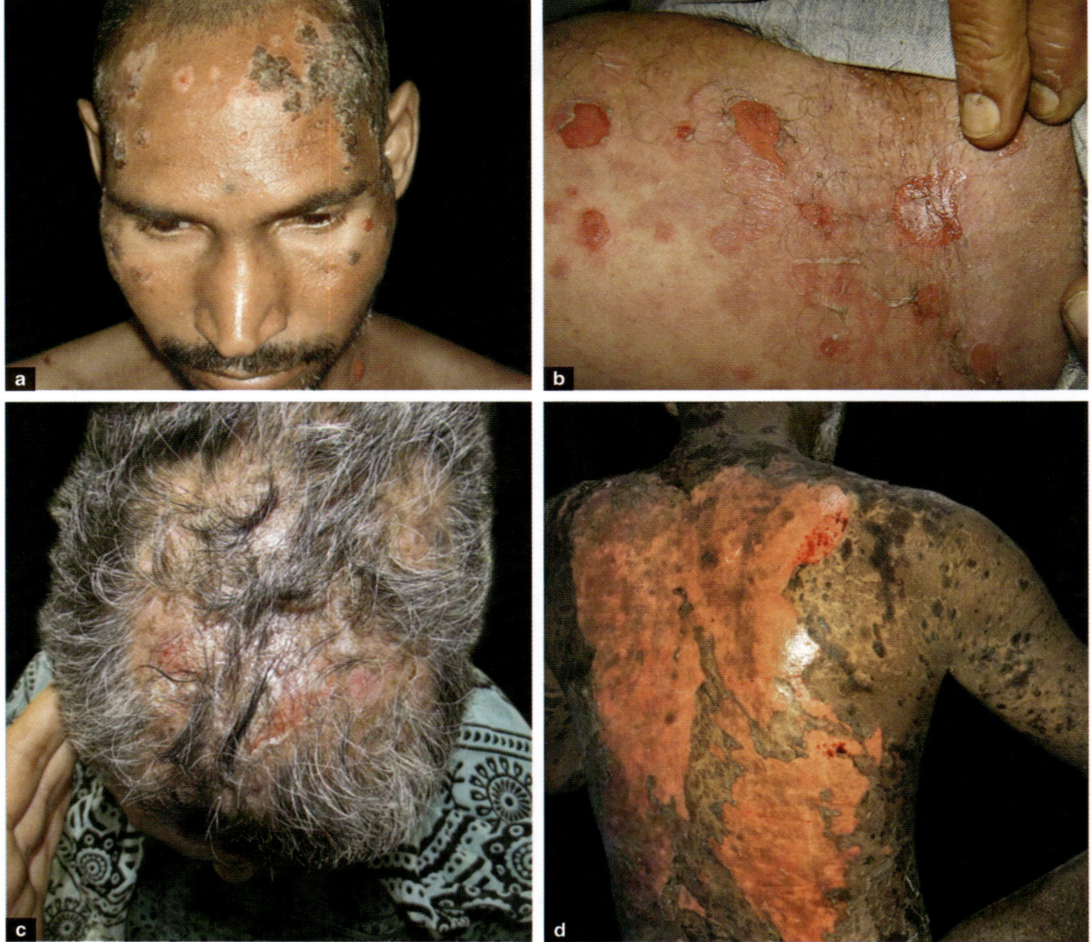

Fig. 7.4: Pemphigus vulgaris with (a) Crusted plaques; (b) Flaccid bullae with erosions and positive Nikolsky sign; (c) Persistent lesions on the scalp; (d) Erythrodermic pemphigus vulgaris

- **Bulla spread sign**—positive (angular margin *vs* rounded margin of BP)
- Most common site—scalp, face, axillae and the oral cavity (buccal and palatal mucosa).
- Nearly all patients have mucosal lesions, and PV presents with oral lesions in 50–70% of patients. Other mucosal surfaces may be involved, including the conjunctiva, nasopharynx, larynx, esophagus, urethra, vulva and cervix.
- **Unusual clinical presentation of PV**
  - Isolated crusted plaque on face or scalp
  - Paronychia and/or onychomadesis
  - Foot ulcers
  - Dyshidrotic eczema or pompholyx
  - Macroglossia

Investigations

1. **Tzanck smear:** Acantholytic cells seen (large round keratinocyte with a hypertrophic nucleus, hazy or absent nucleoli, perinuclear halo, peripherally clumped cytoplasm, and abundant basophilic cytoplasm near the cell membrane ('mourning edge').
   - Other findings—**Sertoli rosettes** (a central necrobiotic keratinocyte with a surrounding leukocyte rosette) and **'streptocytes'** (a chain of leukocytes, joined by a filamentous, glue-like substance).
2. **Histopathology**
   - The earliest histological change—eosinophilic spongiosis followed by intercellular edema with loss of intercellular attachments in the basal layer.
   - The suprabasal epidermal cells separate from the basal cells to form suprabasal clefts and blisters. Basal cells remain attached to the basement membrane but separate from one another and stand like a **'row of tombstones'** on the floor of the blister.
   - Blister cavities contain some acantholytic cells.
   - The superficial dermis has a mild, superficial, mixed inflammatory infiltrate which includes some eosinophils.
   - Useful diagnostic clue in those lesions which lack the roof of the blisteris is that it involves the epithelium of the adnexae.

   Common differential diagnosis of suprabasal acantholysis are given in **Table 7.4**.

TABLE 7.4: Differential diagnosis of suprabasal acantholysis

	Pemphigus vulgaris*	Darier disease*	Hailey-Hailey disease*
Types of lesion	Intraepithelial bullae	Suprabasal clefts	Intraepithelial bullae
Adjacent epithelium	Intact	Intact	Disintegrating, **'dilapidated brick wall'**
Involvement of adnexae	Yes	Yes	**No**
Corps ronds and grains	No	Yes	Rarely
Dermal inflammation	Mononuclear, eosinophils ++	Mononuclear	Mononuclear
IF studies	Positive	**Negative**	**Negative**

*The lesions of Grover disease may mimic any of these conditions and can only be distinguished by IF studies; (IF, immunofluorescence)

3. **Direct immunofluorescence:** The biopsy specimen from perilesional normal skin or mucous membrane shows **IgG and/or C3** deposits at the surface of epidermal keratinocytes **(net-like pattern)**.
   - **DIF of plucked hair (Rao et al., 2009)**
     - **Basis:** Pemphigus antigens are found in the ORS of the hair follicle (structurally analogous to the epidermis) and in dermal bulb matrix. Though hair follicles are present throughout the body, the diameter of scalp terminal hair is almost twice that of vellus hair of body → hence total volume of desmosomal structure is greater per unit area in the scalp → also a reason for the pemphigus predilection for scalp.
     - **Advantage:** Plucked hair DIF can be positive even if no scalp/only mucosal involvement.
4. **Indirect immunofluorescence (IIF):** Circulating pemphigus autoantibodies are detected by IF in over 80–90% of patients. The use of more than one substrate improves sensitivity (esophageal mucosa for **Dsg** 3, whereas normal human skin for **Dsg1**). Titer correlates with disease activity.

Best IIF substrates for pemphigus variants

- PF: Guinea pig esophagus, normal human skin
- PV: Monkey esophagus
- PNP: Rat bladder

5. **ELISA:** Using ELISA, over 95% of PV patients have detectable Dsg 3 antibodies and around 50% have Dsg1 antibodies.

An overview of the **investigations and treatment** will be detailed at the end of this section **(Tables 7.9 to 7.11)**.

PEMPHIGUS VEGETANS

- Pemphigus vegetans is a rare variant of pemphigus vulgaris which is characterized by vegetating erosions, primarily in flexures, but may occasionally involve other body sites, such as the scalp **(Fig. 7.5)**.

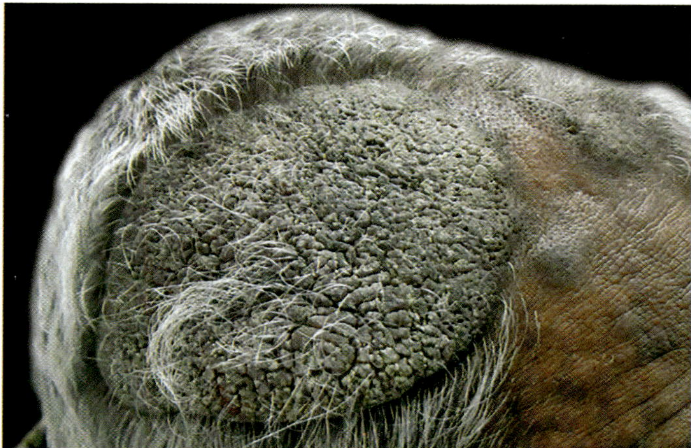

Fig. 7.5: Pemphigus vegetans—a large vegetating plaque involving an atypical site (scalp). This patient had a recurrence annually that highlights the recalcitrant nature of this variant

- The disease affects chiefly middle-aged adults. Two types:
  - **Hallopeau type** (starts as pustules then develops vegetating plaques), better prognosis
  - **Neumann type** (starts as vesicles and bullae which rupture and become vegetative plaques), worse prognosis
- Local moisture, heat and friction may increase number and severity of lesions
- Characteristic glossal changes, termed **'cerebriform tongue'**, may be seen **(Premalatha sign)**.
- **HPE** is similar to PV, but additional findings include pseudoepitheliomatous hyperplasia, increased inflammatory cell infiltrate, intraepidermal microabscesses comprising of eosinophils and neutrophils.
- **DIF** demonstrates intercellular IgG, sometimes with C3.
- Circulating intercellular antibodies can be detected in most patients by **IIF**.

PEMPHIGUS FOLIACEUS (PF)

- Less severe and more superficial than PV.
- **Autoantigen:** Desmoglein 1.
- **Autoantibody:** IgG (IgG4)

The sera from pemphigus foliaceus patients bind to the **extracellular** amino terminal domain of Dsg1, whereas sera from pemphigus vulgaris and pemphigus vegetans patients react with the **intracellular** domain of Dsg1.

Clinical Variants

- Fogo selvagem: Usually seen in Brazil in areas near river banks rich in black flies (*Simulium* spp.)
- Pemphigus erythematosus (Senear–Usher syndrome)
- Pemphigus herpetiformis

Clinical Features

- Small flaccid bullae that readily rupture, resulting in moist erosions and cornflake-like crusts **(Fig. 7.6)**.
- Nikolsky sign—positive.
- The **seborrheic areas** (i.e. face, scalp and upper trunk) are commonly involved, but it may become generalized.
- Mucosal involvement is rare.
- There is a characteristic **musty odor**.
- Although the antibodies in PF can cross the placenta, the neonate is not usually affected.
- It may be exacerbated by sun exposure. The disease is usually chronic but is not life-threatening.
- The disease may stay localized for years or it may rapidly progress, in some cases to generalized involvement and an **exfoliative erythroderma**.

Investigations

1. **HPE:** The bullae are superficial, high in the granular layer or immediately below the stratum corneum (subcorneal bulla). Dyskeratotic cells in the granular layer of older lesions distinguish pemphigus foliaceus from pemphigus vulgaris.
   - PF, pemphigus erythematosus, SSSS, and bullous impetigo all show nearly identical findings on HPE.

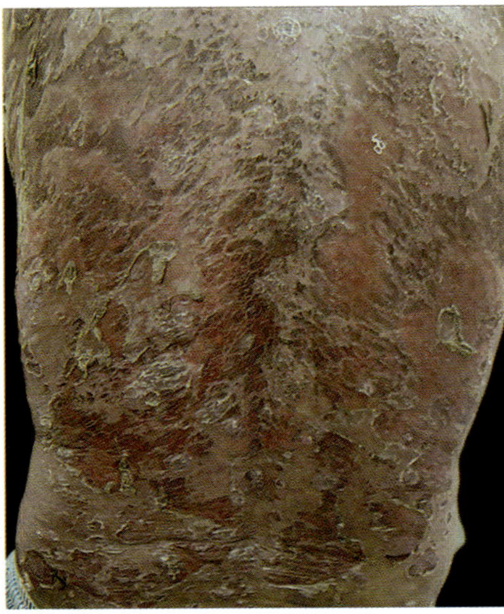

Fig. 7.6: Pemphigus foliaceus—superficial erosions and 'cornflake-like' crusts can be seen and often present as erythroderma

Differential diagnosis of a subcorneal bulla is given in Table 7.5.

2. **Direct and indirect immunofluorescence:** Findings are usually indistinguishable from pemphigus vulgaris with intercellular IgG and C3 throughout the epidermis on DIF. IIF is positive in over 85% of pemphigus foliaceus sera.
3. **ELISA:** Detects antidesmoglein 1 antibodies in up to 71% of patients.

TABLE 7.5: Differential diagnosis of pemphigus foliaceus (conditions characterized by subcorneal pustules)
• Pemphigus foliaceus and variants • IgA pemphigus • Subcorneal pustular dermatosis • Pustular psoriasis • Reiter syndrome • Pustular drug reaction • Bullous impetigo • Staphylococcal scalded skin syndrome • Pustular fungal infection, candidiasis

Treatment

Please *see* pages 144 and 149.

PEMPHIGUS ERYTHEMATOSUS (PE)

- **Senear–Usher syndrome**
- Clinical and serological overlap of **pemphigus foliaceus and lupus erythematosus**. Clinically, the erosio-crusted lesions may typically involve the butterfly/malar distribution. Mucosal involvement is uncommon.
- HPE of PE is similar to that of PF, but in old lesions, follicular hyperkeratosis with acantholysis and dyskeratosis of the granular layer is often pronounced.

- DIF shows the fish-net pattern of intercellular IgG **plus** a linear deposit of IgG and/or C3 at DEJ.
- The patient is also frequently **ANA positive**.

ENDEMIC PEMPHIGUS FOLIACEUS

It is also called *fogo selvagem* (Portuguese for 'wild fire') and is a *Brazilian* variant of pemphigus foliaceus. A striking distribution of lesions on the skin that is exposed to the sun, a 'burnt' appearance of the patient, and a painful burning sensation in lesions. Most of the affected patients live and work close to rivers and streams. Hence, it is believed that endemic pemphigus foliaceus is caused by black fly (*Simulium pruinosum*) or another agent in the environment, with acquired immunity in adulthood.

PEMPHIGUS HERPETIFORMIS

- Rare variant of pemphigus that clinically resembles dermatitis herpetiformis.
- Clusters of pruritic papules and vesicles develop on an erythematous background.
- In general, the clinical course is benign (less severe than pemphigus vulgaris, but may be more chronic).
- **Diagnostic markers**
  - Pruritus
  - Urticated erythema +/– vesicles/bullae/erosions
  - Eosinophilic spongiosis
  - Variable acantholysis
  - Intercellular epidermal IgG deposits on DIF

Investigations

HPE

- HPE findings are widely heterogeneous.
- Subcorneal pustules, intraepidermal vesicles filled with neutrophils and/or eosinophils, neutrophilic and/or eosinophilic spongiosis.
- Acantholysis may be minimal or absent.

Immunofluorescence Studies

- Intercellular Dsg1 or 3, sometimes desmocollin 1 or 3.
- The condition may evolve into classical PF but has also been described preceding PV.
- PH autoantibodies may recognize functionally less important epitopes of Dsg1 or 3 and, therefore, do not lead directly to acantholysis.

Treatment

Dapsone usually effective. Severe cases—oral corticosteroids +/– immunosuppressives.

PARANEOPLASTIC PEMPHIGUS

- Associated with neoplasms (both malignant and benign)—**non-Hodgkin lymphoma (MC)** > chronic lymphocytic leukemia > Castleman disease, thymoma, etc.
- **Prognosis depends on the associated tumor.** Some patients experience rapid improvement after excision of a benign tumor, such as Castleman disease. With malignant tumors, PNP can be severe and unresponsive to treatment.
- As there are multiple epidermal and dermoepidermal antigens targeted, the clinical picture is also typically polymorphic.

- Typically, **the first symptoms include severe painful and intractable oral erosions**, frequently hemorrhagic. Polymorphic lesions—blisters, erosions, papules and plaques. The oral involvement is quite severe and may involve vermilion border of lips, and oropharynx. Oral involvement is almost mandatory for diagnosis.
- **Mucosal involvement:** May involve mucous membranes of the esophagus, stomach, duodenum, intestines and the pulmonary epithelium (bronchiolitis obliterans)—may be extensive and fatal.
- Skin manifestations can be classified into several groups according to the types of alteration **(Box 7.3)** and the diagnostic criteria are listed in **Table 7.6**.

BOX 7.3: Clinical variants of PNP

- Pemphigus-like: Superficial vesicles, flaccid bullae, crusted, erosions
- Bullous pemphigoid-like: Scaly erythematous papules, tense bullae
- Erythema multiforme-like: Polymorphic erythematous papules and plaques, erosions, occasionally hard-to-heal ulcerations
- Graft-versus-host disease: Disseminated dusky-red scaly papules
- Lichen planus-like: Small scaly flat-topped papules and intense mucous membrane involvement

TABLE 7.6: Paraneoplastic pemphigus: Original diagnostic criteria by Anhalt et al. 1990

1. Painful mucosal erosions and a polymorphous skin eruption in the context of an occult or known neoplasm.
2. Intraepidermal acantholysis, dyskeratosis/keratinocyte necrosis, and vacuolar interface changes in histopathology.
3. Deposition of IgG and complement (C3) in intercellular epidermal spaces and linear/granular basement membrane zone seen on direct immunofluorescence.
4. Detection of serum autoantibodies to stratified squamous epithelia and transitional epithelia by indirect immunofluorescence.
5. Serum immunoprecipitation of a characteristic complex of four proteins [desmoplakin 1 (250 kDa), bullous pemphigoid antigen (230 kDa), desmoplakin 2 (210 kDa), periplakin (190 kDa)] on immunoblotting.

Camisa and Helm criteria*

Major

- Polymorphic mucocutaneous eruptions
- Concomitant internal neoplasm
- Serum antibodies with a specific immunoprecipitation pattern

Minor

- Acantholysis observed histologically
- DIF displaying intercellular and basement membrane staining
- IIF staining positive on rat bladder epithelium

*PNP diagnosis requires either 3 major criteria or 2 major and 2 minor criteria.

Investigations

HPE: Variable findings with suprabasal cleavage, basal cell vacuolization, lichenoid infiltrate and necrotic keratinocytes.

DIF: Both intercellular as well as linear or granular IgG and/or C3 at DEJ. DIF can be negative in 50%.

IIF: IgG binding not only to stratified but also to simple and transitional epithelial tissues, e.g. rat bladder epithelium.

Immunoprecipitation and immunoblot: Detection of autoantibodies against the **210 kDa (desmoplakin 2)** and/or the **190 kDa (periplakin)** is both sensitive and specific for PNP. Immunoblot is considered the gold standard for PNP diagnosis.

An extensive **malignancy workup**—blood cell count with peripheral smear, lactate dehydrogenase, stool for occult blood, lymph node aspiration cytology, PAP smear, PSA, flow cytometry, computed tomography of the chest, abdomen, and pelvis. In up to one-third of patients, discovery of the underlying malignancy occurs after onset of PNP.

Treatment

- Usually recalcitrant to therapy and treatment of the underlying neoplasm is paramount.
- Initially, **glucocorticoid** therapy should be implemented—prednisone (0.5–1.0 mg/kg).
- **Steroid-sparing agents—immunosuppressants**, such as cyclosporin, cyclophosphamide, azathioprine and mycophenolate mofetil are often used in combination with prednisone.
- **Rituximab**, a chimeric anti-CD20 monoclonal antibody, has been used in PNP. Lymphoma protocol (375 mg/m^2 weekly for 4 weeks) or RA protocol (1 g repeated in 2 weeks). Additional cycles may be administered every 6–12 months depending on clinical response and recovery of the B cell population.
- **Rituximab** with intravenous immunoglobulin **(IVIG)**—in those patients who do not respond to conventional therapy or rituximab alone. IVIG (2 g/kg per cycle), is repeated on a monthly basis. IVIG can be added into the patient's existing treatment regimen without concern of additional immunosuppression, making it a popular approach among clinicians who treat PNP.

IgA PEMPHIGUS

- A type of pemphigus with intraepidermal IgA deposits
- Middle-aged or elderly
- **Autoantigen:** Desmocollin 1 (SPD type), ± desmoglein 1/3 (IEN type)
- **Clinical:** Two types:
  1. **Subcorneal pustular dermatosis (SPD) type:** Flaccid vesicles or pustules on erythematous or normal skin → tend to coalesce to form an annular or circinate pattern with crusts in the central area **(Fig. 7.7)**. May be associated with underlying IgA gammopathy (may evolve into multiple myeloma).
     Target antigen = Desmocollin 1
  2. **Intraepidermal neutrophilic (IEN) type:** Flaccid pustules and bullae involving intertriginous locations which enlarge forming annular or polycyclic (**sunflower-like**) arrangement.
     Target antigen = Dsg1/Dsg 3
     - **Common sites**—axillae and groins, but the trunk and proximal extremities may be involved
     - About half—pruritus +
     - Mucous membrane—rare.

Investigations

Histology: Subcorneal/suprabasal (respectively in SPD type and IEN type) pustule or vesicles containing neutrophils, neutrophilic infiltration in epidermis, no/slight acantholysis.

DIF: Intercellular IgA deposition (unlike SCPD of Sneddon–Wilkinson) (IgA in upper epidermis in SPD type, IgA throughout epidermis in IEN type)

IIF: + in 50%, intercellular IgA1

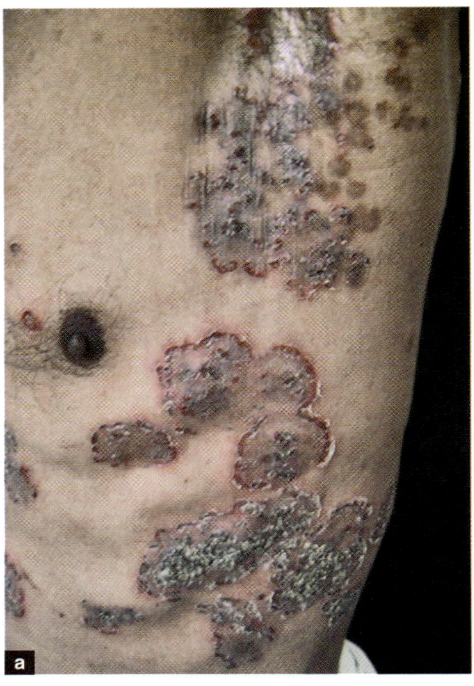

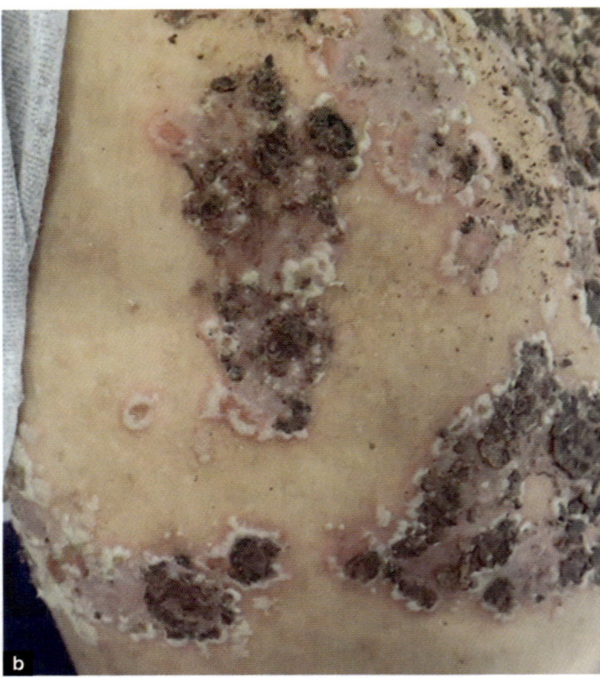

Fig. 7.7: IgA pemphigus showing annular lesions with central crusting—**subcorneal pustular dermatosis variant of IgA pemphigus**

Treatment

- Mainstay for treatment—oral and topical **corticosteroids** (0.5–1 mg/kg prednisolone daily).
- In addition, **dapsone** (100 mg daily) may be very useful due to its effect in suppressing neutrophilic infiltration.
- Colchicine
- Isotretinoin and acitretin

INDUCED PEMPHIGUS

Many factors are believed to induce/trigger the pathogenesis of pemphigus, most importantly drugs **(Box 7.4)**.

BOX 7.4: Mnemonic for causes of induced pemphigus

PE	Pesticides
M	Malignancy
P	Pharmaceuticals/ drugs
H	Hormones
I	Infectious agents
G	Gastronomy/ foods
U	UV radiation
S	Stress

Pesticides

Organochlorine pesticides and organophosphates have been implicated.

Malignancy

PNP has been associated with malignant processes, mainly hematolymphoproliferative diseases such as Hodgkin's lymphoma, non-Hodgkin's lymphoma, chronic lymphocytic leukemia, Castelman disease, and others. Simple coincidental coexistence is also possible with pemphigus.

Pharmaceuticals

- The inciting medications can be classified based on their chemical structure with the main groups being thiol drugs, phenol drugs, and nonthiol/nonphenol drugs. **Pemphigus foliaceus and pemphigus erythematosus are the most common patterns** of pemphigus induced by drugs **(Table 7.7)**.
- **Drug-induced pemphigus**—drug plays a major role in the pathogenesis of the disease, no prior predisposition, caused by **thiol** drugs. Pemphigus foliaceus and pemphigus erythematosus are the most common presentations.
- **Drug-triggered pemphigus**—drug only triggers the disease in patients with a previous predisposition, mostly **pemphigus vulgaris**-like, caused by **phenol drugs** and **non-thiol, nonphenol drugs**.

Hormones

The role of sex hormones, mainly estrogen, in the pathogenesis of pemphigus has not yet been established. An association with pregnancy is possible (aggravation of pemphigus vulgaris during pregnancy and neonatal pemphigus).

TABLE 7.7: Drug-induced pemphigus

Thiol drugs	Phenol drugs	Nonthiol nonphenol drugs
• Contain a sulfhydryl (–SH) group • Thiols may cause acantholysis directly • Mostly **PF or PE-like** • Promote acantholysis by stimulating enzymes like plasminogen activator which disaggregate keratinocytes and inhibiting enzymes that promote keratinocyte aggregation	• Cause acantholysis via immune mechanisms, more likely to cause **PV-like** presentation • Disrupt the integrity of cellular adherence mechanisms by stimulating keratinocytes to release proinflammatory cytokines • The release of TNF-α and IL-1 from cells drives complement and protease activation which contribute to acantholysis	• May cause acantholysis through alternative pathways such as the activation of autoantibodies or altering the target antigen structure on keratinocytes
• Spontaneous recovery in 39.4% with penicillamine-induced and 52.6% with other thiol drugs once the drug is discontinued • Possible that the drug plays the main role and actually induces pemphigus	• Spontaneous recovery in only 15% of the cases • Likely that the drug only triggers pemphigus and does not play a major role—therefore, discontinuation does not help	• Spontaneous recovery in only 15% of the cases • Likely that the drug only triggers pemphigus and does not play a major role—therefore, discontinuation does not help
• **Penicillamine** • **Thiopronine (penicillamine-like drug)**	• Aspirin • Heroin • Rifampicin • Levodopa • Phenobarbital • Cephalosporins	• Nonsteroidal anti-inflammatory drugs • ACE-inhibitors (captopril > enalapril, lisinopril) • Calcium-channel blockers • Glibenclamide • Biologics (few reports) (secukinumab, tocilizumab)

Infection

The most frequently incriminated infectious agents are viruses of the Herpesviridae family, namely HSV, EBV, CMV, and even HHV8.

In addition, bacteria, such as coagulase positive *Staphylococcus aureus*, are capable of inducing pemphigus. Gram-negative bacteria and even *Actinomyces* are possible triggers.

Food

Although rarely mentioned in the literature, certain foods are believed to induce or trigger pemphigus:

- **Phenols**
  - Fruits: Mango, bananas, potatoes, tomatoes
  - Nuts: Pistachio, cashew
  - Food additives: Aspartame, sodium benzoate, tartrazine, vanillin, eugenol, caffeic acid, cinnamic acid, vitamins C and E.
- **Tannins**
  - Nuts: Betel, walnuts
  - Drinks: Tea, fruit juice, beer, wine, liquors, water, coffee, guarana (high tannin content of Brazil river water may explain high occurrence of fogo selvagem).
  - Spices: Ajowan, coriander, cumin, black pepper, red chillies, rosemary, garlic, and ginger
- **Thiols**
  - Vegetables: Garlic, onion, shallot, chive, and leek
- **Isothiocyanates**
  - Mustard oil—allyl/benzyl isothiocyanate (immunologically reactive) and phenyl isothiocyanate (irritant)

Ultraviolet Radiation

Pemphigus is considered a photosensitive disease, mainly the variant pemphigus erythematosus.

Physical factors such as X-ray, radiotherapy, burns, major surgery and cosmetic procedures have also been reported to be capable of inducing pemphigus.

Stress

Several studies and case reports point to the possible contribution of emotional stress as a precipitating factor in pemphigus.

DIFFERENTIAL DIAGNOSIS

An overview of differential diagnoses of different types of pemphigus is given in **Table 7.8**.

INVESTIGATIONS

Table 7.9 provides a comprehensive summary of investigations in pemphigus.

TABLE 7.8: Differential diagnosis of pemphigus	
Pemphigus vulgaris (mucosal)	Acute herpetic stomatitis, erythema multiforme, SJS, aphthous ulcers, oral candidiasis, bullous/erosive lichen planus
Pemphigus vulgaris (cutaneous)	Pemphigoid and its variants, linear IgA disease, dermatitis herpetiformis and erythema multiforme, SJS/TEN overlap
Pemphigus vegetans	Hailey–Hailey disease, blastomycosis-like pyoderma, pyodermatitis-pyostomatitis vegetans, extramammary Paget's disease
Pemphigus foliaceus	Seborrheic dermatitis, impetigo
Pemphigus erythematosus	Seborrheic dermatitis, chronic cutaneous lupus erythematosus
Paraneoplastic pemphigus	Pemphigus vulgaris, erythema multiforme, graft-versus-host disease, lichen planus and viral infections including herpes simplex

TABLE 7.9: Investigations in pemphigus

	Type of investigation	Interpretation/Rationale
Clinical signs and bedside tests	Nikolsky sign	• Positive sign indicates intraepidermal cleavage • A positive direct Nikolsky sign indicates severe activity of the disease • It is the first sign to disappear as the disease responds to therapy
	Bulla spread/Lutz sign (Asboe-Hansen sign)	• Positive in all types of pemphigus and pemphigoid • It has an irregular angulated border in PV and rounded border in subepidermal disorders
	Tzanck smear	• Acantholytic cells seen • **In PV, large round keratinocyte** with a hypertrophic nucleus, increased nucleocytoplasmic ratio (nucleus –7/8th of cell), hazy or absent nucleoli, and hyalinized basophilic cytoplasm • **In PF, oval shaped keratinocyte**, large nucleus (5/8th of cell), basophilic cytoplasm
Baseline investigations	• Complete blood count; • KFT-urea, creatinine, blood electrolytes; • LFT-transaminases, γ-GT, alkaline phosphatase; • Fasting serum glucose • Hepatitis B, C and HIV • Chest X-ray, Mantoux test • BP	• Work-up before corticosteroid or immunosuppressive therapy
Specific investigations	Histopathology	• A biopsy should be taken from a recent (<24 hours) small vesicle or 1/3rd of the peripheral portion of a blister and 2/3rd perilesional skin (placed in 4% formalin solution) for routine histopathological analysis: Intraepidermal suprabasal acantholysis in PV or acantholysis at the granular layer in PF

(Contd.)

TABLE 7.9: Investigations in pemphigus *(Contd.)*

	Type of investigation	Interpretation/Rationale
	Electron microscopy	• Widening of the intercellular space followed by splitting of the desmosome junctions
	Direct immunofluorescence (DIF)	• The biopsy specimen should be taken from perilesional normal skin (up to 1 cm from a recent lesion) or mucous membrane • Ideal transport medium—Michel's medium [citrated buffer 1 M (pH 7.4), magnesium sulphate 0.1 M, N-ethyl maleimide 0.1 M, ammonium sulphate (55 g), distilled water] • Essentially all patients with active PV or PF have a positive DIF – IgG and/or C3 deposits at the surface of epidermal keratinocytes, less frequently IgM and IgA (PV, PF) – Granular IgG and C3 at the basement membrane zone, intercellular IgG and C3 in the epidermis (PE) – IgA deposits with an epithelial cell surface pattern in addition to IgG (IgA pemphigus) – Linear or granular deposits of IgG or C3 along the dermal–epidermal junction along with intercellular fish net pattern (PNP) • The risk of relapse is 13–27% if DIF is negative and 44–100% if DIF is positive
	Indirect immunofluorescence (IIF)	• If both monkey esophagus and normal human skin used as substrate, sensitivity in PV increases to 100% • Rat bladder is used for PNP • A two-fold rise in titer may indicate impending relapse Limitation: Circulating antibodies may not be detectable in early cases and in remission • (The risk of relapse is 24%, if IIF is negative and 57% if IIF is positive)
	ELISA	• Using ELISA, over 95% of pemphigus vulgaris patients have detectable desmoglein-3 antibodies and around 50% have desmoglein-1 antibodies • The desmoglein ELISA has 96–100% sensitivity and specificity • Anti-desmoglein 1 antibody titres tend to show a closer correlation with the course of the disease and activity (as compared with anti-desmoglein 3 antibody titres)
	Immunoblot and immunoprecipitation	• The anti-plakin autoantibodies of PNP can be detected by immunoblot and immunoprecipitation. Gold standard for PNP
	Immunoelectron microscopy	• Helps to detect location of antibody and complement in the epidermis
	Antinuclear antibodies, antibodies to Ro, La and dsDNA antigens	• Supplementary test for pemphigus erythematosus • 30–80% of patients with PE may have circulating ANA with a speckled pattern

(Contd.)

TABLE 7.9: Investigations in pemphigus *(Contd.)*

	Type of investigation	Interpretation/Rationale
Recommended (as per indication)	Thiopurine methyl transferase (TPMT) activity	• If azathioprine is considered
	Abdominal sonography or CT	• For malignancy screening (PNP)
	Quanti-FERON-TB Gold or Mantoux test	• Do for all patients to be started on immunosuppressives
	G6PD	• If dapsone is considered
	Serum IgA deficiency	• Should be ruled out prior to IVIG treatment
	Urinalysis with cytologic examination	• Indicated when the cumulative dose of cyclophosphamide exceeds 50 g, and every 6 months there after, or on any occasion of hemorrhagic cystitis
	Ocular examination (glaucoma, cataract)	• Is recommended prior to glucocorticoid treatment
	Osteodensitometry	• Is recommended prior to glucocorticoid treatment
	ECG	• If rituximab is considered
	Serum Ig levels	
	Anti Dsg 1, 3 levels (preferable)	

TREATMENT OF PEMPHIGUS

Principles of Treatment

The agents that are used are either targeted to the specific cells (T/B cells) or to the antibodies released. In essence, the use of steroids and ISA have a broad range of effects and hence have more side effects and thus the focus is on agents that are specific to the targets.

Published guidelines for pemphigus therapy mostly rely on expert consensus, given the paucity of randomized clinical trials with large sample sizes and rigorous randomization methods. The modalities of treatment of pemphigus foliaceous and vulgaris are similar. We shall briefly discuss some of the important therapeutic modalities in the following section.

The phases of therapy are given in **Table 7.10**, while an overview of the agents is given in **Table 7.11**; details of treatment follow in the text below.

Systemic CS (Boxes 7.5 and 7.6)

- Osteoporosis counselling should be provided if corticosteroid treatment is anticipated to last ≥3 months. Pneumocystis prophylaxis and tuberculosis screening should be considered for patients who will receive high doses of corticosteroids together with another immunosuppressive drug for >1 month.
- At the end of the consolidation phase of therapy, most clinicians begin to taper steroids. Approximately half of patients will relapse during steroid taper, whereas half will achieve complete remission off therapy after a mean treatment duration of 3 years.

Immunosuppressive Agents (ISA)

- Mycophenolate mofetil and azathioprine demonstrate approximately comparable safety and efficacy.
- Mycophenolate mofetil has shown faster and more durable treatment responses than placebo when added to prednisolone regimens.
- Azathioprine is generally preferred for patients with renal failure.

Biologicals

While Rituximab is well accepted as a preferred drug for pemphigus, it is important to focus on its effect on the B-cell activating factor **(BAFF)** which is an important factor for B cell survival, class switch recombination and selection of autoreactive B cells, as well as maintaining long-lived plasma cells. It has been hypothesized that relapses after rituximab might be due to the increase of serum BAFF levels. A study compared this with high dose CS and found that decreased BAFF-R expression after rituximab might be responsible for the delayed generation of memory B cells, resulting in a rather long period of mild pemphigus activity after rituximab therapy. Conversely, the incomplete B cell depletion and persistent BAFF-R expression associated with high BAFF serum levels might explain the high number of relapses in patients treated with CS alone **(Hébert V et al., 2021)**.

Experimental Treatments

Efgartigimod is a neonatal Fc receptor antagonist being developed by argenx for the treatment of autoimmune diseases including myasthenia gravis. In December 2021, intravenous efgartigimod received its first approval in the USA for the treatment of generalized myasthenia gravis in adults who are anti-acetylcholine receptor (AChR) antibody positive. This has been successfully tried in pemphigus.

TABLE 7.10: Phases of treatment of pemphigus

Control	Intensive therapy is given until no new lesions appear for 2 weeks
Consolidation	Treatment is continued until the lesions completely clear
Maintenance	Lowest dose of the drug is given to prevent the appearance of any new lesions
Follow-up	During this period, the patients are advised for regular follow up without any treatment

TABLE 7.11: Topical and systemic therapy

Topical

- Good oral hygiene
- Clobetasol propionate (mild pemphigus). Potent topical or intralesional steroids may reduce the requirement for oral steroids
- Anticholinergic gel (pilocarpine) for oral erosions
- Tacrolimus and cyclosporine
- Intralesional triamcinolone acetonide (2.5–5 mg/mL) for intractable oral ulcers

Systemic

1. **Steroids:** The details of steroids and DCP are explained in **Boxes 7.5** and **7.6**

2. Immunosuppressives:	
Cyclophosphamide	Cyclophosphamide is a potent anti-B cell agent. Dose: 1–3 mg/kg/day
Azathioprine	Dose: 2–3 mg/kg/day
Mycophenolate mofetil	An antimetabolite that inhibits *de novo* pathway of purine synthesis in T and B cells. Dose: 1–3 g/day
Methotrexate	Dose: 10–50 mg/week
Cyclosporine	Dose: 2.5–5 mg/kg/day
3. Anti-inflammatory	
Dapsone	Pemphigus herpetiformis
Acitretin	With prednisolone in pemphigus vegetans
Gold	May have modest effect in pemphigus, though toxic effects limit its utility
Tetracycline, Nicotinamide	Tetracycline and/or nicotinamide in combination with prednisolone may be useful in mild disease.
4. Biologics and IVIG	
IVIG	Unclear mechanism, may have a dilutional effect on pathogenic autoantibodies plus anti-idiotypic effects. Dose: 2 g/kg split over 3–5 days
Rituximab	Chimeric monoclonal antibody against CD20. Dose: 375 mg/m^2 weekly for 4 weeks or two infusions of 1g, 2 weeks apart (*see* **Box 7.7** for details)

5. **Desmoglein-specific immunoadsorption**

   Extracorporeal photophoresis, plasmapheresis, immunoadsorption

   IVIG

6. **Desmoglein-specific B cell depletion**

   Desmoglein 3 chimeric autoantibody receptor T cells (CAARTs) specifically bind to and kill antidesmoglein 3 B cells, leading to disease remission in a pemphigus mouse model without immunosuppression

BOX 7.5: Systemic corticosteroids in pemphigus

- Systemic corticosteroids remain the mainstay of treatment of pemphigus and prednisolone is the preferred drug.
- Improves disease within days despite the same titre of circulating autoantibodies.
- ↑ transcription of desmogleins and other cell adhesion molecules, which counteracts the autoantibody-induced interference with desmoglein adhesive function.
- Prednisolone **(1–1.5 mg/kg/day)** with adjuvant immunosuppression and appropriate topical therapy is sufficient to initiate disease control in most patients.
- Some authors recommend that for mild-to-moderate disease, the starting dose of prednisolone is 60–80 mg/day, whereas for severe disease it is 60–120 mg/day. The initial dose in PV has been seen to predict the chances of relapse by Yamagami et al (greater risk with 0.78 mg/kg *vs* 1.01 mg/kg).
- The steroid dose should be titrated to the clinical response.
- Patients with generalized disease may require more aggressive immunosuppression to suppress blistering. IV pulses of either 1 g methyl prednisolone or 100 mg dexamethasone are safer alternatives that may be used, often together with IVIG, immunoadsorption or plasmapheresis.
- Concomitant immunosuppressives or other adjuvants are advocated,if there are relative contraindications to the use of corticosteroids, serious side effects due to corticosteroids or a reduction in the dose is not possible because of repeated exacerbations in disease activity.

BOX 7.6: Dexamethasone-cyclophosphamide pulse (DCP) therapy

- DCP therapy involves the intravenous administration of 100 mg of dexamethasone (equivalent to 667 mg of prednisolone) with 500 mg of cyclophosphamide in 500 ml of 5% dextrose over 1–2 hours on day 1, followed by daily administration of 100 mg of dexamethasone for the next 2 days.
- These pulses are repeated every 4 weeks.
- On the intervening days, 50 mg of cyclophosphamide is administered orally every day.
- Phase I: DCP is continued till remission is achieved. The lesions start healing soon after the first pulse. If despite pulse, healing does not occur and/or new lesions continue to appear, then daily steroid may be added for initial 2–3 months. The phase I lasts till all the lesions have completely healed and the patient is off daily steroid. This phase is variable from patient-to-patient.
- Phase II: Monthly DCP is continued for 9 more months despite the absence of clinical lesions.
- Phase III: Monthly DCPs are stopped and cyclophosphamide 50 mg daily is continued for another 9 months and then stopped.
- Phase IV: It is the period of observation without medication and patient is kept under follow-up.

Efgartigimod (an engineered Fc fragment that can reduce circulating IgG) has been tried alone/in combination with prednisolone in mild-to-moderate pemphigus vulgaris and pemphigus foliaceus and was found to achieve disease control within 2–41 weeks (Goebeler M, et al., 2022)

Disease Outcome Parameters (Murrell DF et al., 2020)

Some useful terms that help to stratify the disease response are given below.

- **Control of disease activity** (disease control)—time interval from baseline to the time at which new lesions cease to form and established lesions begin to heal.
- **End of the consolidation phase**—no new lesions × 2 weeks and the majority (approximately 80%) of established lesions have healed. Tapering of corticosteroid doses at this point.
- **Complete remission on therapy**—absence of new or established lesions while the patient is receiving minimal therapy (≤10 mg/day of prednisone (or equivalent) and/or minimal adjuvant therapy × 2 months).

BOX 7.7: Rituximab (RTX) in pemphigus

- Initial use—non-Hodgkin B cell lymphoma
- US-FDA approved for pemphigus in June 2018 (also approved for RA, granulomatosis with polyangiitis and microscopic polyangiitis)
- Chimeric murine—human monoclonal antibody against CD20 antigen of B cells (anti-CD20 mAb)
- First biologic to be approved for pemphigus.
- Murrell et al. (JAAD 2020) recommendations—first-line treatment in new onset moderate–severe pemphigus and/or for patients who do not achieve clinical remission with systemic corticosteroids and/or immunosuppressive adjuvants.

Result

- Efficacy—59–100% of patients achieve complete clinical remission after treatment, a mean time to clinical remission of 3–6 months and a median remission duration of 15–19 months. A recent study has noted a 90% remission at 24 months.
- Relapse rates—40% and 81% (depending on the follow-up period) (due to incomplete depletion of the autoreactive clones, long-lived CD20-B cells)
- A PDAI score of 45 or higher (severe pemphigus) and/or persistent anti-DSG 1 antibody values of 20 IU/mL or higher and/or anti-DSG 3 antibody values of 130 IU/mL or higher at 3 months is predictive of relapses [Mignard C]

Mode of action

- CD20 present on all B cells (from pre-B cells to pre-plasma cells) except early pre-B cells, stem cells and plasma cells.
- Leads to up to 90% reduction in B cell counts within 3 days of administration. B cell count remains low for 6 months and returns to baseline by 9–12 months after 4 weekly doses of 375 mg/m^2.

Dose and administration

- 375 mg/m^2 for 4 weeks (lymphoma protocol) or 1 g at interval of 2 weeks [rheumatoid arthritis (RA) protocol] rituximab plus (0.5 or 1.0 mg/kg/day) prednisone tapered over 3 or 6 months. At month 24, 90% achieved complete remission off therapy (Chen et al., 2020). An **ultralow-dose regimen** was described in a recent case series where 2 infusions of 200mg RTX were given 14 days apart. It showed promising results, though relapses were seen with this regimen as well.
- IV infusion over 4–5 hours.
- Premedication—paracetamol, diphenhydramine, intravenous hydrocortisone (1 hr before starting infusion).

Caution

- Immunosuppressive drugs (azathioprine, mycophenolate mofetil, cyclophosphamide, and cyclosporine) are **not** given concomitantly with RTX (except methotrexate).
- **Live vaccine contraindicated, non-live vaccines can be given 4 weeks before RTX administration**. After RTX, vaccination is not recommended sooner than 6 months due to lack of efficacy.
- **Avoid pregnancy** during treatment and for 12 months after the last dose (pregnancy category C).

Maintenance

- In the EU, the recommended maintenance regimen consists of 0.5 g IV infusions at months 12 and 18, and then every 6 months thereafter if needed, based on clinical evaluation.

Adverse effects

- Infusion related- transient fever, headache, nausea, chills, orthostatic hypotension, thrombocytopenia, skin rashes, cardiac arrhythmias.
- Severe cytokine release syndrome—may occur during first infusion
- Infections—more if old age or on concomitant immunosuppression
- Progressive multifocal encephalopathy
- Anemia, thrombocytopenia, neutropenia
- Arrhythmias

- **Complete remission off therapy**—no new and/or established lesions off all systemic therapy × 2 months
- **Relapse/flare**—3 or more new lesions a month that do not heal spontaneously within 1 week, or the extension of established lesions, in a patient who has achieved disease control.
- **Failure of therapy**—failure to control disease activity (i.e. relapse/flare) with full therapeutic doses of systemic treatments.

Course and Prognostic Factors

- Chronic course with average disease duration of 10 years **(Box 7.8)**
- Without steroids—usually fatal and the average mortality was over 73% (because a large portion of the skin loses its epidermal barrier function, leading to the loss of body fluids or to secondary bacterial infections).
- With systemic steroids, it is now 5–15%.
- The most common causes of death are septicemia and pulmonary embolism.

An overview of the latest guidelines of care for pemphigus is given in **Fig. 7.8** (based on JEADV guidelines) (Joly P, 2020).

Scoring Systems

Many systems have been devised to assess severity of pemphigus, but the following two systems have been validated—PDAI **(Fig. 7.9)** and ABSIS **(Table 7.12)**.

PDAI

The PDAI has a total possible score ranging from 0–263, with 250 points representing disease activity and 13 points representing damage.

Extent of pemphigus according to PDAI is as follows (Boulard et al., 2016):

Moderate: 0–15 points

Significant: 15–45

Extensive: >45

ABSIS

The ABSIS has a total posible score of 0–206.

Extent of pemphigus according to ABSIS is as follows (Boulard C, 2016):

Moderate: 0–17 points

Significant: 17–53 points

Extensive: >53 points

BOX 7.8: Prognostic factors*

- Type of pemphigus
- Age of the patient at the time of disease onset (younger is better)
- Initial involvement of mucosa or skin (mucosa has a protracted course)
- Time of institution of therapy (<6 months of onset is better)
- Disease progression before beginning therapy
- Dose of steroids required to control the disease
- Initial dose of prednisolone (<1 mg/kg/day)
- Titre of Dsg antibodies

*Notably not all studies concur on these factors.

Mild pemphigus foliaceous

1st line

- **Dapsone:** 50–100 mg/day (1.5 mg/kg/day)
- **Topical corticosteroids:** Class III and IV
- **Systemic corticosteroids:** Prednisone 0.5–1.0 mg/kg/day
- **Rituximab:** 2 infusions of 1 g 2 weeks apart, alone, or associated with topical corticosteroids or oral prednisone 0.5 mg/kg/day

2nd line

- **Rituximab:** 2 infusions of 1 g 2 weeks apart, alone, or associated with topical corticosteroids or oral prednisone 0.5 mg/kg/day
- **Systemic corticosteroids + ISA:** Azathioprine (1–2.5 mg/kg/day), or mycophenolate mofetil 2 g/day or mycophenolate sodium 1440 mg/day

Mild pemphigus vulgaris

1st line

- **Rituximab:** 2 infusions of 1 g 2 weeks apart, alone, or associated with oral prednisone 0.5 mg/kg/day tapering of steroids to stop then after 6 months with rapid
- **Systemic corticosteroids + ISA:** Azathioprine (1–2.5 mg/kg/day), or mycophenolate mofetil 2 g/day or mycophenolate sodium 1440 mg/day

Control achieved
Taper prednisolone
in 3–4 months

Disease control not achieved
or
Side effects

2nd line

- **If treated with prednisone/ prednisolone alone:** Add rituximab (2 infusions of 1 g 2 weeks apart) with a rapid decrease of oral prednisolone in order to stop corticosteroids after 3 or 4 months
- **If treated with prednisone/prednisolone 0.5–1.0 mg/kg/day plus rituximab:** ↑ the dose of prednisone up to 1 mg/kg/day

Moderate/severe pemphigus vulgaris

1st line

- **Rituximab:** 2 infusions of 1 g 2 weeks apart, alone, or associated oral prednisone 1 mg/kg/day with a rapid decrease in order to stop corticosteroids after 6 months
- **Systemic corticosteroids + ISA:** Azathioprine (1–2.5 mg/kg/day), OR mycophenolate mofetil 2 g/day or mycophenolate sodium 1440 mg/day

Control achieved
3–4 weeks
Continue Rx

Disease control not achieved
OR
Side effects

2nd line

- **If treated with prednisone/prednisolone alone:** (1.0 mg/kg/d): ↑prednisone dose to 1.5 mg/kg/d + add rituximab (2 × 1 g) or add ISA
- **If treated with prednisone (1.5 mg/kg/day) alone:** Add rituximab (2 × 1 g) or add ISA
- **If treated with rituximab and prednisone:** ↑prednisone dose up to 1.5 mg/kg/day or intravenous corticosteroid pulses

Maintenance treatment

At 6 months
- **Rituximab 500 mg or 1 g:** In patients in CR on/off treatment and initially presented with a severe pemphigus and/or still have a high rate of anti-Dsg antibodies at 3 months
- **Rituximab 2 g (2 infusions of 1 g 2 weeks apart):** Without **CR** on/off therapy

12 and 18 months
- **Rituximab 500 mg:** In CR on/off therapy (in particular in patients with persistently positive anti-desmoglein antibodies)

Fig. 7.8: Guidelines for the management of pemphigus vulgaris (Joly P, 2020)

***Mild pemphigus**—PF with BSA <5%, PV with BSA <5% + limited oral lesions, PDAI ≤15.
Moderate and **severe pemphigus**—multiple mucosae, oral lesions with dysphagia, skin lesions >5% BSA, PDAI 15–45 (moderate) and >45 (severe).

Skin	Activity		Damage
Anatomical location	Erosion/Blisters or new erythema		Post-inflammatory hyperpigmentation or erythema from resolving lesion
	0. Absent 1. 1–3 lesions, up to one >2 cm in any diameter, none >6 cm 2. 2–3 lesions, at least two >2 cm diameter, none >6 cm 3. >3 lesions, none >6 cm diameter 5. >3 lesions, and/or at least one lesion 10. >lesions, and/or at least one lesion >16 cm diameter or entire area	Number of lesions if ≤3	0. Absent 1. Present
Ears			
Nose			
Rest of the face			
Neck			
Chest			
Abdomen			
Back, buttocks			
Arms			
Hands			
Legs			
Feet			
Genitals			
Total skin	**/120**		**/12**
Scalp			
Scalp	Erosion/Blisters or new erythema		Post-inflammatory hyperpigmentation or erythema from resolving lesion
	0. Absent 1. In one quadrant 2. Two quadrants 3. Three quadrants 4. Affects whole skull 10. At least one lesion >6 cm	Number of lesions if ≤3	0. Absent 1. Present
Total scalp (0–10)	**/10**		**/1**
Mucous membrane			
Anatomical location	Erosion/Blisters		
	0. Absent 1. 1 lesion 2. 2–3 lesions 5. >3 lesions or 2 lesions >2 cm 10. Entire area	Number of lesions if ≤3	
Ears			
Nose			
Buccal mucosa			
Hard palate			
Soft palate			
Upper gingiva			
Lower gingiva			
Tongue			
Floor of mouth			
Labial bucosa			
Posterior pharynx			
Anogenital			
Total mucosa	**/120**		

Total activity score:

Total damage score:

Fig. 7.9: Pemphigus disease area index (PDAI)

TABLE 7.12: Autoimmune bullous skin disorder intensity score (ABSIS)

Body site of involvement		Parameters assessed by ABSIS
Skin involvement (150 points)		1. Extent (percent of BSA involvement): Score—0–100% 2. Weighting factor (measuring quality of lesions as a multiplier of value for) • Bullae, erosions: Factor 1.5 • Dry erosions: Factor 1.0 • Re-epithelialized erosions: Factor 0.5 Total score: % BSA × weighting factor = 0–150 points
Oral involvement (two independent scores) (11 points and 45 points, recpectively)	Mucosal score 1	Extent (presence of lesions on defined sites): Score: 0–11 points
	Mucosal score 2	Severity (discomfort during eating/drinking): Score: 0–45 points

In the ABSIS and PDAI, skin but not mucosal subscores correlate with the evolution of anti-Dsg1 and anti-Dsg3 ELISA values, respectively. Thus, these are robust tools to accurately assess pemphigus activity.

SUBEPIDERMAL IMMUNOBULLOUS DISEASES

An overview of the antigens is shown in **Table 7.13** and **Fig. 7.10**.

BULLOUS PEMPHIGOID

Epidemiology

- Bullous pemphigoid (BP) is the most common autoimmune subepidermal blistering disease of elderly people. Incidence of BP increases with age.
- Again, the affected age group is younger in Indian patients.
- HLADQB1*0301, DRB1*04, DRB1*1101, and DQB1*0302.

TABLE 7.13: Target antigens and antibodies in subepidermal immunobullous disorders

Conditions	Antigens	Antibodies	DIF	Binding to salt-split skin
Bullous pemphigoid (BP)	• **BP180 NC16A/ collagen** XVII • BP230/BPAG1	IgG (BP180-IgE in more severe disease)	Linear BMZ	Epidermal (few dermal)
Gestational pemphigoid	• **BP180 NC16A** • BP230/BPAG1	IgG	Linear BMZ	Epidermal
Mucous membrane pemphigoid	• **BP180/BPAG2** (C terminal) • **BP230/BPAG1** • **Laminin 332,** (Laminin 5) • Laminin 311# (Laminin 6) • $\alpha_6\beta_4$ integrin (both subunits) • Type VII collagen	IgG, IgA (severe d/s)	Linear BMZ	Epidermal ($\alpha_6\beta_4$ integrin), few dermal (Laminin 332)
Linear IgA bullous dermatosis (LABD)	• **LAD-1 antigen** • BP230/BPAG1 • Type VII collagen	IgA	Linear BMZ	Epidermal (majority) Dermal (minority)
Anti-p200/ laminin γ1 pemphigoid	• **p200 antigen** • **Laminin γ1 (C terminal)**	IgG	Linear BMZ	Dermal
Epidermolysis bullosa acquisita	**Type VII collagen**	IgG	Linear BMZ	Dermal
Bullous SLE	• Type I: Type VII collagen • Type II: BP180, BP230, laminin 332	IgG, IgA	Linear and granular BMZ	Dermal
Lichen planus pemphigoides	• **BP180 NC16A** • BP230	IgG/C3	Linear BMZ	Epidermal
Cicatricial pemphigoid	BP180, BP230, laminin 332	IgG	Linear BMZ	Epidermal/dermal
Dermatitis herpetiformis	Epidermal tissue Transglutaminase	IgG	Granular dermal papillae	Negative

BPAG1e = Epithelial isoform of BPAG1, another term for BP230.
#Laminin 311 shares the α3 chain with Laminin 332 and is co-targated.

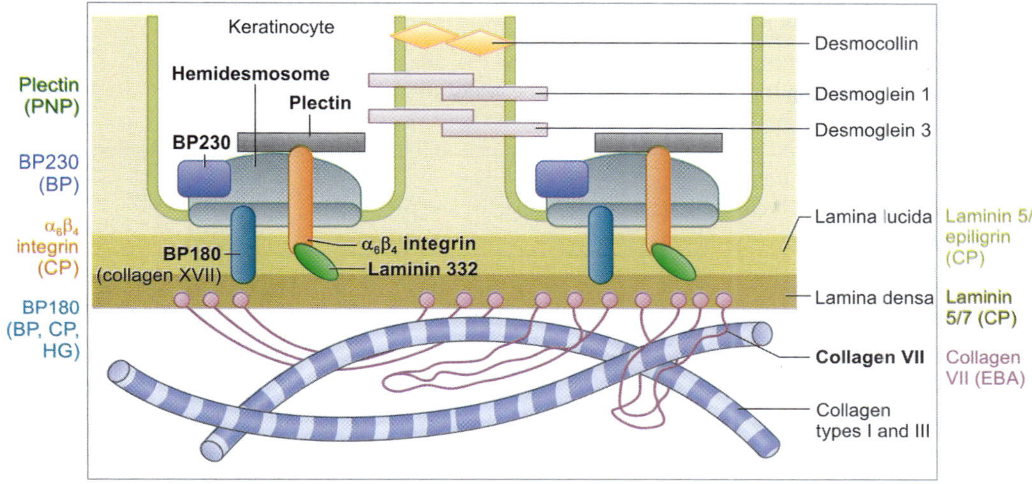

Fig. 7.10: A depiction of the hemidesmosome and BMZ with emphasis on the target antigens in the various structures of the BMZ. The major disorders are listed in brackets with the target antigen

Pathogenesis

- **Antigens:**
  BP180/type XVII collagen/BPAG2 (in 75–90%) and BP230/BPAG1 (in 50–70%)
  - Immunodominant region of BP180—**extracellular portion of the 16th noncollagenous domain (NC16A)** located directly adjacent to the cellular membrane.
    (explains why antibodies to both BP180 and BP230 can be seen in a significant portion of the population without blister formation as these are not against the critical NC16A region of BP180)
  - BP230 (BPAG1): 230 kDa cytoplasmic plaque protein belonging to plakin family; not the primary mediator of BP → antibodies are formed as a secondary phenomenon (epitope spreading)
- **Antibodies: IgG4, IgG1**, also IgE and IgA
- Autoreactive T cells in BP patients produce a Th1/Th2 mixed cytokine profile. Th2 type cytokines are important in human BP. Th17 also plays a role.
- **IgE-anti-BP180 NC16A antibodies**—Circulating IgE against NC16A BP180- seen in 77% of BP sera; Linear deposits of IgE autoantibodies along the DEJ - seen in 41% BP patients. IgE antibodies against the BP180 NC16A are believed to parallel disease activity. High levels of circulating BP180 NC16A IgE and total IgE in serum correlate with higher BPDAI scores (van Beek, 2017). However, there is probably no correlation between serum anti-BP 180 IgE autoantibodies and any specific clinical subtype of BP.
- **Complement activation and mast cell activation—crucial** for neutrophil and macrophage chemotaxis at the DEJ.
- The summary of pathogenesis of BP is depicted in **Fig. 7.11** (*see* **Box 7.9** for key).

Predisposing Factors

- Trauma, burns, skin grafting, radiotherapy
- UV radiation—sunlight, PUVA, PDT
- Influenza vaccination—doubtful role

BOX 7.9: Pathogenesis of BP

1. Binding of autoantibodies against BP180 initiates the cascade.
2. Secretion of interleukin **IL-6** and **IL-8** from basal keratinocytes.
3. Internalization and decreased expression of **BP180** on keratinocytes.
4. **Complement is** activated at the dermal–epidermal junction (DEJ) with **mast cell** degranulation.
5. Inflammatory cells infiltrate into upper dermis.
6. Granulocytes at the DEJ release reactive oxygen species and proteases.
7. Tissue damage and dermal–epidermal separation ensue eventually.

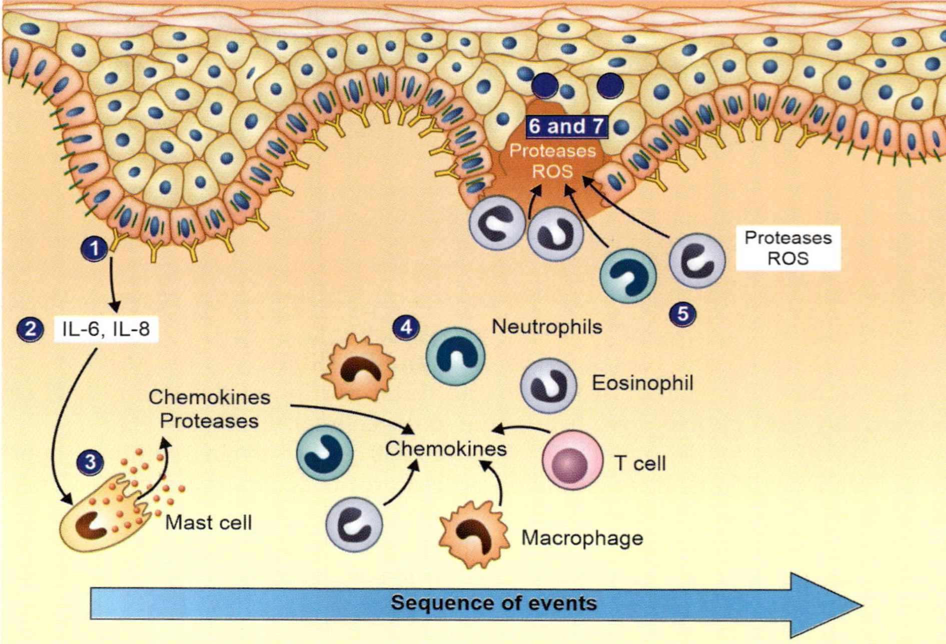

Fig. 7.11: Sequence of events in the pathogenesis of BP (please *see* accompanying text in **Box 7.9**)

- Drugs—**furosemide, spironolactone, phenothiazines,** other loop diuretics, penicillin, ampicillin, penicillamine, ciprofloxacin, potassium iodide, ACE inhibitors, antidiabetics (**dipeptidyl peptidase IV inhibitor—gliptins)**, sulfonamides, clonidine, diclofenac, ibuprofen and practolol, topical anthralin, 5-FU and benzyl benzoate. Usually transient, often localized and generally disappear after discontinuation of the drug. **Box 7.10** summarizes important facts related to gliptin-induced BP.

Clinical Features

The diagnosis is based on certain criterion that inlcude:

1. Age older than 70 years
2. Absence of atrophic scars;
3. Absence of mucosal involvement, and
4. Absence of predominant bullous lesions on the neck and head.

BOX 7.10: Gliptin-induced BP

DPP-4i are significantly associated with BP. The postulated mechanisms include:

a. Inhibition of DPP4 (CO26) on keratinocytes and T cells can increase activity of proinflammatory cytokines.
b. Inhibition of plasmin formation by DPP4 may lead to inappropriate cleavage of NC16A of BP180 (usually cleaved by plasmin) and exposure of epitopes.
c. Inhibition of DPP4 induces the infiltration of eosinophils into the skin through eotoxin (CCL11).

The latency period ranges from 1–48 months.

Vildagliptin has been reported as the most common DPP4i associated with BP. This could be due to the large market share of this drug among the gliptins and its lower selectivity for DPP4 leading to inhibition of DPP8 and DPP9 and subsequent activation of the caspase-1 pathway and triggering of BP. Early cessation of the inciting drug is believed by some authors to lead to rapid improvement/cessation of the disease process. However, the role of gliptins has not been conclusively proven and the effect of cessation of gliptin treatment on the clinical outcome BP remains currently unclear, but a switch of the antidiabetic drug class may be considered in such cases.

- The cutaneous manifestations of BP can be extremely polymorphic.
- Prodromal nonbullous phase—lasts for weeks–months. **Pruritus** (mild to intractable) typical. Excoriations, excoriated papules, eczematous lesions, **urticarial lesions**, hemorrhagic crusts.
- Bullous phase—tense vesicles and bullae arise on erythematous and on normal skin. The blisters are dome-shaped with clear fluid and occasionally hemorrhagic or filled with thick fibrinous fluid **(Fig. 7.12)**. Pruritus present. Nikolsky sign is negative. May persist for several days, leaving eroded and crusted areas and heal with residual post-inflammatory changes including hyper- and hypopigmentation and, occasionally, milia. No scarring unless secondarily infected. The most common of involvement are the lower abdomen, inner thighs, groin and the flexor aspects of the limbs. Mucosal lesions occur less frequently (10–20%).
  - **Childhood BP:** 2 peaks— < 1 year (infantile BP) and 8–9 years.
    - Only about 80 cases of BP in children and adolescents have been described.
    - In some children at least, the IgG subclasses differ from adult disease, consisting of all IgG subclasses or IgG2 in isolation. IgE antibodies are not a feature of childhood disease.
    - Infantile—linked to vaccination, often acral, in particular palms and soles.
    - Childhood—face and genital lesions in 50%.
    - Good prognosis overall. Remission within weeks–months.
    - Treatment: Dapsone/sulfapyridine +/– corticosteroids.

Clinical Variants

Localized BP: Mostly on lower legs—pretibial. Other areas too can have localized lesions. Also around stomata and hemodialysis fistulae. May develop into classical BP later or may remain localized.

BP may also start with **nonclassical lesions in 20%**.

Variants of BP include:

- Dyshidrosiform
- Prurigo nodularis-like/pemphigoid nodularis
- Erythrodermic
- Toxic epidermal necrolysis-like
- Lymphomatoid papulosis-like

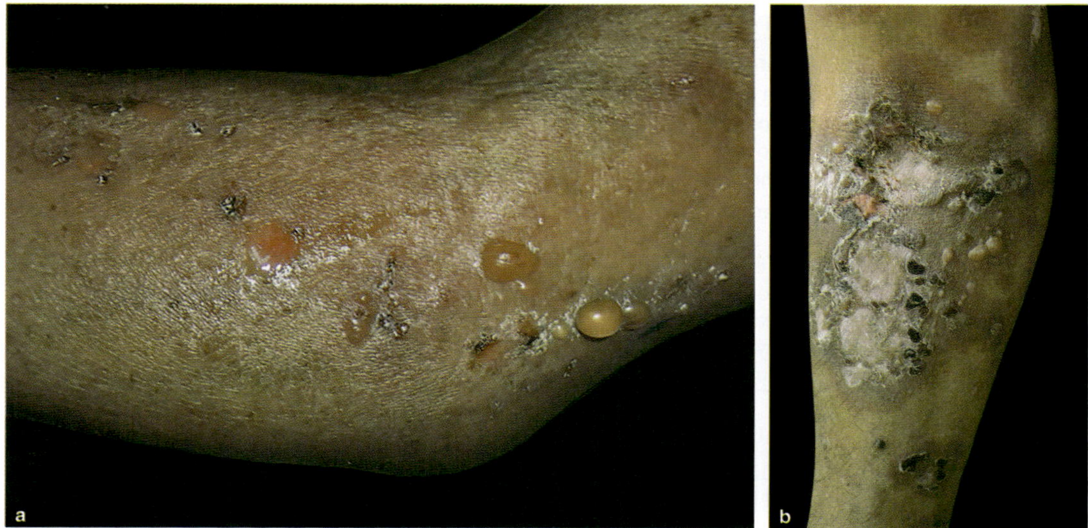

Fig. 7.12: Urticarial plaques with superimposed tense bullae in bullous pemphigoid

- Vegetating/pemphigoid vegetans
- Vesicular pemphigoid
- Ecthyma gangrenosum-like/intertrigo-like/papular/eczematous
- Anti-p105 pemphigoid: Also known as **deep lamina lucida** (anti-p105) pemphigoid which presents as extensive bullae and erosions on mucous membranes and skin resembling toxic epidermal necrolysis or pemphigus vulgaris.
  Target antigen: **105 kDa protein**
  Salt-split skin: IgG binding to dermal side.
- Anti-p450 pemphigoid has been documented in a single patient. The antigen, which has been localized to the basal keratinocyte, belongs to the plectin family.

Differential Diagnosis

- Mucous membrane pemphigoid (MMP)—predominant involvement of mucosal surfaces.
- Linear IgA disease, EBA and anti-p200/laminin γ1 pemphigoid-DIF (for linear IgA disease) and serological analyses (for the latter two entities).
- Dermatitis herpetiformis—DIF, and the serological profile (anti-transglutaminase 1 and 2 as well as antigliadin IgA antibodies).
- Bullous arthropod bites, allergic contact dermatitis, Stevens-Johnson syndrome, bullous drug eruptions, porphyria-histopathology, DIF.
- Inflammatory cell-rich variant of bullous pemphigoid must be distinguished from other subepidermal blistering dermatoses in which a heavy inflammatory cell component is a typical finding **(Table 7.14)**.
- In the non-bullous prodromal stage or in atypical presentations, BP can closely resemble a variety of dermatoses including localized or generalized drug reactions, contact and allergic dermatitis, prurigo, urticaria, urticarial vasculitis, arthropod reactions, scabies, or even pityriasis lichenoides.

TABLE 7.14: Differential diagnosis of cell-rich pemphigoid

Investigations	BP	EBA	BSLE	LAD	DH
DIF	Linear IgG	C3 Linear IgG	C3 Linear IgG	C3 Linear IgA	Granular IgA
IIF	IgG antibodies 75–80%	IgG antibodies 25–50%	IgG antibodies 60%	IgA antibodies 30%	Antitransglutaminase antibodies
Split skin IMF	Roof	Floor	Floor	Roof or floor or both	N/A
EM: Site of split	LL	Sub-LD	Sub-LD	LL, sub-LD or both	Papillary dermis
Western blot	BP180 (180 kDa) BP230 (230 kDa)	290 kDa (type VII collagen)	290 kDa (type VII collagen)	BP180 BP230 200/280 kDa 285 kDa 250 kDa 290 kDa	Antigen uncertain

LL = Lamina lucida, LD = Lamina densa.

Associated Disorders

- Neurological/psychiatric:
  - In one-third to one-half of all patients of BP
  - Cognitive impairment, Parkinson disease, stroke, epilepsy, multiple sclerosis, uni- and bipolar disorders (BP180 and BP230 antigens also expressed in CNS).
- Psoriasis
- Hematological cancers, gastric cancer
- Pulmonary infections and embolism—three times higher risk
- Autoimmune disorders—inflammatory bowel disease, Hashimoto's thyroiditis, rheumatoid arthritis, dermatomyositis, and lupus erythematosus.

  Certain important points that should be elicited in history are detailed below:
  - History of neurological disorders (multiple sclerosis, Parkinson's disease, dementia and stroke).
  - Drugs-(drug intake usually within the 6 months prior to the development of symptoms). The common drugs implicated include diuretics in particular aldosterone antagonists, dipeptidyl peptidase 4 inhibitors, anticholinergics and dopaminergic medications.

    Vildagliptin and linagliptin and immune checkpoint inhibitors are significantly associated with and might cause BP **(Box 7.10)**.
  - Evaluate the impact of BP on patients' quality of life related to the BP lesions.

Investigations

Apart from histology, antibody detection either in the skin or in the blood are used for diagnosis **(Fig. 7.13)**. In the rare cases of BP in which circulating anti-BMZ antibodies are not detectable by either IIF microscopy studies or commercially available ELISA, additional tests can be used to increase the diagnostic sensitivity and to exclude another autoimmune disease like anti-p200 pemphigoid or epidermolysis bullosa acquisita (EBA).

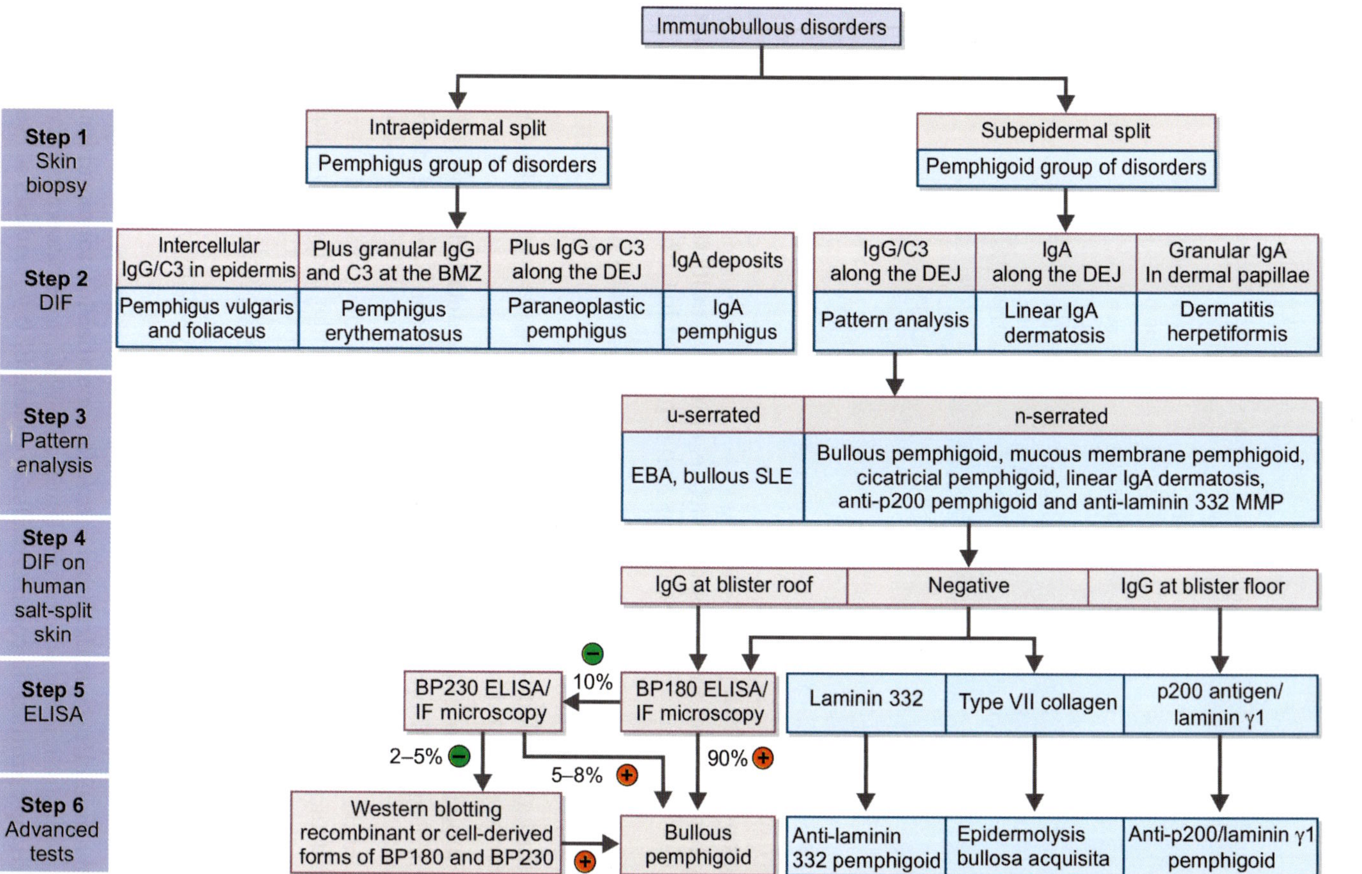

Fig. 7.13: Approach to diagnosis of autoimmune bullous disorders

While binding signals by DIF appear to be mainly due to anti-BP180 antibodies, signals by DIF on esophagus and salt split skin correlate with anti-BP230 antibodies.

1. **Histopathology:** A subepidermal blister containing eosinophils and/or neurophils with a dense eosinophil-rich infiltrate in papillary dermis. Also includes neutrophils, macrophages and T lymphocytes. Margination of eosinophils along the DEJ.
   - If the biopsy is taken from an established blister, the changes are most often those of an inflammatory (cell-rich) variant.
   - A typical finding in bullous pemphigoid is retention of the dermal papillary outline (festooning) which projects into the vesicle cavity.
   - Cell-poor (noninflammatory) features are occasionally seen, if biopsies are taken from lesions arising on non-inflamed skin.
   - Neutrophil dermal papillary microabscesses—may be seen in the vesicular variant.
2. **DIF for tissue bound autoantibodies:** Perilesional uninvolved skin (the biopsy is to be taken form either perilesional erythematous skin 1–2 cm away from an active bullae or from perilesional normal-appearing skin) linear, continuous deposits of IgG (90%) (IgG4 and IgG1) and/or C3 (100%) (sometimes IgE and IgA) along the DEJ. For transportation, skin biopsy specimens should be put either in a 0.9% NaCl solution, into a cryotube in liquid nitrogen or in Michel's fixative.
   - Patients with *in vivo* IgE deposition in the BMZ-Higher Bullous Pemphigoid Disease Area Index (BPDAI) scores took longer to reduce their erosion/blister BPDAI score by 75% after systemic corticosteroid treatment (Kamata A).
   - BP180-specific IgE levels in serum were higher among patients with linear IgE deposition in the BMZ than in those with granular or no IgE deposition.
   - Higher magnification and thinner sections (4 µm)—IgG deposition appears serrated with arches closed at the top ("**n-serrated**") pattern. Mostly correlate with anti-BP180 antibodies.
   - Examination of serration pattern (n-serrated *vs* u-serrated) on standard DIF can be used in lieu of this technique **(Box 7.11)**.
   - Other tests: Salt split DIF and advanced tests like fluorescence overlay antigen mapping (FOAM), double IF labeling—differentiate BP from anti-laminin 332 pemphigoid, anti-p200 pemphigoid and EBA.
3. **Tests for serum autoantibodies:** Circulating autoantibodies can be detected by:
   i. Indirect IF microscopy (IIF), salt-split human skin in a commercial IF BIOCHIP™ mosaic
   ii. Immunoelectron microscopy (IEM)
   iii. Commercial ELISA systems
   iv. Various in-house ELISA, immunoblotting and immunoprecipitation analyses using cell derived or recombinant forms of BP180 and BP230
      - **IIF:** Monkey esophagus—60–75% sensitivity and with salt-split human skin—70–95% sensitivity. Epidermal/roof binding in BP.
      - **IIF** levels do not correlate well with BP disease activity (unlike IIF for PV)

BOX 7.11: Serration patterns in subepidermal blistering diseases

n-serrated linear DIF pattern: BP, linear IgA, MMP, anti-p200 pemphigoid
u-serrated linear DIF pattern: EBA, bullous SLE

- The **salt-split skin** demonstrates—immune deposits in the epidermal side (roof).
  - **Technique:** First use 1M NaCl to split the biopsied skin specimen at lamina lucida → examine with DIF for *in vivo* bound antibodies → determine which side of blister (roof *vs* floor) the antibodies are bound to.
  - Enables differentiation of BP (roof staining) from/"floor-staining" blistering diseases (mainly EBA).
  - The antibodies in pemphigoid variants (with the exception of the anti-p105 and anti-p200 variants) bind to the epidermal side of 1 M NaCl—split-skin, whereas those of inflammatory epidermolysis bullosa and bullous systemic lupus erythematosus bind to the floor.

BIOCHIP® mosaic: IF test allowing simultaneous analysis of several substrates—monkey esophagus, salt-split skin, BP180 NC16A, C-terminal stretch of BP230, Dsg 3, Dsg1 in a single incubation field.

4. **ELISA:** Antigen detection can be done but less frequently employed compared to pemphigus. It is recommended to perform first an ELISA for anti-BP180 IgG, and, if negative, for anti-BP230 IgG. A value of ELISA-BP180 value of <27 U/mL (which is less than two times the upper limit) at day 150 has a good negative predictive value, implying a probability of durable remission of around 90%.
5. **Baseline investigations for initiating therapy** (same as those explained in pemphigus section) **(Table 7.9)**.

Treatment

An overview of the treatment is given in **Table 7.15** and salient definitions are given below (Murrell DF et al., 2012):

Control of disease activity: Time at which new BP lesions cease to form and establised lesions begin to heal/pruritus begins to abate.

End of consolidation phase: Time at which no new lesions for ≥2 weeks and approximately 80% lesions have healed and pruritus is minimal.

Minimal theory: ≤0.1 mg/kg/day prednisolone (or equivalent) or ≤20 g/week clobetasol propionate and/or minimal adjuvant (methotrexate 5 mg/week, azathioprine 0.7 mg/kg/day, MMF 500 mg/day, dapsone 50 mg/day).

Complete remission off theory: No new/establised lesions or pruritus off all BP therapy for at least 2 months.

Relapse/flare: ≥3 new lesions/month or ≥1 large (>10 cm diameter) eczematous/urticarial plaque that do not heal within 1 week, or extension of establised lesions, or daily pruritus in a patient who achieved disease control.

Recent Advances in Therapy

As typical Th2 cytokines, IL-4 and IL-13 contribute to the pathogenesis of BP in multiple ways, such as promoting Th2 cell polarization, driving the immunoglobulin class switching, recruiting eosinophils and basophils, and inducing pruritus it seems that targetting these would be a useful approach in BP.

1. **Biologics in treatment of BP (Cao et al., 2022):** A recent systemic review evaluated rituximab, omalizumab and dupilumab is BP. The findings are summarized below in **Box 7.12**.

   Of these drugs we will focus on Omalizumab as it is often combined with existing therapies. While the role of immunoglobulin E (IgE) antibodies in BP has been studied since the 1970s,

TABLE 7.15: Management algorithm for BP (Borradori et al., 2022)

Mild and moderate BP (BPDAI score <20 and BPDAI score ≥20 <57 respectively)

- **First** choice
  - In localized BP, apply potent or super potent topical corticosteroids on lesions only
  - In nonlocalized mild and moderate BP
    - Superpotent topical corticosteroids applied twice or once a day, on whole body except the face (up to 30–40 g/day)
    - Oral corticosteroids, at an initial dose of **0.5 mg/kg/day** predisone or prednisolone.
- **Second** choice
  - Doxycycline (dose is 200 mg /day and treatment success in 6 weeks was 54%)
  - Dapsone (1.5 mg/kg/day orally, up to a maximum of 150 mg/day)

Severe BP (BPDAI score ≥57)

First choice

- Superpotent topical corticosteroids, twice or once a day, on whole body (except the face), or
- Oral corticosteroids at an initial dose of oral prednisone **0.5 mg/kg/day***
  - *Note*: In patients who do not achieve disease control within 1–3 weeks with 0.5 mg/kg prednisone, two options may be considered:
    - to increase the dose of prednisone up to **0.75 mg/kg**
    - to add superpotent topical corticosteroids

Corticosteroid-dependent or relapsing BP

- Alternative choices as adjunctive therapy:
  - Combination with or introduction of a coventional immunosuppressive drug
    - Methotrexate (10–12.5 mg weekly)
    - Azathioprine (1–3 mg/kg/day)
    - Mycophenolate [(mycophenolate mofetil 2 g/day, mycophenolic acid 1.44 g/day orally)]
- In patients with contraindications to immunosuppresive drugs
  - Doxycycline
  - Dapsone
  - Omalizumab

Treatment-recalcitrant BP (resistant to 0.75 mg/kg/day of prednisone)

- Combination with and/or introduction of conventional immunosuppressants may be considered
  - Methotrexate
  - Azathioprine
  - Mycophenolate mofetil
- Other therapeutic options, which have not been validated in this setting, may be considered (without any prioritization)
  - Rituximab [beneficial effect of rituximab in BP seems <u>lower</u> than in pemphigus in terms of control of disease activity, clinical remission and relapse risk.]
  - Omalizumab (omalizumab may be considered with urticarial inflammatory lesions and high eosinophil and/or serum IgE levels. Dose varies-usual dose is 300 mg/month) **(Fig. 7.14)**
  - Dupilumab
  - Intravenous immunoglobulins (2 g/kg/day)
  - Immunoadsorption

Experimental Drugs

New therapeutic approaches, including blockade of IL-17, IL-12/IL-23, IL-5R alpha, eotaxin, neonatal Fc receptor and LTB4/C5aR

*Steroids can be tapered down to 0.1mg/kg/day which is maintained for 3–6 months and stopped gradually with a total duration of 9–12 months. Total treatment duration including consolidation phase and maintenance treatment is usually between 9 and 12 months.

BOX 7.12: Treatment outcomes with biologics in BP (Cao et al., 2022)

Outcome	Rituximab (n = 122)	Omalizumab (n = 53)	Dupilumab (n = 36)
Complete remission	70.5%	67.9%	66.7%
Average time to remission	5.7 months	6.6 months	**4.5 months**
Recurrence rate	**20.5%**	5.7%	5.6%
Most common adverse effect	Infections	Thrombocytopenia	—

of late there is an increased focus on anti-IgE therapies. A recent reveiw analysed papers on Omalizumab and the vast majority of patients showed varying degrees of improvement after treatment, except for a small number of patients with poor clinical outcomes. Importantly the dosing regimens were variable and dosing frequency had little effect on clinical efficacy with no correlation between the number of doses and clinical efficacy (LingX, 2023).

2. **JAK ib:** A recent paper examined the expression pattern of JAKs and found that patients with DH may benefit especially from targeted JAK3 inhibition. Inhibiting JAK3/STAT3 pathway may result in decreased IL-8 transcription, decreased Th17 cell differentiation, and hence impaired IL-17 production, as well as defective IL-6 signaling. In BP patients, inhibiting JAK2 and JAK3 signaling would result in impaired IL-4, IL-5, and IFN-γ signaling and disrupted IL-17 production. This explains the published cases of upadacitinib and tofacitinib in BP (Juczynska K, 2017).

Box 7.13 summarizes the *prognostic factors* and *severity* and *activity* markers in BP.

The severity score indices are depicted in **Fig. 7.15**.

BOX 7.13: Prognostic factors and markers for severity and activity in BP

Prognosis
- Chronic self-limiting disease
- Relapses frequent in half patients within first 3 months after cessation of therapy (especially if extensive disease, dementia, BP180 Ab)
- Disease duration 3–6 years
- First year mortality rates—10–40%

Risk factors for lethal outcome
- Old age (>80 years)
- Extensive disease
- High doses of prednisolone (>35 mg/day)
- Serum albumin levels <3.6 g/dL
- Karnofsky (performance scale) score of ≤40
- The presence of heart disease, diabetes, or neurological diseases

Severity markers
- BPDAI score (≥57)
- Mucosal involvement
- High concentration of proteins secreted from eosinophils in blister fluid [eosinophil cationic protein (ECP) and major basic protein (MBP)], eosinophil-derived neurotoxin, tryptase levels in blister.
- Eosinophil count in peripheral blood
- D-dimer in serum and blister fluid

Activity markers
- Cytokines (IL-5 and CD-30, IL-31, IL-1β and TNF-α, IL-36, IL-17)
- Chemokines (eotaxin 1 and 3)
- Serum level of soluble CD23
- NLRP3 inflammasome components
- Lactate dehydrogenase and high-mobility group-1 protein in blister fluid
- High heat shock protein (Hsp)-90 in epidermis

(Contd.)

BOX 7.13: Prognostic factors and markers for severity and activity in BP (*Contd.*)

Both activity and severity markers

- IgG and IgE antibody titer against BP180 NC16A
- IL-17, IL-23

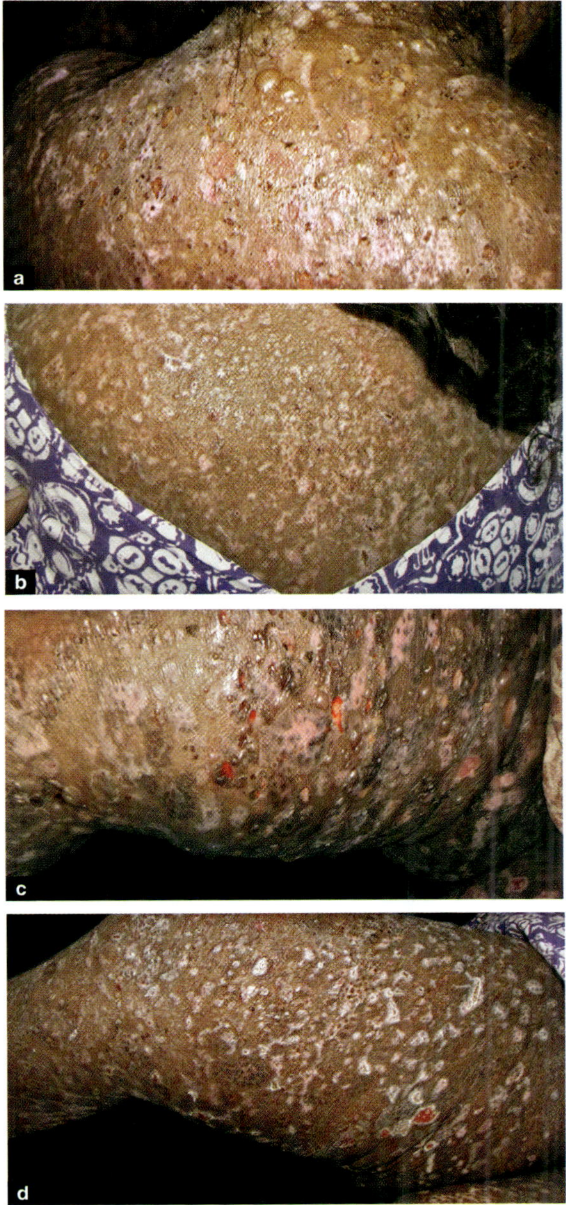

Fig. 7.14: A patient with extensive active BP with multiple tense bullae on the upper back (a) and thigh (c) who achieved rapid control with a single dose of omalizumab (b and d) (*Courtesy*: Surabhi Sinha)

BPDAI Pruritus Component – VAS

Date: ....

☐ Baseline	☐ Beginning consolidation
☐ Consolidation phase	☐ End of consolidation
☐ Tapering phase	☐ Partial remission on minimal therapy
☐ Complete remission on minimal therapy	☐ Partial remission off therapy
☐ Complete remission off therapy	☐ Flare

A. How severe has your itching been over the last 24 hours?

0 1 2 3 4 5 6 7 8 9 10

None Severe

Score out of 10 = ☐

B. How severe has your itching been the past week?

0 1 2 3 4 5 6 7 8 9 10

None Severe

Score out of 10 = ☐

C. How severe has your itching been in the past month?

0 1 2 3 4 5 6 7 8 9 10

None Severe

Score out of 10 = ☐

Average: Intensity score for past month = (A + B + C) = /30

Or

For BP patients with impaired mental functioning:

	No evidence of itch (no excoriations)	0
	Mild itch (isolated excoriations up to two body sites)	10
	Moderate itch (excoriations on ≥3 body sites, impairment of daily activity)	20
	Severe itch (generalized excoriation, sleep impairment)	30
	Total score	**/30**

Fig. 7.15a: Subjective BPDAI (with pruritus VAS score)

BPDAI					
Skin	**Activity**		**Activity**		**Damage**
Anatomical location	Erosion/Blisters	Number of lesions if ≤3	Urticaria/Erythema/other	Number of lesions if ≤3	Pigmentation/ other
	0. Absent		0. Absent		Absent 0, present 1
	1. 1–3 lesions, none >1 cm diameter		1. 1–3 lesions, none >6 cm diameter		
	2. 1–3 lesions, at least one >1 cm diameter		2. 1–3 lesions, at least one lesions, >6 cm diameter		
	3. >3 lesions, none >2 cm diameter		3. >3 lesions, or at least one lesion >10 cm		
	5. >3 lesions, and at least one >2 cm		5. >3 lesions, and at least one lesion >25 cm		
	10. >3 lesions, and at least one lesion >5 cm diameter or entire area		10. >3 lesions, and at least one lesion >50 cm diameter or entire area		
Head					
Neck					
Chest					
Left arm					
Right arm					
Hands					
Abdomen					
Genitalis					
Back/Buttocks					
Left leg					
Right leg					
Feet					
Total skin	**/120**		**/120**		

Mucosa					
	Erosion/Blisters				
	1. 1 lesion				
	2. 2–3 lesions				
	5. >3 lesions or 2 lesions >2 cm				
	10. Entire area				
Eye					
Nose					
Buccal mucosa					
Hard palate					
Soft palate					
Upper gingiva					
Lower gingiva					
Tongue					
Floor of mouth					
Labial mucosa					
Posterior pharynx					
Anogenital					
Total mucosa	**/120**		**/120**		

Fig. 7.15b: Objective BPDAI

MUCOUS MEMBRANE PEMPHIGOID

Epidemiology

- **Oral cavity (85%) >conjunctival** (65%) >nasopharynx, skin (25–30%), anogenital area, larynx, esophagus
- Late middle—old age
- Females > males.

Cicatricial pemphigoid—mucous membranes are not predominantly affected and skin lesions heal with scarring (earlier MMP and cicatricial pemphigoid were used synonymously).

Target antigens and autoantibodies:

- **Target antigens—BPAG2, BPAG1 (75%), laminin 332 (20–25%), $\alpha_6\beta_4$ integrin (both subunits), type VII collagen**
- Serum autoantibodies in low titers, therefore 50% patients have negative IIF on salt-split skin.

Three subgroups of target antigens:

- **Anti-epiligrin MMP:** Target = **laminin 332** (laminin 5, epiligrin); two-thirds cases, salt-split skin shows dermal staining; strongly associated with underlying solid organ malignancy 30% (#1 = adenocarcinoma)
- **Ocular MMP:** Target = β_4 subunit of $\alpha_6\beta_4$ integrin; nearly exclusive ocular involvement
- **Anti-BP antigen MMP:** Target = BP180 (C-terminus); one-third cases, skin and mucosal involvement.

Clinical Features

- At all affected body sites—healing occurs with scarring (except oral cavity).
- Oral lesions—mild to extremely painful erosions, ulcers, desquamative gingivitis.
- Eyes—conjunctivitis (bilateral > unilateral), foreign body sensation, entropion, trichiasis, corneal scarring, symblepharon, blindness.
- Nasal—hemorrhagic crusts, epistaxis, septal perforation.
- Skin involvement (25%): Fewer lesions, different distribution and morphology from conventional BP.
  - Most common sites: Scalp/face/neck and upper trunk
  - Erythematous plaques and recurrent blisters/erosions → heal with atrophic scars (not seen in BP) and milia.
  - Brunsting-Perry variant: Lesions limited to head/neck → scarring alopecia; no mucosal involvement

Clinical Variants

- Oral pemphigoid (target antigen α_6)
- Ocular pemphigoid (target antigen β_4)
- Vulvar pemphigoid

Complications

- Destruction of tear ducts, corneal ulceration, corneal pannus, blindness
- Life-threatening laryngeal stenosis

- Deafness due to middle ear involvement
- Oral and esophageal carcinoma
- Solid organ cancer associated in 30%

Investigations

- **HPE:** Not distinctive (usually performed on erosions as blisters are uncommon). Fewer eosinophils than BP. Later stage: Fibrosis develops
  Conjunctival lesions—epithelial metaplasia, decreased number of goblet cells, lymphocytic infiltrate with plasma cells and mast cells in substantia propria, fibrosis of lamina propria, granulation tissue in submucosa.
- **DIF:** Linear IgG, C3 and/or IgA at DEJ. n-serrated/roof pattern.
- **IIF:** Lower sensitivity even on salt split skin (50–70%)
- **BIOCHIP® mosaic**—may be used, if available.

Prognosis

Chronic and progressive disease, rarely goes into spontaneous remission unlike BP and LAD.

Treatment (Figs 7.16 and 7.17)

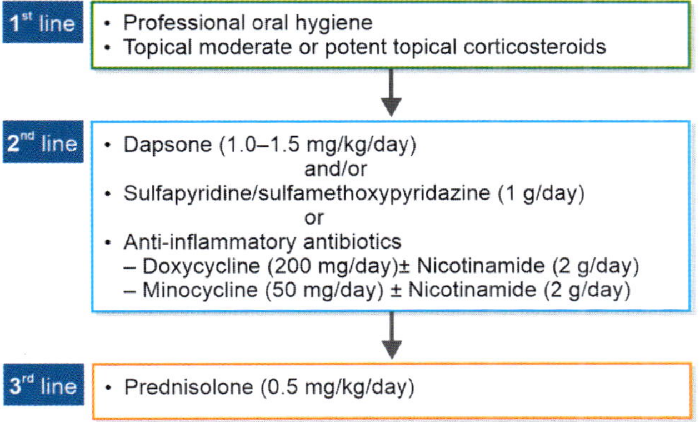

Fig. 7.16a: Management algorithm for MMP (oral pemphigoid)

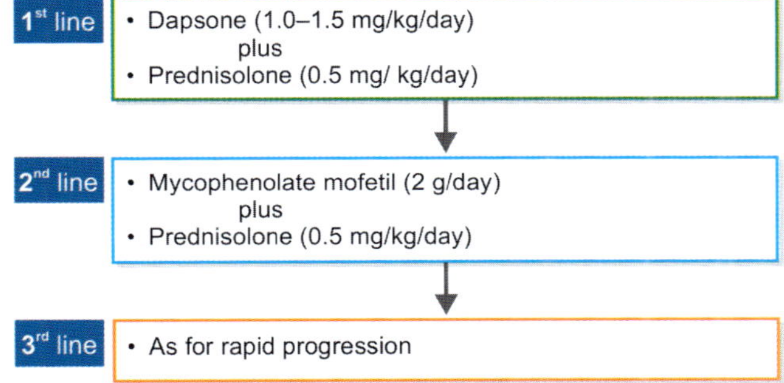

Fig. 7.16b: Management algorithm for generalized MMP without rapid progression

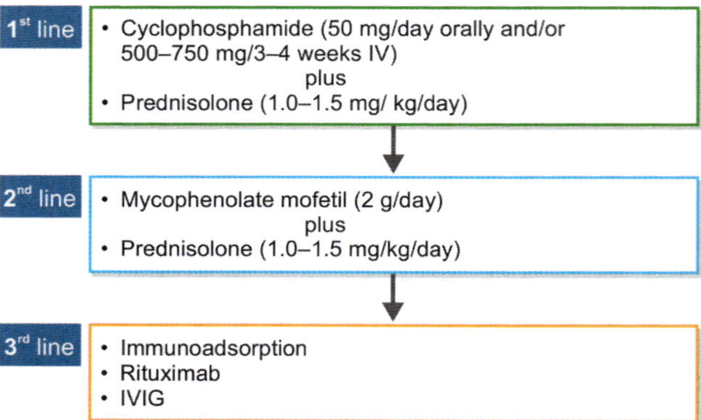

Fig. 7.17: Management algorithm for generalized MMP *with* rapid progression in conjunctivae, larynx or esophagus

LINEAR IgA DISEASE

Rare, subepidermal blistering disease with **IgA deposition at DEJ**.

Clinical types

- **LAD of adults** (around 60 years)—mainly affects trunk, face, perineum, hands and feet.
- **Chronic bullous disease of childhood (CBDC)**—onset around 5 years of age. Most common AIBD in children. Perioral region and perineum are common sites.

Pathogenesis

IgA autoantibodies directed against two related antigens, both derived from C terminal of BPAG2:

- **LAD-1** (120 kDa cleaved portion of BP180 antigen) **[LL (Lamina Lucida) type LAD]**
- **LABD97** (97 kDa cleaved portion of LAD-1) **[LL (Lamina Lucida) type LAD]**
- **Type VII collagen [SD (Sublamina densa) type LAD]**

Predisposing Factors

- **Drugs: Vancomycin, NSAIDs, penicillin**
- Infections, trauma, vaccination, UV radiation exposure
- Building work at home

Clinical Features

- In both children and adults, individual lesions are similar.
- Blisters typically occur in clusters, **crown of jewels or string of pearls appearance** (not pathognomonic for LAD, may be seen in BP too) **(Fig. 7.18)**.
- Pruritus—absent to severe.
  - Children—lesions arise more abruptly, perioral and perineum
  - Adult—trunk and limbs
  - Mucosal involvement is seen in about 70–80% of patients.
  - Heal without scarring usually, milia uncommon
- **SD type LAD has been shown to be more severe and refractory to treatment than LL type LAD.**

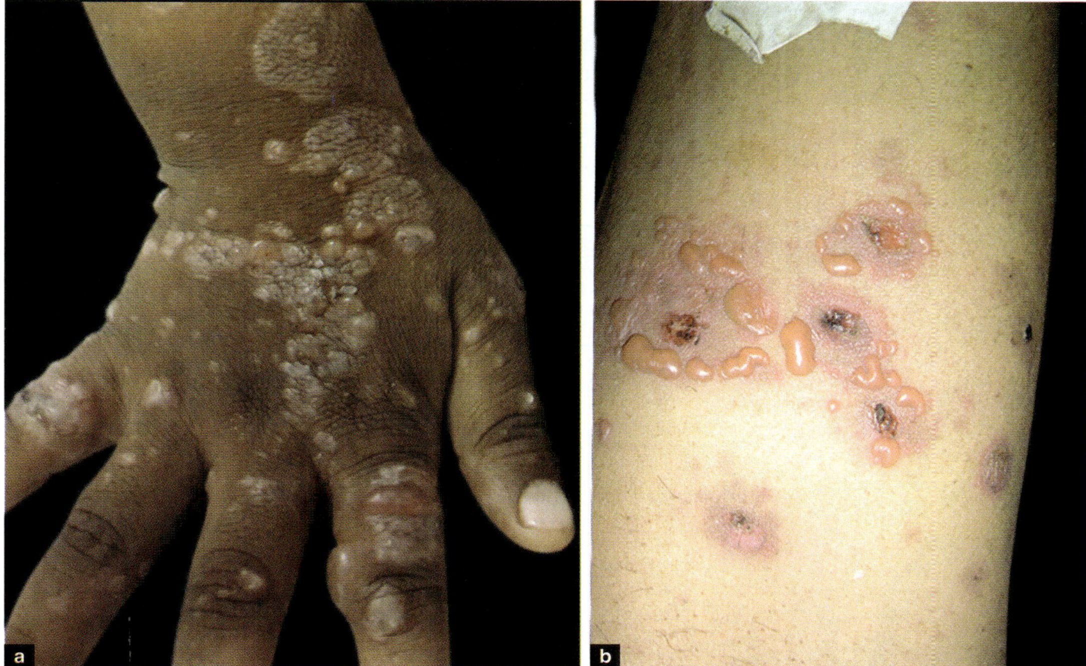

Fig. 7.18: (a) Clustered tense bullae in a string of pearls arrangement in a child with CBDC; and a more classic depiction is seen in (b)

Clinical Variants

In a small number of cases, circulating IgG antibodies are seen and these cases have been referred to as linear IgA/IgG bullous dermatosis (LAGBD). Here the antigen is the ectodomain of BP180.

Investigations

- **Histopathology:** A subepidermal split with superficial dermal infiltrate composed of neutrophils (sometimes forming microabscesses) and a few eosinophils.
- **DIF:** Linear deposition of IgA along the BMZ is pathognomonic. (While IgA is seen in nearly 80% of cases in the rest IgG, IgM, and/or C3 may be present. The deposition of IgA in a linear manner along the basement membrane is not specific for linear IgA bullous dermatosis because it may also be found in several bullous dermatoses and cutaneous diseases. Incidentally, IgA is deposited along the basement membrane of the eccrine secretory coils in patients with alcoholic liver disease based on two cases, it has been suggested that lesions on the volar surface of the forearm may not contain immunoreactants even though they are present in lesions from other body sites thus this site should not be chosen for biopsy).
- **IIF:** Positive in approximately 30% of adults and 80% of children. The sensitivity and titer can be increased by using salt-split skin as the substrate.

  (Circulating IgA antibodies are found more often in childhood than in adult cases. Sera from vancomycin-induced linear IgA dermatosis produces negative results on indirect IF, but coincubation of patient sera with vancomycin does produce positive basement membrane zone IgA staining; it appears that vancomycin mediates IgA autoreactivity against the target antigen, type VII collagen, by modifying IgA rather than the collagen 7 target.)

Treatment

The treatment is depicted in **Fig. 7.19** while the prognosis is given in **Box 7.14**.

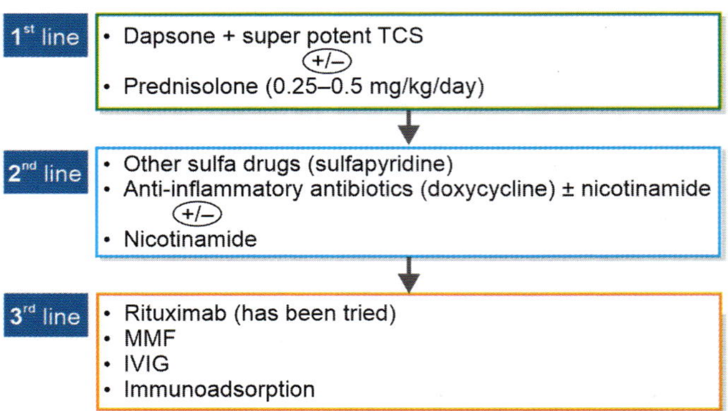

Fig. 7.19: Management algorithm for linear IgA disease

BOX 7.14: Prognosis and course of LAD

- Responds well to treatment
- Relapses over 2–4 years, recurrences are less severe than first episode
- Most children achieve remission within 2 years of disease onset
- Drug-induced LAD—heals within 4–8 weeks of drug discontinuation

Recent Update

As cytokine levels have been estimated it has been seen that there are elevations of IL-6 and C-reactive protein in the blood and extreme elevations of IL-6 in LABD bullous fluid which respond to **tocilizumab** (anti-IL-6 receptor) (Jordan SC, 2023). As the IL 6 pathway is mediated by the JAK1/JAK2 signalling pathway, inhibitors of this pathway, like **tofacitinib** have been tried in Linear IgA BD [Fan B,].

ANTI-p200 PEMPHIGOID

Epidemiology

- First described in 1996.
- Autoantibodies against p200 (200 kDa protein of the DEJ) and against C terminal 245 amino acids of laminin γ1 (90%)
- Label dermal side of salt-split skin (could be mistaken for EBA but better prognosis)
- Old age (but younger than that of BP)
- Males > females
- Psoriasis associated in most Japanese patients

Clinical Features

- Most often present with classic BP eruption. In contrast to conventional bullous pemphigoid, this disorder tends to have more frequent mucous membrane and head and neck involvement and is prone to form milia scars. It is associated with psoriasis in perhaps as many as one-third of cases.
- Heal without scarring, milia infrequent.

Investigations

- HPE—subepidermal split + neutrophils +/– eosinophils in the upper dermis
- DIF—linear deposits of IgG at the DEJ (n-serrated pattern)
- IIF—on 1 M NaCl split, normal human skin autoantibodies label the floor of the artificial split. Thus, on salt-split skin, i misdiagnosis of EBA could be made. In contrast to EBA, patients with anti-p200 pemphigoid usually respond well to topical or medium dose oral corticosteroids.
- Immunoblotting/ELISA-autoantibodies.

Treatment (Fig. 7.20)

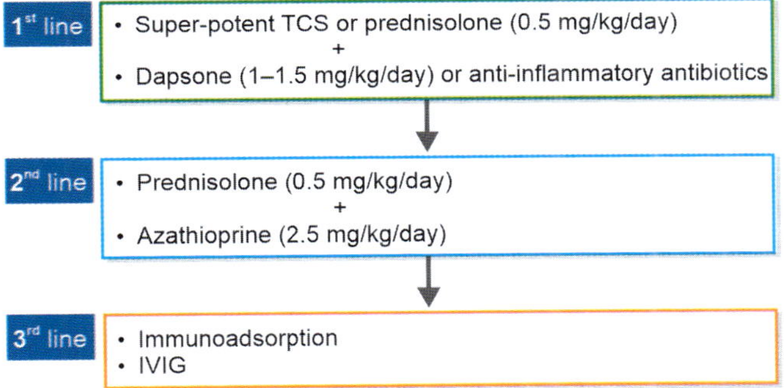

Fig. 7.20: Management algorithm for anti-p200 pemphigoid

EPIDERMOLYSIS BULLOSA ACQUISITA

Epidemiology

- A rare subepidermal acquired, trauma-induced, blistering disease characterized by autoantibody formation against homotrimeric type VII collagen—a constituent of anchoring fibrils.
- **N terminal 145 kDa NC1** domain—immunodominant region
- Age—disease onset at 44–54 years
- 5%—children and adolescents
- Sex—no clear predilection
- Associated with HLA-DR2.

Predisposing Factors

- **Drugs: Penicillin, vancomycin, gentamicin**
- UV radiation
- Contact allergy to metals.

Clinical Types

1. **Classical mechanobullous EBA**—resembles dystrophic EB when severe and porphyria cutanea tarda when mild. Skin fragility, erosions, blisters, crusts followed by formation of scars on trauma-prone areas such as the hands, knuckles, elbows, knees and toes. Scarring alopecia and nail loss may occur.
2. **Inflammatory EBA**—resembles BP (50%)/LAD (5–10%)/MMP (5–10%).
   - Both the patterns may coexist/may interchange in the same patient.
   - Mucosal involvement—50%

Diagnostic Criteria (Roenigk et al., 1971)

- Negative family/personal history for skin blistering
- Adult disease onset
- Resembles hereditary dystrophic EB
- Exclusion of all other bullous diseases

Associated Disorders

- IBD, especially Crohn disease (type VII collagen found in the oral cavity, esophagus, small intestine and colon)
- Hematological malignancies esp. lymphoma

Investigations

HPE: Subepidermal cleavage with variable amount of inflammatory infiltrate

DIF: Linear IgG (±C3) at DEJ. 600-fold magnification shows **'u-serrated' pattern with grass-like appearance**—unique to EBA and particularly important as circulating autoantibodies detected only in 50% patients.

IIF: Positive in only 50%. IIF on SSS shows binding to dermal/floor side of split.

Treatment (Fig. 7.21)

The mainstay is systemic corticosteroids in combination with colchicine and dapsone.

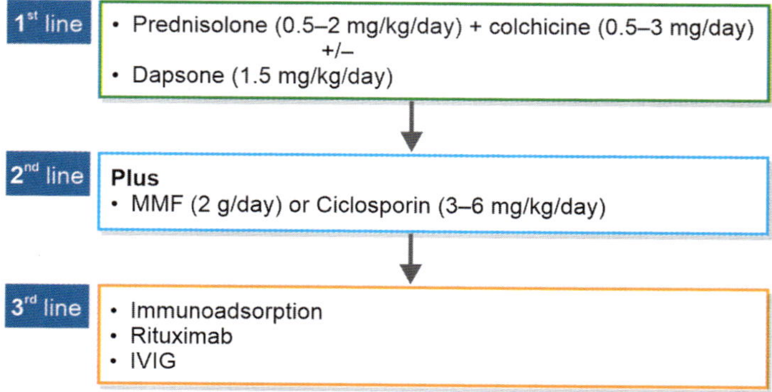

Fig. 7.21: Management algorithm for EB acquisita

Prognosis

- Chronic relapsing disease, difficult to treat.
- Children with EBA—better prognosis than adults.

PEMPHIGOID GESTATIONIS (HERPES GESTATIONIS)

- Pemphigoid gestationis is a rare variant of BP and an intensely pruritic autoimmune polymorphic bullous dermatosis of pregnancy (mainly in 2nd or 3rd trimester) and puerperium.
- Target antigen—BP180 NC16A
- It may recur in subsequent pregnancies.
- Exacerbations of the disease may occur with oral contraceptives intake.
- Intensely itchy condition. Initially, the skin lesion consists of urticated papules, plaques, target lesions and annular wheals, associated with marked pruritus: Subsequently, vesicles and larger blisters appear **(Fig. 7.22)**. It characteristically begins around the umbilicus, and then spreads to the abdomen, thighs, limbs, palms and soles.
- Fetal risk: Risk of prematurity, small for gestational age birth, up to 10% risk of skin involvement.
- DIF: Linear **C3** deposition ± **IgG** at basement membrane
- IIF—positive.
- On salt-split skin study, the autoantibodies bind to the epidermal side.
- IgG antibodies can be detected by ELISA.
- Almost all patients with PG require oral steroids, but mild cases can be successfully treated with potent steroids and systemic antihistamines. Moderate disease responds to 20–30 mg/day of prednisolone, whereas severe disease may need 40–80 mg/day of prednisolone. Plasmapheresis can be considered in the most severe cases.

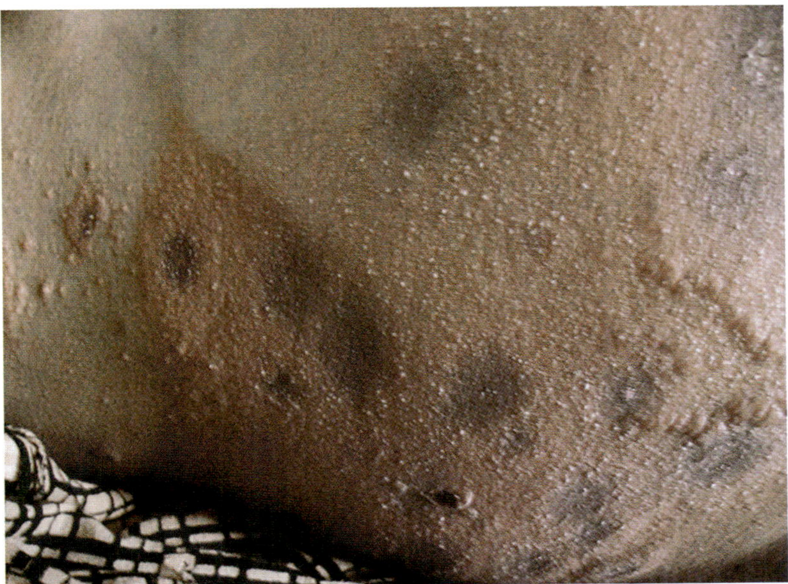

Fig. 7.22: Tense bullae with urticarial lesions in pemphigoid gestationis

BULLOUS SLE

Epidemiology

- Bullous systemic lupus erythematosus (BSLE) is an autoimmune subepidermal blistering disease that occurs in patients with SLE.
- 2nd–4th decade (like SLE)
- Africans ↑↑ (like SLE)
- Females ↑↑ (like SLE)

Predisposing Factors

- Drugs—hydralazine, penicillamine, methimazole
- UVB

Clinical Features

- Two types (Gammon et al., 1993)
  1. BSLE type I—with reactivity against collagen type VII. Both IgG and IgA autoantibodies—against the collagen VII.
     - NC1 domain (like in EBA)—especially the fibronectin-like region.
  2. BLSE type II—with anti-DEJ reactivity against other target antigens (BP180, BP230, laminin 332). No autoantibodies against the collagen VII.
     - Acute onset of widespread tense vesicles and bullae on normal/erythematous skin of SLE patient mostly but not limited to sun-exposed sites.
     - In contrast to other pemphigoid disorders—face often involved
     - May mimic BP/LAD, EBA, and DH
     - Mucosal involvement—rare
     - Pruritus—absent
     - Burning sensation—may be present

Investigations

- **HPE:** Similar to DH. Bullae are subepidermal with a neutrophil-dominant infiltrate, occasionally resulting in microabscesses in the papillary tips. Mucin deposition in reticular dermis and dermal edema (+). **Basal layer vacuolization absent (*vs* bullous lesions of SLE).**
- **DIF:** Shows linear IgG (40%) and granular IgG (60%). IgA, IgM and C3 in the DEJ may be seen. 'u-serrated' pattern in BSLE type I.
- **IIF:** Positive/negative—BSLE type I, negative—BSLE type II.

Diagnostic Criteria

Camisa and Sharma

1. A diagnosis of SLE based on the ACR criteria
2. Vesicles and bullae mainly located on sun-exposed areas;.
3. The histopathology is characterized by subepidermal bullae with microabscesses of neutrophils in the dermal papillae, similar to those found in dermatitis herpetiformis.
4. Linear or granular deposition of IgG, IgM or both, and often IgA and C3 at the basement membrane zone.

Gammon and Briggaman (for BSLE Type I)

1. Meet the criteria for SLE of the American Rheumatism Association
2. Presence of nonscarring acquired bullous eruption on sun-exposed areas, but not limited to these sites
3. Evidence of subepidermal blister with neutrophilic infiltrate in histology
4. Deposition of IgG, IgM, IgA, and C3 at the basement membrane zone
5. Circulating autoantibodies against type VII collagen confirmed by IIF on salt-split skin or immunoprecipitation, and
6. Presence of Ig deposits with anchoring fibrils/type VII collagen by immunoelectron microscopy.

Treatment (Fig. 7.23)

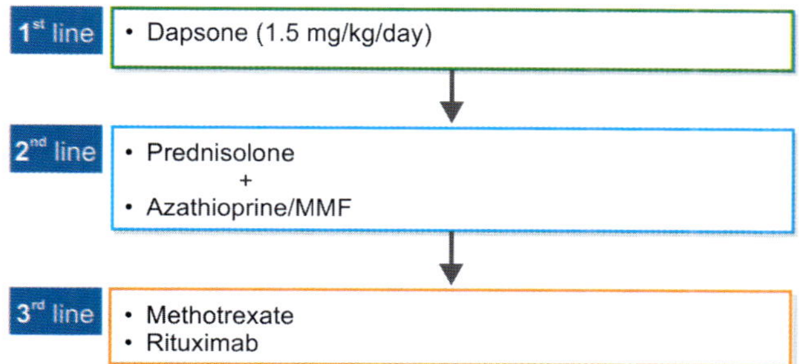

Fig. 7.23: Management algorithm for bullous SLE

Rare Pemphigoid Disorders

Lichen planus pemphigoides

- Very rare
- In conjunction with lichen planus
- Affects younger patients than BP
- On extremities (c.f. BP)
- Targets C-terminal epitopes within the NC16A domain of BP180
- Less severe than BP
- Tense blisters on and outside lichen planus lesions
- DIF—linear IgG +/– C3 at DEJ
- IIF—anti-BP180 NC16A autoantibodies
- Remits only after treatment of lichen planus.

DERMATITIS HERPETIFORMIS (DUHRING-BROCQ DISEASE)

Epidemiology

- Age—adults (4th decade)
- Sex—males:females—1.5–2:1
- A recurrent chronic pruritic disease associated with gluten-sensitive enteropathy (GSE).
- Gluten is found in wheat, rye, and barley and absent in rice, oats or corn.

- GSE antigen—tissue transglutaminase (tTG)
- DH putative antigen—epidermal transglutaminase 3 (eTG3)
- Associated with **HLA-DQ2** (strongest), HLA-DQ8
- Northern Europeans >> (uncommon in Asians)
- In **Asians** (distinct fibrillar pattern of IgA on DIF and not commonly associated with GSE)
- Lower age-adjusted mortality (due to diet modifications).

Associated Disorders

- Increased risk of **small intestine lymphoma**
- Other autoimmune disorders—thyroid (Hashimoto's thyroiditis), type 1 diabetes, Addison disease, vitiligo
- Iodine → flare
- Smoking → improvement (? clinical relevance)

Pathogenesis

- **Celiac disease:** Tissue transglutaminase (tTG2) enzyme, which is present in the gut mucosa, is the autoantigen.
  - DH (Sárdy et al., 2002): Epidermal transglutaminase eTG3 is an autoantigen for IgA deposited in **DH** skin.
  - Studies have shown that almost all untreated patients with CD and 80% of patients with DH have tTG2-targeted IgA deposits in the small bowel mucosa, and that these deposits are gluten-dependent.
  - Subclinical CD in the gut leads to immune complex deposition of high avidity IgA-TG3 antibodies together with TG3 enzyme in the papillary dermis.
  - In *normal skin*, **TG3** is expressed in the **keratinocyte layers** and not in the papillary dermis where the IgA deposits are located in DH.
  - It is hypothesized that release of TG3 occurs from keratinocytes into the papillary dermis, where it is able to bind circulating IgA antibodies; or that circulating complexes of TG3 and IgA are deposited in the skin. Subsequently, neutrophilic infiltration occurs, leading to inflammation and clefting within the lamina lucida.
  - Direct activation of TG3 in dermal aggregates by mechanical force could account for the sites of involvement.
  - The environmental factors relevant to dermatitis herpetiformis include iodine exposure (which can precipitate flares of the disease) and tobacco smoking, which may ameliorate it.
- The steps of pathogenesis are shown in **Fig. 7.24**:
  1. Ingestion of **gluten-containing grains** → gluten broken down into gliadin inside GI lumen → gliadin transported across GI mucosa to lamina propria.
  2. **tTG2** in lamina propria deamidates gliadin → deamidated gliadin forms a covalent bond with TG2 → TG2—gliadin complex is a neoantigen recognized by HLA-DQ2 (or HLA-DQ8) on APCs → specific Th and B cells activated → production of IgA autoantibodies against tTG2 or tTG2–gliadin complex.
  3. **IgA antibodies** bind to tTG2 complexes in lamina propria → neutrophil recruitment, damage to intestinal villi → enteropathy and villous atrophy → later, epitope spreading results in IgA autoantibodies against epidermal transglutaminase **(eTG3)**.

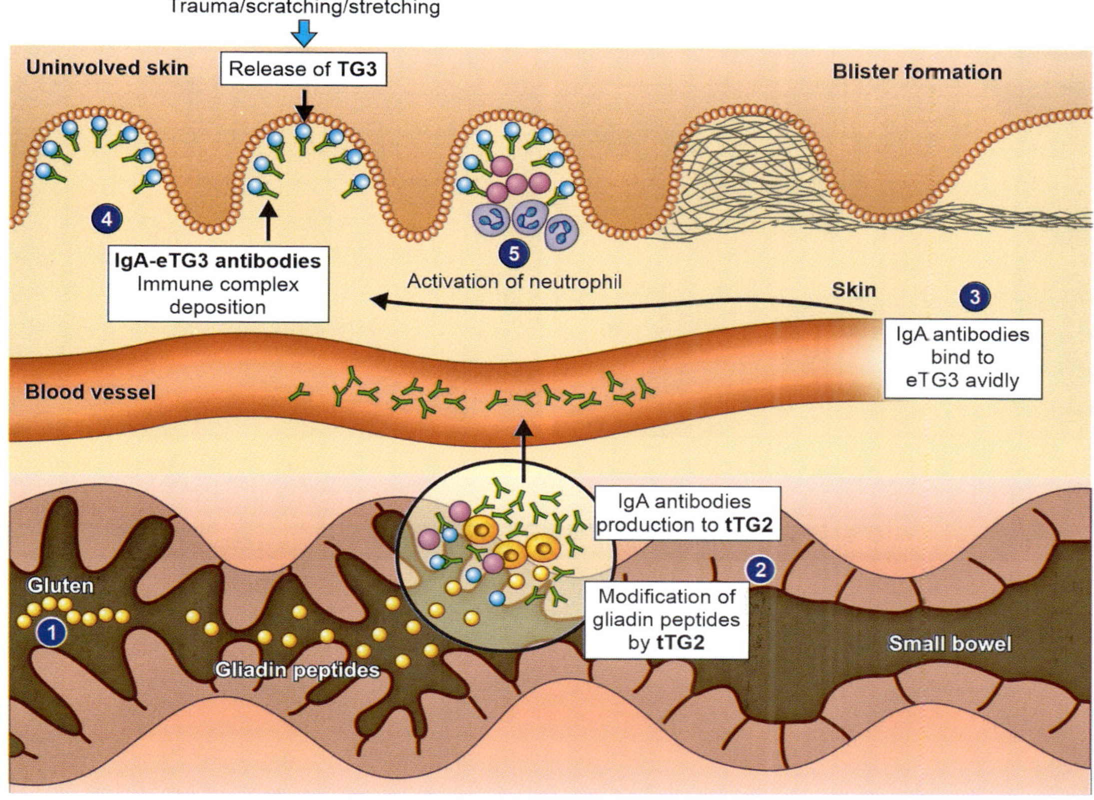

Fig. 7.24: Steps in pathogenesis of DH (explanation given in text)

4. Circulating anti-TG3/IgA binds locally to eTG3 within dermal papillae → neutrophils recruited to dermal papillae (neutrophilic papillitis) → release elastase and MMPs → subepidermal blister most prominent above papillae.

Clinical Features

- Principal symptom—itch
- Pleomorphic, with urticarial plaques, papules, and vesicles.
- Intensely pruritic erythematous grouped papules or vesicles over extensor surfaces—elbows, knees, buttocks **(Fig. 7.25)**.
  - Lesions tend to be symmetrical and heal without scarring.
  - GI symptoms +/–
  - Punctate purpura on palms and soles +/–
  - Dental enamel pits +/–
  - Only **20%** of patients with DH have *symptomatic* GI disease, but **>90%** have some degree of *gluten-sensitive enteropathy* on GI biopsy—the differences are listed in **Table 7.16** and have relevance in serological tests.

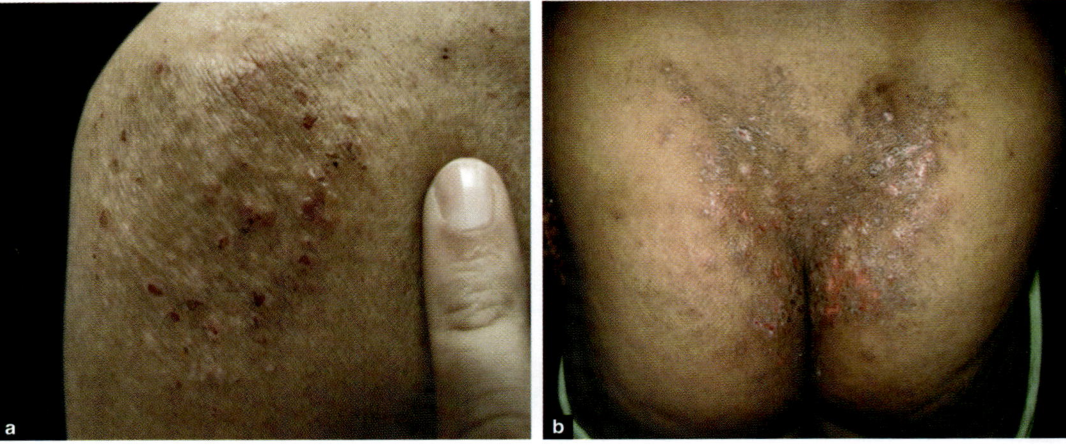

Fig. 7.25: Itchy excoriated papules leaving few intact vesicles on the knee and intergluteal cleft in DH

TABLE 7.16: Comparison of dermatitis herpetiformis (DH) and celiac disease (CD)

	DH	CD
Sex	Slightly more in males	Females predominate
Age at onset	Mainly adults	Children and adults
1st-degree relatives with CD or DH	Yes	Yes
HLA-DQ2	95–100%	95%
IgA deposits in the skin	**100% (by definition)**	**0%**
Small bowel villous atrophy	**70%**	**100% (by definition)**
IgA deposits in bowel mucosa	79%	95–100%
IgA-TG3 antibodies in serum	86%	24%
IgA-TG2 antibodies in serum	86%	92%
IgA-EmA antibodies in serum	89%	95%
Prognosis on a gluten-free diet	Excellent	Decreased all—cause and lymphoma mortality

HLA-DQ2, human leukocyte antigen DQ2; IgA, immunoglobulin A; TG3, epidermal transglutaminase; TG2, tissue transglutaminase; EmA, endomysium.

Differential Diagnosis

Arthropod bites, scabies and urticarial vasculitis, erythema multiforme, bullous SLE, linear IgA disease (LAD), and bullous pemphigoid.

Investigations

- **HPE:** Subepidermal blister formation with neutrophils located at the tips of the dermal papillae.
- **DIF:** Granular/fibrillar (Asians) IgA and C3 deposition in dermal papillae (maximum near active lesion).

- **IIF:** Negative.
- **Serological tests:** Anti-gliadin/anti-endomysial antibodies in DH/celiac disease
  - Useful for clinical follow-up.
  - The sensitivity of (ELISA) for *IgA tissue transglutaminase* antibodies (TG2) is 47–95%, and specificity is >90%.
  - The sensitivity of ELISA for *IgA epidermal transglutaminase TG3* antibodies is 60–81%, and specificity is 93–100%.
  - The measurement of TG3 antibodies does not offer any advantage over the widely used TG2 antibody assay for monitoring treatment.
  - Endomysial antibodies (performed via indirect immunofluorescence)–sensitivity for celiac disease and DH is 52–100% and specificity approximates 100%.
  - Antigliadin antibodies may also be positive, but have high false positive rates.

Thus, a typical serological work-up is:

1. Enzyme-linked immunosorbent assay (ELISA) for IgA tissue transglutaminase antibodies (IgA-TG2Ab)
2. ELISA for IgA epidermal transglutaminase antibodies (when available)
3. Indirect immunofluorescence for IgA endomysial antibodies
4. Total IgA level.

The total IgA level is necessary because selective IgA deficiency, which decreases the likelihood of detecting DH-IgA autoantibodies, occurs at an increased frequency in patients with celiac disease. The assessment of IgG antibodies against tissue transglutaminase and endomysium may be useful in this setting but is not reliable.

Treatment (Fig. 7.26)

- Mainstay-gluten-free diet (reduces GI lymphoma risk too)
- Dapsone and related sulphonamide drugs—highly effective, often suppressing pruritus within 48–72 hours of initiation of treatment. But lesions abruptly recur within 24–48 hours of discontinuation of therapy and drugs have **no effect on GI disease/lymphoma risk.**
- The daily dose can be regulated on a weekly basis to optimize control.
- One to two new lesions per week should be expected on the optimal dose. Higher doses increase toxicity with little added benefit.

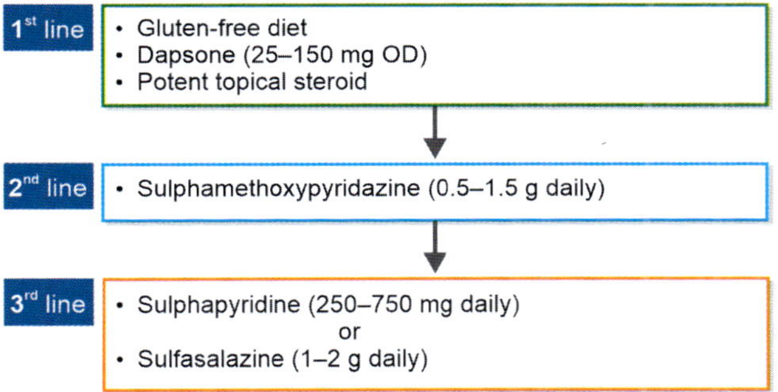

Fig. 7.26: Management algorithm for dermatitis herpetiformis

Disease Course and Prognosis

- Chronic disease, requires a long-term gluten free diet.
- Those that are able to do this, and respond, seem to have excellent long-term survival.

BIBLIOGRAPHY

Books

1. Masayuki Amagai. Pemphigus. Bolognia LJ. Schafler VJ. Cerroni L Editors. In: Dermatology. (4th Edition). London. Elsevier publisher. Ch 29: p 494–509.
2. McKees Pathology of the skin, 4th edn.
3. Philippe Berbard and Luca Borradoi. Pemphigoid Group. Bolognia LJ. Schafler VJ. Cerroni L Editors. In: Dermatology (4th Edition). Elsevier publisher. Ch 30: p 510–26.
4. Rook's Textbook of Dermatology, 9th edn. Chapter 50.

Journals

1. Anhalt GJ, Kim SC, Stanley JR, Korman NJ, Jabs DA, Kory M, et al., Paraneoplastic pemphigus. An autoimmune mucocutaneous disease associated with neoplasia. N Engl J Med 1990;323(25):1729–35.
2. Borroni G, Biagi F, Ciocca O, et al. IgA anti-epidermal transglutaminase autoantibodies: A sensible and sensitive marker for diagnosis of dermatitis herpetiformis in adult patients. J Eur Acad Dermatol Venereol 2013; 27:836.
3. Boulard C, et al. Calculation of cut-off values based on the ABSIS and PDAI pemphigus scoring systems for defining moderate, significant and extensive of pemphigus. Br J Dermatol 2016;175(1):142–9.
4. Chen DM, French Study Group on Autoimmune Bullous Diseases. Rituximab is an effective treatment in patients with pemphigus vulgaris and demonstrates a steroid-sparing effect. Br J Dermatol. 2020 May; 182(5):1111–9.
5. Chrysomallis F, Ioannides D, Teknetzis A, et al. Treatment of oral pemphigus vulgaris. Int J Dermatol 1994; 33: 803–7.
6. Dieterich W, Laag E, Bruckner-Tuderman L, et al. Antibodies to tissue transglutaminase as serologic markers in patients with dermatitis herpetiformis. J Invest Dermatol 1999; 113:133.
7. Fan B, Wang M. Tofacitinib, a JAK1/3 Inhibitor As Treatment for Linear IgA Bullous Dermatosis: A Case Report. Dermatitis. 2023 Mar-Apr;34(2):160–161.
8. Frampton JE. Rituximab: A Review in Pemphigus Vulgaris. American Journal of Clinical Dermatology. 2020 Feb;21(1):149–56.
9. Gach JE, Ilchyshyn A. Beneficial effects of topical tacrolimus on recalcitrant erosions of pemphigus vulgaris. Clin Exp Dermatol 2004;29:271–72.
10. Gammon WR, Briggaman RA. Bullous SLE: A phenotypically distinctive but immunologically heterogeneous bullous disorder. J Invest Dermatol 1993;100(1):28s–34s.
11. Geller S. Interleukin 4 and interleukin 13 inhibition: A promising therapeutic approach in bullous pemphigoid. J Am Acad Dermatol. 2020 Jul;83(1):37–38. doi: 10.1016/j.jaad.2020.03.017. Epub 2020 Mar 13. PMID: 32179081.
12. Gutjahr, et al. Bullous pemphigoid autoantibody-mediated complement fixation is abolished by the low molecular weight heparin tinzaparin sodium.
13. Goebeler M, ARGX-113–1701 Investigator Study Group. Treatment of pemphigus vulgaris and foliaceus with efgartigimod, a neonatal Fc receptor inhibitor: a phase II multicentre, open-label feasibility trial. Br J Dermatol. 2022 Mar;186(3):429–439.
14. Harman KE, Albert S, Black MM; British Association of Dermatologists. Guidelines for the management of pemphigus vulgaris. Br J Dermatol 2003;149:926–37.
15. Hayashida MZ. Biologic therapy induced pemphigus. An Bras Dermatol 2017;92:591–3.
16. Hébert V,. Modifications of the BAFF/BAFF-Receptor Axis in Patients With Pemphigus Treated With Rituximab Versus Standard Corticosteroid Regimen. Front Immunol. 2021 May 14;12:666022

17. Hebert, et al. Large International Validation of ABSIS and PDAI Pemphigus Severity Scores. J Invest Dermatol 2019;139:31–37.
18. Hull CM, Liddle M, Hansen N, et al. Elevation of IgA anti-epidermal transglutaminase antibodies in dermatitis herpetiformis. Br J Dermatol 2008; 159:120.
19. Iraji F, Yoosefi A. Healing effect of Pilocarpine gel 4% on skin lesions of pemphigus vulgaris. Int J Dermatol 2006; 45: 743–46.
20. Joly P, Updated S2K guidelines on the management of pemphigus vulgaris and foliaceus initiated by the european academy of dermatology and venereology (EADV). J Eur Acad Dermatol Venereol. 2020 Aug 24. doi: 10.1111/jdv.16752.
21. Jordan SC,. Linear IgA bullous dermatosis and elevated bullous interleukin-6 levels: Responsive to treatment with Anti-IL-6 receptor monoclonals. Clin Case Rep. 2023 Feb 27;11(2):e6998
22. Juczynska K, Expression of the JAK/STAT Signaling Pathway in Bullous Pemphigoid and Dermatitis Herpetiformis. Mediators Inflamm. 2017;2017:6716419.
23. Kamata A, Kurihara Y, Funakoshi T, Takahashi H, Kuroda K, Hachiya T, Amagai M, Yamagami J. Basement membrane zone IgE deposition is associated with bullous pemphigoid disease severity and treatment results. British Journal of Dermatology. 2020 May;182(5):1221–7.
24. Kanwar AJ, Ajith C, Narang T. Pemphigus in North India. J Cutan Med Surg 2006;10:21–25.
25. Lever W. Pemphigus and pemphigoid. Springfield: Thomas, 1965.
26. Ling X,. Research progress of omalizumab in the treatment of bullous pemphigoid. J Dermatol. 2023 Mar 27.
27. Liu Y, Wang Y, Chen X, Jin H, Li L. Factors associated with the activity and severity of bullous pemphigoid: a review. Ann Med. 2020 May-Jun;52(3-4):55–62. doi: 10.1080/07853890.2020.1742367. Epub 2020 Mar 22. PMID: 32163298.
28. Mascarenhas MF, Hede RV, Shukla P, Nadkarni NS, Rege VL. Pemphigus in Goa. J Indian Med Assoc 1994;92:342–43.
29. Meijer, et al. Assessment of diagnostic strategy for early recognition of bullous and nonbullous variants of pemphigoid. JAMA Dermatol. doi;10.1001/jamadermatol.2018.4390.
30. Mignard C, French Study Group on Autoimmune Bullous Skin Diseases. Factors Associated With Short-term Relapse in Patients With Pemphigus Who Receive Rituximab as First-line Therapy: A Post Hoc Analysis of a Randomized Clinical Trial. JAMA Dermatol. 2020 May 1;156(5):545–52.
31. Murrell DF, Peña S, Joly P, Marinovic B, Hashimoto T, Diaz LA, Sinha AA, Payne AS, Daneshpazhooh M, Eming R, Jonkman MF. Diagnosis and management of pemphigus: Recommendations of an international panel of experts. Journal of the American Academy of Dermatology. 2020 Mar 1;82(3):575–85.
32. Murrell DF, et al. Definitions and outcome measures for bullous pemphigoid: recommendations by an international panel of experts. J AmAcad Dermatol 2012;66(3): 479–82.
33. Roenigk HH, Ryan JG, Borgfeld WF. Epidermolysis bullosa acquisita. Report of three cases and review of all published cases. Arch Dermatol 1971;103:1–10.
34. Rao, et al. Demonstration of pemphigus specific immunofluorescence pattern by DIF of plucked hair. Int J Dermatol 2009;48:1187–9.
35. Sardy M, Karpati S, Merkl B, Paulsson M, Smyth N. Epidermal transglutaminase (TGase 3) is the autoantigien of dermatitis herpetiformis. J Exp Med 2002;195(6):747–57.
36. Sinha S, Agrawal D, Sardana K, Kulhari A, Malhotra P. Complete Remission in a Patient with Treatment Refractory Bullous Pemphigoid after a Single Dose of Omalizumab. Indian Dermatol Online J. 2020 Jul 13;11(4):607–611.
37. Wilgram G, Caulfi eld J, Madgic M. An electron microscopic study of acantholysis and dyskeratosis in pemphigus foliaceous. J Invest Dermatol 1964; 43: 287–99.
38. Wolf R, et al. Drug-Induced versus Drug-Triggered Pemphigus. Dermatologica 1991;182:207–10.
39. van Beek N, Luttmann N, Huebner F, et al. Correlation of serum levels of IgE autoantibodies against BP180 with bullous pemphigoid disease activity. JAMA Dermatol. 2017;153(1):30–38. doi:10.1001/jamadermatol.2016.3357

Chapter

8

Autoimmune Connective Tissue Diseases

Surabhi Sinha, Kabir Sardana, Snigdha Saxena

Autoimmune connective tissue diseases (AICTD) form an important group of multidisciplinary disorders which primarily concerns rheumatologists, but we will discuss them here as the cutaneous manifestations enable an early diagnosis. As ANA is an important test to diagnose certain disorders, including the complications, this is being detailed first.

ANTINUCLEAR ANTIBODY (ANA)

Family of autoantibodies which serves as important diagnostic markers for the systemic autoimmune rheumatic diseases (SARD) and may be directed at one or several of the following nuclear antigens:

a. Extractable Nuclear Antigens (ENAs) (all give a Speckled Pattern on IIF for ANA)

- Sm (Smith)
- Ro (SSA)
- Scl-70 (topoisomerase I)
- RNP (ribonucleoprotein)
- La (SSB)
- Jo-1

b. Non-ENAs

- dsDNA (double stranded)
- Nuclear RNA
- Histone
- **Two types of assays: Indirect IF assay (IIFA) and ELISA:**
  - IIF: Most accurate, on rat liver or Hep-2 epithelial carcinoma cells (due to high nuclear/cytoplasmic ratio), Hep-2 cells considered gold standard in SARD (ACR). Gives pattern of ANA.
  - ELISA: More popular due to lower cost. Considered positive if >1:40. Pattern cannot be obtained.
- 29 Hep-2 IIFA patterns have been described and ascribed alphanumeric codes (AC-1 to AC-29) and are depicted in **Fig. 8.1** and **8.2**, these replace the earlier patterns **(Box 8.1)**
  - AC-0—negative
  - AC-1 to AC-14, AC-29—nuclear
  - AC-15 to AC-23—cytoplasmic
  - AC-24 to AC-28—mitotic
- 5% of normal population—elevated ANA but insignificant; ANA increases with age (i.e. 15% patients >55 years of age have increased ANA titer but no clinical significance).

Rates of ANA positivity

- SLE: 99%
- SJS: 70%
- SSc: 90%
- DM/PM: 40–65%

A summary of auto-antibodies found in various disorders is depicted in **Fig. 8.3** and **Table 8.1**.

BOX 8.1: The important nuclear patterns on Hep-2 IIFA [International Consensus on ANA Patterns (ICAP)]

Earlier nomenclature	Code	Pattern	Clinical relevance	Autoantibodies to
Homogeneous	AC-1	Diffuse, homogeneous	• SLE	• dsDNA
Speckled	AC-2	Dense fine speckled (DFS)	• Apparently healthy individuals without SARD	• DFS70
	AC-4	Fine speckled	• SJS, NLE, SCLE • SLE • DM, SSc	• SS-A/Ro • Mi-2, TIF1γ, Ku
	AC-5	Coarse speckled	• SLE • SSc • MCTD • SSc-AIM overlap	• Sm, U1-RNP • RNA-pol III • U1-RNP • Ku
	AC-29	TOPOI-like	• dSSc (highly specific)	• Topoisomerase I (Scl-70)
Centromere	AC-3	Centromere	• lSSc	• CENP—A, B, C
Nuclear dots	AC-6	Multiple nuclear dots	• PBC • AIM (DM)	• Sp-100 • MJ/NXP-2
	AC-7	Few nuclear dots	• Low predictive value	
Nucleolar	AC-8	Homogeneous nucleolar	• SSc • SSc-AIM overlap	• Th/To • PM/Scl
	AC-9	Clumpy nucleolar	• SSc	• U3-RNP/fibrillarin
	AC-10	Punctate nucleolar	• SSc • SJS	

*AC-11-14 are less well defined and not included here. SLE, systemic lupus erythematosus; SJS, sjogren syndrome; NLE, neonatal LE; SCLE, subacute LE; DM, dermatomyositis; AIM, autoimmune myositis; SSc, systemic sclerosis; PBC, primary biliary cholangitis; MCTD, mixed connective tissue disease. SARD, systemic autoimmune rheumatic diseases.

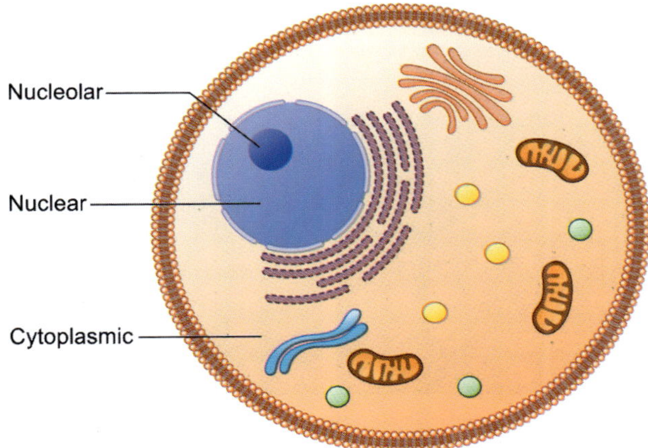

Fig. 8.1: An artistic depiction of the sites of various ANA patterns on IIF

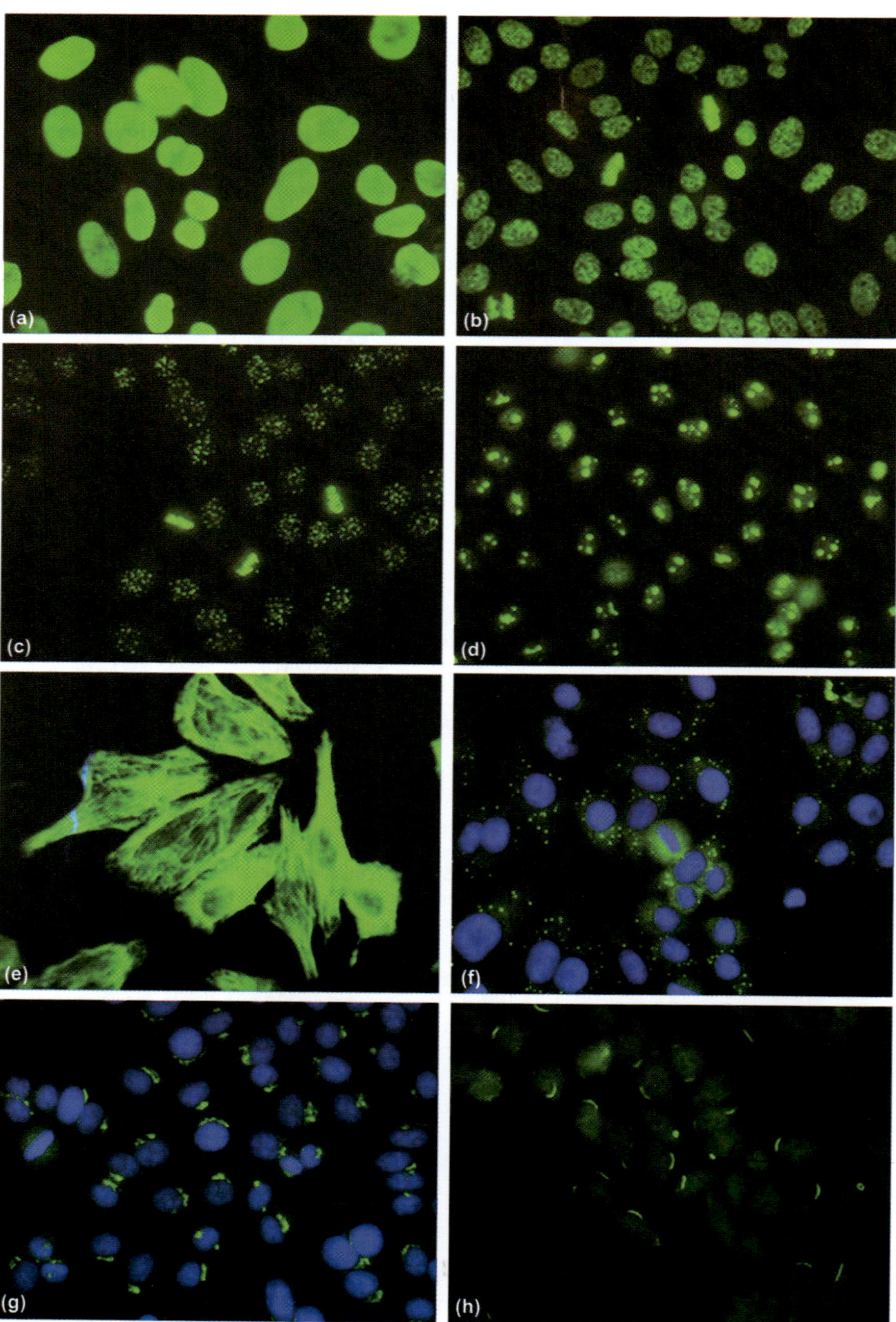

Fig. 8.2: Hep-2 cell patterns: (a) Homogeneous nuclear (AC-1); (b) Nuclear dense fine speckled (AC-2); (c) Centromere (AC-3); (d) Homogeneous nucleolar (AC-8); (e) Cytoplasmic fibrillar linear (AC-15); (f) Cytoplasmic discrete dots (AC-18); (g) Polar/Golgi-like (AC-22); (h) Rods and rings (AC-23)

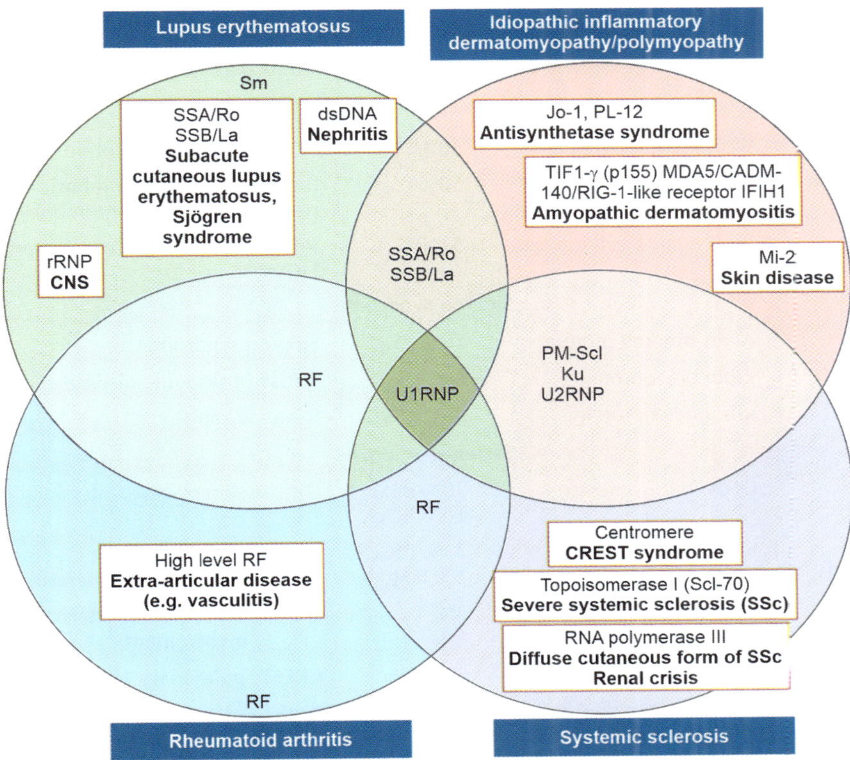

Fig. 8.3: A depiction of autoantibodies in various CTDs (boxed antigens are specific to the listed associations)

TABLE 8.1: Overview of autoantibodies in CTD

Antibody	Antigen	Prevalence	Clinical associations
	Systemic lupus erythematosus (SLE)		
Anti-dsDNA	Native DNA	40–90%	Highly specific, **lupus nephritis,** correlates **with disease activity, early/severe** disease
Anti-Sm	Ribonucleoprotein	10–30%	Highly specific, **lupus nephritis**
Anti-rRNP	Ribosomal P protein	10%	Highly specific, **neuropsychiatric LE**
Anti-Ro (SSA)	Ribonucleoprotein	40–60%	Mild SLE, **photosensitivity, SCLE, neonatal LE/congenital heart block**
Anti-La (SSB)	Ribonucleoprotein	20–30%	Same as anti-Ro associations
Anti-U1RNP	Ribonucleoprotein	30–60%	SCLE, mild SLE with limited systemic involvement
Anti-histone	Histone	40%	**Drug-induced** SLE mainly but can also be seen in SCLE
Anti-Ku	p70/p80 nucleolar protein (DNA repair)	10%	SLE with **polymyositis**
Anti-ssDNA	Denatured DNA	70%	Possible risk for SLE in DLE patients

(Contd.)

TABLE 8.1: Overview of autoantibodies in CTD *(Contd.)*

Antibody	Antigen	Prevalence	Clinical associations
		Systemic lupus erythematosus (SLE)	
Anti-C1q	C1q of complement	60%	Severe SLE, lupus nephritis
Anticardiolipin	Cardiolipin (phospholipid)	50%	Increased risk of **thrombotic events**, recurrent fetal loss, thrombocytopenia
Anti-PCNA	Proliferating cell nuclear antigen	5–10%	Renal disease, hypocomplementemia, HBV, HCV
		Sjögren syndrome	
Anti-α-fodrin	Actin-binding protein	70%	Sjögren syndrome
Anti-Ro	Ribonucleoprotein	60%	↑ Risk of systemic disease and lymphoma
Anti-La	Ribonucleoprotein	35–85%	Same as anti-Ro
		Systemic sclerosis	
Anti-Scl-70	DNA topoisomerase I	30% dSSc 10% lSSc	Diffuse skin disease, interstitial lung disease
Anti-RNA polymerase III	RNA polymerase III	25% dSSc 2% lSSc	Rapid-onset and **severe** disease with major organ and **diffuse cutaneous** involvement
Antifibrillarin	U3RNP	5%	Diffuse skin disease, **internal organ involvement**
Anti-centromere	CENP-B	50% lSSc 5–7% dSSc	**CREST, pulmonary HTN**
		Dermatomyositis	
Anti-p155	TIFγ1 nuclear proteins	80% CADM, 20% classic	**MSA, amyopathic** dermatomyositis, **cancer-**associated dermatomyositis
Anti-Jo1 pulmonary	Histidyl tRNA synthetase	20%	**MSA, antisynthetase syndrome** (Raynaud phenomenon, mechanic's hands, fibrosis, arthritis, myositis)
Anti-EJ	Glycyl-tRNA synthetase	rare	MSA, antisynthetase syndrome
Anti-OJ	Isoleuecyl-tRNA synthetase	rare	MSA, antisynthetase syndrome
PL-7, PL-12	tRNA synthetase	3–5%	MSA, antisynthetase syndrome
MDA-5/ CADM-140	MDA5/IFIH1	10–45%	MSA, CADM, ILD, vasculopathy
Anti-NXP-2	Nuclear matrix protein	20–25% JDM	MSA, associated with calcinosis in JDM, associated with cancer in adults
Anti-SRP	Signal recognition particle	5%	**MSA, cardiac** involvement, severe and poor prognosis
Anti-Mi2	Nuclear helicase	15%	MSA, Hallmark **skin lesions, good prognosis**
Anti-Ku	p70/p80 protein	<5%	MAA, DM/PM overlap with SLE or scleroderma
Anti-PM/Scl	Nucleolar proteins	<10%	MAA, DM/PM overlapping with **scleroderma**
		Mixed connective tissue disease (MCTD)	
Anti-U1RNP	Ribonucleoprotein	100%	MCTD

MAA, myositis-associated autoantibody; MSA, myositis specific autoantibody.

CHRONIC CUTANEOUS LE (CCLE/DLE)

Epidemiology

- Age-adults mostly
- F > M
- More common and more severe in Asians and other skins of color
- Around half patients—fulfills ACR criteria for SLE.

Pathophysiology

- UVR (UVB > UVA) → increases SS-A/Ro antigen expression on keratinocyte surface (further increased by estrogen) → antibody binding → disease
- Type I interferon signature suggestive of CD4+ T-helper 1 (Th1) cells and CD8+ cytotoxic T cell recruitment and activation.

Predisposing Factors

- Genetic
- UV exposure
- Trauma (including X-rays and diathermy), stress, infections (including herpes zoster).
- Drugs: Thiazides, isoniazid, penicillamine, CCBs, terbinafine, griseofulvin, dapsone.
- Tobacco: Risk factor for recalcitrant disease.

Clinical Types

- Localized DLE → SLE (1.3–6.5%)
- Disseminated DLE → SLE (22%)

1. *Localized (lDLE)*

Face and scalp are most commonly affected and circumscribed or discoid form is the most frequent type.

- Occurs predominantly on cheeks, bridge of nose, concha or triangular fossa of ears, **(Fig. 8.4a** and **b)**, side of neck and scalp.
- Scarring alopecia in scalp—in one-third of patients (*see* Chapter 11: CCLE scalp)
- Adherent scale which, when removed, shows horny plugs on under surface occupying dilated pilosebaceous canals—**'tin-tack'** sign (also sometimes seen in localized pemphigus foliaceous).
- Scarring is common and may be **atrophic, hypertrophic, cribriform or acneiform**.
- Pigmentary disturbances (central depigmentation and peripheral hyperpigmentation) **(Fig. 8.4c)**.
- Relapses start in the erythematous zone surrounding the scar **(Fig. 8.4d)**.

2. *Disseminated (dDLE)*

- Widespread pattern on trunk and limbs.
- Mostly in women, usually cigarette smokers.
- Six types:
  i. **Papulosquamous:** Resembling papulosquamous type of SCLE but scarring occurs. Persistent and resistant to therapy.

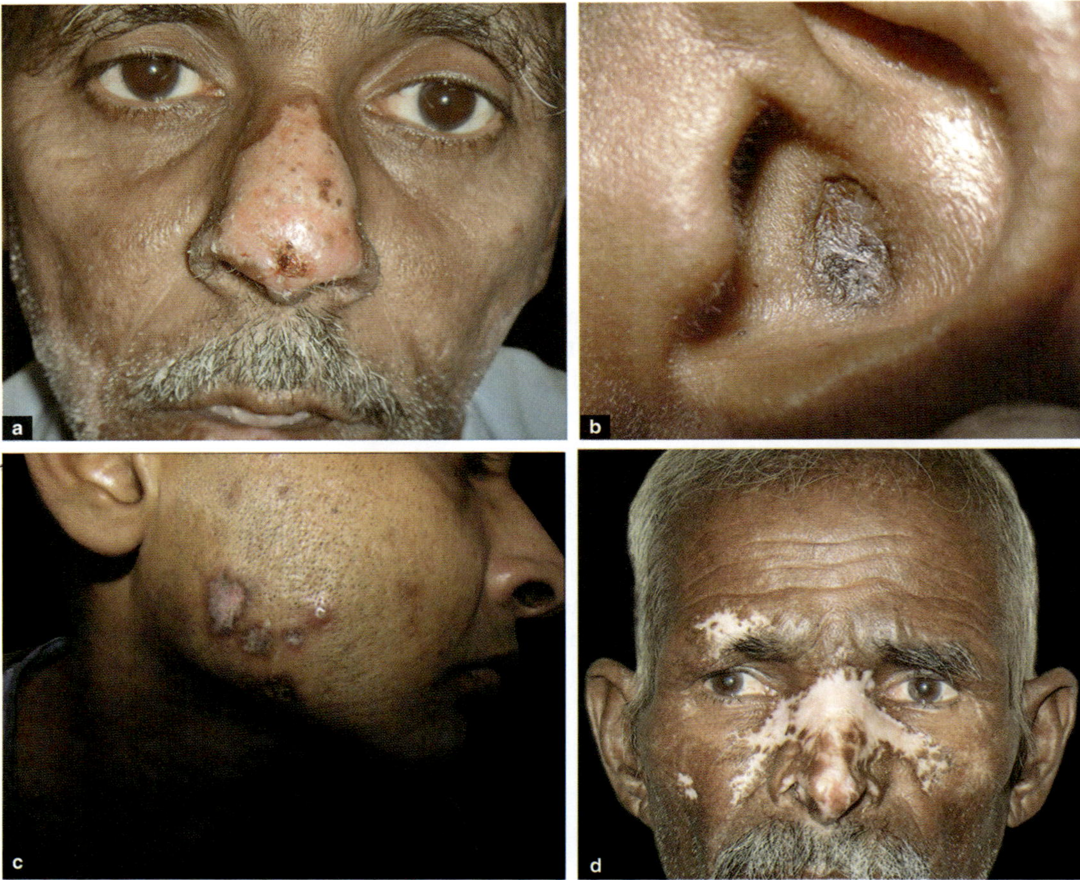

Fig. 8.4a to d: (a) DLE plaque on the nose, note the follicular plugging; (b) DLE with follicular plugging and scarring in the concha of the ear (Shuster sign); (c) A case of DLE with the prominent peripheral pigmentation and central scarring depigmentation and follicular plugging; (d) DLE healing with marked pigmentary loss

ii. **Reticulate telangiectasia/lupus erythematosus telangiectoides:** Usually seen on arms, legs and back of the calves but may be widespread.
iii. **Annular variant/lupus erythematosus gyratum repens:** Consists of migratory gyrate annular erythema.
iv. **Bullous:** Rare
v. **Arteritic:** Resembles Degos syndrome or disseminated atrophie blanche.
vi. **Linear lesions:** Follow Blaschko lines.

Clinical Variants of DLE

a. Chilblain lupus

- In 6%, predominantly females, chilblain-like lesions mainly on toes and fingers.
- Precipitated by pregnancy

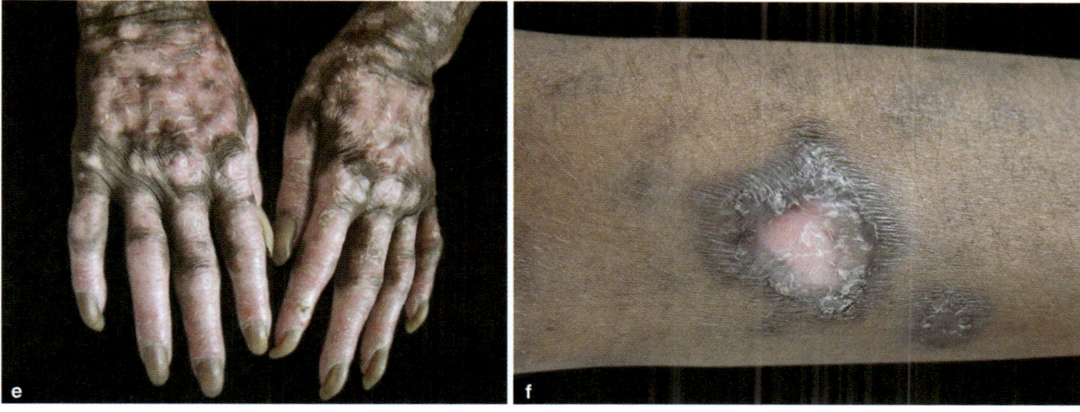

Fig. 8.4e and f: (e) Chilblain lupus; (f) Hypertrophic DLE

- Some patients have cryofibrinogenemia or cold agglutinins.
- Often anti-Ro antibody positive (may be negative)
- The fingers and toes **(Fig. 8.4e)** may become markedly atrophic, with patchy erythema and tuft resorption on X-ray.
- 15% patients develop SLE
- Persist year-round (*vs* non-lupus-associated chilblains)

b. Lupus erythematosus (LE) profundus (panniculitis) (Kaposi–Irgang disease):

- Unusual
- Cutaneous infiltrate present primarily in deeper portions of the dermis giving rise to firm, sharply defined nodules, lying beneath clinically normal skin and followed by atrophy of fat.
- Clinical LE profundus occurs in 3–5% of patients with DLE while histologically in up to 30%.
- Antimalarials effective
- 15% may be associated with SLE (panniculitis may be first sign)

c. Hypertrophic (verrucous) LE

- Thick, hyperkeratotic and verrucous scaling plaques with indurated border **(Fig. 8.4f)**
- ↑ risk of SCC (akin to hypertrophic LP)
- Typical locations: Extensor forearms, face, and upper trunk (sun-exposed sites)
- Usually accompany typical discoid lesions
- Topical and systemic retinoids are the drugs of choice.

d. Annular atrophic plaques

- Depressed atrophic centre of raised annular plaque
- D/D—morphea/lichen sclerosus

Diagnosis and Severity Scoring

Classification criteria for DLE (Elman, et al., 2017) is given in **Table 8.2** and is mostly for use in clinical trials. Cutaneus Lupus Erythematosus Disease Area and Severity Index (CLASI) is used to score disease activity and damage.

TABLE 8.2: Classification criteria for DLE (Elman, et al., 2017)	
Clinical feature	**Points assigned**
Atrophic scarring	3
Location in the conchal bowl	2
Preference for head and neck	2
Dyspigmentation	1
Follicular hyperkeratosis/plugging	1
Erythematous to violaceous in color	1

*A score of 5 points yields classification as DLE with 84.1% sensitivity and 75.9% specificity, while a score of 7 points yields 73.9% sensitivity and 92.9% specificity.

Differential Diagnosis

Table 8.3 lists the common differential diagnoses of DLE.

Investigations

Table 8.4 lists the important investigations in DLE while a comparison of clinical features and serological tests of DLE and SLE is given in **Table 8.5**.

Histopathology of cutaneous LE is important and detailed below:

1. Epidermal atrophy
2. Keratotic plugging
3. Liquefactive degeneration of the basal layer
4. Lymphocytic interface dermatitis
5. Apoptotic keratinocytes
6. Edema and hyalinization and thickening of the basement membrane
7. Dermal mucinosis
8. Marked perivascular and periadnexal inflammatory infiltrate.

Lupus band test (LBT): LBT (+) on lesional skin in 75%; ideal to choose lesion that has been present for a few months or more. More likely to be positive on head/neck and extremities compared with trunk.

TABLE 8.3: Differential diagnosis of DLE	
Disease	**Differentiating features**
Rosacea	Pustules +, episodic flushing + (absent in DLE)
Jessener lymphocytic infiltrate	No immunoglobulin deposition at dermoepidermal junction on DIF (present in DLE)
Lupus vulgaris	Early age of onset, may be ulcerated and usually has apple-jelly nodules on diascopy
Morphea and lichen sclerosus	• Morphea—bruise like → sclerotic → atrophic Collagen hyalinization on biopsy • LSeA—porcelain white, atrophy Characteristic 3 zones on biopsy

TABLE 8.4: Investigations in DLE

- Diagnosis is clinical—demonstrate 'Tin-Tack' sign
- ANA and extractable nuclear antigens (ENAs) to assess the possibility of having systemic form of disease
- Routine hematology and biochemistry
- Urine testing for proteinuria
- Visual acuity and visual fields for those requiring antimalarials
- Histopathology
- Lupus band test

TABLE 8.5: Comparison of clinical features and serological tests of DLE and SLE

	DLE (n = 120) (%)	SLE (n = 40) (%)
Rash	**100**	80
Joint pains	23	**70**
Fever	0	40
Raynaud phenomenon	14	35
Chilblains	22	22
Poor peripheral circulation	26	32
ESR >20 mm/h	20	85
Serum globulin >3 g (%)	29	76
LE cells	1.7	**83**
Antinuclear antibody (ANA)	35	**87**
Homogeneous	24	74
Speckled	11	26
Nucleolar	0	5.4
Precipitating autoantibodies	4	42
WR positive	5	22
Rheumatoid factor positive	15	37
Direct Coombs test positive	2.5	37
Leukopenia	12.5	37
Thrombocytopenia	5	21

WR, Wassermann reaction

A summary of the salient histopathological features of clinical variants of DLE is given in **Table 8.6**.

Treatment

General Principles

- Appropriate sun protection against UVA and UVB.
- Avoid smoking, stress

  For Raynaud's phenomenon and chilblains—vasodilators like calcium channel blockers—nifedipine and intravenous prostacyclin.

TABLE 8.6: HPE of variants of DLE	
Hypertrophic (verrucous) LE	• Orthohyperkeratosis and **endophytic buds of hyperplastic follicular epithelium** • Dense lymphatic infiltrate
Chilblain LE	• Demonstrates features of both chilblains (papillary edema, perivascular and dermal lymphohistiocytic infiltration) and DLE • DIF: Positive
Tumid LE	• Epidermis is normal • Massive mucin deposition in dermis (more than classic DLE) • DIF: Should be negative by definition but a study showed +ve DIF in 16/19 patients
LE panniculitis	Subcutaneous findings: • Lymphocytic lobular panniculitis • Hyaline ('waxy/pink') fat necrosis • Nodular lymphoid aggregates • Fat lobules may be rimmed by lymphocytes

Flowchart 8.1: Treatment of DLE

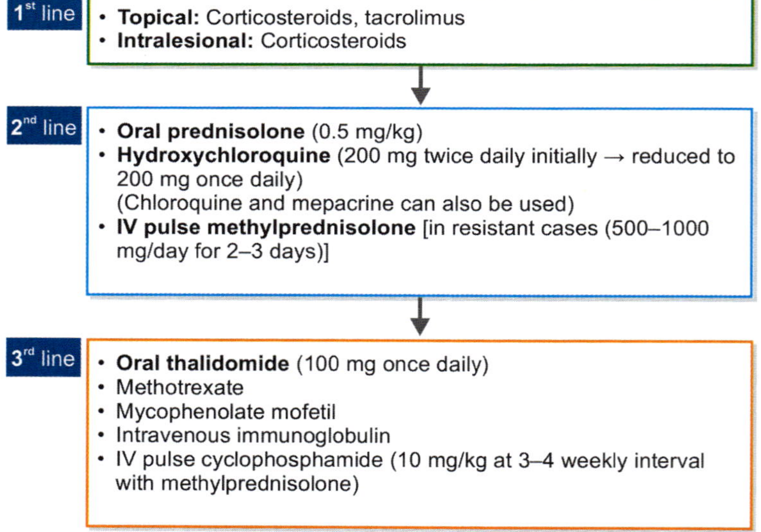

- **Flowchart 8.1** depicts a treatment algorithm for DLE.
- Other drugs: Acitretin, auranofin, dapsone, cyclosporine, sulfasalazine, isotretinoin, clofazimine, phenytoin, azathioprine.

Therapy Update

Recent drugs have been used targeting the main pathogenic steps that mediate DLE. It has been shown that the main cytokine that plays a dominant role in LE is type I IFNs and this has been shown by gene expression analyses in both SLE and CLE and their role is depicted in **Fig. 8.5**. This lead to the use of development of anti-IFN directed therapeutic strategies of LE

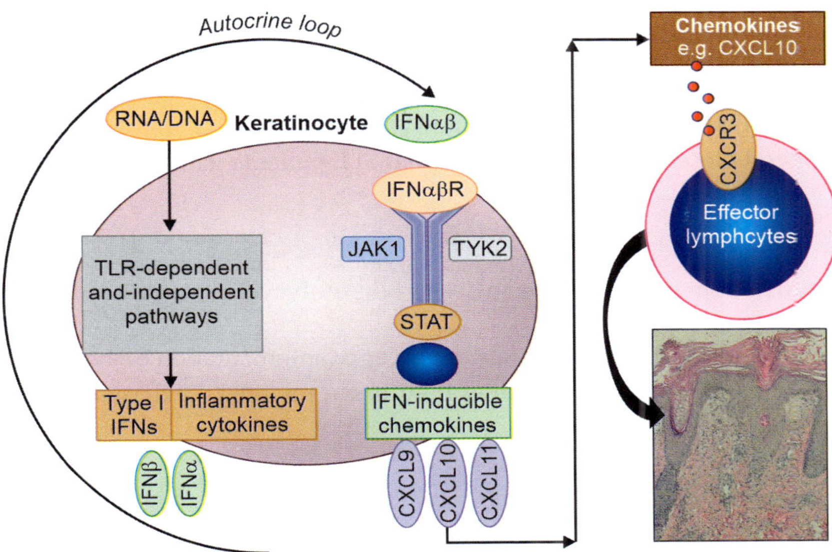

Fig. 8.5: Endogenous nucleic acids (RNA/DNA) activate TLR-dependent and -independent pathways to produce proinflammatory cytokines and type I interferons (IFN) which by a autocrine loop activate JAK1/TYK2-signaling by binding to IFN-α/β receptor thus enhancing CXCL chemokine production (e.g. CXCL10). Chemokines recruit CXCR3 + effector cells into lesional skin, which induce keratinocyte cell death and again release of proinflammatory mediators. JAK1-inhibitors prevent JAK/STAT-mediated signal transduction and significantly reduce chemokine gene expression by functionally targeting JAK1.

patients inlcuding sifalimumab and rontalizumab but while they reduced the IFN signature in the blood but had limited effect on disease activity. This was possibly due to the high variability of the different type I IFNs, including not only IFNα but also IFNβ and IFNκ binding to the same receptors. Thus a specific anti-IFNαβ-receptor antibody **anifrolumab** was used and it significantly reduced the CLASI skin score in LE patients (Carter LM, 2023).

The other agents that can be used include "indirect" inhibition of the IFN system by (i) targeting the IFN-producing cells or (ii) the intracellular IFN-pathway. In skin and blood plasmacytoid DCs are regarded as the main IFN-producing cells and the pDC-specific antibodies BIIB059 and VIB7734 are now in clinical trials with first results indicating a decline of the CLASI-activity score.

As the IFN-pathway, is mediated by **JAK1/TYK2** signaling, JAK inhibitors are emerging as a potential tool in DLE and SLE.

Lupus Erythematosus Tumidus (LET)

- Some authors call this as: 'Intermittent cutaneous LE' (in Duesseldorf classification of cutaneous LE).
- Considered to be on a clinical spectrum with Jessner lymphocytic infiltrate (JLI) and reticular erythematous mucinosis (REM), with similar findings on histology.

- Lupus tumidus (LET) and Jessner lymphocytic infiltrate are not part of LE spectrum because of:
    - Lack of interface dermatitis (histological hallmark of LE).
    - Also, no 'IFN signature' (large number of IFN-inducible genes are upregulated in peripheral blood mononuclear cells from SLE patients with active disease).

- ***Extreme photosensitivity***, M > F
- Face
- Erythematous edematous smooth urticaria-like polycyclic plaques with sharp raised borders
- No follicular plugging, no scaling, no scarring or dyspigmentation on healing.
- HPE—dense perivascular and periadnexal infiltrate, no interface dermatitis
- DIF—negative
- ANA +ve in only 10%.

SUBACUTE CUTANEOUS LE (SCLE)

- 10% of LE
- Mostly females

Clinical Features

- Papulosquamous (two-thirds) or annular/polycyclic (one-third) erythematous scaly plaques above the waist on shoulders, trunk, extensor arms; face typically spared; heal without scarring but telangiectasia and hypopigmentation are common; fatigue and arthralgias common but limited organ involvement **(Fig. 8.6)**. Diffuse nonscarring alopecia and photosensitivity in 50%.
- **Drug-induced SCLE:** Most important implicated drugs—hydrochlorothiazide, terbinafine, diltiazem, ACE inhibitors, NSAIDs, griseofulvin, antihistamines, IFN, PUVA, TNF-α.

Associations

HLA-B8 (strongest), HLA-DR3 (annular SCLE, anti-Ro), HLA-DR2 (papulosquamus SCLE), HLA-DRw52, HLA-DQ1.

Differential Diagnoses

Dermatomyositis, SLE, annular erythemas, granuloma annulare, lichen planus, psoriasis, tinea corporis.

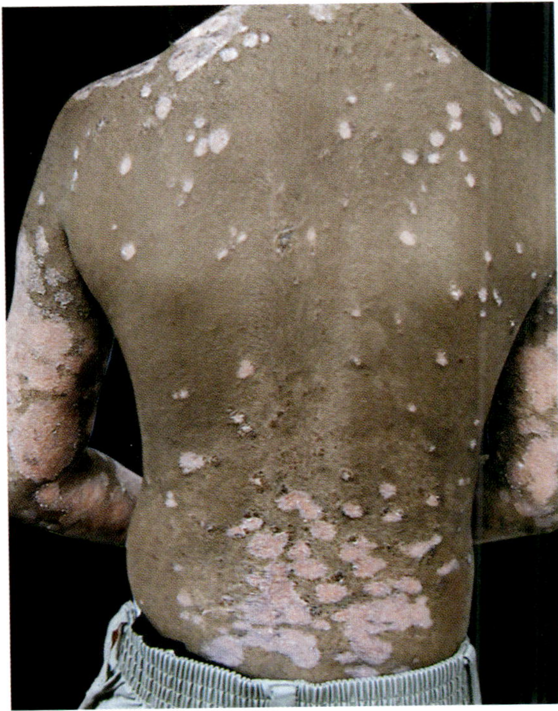

Fig. 8.6: Annular lesions of subacute LE

Investigations

60–80% +ve ANA, 60–90% **+ve anti-Ro**, histopathology similar to DLE but SCLE has more epidermal atrophy and lesser hyperkeratosis, basement membrane thickening, follicular plugging, inflammatory infiltrate and pilosebaceous atrophy.

Course

Persistent with intermittent flares, up to 50% will eventually meet SLE criteria (but milder disease).

Treatment

Sun protection, topical steroids and tacrolimus, antimalarials, oral corticosteroid, dapsone or other immunosuppressive agents.

Neonatal LE

This is being mentioned here as it is usually associated with the same autoantibodies as subacute cutaneous LE (**Fig. 8.7)** though it is detailed later (under SLE).

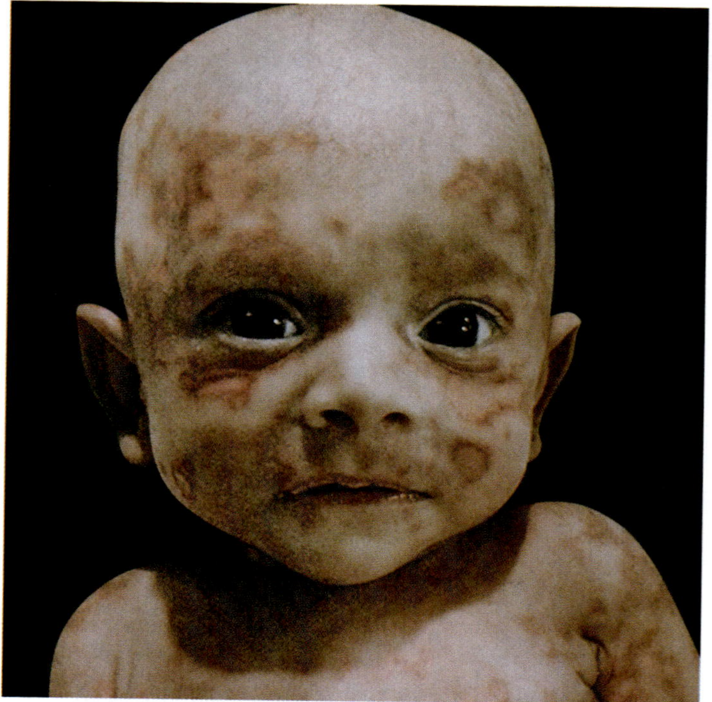

Fig. 8.7: Annular lesions of neonatal LE (*Courtesy:* Dr Chanchal Singh, MD, MRCOG)

SYSTEMIC LUPUS ERYTHEMATOSUS

A combination of history, clinical findings, and laboratory values were used by Gilliam and Sontheimer to classify LE—**Gilliam classification (Fig. 8.8a)**.

Criteria for SLE

- ARA (1971)
- ACR (earlier ARA) (1982) (1997—further modification)
- SLICC (Systemic Lupus International Collaborating Clinics) (2012)—higher sensitivity (96.7%) but lower specificity (83.7%) **(Fig. 8.8b)**.
- The recent ACR/EULAR criteria for classification of SLE (2019) state that ANA of at least 1: 80 on HEP-2 cells or an equivalent positive test is imperative for diagnosis of SLE **(Fig. 8.8c)**. Sensitivity (96.1%) and specificity (93.4%).

Epidemiology

- African-Americans-highest rate of internal organs damage, especially kidney.
- **F:M** = 7:1 to 15:1
- Earlier onset in F *vs* M (38 years *vs* 44 years)

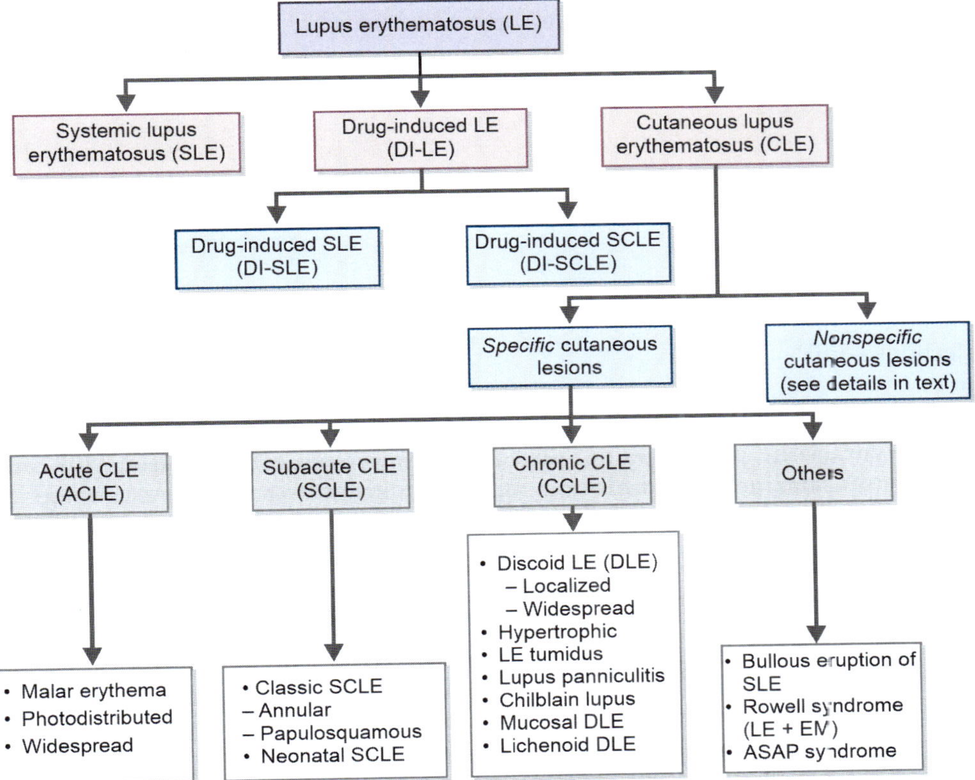

Fig. 8.8a: Classification of LE (based upon the system originally proposed by Gilliam and Sontheimer in1981)

2012 SLICC Classification Criteria for SLE

CLINICAL	IMMUNOLOGIC
• Acute cutaneous lupus	• ANA
• Chronic cutaneous lupus	• Anti-dsDNA
• Oral nasal ulcers	• Anti-Sm
• Non-scarring alopecia	• aPL antibodies
• Synovitis ≥2 joints	• Low complement
• Serositis	• Direct Coombs test
• Renal	
• Neurologic	
• Hemolytic anemia	
• Leucopenia/lymphopenia	
• Thrombocytopenia	

Fig. 8.8b: SLICC criteria for SLE (2012)
(Need at least 4 criteria with ≥1 clinical + ≥1 immunological criteria or biopsy proven lupus nephritis compatible with SLE along with ANA/anti-ds-DNA antibodies.)

- Late-onset SLE: Onset at **>50 years of age**
- Serositis and Sjögren syndrome < in elderly
- Renal, serositis, neurological, vasculitis, thrombosis, cytopenias < in males.

Predisposing Factors

Genetic factors

- HLA-DR2, DR3—most evidence.

Environmental factors

- Sunlight
- UV radiation
- Smoking
- Infections—EBV
- Stress
- Hormones—estrogen-containing OCPs, postmenopausal estrogen, prolactin
- Drugs: **Hydralazine, procainamide, quinidine, minocycline, captopril, isoniazid, carbamazepine, sulfasalazine, TNF inhibitors** (arthritis > rash). (*Note*: If ANAs develop in such patients without symptoms—no treatment is required).
- Silica and solvents.

Pathogenesis

The development of SLE is a multistep, multifactorial process that involves a complex interplay among genetic, hormonal, and environmental factors leading to profound alterations in immune function and regulation. Aberrant cell death processes promote immunostimulatory pathways in SLE, leading to activation of innate and adaptive immune responses. Tissue-specific factors modulate the organ-specific immune responses, resulting in varying manifestations of the disease. **"IFN signature" (elevated expression of type I IFN-regulated genes) is a characteristic of SLE**. An overview of the steps in pathologenesis is shown in **Fig. 8.9a**. (Lu R, et al., 2016)

Entry citerion
Antinuclear antibodies (ANA) at a titer of ≥1:80 on HEP-2 cells or an equivalent positive test (ever)

↓

If absent, do not classify as SLE
If present, apply additive criteria

↓

Additive criteria
Do not count a criterion if there is a more likely explanation than SLE.
Occurrence of a criterion on at least one occasion is sufficient.
SLE classification requires at least one clinical criterion and ≥10 points.
Criteria need not occur simultaneously.
Within each domain, only the highest weighted criterion is counted toward the total score§.

Clinical domains and criteria	Weight	Immunology domains and criteria	Weight
Constitutional		***Anti-phospholipid antibodies***	
• Fever	2	• Anti-cardiolipin antibodies or	
		• Anti-β2GP1 antibodies or	
		• Lupus anticoagulant	2
Hematological		***Complement proteins***	
• Leukopenia	3	• Low C3 or low C4	2
• Thrombocytopenia	4	• Low C3 and low C4	4
• Autoimmune hemolysis	4		
Neuropsychiatric		***SLE-specific antibodies***	
• Delirium	2	• Anti-dsDNA antibody* or Anti-Smith antibody	6
• Psychosis	3		
• Seizure	5		
Mucocutaneous			
• Non-scarring alopecia	2		
• Oral ulcers	2		
• Subacute cutaneous or discoid lupus	4		
• Acute cutaneous lupus	6		
Serosal			
• Pleural or pericardial effusion	5		
• Acute pericarditis	6		
Musculoskeletal			
• Joint involvement	6		
Renal			
• Proteinuria >0.5g/24h	4		
• Renal biopsy Class II or V lupus nephritis	8		
• Renal biopsy Class III or IV lupus nephritis	10		
Total score			

↓

Classify as systemic lupus erythematosus with a score of 10 or more and one or more clinical criteria if entry criterion fulfilled

§ = Additional criteria within the same domain will not be counted; * = In an assay with 90% specificity against relevant disease controls.
Anti-β2GPI = Anti-β2-glycoprotein 1; Anti-dsDNA = Anti-double-stranded DNA.

Fig. 8.8c: ACR classification criteria for systemic lupus erythematosus (SLE) (2019)

The interrelationship between cytokine expression and the autoimmunity and tissue damage is depicted in **Fig. 8.9b**. It is highlighted by a <u>Th2 response</u> mediated by (IFN-γ), which leads to an augmented B cell response.

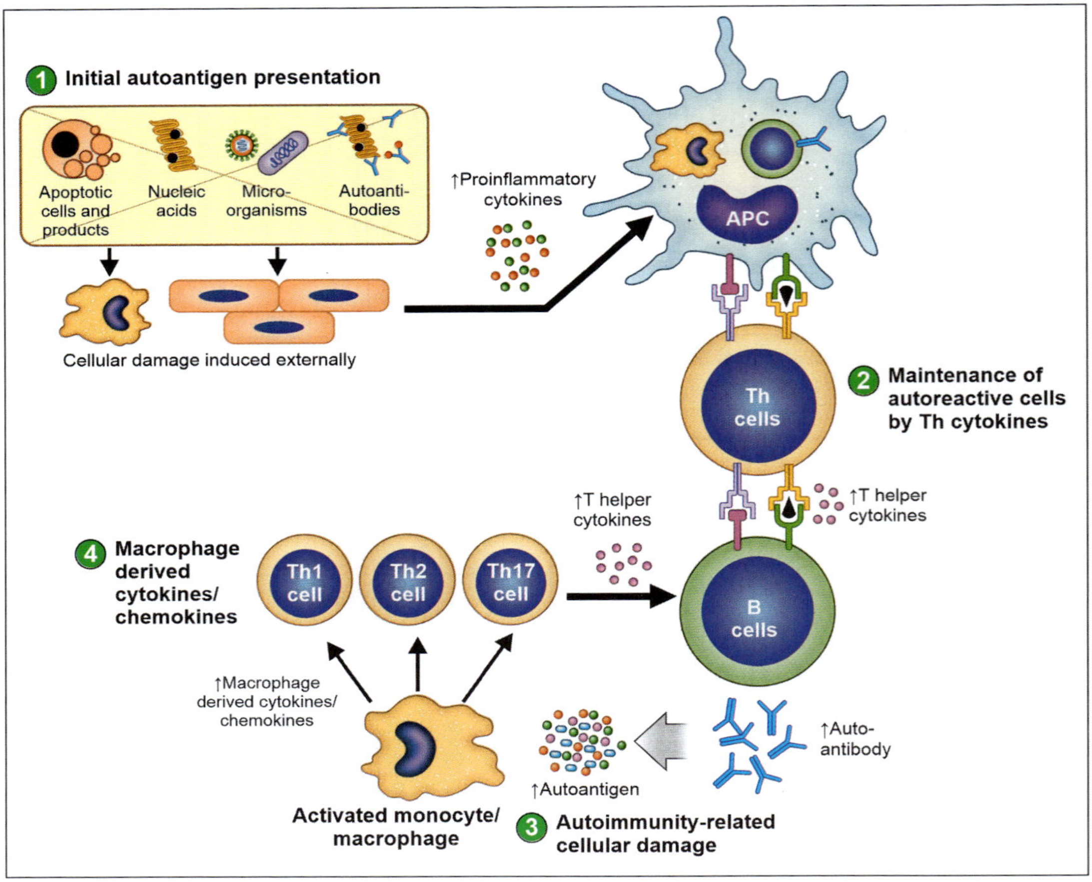

Fig. 8.9a: Pathogenesis of SLE: (1) Genetic predisposition affects apoptotic clearance, antigen presentation, and lymphocyte responses; (2) Aberrant elevation of T helper (Th)-type cytokines, which provides further costimulatory signals for the expansion of autoreactive cells and potentiates the formation of lupus-associated autoantibodies; (3) Immune dysregulation results in tissue damage and further exposure to intracellular autoantigens, which may result in hyperactivation of innate immune cells; (4) Further dysregulation of soluble mediators contributes to enhanced apoptosis and intracellular autoantigen exposure, perpetuating the cycle of autoimmunity (J Autoimmun, 2016).

Clinical Features

- Fever (90%)
- Arthritis and arthralgias (90%)
- Skin lesions (80%):

  A. **LE specific**

  i. **CCLE**—localized DLE, generalized DLE, hypertrophic DLE, lupus profundus/panniculitis, lupus tumidus, chilblain lupus, DLE/LP overlap

  ii. **SCLE**—annular, psoriasiform, mixed (in 16%).

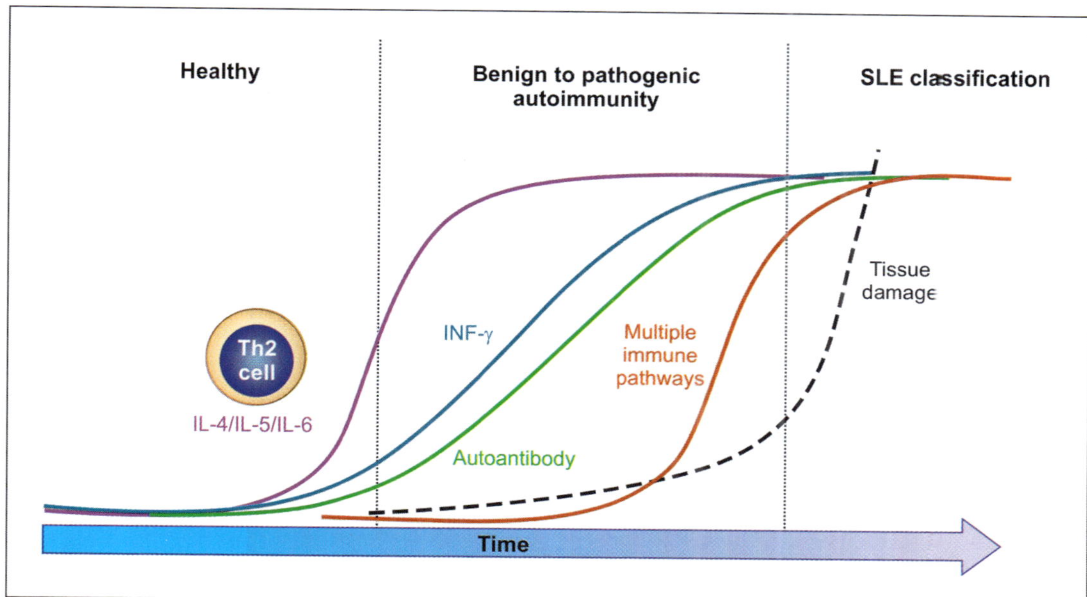

Fig. 8.9b: A depiction of the course of cytokine expression antibody response and tissue response in SLE

iii. **ACLE**

- Widespread photo-distributed erythema **(Fig. 8.10a** and **b)**
- TEN-like ACLE (acute syndrome of apoptotic panepidermolysis or ASAP) **(Fig. 8.10c)**—widespread TEN-like cleavage following a trigger in SLE patients.

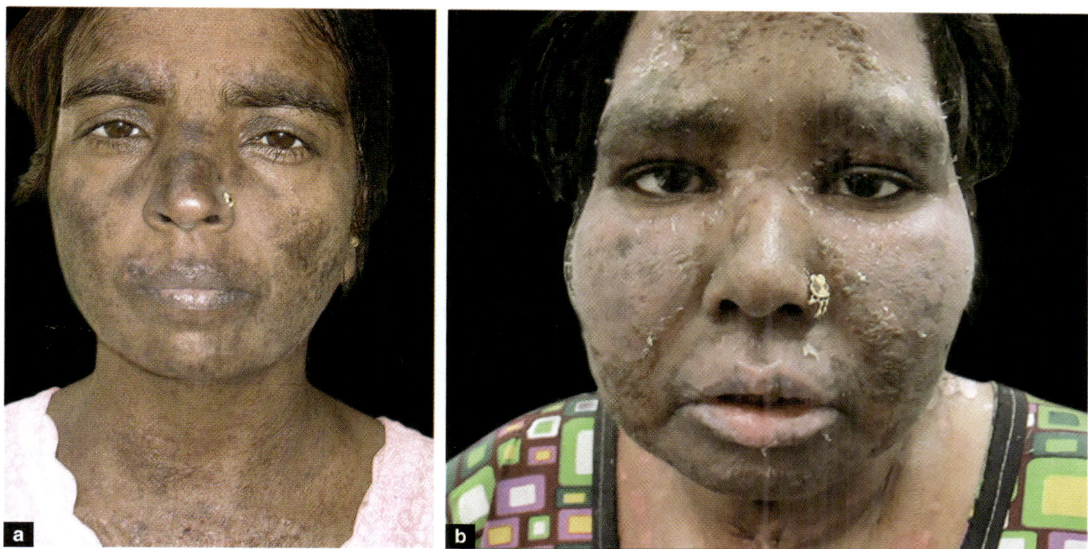

Fig. 8.10a and b: SLE—acute erythematous rash (malar rash) with post-inflammatory hyperpigmentation

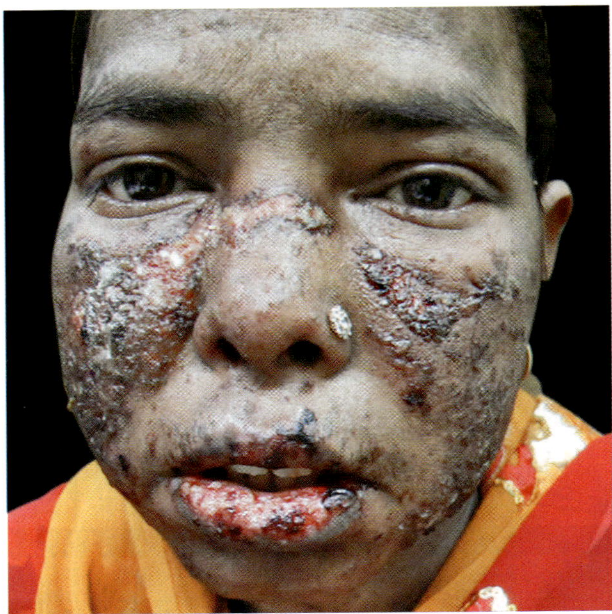

Fig. 8.10c: ASAP syndrome—acute syndrome of panepidermolysis and thrombotic storm arising in a patient with systemic lupus erythematosus, a condition that closely mimics TEN

- **Bullous ACLE**—SLE + vesicobullous eruption on sun-exposed sites. Subepidermal bulla with PMN infiltrate + IgG, IgA, IgM and C3 deposition at the BMZ. Dapsone +/– prednisolone—treatment of choice.

B. **LE non-specific**
- **Erythema** over thenar and hypothenar eminences **(Fig. 8.11a)**
- **Nail**
  - Nail-fold erythema, splinter hemorrhages, red lunulae, nail-fold hyperkeratosis, ridging, onycholysis, onychomadesis, punctate/striate leukonychia, blue-black nail pigmentation (due to antimalarials).
  - Nail-fold capillaroscopy—glomerulization of capillaries usually. Capillary drop-outs and dilatations +/–, usually with anti-U1RNP antibodies. **"Wandering" dilated glomeruloid loops**.
- **Hair**
  - **Nonscarring telogen effluvium**—most common non-specific skin manifestation of SLE (60%).
  - **Lupus hair**—due to disease activity, nonscarring, coarse dry fragile hair along hairline.
  - **Alopecia areata**
  - **Scarring alopecia**—similar to that seen in DLE
- **Vasculitis and vasculopathy**
  - **Vasculitis**—CSVV most common palpable purpura in dependent areas. Also digital gangrene, periungual infarcts, splinter hemorrhages, urticaria, bullous lesions.

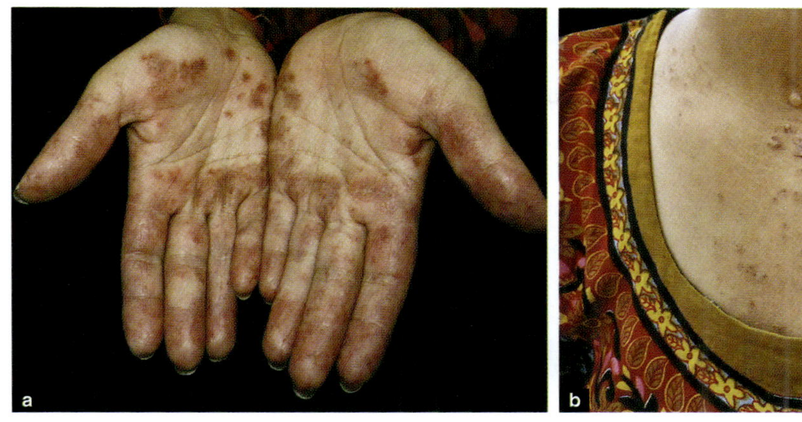
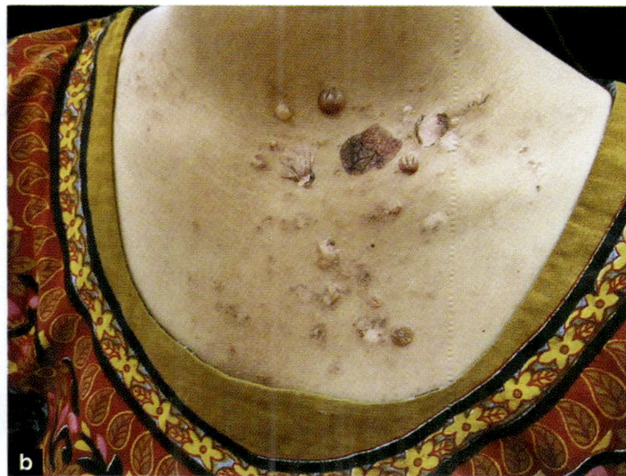

Fig. 8.11: (a) Erythema over the palms; (b) Bullous lesions on the exposed V of the neck

  - **Vasculopathy**—Raynaud's phenomenon—one of the most common nonspecific findings. Livedo reticularis, atrophic blanche-like lesions, Degos disease (malignant atrophic papulosis) like lesions.
- **Urticaria**—both urticaria and urticarial vasculitis (hypocomplementemic) may occur.
- **Mucinosis**—papulonodular mucinosis (differential diagnosis—lupus tumidus)
- **Dystrophic calcinosis**—mostly with lupus panniculitis, may occur in SLE too. Seen on extremities and buttocks. Asymptomatic nodules/ulcerated nodules extruding chalky material.
- **Bullous lesions (nonspecific)—two types:**
  - **Subepidermal bullae** due to severe liquefactive degeneration of basal layer and dermal edema, DIF –ve. **(Fig. 8.11b)**
  - **Other autoimmune bullous diseases** can be associated with SLE—including pemphigus erythematosus and other intra- and subepidermal bullous diseases, DIF +ve.
- **Pigmentary changes**
  - Hypopigmentation following DLE/ACLE lesions
  - Bluish black discoloration due to antimalarials
  - Yellow discoloration due to mepacrine
- **Mucosal lesions**
  - **Oral and nasopharyngeal ulcers**—nonspecific, shallow, in crops, not painful, on hard palate.
  - **Recurrent aphthous stomatitis**—painful

Chances of conversion to SLE

- Localized DLE—5%
- Disseminated DLE—20%
- SCLE—50%
- Chilblain DLE—20%
- Lupus panniculitis—35% (very high)
- Lupus tumidus—rare

The general physical and systemic findings in SLE are summarized in **Tables 8.7** and **8.8**.

TABLE 8.7: General physical examination findings in SLE

GPE finding	Possible causes in SLE
Hypertension	Chronic kidney disease, myocardial involvement, pulmonary hypertension
Pallor	Anemia of chronic disease. Also due to AIHA, iron deficiency, chronic kidney disease, hemolytic anemia, and PRCA (rare)
Icterus	Lupoid hepatitis, autoimmune hepatitis
Pedal edema	Hypoproteinemia, anemia, CHF, nephritic syndrome
Lymphadenopathy	Kikuchi disease

TABLE 8.8: Systemic findings in SLE

System involved	Symptoms and signs
Joints (90%)	• Arthralgias > arthritis • RA-like deformity (less erosive than RA, anti-CCP –ve) • **Rhupus** (SLE + RA, rare, erosive like RA, anti-CCP +ve) • Jaccoud arthropathy • Dystrophic calcinosis
Muscle	• Muscle pain • Inflammatory myopathy • Steroid myopathy
Bone	• AVN—osteoporosis
Heart	• <u>CAD—most common cause of death in long-standing SLE</u> • Pericarditis • Valvular dysfunction of left heart
Lungs	• Pleuritis • Acute pneumonitis (rare) • Shrinking lung syndrome (typical)—restrictive without parenchymal involvement, due to diaphragmatic fibrosis • Pulmonary hypertension (rare)
Kidney	• Important for prognosis, cause of mortality • Nephritis usually develops in first 3 years • More in younger patients
GIT	• Anorexia, vomiting, abdominal pain, esophageal dysmotility, pancreatitis (due to steroids), ascites
Liver	• Type I autoimmune hepatitis (lupoid hepatitis) • Cirrhosis • Granulomatous hepatitis • Chronic active hepatitis
Thyroid	• Hyperthyroidism, hypothyroidism
CNS	• Cognitive dysfunction • Mood disorders • Seizures • Anxiety, psychosis • Headache • Cerebrovascular disease • Polyneuropathy
Eyes	• Keratoconjunctivitis sicca • Cotton wool spots • Retinal vasculopathy • Optic neuritis (rare)
Ears	• SNHL (with antiphospholipid syndrome)

Clinical Types/Variants

- **Drug-induced SLE (DILE)**
  - ***High risk*: Procainamide, hydralazine**
  - Low risk: Quinidine, methyldopa, isoniazid, chlorpromazine, D-penicillamine, propylthiouracil, PUVA, minocycline, TNF-α inhibitors
  - Usually develops >1 year after drug initiation, typically resolves within 4–6 weeks of discontinuation of offending drug.
  - Less in blacks, more in elderly, renal and CNS uncommon.
  - Antihistone antibodies (+), anti-DNA antibodies (–), serum complement—normal
    Exceptions: Minocycline → negative antihistone, positive ANCA (against MPO or elastase).
    Also TNF-α inhibitors: Anti-dsDNA antibodies frequently positive (>antihistone) and more skin involvement.
  - DILE typically **lacks skin findings** and has milder systemic involvement. MC symptom is **arthritis/arthralgia** (90%)
- **SLE in elderly:** 12–18%
  - Raynaud's phenomenon, sicca symptoms, pleuritis—more common
  - Renal disease—less
  - Anti-Ro, anti-La, HLA-DR3—more common
- **SLE in childhood:** 15–20% onset in childhood
  - **More severe** overall
  - Malar rash, mucocutaneous lesions, hematological abnormalities, seizures, renal involvement, urinary cellular casts, proteinuria, lymphadenopathy, fever—more common
- **SLE in females**
  a. **SLE and pregnancy**
     - Clinical remission/minimal activity in preceding 6 months before conception lowers chances of disease flare during pregnancy. But SLE increases chances of complicated pregnancy even if no flare
       - Active lupus nephritis—highest risk of fetal loss (8–36% risk)
       - Other major risk factors for adverse maternal/fetal outcome-active/flaring SLE, history of lupus nephritis, presence of antiphospholipids (aPL)/antiphospholipid syndrome (APS)
       - APS—if untreated, 45–90% pregnancies may have fetal loss, 30% on treatment.
       - Monitor with:
         - KFT
         - Serological markers—C3/C4, anti-dsDNA titers
         - Fetal Doppler (in T3)—if SLE with APS
         - Fetal echo-suspected fetal dysrhythmia/myocarditis, esp. if anti-Ro/anti-La +ve
       - Pregnancy outcome:
         - 20%—preeclampsia
         - 30%—preterm delivery
         - 30%—cesarean section
       - Treatment of SLE in pregnancy
         - BP monitoring/control

- Low-dose aspirin (LDA)
- LMWH
- HCQS—safe, may reduce disease flares, may reduce neonatal lupus and heart block—start preconception and continue throughout pregnancy
- Oral prednisolone (<10% crosses placenta)—safe
- Azathioprine—safe
- Cyclosporine—safe
- Severe flare—IV pulse steroids, IVIG, plasmapheresis
- MMF, MTX, cyclophosphamide, leflunomide—contraindicated
- Calcium, vit. D, folic acid supplementation

- Vaccination
  - HPV vaccination—if stable/inactive SLE, SLE with APS

b. **Contraception and SLE**
   - Barrier/Copper IUD—safe
   - Combined OCP, levonorgestrel-containing IUD—may be given in stable/inactive SLE, avoid in aPL/APS
   - Progestin—only pills—safe in stable/inactive SLE, may be given in aPL/APS if benefit outweighs risk of thrombosis
   - Progestin—only emergency contraception—may be given in SLE, APS

c. **Fertility in SLE**

   Fertility normal if renal function good and not on alkylating agents. It may be reduced due to increasing age while waiting for disease to stabilize and due to alkylating agents.
   - Fertility preservation with GnRH analogs for all women on alkylating agents
   - Assisted reproductive techniques—safe in stable/inactive disease

d. **SLE and lactation**
   - Azathioprine safe—majority excreted within 4 hours. So, breastfeed after 4 hours of dose.
   - Aspirin—safe
   - HCQS—safe
   - Low dose steroids—safe

- **Neonatal LE**
  - Autoimmune disease caused by transplacental passage of maternal autoantibodies against Ro/SS-A (>90%), La/SS-B and less commonly U1-RNP. Associated with high mortality and morbidity.
    - Women with SLE or another defined CTD with anti-Ro/SS-A-antibodies—**15%** risk having a child with NLE
    - Women who have a prior child with NLE—**25%** risk of NLE in subsequent children
  - Annular scaly red plaques involving head and extremities, periorbital erythema "raccoon eyes" **(Fig. 8.5)**.

    Lesions resolve spontaneously within 6 months without scarring; associated with **congenital heart block (30–40%)**, thrombocytopenia and transaminitis.
  - Investigations: Anti-Ro positive (maternal autoantibodies)

Prevention of cardiac disease *in utero*:

- Prenatal systemic corticosteroids may ↓risk of developing **congenital heart block**, but do not decrease rate of **cutaneous NLE**.
- Hydroxychloroquine throughout pregnancy ↓risk of a child with cardiac NLE.

Associated Diseases

- **Kikuchi–Fujimoto disease**
  - Benign self-limiting histiocytic necrotizing lymphadenitis
  - Females > males
  - Tender cervical lymphadenopathy
  - Fever, weight loss, night sweats

Investigations

Table 8.9 details the investigations in a patient of SLE while **Table 8.10** lists the autoantibodies and their associations in SLE.

TABLE 8.9: Investigations in SLE

Bedside tests	• Urine for proteins • Tests for Raynaud's phenomenon
Routine tests	• Hemogram with ESR and CRP • LFT, KFT • Urine routine/microscopy • Complement levels
Histopathology	• Liquefactive degeneration of the stratum basale and upper dermal edema with interface vacuolar dermatitis and perivascular lymphocytic infiltrate • Fibrinoid necrosis • Collagen sclerosis and necrosis • Mucin in reticular dermis • **LE cells**—PMNs that have engulfed nuclear material from dying cells • **Hematoxylin/basophilic bodies**—blue staining homogeneous material (stains for DNA by Fuelgen technique)—from nuclei of dying cells • Increase in plasmacytoid dendritic cells (PDCs) and expression of type I IFN-related proteins
DIF	• **IgG > IgM > IgA with C3 and C1q —at DEJ** (2 or more Igs—more suggestive of SLE) • Lupus band test – Involved skin—>80% – Exposed uninvolved skin—75% – Unexposed uninvolved skin—50%
Serology (see also Table 8.10)	• Non-organ-specific Ab • ANA—95–100% sensitive for SLE. May be positive around 3 years prior to eventual clinical diagnosis. 1–5% → ANA negative SLE • **Anti-DNA and anti-RNA antibodies**—unlikely to be pathogen c
Others	• Cryoglobulins (11%) • Cold agglutinins (6%)

TABLE 8.10: Associations of autoantibodies in SLE

Parameter	Prevalence in SLE (%)	Role
ANA	99	No correlation with activity/severity
Anti-dsDNA	60–70	• Not sensitive, but highly specific • Levels correlate with active SLE (esp. >200 IU/mL) • Monitoring disease activity • Lupus nephritis
Anti-Sm	30	Specific for SLE, not correlate with activity
Antihistone	40	Drug-induced LE
Anti-rRNP (anti-ribosomal P protein)	25–40	• Higher in African–Americans • Neuropsychiatric SLE
Anti-Ro	30–40	Rash, heart block in NLE, photosensitivity, Sjögren's syndrome, interstitial pneumonitis, shrinking lung syndrome, deforming arthropathy, ANA negative SLE, lupus-like syndromes, SCLE (75–90%)
Anti-La	10–15	With anti-Ro, Sjögren's syndrome, SCLE (30–40%)
Anti-cardiolipin		APL syndrome
Lupus anticoagulant		Thrombosis, abortion
Antiphospholipid		Thrombosis, abortion
Anti-U1RNP	50	Overlap syndrome, MCTD (100%)

Treatment

The treatment of SLE is difficult to compress into a section; hence we have detailed in **Table 8.11** the treatment of SLE according to disease severity and in **Table 8.12** as per the predominant organ involved. An algorithmic approach to treatment of nonrenal SLE (EULAR 2019) is depicted in **Fig. 8.12** and can serve as a visual overview of the treatment of SLE.

TABLE 8.11: Treatment of SLE according to disease severity (EULAR 2019)

Severity of disease	Treatment options
All patients	• Smoking cessation • Photoprotection—broad spectrum sunscreens, broad brimmed hats • HCQ (up to 5 mg/kg real BW)
Treatment for Raynaud's phenomenon	• *See* section on systemic sclerosis
Mild disease	• Potent TCS • HCQ/CQ/mepacrine/quinacrine*
Moderate–severe disease (not responding to HCQ alone)	**ADD** • IV pulsed methylprednisone (250–1000 mg/day for 1–3 day) → taper to oral prednisolone (<7.5 mg/day)
Severe–active disease (not responding to HCQ +/– CS or Unable to taper CS or organ-threatening disease)	**ADD** • MTX/azathioprine/MMF

(*Contd.*)

TABLE 8.11: Treatment of SLE according to disease severity (EULAR 2019) (*Contd.*)

Severity of disease	Treatment options
Severe organ-threatening SLE or not responding to other immunosuppressives (rescue therapy)	• Cyclophosphamide
Inadequate response to standard-of-care (HCQ + CS +/– immunosuppressive), defined as residual disease activity not allowing tapering of CS and/or frequent relapses	Consider • Belimumab
Organ-threatening disease refractory or with intolerance/ contraindications to standard immunosuppressive agents	Consider • Rituximab

*Maximum dose of HCQ–5 mg/kg/day, CQ–2.3 mg/kg/day.

TABLE 8.12: Treatment of SLE according to organ involvement (EULAR 2019)

Organ involved	Treatment option
Skin	• Topical—CS/TCI • Systemic—HCQ +/– CS
Neuropsychiatric (inflammation-related symptoms)	CS/immunosuppressives
Neuropsychiatric (aPL-related symptoms)	• Anti-platelet (aspirin) • Anti-coagulant (LMWH)
Hematological (acute thrombocytopenia)	• High dose CS/IV pulsed methylprednisiolone +/– • IVIG
Hematological (maintenance)	Immunosuppressives—MMF/Aza/Cyc
Renal (induction treatment)	• MMF or • Low-dose cyclophosphamide
Renal [high risk of renal failure (less GFR, fibrous crescents or fibrinoid necrosis, tubular atrophy or interstitial fibrosis)]	• MMF +/– • High dose cyclophosphamide
Renal (maintenance)	• MMF or • Azathioprine
Renal (incomplete response/severe nephrotic syndrome/ high chronicity index/reduced GFR (rule out uncontrolled hypertension)	• MMF + Low dose cyclosporine/tacrolimus
Antiphospholipid syndrome (APS)—prophylaxis	Anti-platelet drugs
Infections	• Immunization • Early recognisiton and treatment
Cardiovascular	• Low-dose aspirin • Lipid lowering agents

Prognosis

The survival of SLE patients has considerably increased on treatment. The prognosis and causes of death are given in **Box 8.2**.

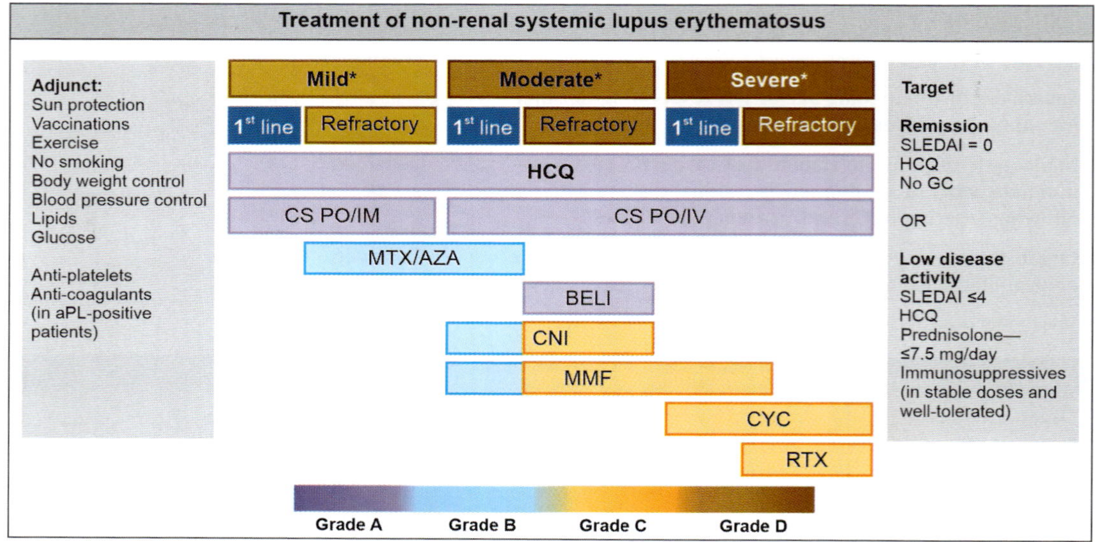

Mild: Constitutional symptoms/mild arthritis/rash ≤9% BSA/PLTs 50–100 × $10^3/mm^3$; SLEDAI ≤6; BILAG C or ≤BILAG B manifestation

Moderate: RA-like arthritis/rash 9–18% BSA/cutaneous vasculitis ≤8% BSA; PLTs 20–50 × $10^3/mm^3$/serositis; SLEDAI 7–12; ≥2 BILAG B manifestations

Severe: Major organ-threatening disease (nephritis, cerebritis, myelitis, pneumonitis, mesenteric vasculitis; mesenteric vasculitis; thrombocytopenia with platelets < 20 × $10^3/mm^3$; TTP-like disease or acute hemophagocytic syndrome; SLEDAI >12; ≥1 BILAG A manifestations

HCQ = Hydroxychloroquine; CS = Steroids; MTX = Methotrexate; AZA = Azathioprine; BELI = Belimumab; Cyc = Cyclophosphamide; CNI = Calcineurin inhibitors; MMF = Mycophenolate mofetil

Fig. 8.12: Treatment algorithm of nonrenal SLE (EULAR 2019)

BOX 8.2: Prognosis of SLE

- Childhood onset—↑ risk of lupus nephritis and mortality
- 10 year survival approx. 90%
- Most common cause of death:
  - **First** 5 years: Inflammatory lesions of SLE and infection
  - **Beyond** 5 years: Arterial (e.g. MI) and venous (i.e. DVT/PE) thromboses

Disease Activity Index

- SLEDAI is used to assess disease activity and monitor the patient on treatment.
- Patient reported outcomes (PRO)—now being used more frequently as QoL becomes increasingly relevant.

WHAT IS NEW?

Biomarkers of Specific Organ Involvement

- Alpha-1—antichymotrypsin (ACT) and haptoglobulin (HAP)—only detected (by ELISA) in urine with active renal disease. Also correlates with SLEDAI.
- Retinol binding protein (RBP)—also reliable marker.
- CCL-10 and IP-10-increased with lung involvement.
- Anti-carbamylated protein antibodies (anti-CarP)—recently described biomarker for RA. Also seen to be increased in SLE patients with arthritis.

Recent Therapies for SLE

1. **Anti-BAFF-(anti-B cell activating factor)**
   - **Belimumab**
     - Is a monoclonal Ab that binds to BAFF and blocks its binding to its B cell receptors.
     - Is the first biologic approved for SLE (2017)—USFDA approved at dose of 200 mg subcutaneous weekly for active autoantibody positive SLE on standard therapy.
     - Skin and musculoskeletal symptoms—benefit most
     - High disease activity, anti-DNA +ve, hypocomplementemia, on high steroid doses—better response
     - Smoking—decreases belimumab effect
   - **Blisibimod**
     - Binds to both soluble and membrane bound BAFF
     - Phase III trials concluded that it had a steroid-sparing effect though did not have very encouraging effects.
   - **Atacicept**
     - Anti-BAFF monoclonal antibody
     - Is a fusion protein between BAFF receptor and Fc of IgG1
     - Led to higher infection rates in SLE, failed to show an effect in trials.
2. **Anti-B cell**
   - **Rituximab**
     - Anti-CD20
     - Seen to be effective in SLE, especially lupus nephritis.
     - Increases BAFF levels—so belimumab could be used after RTX.
3. **Anti-IFN-1**
   - SLE is a prototypical IFN-1-mediated autoimmune disease.
   - High levels relate to high disease activity.
   - Over-expression of type I IFN-regulated genes—IFN signature due to continuous stimulation of pDCs.
   - Even HCQ blocks IFN by blocking TLR7, 9 activation
   - **Sifalimumab**
     - Monoclonal AB to IFN-α seen to improve SLE
   - **Anifrolumab**
     - Monoclonal AB against IFNAR1 (blocks IFN-α and IFN-β)
4. **JAK inhibitors**
   - The use of JAK inhibitors in SLE is currently being assessed and is due to the fact that there are cytokines that bridge the innate and adaptive immune systems, such as type I interferons, IL-12 and IL-23, as well as those that activate T cell–B cell interaction, such as IL-21, IL-6 and IL-4, which can be targets of JAK inhibitors as they are mediated by JAK TYK signalling pathway.

     The drugs tried include tofacitinib, baricitinib and brepocitinib.

SYSTEMIC SCLEROSIS

A spectrum of disorders are described under the umbrella term "sclerosing disorders" **(Fig. 8.13)** but here we will focus on systemic sclerosis, which is now diagnosed based on the modified ACR/EULAR criteria as given in **Table 8.13**. However, readers should keep in mind that these criteria are not applicable to:

a. Patients having a SSc-like disorder better explaining their manifestations, such as: nephrogenic systemic fibrosis, generalized morphea, eosinophilic fasciitis, scleredema diabeticorum, scleromyxedema, erythromelalgia, porphyria, lichen sclerosus, graft versus host disease, and diabetic cheiropathy.
b. Patients with 'skin thickening sparing the fingers'.

(Updated ACR/EULAR criteria are more sensitive—can pick up some early diffuse or limited SSc cases that were missed by earlier ACR criteria. However, they still miss very-early to early disease!)

Epidemiology

- Higher incidence and more severe in **African–Americans** (highest in Choctaw Native Americans)
- **F:M = 4:1**
- 20% cases—SSc overlap
- Rare—SSc sine scleroderma (only diffuse/salt and pepper pigmentation may be present)
- **SSc—highest mortality of any SARD**
- Two age peaks—30–40 years and 50–60 years (men—younger age of onset)
- **Hypertension, cardiac disease** > in elderly

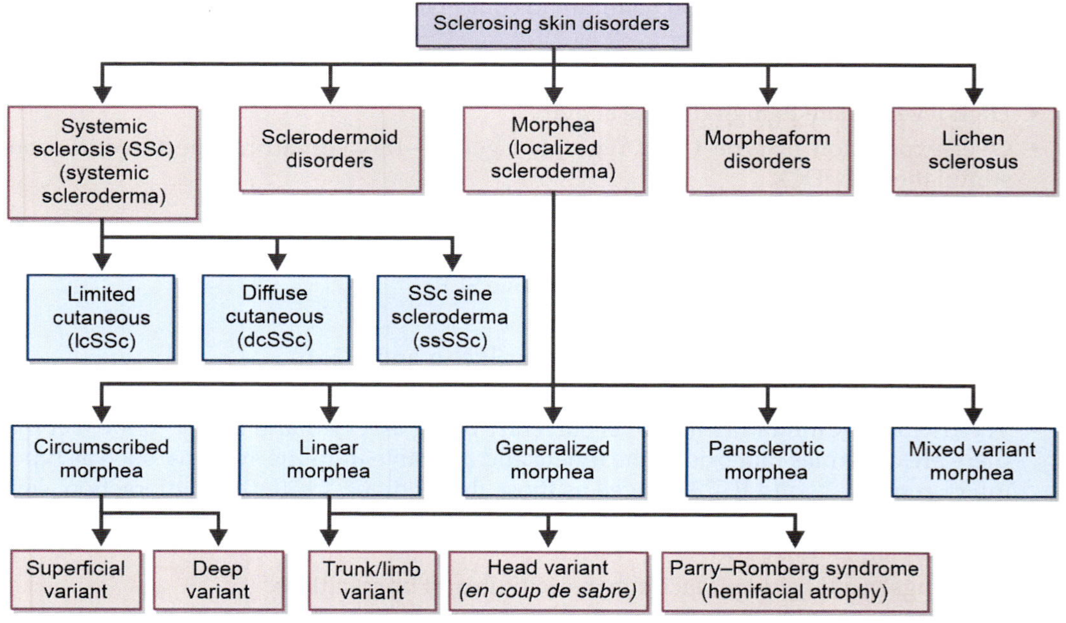

Fig. 8.13: Spectrum of sclerosing skin disorders

TABLE 8.13: ACR/EULAR classification criteria for SSc (van den Hoogen et al., 2013)

Item	Subitem(s)	Weight/score
Skin thickening of the fingers of both hands extending proximal to the metacarpophalangeal joints **(sufficient criterion)**	–	9
Skin thickening of the fingers **(*only count the higher score*)**	Puffy fingers, sclerodactyly of the fingers (distal to the MCPs but proximal to the proximal interphalangeal joints)	2 4
Fingertip lesions **(*only count the higher score*)**	Digital tip ulcers Fingertip pitting scars	2 3
Telangiectasia	–	2
Abnormal nail-fold capillaries	–	2
Pulmonary arterial hypertension and/or interstitial lung disease **(*maximum score* is 2)**	Pulmonary arterial hypertension—interstitial lung disease	2 2
Raynaud's phenomenon	–	3
SSc-related autoantibodies **(*maximum score is 3*)**	ACA, Scl-70, RNA Pol-III	3

Note: The total score is determined by adding the maximum weight (score) in each category. Patients with a total score of ≥9 are classified as having definite SSc. ACA, anti-centromere; MCPs, metacarpophalangeal joints; RNA Pol, RNA polymerase III, Scl-70, antitopoisomerase 1; SSc, systemic sclerosis. [Modified from van den Hoogen F, Khanna O, Fransen, et al., 2013 classification criteria for systemic sclerosis: an American College of Rheumatology/European League Against Rheumatism collaborative initiative. *Arthritis Rheum* 2013; 65:2737–47.]

- **Limited SSc, SSc overlap, better prognosis** > in children
- **Diffuse SSc, ILD, malignancy, higher mortality** > in males

Predisposing Factors

- **Genetic**
  - HLA-DPB1, -B, -DOA, -DRB1, -DQA1
- **Environmental**
  - Occupational—silica, organic solvents (especially PVC), white spirit, aromatic solvents, trichloroethylene, ketones, welding fumes (no association with silicone breast implants)
  - Smoking—increases severity, especially of vasculopathy.

Pathogenesis

- Four major factors—Vasculopathy + Inflammation + Fibrosis + Autoimmunity **(Fig. 8.14a)**.
- **Vascular dysfunction**, primarily of microcirculation, is the earliest feature with endothelial injury and endothelial cell activation. (Abraham DJ, et al., 2005)
- Major cytokines—**Th2**-predominant profile and ↑ production of **profibrotic cytokines** growth factors (IL-4, –6, –8, –10, –13, –17, TGF-α, PDGF, and endothelin-1) → accumulation of myofibroblasts in affected tissues → excess collagen production (predominantly types I and III) and other ECM proteins.
- **Three phases**—edematous (6–12 months) → indurative (1–4 or more years) → atrophic (rest of life).

  A detailed overview of pathogenesis is shown in **Fig. 8.14b**.

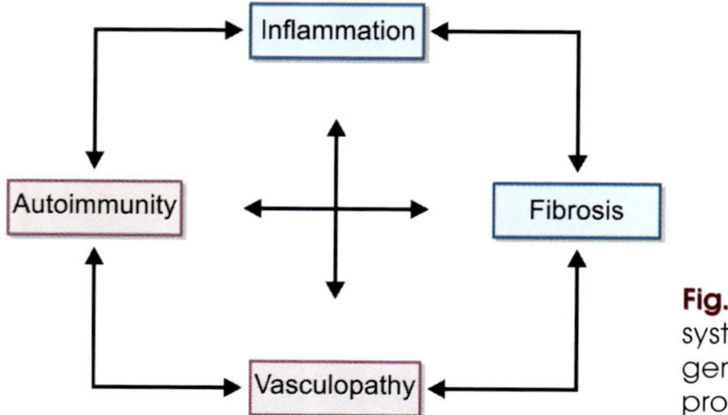

Fig. 8.14a: The pathophysiologic **quartet** underlying systemic sclerosis. Autoimmunity and vasculopathy generally precede the onset and contribute to the progression of fibrosis

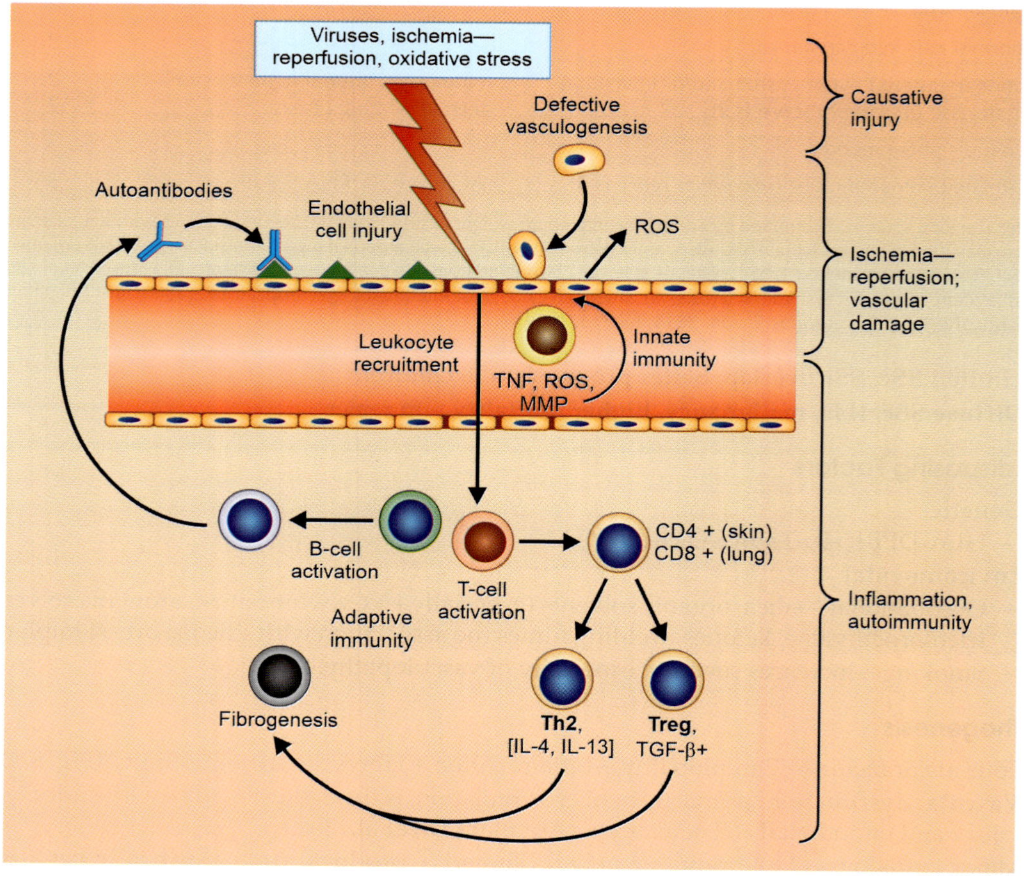

Viruses, ischemia—reperfusion, oxidative stress
Defective vasculogenesis
Causative injury
Autoantibodies
Endothelial cell injury
ROS
Ischemia—reperfusion; vascular damage
Leukocyte recruitment
Innate immunity
TNF, ROS, MMP
B-cell activation
T-cell activation
CD4 + (skin)
CD8 + (lung)
Adaptive immunity
Inflammation, autoimmunity
Fibrogenesis
Th2, [IL-4, IL-13]
Treg, TGF-β+

Fig. 8.14b: Vascular injury in systemic sclerosis (SSc) leads to injury to vascular endothelium that initiates a sequence of events, including release of proinflammatory mediators, growth factors, chemokines, and reactive oxygen species (ROS), that activate a repair processes. Transition from innate (macrophages) to adaptive immune responses is associated with a type 2 helper T-cell (Th2) response which has a profibrotic activity and orchestrates tissue repair. (Regulatory T cells (Tregs) produce transforming growth factor-β (TGF-β) and suppress effector T cell function). B-cell stimulation leads to the generation of specific autoantibodies that may directly contribute to tissue damage

Clinical Features

Two types of SSc—**limited** and **diffuse** (differentiated in **Table 8.14**).

Two more types have been described in rheumatology textbooks:

- **Sine SSc**
  - Features of RP with scleroderma-associated ANA reactivity and at least one internal organ manifestation of SSc
  - Frequency uncertain because of likely underdiagnosis
- **Overlap SSc**
  - Cases that fulfill classification criteria for SSc and are diagnosed as SSc but also show features of another autoimmune rheumatic disease
  - Most often myositis
  - Other cases of lupus, arthritis, or vasculitis
  - Comprise up to 20% of SSc cohorts

Presenting Features

a. Raynaud phenomenon (RP)
   - Triphasic/biphasic
   - Suspect in any new RP after age of 40 years, especially if ANA/ACA+
   - Longer history prior to skin sclerosis in lSSc

b. Swollen digits—nonpitting edema and puffiness

c. GERD/dysphagia

Cutaneous Manifestations

- The most important and frequent manifestation is skin thickening, and this can be assessed using the modified Rodnan skin score **(Fig. 8.15)**.

TABLE 8.14: Clinical types of SSc—limited versus diffuse

Clinical/laboratory feature	Limited SSc	Diffuse SSc
Skin sclerosis extent	Distal to elbows and knees, face	Proximal limbs, trunk, face
Raynaud's phenomenon	Long history prior to skin sclerosis	Short history/concomitant
Rate of skin sclerosis progression	Slower	Rapid in first 6–18 months
Peak MRSS score	<14	>14
PAH	Primary (isolated)	Secondary
Interstitial lung disease/ Pulmonary fibrosis	Half as common	Common, especially in ATA+ group
Gastrointestinal disease	Universal, especially GERD	May be present
Scleroderma renal crisis	Low-risk	Higher risk, especially in RNAP+ group
Cardiac disease	Low-risk	Higher risk
Autoantibodies	ACA+ in 50% (ATA+ in 10%)	ATA+ in 30%, ARA/ RNAP+ in 25%

MRSS, modified Rodnan skin score; ACA, anticentromere antibody; ATA, antitopoisomerase antibody; ARA/RNAP, anti-RNA polymerase

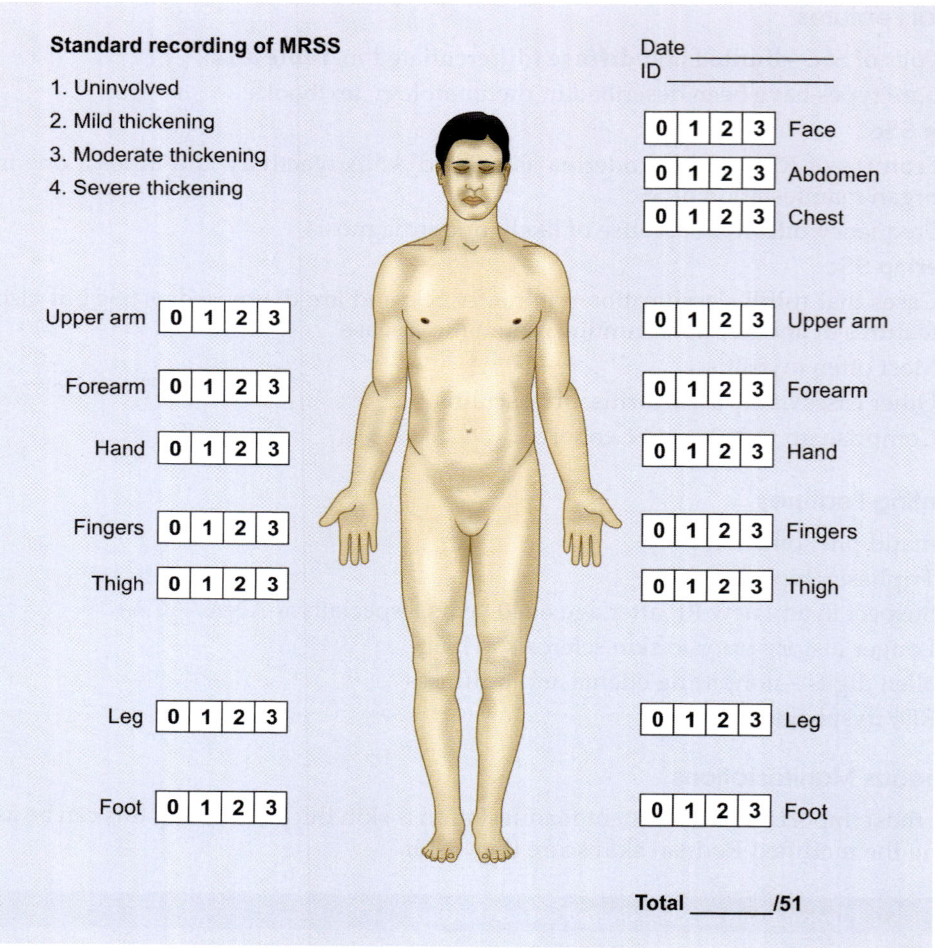

Fig. 8.15: Modified Rodnan skin score (MRSS). The MRSS is used in routine assessment of SSc and in clinical trials in which it is a validated endpoint for diffuse SSc. The score assesses estimated skin thickness, which correlates with the skin biopsy—thickness, weight, and collagen content. The thickness is assessed by palpation at 17 sites

- Itch (in 40%)—hallmark of diffuse skin involvement
- Swollen fingers → sclerosis of skin → atrophy
- Round finger pad sign **(Mizutani sign)**
- Mask-like facies pursed lips **(Fig. 8.16a)**
- Younger looking—d/t loss of wrinkles
- Nasal beaking
- Dental crowding, perioral radial furrowing, reduced mouth opening
- Pigmentation—diffuse, Addisonian, acanthosis nigricans-like, salt and pepper (perifollicular maintenance of blood supply to melanocytes) **(Fig. 8.16b)**.
- Ulceration, gangrene, and telangiectasia **(Fig. 18.16c to e)**.

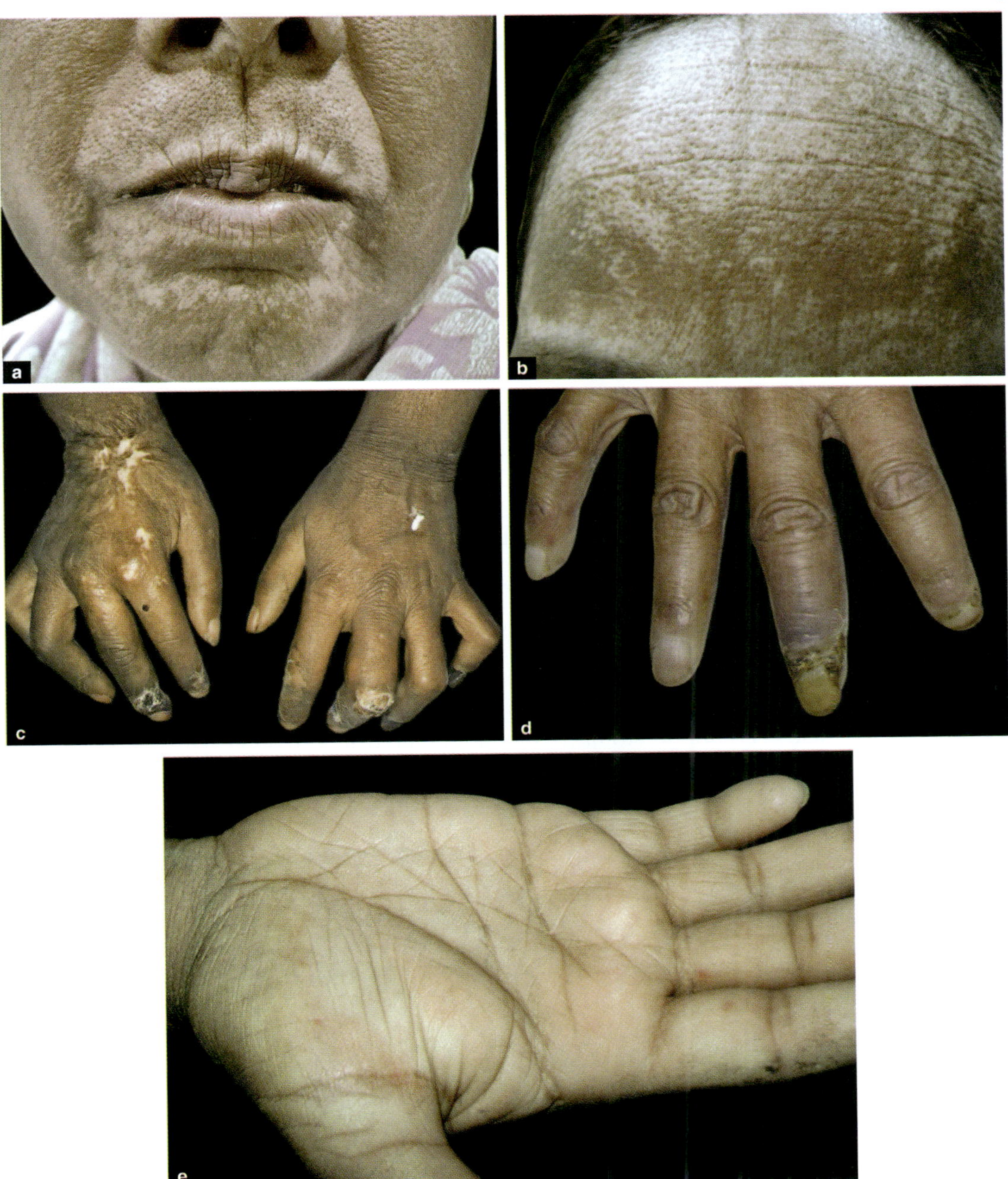

Fig. 8.16: (a) Pursed lips; (b) Salt and pepper pigmentation; (c) Clawing of fingers, ulceration over joints, and distal gangrene; (d) Digital gangrene; (e) Mat-like telangiectasia

A detailed list of cutaneous manifestations and relevant investigations is given in **Table 8.15**.

TABLE 8.15: Cutaneous manifestations in systemic sclerosis

Skin symptom	Sites	Investigations
Raynaud phenomenon	Digits, ears, nose	Cold challenge test, thermography, nail-fold capillaroscopy, nail-fold dermoscopy, serology
Skin sclerosis (Fig. 8.16c)	Distal (lSSc), proximal (dSSc)	mRss, durometry, 20 MHz USG, optical coherence tomography (OCT)
Digital ulcers (DU) (Fig. 8.16c and d)	Fingertips (**DU predictors**—dSSc, lung and cardiac disease, IL-6 level > 2 pg/mL, lupus anticoagulant +, avascular areas on NVC)	Swab, culture, X-ray, MRI
Pruritus		
Mat-like telangiectasia (Fig. 8.16e)	Late feature. Face, lips, palms, mucosae	Dermoscopy
Calcinosis cutis	Dystrophic, late feature Palmar tips of fingers, finger joints and pressure points	X-ray, MRI

MRSS, modified Rodnan skin score; GTN, glyceryl trinitrate; NVC, nail-fold video capillaroscopy.

Systemic Manifestations

Fatigue and weight loss are very common—due to reduced appetite, dysphagia, sicca symptoms, less acid secretion in stomach, bloating, diarrhea. The other features along with relevant investigations are listed in **Table 8.16**.

Associated Disorders

SSc Overlap

- In 20%
- 2 or more CTDs
- Different autoantibody profile from dSSc and lSSc and slightly different clinical course from SSc
- Most common CTDs:
  - Myositis (anti-PM-Scl, Jo1, anti-Ku)
  - RA (anti-CCP)
  - Sjögren's syndrome (ACA, anti-Ro)
  - SLE (U1-RNP)

Malignancy and SSc

- In 3.6–10.7% SSc patients
- Associated with anti-RNA polymerase III autoantibodies—unique nucleolar pattern
- Lung, breast, NHL, hematopoietic, GIT, gynecological malignancies

8

TABLE 8.16: Systemic features of systemic sclerosis		
System	**Symptoms/Signs**	**Risk predictors/Risk factors**
GIT	• Mouth—sicca symptoms, dental crowding, fibrosis of frenulum	
	• Esophagus—>90% have reduced motility → **dysphagia**, GERD	• MC site of visceral disease • Causes morbidity but not mortality
	• Stomach—impaired acid secretion, reduced gastric emptying, mucosal atrophy, GAVE (gastric antral vascular ectasia)	
	• Small intestine—more in lSSc, atonic dilatation and bacterial over-growth → bloating, malabsorption, malodorous diarrhea, pseudo-obstruction	
	• Large intestine—more in lSSc, constipation, fecal incontinence, weight loss	
Lungs	• **Interstitial lung disease** → pulmonary fibrosis **Dyspnea,** cough, moist basilar rales	—
	• **Pulmonary artery hypertension** (PAP of 25 mm Hg at rest with normal PCWP <15 mm Hg) • Overlapping symptoms with ILD/cardiac—**dyspnea,** fatigue, cough [15–35% SSc (isolated in lSSc and with PF in dSSc)]	Age, low FVC, **low DLCO/VA** (reflects capillary gas exchange), **high NT-proBNP** (reflects cardiac wall stress)
Heart	Ventricular dysfunction, arrhythmias, myocardial fibrosis, pericardial effusion—palpitations, syncope, pericardial rub	
Kidneys	Scleroderma renal crisis (SRC)—5–10%, usually within first 5 years: • Abrupt onset of hypertension, acute renal failure, headaches, fever, malaise, hypertensive retinopathy, encephalopathy, and pulmonary edema	dSSc, rapidly progressive disease, recent onset disease without RP, recent high dose steroids, tendon friction rubs
Musculoskeletal	• Muscle weakness—90% • Low grade myopathy (more common) or inflammatory myositis (in overlap syndrome) • Tendon friction rubs—10%	

ERB, endothelin receptor blocker; PDE5, phosphodiesterase 5, PC, prostacyclin; DL_{CO}/VA, lung diffusion capacity/alveolar volume; NT, proBNP: N-terminal pro-B-type natriuretic peptide; AHST, allogeneic hematopoietic stem cell transplantation; RP, Raynaud's phenomenon.

Differential Diagnosis

Other scleroderma-like disorders can be differentiated from SSc on the basis of:

- Lack of Raynaud's phenomenon
- EULAR classification criteria not met
- Lack of internal organ involvement
- Distribution/characteristics of skin involvement atypical: Asymmetric, hands and fingers spared, regional, patchy skin involvement, papular, nodular, orange-peel like skin.

Table 8.17 lists the common differential diagnosis (D/Ds) of SSc.

TABLE 8.17: List of scleroderma-like disorders (pseudoscleroderma)

SSc-like disease	Overlap syndromes
• Localized scleroderma variants (pansclerotic morphea) • Acrodermatitis chronica atrophicans • Stiff skin syndrome • Eosinophilic fasciitis	• Dermatomyositis • Systemic lupus erythematosus
Deposition disorders • Scleredema adultorum • Scleromyxedema • Nephrogenic fibrosing dermatopathy • Systemic amyloidosis	**Occupational factors** • Polyvinyl chloride • Organic solvents • Epoxy resins • Silica • Radiation fibrosis • Pressure hammer
Genetic disorders • Progeria • Acrogeria • Werner syndorme	**Exogenous factors (drugs)** • Vitamin K1 • Bleomycin • Pentazocine
Metabolic disorders • Phenylketonuria • Porphyria cutanea tarda • Diabetes mellitus (diabetic scleredema) • Carcinoid syndrome • Graft versus host disease	**Carbidopa** • L-tryptophan (eosinophilia—myalgia syndrome) • Aniline—contaminated rapessed oil (toxic oil syndrome) • Silicon

Diagnosis

Box 8.3 lists the important investigations in SSc. While **Table 8.18** lists the varied autoantibodies and their interpenetration

BOX 8.3: Investigations in systemic sclerosis

1. **Bedside tests**
   a. Test for Raynaud's phenomenon
   b. Modified Rodnan Skin Scoring (17 sites—score 0–51)
      - Validated and correlates with clinical severity
      - 0—no sclerosis, 1—mild thickness, 2—moderate thickness and difficult to pinch up skin, 3-severe thickness and impossible to pinch up skin
   c. Urine for proteins
   d. Nail-fold capillaroscopy/video capillaroscopy: Scleroderma pattern (differential diagnosis with similar NVC—dermatomyositis, polyarteritis nodosa)
2. **Measurement of skin thickness**
   mRss, durometry, 20 MHz USG, optical coherence tomography (OCT)
3. **HPE**
   - Thinning of epidermis with reduced appendages
   - Lymphocytic inflammatory infiltrate
   - Homogenization of collagen bundles
   - Fibrosis in the papillary and/or reticular dermis

(Contd.)

(Contd.)

4. **Serology (Table 8.18)**
5. **GIT**
   Stomach /Esophagus: Endoscopy, barium swallow, manometry, MUST evaluation (malnutrition universal screening tool)
   Small bowel: Hydrogen breath test, plain abdominal radiography, colonoscopy, sigmoidoscopy
   Large bowel: Barium enema, CT of abdomen, plain abdominal radiography
6. **Lung**
   ILD-HRCT, serial PFTs; **PAH-**ECG, troponin T, %FVC DLCO (ratio is usually >1.6)
7. **CVS**
   Echocardiogram,24-hours Holter, cardiac catheterization, cardiac MRI, endomyocardial biopsy
8. **Renal**
   BP, urine R/M, KFT, GFR, renal USG, renal echo
9. **Raynaud's**
   Cold challenge test, thermography, nail fold capillaroscopy, serology.

TABLE 8.18: Associations of autoantibodies in SSc

Autoantibody	Target antigen	Frequency	Clinical features
Antitopoisomerase (ATA/ Scl-70)	Topoisomerase 1	30% dSSc, 10% lSSc	• dSSc > lSSc, **severe digital vasculopathy** • ILD, PF • Severe cardiac disease • Secondary PAH • **Highest overall mortality, 57% 15-year survival**
Antiribonucleoprotein (ARA/RNAP)	RNA polymerase III	25% dSSC, 2% lSSc	• **Rapid progression of skin sclerosis, scleroderma renal crisis (SRC)** • Associated with malignancy with 3 years of diagnosis • Lower overall mortality, 93% 15-year survival
Anticentromere (ACA)	CENP-B protein	50% lSSC, 5% dSSc	• **lSSc, severe GI disease** • **Isolated PAH** • Predictive for PF and SRC • 78% 15-year survival
Antipolymyositis-scleroderma (anti-PM-Scl)	PM-Scl-75 and -100	33% SSc/myositis overlap	Myositis, mild skin
Anti-U1RNP	nRNP	44% SSc/SLE overlap	lSSc > dSSc, overlap with SLE
Antifibrillarin (U3-RNP) Th/To	Fibrillarin ribonucleoprotein	5% SSc 5% SSc	lSSc, poor prognosis

Monitoring of SSc Patients

- Nail-fold video capillaroscopy—6 monthly or yearly **(Box 8.4 and Fig. 8.17)**.
- Lung: PFT, HRCT, echocardiography, DLCO/VA, NT-pro BNP (N+ terminal prohormone of brain natriuretic peptide)—PAH and ILD.

BOX 8.4: Nail-fold capillaroscopy changes (SSc)

Early	• Few enlarged/giant capillaries • Few capillary hemorrhages • Relatively well-preserved capillary distribution • No evident loss ('drop out') of capillaries
Active	• Frequent giant capillaries • Frequent capillary hemorrhages • Moderate loss of capillaries • Mild disorganization of capillary architecture • Absent/mild ramified capillaries
Late	• Irregularly enlarged capillaries • Few/absent giant capillaries and hemorrhages • Severe loss of capillaries with extensive avascular areas • Disorganization of normal capillary array • Ramified/bushy capillaries

- CVS: Ambulatory ECG, echocardiography, Holter ECG, MRI—cardiac pathology
- Kidney: Creatinine clearance, renal USG, Doppler—renal.

Disease Course and Prognosis

Box 8.5 lists the prognostic markers and mortality indices in SSc.

BOX 8.5: Poor prognostic factors and mortality in SSc

Poor prognostic factors in SSc

- Black skinned males
- Onset—late age at disease onset and/or diagnosis
- Disease—dSSc
- Characteristics
  - ILD/low DLCO
  - PAH
  - Renal disease
  - Worse cardiac functional class (III/IV)
- Serology—anti-Scl-70 +

Mortality in SSc

- 10-year survival:
  - dSSc: 50%
  - lSSc: 70%
- Due to use of ACE inhibitors, now **ILD** is the most common cause of death (ahead of scleroderma renal crisis)
- Causes of death:
  - Pulmonary fibrosis—35%
  - Pulmonary arterial hypertension—26%
  - Cardiac causes (CHF, arrhythmias)—26%
  - Non-SSc-related deaths—infection, malignancy

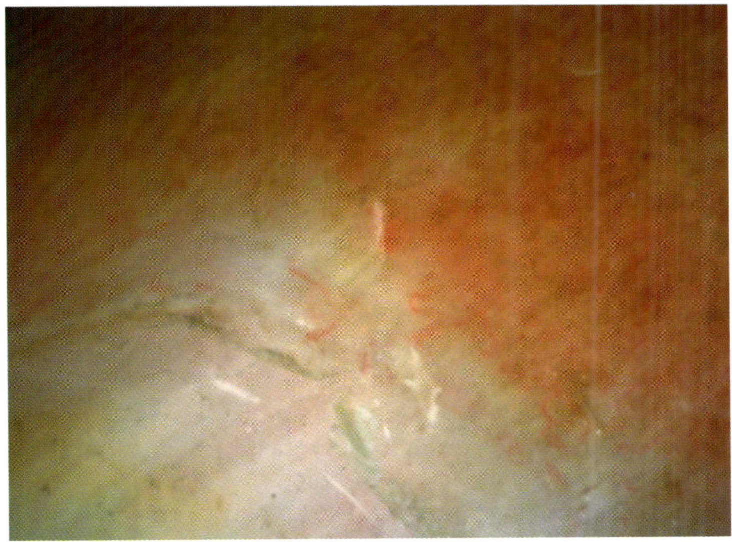

Fig. 8.17: Giant loops and ischemic areas with capillary dropouts in a patient with systemic sclerosis (*Courtesy*: Dr Ananta Khurana)

Other Scoring Recommendations

European scleroderma trials and research group (EUSTAR): VEDOSS (very early diagnosis of systemic sclerosis).

Why is it needed? To pick up disease before microvascular damage, tissue fibrosis/atrophy become irreversible.

'Red flags'—to raise suspicion of SSc

1. Raynaud's phenomenon
2. Puffy swollen digits (turning into sclerodactyly later)

Confirm diagnosis of VEDOSS with

1. Specific SSc antibodies—ACA, ATA
2. Abnormal nail-fold capillaroscopy with scleroderma pattern
3. EUSTAR 10-point revised disease activity criteria (2017) **(Box 8.6)**

BOX 8.6: EUSTAR 10-point revised disease activity (2017)

Criteria	Points
Patient assessed skin worsening during past 1 month	1.5
mRss >18	1.5
Digital ulcers	1.5
Tendon friction rubs (TFR)	2.25
CRP >1 mg/dL	2.25
DLCO <70%	1.0
Total	**≥2.5 → active disease**

Treatment

There is marked clinical heterogeneity in scleroderma with a range of disorders from pre- or possible scleroderma to rapidly progressive diffuse cutaneous SSc with multiorgan failure. There is also the limited cutaneous SSc with and without organ involvement, diffuse cutaneous disease with less rapidly progressive skin manifestations but more organ involvement, and extensive diffuse cutaneous disease without organ involvement. To add to the complexity there are the overlap syndromes with features of other autoimmune rheumatic disorders. This necessitates an individualized approach to treatment.

The principles of therapy are:

- Establishing an accurate diagnosis at the earliest opportunity.
- Staging disease by onset and rate of symptom progression and determining subset based on autoantibodies and organ system involvement so that appropriate screening, organ diagnosis, and treatment can be achieved in every patient.
- Addressing all potential problems through early identification, appropriate therapy, and aggressive intervention for the more serious organ problems.
- Educating patients regarding their own risk factors and prognosis and allowing them to participate in treatment with a holistic approach that recognizes the impact of the disease on lifestyle and relationships.

The ideal method of treatment is to identify the potential and major systemic involvement and decide which would need specific therapy **(Flowchart 8.2)**. In general, to treat the whole scleroderma patient, it is important to remember that the 'whole is the sum' of all the different components and as no drug has been shown to be disease-modifying treatments it is not justified to "over treat" limited cutaneous SSc, or even stable late-stage diffuse disease. Thus **organ-based treatment strategies** directed toward complications such as renal disease, pulmonary hypertension, or ILD will have more immediate effect on mortality than the development of generalized disease-modifying strategies. A summary of the agents used for cutaneous manifestations is detailed in **Table 8.19**.

The two drugs used for ILD (cyclophosphamide and MMF) help in halting progression rather than any reversal of existing fibrotic disease even though JAK inhibitors hold potential in the future.

The organ specific treatment is classified according to the underlying pathogenic process that they target, including immunomodulatory, vasodilatory, or antifibrotic therapies. and are listed in **Table 8.20**.

JAK inhibitors in Systemic Sclerosis

The role of JAKinibs on ILD pathogenesis may be intimately linked to the JAK/STAT signaling pathway, which is crucial for several cellular processes and, when altered, may play a role in the development of inflammatory and autoimmune diseases. The JAK/STAT pathway is usually activated when a ligand, typically a cytokine (e.g. IL-4, IL-13, IL-6, IL-11, IL-31), growth factor (e.g. TGF-β1, EGF, PDGF, VEGF), or interferon, binds its receptor leading to its dimerization. Subsequently, receptor-associated JAKs get activated causing the phosphorylation of the tyrosine residues of the intracellular tail of their receptors, creating the docking sites for STATs. The activated STATs then translocate to the nucleus and modulate gene expression.

TABLE 8.19: Management of digital vasculopathy and skin manifestations in systemic sclerosis

Clinical presentation	Management
Raynaud's phenomenon	• General measures—hand warmers, protective clothing • **Topical nitrates:** Topical glyceryl trinitrate (GTN) • **Calcium channel blockers (CCB):** Nifedipine10 mg TDS (oral nifedipine 1st line therapy); Diltiazem 60 mg BD/TDS • **PDE-5 inhibitors:** Sildenafil (50 mg BD), tadalafil (20 mg on A/D) for severe RP and/or unsatisfactory response to CCB • **Angiotensin receptor blockers:** Losartan 25–50 mg/day • **SSRI:** Fluoxetine (20 mg/day) in patients intolerant/unresponsive to vasodilators • **Prostanoids:** IV Iloprost (IV 0.5 ng/kg/min × 3–5 days) for severe RP after failure of oral therapies with CCB and PDE 5 inhibitors • **Others:** Botulinum toxin, sympathectomy
Digital ulcers	• Wound care • **Prostanoids:** IV iloprost promotes healing • **PDE-5 inhibitors:** Promote healing and may prevent new digital ulcers (sildenafil 25–50 mg TDS) • **Endothelin receptor blockers:** Bosentan has confirmed efficacy in reduction of new ulcers. (125 mg twice a day) • **Statins:** Atorvastatin 40 mg/day • **Anti-thrombotic therapy:** Clopidogrel, aspirin, LMW heparin • **Others:** Botulinum toxin, sympathectomy
Diffuse skin sclerosis <u>without</u> lung involvement	• **Methotrexate (MTX):** Improves skin score. Efficacy in early diffuse SSc. (MTX 15–25 mg/week) • Mycophenolate mofetil (MMF) 2–3 g/day • Azathioprine (AZA) if intolerant to MTX or MMF (AZA 2–3 mg/kg/day) • Tyrosine kinase inhibitors (imatinib, nilotinib, dasatinib) • UVA1 role?
Pruritus	• Ketotifen 6 mg/day • Naltrexone 2–4.5 mg/day • Antihistamines; montelukast; steroids • TLO1/PUVA
Mat like telangiectasia	• Pulse dye laser (PDL) • Intense pulsed light (IPL)
Calcinosis cutis	• Diltiazem (1st line); colchicine (2nd line); minocycline; aluminum hydroxide • Surgery • CO_2 Laser
Skin sclerosis with myositis	• IV immunoglobulin (IVIG) 2 g/kg over 2–5 days monthly • Ciclosporin

?, questionable efficacy

TABLE 8.20: Management of noncutaneous organ-based complications in systemic sclerosis

Clinical presentation	Management
GIT: Diarrhea/constipation	• Loperamide, opiates • **Laxatives**—nonstimulant • **Rotational antibiotics**, metronidazole, ciprofloxacin, rifaximin, octreotide (low dose) for severe disease
Musculoskeletal	• MTX; MMF; AZA • Rituximab • IVIG
Interstitial lung disease/ pulmonary fibrosis	• **Cyclophosphamide (CYC):** Pulse IV or oral CYC with dose and duration tailored individually. For induction pulse IV CYC 600 mg/m^2 with MMF or AZA • **Mycophenolate mofetil (MMF)** oral 2 g/day for induction (in addition to CYC)/maintenance • **Azathioprine (AZA)** oral 150 mg/day for induction (in addition to CYC)/ maintenance • **Steroids:** Prednisolone 10 mg OD for induction • **Rituximab:** For refractory progressive disease • **Autologus hematopoietic stem cells transplant (AHST)** for rapid progressive disease at risk of organ failure • Oxygen therapy • **Pirfenidone and nintedanib**
Pulmonary artery hypertension	• **Endothelin receptor blockers:** Ambrisentan, bosentan, macitentan • **Nitric oxide stimulation** – **PDE-5 inhibitors:** Sildenafil, tadalafil – **Guanylate cyclase stimulator:** Riociguat • **Prostacyclin analogues:** Epoprostenol IV for severe class III and IV PAH; iloprost inhaled or IV; treprostinil S/C or IV
Cardiac dysfunction	• **Diastolic dysfunction:** Diuretics • **Systolic dysfunction:** ACEi, ± carvedilol, ± selective β-blocker • **If ↑ troponin T:** Immunosuppression—CYC, MMF or AZA, prednisolone • Pacemaker/ implantable defibrillator
GIT: GERD/dysphagia	• **PPI:** Omeprazole, lansoprazole • **H_2-receptor blocker** (ranitidine 150–300 mg BD) • **Prokinetics** (domperidone/metoclopramide/erythromycin short courses)
Scleroderma renal crisis	• **ACE inhibitors/angiotensin receptor blockers** • **Additional antihypertensives: CCB, α-blockers** • **Iloprost IV** • **Avoid steroids** • **Blood pressure and KFT monitoring**

Flowchart 8.2: An approach to the treatment of systemic sclerosis

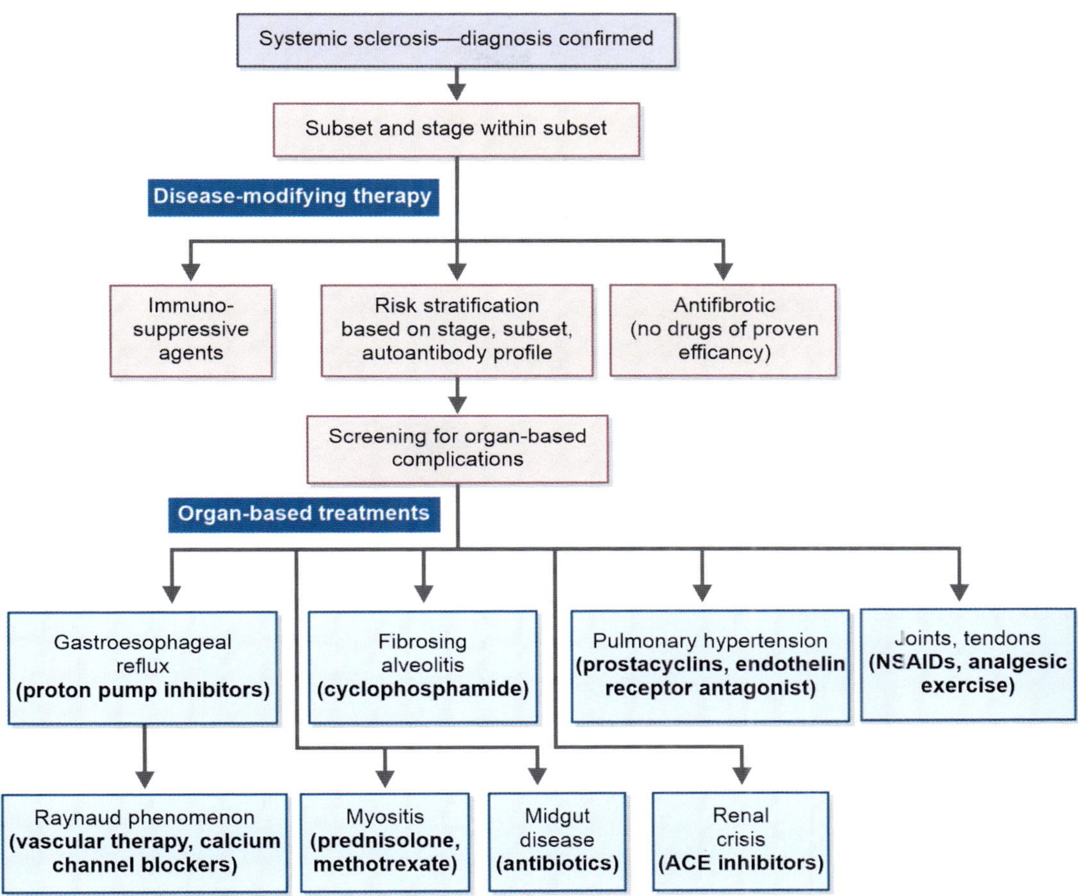

Overexpression of profibrotic and proinflammatory cytokines and growth factors is common in different ILDs. It has been noted that the JAK/STAT pathway in turn triggers polarization of the macrophages which, depending on their surrounding microenvironment and cytokine stimuli, can adopt various activation profiles. Thus JAKib have been found to be useful and impact both on the ILD and the mRSS by inhibiting cytokines and macrophages that mediate fibrosis **(Fig. 8.18)**. More studies are needed to understand the correct stage at which these drugs can be used to halt or reverse the progression of the disease [Moriana C, 2022].

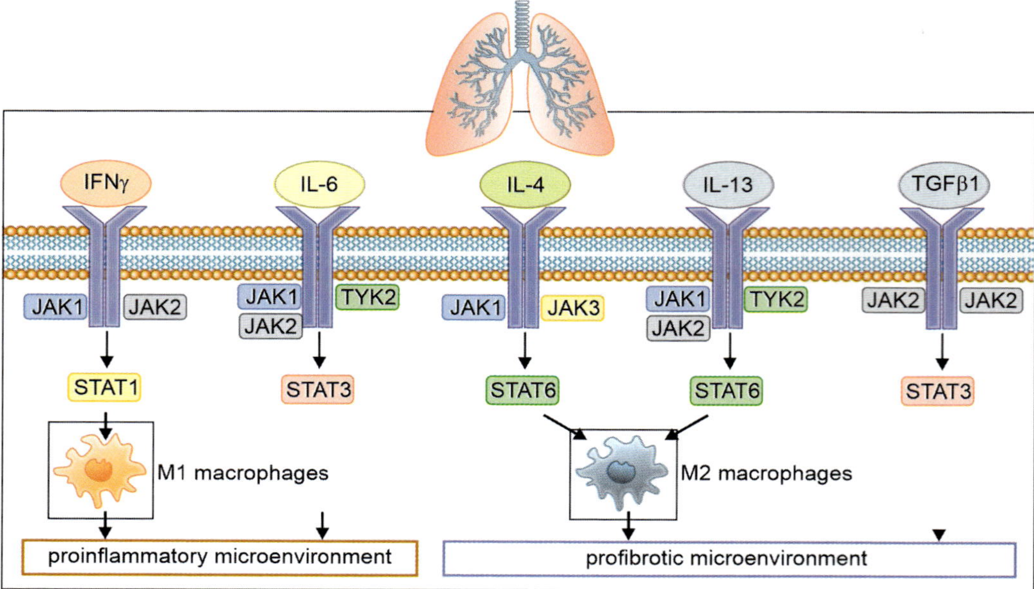

Fig. 8.18: A depiction of the role of cytokines that activate the JAK STAT pathway and macrophages and in turn lead to fibrosis

DERMATOMYOSITIS (IDIOPATHIC INFLAMMATORY MYOPATHY—IIM)

Definition

Dermatomyositis (DM) is an autoimmune disorder affecting, predominantly, the skin and skeletal muscle. It is classified alongside polymyositis in the idiopathic inflammatory myopathies (IIMs) or autoimmune myositis (AIM).

The classification of **Bohan** and **Peter** is still relevant in diagnosis of DM and is given in **Table 8.21**.

Drawback: Does not cover amyopathic DM, does not distinguish inclusion body myositis from PM.

Epidemiology

- Female predominance
- UV radiation may have an influence on the presentation and phenotype of DM
- Bimodal peaks: Childhood (5–14 years) and adulthood (45–65 years).

Pathogenesis

- Environmental factors (e.g. malignancy, viral infections) trigger an immune-mediated process in susceptible individuals.
- Genetic predisposition: Polymorphisms in various HLA alleles.
  TNF-α308A polymorphism (associated with juvenile DM) →↑ thrombospondin-1 (a potent anti-angiogenic factor) →↑ occlusion of capillaries.
- Three major effector mechanisms have been proposed to be important for the development of chronic muscle inflammation and the major clinical symptoms, muscle weakness, and muscle fatigue:
  - Direct effects of infiltrating leukocytes, mainly T lymphocytes and macrophages, on muscle cells (e.g. by means of cytotoxicity)
  - Indirect effects of molecules from the immune system (cytokines and others) on muscle metabolism and function
  - Involvement of microvessels and a disturbed microcirculation, which could lead to acquired metabolic disturbances and thereby cause reduced muscle function
- DM: Humorally-mediated microvasculopathy, PM: Cell-mediated cytotoxicity with CD8+ T cells invading muscle fibers.
- JAK STAT pathway: There is an active role of IFNs which mediate their action via JAK1 and 2, IFN α/β (JAK1, TYK2) and IL6, with a minor role of TGFβ. STAT have a prominent role with STAT1 involved in inflammation, STAT2 in the promotion of apoptosis and STAT3 in the production of angiotensinogen.

TABLE 8.21: Bohan and Peter classification of idiopathic inflammatory myopathies

	Polymyositis	Dermatomyositis
1. Symmetrical proximal muscle weakness 2. Muscle biopsy evidence of myositis 3. Elevation in serum skeletal muscle enzymes 4. Characteristic electromyography pattern of myositis 5. Typical rash of dermatomyositis	Definite: All of 1–4 Probable: Any three of 1–4 Possible: Any two of 1–4	Definite: 5 plus any three of 1–4 Probable: 5 plus any two of 1–4 Possible: 5 plus any one of 1–4

TABLE 8.22: Myositis-specific antibodies	
Antisynthetase antibodies **Jo-1, EJ** **OJ, PL-7, PL-12**	• Antisynthetase syndrome (myositis, ILD, arthritis, RP, mechanic's hands, fever) • Poor prognosis • ILD more common in non-Jo-1 anti-ARS polymyositis
Mi2	• 'Classic' skin and muscle disease • Elevated CK • Good prognosis • Low prevalence of ILD/cancer
TIF1γ	Severe skin disease and a high incidence of cancer
MDA-5	CADM (85–100%) and ILD (92%), with vasculitic ulcers
SUMO	Skin disease with increased frequency of dysphagia
NXP2	JDM (11–23%) where they are associated with calcinosis, a/w cancer in adults
SRP	PM, severe disease, cardiac, poor prognosis

- Two types of antibodies
  - **Myositis specific (Table 8.22)** and **myositis associated** (such as anti-52kD Ro, U1-RNP, U3-RNP, PM-Scl and Ku). MDA-5 and ant-Jo-1 can correlate with **activity of disease**.
  - Antinuclear or anticytoplasmic antibodies are detected in more than **90%** of patients with myositis. A negative antinuclear antibody (ANA) test does not exclude the presence of MSAs in myositis because many antigen targets are cytoplasmic in location with subtle immunofluorescence staining patterns.

Drug-induced dermatomyositis

- Hydroxyurea (most common >50%)
- Statins
- D-penicillamine
- Cyclophosphamide
- BCG vaccine
- TNF-α inhibitors.

Clinical Features

Pruritus—often severe (especially on scalp)—this helps differentiate DM from lupus and psoriasis, which do not tend to itch.

A. **Muscle disease**
   - Slowly progressive, symmetric proximal muscle weakness (**extensors** > flexors)
   - Generally lacks muscle pain (myalgias)
   - Typically affects shoulders, hip girdle, and neck flexors → difficulty walking upstairs, standing up from sitting position, or brushing hair.
   - Esophageal oropharyngeal muscles → dysphagia, aspiration pneumonia

B. **Dysphagia** occurring early in the disease indicates an aggressive course and is associated with a poor prognosis. Patients can have swallowing problems.

C. **Cardiac disease (common)**
   - Mostly subclinical ECG abnormalities
   - Clinically overt disease (CHF, complete heart block, dangerous arrhythmias, and coronary artery disease) is rare but life-threatening.

D. **Diaphragm weakness (rare but life-threatening)**

E. **Classic skin findings (Fig. 8.19)**

1. **Gottron papules (pathognomonic)**
   - Lichenoid papules overlying knuckles (> other extensor joints) **(Fig. 8.20a)**. On the palmar surfaces of the finger creases, they are referred to as *inverse Gottron papules*.
   - Less common than *Gottron sign* (macular erythema overlying joints) **(Fig. 8.20b)**.
2. **Symmetric confluent macular violaceous erythema (CMVE)**

   This can be localized at various sites with different names ascribed to the distribution:
   - Facial erythema and malar involvement, usually involving the melolabial folds (*vs* lupus). Also more violaceous (*vs* red color of SLE).
   - Eyelids = **Heliotrope sign** +/– periorbital edema **(Fig. 8.20c)**

     (Arises as a result of inflammation of underlying orbicularis oculi muscle and affects the upper eyelid)
   - Lateral thigh = **Holster sign**
   - Overlying joints (elbows, knees, DIP, PIP and MCP joints)—**Gottron sign (Fig. 8.20b)**
   - Overlying extensor tendons of hands and forearms = Linear extensor erythema
   - Photodistributed CMVE or poikiloderma (hyperpigmentation, hypopigmentation, telangiectasias, and atrophy) involving chest/upper back = **'V-sign'/'Shawl sign' (Figs 8.20d and e).**

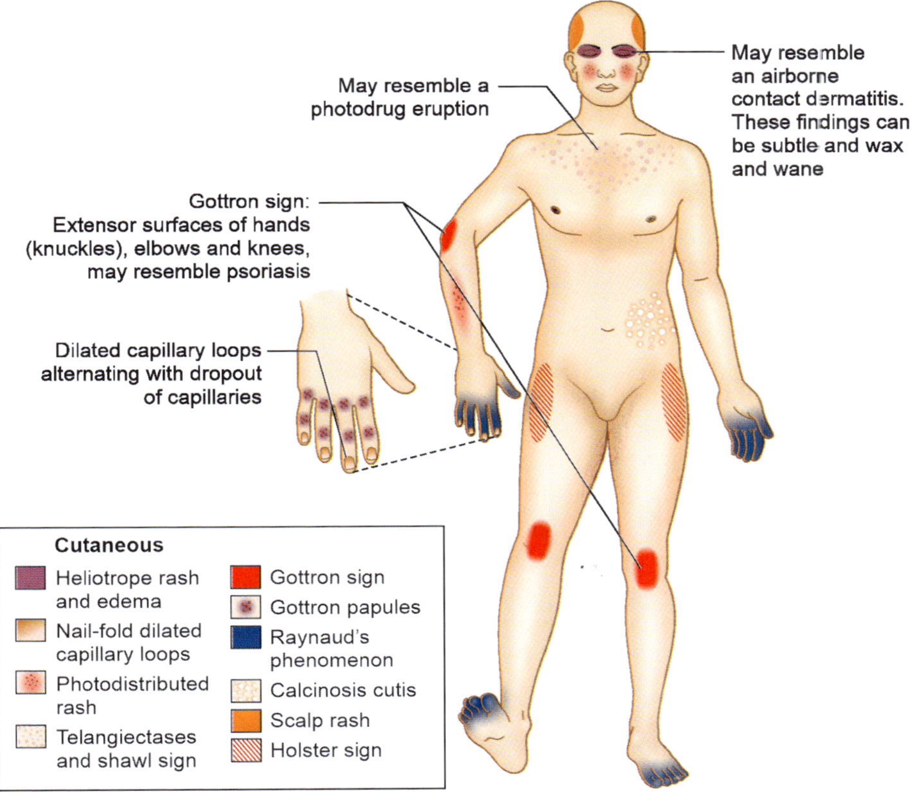

Fig. 8.19: A depiction of cutaneous features of dermatomyositis

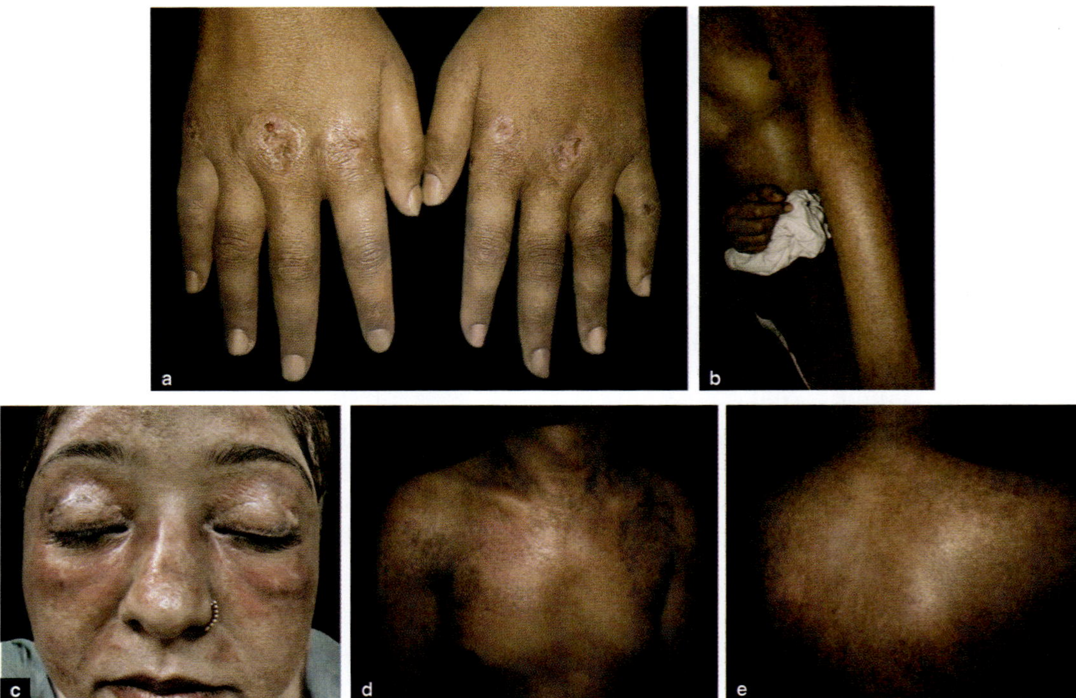

Fig. 8.20: (a) Gottron papules; (b) Gottron sign; (c) Heliotrope sign; (d and e) Photodistributed CMVE involving V of the neck and the exposed upper back 'Shawl sign'

3. **Other skin findings**
   - **Mechanic's hands:** Rough, hyperkeratosis and fissuring of the *lateral* and *palmar* side of fingers, usually more radial digits involved. Look like callosities. Strongly associated with *antisynthetase syndrome*
   - Nail changes
     - 'Ragged' and dystrophic cuticles (Samitz sign)
     - Proximal nail-fold-dilated capillary loops alternating with areas of vessel dropout
     - Periungual erythema
     - Splinter hemorrhages.
   - Seborrheic dermatitis-like scaling on the scalp
   - **Vasculopathy:** Ulcers, which tend to be punched out and surrounded by a zone of dusky erythema, may occur on the fingers, dorsal aspect of the hands and extensor surfaces of the elbows and knees associated with the presence of **anti-MDA-5 antibody**. [TIF1γ—in adults associated with malignancy, JDM with severe systemic vasculitis (Banker variant)].
   - **Calcinosis cutis**
     Much more common in *juvenile DM* (25–70%) than adults (<20%), **associated with anti-p140 (NXP-2)** autoantibodies

F. **Lung:** Diffuse interstitial lung disease (ILD) of varying severity
Rapidly progressive ILD → associated with anti-synthetase and anti-CADM-140 autoantibodies.

Classification (Box 8.7)

1. **Adult-onset DM:** Classic DM—slowly progressive symmetric, proximal muscle weakness, with classic skin findings.
2. **Amyopathic DM** (amyopathic or hypomyopathic)
   - A subset of DM characterized by biopsy confirmed hallmark cutaneous manifestations of classic DM occurring for **6 months or longer** with no clinical evidence of proximal muscle weakness and no serum muscle enzyme abnormalities.
   - Subclinical myopathy: Hypomyopathic
   - Associated with ILD
   - Associated with anti-CADM-140/(MDA-5) autoantibodies
   - Exclusion criteria for amyopathic DM:
     i. Treatment with systemic immunosuppressive therapy for two consecutive months or longer within the first 6 months after skin disease onset.
     ii. The use of drugs known to be capable of producing DM-like skin changes (e.g. hydroxyurea)
3. **Antisynthetase syndrome**
   - Acute disease onset
   - Constitutional symptoms
   - Raynaud's phenomenon
   - ***Mechanic's hands***
   - Nonerosive arthritis
   - ILD
   - Anti-synthetase autoantibodies
4. **Juvenile DM**
   - Less risk of malignancy, more calcinosis and vasculitis
   - Important autoantibodies in JDM:
     1. Anti-CADM-140 (MDA5) → associated with ILD
     2. Anti-p155/140 → associated with extensive skin disease
     3. Anti-p140 (recognizes nuclear matrix protein NXP-2) → associated with calcinosis and contractures.
     4. Anti-TIF1γ is associated with cancer in adult disease; whereas in juvenile disease there is an association with ulcerating skin lesions.
5. **Cancer-associated myositis**
   Associated with: ↑Age (5th to 6th decades most common), rapid disease onset, skin necrosis, periungal erythema, markedly elevated ESR or CK, anti-p155/140 autoantibodies, lack of antisynthetase syndrome features, and lack of Raynaud phenomenon.

Most common cancers:

- **Adenocarcinoma. In♀ breast and ovary, in♂ lung, overall lung.**
- Nasopharyngeal carcinoma overrepresented in Asians.

BOX 8.7: Classification of DM

Adult-onset
- Classic DM
- Cancer-associated myositis (CAM)
- Clinically amyopathic DM (CADM)
  - Amyopathic DM
  - Hypomyopathic DM

Juvenile DM
- Classic DM
- Clinically amyopathic DM (CADM)
  - Amyopathic DM
  - Hypomyopathic DM

- *Timing*: Malignancy may be discovered before, after, or at the same time as the diagnosis of DM patients (one-third in each scenario). Cancers diagnosed before DM precede diagnosis by ≤2 years.

Prognosis

Shorter survival is associated with certain cohorts, including myositis-associated malignancy, but populations enriched with overlap myositis, JDM, and those with a lower mean age at onset have better survival. The reasons for improved survival likely include earlier diagnosis, detection of milder cases, better general medical care, and more judicious use of immunosuppressive drugs. Although poor survival in JDM relates to GI vasculitis and sepsis, children generally do well, *see* **Box 8.8** for prognostic factors of DM.

BOX 8.8: Prognosis of DM

- **Poor prognostic factors:**
  - Delay in diagnosis
  - Malignancy
  - Delayed initiation of immunomodulatory treatment
  - Pharyngeal dysphagia with aspiration pneumonia, ILD, myocardial involvement, and treatment-related complications
  - Previous lack of response to immunosuppressive therapy
  - Antisynthetase, antisignal recognition particle (SRP), antitranscriptional inhibitory factor 1 (p155/140), and antimelanoma differentiation-associated protein 5 (MDA-5) autoantibodies
- MC cause of **death** in adult DM: Ischemic heart disease, malignancy, pulmonary complications
- Juvenile DM: With corticosteroid therapy, majority have favorable outcomes with minimal/no sequelae

Investigations

Box 8.9 lists the important investigations in DM.

BOX 8.9: Investigations in dermatomyositis

- Complete blood count and biochemistry profile
- Muscle enzymes—CK-MB, aldolase, SGOT, SGPT, LDH
  - Serum CK is the most reliable enzyme for muscle involvement in DM, positive early in the disease, may be normal in DM, and reduced in IBM.
- Serology—ANA (+ in 80%), ENA, dsDNA, lupus-anticoagulant, complement levels, anticardiolipin antibodies and $\alpha 2$ glycoprotein-1-antibodies, myositis specific and myositis associated autoantibodies (MSA and MAA).
- EMG
  - relatively sensitive but nonspecific test
  - 90% of patients with active myositis have abnormal EMG findings
  - helpful in selecting a muscle for biopsy
  - can help distinguish myopathy from neuropathic causes of muscle weakness.
- MRI/USG
- Muscle biopsy **(gold standard) percutaneous needle muscle biopsy is as good as an incisional biopsy**
  - HPE: Subtle vacuolar interface dermatitis with rare scattered necrotic keratinocytes, epidermal atrophy, sparse perivascular/periappendageal lymphocytic inflammation, massive dermal mucin deposition.
  - DIF (non-specific): Granular deposition of immunoglobulins and C3 at DEJ (50%) and colloid bodies.

Treatment

An overview of the approach to treatment with the salient drugs is given in **Flowchart 8.3** and the lines of management is given in **Fig. 8.21** due to marked cytokin pathways that are meaited by IFN and IL 6 JAK ib have a role and clinical improvement was most striking in adult patients with pronounced skin involvement (Paik JJ, et al., 2023).

Flowchart 8.3: Treatment algorithm for adult patients with polymyositis (PM) or dermatomyositis (DM)

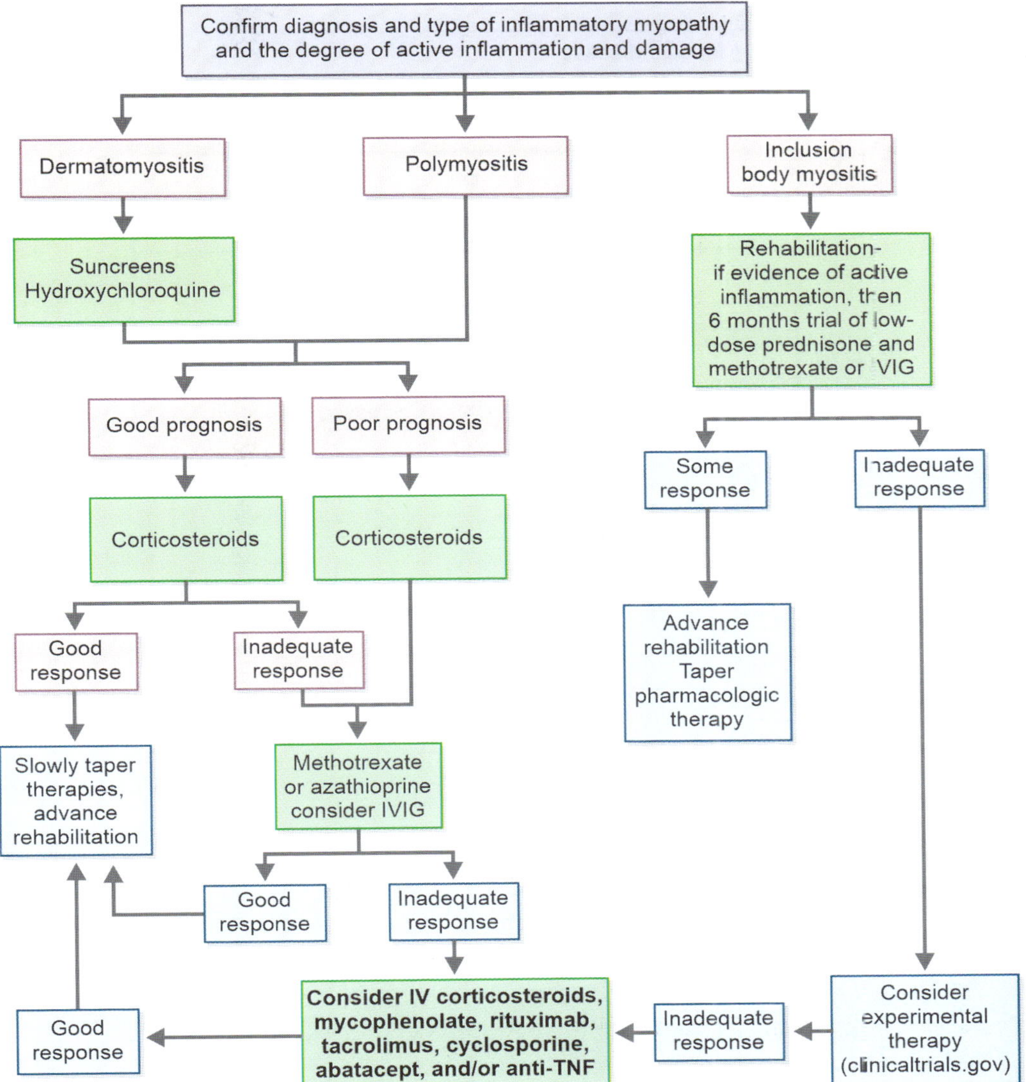

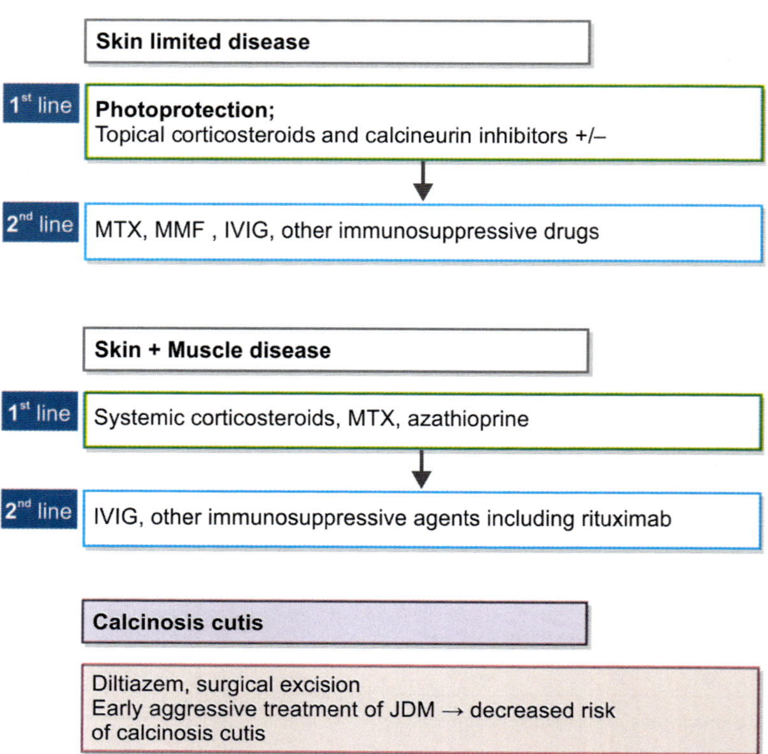

Fig. 8.21: Treatment of cutaneous involvement in DM

MCTD/OVERLAP SYNDROME/SHARP SYNDROME

Epidemiology

- One third may evolve into more differentiated AICTDs later in the course—usually **SLE/SSc**.
- Hence considered as one of the 'undifferentiated' CTDs.
- Some authors believe it may not be a distinct entity.
- Age—middle aged
- Children—rare, more severe, cardiac, renal and joint disease more common
- Sex—females > males

Clinical Features

- Presenting symptoms—Raynaud phenomenon, arthralgias/arthritis, sausage digits, swelling of hands and feet
- Variable symptoms—corresponding to the CTDs in the overlap

Investigations

Serology

- **Classic MCTD—all have speckled ANA+**
- **Ab to ENA (high titers)**
- **U1RNP+**
- Anti-Ro, anti-La → sicca symptoms
- PM-1 and Ku → polymyositis/SS coverlap
- SL-Ki → SLE + SSc + Sicca syndrome
- Complement levels—normal
- Anti-endothelial Ab—50%
- Anti-dsDNA—low titers, uncommon, disappear on treatment

Treatment

- **First line**
  - Corticosteroids—use early (0.5 mg/kg)
  - Treat Raynaud phenomenon
- **Second line**
  - HCQS
  - Methotrexate

BIBLIOGRAPHY

Books

1. Dana P Ascherman, Rohit Aggarwal, Chester V. Oddis Classification, epidemiology, and clinical features of inflammatory muscle disease. https://expertconsult.inkling.com/read/hochberg-rheumatology-2-vol-set-7e. [Hochberg Rheumatology]
2. Kelly Textbook of Rheumatology, 10th edition.
3. Rook's Textbook of Dermatology 9th edn. 2016 John Wiley and Sons Ltd.
4. Virginia D. Steen. Management of systemic sclerosis, https://expertconsult.inkling.com/read/hochberg-rheumatology-2-vol-set-7e. [Hochberg Rheumatology]

Journals

1. Abraham DJ, Varga J. Scleroderma: from cell and molecular mechanisms to disease models. Trends Immunol. 2005 Nov; 26 (11): 587–95. doi: 10.1016/j.it.2005.09.004.
2. Andreoli L, Bertsias GK, Agmon-Levin N, Brown S, Cervera R, Costedoat-Chalumeau N, et al. Eular recommendations for women's health and the management of family planning, assisted reproduction, pregnancy and menopause in patients with systemic lupus erythematosus and/or antiphospholipid syndrome. Ann Rheum Dis. 2017 Mar;76 (3): 476–85. doi: 10.1136/annrheumdis-2016-209770. Epub 2016 Jul 25. PMID: 27457513; PMCID: PMC5446003.
3. Carter LM, Rapid efficacy of anifrolumab across multiple subtypes of recalcitrant cutaneous lupus erythematosus parallels changes in discrete subsets of blood transcriptomic and cellular biomarkers. Br J Dermatol. 2023 Mar 22:ljad089.
4. Chan EK. Report of the First International Consensus on Standardized Nomenclature of Antinuclear Antibody HEp-2 Cell Patterns 2014–2015. Front Immunol. 2015 Aug 20;6: 412.
5. Damoiseaux J, Andrade LEC, Carballo OG, et al. Clinical relevance of HEP-2 indirect immunofluorescent patterns: the International Consensus on ANA patterns (ICAP) perspective. Annals of the Rheumatic Diseases 2019;78: 879–89.
6. Denton CP, Khanna D. Systemic sclerosis. Lancet. 2017 Oct 7;390 (10103): 1685–99.
7. Di Battista, et al. One year in review 2018: SLE. Clin Exp Rheumatol 2018;36 (5): 763–77.
8. EKL Chan, J Damoiseaux, G Carballo, K Conrad, W de Melo Cruvinel, PLC Francescantonio, et al. Report of the First International Consensus on Standardized Nomenclature of Antinuclear Antibody HEP-2 Cell Patterns (ICAP) 2014–2015. Front. Immunol. 2015, Aug 20;6: 412.
9. Elman SA, Joyce C, Braudis K, et al. Creation and Validation of Classification Criteria for Discoid Lupus Erythematosus. JAMA Dermatol. 2020;156 (8): 901–6.
10. Elman, SA. et al. Development of classification criteria for discoid lupus erythematosus: Results of a Delphi exercise. AJ Am Acad Dermatol 2017;77: 261–7.
11. Fanouriakis A, Kostopoulou M, Alunno A, et al. 2019 update of the EULAR recommendations for the management of systemic lupus erythematosus. Annals of the Rheumatic Diseases 2019;78: 736–45.
12. Jordan S, Distler JH, Maurer B, Huscher D, van Laar JM, Allanore Y, Distler O; Eustar Rituximab Study Group. Effects and safety of rituximab in systemic sclerosis: Analysis from the European Scleroderma Trial and Research (Eustar) group. Ann RHEUM Dis. 2015J;74 (6): 1188–94.
13. Kafaja S, Clements P. Management of Widespread Skin Thickening in Diffuse Systemic Sclerosis. Curr Treat Options in Rheum. 2016;2 (1): 49–60.
14. Keyal U, Bhatta AK, Wang XL. UVA1 a promising approach for scleroderma. Am J Transl Res 2017;9 (9): 4280–87.
15. Kowal-BieleckaO, FransenJ, AvouacJ, et al. Update of EULAR recommendations for the treatment of systemic sclerosis. Ann Rheum Dis. 2017;76:1327–39.
16. Lu R, Munroe ME, Guthridge JM, Bean KM, Fife DA, Chen H, Slight-Webb SR, Keith MP, Harley JB, James JA. Dysregulation of innate and adaptive serum mediators precedes systemic lupus erythematosus classification and improves prognostic accuracy of autoantibodies. J Autoimmun. 2016 Nov; 74: 182–93.
17. Moriana C,. JAK inhibitors and systemic sclerosis: A systematic review of the literature. Autoimmun Rev. 2022 Oct;21(10):103168
18. NagarajaV, Denton CP, Khanna D. Old medications and new targeted therapies in systemic sclerosis. Rheumatology (Oxford). 2015;54 (11):1944–53.
19. Paik JJ, Lubin G, Gromatzky A, Mudd PN Jr, Ponda MP, Christopher-Stine L. Use of Janus kinase inhibitors in dermatomyositis: a systematic literature review. Clin Exp Rheumatol. 2023 Mar;41(2):348–358.
20. Sullivan KM, et al. Myeloablative Autologous Stem Cell Transplantation for Severe Scleroderma. N Engl J Med. 2018;378: 35–47.
21. Valenzuela A, Chung L. Management of Calcinosis Associated with Systemic Sclerosis. Curr Treat Options in Rheum 2016;2: 85–96.
22. van den Hoogen F, Khanna O, Fransen, et al. 2013 classification criteria for systemic sclerosis: an American College of Rheumatology/European League Against Rheumatism collaborative initiative. Arthritis Rheum. 2013; 65: 2737–47.

Chapter

9

Cutaneous Mosaicism

Kabir Sardana, Surabhi Sinha, Sinu Rose Mathachan, Aastha Agarwal

HISTORY

- Systematic phenotypic observations of Blaschko in 1901.
- Jackson in 1976 observed that patterns were due to the genetic mechanism of mosaicism.
- Happle suggested 6 phenotypes (**Table 9.1; Figs 9.1** and **9.2**)
- Two early discoveries of molecular proof for mosaicism—McCune–Albright syndrome and mosaic epidermolytic hyperkeratosis.

TABLE 9.1: Patterns of cutaneous mosaicism as described by Happle

Type 1a	Narrow bands	• Hypomelanosis of Ito • Epidermal nevi • Incontinentia pigmenti
Type 1b	Broad bands	McCune-Albright syndrome.
Type 2	Checkerboard pattern (also called flag-like) characterized by alternating squares of hyperpigmentation with a sharp midline separation	1. Speckled lentiginous nevi 2. Becker's nevi 3. Port-wine stains 4. Cutis marmorata telangiectatica congenita 5. X-linked congenital generalized hypertrichosis 6. Segmental NF1 7. Café au lait macules 8. Nevus depigmentosus 9. Segmental vitiligo
Type 3	Phylloid pattern with leaf-like or oblong macules showing a dorsal and ventral midline separation	Phylloid hyperpigmentation
Type 4	Patchy pattern without midline separation	Large congenital melanocytic nevi
Type 5	Lateralization pattern	CHILD syndrome
Type 6	Sash-like pattern	

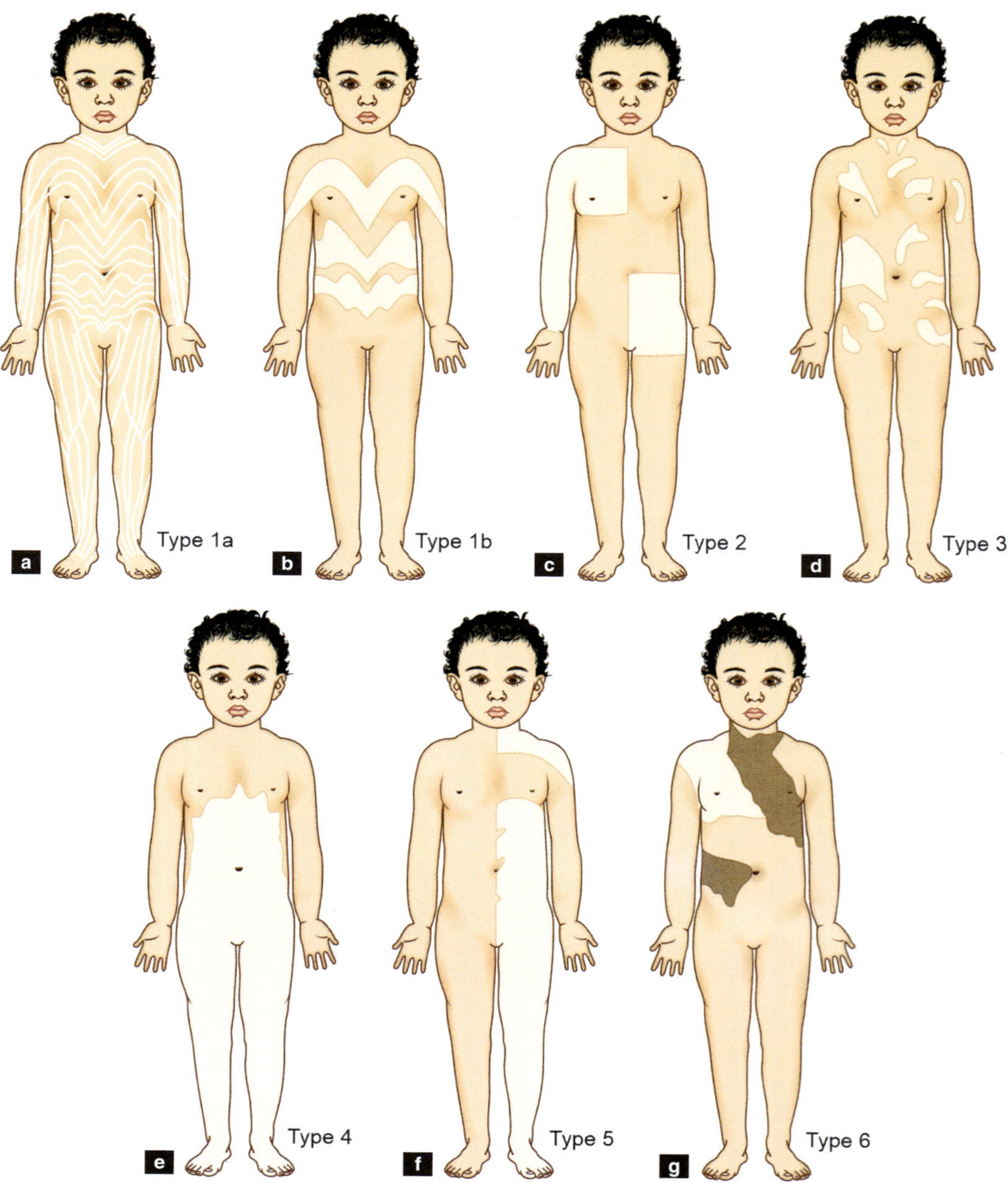

Fig. 9.1: The six archetypical patterns of cutaneous mosaicism: (a) Type 1a, **narrow bands**: (b) Type 1b, **bands**; (c) Type 2, **block-like** pattern (also called checkerboard, flag-like or segmental pattern). This pattern is characterized by unilateral of bilateral quadrilateral shaped with a sharp midline demarcation; (d) Type 3, **phylloid** pattern, which is evocative of a floral ornament with oblong, leaf-like, or pear-shaped lesions; (e) Type 4, **patchy** pattern without midline demarcation, with a broad garment-like, bathing trunk, or cape-like distribution; (f) Type 5 **lateralization** pattern, with diffuse unilateral involvement and a clear midline separation; (g) Type 6, **sash-like** pattern, characterized by large oblique patches or round areas reminiscent of a swathed scarf or belt

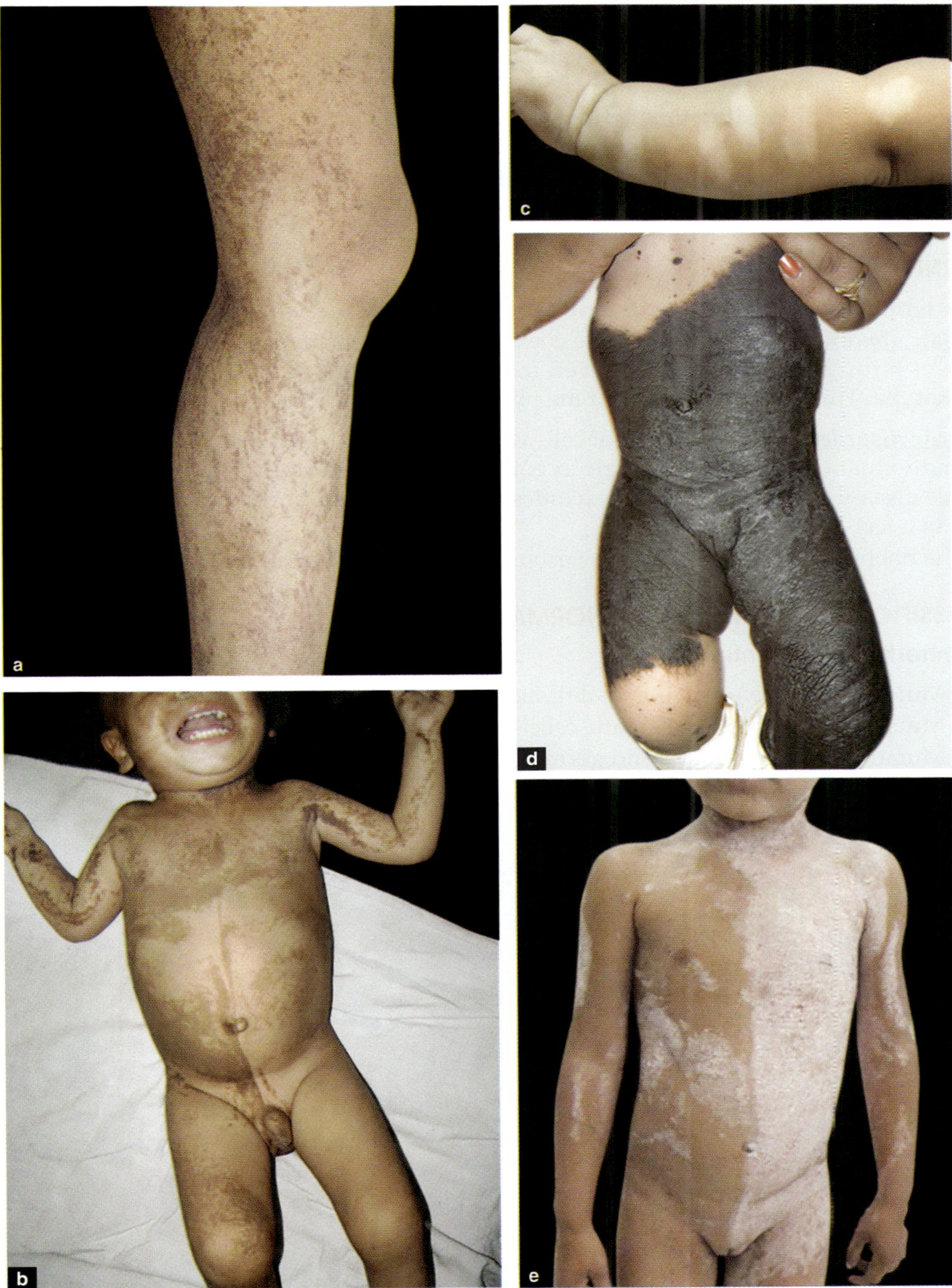

Fig. 9.2: (a) Linear whorled hypermelanosis—type 1a pattern; (b) Type 1b pattern in a case of systematized epidermal nevus; (c) Type 3 or phylloid pattern; (d) Type 4 bathing trunk congenital melanocytic nevi; (e) Type 5—lateralization pattern in a case of nevoid psoriasis

INTRODUCTION

- **Traditional definition:** The coexistence of cells with at least two genotypes, in an individual derived from a single zygote
- **Reasons for discarding this definition**
  - We all have mutations *in utero* all the time
  - We all have mutations after birth all the time—naevi, cancer, etc.
  - Hence—we are all mosaic by this definition.

DEFINITION

Two terms have been used to describe the spectrum of these disorders.

Mosaic *abnormality* of the skin: The coexistence of cells with at least two genotypes, by the time of birth, in an individual derived from a single zygote, and which leads to a disease phenotype. This does not mean that the phenotype has to be present at birth.

Mosaic *disorder*: The coexistence of cells with at least two genotypes, by the time of birth, in an individual derived from a single zygote, where the postzygotic mutation has led to the whole disease phenotype at birth (excludes type 2 mosaicism and revertant mosaicism which occurs later).

The phenotype is determined by various factors as depicted in **Fig. 9.3**.

CLASSIFICATION OF MOSAIC ABNORMALITIES OF SKIN

a. Inheritance Potential

i. Mutation exclusively in gonadal tissue—**gonadal mosaicism**
ii. Mutation exclusively in somatic cells—**somatic mosaicism**
iii. Mutation in both somatic and germline cells—**genosomal mosaicism**

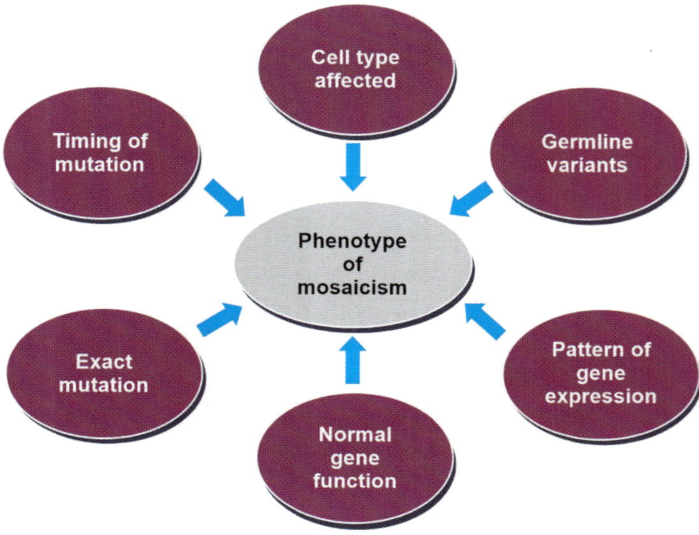

Fig. 9.3: Various aspects that determine the phenotype of a mosaic disorder

While gonadal mosaicism is important, it is only really of value if it is known that the mutation in question is not lethal, as lethal mutations affecting the gonads could be passed onto the zygote but would lead to a miscarriage. If the underlying mutation acts as a lethal factor, the risk for the next generation is virtually nil, whereas children of a patient showing mosaicism of a nonlethal mutation run an increased risk that the same phenotype may diffusely affect the entire body.

Hence, a more useful classification is dividing the conditions into germline lethal or germline heritable, on the basis of the literature **(Table 9.2)**.

b. Pathogenesis

The cause of mosaic abnormalities of the skin by the definition above is consequent to a genetic mutation arising *in utero*, whether or not the resultant abnormality is visible at the time of birth. A classification that combines the type of mutation and the inherited (germ-line) genotype is useful as it helps in genetic counseling. Here, it is to be noted that only the Mendelian disorders can be transmitted specially the one with a dominant inheritance **(Fig. 9.5)**. In **Fig. 9.4**, the second and third variants have also been described as nonlethal mutations of type 1 and type 2. In a type 1 segmental involvement, the remaining skin is healthy **(Fig. 9.5)**. By contrast, a type 2 segmental manifestation is rather pronounced and superimposed on the nonsegmental disorder, which means that the remaining skin is affected to a degree as noted in the ordinary, nonmosaic phenotype. This dichotomy of mosaic manifestations is important for genetic counselling because in the type 2 segmental involvement, the next generation runs a 50% risk of occurrence of the nonsegmental trait, whereas in the type 1 this risk is much lower.

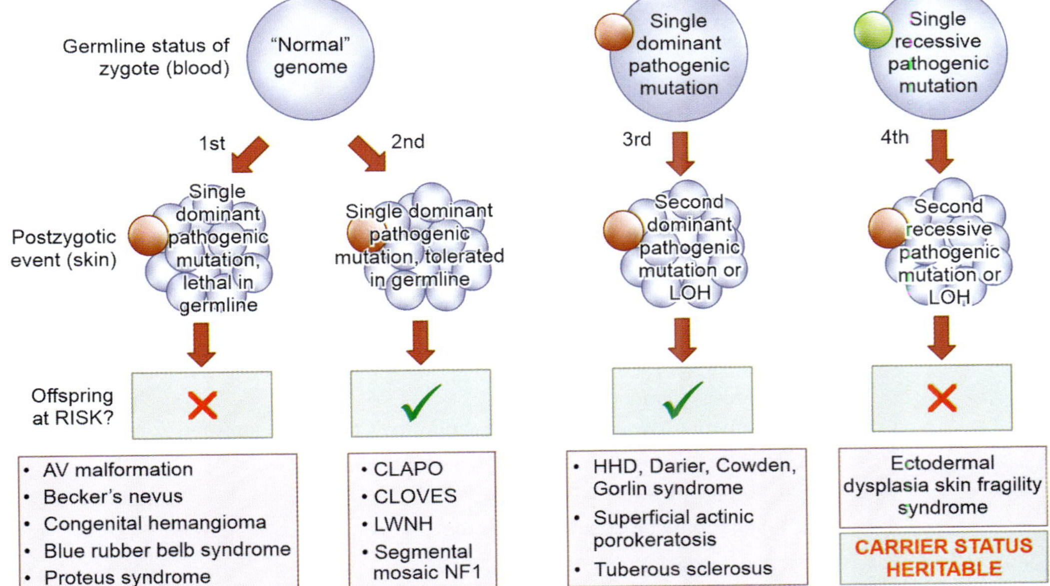

Fig. 9.4: A depiction of the molecular mechanisms that predict mosaic abnormalities of the skin. This helps to determine risk to offspring as sporadic mosaic disorders cannot be passed on as a disease phenotype to future generations, whereas the two types involving Mendelian disorders are passed on

TABLE 9.2: Summary of established mosaic disorders affecting the skin with their mutation and inheritance potential

	Mosaic disorders	Mutation
Germline lethal	Arteriovenous malformation (HRAS, BRAF)	HRAS, BRAF
	Becker's nevus and syndrome	ACTB
	Blue rubber bleb nevus syndrome	TEK
	Congenital hemangioma	GNAQ
	CLAPO syndrome	PIK3CA
	CLOVES syndrome	PIK3CA
	Dermal melanocytosis	GNAQ
	Keratinocytic *KRAS* epidermal nevus syndrome	KRAS
	Linear syringocystadenoma papilliferum	BRAF
	McCune-Albright syndrome	GNAS
	Congenital melanocytic nevi (CMN) syndrome	NRAS/BRAF
	Phakomatosis pigmentovascularis	GNA11/GNAQ
	Proteus syndrome	AKT1
	Sturge–Weber syndrome	GNAQ
Germline heritable	Linear and whorled nevoid hypermelanosis (LWNH)	KITLG
	Hypomelanosis of Ito (passed on as Smith–Kingsmore syndrome)	MTOR
	Keratinocytic FGFR3 epidermal nevus syndrome (passed on as thanatophoric dwarfism)	FGFR3
	Linear nevus comedonicus (passed on as Apert syndrome)	FGFR2
	Lymphatic malformations	*PIK3CA*
	Macrocephaly-capillary malformation syndrome	*PIK3CA*
	Mosaic dominant dystrophic epidermolysis bullosa (passed on as germline EB)	*COL7A1*
	Mosaic Legius syndrome (passed on as germline Legius syndrome)	*SPRED1*
	Mosaic neurofibromatosis type 1 (NF1) (passed on as germline NF1)	NF1
	Nevoid epidermolytic hyperkeratosis (passed on as epidermolytic ichthyosis)	KRT10/KRT1
	Parkes–Weber syndrome	RASA1
	Phakomatosis pigmentokeratotica (passed on as cardiofaciocutaneous syndrome/Costello syndrome)	HRAS/KRAS
	Porokeratotic eccrine ostial and dermal duct nevus (passed on as KID syndrome)	GJB2
	PTEN hamartoma or Cowden syndrome	PTEN
	Sebaceous nevus syndrome/Schimmelpenning syndrome (passed on as Costello syndrome)	*HRAS, KRAS*
	Woolly hair nevus (passed on as cardiofaciocutaneous syndrome/Costello syndrome	HRAS/BRAF

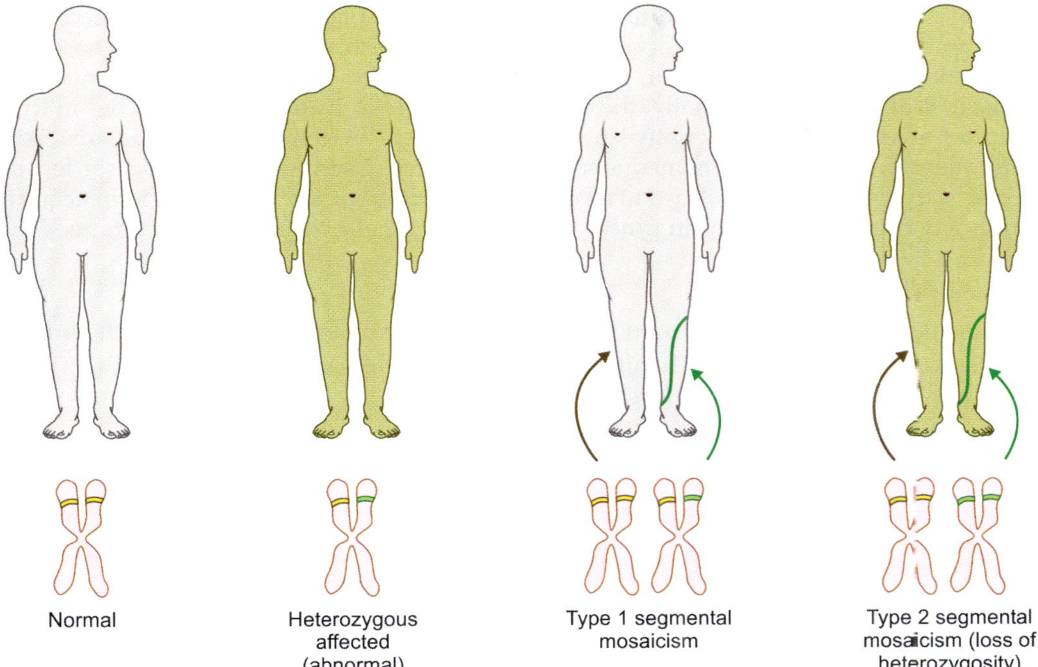

Fig. 9.5: Types of segmental mosaicism. Segmental mosaicism refers to the Blaschko-linear patterning of cutaneous lesions that respect the midline: Single postzygotic mutations leading to segmental lesions reflect type 1 segmental mosaicism, by which the mutation is limited to lesional tissue in an otherwise wild-type individual. Type 2 segmental mosaicism occurs when a second mutagenesis event—such as loss of heterozygosity—occurs in individuals already carrying heritable mutations, leading to segments with more severe phenotype

A **third category** of mosaicism develops at a later stage of fetal development or during postnatal life. It is by far the most common type of mosaicism occurring in autosomal dominant traits and consists in a nonsegmental, disseminated arrangement of neoplastic or nonneoplastic skin lesions. For example, all neurofibromas and café au lait macules of neurofibromatosis.

When a mosaic abnormality of the skin is consequent to epigenetic alterations it is not a mosacism as it does not alter the DNA genotype. Epigenetic mosaicism results in a modified gene expression due to activation or silencing of genes and is exemplified by lyonization, the random inactivation of one X chromosome in every cell of the female embryo.

The phenomenon of **revertant mosaicism (RM)** is also known as natural gene therapy. Cutaneous RM was first described in a case of generalized atrophic benign epidermolysis bullosa (GABEB), now known as generalized intermediate junctional EB (JEB), caused by mutations in *COL17A1* or *LAMB3*. While less common than in JEB, somatic reversion in both recessive and dominant subtypes of EB simplex, as well as recessive dystrophic EB (RDEB) has also been reported. Another disorder with RM is ichthyosis with confetti (IWC). Understanding mechanisms of revertant mosaicism holds potential for therapeutic reversion of inherited and acquired disorders. Autologous transplantation of revertant skin from a patient with generalized intermediate JEB has successfully reepithelized healthy skin in both the donor and grafted areas, suggesting expansion of revertant skin for clinical use as potential strategy against genetic blistering disorders. Revertant keratinocytes from an RDEB patient has also been successfully reprogrammed into induced pluripotent stem cells, suggesting the potential to generate an inexhaustible supply of functional, patient-specific cells for therapeutic transplantation in various end-organ systems. Finally, the efficacy of BMT to induce revertant patches in RDEB implicates a yet-unknown link between the hematopoietic system and cutaneous reversion. The frequent, widespread spontaneous self-correction we observe in blistering disorders and IWC raises a promising possibility that any dominant mutation, whether inherited or acquired, including oncogenic mutations in cancer, is capable of genetic reversion to wild type.

CLINICAL ASSESSMENT

The important features to be assessed that can confirm the diagnosis of a mosaic disorder are

a. Sporadic occurrence—no family history, even of a mild phenotype
b. Congenital or early-childhood onset
c. Mosaic patterning on the skin
d. Variability/patchiness of the overall body phenotype

While Blaschko's description of linear and whorled patterning is the most familiar image of cutaneous mosaicism, which was extended to the head by Happle and Assim. The most familiar classification is proposed by Happle **(Fig. 9.6)** who expanded and classified the mosaic cutaneous patterns into between five and seven types, six of which have now been proven to be the result of at least one mosaic disorder (with the sash pattern being the only one outstanding at this time). They may be used for phenotypical classification but may not be different genotypically. Notably pigmentary disorders that follow this pattern are also described and this is know as pigmentary mosacism.

Cutaneous pigmentary mosaicism refers to various patterns of hyper- or hypopigmentation due to the genetic heterogeneity and altered ability of mutated cells to produce melanin. Mosaic or nevoid hypopigmentation comprises, among others, nevus depigmentosus (nevus achromicus) and the six archetypal patterns of cutaneous mosaicism, which are well described in the literature. Hypomelanosis of Ito is now reserved for extensive hypopigmented blaschkoid mosaicism associated with extracutaneous anomalies **(Fig. 9.7)**. As extracutaneous manifestations are important for the clinician, a summary of the clinical presentations of pigmentary mosaicism that predict extracutaneous involvement are depicted in **Box 9.1**. Notably 14–33% of patients have extracutaneous findings.

The important considerations are a **full body photography** and to look for **extracutaneous features**.

Investigations

Investigations in cutaneous mosaicism are done based on **Table 9.3**.

BOX 9.1: Predictors of extracutaneous manifestations

- Block-like pattern
- Facial involvement (mostly centrofacial lesions)
- Numerous sites of involvement (≥4)
- Phylloid hypomelanosis (chromosome 13)

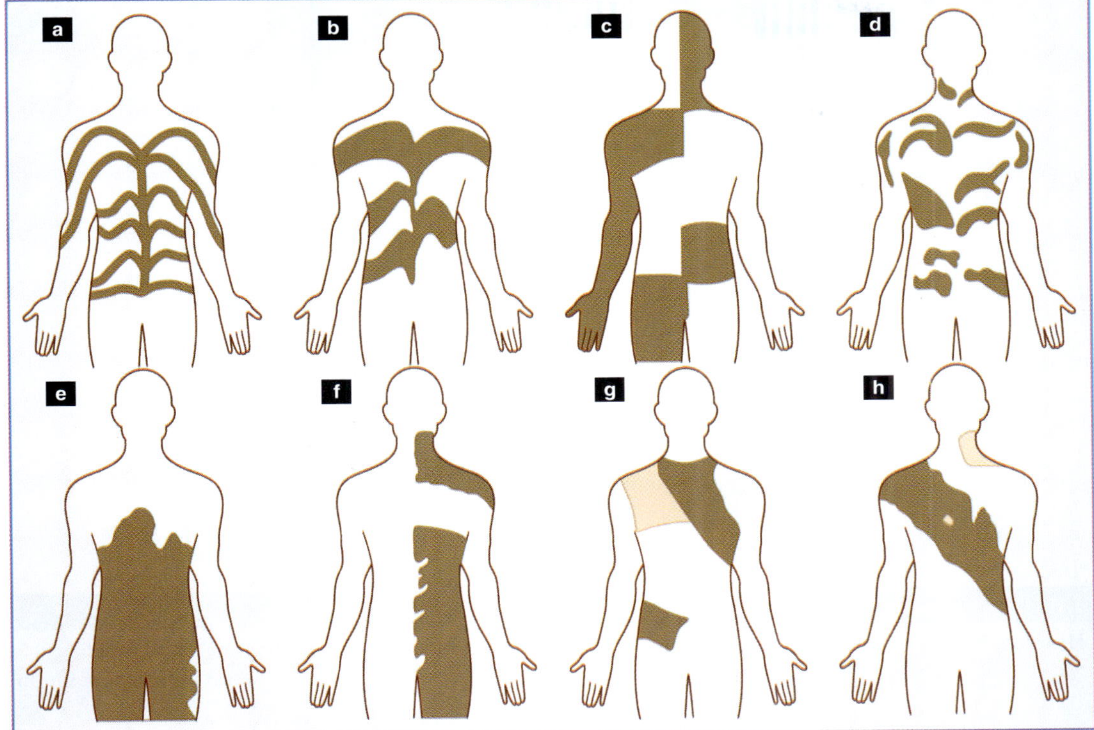

Fig. 9.6: Patterns of pigmentary mosaicism as described by Happle: (a) Type 1a, narrow bands; (b) Type 1b, broad bands; (c) Type 2, block-like pattern (also called checkerboard, flag-like or segmental pattern); (d) Type 3, phylloid pattern, which is evocative of a floral ornament with oblong, leaf-like, or pear-shaped lesions; (e) Type 4, patchy pattern without midline demarcation, with a broad garment-like, bathing trunk, or cape-like distribution; (f) Type 5, lateralization pattern, with diffuse unilateral involvement and a clear midline separation; (g and h) Type 6, sash-like pattern, characterized by large oblique patches or round areas reminiscent of a swathed scarf or belt (anterior and posterior views)

TREATMENT

- Involving multidisciplinary team
- Malignancy screening for certain mosaic abnormalities of the skin (like PTEN hamartoma, CMN, sebaceous nevi)
- To provide psychological support services and patient support groups
- Genetic counseling (depending on the inheritance potential (germline lethal/heritable) of mosaic disorders as given in **Table 9.2**, as AD disorders with a superimposed mosaic phenotype have a 50% chance of inheritance (similar to any other mendelian AD disorder) while for AR mosaic disorders, the offspring could inherit a heterozygous carrier status, but would be highly unlikely to have the second somatic hit in required to produce a phenotype, **(*refer* to Fig. 9.5)**.
- Targeted therapies for mosaic skin disorders **(Table 9.4)**.

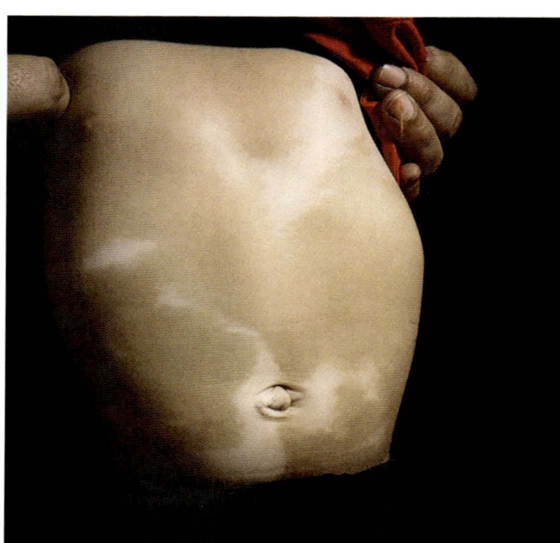

Fig. 9.7: Cutaneous pigmentary mosaicism in Hypomelanosis of Ito

TABLE 9.3: Investigations in cutaneous mosaicism

Histology	• Helps distinguish between epidermolytic, nonepidermolytic VEN and ILVEN • To differentiate between congenital hemangioma, tufted hemangioma and kaposiform hemangioendothelioma
Radiology/Imaging	• MRI of the central nervous system (CNS)—multiple congenital melanocytic nevi, PIK3CA-related overgrowth spectrum, Sturge–Weber syndrome • Doppler USG and/or MRI/MR angiography—vascular malformations/vascular tumors
Genetic testing	• Mosaic mutation—fresh **skin biopsy** from affected skin taken immediately to the genetics laboratory on saline-soaked gauze (not to be kept in formalin) • Germline mutation—**blood sample** for next generation sequencing (NGS), and whole-genome copy number analysis
Blood sampling	• Blood (and urine) for calcium, phosphate, vitamin D and fibroblast growth factor 23 (to rule out metabolic bone disease associated with Schimmelpenning syndrome, phakomatosis pigmentokeratotica) • Platelets, fibrinogen and D-dimers (in disorders like CLOVES, Klippel–Trenaunay or Proteus syndrome, venous, lymphatic, arterial or complex vascular malformations)

TABLE 9.4: Targeted therapies used as a part of clinical trial/compassionate-usage study in mosaic cutaneous disorders

Vascular malformations	mTOR inhibitor **rapamycin**
PIK3CA-mutation positive patients with overgrowth	Targeted inhibitor, which inhibits **p110α** activity
Proteus syndrome	**Protein kinase B** (AKT) inhibitors
Congenital melanocytic nevus syndrome with primary CNS melanoma FGFR1-mosaic encephalocraniocutaneous syndrome	Mitogen-activated protein kinase inhibition **(Trametinib)**

BIBLIOGRAPHY

1. Belzile E, McCuaig C, Le Meur JB, Coulombe J, Hatami A, Powell J, Rivière JB, Marcoux D. Patterned cutaneous hypopigmentation phenotype characterization: A retrospective study in 106 children. Pediatr Dermatol. 2019 Nov;36(6):869–875.
2. Kinsler VA, Boccara O, Fraitag S, Torrelo A, Vabres P, Diociaiuti A. Mosaic abnormalities of the skin: review and guidelines from the European Reference Network for rare skin diseases. Br J Dermatol. 2020;182(3):552–563.
3. Molho-Pessach V, Schaffer JV. Blaschko lines and other patterns of cutaneous mosaicism. Clin Dermatol. 2011;29(2):205–225.
4. Ruiz-Maldonado R, Toussaint S, Tamayo L, Laterza A, del Castillo V. Hypomelanosis of Ito: Diagnostic criteria and report of 41 cases. Pediatr Dermatol. 1992;9(1):1–10.
5. Taibjee SM, Bennett DC, Moss C. Abnormal pigmentation in hypomelanosis of Ito and pigmentary mosaicism: The role of pigmentary genes. Br J Dermatol. 2004;151(2):269–282.

Chapter

10

Dermatitis

Ananta Khurana, Seema Rani

Though dermatitis is a vast chapter, we shall be covering only topics relevant to examinations. We shall start with phytodermatitis, focusing on parthenium dermatitis, a very commonly encountered clinical case, and will later discuss airborne contact dermatitis.

PHYTODERMATITIS

- Phytodermatitis is described as a cutaneous adverse reaction to plants and their derivatives.
- The basic clinical patterns of phytodermatitis include:
  1. Allergic phytodermatitis
  2. Phytophotodermatitis
  3. Irritant contact dermatitis
  4. Pseudophytodermatitis, and
  5. Pseudophytophotodermatitis

  In addition, mechanical injury due to plants, and pharmacological injury due to pharmacologically active substances present in some plants (histamine, acetylcholine, serotonin) which get "injected" into the skin after accidental injury with thorns and bristles, are also classified as phytodermatitis by some authors.
- **Allergic phytodermatitis** occurs due to oleoresins produced by various plants. These are complex mixtures of aldehydes, aromatic alcohols, terpenic compounds, aliphatic and aromatic esters, and phenols (catechols, resorcinols, and hydroquinones). These low-molecular-weight compounds behave as haptens and induce a cell-mediated inflammatory reaction that requires prior sensitization and priming of memory and effector T lymphocytes similar to other contact allergic dermatitis. Common causative plants include Anacardiaceae family (poison ivy, mango tree and Indian marking nut tree), Ginkypaceae family and Proteceae family. In mangoes, allergenic catechols are found in the skin of the fruit. A severe perioral dermatitis can occur when one bites into an unpeeled mango.
- **Phytophotodermatitis** occurs due to psoralens or furocoumarins in some plants that trigger a phototoxic eruption when activated by exposure to ultraviolet A light after contact with the skin. The pattern is most often caused by contact with plants of the Apiaceae, or

Umbelliferae family. They include weeds and edible plants, such as hogweed, cowbane, carrot, parsnip, dill, fennel, celery, and anise.

- **Irritant contact dermatitis** occurs due to certain substances in plants that cause direct toxic effects on the skin, similar to a chemical burn. Some are secreted directly at the surface of the plant and others are released only when the plant is crushed or cut. The reaction occurs within minutes to hours with a burning sensation, erythema, edema, blisters, and sometimes necrosis. The causative plant families include Araceae, Amaryllidaceae and Liliaceae, Euphorbiaceae, Ranunculaceae and Brassicaceae.
- **Pseudophytodermatitis** is caused by arthropods or pesticides present on plants, rather than any intrinsic plant component.
- **Pseudophytophotodermatitis** results from a furocoumarin-containing substance in the plant but not made by it. Celery, in the family Umbelliferae, is the most frequent species producing this pattern. Dermatitis results not from the celery itself but from a furocoumarin manufactured by a fungus (*Sclerotinia sclerotiorum*) infecting the celery.
- The most prominent phytodermatitis in India is an allergic contact dermatitis due to Parthenium ("Congress grass" or "Congress weed").

PARTHENIUM DERMATITIS (PD)

- *Parthenium hysterophorus* belongs to the family Asteraceae (Compositae).
- It is an annual plant, growing all round the year except in extreme winters **(Fig. 10.1)**.
- It has detrimental effects on vegetation in its vicinity (allelopathic effects) and also the livestock consuming it. Thus, it is aptly called the "Scourge of India".
- The most important allergens responsible are ***sesquiterpene lactones*** (SQLs) **(Box 10.1)**.
- SQLs are present in the leaf, stem, flower and pollen, but the highest concentrations are present in the small glandular hairs (trichomes) present on the undersurface of the leaves and stem.
- SQLs are classified on the basis of their carbocyclic skeletons into germanocranolides, guaianolides, eudesmanolides, pseudoguaianolides and xanthonolides.
- ***Parthenin*** is the major SQL in *P. hysterophorus* seen in India.
- Other members of the Compositae family in North India include *Xanthium strumarium*, *Chrysanthemum morifolium* (chrysanthemum), *Dahlia pinnata* (dahlia) and *Tagetes indica* (marigold). *P. hysterophorus* and *X. strumarium* have shown a high rate of cross-sensitivity in Indian patients, whereas the prevalence of cross reaction with chrysanthemum is generally low.

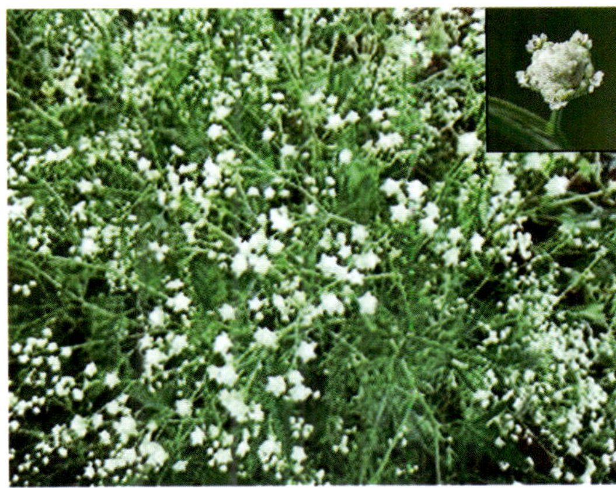

Fig. 10.1: Mature plant of *Parthenium hysterophorus* with flowering. Each flowerhead (capitulum) is borne on a stalk (pedicle) and has five tiny 'petals' (ray florets). Inset shows numerous tiny white flowers (tubular florets) in the center which are surrounded by two rows of small green bracts (involucre)

Skin sensitization by parthenium antigen propagates as a cell-mediated hypersensitivity immune response with an early sensitization phase and a subsequent elicitation phase, if antigen exposure persists. Antigen presentation to T lymphocytes in the regional lymph nodes is followed by T cell proliferation and production of effector and memory T cells. There is subsequent infiltration of these T cells into re-exposed skin sites leading to cutaneous inflammation. Elevated levels of TNF-α, IL-6, IL-8 and IL-17 and reduced levels of anti-inflammatory cytokines IL-4 and IL-10 have been demonstrated in patients with PD.

BOX 10.1: Allergens in *Parthenium Hysterophorus*

- Parthenin (major allergen in India; belongs to pseudoguaianolide class of SQLs)
- Coronopilin
- Tetraneurin A
- Hymenin
- Hysterin
- Ambrosin
- Dihydroisoparthenin

- In addition to this well-accepted model of type IV delayed type hypersensitivity, some authors have postulated that type I hypersensitivity may also be playing a role, especially in those with an atopic diathesis. This may be demonstrated by a positive skin prick test.
- SQLs are *not photosensitizers*, they have neither phototoxic nor photoallergic properties. Reduced minimal erythema dose (MED) to UVB, and reduced minimal phototoxic dose (MPD) to UVA has been well-described with parthenium dermatitis and may contribute to the chronic actinic dermatitis (CAD) pattern.

Clinical Features

- Males are more commonly affected than females. The difference is related to outdoor exposure and nature of clothing but cannot be completely explained by these alone, as women also work in fields.
- Parthenium dermatitis is rare among teenagers and children.
- In sensitized individuals, the clinical manifestations usually start within 24 hours of exposure, but may be delayed for up to 2–3 days or even longer in milder cases. The severity varies from brief periods of erythema and itching to persistent erythema, swelling, papules or papulovesicles with itching and burning in moderate cases and extensive vesiculation and exudation associated with edema in severe ones.

  Contact sensitivity to parthenium is everlasting. The disease runs a chronic course with exacerbation during summers initially and some reduction in winters. The *seasonal* pattern, however, gradually evolves over years into a *persistent eruption* with pruritic lichenified dermatitis.
- Parthenium dermatitis may present with a variety of morphologies **(Box 10.2) (Fig. 10.2)**. A few of them are as follows:
  1. **Airborne contact dermatitis (ABCD) pattern** is the most characteristic (discussed later).
  2. **Chronic actinic dermatitis (CAD) pattern** presents with lichenified papules, plaques, or nodules over the exposed areas.

BOX 10.2: Clinical patterns of parthenium dermatitis

- Airborne pattern contact dermatitis (ABCD)
- Chronic actinic dermatitis (CAD)
- Mixed pattern dermatitis (combination of air-borne and CAD)
- Pseudophotodermatitis
- Exfoliative dermatitis
- Hand and feet dermatitis
- Photosensitive lichenoid eruption
- Prurigo nodularis like
- Perianal dermatitis
- Vesicular hand eczema
- Seborrheic pattern
- Dermatitis simulating lichen nitidus
- Atopic pattern
- Polymorphic light eruption like

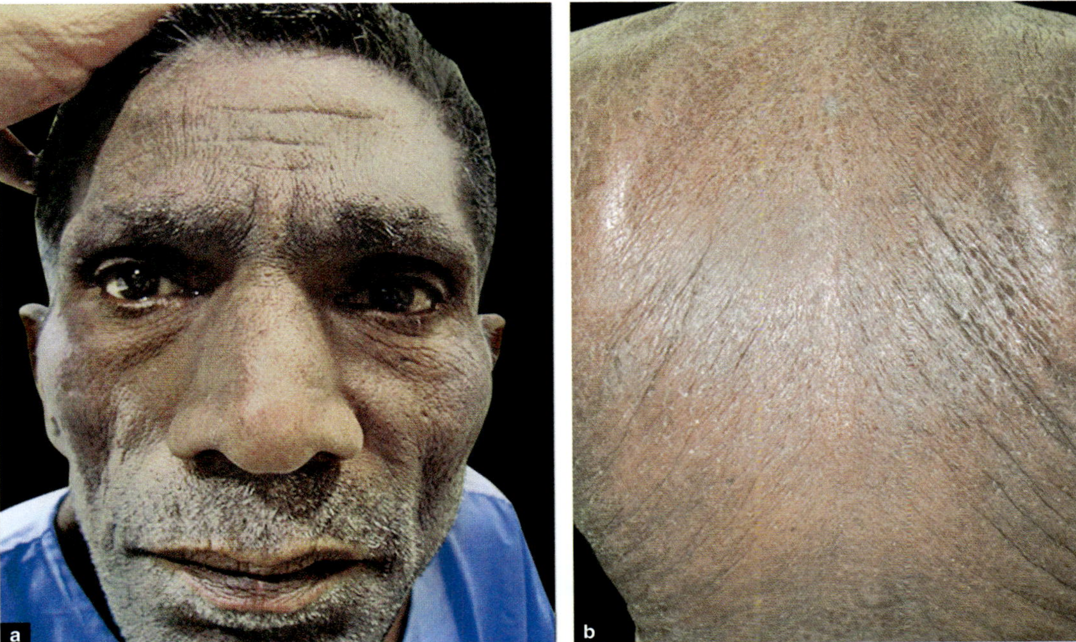

Fig. 10.2: (a) Parthenium dermatitis involving the folds of the forehead; (b) Diffuse involvement in a severe case

3. The **photosensitive lichenoid eruption** pattern presents with pruritic, discrete, flat, violaceous papules and plaques over sun-exposed parts such as forehead, ears, cheek, upper chest and back, extensor aspect of forearms and dorsae of hands.
4. **Exfoliative dermatitis**, with widespread erythema and scaling, can develop in severely affected patients.
5. Recurrent **erythroderma**
   - A study reported frequency of different patterns seen with parthenium dermatitis as—ABCD pattern (46%), mixed pattern (30%), erythroderma (14%) and chronic actinic dermatitis (10%). The pattern of involvement with parthenium dermatitis also changes over time. An ABCD pattern at the outset can change to mixed or CAD pattern.
   - Vitiliginous skin is thought to be spared due to the vacuolization of Langerhans cells of the area.

Diagnosis

1. **Patch testing:** Patch test detects the delayed type (IV) hypersensitivity to tested antigens. It is carried out with the plant material "as is". In addition, parthenium antigen from the Indian Standard Series (ISS) may also be applied (but is less sensitive).
2. **Photopatch testing:** Perfomed in PD confined to exposed parts but is uncommonly positive.
3. **Prick test:** Detects the immediate (type I) hypersensitivity, which is also proposed to play a role.
4. **Optional tests:** RAST (radioallergosorbent test); serum IgE levels, histopathology (to differentiate from other dermatoses if required).

Treatment

While the existent treatment is given below, in recalcitrant cases Tofacitinib is a useful drug, as it effectively inhibits the cytokines that play a predominant role in parthenium dermatitis (Muddebihal A, 2023).

General measures
- Removal of the plant from immediate vicinity
- Protection with appropriate clothing
- Repeated application of barrier creams after washing the exposed parts
- Drying clothes indoors
- Sun protection if photoexaggeration
- Bathing and changing into fresh clothes following outdoor exposure

Topical drugs: Steroids (for limited involvement), tacrolimus and pimecrolimus (mainly for CAD due to parthenium.

Systemic drugs

Oral steroids	Prednisolone: 0.5–1 mg/kg/day Betamethasone: 2–3 mg/day	Mainstay for acute flares
Azathioprine (AZA)	1–2 mg/kg/day **Daily regimen:** Daily AZA±monthly 300 mg boluses **Weekly regimen:** 300 mg once a week	Mainstay of long term maintenance
Cyclosporine	2.5 mg/kg/day	Very quick remission reported in atopics with PD. Unpublished observations support the role in rapid clearance of flares
Methotrexate (MTX)	15 mg/week	MTX + tapering steroids showed faster clearance than AZA +tapering steroids

AIRBORNE CONTACT DERMATITIS (ABCD)

Though the most common cause remains *Parthenium*, an overview of the whole spectrum of ABCD will be given here.

Epidemiology

- ABCD can be classified into *occupational* and *nonoccupational* ABCD.
- It can affect any individual, at any age, and both men and women are affected by this condition.
- It is believed that *airborne irritant dermatitis* is much common than the *allergic type.*

An overview of the common allergens reported is given in **Box 10.3** and the implicated allergen varies depending on the area of study with a difference between the urban and rural areas.

Etiopathogenesis

- Airborne contact dermatitis denotes a unique subtype of contact dermatitis.
- Both irritants as well as allergens may cause volatile or airborne contact dermatitis **(Tables 10.1** and **10.2)**.
- Nature of airborne reactions may be irritant, allergic, phototoxic, photoallergic or contact urticarial.

BOX 10.3: Salient studies on ABCD

Author	Results
Handa S, et al. (2011)	Perfumes, metals, many industrial and pharmaceutical chemicals, pesticides, fungicides, animal feed additives, textile dyes and matches
Hostetler SG	Housedust mite antigens
Sharma et al. and Agarwal et al. (2009)	*Parthenium*
Nandakishor et al. (1994) and Pasricha et al. (1995)	*Parthenium hysterophorus, Xanthium strumarium, Chrysasanthemum coronarium, Heli anthus anovus* and *Dahlia pimrata*
Ghosh and Johnson	Cement, perfumes, deodorants, volatile paints
Singhal et al. (2000)	*Parthenium* (20%), potassium dichromate (16%), xanthium (13.3%), nickel sulfate (12%), chrysanthemum (8%) and mercaptobenzothiazole (6.7%)

TABLE 10.1: Antigens contributing to allergic airborne contact dermatitis

Plants and natural resins	Plastics, rubber and glues	Metals	Industrial chemicals and drugs	Miscellaneous
• *Parthenium hysterophorus*	• Epoxy resins	• Chromate • Cobalt • Gold	• Organophosphorus pesticides	• Agricultural dust
• *Eucalyptus pulverulenta* • Cedar pollen • Citrus fruits • Compositae • Cinnamon	• Formaldehyde and formal-dehyde resins	• Mercury • Nickel • Silver	• Animal feed • Antibiotics • Paraphenylenedi-amine	• Disperse dyes • Cigarettes
• Chrysanthemum • Sunflower • Garlic	• Rubber additives • Fragrance mix		• Potassium metabisulfite • Quaternerium-15 • Potassium dichromate	
• Essential oils • Tropical and domestic woods • Latex • Psyllium	• Colophony • Fiberglass		• Metaproterenol • Rhodium solution	

TABLE 10.2: Specific antigens contributing to ICD, photoallergic and contact urticaria (Santos R et al and Huygen S)

ICD	Photoallergic reaction	Contact urticaria
Phosphates	Carprofen	Amoxycillin
Synthetic fibers	Chlorpromazine	Epoxy resins
Mustard gas, ethylene oxide	Olaquindox	Hyacinth
Metal dust	Pesticides	Pine processes
Carbon dust		Weeping fig

- Most common allergens are plants, especially Compositae allergens.
- In India, most common cause of ABCD is *Parthenium hysterophorus* (Congress weed).
- Other allergens are natural resins, woods, cement, plastic, rubber, glues, metals, pharmaceutical chemicals, insecticides and pesticides.
- In India, ABCD affects adult men more than adult women or children, male-to-female ratio being 20:1.

Historically ABCD in Indian patients has been attributed exclusively to pollens of plants like *Parthenium hysterophorus, Xanthium strumarium, Chrysanthemum coronarium, Helianthus annus* and *Dahlia pimrata*. Recent reports by Ghosh and Johnson et al have however shown that the scenario has been changing rapidly in *urban* and *semiurban* perspective where **cement, perfumes, deodorants, volatile paints, etc.** have become **the commonest allergens** contributing to ABCD.

Clinical Features

Dooms-Goossens and Deleu classified airborne dermatitis into 5 types:

1. Airborne irritant contact dermatitis
2. Airborne allergic contact dermatitis
3. Airborne phototoxic reactions
4. Airborne photoallergic reactions
5. Airborne contact urticaria

Clinical Presentation

- Commonly involves face, 'Wilkinson's triangle', eyelids, nasolabial folds and area under the chin, neck, V-area of chest as well as non-exposed skin such as axilla and waist lines **(Fig. 10.3a)**.
- Later, all exposed areas develop a chronic pruritic and lichenified dermatitis.
- Photoallergic dermatitis: Submental and postauricular area is spared (Ghosh, 2011).
  - Some agents, such as *P. hysterophorus*, can produce both allergic and phototoxic dermatitis.
  - Mixed pattern is also seen in formaldehyde and phosphorus sesquisulfide where allergic CD can coexist with contact urticaria (Dooms-Goossens and Deleu).

Some common causes and their clinical features are given in **Box 10.4.**

BOX 10.4: Common causes of ABCD and their clinical features

Parthenium dermatitis	ABCD, occasionally presents with other morphologies **(see Box 10.2)**
Wood dust	• Starts on the eyelids or the lower half of the face—swelling and redness spread to the neck, hands and forearms • Limited at the margins of the sleeves and collar • Elbow flexures and the skin under a tight collar are often lichenified
Cabinet makers	• Genital dermatitis • Swelling and redness of the eyelids
Cement dust	• Dry lichenified dermatitis
Household sprays, insecticides	• Eyelid dermatitis
Pesticide	Airborne contact dermatitis seen in 20%

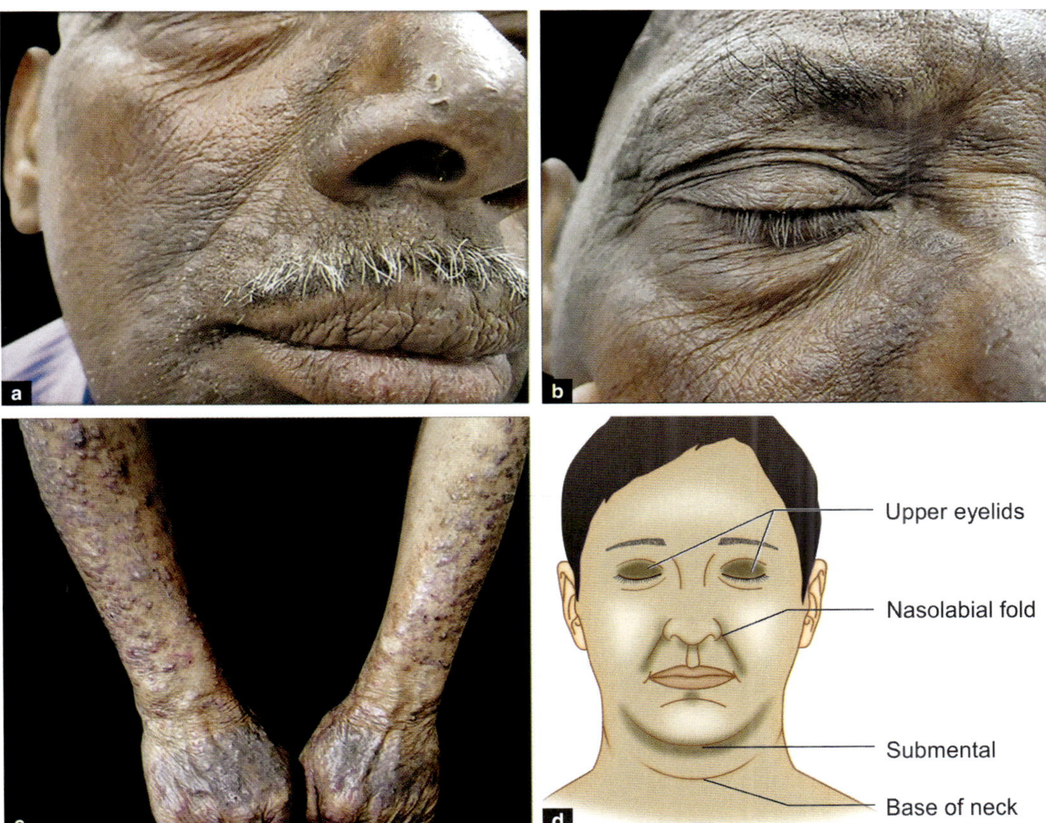

Fig. 10.3: (a) Face affected by airborne contact dermatitis: Note the involvement of the folds of the skin; (b) Marked involvement of the eyelids; (c) Forearm affected by airborne contact dermatitis (lichenoid morphology); (d) Submental area, nasolabial fold and eyelids affected by airborne contact dermatitis (contrasting from photoallergic dermatitis)

Diagnosis

- On the basis of history, morphology and distribution of lesions
- Proved by allergic patch test, prick test or radioallergosorbent test.

Differential Diagnosis

- Contact dermatitis, either by directly applied allergens or by transfer of allergens
- Id reaction
- Systemic contact dermatitis
- Photo-induced dermatosis
- Atopic dermatitis
- Seborrheic dermatitis

Treatment

- Preventive management:
  - Avoiding going outdoors on days when pollen are present in high concentration specially in summers and in the month of September to November.
  - Air-conditioning also reduces the indoor pollen loads
  - Simple routine-like taking a bath after coming indoors, wearing fresh clothes is helpful
  - Eliminating grasses and weeds in the house garden
  - Photoprotection
  - Addition of ferrous sulfate to cement converts the hexavalent chromates into trivalent ones, thereby reducing the sensitizing potential of cement.
  - Change of job or place, if possible
- Treatment of existing dermatitis:
  - Topical steroids
  - Use of emollients especially for dry, lichenified skin lesions
  - Systemic steroids when more than 25% of body surface area involved
  - Phototherapy—PUVA, UVB
  - Other immunosuppressives like methotrexate, azathioprine, cyclosporine
  - JAKi like tofacitinib have also been used successfully
  - Oral hyposensitization is an alternative therapeutic option

BIBLIOGRAPHY

Books

1. Ghosh S. Airborne contact dermatitis: An urban perspective. Perilsofurban pollution: Proceedings National Seminaron Pollutionin Urban Industrial Environment. In: Mitra AK, Editor. Kolkata: St Xavier's College; 2006 p.9–12.
2. Khurana A. Parthenium dermatitis. In Sardana K, Khurana A, Rani S. Handbook of eczema for dermatologists. CBS publishers, New Delhi, 2018.
3. Rook's Textbook of Dermatology, 9th ed. Chapter 39: Eczematous Disorders.
4. Seema Rani, Sanjay Ghosh, Saurav Kundu. Air Borne Contact Dermatitis. In Kabir Sardana, Ananata Khurana, Seema rani. Handbook of Eczema, 2nd edn, CBS.

Journals

1. Agarwal KK, Souza MD. Airborne contact dermatitis induced by parthenium: A study of 50 cases in South India. Clin Exp Dermatol 2009; 34:e4–6.
2. Akhtar N, Verma KK, Sharma A. Study of pro- and anti-inflammatory cytokine profile in the patients with parthenium dermatitis. Contact dermatitis 2010;63:203–8.
3. Christophe J, LeCoz, Ducombs G. Plants and plant product contact dermatitis. In: Frosch PJ, Menne T, Lepoittevin JP, Editors, Contact Dermatitis 4th ed. Heidelberg: Springer; 2006.p.751–800.
4. De D, Sarangal R, Handa S. The comparative efficacy and safety of azathioprine *vs* methotrexate as steroid-sparing agent in the treatment of airborne-contact dermatitis due to Parthenium. Indian J Dermatol Venereol Leprol. 2013 Mar–Apr;79(2):240–1.
5. Ghosh S. Airborne contact dermatitis of non-plant origin: An overview. Ind J Dermatol 2011; 56:(6)711–4.
6. Handa S, De D, Mahajan R. Airborne contact dermatitis current perspectives in etiopathogenesis and management. Indian J Dermatol 2011; 56: 700–706.
7. Lakshmi C, Srinivas CR, Jayaraman A. Ciclosporin in parthenium dermatitis—a report of 2 cases, Contact Dermatitis, 2008;59:245–248.

8. Lakshmi C, Srinivas CR. Parthenium the terminator: An update. Indian Dermatol Online J. 2012 May–Aug; 3(2):89–100.
9. Muddebihal A, Tofacitinib in refractory Parthenium-induced airborne allergic contact dermatitis. Contact Dermatitis. 2023 Feb;88(2):150–152.
10. Nandakishore TH, Pasricha JS. Pattern of cross- sensitivity between four Compositae plants Partheniumhysterophorus, Xanthiumstrumarium, Chrysanthemum coronarium, Helianthusannus in Indian patients. Contact Dermatitis 1994;30:162–7.
11. Nousari HC, Anhalt GJ, Morison WL. Mycophenolate in psoralen-UV-A desensitization therapy for chronic actinic dermatitis, Arch. Dermatol., 1999; 135:1128–29.
12. Pasricha JS, Verma KK, D'souza P. Airborne contact dermatitis caused exclusively by Xanthium strumarium. Indian J Dermatol Venerol Leprol 1995; 61:354–5.
13. Santos R, Goossens AR. An update on airborne contact dermatitis: 2001–2006. Contact Dermatitis 2007;57: 353–60.
14. Sasseville D. Clinical patterns of phytodermatitis. Dermatol Clin. 2009;27(3):299–308.
15. Sasseville D. Phytodermatitis. J Cutan MedSurg. 1999;3(5):263–79.
16. Sharma A, Mahajan VK, Mehta KS, Chauhan PS, Sharma V, Sharma A, Wadhwa D, Chauhan S. Pesticide contact dermatitis in agricultural workers of Himachal Pradesh (India). Contact Dermatitis. 2018 Oct;79(4): 213–7.
17. Sharma VK, Bhat R, Sethuraman, Manchanda Y. Treatment of parthenium dermatitis with methotrexate, Contact Dermatitis, 2007; 57:118–9.
18. Sharma VK, Sethuraman G, Bhat R. Evaluation of clinical patterns of Parthenium dermatitis: Astudy of 74 cases. Contact Dermatitis 2005;44:49–50.
19. Sharma VK, Verma P, Maharaja K. Parthenium dermatitis. Photochem. Photobiol. Sci., 2013;12: 85–94.
20. Sharma VK, Verma P. Parthenium dermatitis in India: Past, present and future. Ind J Dermatol Venereol Leprol. 2012;78(5):560–8.
21. Singhal V, Reddy BS. Common contact sensitizers in Delhi. J Dermatol 2000;27:440–5.
22. Verma KK, Mahesh R, Srivastava P, Ramam M, Mukhopadhyaya AK. Azathioprine versus betamethasone for the treatment of parthenium dermatitis: a randomized control ledstudy, Indian J. Dermatol., Venereol. Leprol., 2008,74,453–457.
23. Verma KK, Bansal A, Sethuraman G. Parthenium dermatitis treated with azathioprine weekly pulse doses. Indian J Dermatol Venereol Leprol. 2006 Jan-Feb;72(1):24–7.

Chapter

11

Erythroderma

Pooja Arora Mrig, Seema Rani, Snigdha Saxena

Erythroderma (Hebra, 1868) is a term applied to any inflammatory skin disease that affects more than 90% of the body surface.

EPIDEMIOLOGY

Men are more commonly affected (M:F = 2:1 to 4:1).
Mean age: 46 years

ETIOPATHOGENESIS

Causes of erythroderma in neonates and infants are listed in **Box 11.1** and **Table 11.1** lists common causes in adults.

BOX 11.1: Causes of neonatal erythroderma

Non-syndromal ichthyosis
- ARCI (including lamellar ichthyosis, congenital ichthyosiform erythroderma, Harlequin ichthyosis), ichthyosis with confetti
- Epidermolytic ichthyosis (including ichthyosis bullosa of Siemens)
- Ichthyosis prematurity syndrome
- Peeling skin syndrome type B
- Self-healing collodion
- X-linked recessive ichthyosis

Syndromal ichthyosis
- Netherton syndrome
- Sjögren–Larsson syndrome
- Chanarin–Dorfman syndrome
- Conradi–Hünermann–Happle syndrome
- Keratitis-ichthyosis-deafness syndrome (KID), KID-AR, and ichthyosis hystrix of Curth–Macklin
- IFAP syndrome

Ectodermal dysplasia
- Ankyloblepharon-ectodermal defects-Cleft lip/palate syndrome (AEC)

Metabolic disorders
- Multiple carboxylase deficiency (holocarboxylase synthetase deficiency and biotinidase deficiency)
- Amino acid disorders (methylmalonic acidemia, propionic acidemia and maple syrup urine disease)
- Urea cycle disorders (citrullinemia)
- Menkes' disease

Infections
- Staphylococcal scalded skin syndrome
- Congenital cutaneous candidiasis

Immunodeficiencies
- Omenn syndrome
- SCID
- Wiskott–Aldrich syndrome (WAS)

(Contd.)

(Contd.)

- Immunodysregulation, polyendocrinopathy and enteropathy. X-linked, syndrome (IPEX)
- Maternal graft-versus-host disease
- Severe dermatitis, multiple allergies, and metabolic wasting syndrome (SAM). SAM-like phenotype
- Digeorge syndrome
- Selective IgA deficiency
- Gaucher syndrome type 2
- AD/AR-hyper IgE syndrome
- X-linked agammaglobulinemia
- CVID

Drugs

- Stevens–Johnson syndrome
- Toxic epidermal necrolysis
- Drug-induced hypersensivity syndrome (vancomycin, phenyloin and ceftriaxon)
- Toxic shock syndrome

Other

- Atopic dermatitis
- Psoriasis
- Seborrheic dermatitis
- Pityriasis rubra pilaris
- Diffuse cutaneous mastocytosis
- COFS syndrome
- Kindler EB
- After cow milk consumption
- Scabies
- Hemophagocytic lymphohistiocytosis
- Congenital lues
- Acrodermatitis enteropathica

AD, autosomal dominant; AR, autosomal recessive; ARCI, Autosomal recessive congenial ichthyosis; COFS, Cerebro-oculo-facio-skeletal syndrome; CVID, combined variable immunodeficiency; EB, epidermolysis bullosa; IFAP, Ichthyosis follicularis atrichia and photophobia; SCID, severe combined immunodeficiency. (Cuperus et al., 2022)

TABLE 11.1: Causes of erythroderma in adults

Conditions causing erythroderma	Relative prevalence (%)
Eczema (atopic dermatitis, contact dermatitis, ABCD, seborrheic dermatitis, chronic actinic dermatitis)	40
Psoriasis	25
Lymphoma (both HL and NHL) and leukemia	15
Drugs • Allopurinol • Beta-lactam antibiotics • Carbamazepine/oxcarbazepine • Gold • Phenobarbital • Phenytoin • Sulfasalazine • Sulfonamides • Zalcitabine	10
Unknown	8
Hereditary disorders (ichthyosiform erythroderma, pityriasis rubra pilaris)	1
Bullous dermatoses (pemphigus foliaceus, bullous pemphigoid, paraneoplastic pemphigus)	0.5
Other skin diseases (lichen planus, dermatophytosis, crusted scabies, dermatomyositis, sarcoidosis, mastocytosis, GVHD, acute or subacute cutaneous lupus erythematosus)	0.5

Source: Rook's Textbook of Dermatology.

Erythroderma in HIV/AIDS

- Erythroderma has occasionally been reported with sero-conversion following HIV infection. In established AIDS, erythroderma may arise from a variety of causes including seborrheic dermatitis, lymphoma or an unknown cause. CD4+ T lymphocytopenia has been associated with erythroderma in the absence of HIV infection.

CLINICAL FEATURES

- In **acute stage (<6 weeks)**, scales are usually large and crusted, whereas in **chronic stage (>6 weeks)**, scales are smaller and drier **(Figs 11.1a** and **b)**.
- Erythroderma developing in primary eczema or associated with a lymphoma is often of sudden onset.
- Patchy erythema which soon becomes generalized in 12–48 hours **(Fig. 11.1c)**.
- Scaling appears after 2–6 days, often first in the flexures.
- The periorbital skin may be inflamed and edematous, resulting in ectropion, with consequent epiphora and is specially pronounced in CIE.
- Pruritus in 90% cases, nail changes in 40%
- Associated symptoms are fever, shivering and even hypothermia
- **Hair:** In persistent cases of erythroderma, scalp and body hair may be shed. **Diffuse nonscarring alopecia** appears in 20% of patients with chronic erythroderma.
- **Nails** become shiny (nail polish sign)
  - Other changes are discoloration, brittleness, dullness, subungual hyperkeratosis, Beau's lines, paronychia and splinter hemorrhages may be observed.
  - Shorenails (alternate bands of nail plate discontinuity)—seen in drug-induced erythroderma.
  - There can be total shedding of nails.
- **Systemic manifestation** in the form of pedal edema (50%), tachycardia (40%), high output cardiac failure, hyperthermia (37%) more often than hypothermia (4%), anemia of both iron deficiency and of chronic disease.
- **Dermatopathic lymphadenopathy**
  - Lymph nodes usually slightly or moderately enlarged and of rubbery consistency.

The clues to certain disorders causing erythroderma in adults are given in **Table 11.2**. While we will discuss neonatal erythroderma in detail in the next section (below).

Neonatal Erythroderma

Collodion Membrane and Scaling

A collodion membrane is a descriptive term for a transient condition in newborns, without implicating a specific diagnosis or disorder. It can occur with erythroderma or the erythroderma appears when the collodion membrane disappears. It is shed within 3–4 weeks after birth.

In 10% of cases the collodion membrane sheds, without leaving any sign of ichthyosis and is known as self-healing collodion baby (SHCB), also known as self-improving congenital ichthyosis or lamellar ichthyosis of the newborn) **(Fig. 11.1d)**. The most common related disorders associated with the collodion membrane are inherited ichthyoses **(Box 11.1)**.

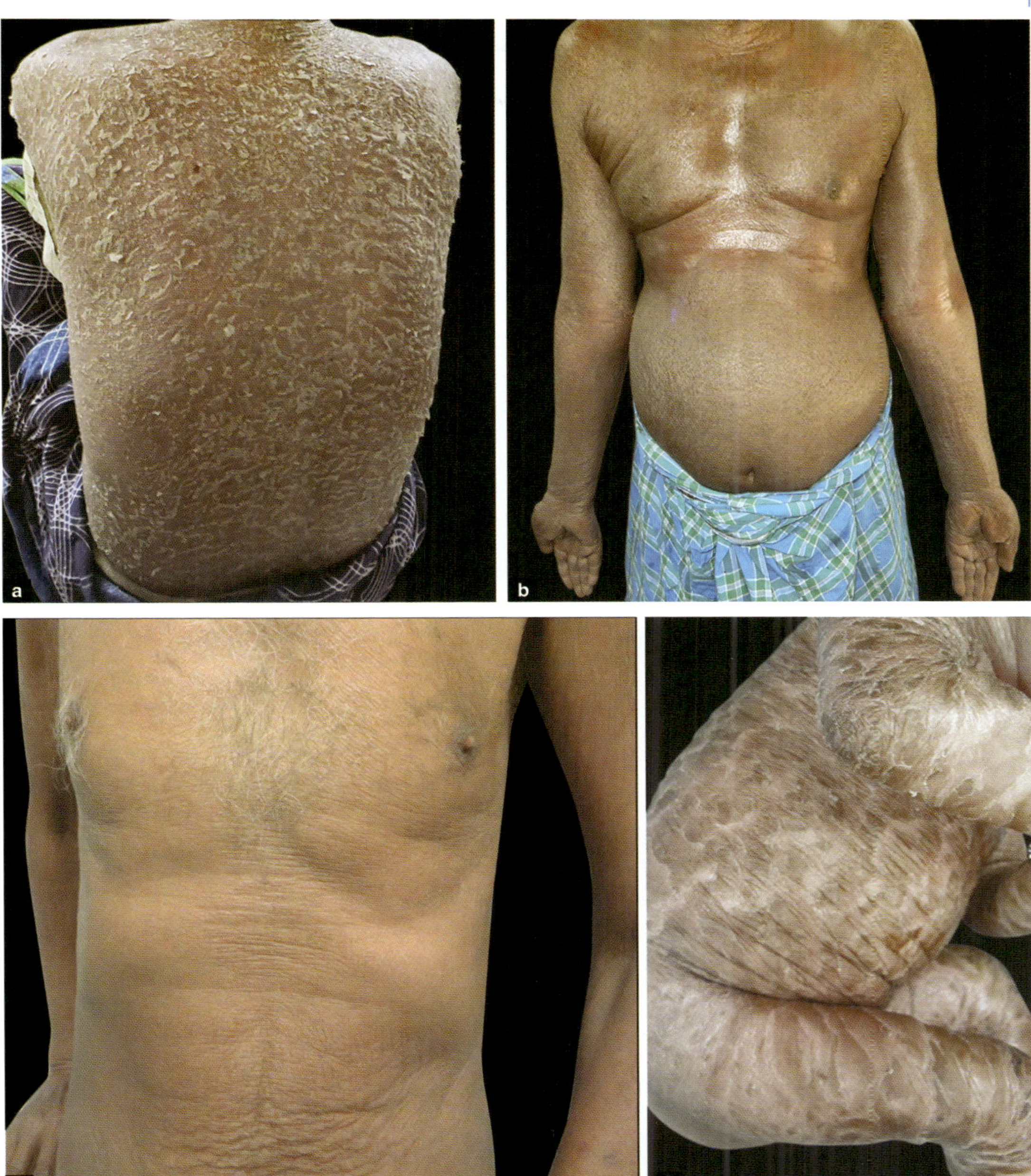

Fig. 11.1: (a) Acute case of psoriatic erythroderma—note the large scales; (b) Chronic idiopathic erythroderma with flexural maceration in a suspect case of airborne contact dermatitis—note the relatively finer scaling; (c) Diffuse involvement of the skin with erythema and scaling in a suspected psoriatic erythroderma patient; (d) Ichthyosiform erythroderma with large lamellar plate-like scales in a 3-week-old baby. The baby had a history of collodion membrane at birth

TABLE 11.2: Clinical clues for diagnosis of common causes of erythroderma

Atopic dermatitis	• Lesions in flexures • Severe pruritus, excoriations • Lichenification, including eyelids, with prurigo nodularis • Elevated serum IgE, eosinophilia • Personal or family history of atopy
Dermatitis (nonatopic)	• Preexisting localized disease • Distribution of initial lesions • Occupation and hobbies • Patch testing • Review oral medications (systemic contact dermatitis)
Drugs	• Most common cause in HIV patients • Preceded by generalized eczema, or scarlatiniform or morbilliform erythema, often accompanied by some irritation, which increases steadily in severity. Erythema may first appear in the flexures, or over the whole skin • Lesions may become purpuric in ankles and feet • Associated features: Fever, lymphadenopathy, organomegaly • Leukocytosis, eosinophilia, liver and renal dysfunction • Shorter duration than other erythrodermas (resolves 2–6 weeks after drug withdrawal) Except—DRESS/DIHS • Most common drugs: Allopurinol, sulfa drugs (TMP-SMX, dapsone), antiepileptics, INH, minocycline, and antiretrovirals
Idiopathic erythroderma	• Elderly men • Chronic, relapsing with severe pruritus Also known as—red man syndrome (marked palmoplantar keratoderma, dermatopathic lymphadenopathy and raised serum IgE) • 3 most common causes are atopic eczema of the elderly, intake of drugs overlooked by the patient and prelymphomatous eruptions • Continue to reevaluate for cutaneous T cell lymphoma
Psoriasis	• Usually preceded by typical plaques • 25% appear de novo; less scaly than typical psoriasis lesions, occasionally pustules may be present • Precipitating factors—emotional stress, intercurrent illness and phototherapy overdosage, drug withdrawal (steroid, MTX, cyclosporine) • Nails may show characteristic psoriasis findings
Pityriasis rubra pilaris	• Begins in childhood or adult life • Follicular, horny plugs on the knees and elbows, and on the backs of the fingers and toes • Islands of sparing are very suggestive of the diagnosis • Skin on the palms and soles often has an orange discoloration, keratoderma +/–
Lichen planus	• After the initial erythema and edema subside, individual violaceous papules may be revealed
Papuloerythroderma of Ofuji	• Widespread, pruritic, red brown, flat-topped papules; may become confluent • Sparing of skin folds ('deck chair' sign) • Favors elderly men • May be associated with lymphoma or HIV infection

(Contd.)

TABLE 11.2: Overview of clinical features of common causes of erythroderma (Contd.)	
CTCL (Sézary and erythrodermic MF)	• **Lymphoma:** Pruritus is often very severe. Rubbing and scratching may produce secondary lichenification. Eosinophilia may suggest Hodgkin's lymphoma • **Sézary syndrome:** Leonine facies, painful fissured keratoderma, alopecia, lymphadenopathy, hepatosplenomegaly. Primary erythroderma; T cell clone in blocd plus one of the following: 1. ≥1000 Sézary cells/μL; 2. CD4:CD8 ratio of ≥10:1; or 3. ↑percentage of CD4+ cells with abnormal phenotype (loss of CD7 or CD26) • **Erythrodermic MF:** Secondary erythroderma; due to progression from classic MF

Alopecia, Bullae, and Pustules

Alopecia is common (45–46% of cases) and is considered as a complication of any severe type of NE. It frequently occurs in PIDs (primary immunodeficiency syndrome), particularly in OS (Omenn syndrome), but also presents in metabolic disoders. Alopecia is seen trichothiodystrophy (TTD), Netherton syndrome (NS), OS and AEC syndrome. Alopecia totalis or alopecia of eye brows and eyelashes is suggestive of a PID.

Bullae can be seen in epidermolytic ichthyosis (EI) (formerly known as bullous ichthyosis, keratinopathic ichthyosis or epidermolytic hyperkeratosis), staphylococcal scalded skin syndrome (SSSS) and DCM (diffuse cutaneous mastocytosis). In EI, the bullae will diminish over time and are replaced by diffuse hyperkeratosis. In SSSS, the skin is usually painful, and the child can present with fever, general malaise and irritability. The erythroderma starts abruptly with bullae developing within the erythematous area within 24–48 hours. Also in addition there is desquamation with scalded appearance, mainly in friction zones, periorificial cracking and a positive Nikolsky sign. Mucosae are usually not affected and the erythema often starts in the umbilical area (omphalitis) and diaper area (e.g. pustules, impetigo and cellulitis). In neonatal DCM, a red skin and blistering was reported in 79% of cases and in case of diffuse affliction there is a classical indurated, appearance likened to peau d'orange. Extensive blistering with positive Darier sign is a more frequent presentation.

In congenital cutaneous candidiasis (CCC), papules and pustules may evolve into NE and will usually spare the oral cavity and diaper area but may include palms and soles. Widely scattered spots on placenta and umbilical cord are a clue to the diagnosis. In CCC, one must look for an underlying PID such as severe combined immunodeficiency (SCID).

Systemic

Extracutaneous involvement and systemic symptoms. Extracutaneous symptoms can occur in other organ systems and are often present in syndromic ichthyoses, PIDs and metabolic disorders. Common systemic symptoms in NS are failure to thrive (FTT) and hypernatremic dehydration. FTT is absent in atopic dermatitis, minimal in ichthyosis but was described in 69% of erythrodermas, predominantly in NS and all PIDs.

However, due to a protective effect of maternal antibodies, PIDs rarely give systemic symptoms at birth. NS is highly suspected when FTT is combined with a mild to severe erythroderma, sepsis and hypernatremic dehydration. A PID (OS or severe combined immunodeficiency (SCID)) should be suspected with lymphadenopathy and hepatosplenomegaly in combination with diarrhoea and/or FTT. Opportunistic infections and candidisis are mainly seen in PIDs.

Metabolic diseases are suspected when desquamative erythroderma is accompanied with neurological manifestations such as coma.

INVESTIGATIONS

Bedside tests and laboratory investigations in a case of erythroderma are summarized in **Tables 11.3** and **11.4**, respectively. We will detail certain investigations which can be of value in adult cases and in cases of neonatal erythroderma.

Blood Investigations

Certain specific tests are needed in neonatal erythroderma and are listed in **Box 11.2**.

Hair Analysis

Hair abnormalities are seen in genetic disorders, such as NS, Menkes disease, TTD, uncombable hair syndrome and loose anagen hair syndrome. The features seen are trichorrhexis invaginata, pili torti and trichorrhexis nodosa. In NS, pili torti and trichorrhexis nodosa can be seen.

BOX 11.2: Special investigations for neonatal erythroderma

Capillary blood gas	Ketoacidosis
Natural killer (NK-) cells	↓, NS
Immunoglobulins IgE, IgG, and IgA	↓↑-NS, Omenn, AD, WAS, IPEX, IgA deficiency
T and B lymphocytes	↓-PID
Serum zinc and alkaline phosphatase	↓ Acrodermatitis enteropathica
Biotinidase and holocarboxylase essays	↓ Biotinidase and holocarboxylase deficiency
Serum tryptase	↑ Diffuse cutaneous mastocytosis
Serum creatin kinase	↑ CDS
Ceruloplasmin and serum copper	↑ Menkes' disease
Glucose	↓ Common
Ammino acids (urine)	↑ NS
Serum ammonia	↑ Metabolic diseases
Serum calcium	↓ DiGeorge

[AD, atopic dermatitis; CDS, Chanarin-Dorfman syndrome; IPEX, immunodysregulation polyendocrinopathy enteropathy X-linked; NS, Netherton syndrome; OS, Omenn syndrome; PID, primary immunodeficiency; WAS, Wiskott-Aldrich syndrome.]

TABLE 11.3: Bedside investigations in a case of erythroderma

Name of test	Remarks
1. Auspitz sign (plaques with scaling)	May be negative in psoriatic erythroderma
2. Gram's stain (pustular, crusted lesions)	Pustular psoriasis (sterile), infection (SSSS, *Candida*)*
3. Tzanck smear (vesicles, bullae, erosions)	Acantholytic cells (pemphigus), eosinophils (bullous pemphigoid)
4. KOH mount (fine scaling)	Dermatophytoses

*If local *S. aureus* or another infection such as SSSS is suspected, skin swabs from infected sites or from eyes, nose,umbilicus and the vagina of the mother should be sent for bacterial culture.

TABLE 11.4: Laboratory investigations in a case of erythroderma	
Investigations	**Interpretation**
CBC with ESR	Anemia (anemia of chronic disease, dermatogenic enteropathy, iron deficiency) Leukocytosis (due to erythroderma, steroid induced, sepsis, hematological malignancy) Eosinophilia (nondiagnostic, seen in 20% erythroderma, highly elevated—Hodgkin's disease) ↓ESR
Peripheral smear	Normocytic normochromic anemia, microcytic hypochromic anemia; Sezary cells
S Ig E levels	May be elevated in patient with erythroderma unrelated to AD, 81% of psoriatic erythroderma
Kidney function tests (urea, creatinine)	Elevated in drug reactions with renal dysfunction, CTDs, acute renal failure due to sepsis, drug induced, e.g. cyclosporine
Serum electrolytes	Imbalance due to fluid loss, poor intake
Liver function tests	May be deranged in CTDs, drug reaction with liver dysfunction
Serum proteins	↓ due to loss in scales, protein losing enteropathy
Urine routine microscopy	To look for pus cells, RBCs, proteins in c/o CTD, renal dysfunction in drug reactions
HIV serology and viral markers	Should be done in all patients and before starting immunosuppressives
Cultures	Blood (on admission/ suspected sepsis), pus (secondary infection, crusted lesions , pustular lesions)
Chest X-ray/ECG	Lung involvement due to underlying disease (sarcoidosis, CTD, malignancy), secondary infection—pneumonitis
Sezary cell counts, CD4:CD8 cell ratio, TCR gene analysis, immuno-phenotyping	If CTCL is suspected
Malignancy screen in suspected cases	Atypical cells, stool for occult blood, USG abdomen and pelvis, Pap smear. mammography
Skin biopsy	Multiple biopsies may be needed; diagnostic in 50–60% cases, features of underlying dermatoses may be masked
DIF	Immunobullous diseases
FNAC (lymph node) Lymph node biopsy	FNAC may show findings of reactive LAP Biopsy may be required in suspected CTCL
Patch test	After subsidence of active disease in suspected parthenium dermatitis

HPE

- Nonspecific features of erythroderma mask features of underlying dermatoses.
- Histopathology can diagnose the cause in 50–60% cases.
  The diagnosis of CTCL will depend on how carefully it is looked for (serial biopsies, multiple biopsies)

- In the ***acute stage***, spongiosis and parakeratosis are prominent, and a nonspecific inflammatory infiltrate permeates a grossly edematous dermis to a variable depth. In the ***chronic stage***, acanthosis and elongation of the rete ridges become more prominent.
- Erythroderma due to lymphoma—the infiltrate may become increasingly pleomorphic with atypical cerebriform mononuclear cells and Pautrier's microabscesses.
- In NS Kazal-type related inhibitor (LEKTI) is recommended particularly in psoriasiform epidermal hyperplasia. In NS, different histology patterns are seen, based on different phases within the spectrum.
- The diagnosis of PID is made based on a spongiotic reactions pattern with keratinocytic necrosis, satellite cell lymphocytes and infiltrates of lymphocytes with or without eosinophils.
- In ichthyoses, a biopsy is helpful in ~50% of cases.
- EI can be differentiated from SSSS and hereditary epidermolysis bullosa (EB).

Advanced Tests

These include imaging and molecular tests.

Complications and Comorbidities

- Hemodynamic and metabolic disturbances
- Hypothermia
- Hypoalbuminemia is in part due to increased protein loss from exfoliated scale, which may reach 9 g/m^2 of body surface or more each day.
- Fluid loss by transpiration is much increased and is roughly proportional to the basal metabolic rate.
- Altered immune response, increase in globulins or CD4+ T lymphocytopenia in the absence of HIV infection.

COURSE AND PROGNOSIS

The disease course and prognosis are given in **Box 11.3**.

BOX 11.3: Disease course and prognosis

- Potentially fatal condition with mortality varying from 18–64%
- Prognosis depends on various factors—etiology, age, comorbidities, speed of onset and early therapy.
- Cutaneous, subcutaneous, respiratory infections common
- Causes of death—sepsis, pneumonia and cardiac failure
- More frequent forms of erythroderma, i.e. eczematous, psoriatic, idiopathic—may continue for months/years following relapsing remitting course.

APPROACH TO DIAGNOSIS

An approach to the diagnosis of erythroderma is given in **Flowchart 11.1** while **Flowchart 11.2** shows a step by step approach to diagnosis of neonatal erythroderma.

Neonatal Erythroderma

Step 1: A combined multi speciality approach of dermatologists and pediatricians is recommended with a complete medical history (pregnancy, complications and miscarriages,

Flowchart 11.1: Approach to the diagnosis of erythroderma

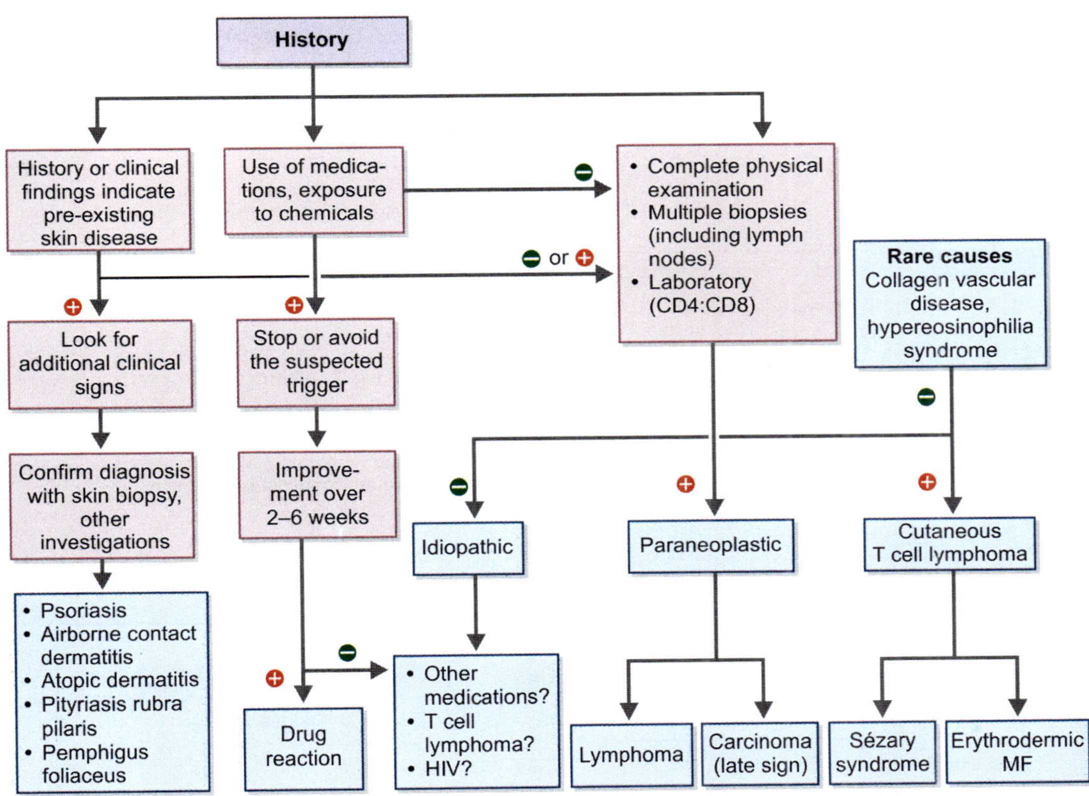

recent medication use, consanguinity, family history of PID, ichthyosis, atopy and psoriasis) and physical examination with special attention to the presence of collodion membrane, alopecia, blisters and pustules. In case blisters are present, DIF is recommended. One must exclude bacterial or fungal infections such as SSSS or CCC by taking swabs.

Step 2: As a first step, basic blood tests must be ordered.

Step 3: If no diagnosis is found, special blood tests are needed along with biopsy and trichoscopy. Specialized tests needed include whole blood samples (or DNA) that can be sent for molecular genetic testing (e.g. Sanger sequencing, targeted NGS panel, WES and WGS).

Step 4: Investigate for extracutaneous, syndromic and/or systemic symptoms.

The combination of neurological signs, hair abnormalities and specific extracutaneous symptoms can narrow down the possible diagnosis towards types of syndromic ichthyosis such as NS. PIDs and metabolic diseases should be excluded, especially in cases with failure to thrive,superimposed infections or lack of response to therapy.

Step 5: When step 4 shows no abnormalities, consider an inherited ichthyosis. Also consider benign inflammatory skin disorders, such as atopic dermatitis, psoriasis and seborrheic dermatitis, which are rare in the neonatal period and when erythrodermic, mainly manifest after three months of age.

Flowchart 11.2: Approach to diagnosis of neonatal erythroderma

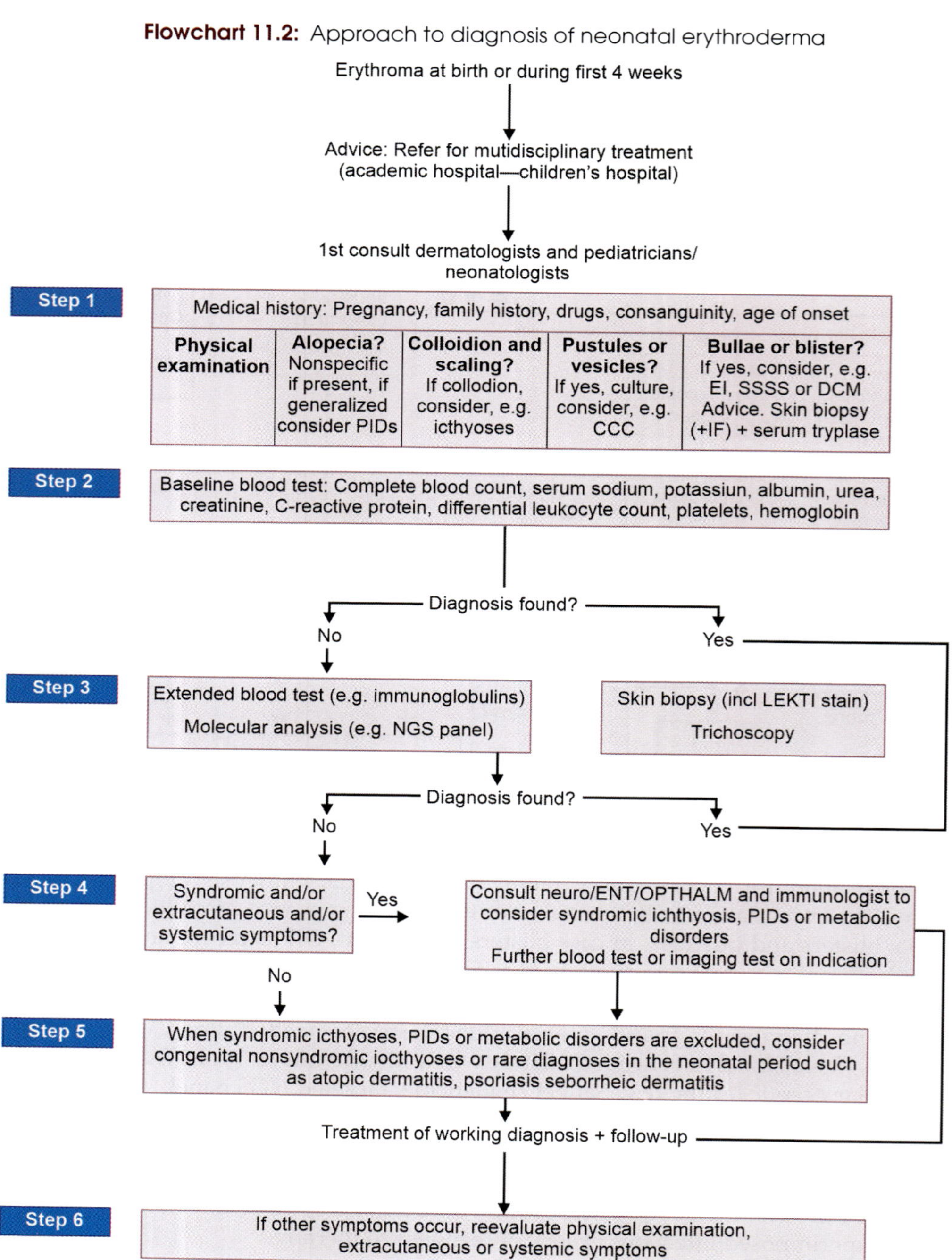

MANAGEMENT

Tables 11.5 and 11.6 summarize the management of erythroderma.

TABLE 11.5: General measures in erythroderma

- Admission in hospital
- Provide warm and humid environment
- Monitoring of pulse, BP, temperature
- Withdraw or switch medications that may be implicated as a cause/stop all unnecessary medications
- Monitor and correct temperature, fluid balance and nutritional assessment
- High protein diet, folate supplementation
- Treat any secondary infection

TABLE 11.6: Specific treatment of erythroderma

Topical	• Open wet dressings • Bland emollients • Low to mid-potent topical corticosteroids (ointments > creams) • Wet dressings **Avoid**: High potency steroids, irritants such as coal tar and anthralin, topical immunomodulators, vitamin D analogues
Systemic	• Treatment of underlying disorder • Immunosuppressive agents (use depends on underlying etiology, should be used only after ruling out CTCL) – Systemic CS—start dose of prednisolone: (1 mg/kg with maintenance dose of ≤0.5 mg/kg day with slow tapering) – Methotrexate (7.5–10 mg/week) – Cyclosporine (initial dose of 4–5 mg/kg/day with reduction to 1–3 mg/kg/day) – Azathioprine—for AD and ABCD • Oral antihistamines • Oral antibiotics (if needed)
Psoriatic erythroderma	Methotrexate, acitretin, cyclosporine, biologics

BIBLIOGRAPHY

1. Cuperus E, Bygum A, Boeckmann L, Bodemer C, Bolling MC, Caproni M, et al. Proposal for a 6-step approach for differential diagnosis of neonatal erythroderma. J Eur Acad Dermatol Venereol. 2022 Jul;36(7): 973–986.
2. Rook's Textbook of Dermatology, 9th ed. Chapter 39: Eczematous disorders.

Chapter

12

Follicular Disorders

Ananta Khurana

- A group of disorders presenting with small papules localized around follicles and appendages.
- **True follicular disorders:** Present clinically with keratotic papules or papules with prominent spine and follicular plugging on histopathology (Sardana K, 2014).
- Typically, follicular lesions do not have a tendency to coalesce.

Classification

An approach to the diagnosis of the follicular disorders is given in **Flowchart 12.1**. These are conveniently divided into three broad types—keratotic papules, lichenoid papules and the Id eruptions. A regional classification is given in **Flowchart 12.2**. **Table 12.1** gives an etiological classification of the common follicular disorders.

The details of the common disorders seen are listed in **Table 12.2** and some are discussed in the text that follows.

KERATOSIS PILARIS (KP)

Etiopathogenesis: Not well understood but many factors, including histopathologic findings, the tendency to improve during adolescence, the association with filaggrin mutations and 18p monosomy, the effects of androgen and insulin dysregulation, and reduced prevalence in patients with acne vulgaris, support KP as a disorder of the sebaceous gland, which disrupts the permeability barrier of the SC and causes aberrant keratinization and hair abnormalities.

Onset: First two decades of life (peak at puberty)

Family history: Positive in 39%

Clinical Presentation

- 'Chicken skin,' appearance.
- Keratotic papules in a folliculocentric distribution; **'antenna sign'** positive **(Fig. 12.1a)**.
- Distributed on the extensor surfaces of the proximal extremities.
- Variable amount of perifollicular erythema—present.
- Mild KP may have coiled or twisted vellus hairs, either single or in groups of 2–3, surrounded by peripilar casts.

Flowchart 12.1: An overview of the common follicular disorders based on the prominent morphology

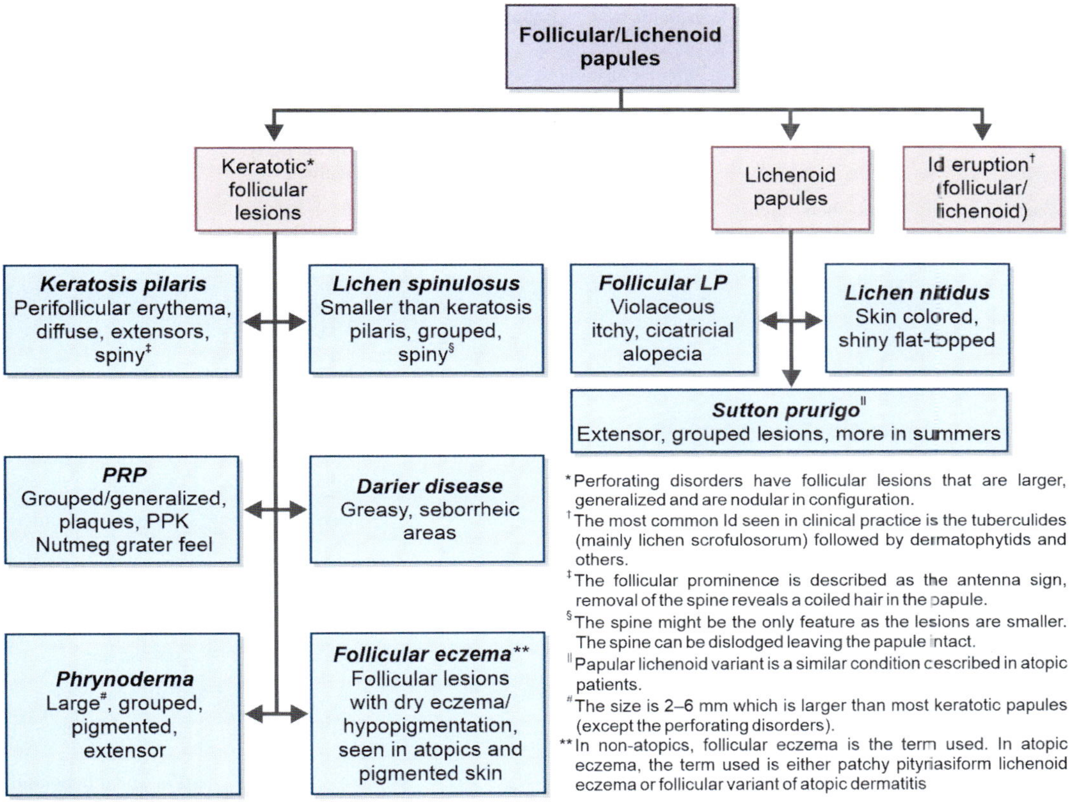

Follicular/Lichenoid papules

- **Keratotic* follicular lesions**
  - ***Keratosis pilaris*** — Perifollicular erythema, diffuse, extensors, spiny‡
  - ***Lichen spinulosus*** — Smaller than keratosis pilaris, grouped, spiny§
  - ***PRP*** — Grouped/generalized, plaques, PPK, Nutmeg grater feel
  - ***Darier disease*** — Greasy, seborrheic areas
  - ***Phrynoderma*** — Large#, grouped, pigmented, extensor
  - ***Follicular eczema***** — Follicular lesions with dry eczema/hypopigmentation, seen in atopics and pigmented skin
- **Lichenoid papules**
  - ***Follicular LP*** — Violaceous itchy, cicatricial alopecia
  - ***Lichen nitidus*** — Skin colored, shiny flat-topped
  - ***Sutton prurigo*‖** — Extensor, grouped lesions, more in summers
- **Id eruption† (follicular/lichenoid)**

*Perforating disorders have follicular lesions that are larger, generalized and are nodular in configuration.

†The most common Id seen in clinical practice is the tuberculides (mainly lichen scrofulosorum) followed by dermatophytids and others.

‡The follicular prominence is described as the antenna sign, removal of the spine reveals a coiled hair in the papule.

§The spine might be the only feature as the lesions are smaller. The spine can be dislodged leaving the papule intact.

‖Papular lichenoid variant is a similar condition described in atopic patients.

#The size is 2–6 mm which is larger than most keratotic papules (except the perforating disorders).

**In non-atopics, follicular eczema is the term used. In atopic eczema, the term used is either patchy pityriasiform lichenoid eczema or follicular variant of atopic dermatitis

Flowchart 12.2: A regional classification of follicular disorders

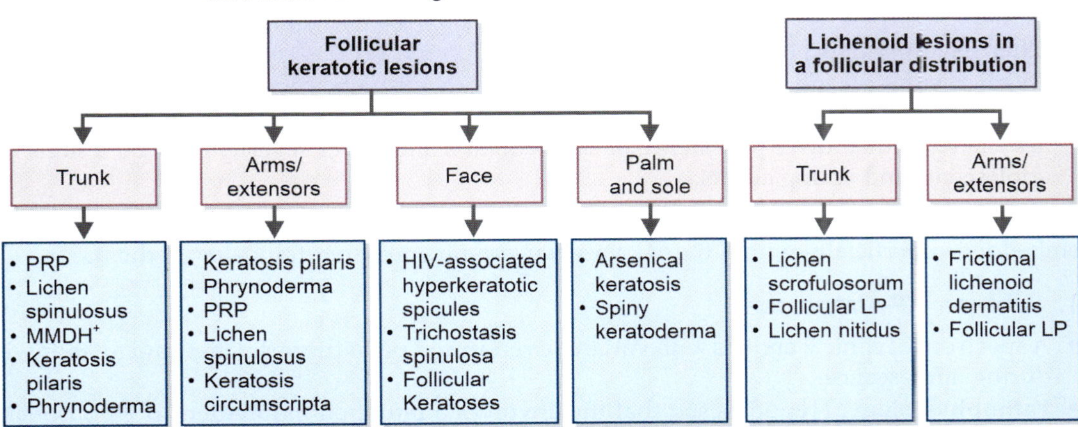

PRP, pityriasis rubra pilaris; LP, lichen planus; MMDH+, multiple minute digitate hyperkeratoses (typically nonfollicular)

TABLE 12.1: Classification of common follicular disorders

Keratinization disorders	Follicular lichenoid dermatoses	Eczematous dermatoses	Papulosquamous disorders	Infective	Miscellaneous
Keratosis pilaris	Lichen plano-pilaris	Follicular eczema	Follicular psoriasis	Follicular Id eruption (lichen scrofulosorum, dermatophytid, scabies)	Trichostasis spiunulosa
Lichen spinulosus	Lichen nitidus		Follicular pityriasis rosea	Bacterial folliculitis, viral folliculitis (*Molluscum contagiosum*, HSV)	Granulosa rubra nasi
Phrynoderma	Follicular LP		Pityriasis rubra pilaris	Secondary syphilis (folli-cular variant)	Follicular mycosis fungoides
Darier disease	—	—	—	Pityrosporum folliculitis	Follicular mucinosis
Follicular ichthyosis/ ichthyosis follicularis with alopecia and photophobia (IFAP)	—	—	—	Demodicidosis	Perforating disorders
Keratosis follicularis squamosa (Dohi)	—	—	—	—	Follicular lesions in sarcoidosis
Disseminated and recurrent infundi-bulofolliculitis	—	—	—	—	Follicular nevi
Pityriasis rubra pilaris	—	—	—	—	Frictional lichenoid dermatitis
Familial dyskeratotic comedones	—	—	—	—	—

- In more severe KP: Coiled vellus hair are impacted in the horny layer.
- Often asymptomatic, but may be pruritic.
- Dyspigmentation and erythema make it a significant cosmetic concern in some.
- One study suggests that the presence of moderate-to-severe keratosis pilaris on the arms is associated with a lower prevalence of acne vulgaris and lower severity of facial lesions in adolescents and young adults.

Dermatoscopy: Abnormal hair shaft structure—thin and short, coiled or semicircular hair, embedded superficially within the SC; vascular prominences; perifollicular erythema.

1. *Subtype: KP Atrophicans*

- A spectrum of clinical entities with variable overlap and pediatric onset that tend to improve during adolescence.
- **Pathophysiology:** Hypothesised that this involves a mutation in low-density lipoprotein (LDL) receptor-related protein 1 (LRP1), causing keratinocytes to release cytokines in

TABLE 12.2: Salient features of common follicular disorders

	Keratosis pilaris	Lichen spinulosus	Lichen scrofulosorum	Phrynoderma
Site	Extensors of proximal extremities (Less: distal extremities, face, trunk, buttocks)	Abdomen, neck, thighs, extensor arms, buttocks, trochanteric region	Trunk	Elbows, knees Buttocks, extensors (Friction prone sites)
Morphology	Keratinous plugs in follicular orifices~1 mm size **"Antenna sign"** positive	• Minute skin colored follicular papules • 1–2 mm • Central horny spine • Rough feel on palpation • May be symmetrical	• Skin colored to erythematous to reddish brown • Follicular or perifollicular • Flat topped • Surface: Scaling/horny spines/micropustules • Variant presentations: Lichenoid/psoriasiform	• Large (2–3 mm) keratotic follicular papules • Adjacent skin: may be hyperpigmented, scaly • Bilateral symmetrical arrangement
Grouping	None	Grouped	Grouped	None
Erythema	Variable **perifollicular erythema (+)**	None	May be erythematous	None
Histopathology	• Orthokeratotic follicular plugs • May have 1/more twisted hair • Dilated infundibulum • May be associated with a mild inflammatory infiltrate • Sebaceous glands strikingly absent from lesions but present in unaffected skin	• Orthokeratotic follicular plugging • Perifollicular mononuclear infiltrate	• Non-caseating, epithelioid cell granulomas in the superficial dermis around hair follicles or eccrine glands • Acid fast bacilli absent	Orthokeratotic follicular plugging

response to follicular plugs, leading to perifollicular inflammation that promotes fibrosis, alopecia, atrophy, and hair bulb shrinkage.

Includes clinical variants such as:

a. *Keratosis follicularis spinulosa decalvans*: Keratotic papules, occasionally erythematous; involve malar regions, eyebrows, eyelashes, neck, extremities, scalp, axillae and pubic regions; scarring +; widespread KP, palmopantar keratoderma, prominent cuticles, hyperkeratosis of heels and knees; blepharitis; keratitis; corneal dystrophy; photophobia; enamel hypoplasia. X-linked dominant KFSD tends to remit after puberty.

b. *Keratosis rubra pilaris faciei atrophicans/ulerythema ophryogenes*: Small, follicular, keratotic papules and erythema on the lateral third of the eyebrows, extending to the forehead and cheeks and eventually leading to scarring alopecia. KP is often present on extensor surfaces. Follicular atrophy may occur. Disease course typically ends at puberty but for the permanent alopecia and atrophy which may have already developed.

c. *Atrophoderma vermiculatum* **(honeycomb-atrophy)**: Begins with follicular, keratotic papules, erythema, and milia on the cheeks and heals with reticular, atrophic pitting of the cheeks, creating a worm-eaten or honeycomb appearance. Inflammation stops after puberty while the erythema and reticulated atrophy tend to improve spontaneously and gradually.

d. *Folliculitis spinulosa decalvans*: It is an autosomal dominant condition seen at puberty. It is characterized by formation of follicular pustules on the scalp with alopecia.

2. *Subtype*: *Erythromelanosis Follicularis Faciei et colli*

- A rare pigmented subtype of KP, without scarring or atrophy.
- Presents with bilateral hyperpigmentation, follicular papules, and erythema on the cheeks and temples, potentially progressing to the submandibular neck and preauricular areas **(Fig. 12.1b)** (Sardana K, 2012).
- Affected skin is rough with fewer vellus hairs, but there is neither scarring nor atrophy.
- Associated KPs can be seen in 88%.

3. *Subtype*: *Keratosis Pilaris Rubra*

- KP with more overt erythema and a larger distribution of skin involvement, most often the lateral cheeks and proximal extremities.
- Erythema persists during puberty and can even worsen.

Associations of Keratosis Pilaris

- Icthyosis vulgaris (with or without atopic dermatitis)
- Atopy (present in up to 37% of patients)
- Endocrinological and metabolic disorders: Obesity, type 1 diabetes mellitus, pregnancy
- Follicular hyperkeratosis: monelithrix, pachyonychia congenita, ectoderma dysplasias
- Renal insufficiency
- Syndromes: Down, Noonan, Olmsted, neurocardiofacial-cutaneous syndromes (RASopathies), Graham Little Picardi.
- Drugs inducing widespread KP like eruptions: Steroids, lithium, cyclosporine, targeted inhibitors of B-Raf, tyrosine kinase inhibitors.
- Filaggrin (*FLG*) mutations; in some—independent of atopic dermatitis/icthyosis as well. Filaggrin mutations may contribute to KP by down regulating sebocyte proliferation, causing atrophy of the sebaceous glands, and disrupting the epithelial barrier.

Histopathology: ***See*** **Table 12.2 and Fig. 12.1c.**

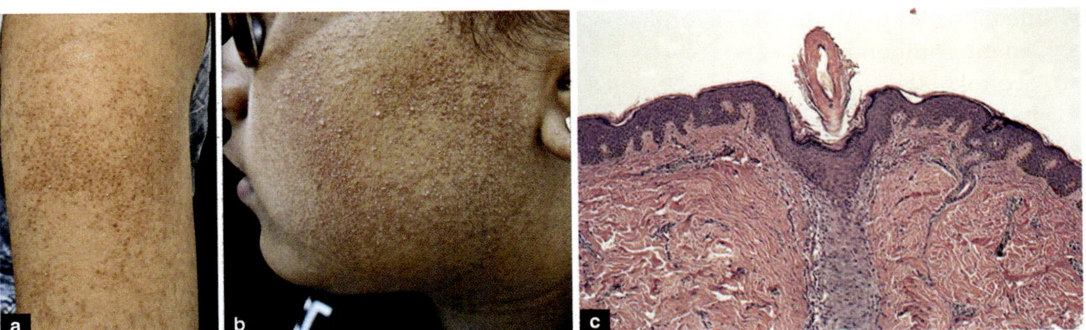

Fig. 12.1: (a) Keratosis pilaris-follicular erythematous lesions with some showing a protruding spine—the so-called antenna sign (*Courtesy*: Dr Kabir Sardana); (b) Erythromelanosis follicularis faciei et colli (*Courtesy*: Dr Kabir Sardana); (c) Keratin plug fills the infundibulum of the hair follicle and this represents the "keratotic spne" of keratosis pilaris

Course and Prognosis

- Persistence into adulthood in 43%, improvement with increasing age in 35%, worsening with age in 22%.
- In about half: KPs improve in summer; worsen in the winter.

Treatment

- Partial effect; recurrences common
- Gentle cleansing, mild hydration of skin
  - Avoid washing the skin too often
  - Take warm showers rather than hot baths
  - Use lipid enriched soaps and keep the atmosphere humid
  - Apply any treatments to damp skin.
- Keratotic component: Topical lactic acid, salicylic acid, urea, retinoids (tazarotene)
  - "Salicylated vaseline": Salicylic acid 3 g and Vaseline 100 g.
  - 10–30% urea, acts both as a moisturizer and a keratolytic.
- Erythema: Topical tacrolimus and topical steroids. Steroids should be only used to reduce the inflammation if any, while tacrolimus has been found to be as good as a moisturizer in studies.
- Lasers have been used for the erythematous component (KTP, PDL, IPL); and for dyspigmentation (1064 nm QsNd:YAG).

The treatment approach is to use a mild steroid initially and maintain the patient with a keratolytic or topical urea.

LICHEN SPINULOSUS

Etiology: Not precisely defined; probably represents a follicular reaction pattern of more than one origin.

Reported associations include

- Atopic diathesis

- Infections: Id to fungi, HIV, syphilis
- Genetic components
- Alcohol
- Hodgkin's disease, Crohn's disease
- Seborrheic dermatitis
- Drugs: Thallium, omeprazole, gold, diphtheria toxin, arsphenamine.

Age of onset: Children and adolescents; rarely adults

Clinical Presentation

- Grouped follicular lesions erupt in crops, grow rapidly and then remain stationary.
- Two variants have been described **(Fig. 12.2)**.
  - The first has lesions consisting of grouped, symmetrical, minute, filiform, keratotic papules. The follicular lesions are initially red, but later on, they acquire a skin colored tone. Unlike keratosis pilaris they are grouped and do not have perifollicular erythema. It is possible to remove the spine of the lesions without removing the papule, which is an important feature distinguishing it from keratosis pilaris.
  - The second type has horny spines, which are follicular but independent of any papules. The lesions appear in crops and are symmetrically distributed over the neck, buttocks, trochanteric region, abdomen, thighs, popliteal spaces and extensor aspects of the arms. The face is usually spared.

    A long strand of keratin glinting maybe seen when examined in side light.

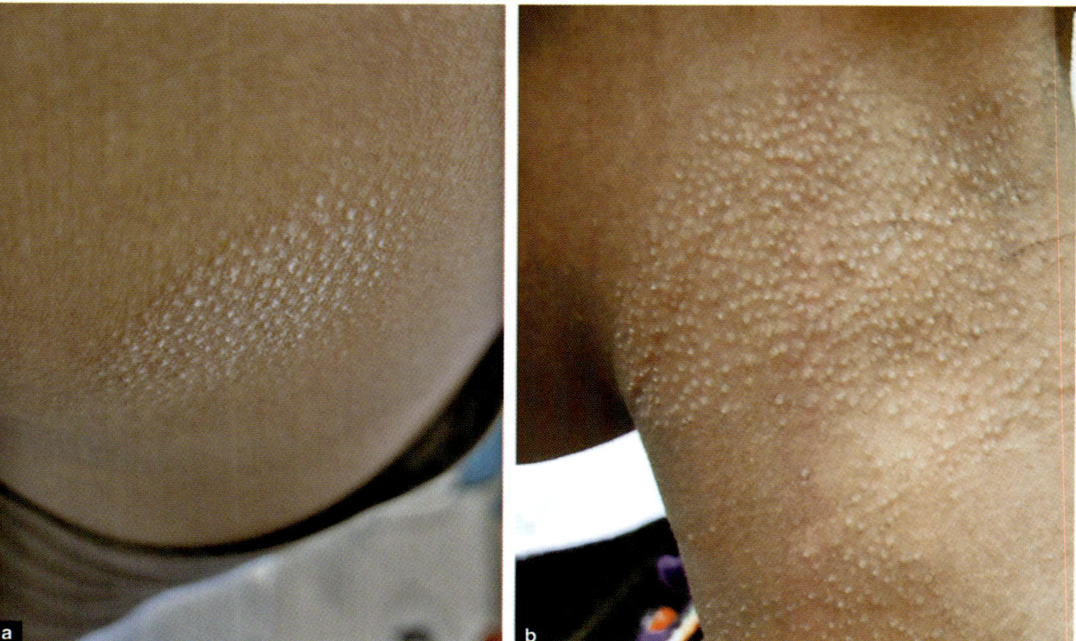

Fig. 12.2: Lichen spinulosus-grouped follicular papules with a keratotic spine (*Courtesy*: Dr Kabir Sardana)

Treatment

- Keratolytics [topical salicylic acid (3–6%), lactic acid (12%) and urea (20–40%)], emollients, and mid-potency corticosteroid are usually effective, along with removal of the trigger if identifiable.
- Tendency to disappear spontaneously at puberty in childhood onset type.

Histopathology

While there is a keratotic plug in the follicular infundibulum akin to keratosis pilaris there is also a heavier perifollicular infiltrate of lymphocytes in lichen spinulosus, particularly adjacent to the infundibulum of the follicle, which is often dilated.

PHRYNODERMA (Fig. 12.3)

- **Phryno** (Greek: Toad)
- **Etiology:** Various nutritional deficiencies have been associated. Local factors like pressure and friction may also play a role.

  Postulated nutritional deficiencies include:
  - Malnutrition (strongest association)
  - Vitamin A
  - Vitamin B complex
  - Vitamin C
  - Vitamin E
  - Essential fatty acid (EFA)
  - Malabsorption from various etiologies

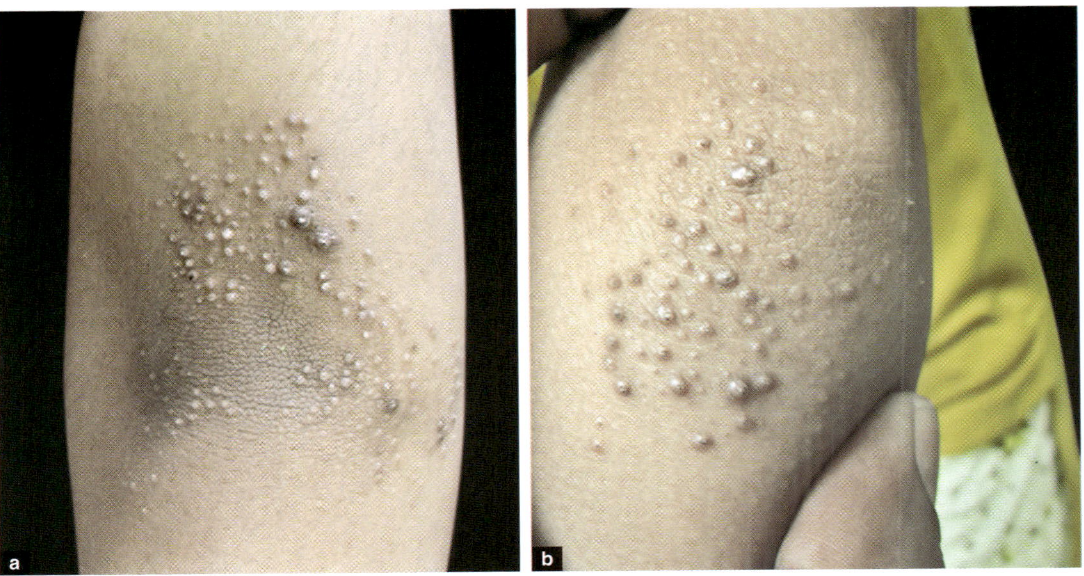

Fig. 12.3: Phrynoderma—large, pigmented, follicular papules with a discrete keratotic plug (*Courtesy*: Dr Kabir Sardana)

- But the prevalent hypothesis is that multiple nutrients may play a role rather than one isolated nutritional deficiency. Impaired balance or threshold levels of these nutrients with or without a deficiency state seem to alter the intersecting biochemical pathways and the local milieu of these nutrients resulting in phrynoderma.
- **Onset:** Young children and adolescents
- **Clinical appearance:** Discrete, brown or skin colored, acuminate, keratotic papules with central keratin plug predominantly distributed over elbows, knees, extensor extremities, and/or buttocks. Surrounding skin is often dry and scaly **(Fig. 12.3)**.
- Biopsy shows hyperkeratosis and prominent keratotic follicular plug-ging. Sweat glands may be atrophic; in severe cases, they show squamous metaplasia.
- **Treatment:** Multifactorial disease; thus a combination therapy with vitamins and EFA along with adequate nutrition.

  Clinical improvement follows nutritional intervention.

BIBLIOGRAPHY

Books

1. Acquired Disorders of Epidermal Keratinization. Rook's Textbook of Dermatology, 9th edition. Part 8, Chapter 87:http://www.rooksdermatology.com/
2. Sardana K: Disorders with Follicular Morphology. In. Diagnosis and Management of Skin Disorders: An Evidence Based approach Paperback-1, January 2012. 1st Edn LWW. Delhi.

Journals

1. Gerbig AW. Treating keratosis pilaris. J Am Acad, 2002;47:457.
2. Sardana K, et al. An observational analysis of erythromelanosis follicularis faciei et colli. Clin Exp Dermatol. 2008 May;33(3):333–6.
3. Sardana K. Follicular disorders of the face. Clin Dermatol. 2014 Nov-Dec;32(6):839–72.
4. Wang JF, Orlow SJ. Keratosis Pilaris and its Subtypes: Associations, New Molecular and Pharmacologic Etiologies, and Therapeutic Options. Am J Clin Dermatol. 2018 Oct;19(5):733–757.

Chapter 13

Genetic Skin Disorders

Kabir Sardana, Surabhi Sinha, Sinu Rose Mathachan, Rahul Mahajan

INTRODUCTION

Genetic skin disorders often are difficult to comprehend, diagnose and treat and in certain countries form a major OPD concern, though the same may not be true in tropical countries. Nevertheless they remain a core domain of dermatologists and most texts are either too verbose or conversely too compact to comprehend.

While we discuss the disorders under various headings, we have also made 'full body' artist diagrams to make them easy to comprehend and possibly diagnose. Most of the clinical features have been depicted in the diagrams while additional features can be added in these by the readers themselves!

These can be broadly divided into the following types:

1. **Collagen defect:** EDS and OI
2. **Elastic fibers defect**
   a. **Elastinopathies:** Cutis laxa, Michelin tyre baby
   b. **Fibrinillopathies:** Marfan syndrome
3. **Ectopic calcification:** PXE
4. **Infantile stiff skin syndromes:** Hyaline fibromatoses, restrictive dermopathy, stiff skin syndrome
5. **Others:** Lipoid proteinosis, focal dermal hypoplasia (Goltz syndrome).

1. EHLERS-DANLOS SYNDROME (EDS)

An overview of clinical features in EDS is depicted in **Figs 13.1** and **13.2**.

- Heterogeneous group characterized by abnormal collagen structure and/or function within the skin, joints, and vasculature. **Table 13.1** depicts a summary of all 8 types:
  - *Most common* is the *hypermobility* type, followed by *classical* and then the *vascular* type.
  - Most patients present late in childhood as the diagnosis can be difficult to make, particularly in classical and hypermobile types, until the child starts to walk.
  - Skin histology is variable and often within normal limits.

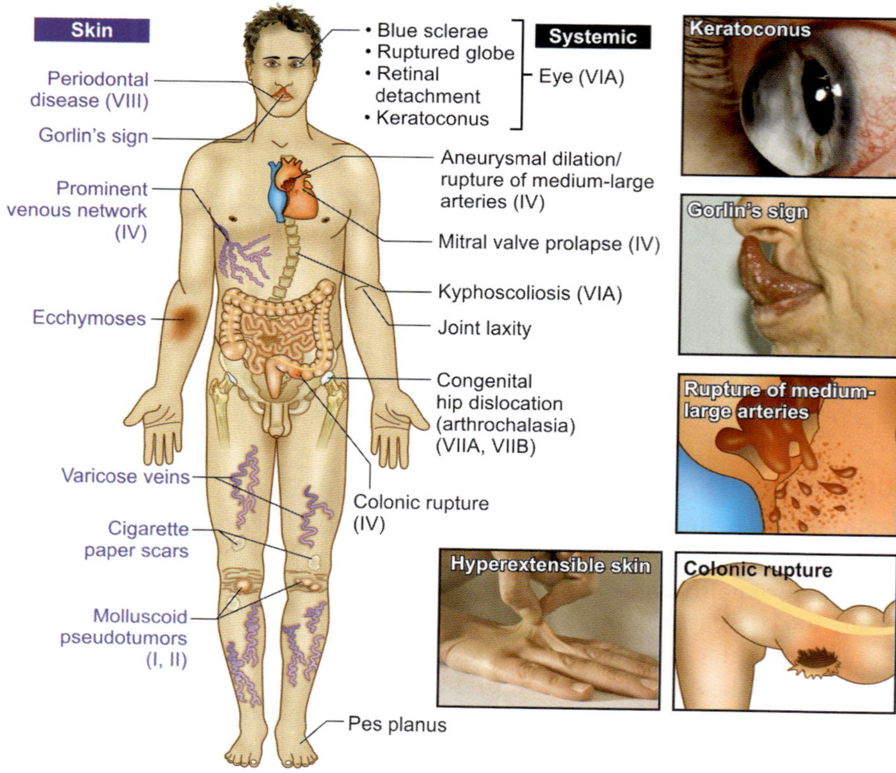

Fig. 13.1: Artistic depiction of features of EDS

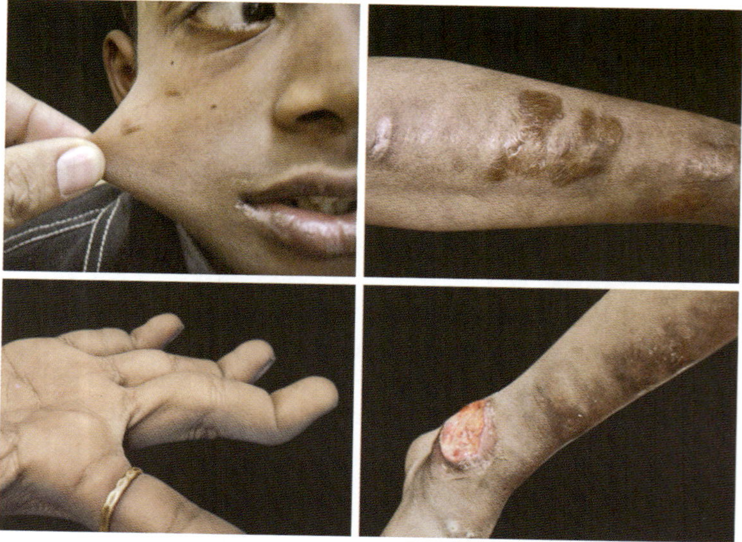

Fig. 13.2: Depiction of varied features of EDS: Hyperextensibility of skin, cigarette paper scars, hypermobile joints and delayed healing of wounds

TABLE 13.1: Clinical and molecular subtypes of EDS (Villefranche classification)

EDS type	Molecular defect and mode of inheritance	Skin	Joints	Other systemic features
Classical (Type I, "gravis" and Type II, "mitis")	COL5A1, COL5A2 ***AD*** ("cauliflower" fibrils on EM)	• Hyperextensibility • Easy bruising • **Fragile skin** Widened wounds ("fish mouth" wounds) and "cigarette paper" scars • **Molluscoid pseudo-tumors** (overlying joints and pressure points) • Spheroids (shin, forearms)	**Hypermobility** and joint dislocations	Gor in's sign +
Hypermobility (formerly Type III)	TNXB ***AD***	Mild	• Hypermobility • Chronic joint pain + • Arthritis • Recurrent dislocations and subluxations	—
Vascular/ Acrogeric (formerly Type IV)	COL3A1 ***AD*** Small variable fibrils	• Thin, translucent skin • Extensive bruising • Early varicosities (can visualize veins under skin easily) • **Acrogeria**	**Small joint Hypermobility**	• Rupture of bowel, uterus, or arteries • **Most life-threatening** form
Other form (formely type V)	XLR	Resembles mild classical, bruising	—	—
Kyphoscoliotic (VIA)	Lysyl hydroxy-lase 1 (PLOD1) ***AR***	• Mild	**Hypermobility Severe scoliosis**	• Severe muscle hypotonia • **Ocular fragility** Ruptured globe, blindness, retinal detachment, or keratoconus • Marfanoid features • Osteopenia • Ascorbic acid supplementation may help
Arthrochalasic (formerly types VIIA and VIIB)	COL1A1, COL1A2 AD	• Mild • Criss-crossing of palm and sole skin (+/–)	**Floppy infant, Most severe hyper-mobility with** recurrent subluxations/dislocations (much *more severe* than hypermobility type)	• Congenital hip dislocation • Short stature

(Contd.)

TABLE 13.1: Clinical and molecular subtypes of EDS (Villefranche classification) *(Contd.)*

EDS type	Molecular defect and mode of inheritance	Skin	Joints	Other systemic features
Dermatosparaxis (formerly type VIIC)	Procollagen N-proteinase (ADAMTS2) ***AR***	• Severe fragility • Sagging, redundant skin and bruising	Markedly hypermobile joints	• Umbilical/ inguinal hernias • Premature rupture of fetal membranes
Periodontal type (formerly type VIII)	***AD***	• Hyperextensible skin with scarring (esp. pretibial) and bruising	Mild	• Severe periodontitis → teeth loss

Differential Diagnosis

- **Cutis laxa:** Skin hangs in flaccid redundant folds, slow recoil.
- **EDS:** Redundant skin folds may develop in late adult life, but they are usually limited to the elbows and around the eyes (blepharochalasis), normal recoil.

Investigations

Echocardiogram	For valvular prolapse. Views of the aortic arch should also be obtained to look for aortic dilatation
DEXA scan	In patients with significantly reduced physical activity
HPE	Loose disordered dermal collagen network. Elastic fibers increased and irregular
EM	Irregular fibrils size and shape of collagen

a. Classical EDS

May deliver/be delivered preterm as a result of early rupture of fetal membranes; normal lifespan.

Mucocutaneous Manifestations

Velvety, soft, and **doughy consistency** of skin. The facies may be distinctive, with widely spaced eyes, a wide nasal bridge and epicanthic folds.

- Marked hyperextensibility of skin—but **normal recoil** (versus elastinopathies)
- Poor wound healing (**"fish mouth"** wounds)
- Widened atrophic cutaneous scars (**"cigarette paper"** scars)
- Piezogenic pedal papules
- Fragile blood vessels → hematomas and easy bruising
- **Subcutaneous spheroids** (fat lobules that have calcified after losing their blood supply)
- **Molluscoid pseudotumors** (blue gray spongy) associated with scars over knees and elbows
- Blue sclerae
- Signs:
    i. **Gorlin's sign:** Ability to touch tip of nose with tongue (50%)

ii. **Metenier sign** (easy eversion of upper eyelid)
iii. **Reverse *namaskar* sign** (described by Premlatha)—hands can be joined in *namaskar* position behind the back.

Musculoskeletal Manifestations

- Generalized joint hypermobility
- Double-jointed fingers
- Frequent subluxation of larger joints
- Chronic joint and limb pain
- Kyphoscoliosis
- Pes planus.

GI Manifestations

- Hiatal/inguinal hernia, postoperative hernias, and anal prolapse
- GI bleeding/rupture.

Cardiac Manifestations

- Mitral valve prolapse
- Aortic root dilation.

b. Hypermobile EDS

The skin is *minimally affected*

- Not prone to life-threatening complications
- Severe joint laxity, recurrent dislocations/subluxations, and chronic joint pain +/– arthritis
- Mitral valve prolapse
- Symptoms of autonomic dysfunction, including postural orthostatic tachycardia syndrome (POTS). There is a failure to respond to local anesthetics
- GI and urinary symptoms.

c. Vascular EDS

Tissues rich in type III collagen, notably arterial media, bowel and uterus are mainly affected.

- *Life-threatening risk* of blood vessel and organ rupture → sudden death in third/fourth decade (arterial or colonic rupture; maternal death may occur as a result of uterine or arterial rupture during pregnancy).
- *Cutaneous manifestations*
  - Easy bruising
  - Thin and translucent skin with visible underlying blood vessels
  - Skin is not hyperextensible, but can be fragile
  - Lack of subcutaneous fat.
- *Facial features*: Thin, pinched nose; prominent sunken eyes; thin upper lip; and lobeless ears
- Blue sclera (>90%)
- Acrogeria
- Hypermobility limited to digits

- Congenital talipes (clubfoot)
- Recurrent pneumothorax
- Arterial (including aorta) dissection, rupture, and aneurysm of medium-sized vessels
- Intracranial aneurysms associated with cerebrovascular accidents
- Obstetric complications, including uterine and arterial rupture, massive postpartum hemorrhage, and severe laceration from tearing at vaginal delivery.
- Short stature.

Treatment

An overview is given in **Table 13.2**.

TABLE 13.2: Treatment of EDS

Skin	• Avoid contact sports • Avoid sunlight • (1–4 g/day) ascorbic acid (vitamin C)—kyphoscoliosis type EDS • Wound stitch protocol to be modified
Joints	• Avoid excessive activities • Physiotherapy is aimed at increasing tone and strength
Vascular EDS	• Avoid trauma, including physical contact sports, and to avoid activities which raise intracranial pressure by the Valsalva effect • Celiprolol, long-acting β_1 antagonist is helpful

2. OSTEOGENESIS IMPERFECTA (OI)

This disorder is characterized by osteoporosis with fractures, due predominantly to type I collagen abnormalities.

Defect: Mutations in type I collagen → fragile bones (poor cortical modeling and less trabecular bone formation).

Mutations in *COL1A1* and *COL1A2* genes.

Clinical types: There are at least 8 well-defined types of OI, but types I–IV account for 90%.

Clinical features: Fractures, blue sclerae, deafness, skeletal deformity, abnormal dentine formation (dentinogenesis imperfecta), mild joint hypermobility, hernias, mitral valve prolapse, microvascular fragility leading to bruising and thin fragile skin **(Fig. 13.3** and **Table 13.3)**.

- **Type I** (most common form, AD, accounts for 50% of OI; generally mild; fractures in childhood and adolescence, but skeletal deformity is absent or nil)
- **Type II** (**most severe form**, fatal in perinatal period, crumpled humeri and femora, beaded ribs)
- **Type III** (progressive scoliosis and deforming bowing of long bones)
- **Type IV** (mild form with normal sclera)
- **Types V–XV** molecular heterogeneity, rarer types.

Prognosis

- Types I and IV: Normal life span
- Type II: Death in perinatal period
- Type III: Increased mortality in 3rd/4th decade due to respiratory failure (secondary to kyphoscoliosis) or head trauma.

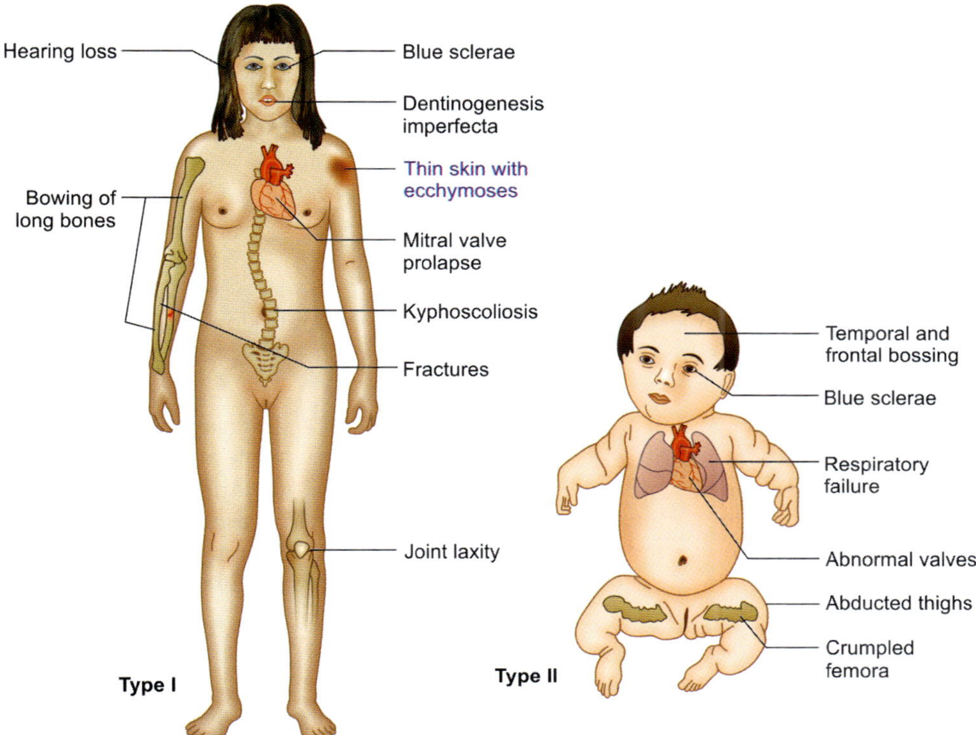

Fig. 13.3: Artistic depiction of the clinical features of osteogenesis imperfecta (text in blue depicts skin manifestations)

TABLE 13.3: Extracutaneous features of OI	
Musculoskeletal	• Hyperlaxity of ligaments and hypermobility of joints • Brittle bones + fractures (skull, long bones, and vertebrae; occurs *in utero* in severe forms) • Scoliosis • Beaded ribs • Limb deformities
Eye	• Blue sclera
Ear	• Otosclerosis with hearing loss (may begin during adolescence)
Teeth	• Fragile/discolored teeth • Dentinogenesis imperfecta (DI)
CVS	• Mitral and aortic valve prolapse/dilatation and regurgitation • Cystic medial necrosis of the aorta

Treatment

The treatment revolves around enhancing the bone mineral density. Bone mineral density (BMD) can be reduced in OI but the magnitude of increase in fracture risk is far greater than can be accounted for by low BMD, highlighting that a key mechanism of bone fragility is reduced bone quality due to defects of bone matrix and mineralization. Bisphosphonates form the mainstay of treatment. A summary of the agents is listed in **Box 13.1**.

BOX 13.1: Treatment for OI (Ralston SH)

Bisphosphonates	Pamidronate, alendronate, neridronate
Denosumab	Monoclonal antibody directed against receptor activator of nuclear factor kappa-B ligand (RANKL), a molecule that plays an essential role in osteoclast activation
Bone anabolic agents	Teriparatide
Sclerostin inhibitors	Romosozumab
Others	Gene therapy and cell therapy

3. CUTIS LAXA, HEREDITARY GENERALIZED

Cutis laxa is characterized clinically by lax pendulous skin that only slowly recoils when pulled (versus normal recoil of EDS).

Types

- AR forms **(most common)**: FBLN5, EFEMP2/FBLN4, LTBP4, ATPase, ATP6V0A2, PYCR1, and ALDH18A1; present at birth to early childhood; skin + severe internal organ involvement.
- XLR form (**occipital horn syndrome**, previously EDS IX): Mutations in ATPase, Cu^{2+}–transporting, alpha polypeptide (ATP7A) (allelic to Menkes disease).
- AD forms (less common): Elastin gene (ELN) or fibulin 5 (FBLN5) mutations → dysregulation of elastic fiber network in the skin mainly (internal involvement uncommon); presents in early adulthood.

Clinical Features

Classical clinical features are depicted in **Fig. 13.4**.

- **Typical facies:** Downward slanting palpebral fissures **(hound-dog facies)**, a broad flat nose, sagging cheeks and large ears. There are prominent skin folds around the knees, abdomen and thighs. Loose, sagging skin with reduced elasticity and recoil.
  Deep voice due to vocal cord laxity.
- **Types of cutis laxa:**
  1. **AR cutis laxa (ARCL)**
     a. ARCL type I
        - Potentially fatal involvement of **lungs** (hypoplastic lungs and emphysema)
        - Cardiovascular abnormalities (aortic tortuosity and aneurysms)
        - Inguinal/diaphragmatic/umbilical hernias
        - **GI/genitourinary diverticula**
        - Joint laxity, arachnodactyly, and fractures (variable).
     b. ARCL type II
        - This type has **prominent neurological manifestations** and structural abnormalities of brain **(De Barsy syndrome)** distinguished by developmental delay and corneal clouding due to degeneration of the tunica elastica of the cornea.
  2. **XLR cutis laxa** (now termed **occipital horn syndrome**). It is considered a less severe form of Menkes syndrome, and both conditions are caused by mutations in the *ATP7A gene*
     - Easy bruising and coarse hair (variable)
     - Tortuous arteries
     - Genitourinary diverticula
     - Inguinal, diaphragmatic and umbilical hernias

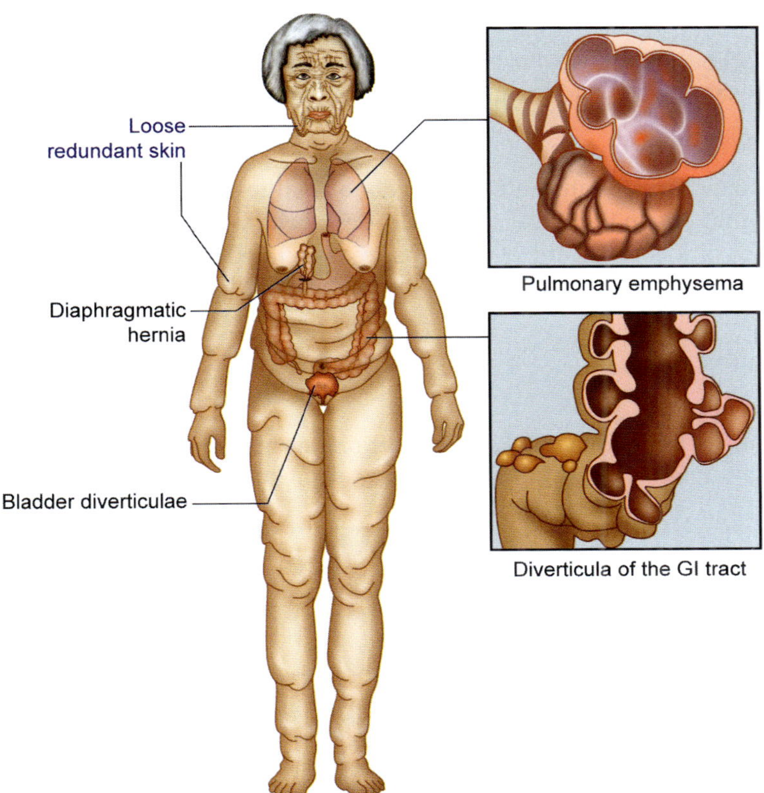

Fig. 13.4: Artistic depiction of the features of cutis laxa (text in blue depicts skin manifestations)

- Long face with high forehead and hooked nose
- **Wedge-shaped occipital calcifications (occipital horns)**
- Hip dislocations (joint laxity).

3. **AD cutis laxa:** Primarily generalized cutaneous findings, cardiac valve abnormalities, aortic dilatation (variable), emphysema (uncommon), and hernias.

Differential Diagnosis

- In **EDS**, the skin is hyperextensible but not lax, and it recoils quickly.
- In **PXE**, the skin may be lax, but it is *yellowish* and the face is usually *spared*. It is distinguished histologically by the presence of **calcification**.
- **Acquired cutis laxa:**
  - Primarily adults with sagging of skin and little associated internal involvement.
  - Cutaneous involvement may be primarily acral; generalized involvement typically begins on the face/neck.
  - May occur in association with drugs (penicillamine and isoniazid), other cutaneous disorders (e.g. cutaneous lymphoma, Sweet syndrome like eruption, interstitial granulomatous dermatitis, and cutaneous mastocytosis) or systemic disease (rheumatoid arthritis, sarcoidosis, SLE, and infectious disorders).

Investigations

Skin biopsy, echocardiogram, chest X-ray and lung function testing should be performed. Neurological examination and imaging is mandatory in autosomal recessive cutis laxa type 2.

4. MARFAN SYNDROME

Aortic dilatation, ectopia lentis and skeletal abnormalities.

Defect: AD mutations in the FBN1 gene (encodes fibrillin-1).

Fibrillin 1 is one component of the elastin-associated microfibrils which is especially important in the ciliary zonule of the eye (the suspensory ligament of the lens). It also affects the function of TGF-β.

Clinical Features

Skin

Often exceptionally *tall*, and the skeletal proportions are abnormal. The limbs are longer distally giving rise to *arachnodactyly* **(Fig. 13.5)** and they also feature elastosis perforans serpiginosa.

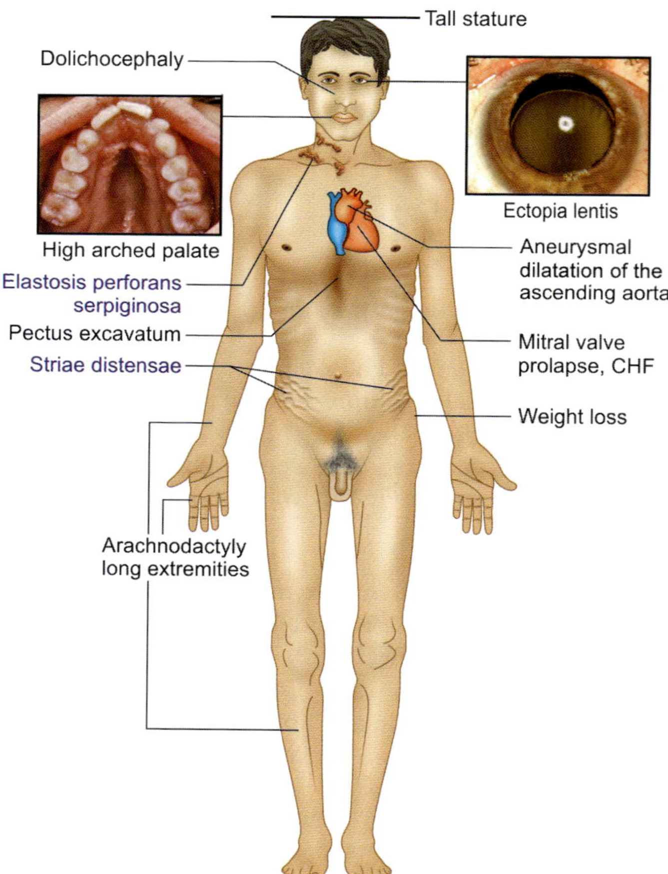

Fig. 13.5: Artistic depiction of Marfan syndrome (text in blue depicts skin manifestations)

Screening tests

"Thumb sign" (positive if the thumb, when completely opposed in the clenched hand, projects beyond the ulnar border).

"Wrist sign" (positive if the thumb and little finger overlap when wrapped around the opposite wrist). Ratio of lower segment (pubic rami to floor) to upper segment (height minus lower segments) may vary with age and sex.

Other features of Marfan syndrome are given in **Table 13.4**.

TABLE 13.4: Extracutaneous features of Marfan syndrome	
Skeletal manifestations	• Kyphoscoliosis, pectus excavatum, and dolichocephaly • Pes planus • Joint laxity, patellar dislocation, and hip dislocation
Eye	• **Ectopia lentis** (upward lens displacement; 60% of patients) • **Ocular globe elongation** leading to myopia (~40%) • Retinal detachment, cataracts, glaucoma
CVS	• Dilatation of **ascending aorta** → regurgitation, CHF, dissection/aneurysm, and rupture • **Mitral valve prolapse** • Left ventricular dilation—cardiac complications may → death
Lung	• Spontaneous pneumothorax, apical blebs, and bullous emphysema

Prognosis

Aortic dissection is the most common cause of mortality.

Treatment

The standard treatment includes prophylactic beta-blockers in order to slow down dilation of the ascending aorta, and prophylactic aortic surgery. The success of current medical and surgical treatment of aortic disease in Marfan syndrome has substantially improved mean life expectancy, extending it beyond 72 years.

Also angiotensin converting enzyme inhibitors have been used. They are used as they inhibit the circulating TGF-β. A trial showed that the addition of **Losartan** reduces aortic root dilatation and, after aortic root replacement, it reduces the dilatation rate of the aortic arch.

Surgical interventions are needed for aortic root dissection and rupture.

5. INFANTILE STIFF SKIN SYNDROMES

Hyaline fibromatosis includes both infantile systemic hyalinosis (ISH) and juvenile hyaline fibromatosis (JHF).

- This is characterized by hard stiff skin and joint contractures in the first few weeks of life.
- Allelic autosomal recessive (AR) diseases caused by mutations in ANTXR2/CMG2 (Anthraxtoxin receptor 2 gene)/(capillary morphogenesis protein-2) → abundance of hyalinized fibrous tissue in skin and internal organs.
- ISH is more severe than JHF.

Clinical Features

Cutaneous Manifestations (Fig. 13.6)

- Diffusely thickened skin and hyperpigmentation overlying bony prominences is characteristic of ISH
- Perianal nodules
- Small pearly papules on ears and face (perinasal and perioral)
- **Scalp nodules** are characteristic of JHF

Oral Manifestations

- Thickening of oral mucosa, gingival hypertrophy and marked curvature of dental roots
- Replacement of periodontal ligament by hyaline fibrous material
- Feeding difficulties.

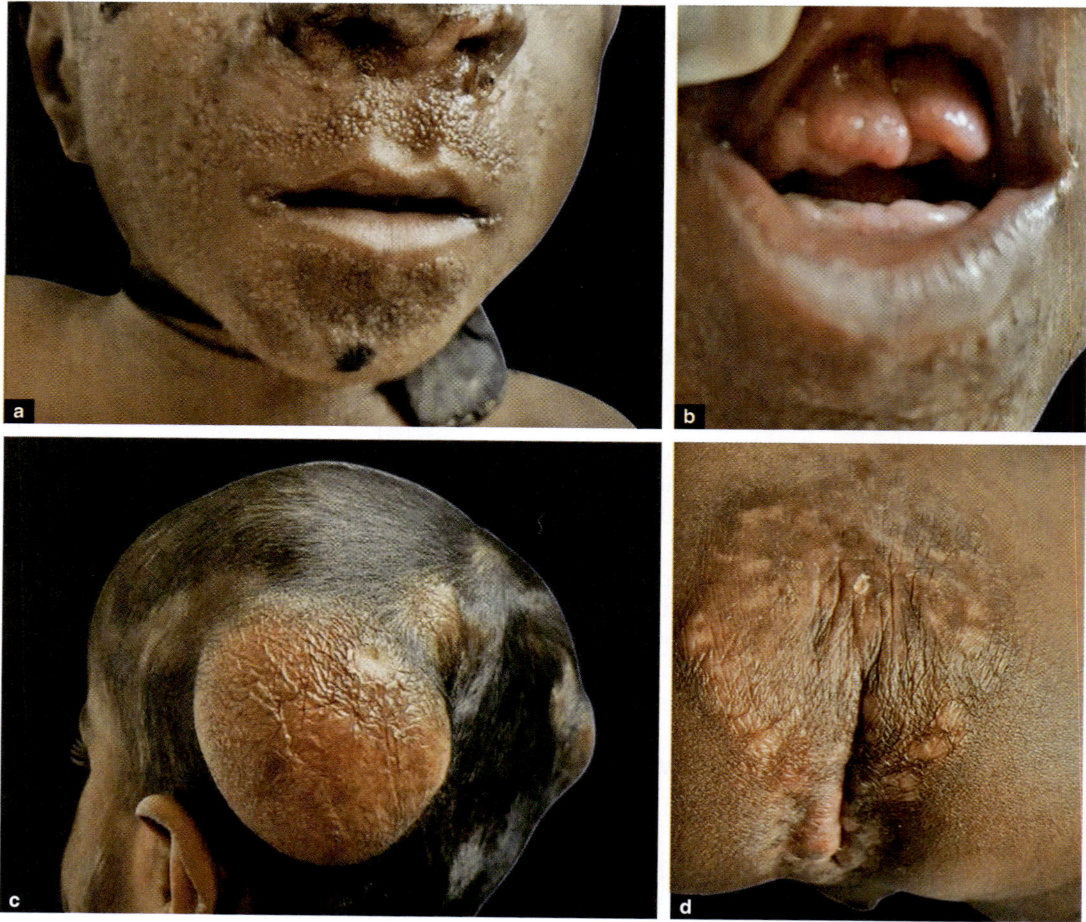

Fig. 13.6: Perioral facial papules, gingival hypertrophy, scalp nodules and vulval papules seen in a case of juvenile hyaline fibromatosis (*Courtesy*: Dr Rakhi Ghodge, Associate Professor, Goa Medical College, Bambolim, Goa)

Musculoskeletal Manifestations

- Debilitating joint contractures and tumors
- **Osteolytic bone lesions** are characteristic of JHF
- Normal intelligence.

Visceral Involvement (ISH Only)

Hyaline deposits develop in multiple internal organs with recurrent infections, malabsorption, protein-losing enteropathy, and failure to thrive.

Histology: ↑fibroblasts embedded in hyalinized connective tissue stroma that is homogeneous, amorphous, and acidophilic (PAS-positive).

Prognosis

- ISH presents within first **6 months of life** with cutaneous, mucosal, skeletal, and internal organ involvement and death in early childhood. The death is due to recurrent pulmonary infections and GI complications and occurs by 2 years usually.
- JHF presents during **early childhood** with cutaneous, mucosal, and skeletal/joint (often debilitating) involvement only; survival into adulthood is usual.

Other Syndromes

- *Stiff skin syndrome* is one of several rare syndromes causing hard stiff skin and joint contractures in early life.
- *Restrictive dermopathy* is a very rare autosomal recessive lethal laminopathy that presents at birth with a taut shiny skin restricting movement of the joints.

6. LIPOID PROTEINOSIS (HYALINOSIS CUTIS ET MUCOSAE, URBACH-WIETHE DISEASE)

AR disorder due to mutations in the **extracellular matrix protein 1 (ECM1)** gene; ↑in South Africa.

Thickening of basement membrane and deposition of hyaline material in dermis → characteristic thickening of the skin, mucous membranes, and certain viscera.

Clinical Features

Oral: Hoarse cry or weak cry from infiltrated vocal cords—first clinical sign (occurs in infancy and persists for life). Infiltration of mucosa of pharynx, soft palate, tonsils, and lips, thickened "woody" tongue; inability to protrude tongue (due to shortened frenulum).

Cutaneous lesions develop during first 2 years of life in two overlapping stages:

- **First stage: Vesicles and hemorrhagic crusts** involving the face, extremities, and oral mucosa develop in association with trauma and resolve with acneiform, **"ice-pick"** scars.
- **Second stage:** ↑Hyaline material deposition within the dermis → yellow, waxy, and coalescing papules and nodules on the face/neck and extremities; beaded eyelid papules resembling **"string of pearls"** (50%–moniliform blepharosis); verrucous nodules on elbows, knees, hands.

Respiratory difficulty associated with upper respiratory tract infections and may require tracheostomy; occasionally fatal in infancy (major cause of early death).

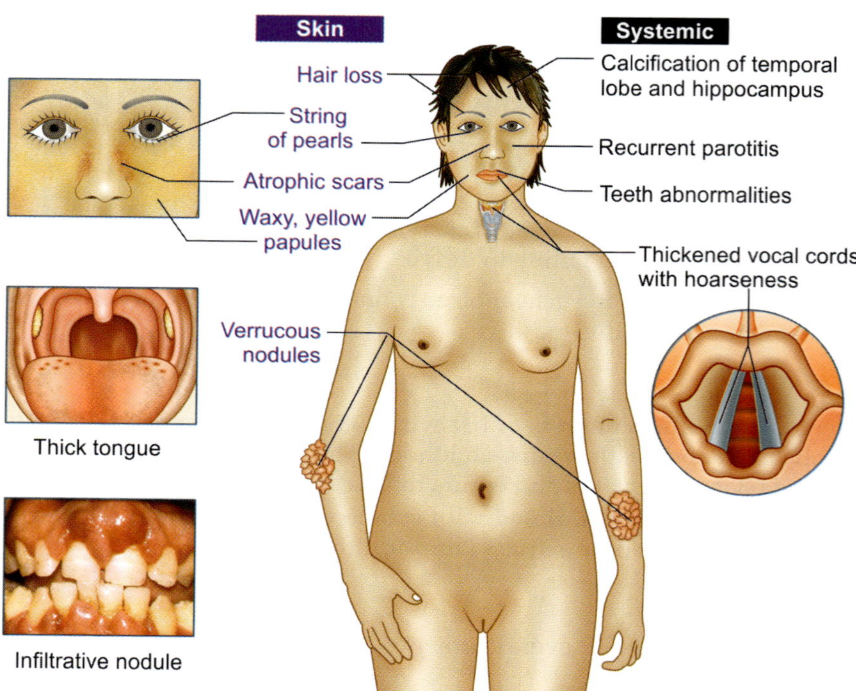

Fig. 13.7: Artistic depiction of lipoid proteinosis

Neurologic manifestations include seizures and neuropsychiatric symptoms, associated with pathognomonic **sickle or "bean-shaped" calcifications in temporal lobes or hippocampus. Fig. 13.7** shows a diagrammatic representation of the clinical features.

Investigations

- **Initial:** Dermoscopy; ophthalmoscopy+ OCT; ECG + heart ultrasound; thoracic CT; video-EEG; abdominal + pelvic ultrasonography; brain MRI/MRA; IQ testing.
- **Genetic testing:** ECM1 gene.

Histology

Deposition of amorphous or laminated basement membrane-like material containing collagen (types II and IV) and laminin around blood vessels, dermal-epidermal junction, adnexal epithelia, and in connective tissues (appears as vertically oriented pink dermal deposits).

Deposits are PAS (+) and diastase-resistant.

Differential Diagnosis

- **Erythropoietic protoporphyria** causes waxy papules and depressed scars but the scars are confined to sun-exposed skin.
- Xanthomatosis and amyloidosis are also excluded by the histological appearances.
- In adults, other differential diagnoses include lichen myxedematosus and myxedema with hoarseness.

7. PSEUDOXANTHOMA ELASTICUM

Ectopic mineralization disorders are due to gene defects and include pseudoxanthoma elasticum (PXE), generalized arterial calcification of infancy (GACI), and arterial calcification due to deficiency of CD73 (ACDC). We will focus on PXE.

Defect: AR disorder as a result of mutations in **ABCC6** (ATP-binding cassette, subfamily C, member 6) gene leading to mineralization of the elastic tissue of the eyes, skin, and arteries.

Leads to reduced levels of inorganic pyrophosphate (PPi) in plasma. Because PPi is a powerful anti-mineralization factor, it has been postulated that reduced PPi is a major determinant for ectopic mineralization in these conditions.

Clinical Features

Cutaneous Manifestations

- Thin, **yellowish papules** in flexural areas arise during first or second decade of life:
  - Typically first appear on the lateral aspects of the neck.
  - Antecubital and popliteal fossae, wrists, axillae, groin, and periumbilical area (in multiparous women) are involved.
  - Papules coalesce to form cobblestone-like plaques resembling **"plucked chicken skin"** or **"Moroccan leather" (Fig. 13.8)**.

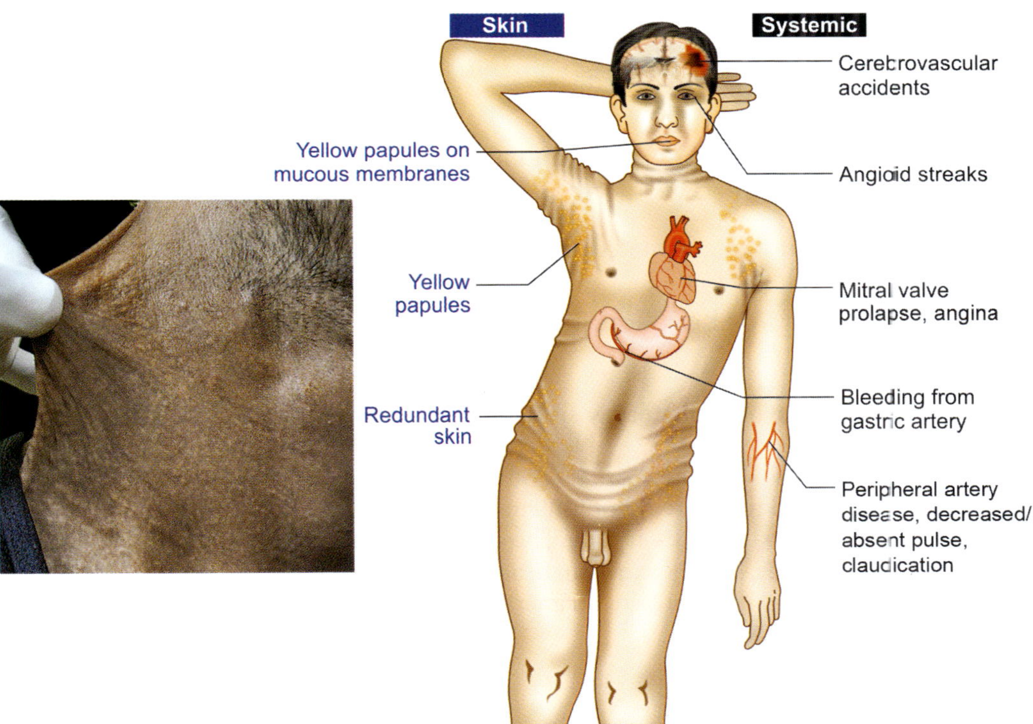

Fig. 13.8: Artistic depiction of PXE and the typical cobblestone-like plaques resembling "plucked chicken skin"

- **Loss of recoil** and **sagging skin** in axillae and groin
- Yellow papules (resembling Fordyce spots) may develop in oral/anogenital mucosa
- Perforating PXE: In advanced disease, ↑dermal calcium deposition and extrusion of this yellowish material through the epidermis may occur (transepidermal elimination).
- An exaggerated mental (chin) crease is highly sensitive and specific for PXE in age <30 years.

Ocular Manifestations

- Asymptomatic angioid streaks **(Bruch's membrane rupture)** usually in first decade. Angioid streaks are also seen in Paget's disease of bone, sickle cell anemia, thalassemia, EDS, lead poisoning, and age-related degeneration.
- Macular degeneration, optic drusen, and retinal hemorrhage (blindness).
- **Mottling of retinal pigment epithelium.** This is the most prevalent ophthalmologic finding; may precede development of angioid streaks.
- **"Owl's eyes":** Paired areas of hyperpigmented spots straddling an angioid streak.

Cardiovascular Manifestations

- Intermittent claudication, loss of peripheral pulses, renovascular hypertension, mitral valve prolapse, angina/myocardial infarction, and stroke.
- Progressive calcification of elastic media and intima → atheromatous plaques involving predominantly medium-sized arteries (especially in extremities).

GI Manifestations

Gastric artery hemorrhage, hematemesis, epistaxis.

Obstetric Complications

Increase risk of first trimester miscarriage and maternal cardiovascular complications.

Histopathology

Distorted, basophilic, and fragmented calcified elastic fibers in mid/deep reticular dermis.

Special stains for PXE

- VVG (elastin) and
- Von Kossa (calcium)

Differential Diagnosis

- The disseminated form of **dermatofibrosis lenticularis** (Buschke–Ollendorff) can be clinically similar.
- **Papular elastorrhexis** is an uncommon acquired disorder of elastic fibers that presents as multiple, whitish or skin colored, nonfollicular papules, with symmetrical distribution on the trunk and upper extremities and may be confused with PXE.
- If laxity of the involved skin is extreme, **other forms of cutis laxa** must be excluded. The diagnosis can be difficult in the presence of marked solar elastosis and/or macular degeneration.

Investigations

- **Calcium and phosphate levels.**
- **HPE** of PXE are often distinctive (site—from the side of the neck)
- **Radiologically**—soft tissue or vascular calcification
- Baseline **echocardiogram**

- If a GGCX gene deficiency—vitamin K and clotting factors
- **Molecular analysis** of the ABCC6 gene—definitive diagnosis.

Prognosis

Morbidity and mortality secondary to GI hemorrhage, cerebral hemorrhage, atherosclerotic disease, and myocardial infarction.

Treatment

Flowchart 13.1 depicts the treatment of PXE.

Flowchart 13.1: Treatment of PXE

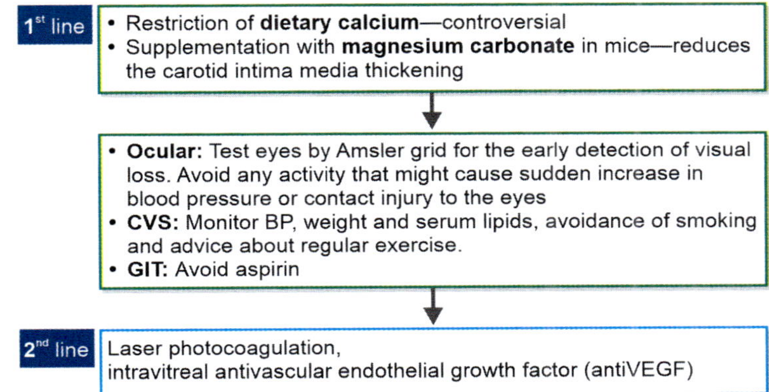

8. FOCAL DERMAL HYPOPLASIA (GOLTZ SYNDROME, GOLTZ-GORLIN SYNDROME)

Inheritance: X-linked dominant (XLD) disorder due to mutations in the PORCN (porcupine) gene (regulator of Wnt signaling proteins, which are critical for embryonic development of skin, bone, teeth, and other structures). In Rook's textbook, the disorders is listed under **ectodermal dysplasias**.

Majority of patients are heterozygous females (90%); lethal in males.

Clinical Features

FOCAL has been suggested as an "acronym" that incorporates the key clinical features of this disorder:

- **F**emale, XLD
- **C**olobomas
- **L**obster claw deformity.
- **O**steopathia striata
- **A**plasia of ectodermal elements

Cutaneous Manifestations (Fig. 13.9)

- Widely distributed **linear/blaschkoid** areas of **hypoplasia/atrophy** (cribriform atrophic lesions) of **the skin, with telangiectasia**.
- Soft, yellow to reddish nodular outpouchings caused by herniation of subcutaneous fat through thinned dermis.
- Dysmorphic facies (notched nasal ala and malformed ears)
- Large cutaneous ulcers (from a congenital absence of skin) that heal with atrophic scarring
- Streaky hyper- and/or hypopigmentation.
- Red ("raspberry-like") papillomas; favors lips, anogenital region, larynx and acral skin.

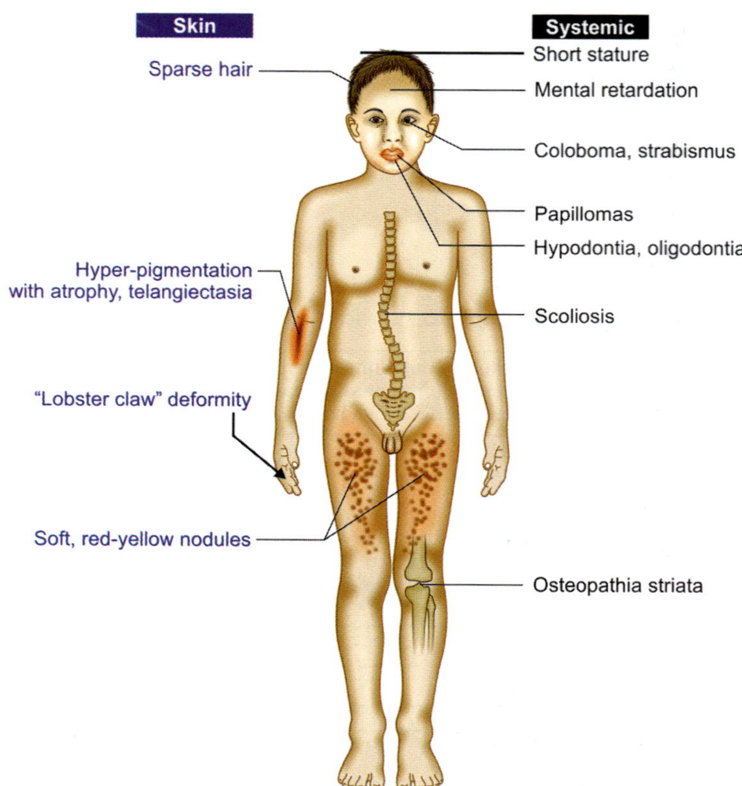

Fig. 13.9: Artistic depiction of Goltz syndrome

- Hair is thin or absent.
- Dystrophic or completely absent nails.

Differential diagnosis: Focal facial dermal dysplasia types 1–4 and MIDAS syndrome.

Systemic Features (Table 13.5)

TABLE 13.5: Extracutaneous features of Goltz syndrome

Skeletal manifestations	• Oligodactyly, syndactyly, ectrodactyly **(Lobster claw deformity)**, and polydactyly • Microcrania, asymmetric development of skull, pointed mandible, and deviated nasal septum • Scoliosis, kyphosis, spina bifida occulta, rudimentary tail, and fusion of vertebral bodies • Osteopathia striata: Vertical striations in long bone metaphyses on X-ray
Ophthalmologic manifestations (40%)	• Colobomas of iris/choroid/retina/optic disc • Strabismus • Anophthalmia, microphthalmia, and incomplete development of the retina and optic nerve • Hypopigmented/hyperpigmented retina, cloudy vitreous, and subluxation of lens
Dental manifestations	• Underdeveloped, dysplastic, or absent teeth • Delayed eruption of primary dentition • Notched incisors • **Linear enamel hypoplasia** • Severe malocclusion if mandible is malformed

ICHTHYOSIS

The term 'ichthyosis' was first introduced more than 200 years ago by Robert Willan. It is derived from the Greek word *ichthys*, which means fish.

The majority of keratinization disorders are now referred to as Mendelian disorders of cornification (MeDOC). Thus, ichthyoses are known as **MeDOCs ichthyoses**. In the Ichthyosis Consensus Conference (in Sorèze, 2009), it was decided not to make a distinction between the group of erythrokeratodermas and ichthyoses, but to group them together.

CLASSIFICATION

Ichthyosis results in abnormal differentiation and/or abnormal desquamation showing impaired corneocyte shedding (retention hyperkeratosis) or accelerated keratinocyte production (epidermal hyperplasia/hyperproliferative hyperkeratosis). The development of hyperkeratosis in these diseases may be understood as a homeostatic repair response aimed at compensating for an abnormal epidermal barrier.

The classification that is now followed is given in **Table 13.6** where two types are described—**syndromic** and **nonsyndromic**.

TABLE 13.6: Clinical classification of inherited ichthyosis: Nonsyndromic and syndromic forms

Nonsyndromic	
Common ichthyoses	• Ichthyosis vulgaris (IV)* • Non-syndromic recessive X-linked ichthyosis (RXLI)*
Autosomal recessive congenital ichthyosis (ARCI)	• Harlequin ichthyosis (HI) • Lamellar ichthyosis (LI)* • Congenital ichthyosiform erythroderma (CIE)* • Self-healing collodion baby (SHCB) • Acral self-healing collodion baby • Bathing suit ichthyosis (BSI)
Keratinopathic ichthyosis (KPI)	• Epidermolytic ichthyosis* (EI) • Superficial epidermolytic ichthyosis (SEI) • Congenital reticular ichthyosiform erythroderma (CRIE) • Annular epidermolytic ichthyosis (AEI) • Ichthyosis Curth–Macklin (ICM) • Autosomal recessive epidermolytic ichthyosis (AREI) • Epidermolytic naevi
Others	• Loricrin keratoderma (LK) • Erythrokeratodermia variabilis (EKV) • Inflammatory peeling skin disease (PSS type B) • Exfoliative ichthyosis (*PPK, aggravated by sweating, generalised moulting*) • Keratosis linearis-ichthyosis congenita and sclerosing keratoderma (KLICK) (*keratotic papules, linearly arranged on flexures*)

(*Contd.*)

TABLE 13.6: Clinical classification of inherited ichthyosis: Nonsyndromic and syndromic forms *(Contd.)*	
Syndromic	
X-linked ichthyosis syndromes	• Recessive X-linked ichthyosis (RXLI) • Ichthyosis follicularis, alopecia and photophobia (IFAP) • Conradi-Hünermann-Happle syndrome (CDPX2) • Congenital hemidysplasia with ichthyosiform erythroderma and limb defects **(CHILD)** syndrome
Autosomal syndromes with prominent hair abnormalities (AR)	• Netherton syndrome (NS) • Severe dermatitis, multiple allergies, metabolic wasting (SAM) • Ichthyosis with hypotrichosis • Neonatal ichthyosis-sclerosing cholangitis (NISCH) • Trichothiodystrophy • Sabinas brittle hair syndrome
Autosomal syndromes with prominent CNS defects (AR)	• Refsum syndrome (HMSN4) • Gaucher syndrome type 2 • Sjögren–Larsson syndrome (SLS) • Neutral lipid storage disease (NLSD) with ichthyosis • CHIME syndrome
Syndromes with prominent deafness	• Keratitis-ichthyosis-deafness (KID) (AD) • Mental retardation, enteropathy, deafness, neuropathy, ichthyosis, keratodermia (MEDNIK) (AR)
Ichthyosis syndromes with transient neonatal respiratory distress (AR)	• Ichthyosis-prematurity syndrome (IPS)
Autosomal recessive ichthyosis syndromes with fatal disease course	• Gaucher syndrome type 2 • Multiple sulfatase deficiency • Cerebral dysgenesis, neuropathy, ichthyosis, palmoplantar and keratoderma (CEDNIK) syndrome • Arthrogryposis-renal dysfunction-cholestasis (ARC) syndrome

*Commonly seen

Principles of Treatment

An overview of the treatment options is listed in **Table 13.7**. Oral retinoids may be considered in addition to topical therapy when topical therapy is insufficient to reduce the scaling or hyperkeratosis. The efficacy of acitretin in children is documented in a few small case series of various disorders of keratinization, essentially in LI, congenital ichthyosiform erythroderma or HI. It is recommended to reserve retinoids for those with a severe phenotype and functional impairment. As acitretin is the most common systemic agent used, an overview of its use is given in **Box 13.1**. No significant skeletal toxicity in children has been noted between ages of 6 months to 16 years and 6 monthly skeletal scans can be performed. Isotretinoin is not preferred in ichthyosis due to the skeletal toxicity, which in contrast to acitretin, is clearly reported for isotretinoin. To avoid longterm side effects of acitretin, **alitretinoin** may provide a safer alternative, as evidenced by a study where alitretinoin 10–30 mg once daily, increasing to a maximum of 40–60 mg daily, was found to be effective in treating patients with lamellar ichthyosis (LI). While the various treatments are listed below, the **basic principles** for care are as follows:

TABLE 13.7: Topical therapy of ichthyosis*

Agent	Concentration (%)	Comment
Emollients	Petrolatum occlusive	• Several times a day (at least twice) and ideally after bathing • Urea is not recommended on inflamed skin, flexural areas or erosions
	• Propylene glycol (<20%) • Dexpanthenol (5–10%) • Glycerol (i.e. glycerin)	Moisturizer effect
Keratolytics	Urea (20%–40%)	• Localized areas of thick scale or hyperkeratosis • Application on the face, flexures and areas of fissuring is not recommended • Urea (≥10%) is not recommended before the age of 1 year
	Lactic acid (5–12%)	Alternative to urea. Commercial preparations are often optimized by buffering
	Propylene glycol (15–20%)	Moisturizer and keratolytic
Retinoids	Tazarotene Adapalene	In CIE, severe X-linked recessive ichthyosis
Other agents	Calcipotriol N-Acetylcysteine	High-risk of systemic absorption, treat less than 10% of body surface
Targeted topical therapy	Topical cholesterol with a topical statin to reverse the ichthyotic phenotype	CHILD syndrome
Bathing	• Bathing once or twice a day with mild soap is recommended • Additives and mechanical removal of scales may be used	• Moisturizing additives, colloidal preparations, baking soda (3–6 g L) or saltwater baths (normal saline 0.9%) • Routine use of antiseptics is not recommended. If recurrent infections, they can be used 2–3 times a week in KID syndrome or Netherton syndrome [chlorhexidine-dilution 5 parts in 1000–10 000; 0.1%, potassium permanganate-dilution 1 part in 10000; diluted bleach baths (0.005% solution)]
Scalp	Foams, solutions and shampoos are cosmetically more acceptable	Application of emollient or keratolytic (washable preparation) before shampooing and gentle removal of scales
Palmoplantar keratoderma	Keratolytics in ointment formulations (salicylic acid up to 25% or urea up to 40%)	• Once or twice daily after protection of fissures and surrounding skin (using petroleum jelly) • Mild case respond to tazarotene gel

*Management of congenital ichthyoses: European guidelines of care, part one. Br J Dermatol. 2019 Feb;180(2):272–281.

Ichthyosis with Prominent Erythroderma

- No keratolytics
- Oral retinoids may be used but with caution and at a low dosage. Alitretinoin may reduce erythema.

Ichthyosis with Prominent and Severe Scales

- Keratolytics
- Oral retinoids

Box 13.2 depicts acitretin use in ichthyosis.

BOX 13.2: Acitretin in ichthyosis*

Actions	↓Hyperkeratosis, improvement of hypohidrosis, hair regrowth, improvement of ectropion and eclabium, improvement of hearing and shortening of the daily time spent on skin care Retinoids have been used successfully in most ichthyosis with the exception of autosomal dominant ichthyosis vulgaris.
Indications	• Ichthyosis with thick scales, i.e. LI and HI • Milder forms such as severe X-linked recessive ichthyosis • In EI the results are much better for patients with KRT10 mutations than those with KRT1 mutations
Dose	• 10–75 mg • Start at a low dose (i.e. 10 mg for adults) once daily or every second day • 0.5 mg/kg ideal dose • 1 mg/kg in Lamellar ichthyosis • **Avoid** in marked erythroderma **(EI and NS)** • After optimal effect taper down to optimal dose • Stop therapy in hot and humid months • Effect does not last on stopping the drug
How to administer in children	Light sensitive, capsules should be opened away from daylight or added to breast milk in a bottle protected by aluminium foil.

*Risk-benefit analysis of acitretin shows it to be favorable, even though potential adverse effects may be problematic; (Management of congenital ichthyoses: European guidelines of care, part one. Br J Dermatol. 2019 Feb;180 (2):272–281).

Complications

There are numerous complications that can be seen in ichthyosis and a summary of these with their management is given in **Table 13.8**.

TABLE 13.8: Common complications and their management

Eye complications	Ocular lubrication Regular and long term ocular lubrication with preservative-free topical medication if lagophtalmos (from once daily to half-hourly) *Ectropion* • Emollients and massage of the eyelid • Other topical agents (urea or N-acetylcysteine or topical tazarotene) applied on the eyelid may be helpful • Oral retinoids: Second line therapy in case of moderate to severe ectropion help to reduce moderate to severe ectropion and prevent worsening • Eyelid skin grafting: Third line therapy, may only be considered when symptomatic corneal exposure or epiphora persists despite adequate conservative treatments

(Contd.)

TABLE 13.8: Common complications and their management *(Contd.)*	
Ear complications	• Removal of ear wax/cerumen by using ear drops, oil and mechanical techniques once to four times a year • External otitis: Cleansing and debridement measures with use of antibiotic drops
Pruritus	• Local skin care • Antihistamines, oral retinoids
Cutaneous infections	• Treatment of bacterial superinfections • Treatment of dermatophyte infection • Scabies treatment
Vitamin D	Estimate 25-hydoxyvitamin D in all forms, yearly or twice yearly if risk factors • In case of severe deficiency, check parathyroid hormone, calcium, phosphorus, bone mineral density and X-rays (if skeletal symptoms) • Supplementation methods follow the general recommendations for adults and children
Reactions to hot or cold atmospheres	Topical therapy may help to reduce the hyperkeratotic plugging of sweat glands

NONSYNDROMIC VARIANTS

1. Ichthyosis Vulgaris

Gene: FLG, **autosomal semidominant**

The number of FLG mutations dictate the clinical features. If there are two mutations the clinical features are marked.

Onset: Infancy/childhood **(Fig. 13.10a)**.

Clinical

- Fine, **light gray, adherent** scales on extremities and trunk with **sparing of flexures** and abdomen (cf RXLI)
- Larger scale on lower legs.
- Groin and larger flexures are always spared.
- Decrease in summers due to seasonal variation and increased humidity.
- **Hyperlinear palms/soles** and furrowed heels.
- Keratosis pilaris; atopic diathesis, hypohidrosis.

Histopathology: Diminished/absent **stratum granulosum** with overlying **orthohyperkeratosis**.

Immunostaining: Absent/reduced filaggrin.

Treatment

- Creams containing glycerol.
- If there is no feature of AD, urea containing creams (up to 10%) or creams containing lactic acid (up to 12%) also work well.
- Also *see* **Table 13.7** for details of various therapeutic modalities.

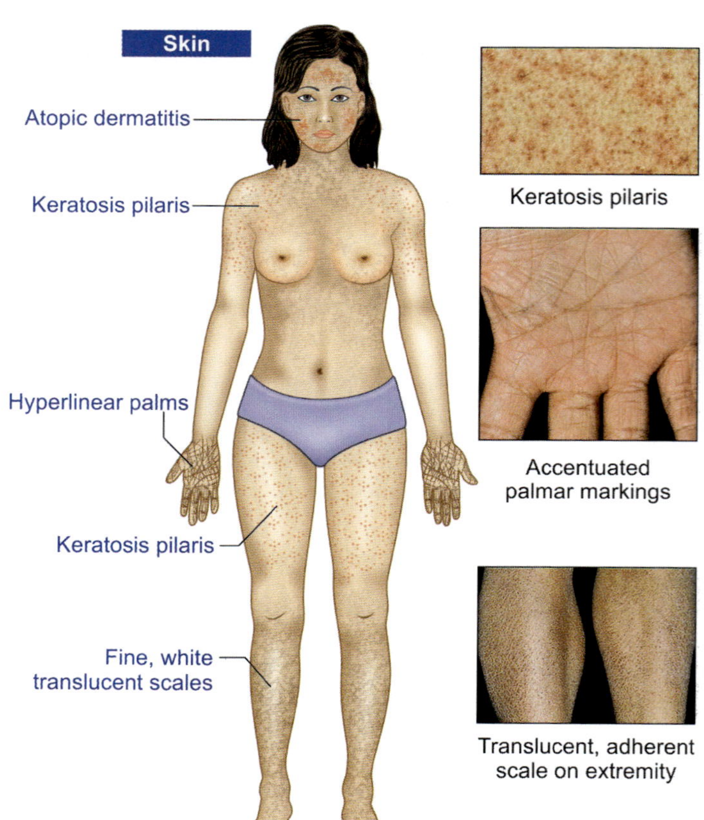

Fig. 13.10a: Artistic depiction of ichthyosis vulgaris

2. X-linked Recessive Ichthyosis (Steroid Sulfatase Deficiency)

Gene: STS, increased severity with FLG mutation. Retention HK but paradoxical increase in TEWL.

Inheritance: XLR, contiguous ANOS1 gene deletion may be seen in **Kallmann syndrome** (hypogonadism + anosmia).

Clinical Features

Onset: Infancy (2–6 months).

- Fine to large, **dark/brown, adherent scales** on extremities, trunk (abdomen involved) neck, and lateral face **(Figs 13.10b** and **c)**
- **Dirty look** of neck and back
- Spares flexures, palms, soles, and face
- Corneal comma-shaped opacities; **cryptorchidism** (20%); ↑risk of testicular cancer, and hypogonadism
- Attention deficit hyperactivity syndrome (ADHD) in up to 40% or autism in around 25%.

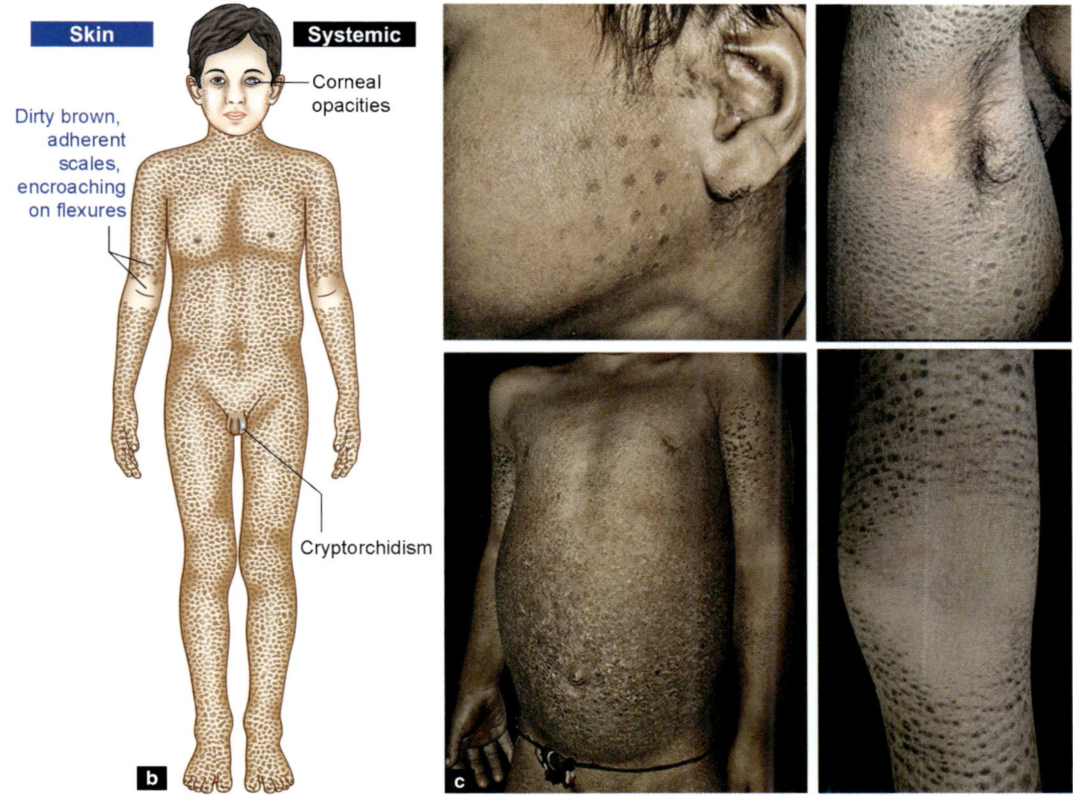

Figs 13.10b and c: (b) A depiction of XLRI; (c) XLRI-dark brown scales with sparing of flexures with a characteristic preauricular involvement

- Female carriers: **Corneal opacities**; ***prolonged labor with affected child*** (due to placental sulfatase deficiency)
- Other associations: X-linked chondrodysplasia punctata, ocular albinism, intellectual disability, and short stature.

Histopathology

Retained corneodesmosomes within stratum corneum

Reason: ↑Cholesterol sulfate → inhibits proteases (kallikrein 5, 7) required for normal degradation of corneodesmosomes.

Investigations

- Lipoprotein electrophoresis (↑mobility of α-fraction); plasma cholesterol sulfate increased
- Decreased steroid sulfatase activity in leukocytes
- FISH, array CGH, genetic testing
- Maternal carriers may have abnormal triple/quad screen during affected pregnancy with decreased serum estriol.
- Electron microscopy: Increased size and number of keratohyalin granules.

Treatment

- Treatment with moisturizers does not normalize the transepidermal water loss but rather tends to further increase it, but the skin dryness does improve.
- Oral retinoids for winter flares.

3. Autosomal Recessive Congenital Ichthyosis

Autosomal recessive congenital ichthyosis (ARCI) is an umbrella term associated with mutations in a number of genes which code for multiple proteins involved in lipid transport, such as ABCA12 and CERS3 involved in fatty acid metabolism and have a role in assembling suprastructures such as the cornified envelope.

a. *Collodion Baby*

Most ARCI manifest as a **collodion baby (Fig. 13.11)**. In this the neonate is encased in a shiny parchment-like membrane which cracks within a few days after birth. The various ichthyoses that can present with a collodion baby are listed in **Box 13.3**.

- Parchment-like membrane covering the body surface
- It peels off within the first 4 weeks of life.
- In around **80% of cases**, collodion baby is followed by the onset of an ARCI subtype
- The various morphological types that develop include BSI, LI or CIE (in 80%).
- Around 10–20% of cases develop self-healing collodion baby (SHCB) or self-improving congenital ichthyosis (SICI).

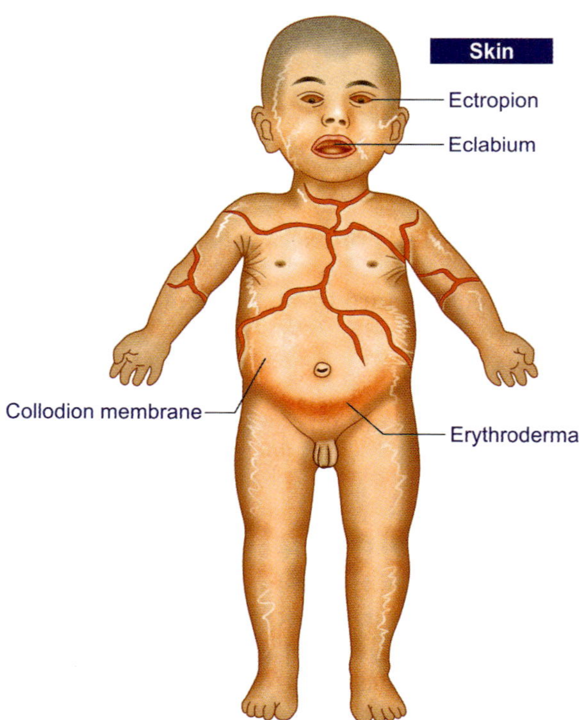

Fig. 13.11: Artistic depiction of collodion baby

BOX 13.3: Ichthyoses that can present with collodion membranes at birth*

- Lamellar ichthyosis (LI)
- Congenital ichthyosiform erythroderma (CIE)
- Self-improving collodion ichthyosis (SICI)
- Bathing suit ichthyosis (BSI)
- Recessive X-linked ichthyosis (RXLI)
- Neutral lipid storage disease with ichthyosis
- Trichothiodystrophy with ichthyosis
- Conradi-Hünermann-Happle syndrome
- Loricrin keratoderma (very mild)
- Arthrogryposis-renal dysfunction-cholestasis (ARC) syndrome
- Ichthyosis with confetti
- KLICK syndrome
- Holocarboxylase synthetase deficiency
- Gaucher disease type 2
- Congenital hypothyroidism

*Management of congenital ichthyoses: European guidelines of care, part two. Br J Dermatol. 2019 Mar;180 (3):484–495.

Shedding of the collodion membrane is followed by the development of large dark grey/brownish scales affecting *the trunk and the scalp*, usually sparing the face and extremities. *Hyperkeratoses can develop in the ear canal* affecting the ability to hear.

BSI (a temperature dependent ichthyosis)—mutation in TGM1, patients benefit from temperature <31°C.

b. *Lamellar Ichthyosis (LI) and Congenital Ichthyosiform Erythroderma (CIE)*

LI was named by Frost. These two disorders are mediated by a series of genes with a clinical spectrum ranging from LI to CIE.

Gene defects and phenotypes

- **TGM1:** Critically contributes to the assembly of the cornified envelope
- **ABCA12**
- CYP4F2: Manifests as CIE
- CERS3: Forms ceramide—manifest as CIE often with improvement of the ichthyosis phenotype in the summer time
- LIPN: Late onset around 5 years
- ALOXE3
- ALOX12B: PPK
- NIPAL4 (ichthyin) CIE/LI overlapping phenotype
- PNPLA1.

Clinical Features

LI: After collodion membrane peels, there occur large, thick, plate-like brown scales in generalized distribution with significant flexural involvement and variable palm/sole involvement (PPK) **(Fig. 13.12)**.

There are various genotypes which determine the varied phenotypic expression and are listed in **Box 13.4**.

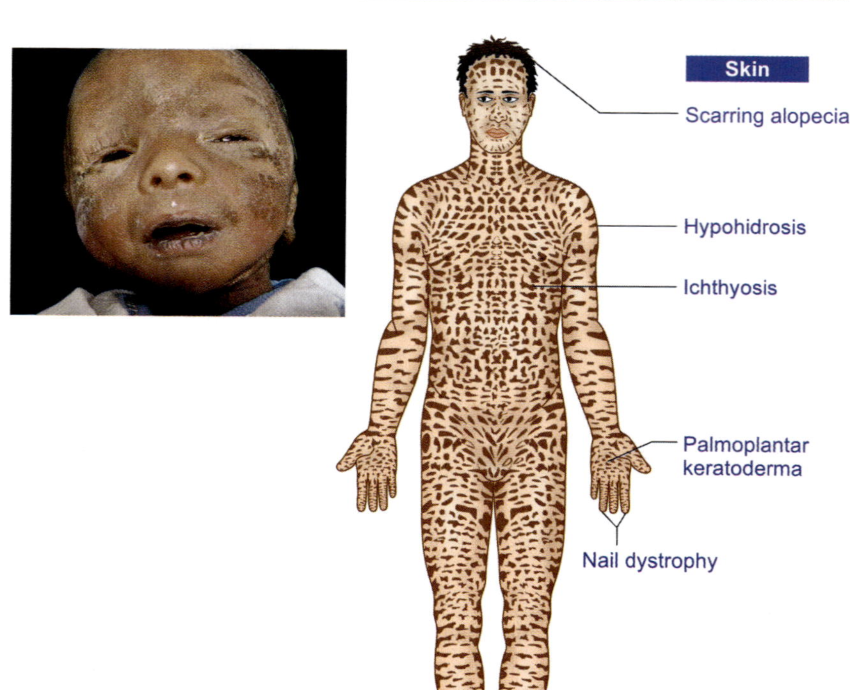

Fig. 13.12: Artistic depiction of lamellar ichthyosis. The image shows an infant with collodion baby which may be followed by LI phenotype (Note the thick scales and ectropion)

BOX 13.4: Phenotype genotype correlation

Neonates	Premature birth	ABCA12, SLC27A4
	Absent retroauricular fold	ABCA12
	Anteriorly overfolded ear	ALOX12B
	Eclabium/ectropion at birth	TGM1, ABCA12
Older children	Moderate-to-severe erythema on body	ABCA12, NIPAL4
	Larger plates of scale on lower body	TGM1
	Ectropion persisting, hair loss	TGM1, ABCA12
	Favorable retinoid usage	TGM1, ABCA12, NIPAL4
	Self-improving phenotype	TGM1, ALOX12B, SLC27A4

*Genotype–phenotype correlation in a large English cohort of patients with autosomal recessive ichthyosis. Br J Dermatol. 2020 Mar; 182 (3):729–737.

- *Heat intolerance* (hypernatremic dehydration); frequent scarring alopecia; dystrophic nails
- Hypohidrosis

CIE: After collodion membrane peels, **fine white scales** in generalized distribution (*flexures involved*); erythroderma; variable palm/sole involvement is seen in **Fig. 13.13**.

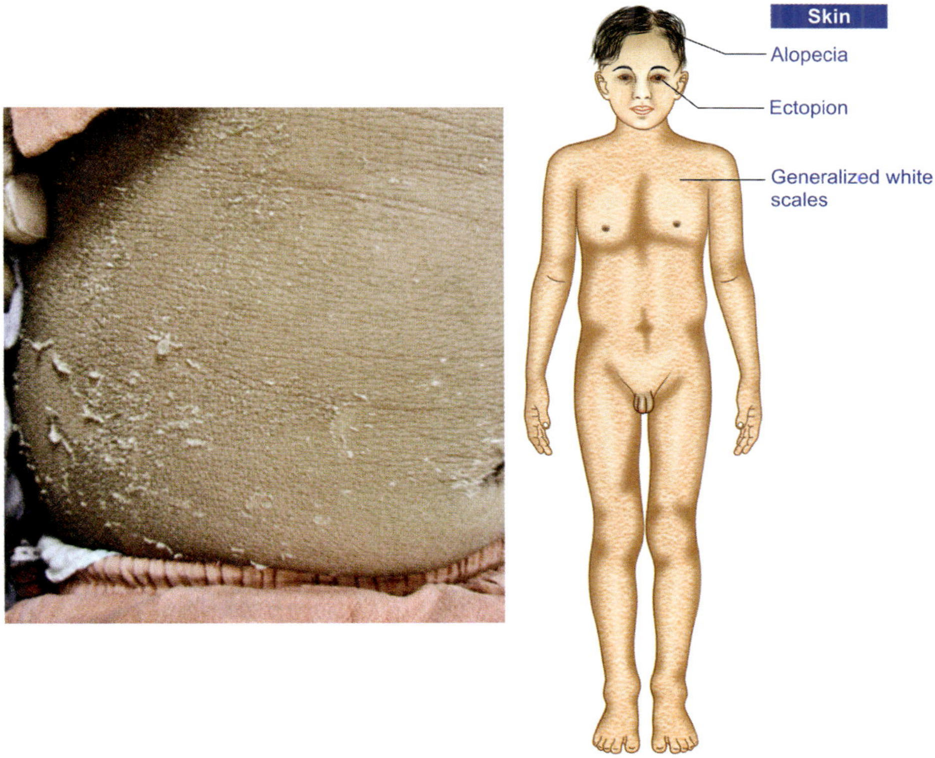

Skin
Alopecia
Ectopion
Generalized white scales

Fig. 13.13: Congenital ichthyosiform erythroderma (CIE). The image on the left shows diffuse fine scaling involving the whole body

Histopathology

Depends on the gene defect.

TGM1: Thin cornified envelope and disorganized lamellar bilayers.

ABCA12: Absence of lamellar body content.

NIPAL4: Defective lamellar bodies and perinuclear membranes within stratum granulosum.

Treatment

There is an emergent need for special care in the neonatal period in collodion baby, neonates with HI, congenital ichthyosiform erythroderma, NS, EI and ichthyosis prematurity syndrome (IPS). The problems include transepidermal water loss (TEWL), infections, electrolyte imbalance, disrupted thermoregulation and/or metabolic wasting and respiratory distress **(Table 13.9)**.

As long as no targeted therapy is available for patients, most treatments have the goal of reducing scaling, but this will enhance the barrier defect to some degree. Transepidermal water loss increases after successful treatment of ARCI with either systemic retinoids or topical keratolytics:

- Add sodium bicarbonate to bath (two handfuls of baking soda to a bathtub)
- Topical agents **(Table 13.7)**
- Systemic treatment **(Box 13.1)**

Retinoids may be useful in case of mutations with TGM1, ABCA12, NIPAL4 genes.

TABLE 13.9: Care of collodion baby (CB) and harlequin ichthyosis (HI) in the neonatal period	
Incubator	• Highly humidified incubator (>60%), ↓ every 3–4 days to reach normal conditions (↑ humidity causes *Pseudomonas* or fungal infections—candidiasis.) • Monitoring of body temperature, weight, water and electrolyte balance
Nutritional support	Regular assessment and caloric supplementation, oro or nasogastric tube feeding if necessary
Topical therapy	• Bathing f/b emollient 3–8 times a day, avoid other topical medication • Antiseptics (chlorhexidine 0.05%) may be used in erosive lesions and antifungal cream in macerated areas • The application technique should avoid contamination (latex-free gloves, single-use packets) • Monitoring, standard precautions, regular bacteriological samplings. • No prophylactic antibiotic treatment for CB, it may be an option in HI (AVOID—urea, lactic acid or silver sulfadiazine, salicylic acid)
Ear	Removal of ear scales
Constriction bands	• Massages as preventative measure • Simple emollient or 10% urea in limited areas, tazarotene 0.1% • Surgery if ischemia, oral retinoids to be considered
Retinoids	May be used in HI, NOT in CB

4. Keratinopathic Ichthyosis

The term 'keratinopathic' was coined at the Sorèze Consensus Conference as an umbrella term for all types of ichthyoses which are caused by mutations in one of the keratin genes.

- Epidermolytic ichthyosis (bullous CIE)—AD; KRT1/KRT10)
- Superficial epidermolytic ichthyosis—AD; KRT2

Gene defect: KRT1 and KRT10 (palms and soles spared)

KRT1 has severe involvement of the palms and soles—**avoid** retinoids.

AD: May have somatic mosaicism with extensive epidermal nevi **(ichthyosis hystrix)**; if it is gonadal mosaicism, then may have offspring with full blown disease.

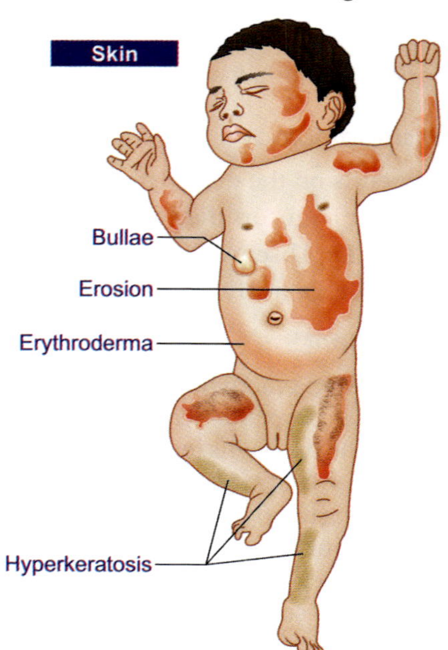

Fig. 13.14: Epidermolytic ichthyosis ("Burnt child" appearance at birth)

Clinical Features

- Birth: Erythroderma, blistering, and erosions **(Burnt child appearance) (Fig. 13.14)**.
  Later: Hyperkeratosis develops instead of blistering, with cobblestone pattern (most prominent over joints) with pronounced ridging of the flexures **(Fig. 13.15)** (the severe involvement correlates with skin regions where the body temperature is somewhat elevated and thus this aggravation may be induced by differences in body temperature).

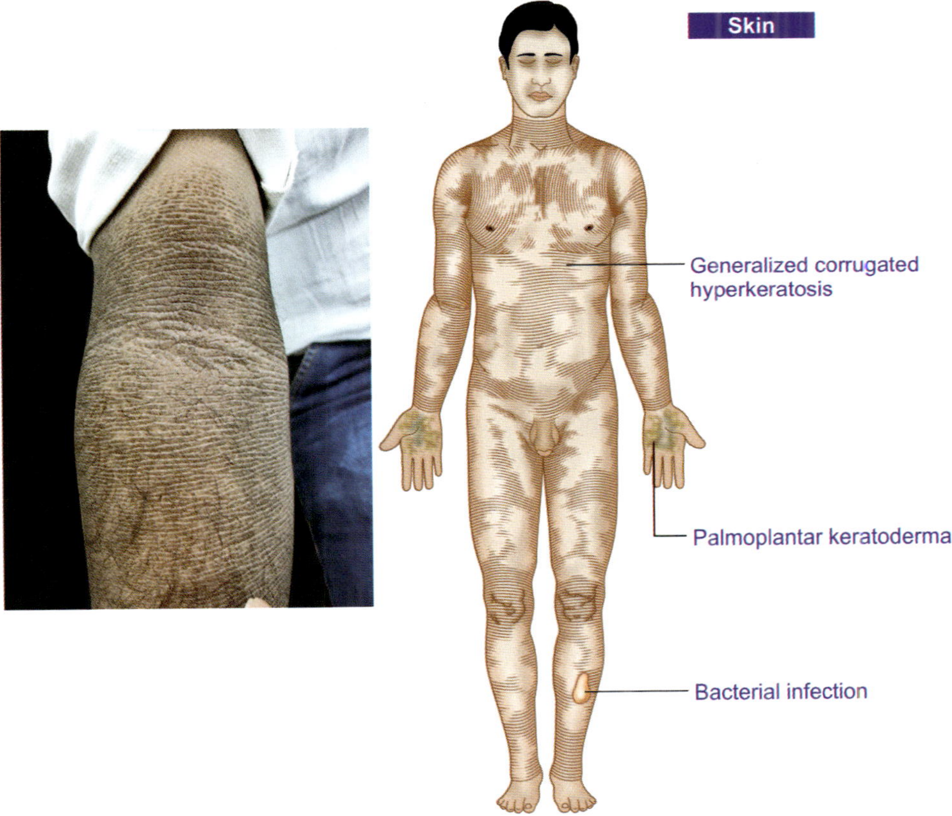

Fig. 13.15: Epidermolytic ichthyosis in later stages there is marked hyperkeratosis with cobblestone pattern (most prominent over joints)

- Variable degree of erythroderma, palmoplantar involvement, and blistering/bullae.
- Frequent skin infections; malodor; gait and posture abnormalities.
- Worsened by systemic retinoids.

Histopathology

- Hyperkeratosis, keratinocyte vacuolization, and a **prominent granular layer** with clumped keratin in suprabasal cells; **lamellar body accumulation.**
- Tonofilaments are lost—promote blistering.

Treatment

- Neontal period: Skin fragility and erosions
- Bacterial colonization responsible for bad odor: Regular use of antiseptics during bathing
- Hyperkeratosis and palmoplantar keratoderma
- Oral retinoids with caution and at low dosage (risk of exacerbation of blistering)
- High concentration keratolytics
- Retinoids—as a general principle, useful in LI, HI, and EKV, *avoid* in CIE.

- Those with a **KRT10 mutations** may benefit when given a low dosage. As complete inhibition of *KRT2* occurs during retinoid treatment, patients with **superficial EI** caused by *KRT2* mutations are ideal candidates for retinoids. In contrast, EI patients with *KRT1* **mutations** may actually **worsen** during retinoid therapy because wild-type keratin 2 is needed to partially replace mutated keratin 1 during dimerization with keratin 10.
  Acitretin dose = less than 0.5 mg/kg to 1 mg/kg
- There is a variation in preferred retinoid (Europe acitretin; USA = low dose isotretinoin >16 years of age).

5. Erythrokeratoderma

In the Sorèze Consensus Conference, it was decided that the various conditions that still carry the name erythrokeratoderma should also be considered as 'ichthyosis'.

a. **Erythrokeratoderma variabilis (Mendes da Costa syndrome)**
   - Gene: GJB3, GJB4 (encode connexin 31 and 30.3, respectively)/AD
   - Gene predicts function of gap junctions in skin, CNS, CVS and muscle.

   Clinical features
   Onset-birth/infancy
   - Transient, polycyclic/comma-shaped, erythematous macules at any site.
   - More **stable**, geographic, hyperkeratotic plaques over knees, elbows, Achilles tendon, extremities, buttocks, and lateral trunk:
     - Palmoplantar keratoderma in ~50% of patients
     - Burning or stinging sensation preceding or accompanying erythema

   Histopathology: Nonspecific; may reveal reduced lamellar bodies in stratum granulosum and reduced keratinization.
   Treatment: Acitretin treatment and low-dose isotretinoin.

b. **Progressive symmetric erythrokeratoderma (Gottron's syndrome)**
   - Gene: **LOR**, GJB4 and other unknown gene
   - AD/AR

   Clinical Features
   Onset: Infancy/childhood
   - Fixed, slowly progressive, nonmigratory, erythematous, hyperkeratotic plaques with sharp, figurate borders **(Fig. 13.16)**.
   - On cheeks, knees, elbows, extremities, and rarely trunk.
   - Palmoplantar keratoderma common.

6. Peeling Skin Syndromes

Clinical, ultrastructural, genetic and pathophysiological aspects demonstrate a relation between LEKTI deficiency (Netherton syndrome), desmoglein-1 deficiency (SAM syndrome) and corneodesmosin deficiency (inflammatory peeling skin disease).

a. **Peeling skin syndrome type A (noninflammatory)**
   First reported by FOX. gene: Mutation in CHST8
   Clinical Features
   Onset: 3–6 years of age
   - Asymptomatic, generalized skin peeling with areas of hyperpigmentation **(Fig. 13.17)**.

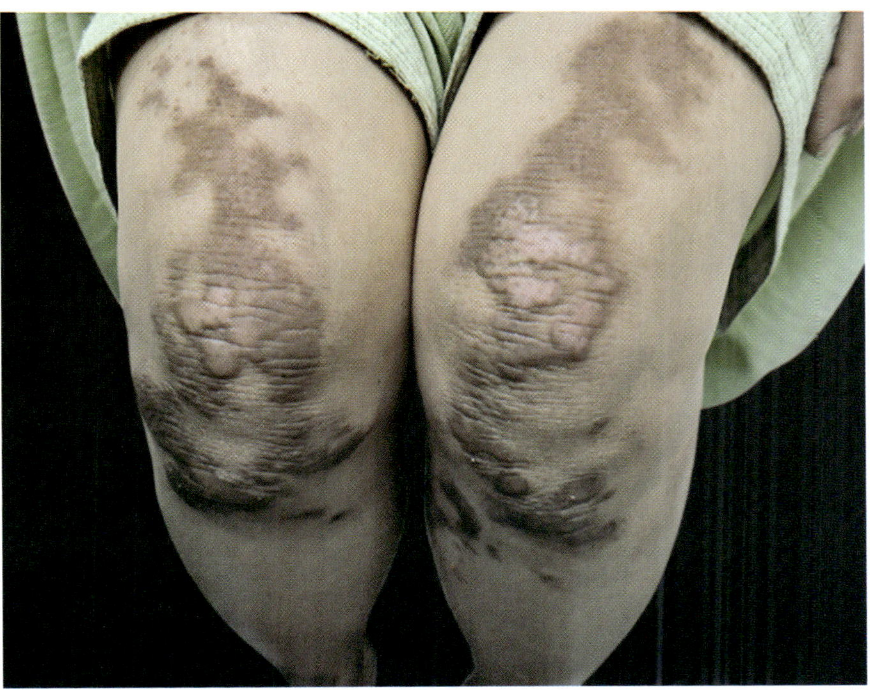

Fig. 13.16: EKV showing nonmigratory, erythematous, hyperkeratotic plaques with sharp, figurate borders

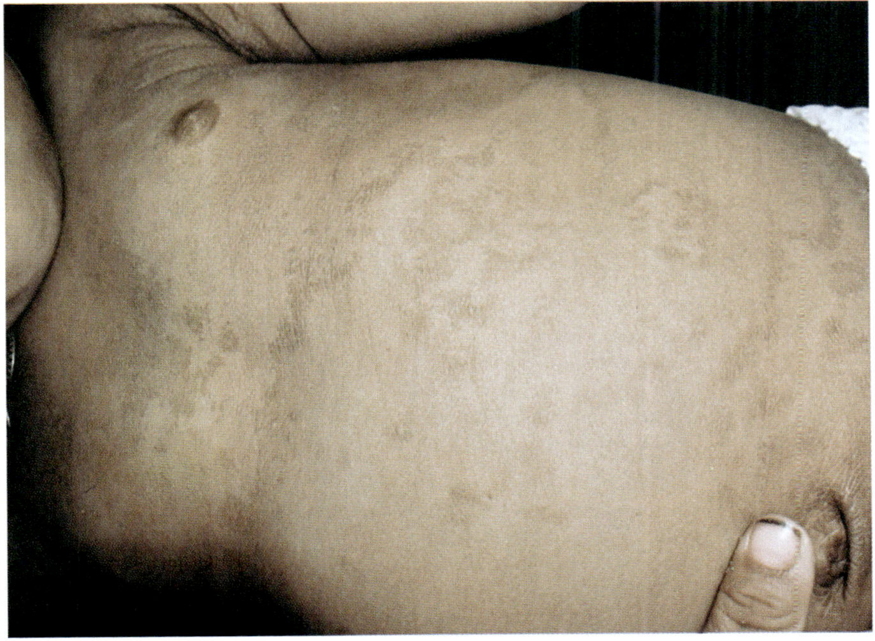

Fig. 13.17: Areas of peeling of skin in a child with peeling skin syndrome (type A)

b. **Inflammatory peeling skin disease**

Gene: Mutations in CDSN (encoding corneodesmosin).

Clinical features

Onset: Birth or a few days later.

- Infants develop ichthyosiform erythroderma
- Patchy peeling affecting the entire skin
- Aggravated by mechanical stress, environmental factors, e.g. low humidity or temperature changes.

Histopathology

- Subcorneal splitting and/or enhanced detachment of corneocytes.

c. **Acral peeling skin syndrome**

Acral peeling skin syndrome (APSS) has been reclassified as a type of epidermolysis bullosa.

Gene: TGM5 (encoding transglutaminase 5).

Clinical features

- Superficial painless peeling of the skin predominantly on the dorsal aspects of the hands and feet.
- In infants, it frequently manifests with blistering on the palms and soles.
- Aggravated by mechanical factors and by humid warm environments.

While the major ichthyoses have been discussed above, the rare variants and syndromic ichthyosis are listed in **Table 13.10**.

TABLE 13.10: Summary of selected ichthyoses

Types	Name/gene and inheritance	Clinical features	Histopathology	Comments
ARCI	**Harlequin ichthyosis** • ABCA12/AR	• Very thick, yellow-brown plates of scale (with large, deep and bright red fissures) that tightly encase the neonate • Massive armour-like hyperkeratosis with fissuring, severe erythroderma **(Fig. 13.18)** • Extreme *ectropion, eclabium,* and ear deformities. • Survivors develop severe CIE-like phenotype • Often neonatal death from sepsis or respiratory insufficiency	Vesicular *lamellar body "ghosts"*, paucity of secreted lamellar structures in stratum corneum	Early initiation of systemic retinoids
Keratinopathic ichthyosis	Superficial epidermolytic ichthyosis **(ichthyosis bullosa of Siemens)** • KRT2/AD	**Birth:** Erythroderma and superficial blistering **Later:** Hyperkeratosis with accentuation over joints, flexures, and dorsal hands/feet; "**molting**" of the skin; palms and soles spared	Cytolysis of granular cells	

(Contd.)

TABLE 13.10: Summary of selected ichthyoses *(Contd.)*

Types	Name/gene and inheritance	Clinical features	Histopathology	Comments
Keratinopathic ichthyosis	**Ichthyosis hystrix (Curth-Macklin)** • KRT1/AD	• Mutilating palmoplantar keratoderma • Hyperkeratosis with verrucous, cobblestone, **hystrix-like** pattern on extremities and trunk • Pseudoainhum; digital contractures	Binuclear cells; particular concentric perinuclear "shells" of aberrant, putatively keratin material	
	Congenital reticular ichthyosiform erythroderma (CRIE) (Ichthyosis en confetti) • KRT10/AD	• Birth-erythroderma and scaling • Later, confetti-like areas of scaling (result from **revertant mosaicism—natural gene therapy)** • Palmoplantar keratoderma • Joint contractures	Binuclear cells and perinuclear vacuolization	
Syndromic with hair defect	**Netherton syndrome** • SPINK5 (encodes LEKT1, serine protease inhibitor) • AR	• Congenital erythroderma and scaling • **2 morphologies: Ichthyosis linearis circumflexa** (annular or serpiginous plaques with double-edged scale) and **CIE-like** pruritus and eczematous plaques **(Fig. 13.19)** • **Trichorrhexis invaginata** • ↑IgE; neonatal temperature instability, electrolyte imbalance (hyponatremia), and failure to thrive, **atopic dermatitis** • Recurrent infections; food and other allergies/anaphylaxis	Psoriasiform histopathology; ("bamboo hair")	IVIG, infliximab. Retinoid therapy is generally not recommended
Syndromic with hair defect	**Sjögren-Larsson syndrome** ALDH3A2/ FALDH • AR	• Birth: Erythema and hyperkeratosis • Later, fine to plate-like/dark scaling or nonscaling hyperkeratosis; favors abdomen, neck, flexures **(Fig. 13.20)** • Palmoplantar keratoderma • Pruritus can be severe	Nonspecific; hyperkeratosis, acanthosis, and preservation of granular layer	Major extracutaneous features • Progressive spastic **di-** and **tetraplegia (2 years of life)** • **Perifoveal glistening** white dots • **Photophobia** • Rx: **Benzafibrate** (+FALDH) • Acitretin 10 mg weekly to 25 mg daily. (↓ pruritus)

(Contd.)

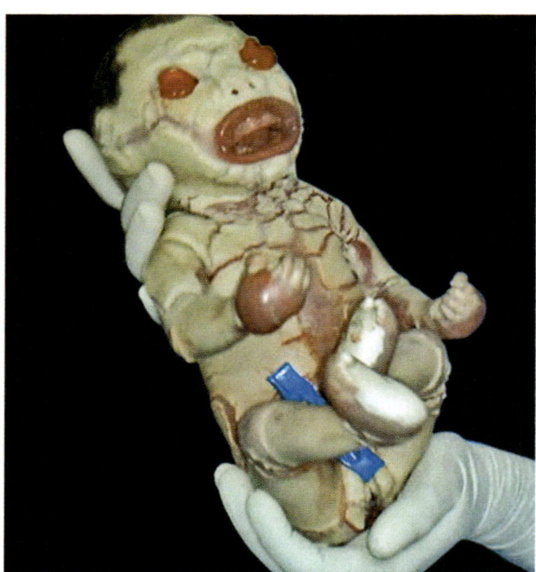

Fig. 13.18: A case of Harlequin ichthyosis (*Courtesy*: CNBC Pediatric Hospital, Delhi)

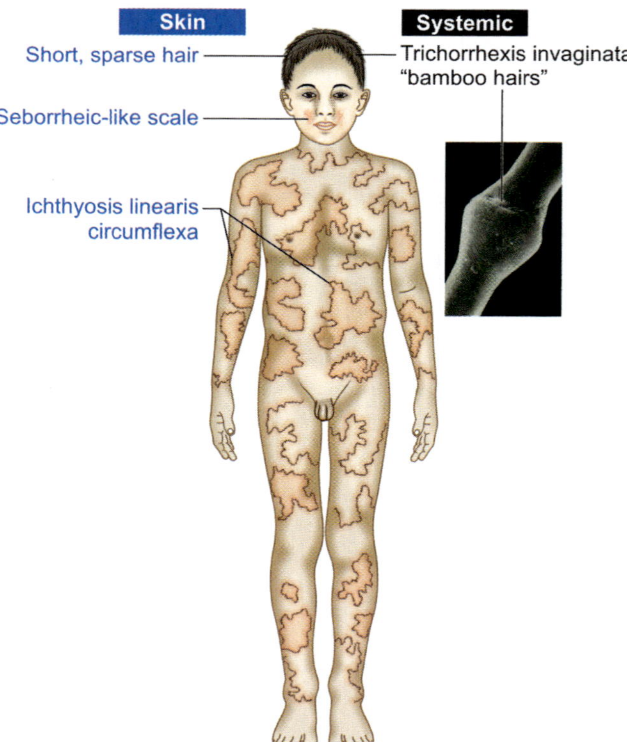

Fig. 13.19: Netherton syndrome

TABLE 13.10: Summary of selected ichthyoses *(Contd.)*

Types	Name/gene and inheritance	Clinical features	Histopathology	Comments
Syndromic with hair defect	**Neutral lipid storage disease with ichthyosis/ (Chanarin-Dorfman syndrome)** • ABHD5 (CGI-58) • AR	• Generalized, fine, white scales with variable erythema • **Developmental delay; Hepatomegaly** • Myopathy; hearing impairment; cataracts	**Globular electron-lucent** inclusions in epidermis	Peripheral blood smear to detect **lipid vacuoles** in eosinophils, and monocytes • Rx: Acitretin (0.5 mg/kg day)
	Refsum syndrome • PHYH, PEX7 • AR	• Fine, white scales on extremities and trunk, **resembling ichthyosis vulgaris** (50%) • Peripheral motor and sensory **neuropathy;** cranial nerve dysfunction (deafness, anosmia); cerebellar ataxia; atypical **retinitis pigmentosa** ("salt and pepper pigment")	• Orthokeratotic hyperkeratosis and lipid-containing vacuoles in basal keratinocytes • Increased plasma phytanic acid	**Rx:** • Exclusion of chlorophyll, dairy products, fats • Lipid apheresis
X-linked ichthyosis syndromes	**Congenital hemidysplasia with ichthyosiform erythroderma and limb defects (CHILD) syndrome** • NSDHL (3β-hydroxysteroid-dehydrogenase) • **XLD**	• At birth, **unilateral** (right >left-sided) erythema and waxy, yellowish adherent scale on 1/2 of the body. Later on hyperkeratosis **develops (Fig. 13.21)** • Ipsilateral alopecia, ipsilateral organ aplasia/agenesis, cleft palate • Ipsilateral skeletal defects such as hypoplasia of digits or ribs to complete amelia, **stippled epiphyses**	Nonspecific	Ointment composed of 2% lovastatin and 2% cholesterol twice daily
	Conradi-Hünermann-Happle syndrome • EBP (emopamil-binding protein) • **XLD**	• At birth, ichthyosiform erythroderma (generalized *vs* unilateral in CHILD syndrome) with feathery, adherent scales along Blaschko's lines **(Fig. 13.22)** • Erythema resolves in first few months of life (unlike CHILD syndrome) and is replaced by follicular atrophoderma		Unilateral cataracts; stippled epiphyses/ chondrodysplasia punctata seen only during infancy
	Ichthyosis follicularis, alopecia photophobia (IFAP) syndrome • **MBTPS2, XLR**	• Erythroderma, scaling, and follicular hyperkeratosis • **Generalized alopecia**, including eyebrows and eyelashes	Follicular plugging and hypoplastic pilosebaceous structures	Growth retardation and microcephaly; corneal opacities and ulcerations

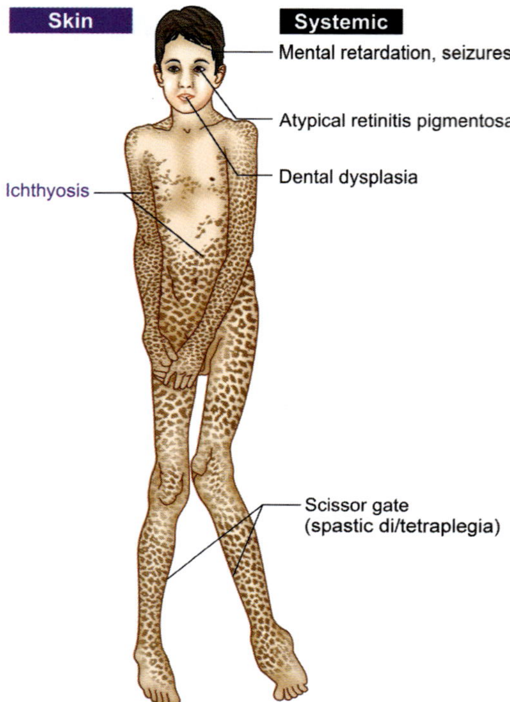

Fig. 13.20: Sjögren–Larsson syndrome

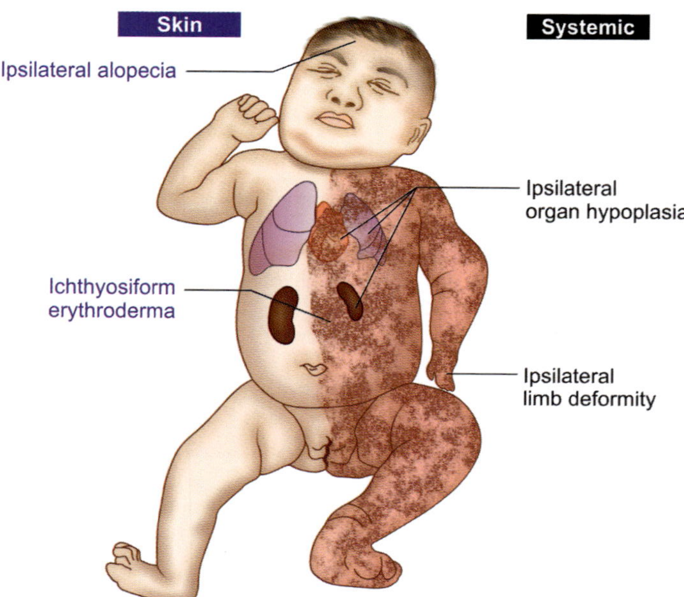

Fig. 13.21: A depiction of CHILD syndrome

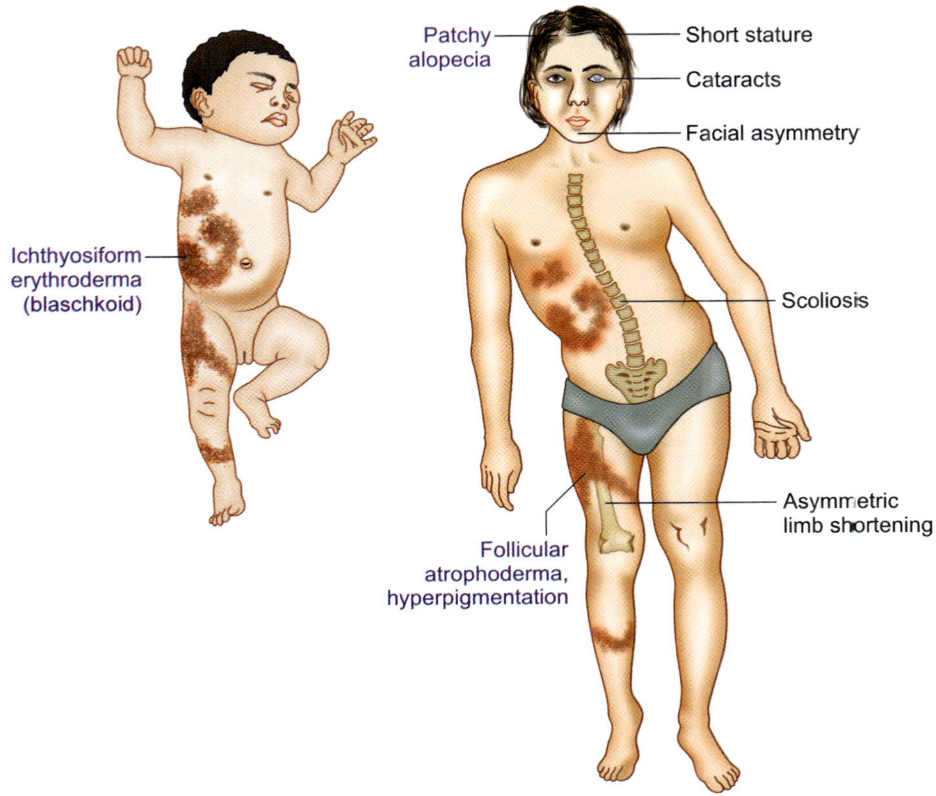

Fig. 13.22: Conradi–Hünermann–Happle syndrome

NEUROCUTANEOUS/HAMARTONEOPLASTIC SYNDROMES

Phacomatoses are a heterogeneous group of conditions (mainly) affecting the skin (with congenital pigmentary/vascular abnormalities and/or tumors), the central and peripheral nervous system (with congenital abnormalities and/or tumors) and the eye (with variable abnormalities). They have been relabelled as hamartoneoplastic syndromes and include neurofibromatosis type 1, tuberous sclerosis complex, Gardner syndrome and Cowden syndrome.

The pathogenesis is believed to be consequent to an interplay between intra- and extra-neuronal signalling pathways encompassing receptor-to-protein and protein-to-protein cascades involving RAS, MAPK/MEK, ERK, mTOR, RHOA, PI3K/AKT, PTEN, GNAQ and GNA11 pathways, which explain the phenotypic variability and overlapping features. A brief overview of the history and nomenclature is given in **Box 13.5**.

BOX 13.5: Nomenclature of neurocutaneous syndromes

Jan van der Hoeve (ophthalmologist) 1920	Phakoma/phakomata (from the old Greek word "axaa" = lentil, spot, lens-shaped)—to describe retinal lesion in NF & TSC
American neurologist Paul Ivan Yakovlev and psychiatrist **Riley H. Guthrie** (1931)	Neurocutaneous syndromes

The various categories include:

1. Those predisposing to development of *tumors* (i.e. neurofibromatoses and allelic/similar disorders and schwannomatosis; tuberous sclerosis complex; Gorlin–Goltz syndromes).
2. *Vascular* malformations (i.e. Sturge–Weber and Klippel–Trenaunay syndromes; CLOVES, Wyburn–Mason syndrome; blue rubber bleb nevus syndrome; hereditary hemorrhagic telangiectasia);
3. *Vascular* tumors (von Hippel–Lindau disease; PHACE(S)
4. *Pigmentary/connective tissue mosaicism* (incontinentia pigmenti; pigmentary/Ito mosaicism; neurocutaneous melanocytosis; epidermal/papular spilus/Becker's nevi syndromes;
5. *Twin spotting* or similar phenomena (phacomatosis pigmentovascularis and pigmento-keratotica; and cutis tricolor).

RASOPATHIES

The term **'RASopathies'** covers a group of AD diseases that have mutations in the genes that code for the proteins of **the RAS/MAPK pathway**.

- Neurofibromatosis type 1, Noonan syndrome, Legius syndrome, LEOPARD syndrome, Costello syndrome, capillary malformation-arteriovenous malformation syndrome and cardiofaciocutaneous syndrome.
- Involvement of the RAS/MAPK pathway not only increases predisposition to tumors, but also determines the presence of phenotypic anomalies and alterations in learning processes.
- Drugs that act on the membrane receptors, such as tyrosine kinase inhibitors in the mTOR pathway or MEK inhibitors can be used for these disorders.

An overview of the varied drugs that can be used in RASopathies is listed in the **Fig. 13.23**.

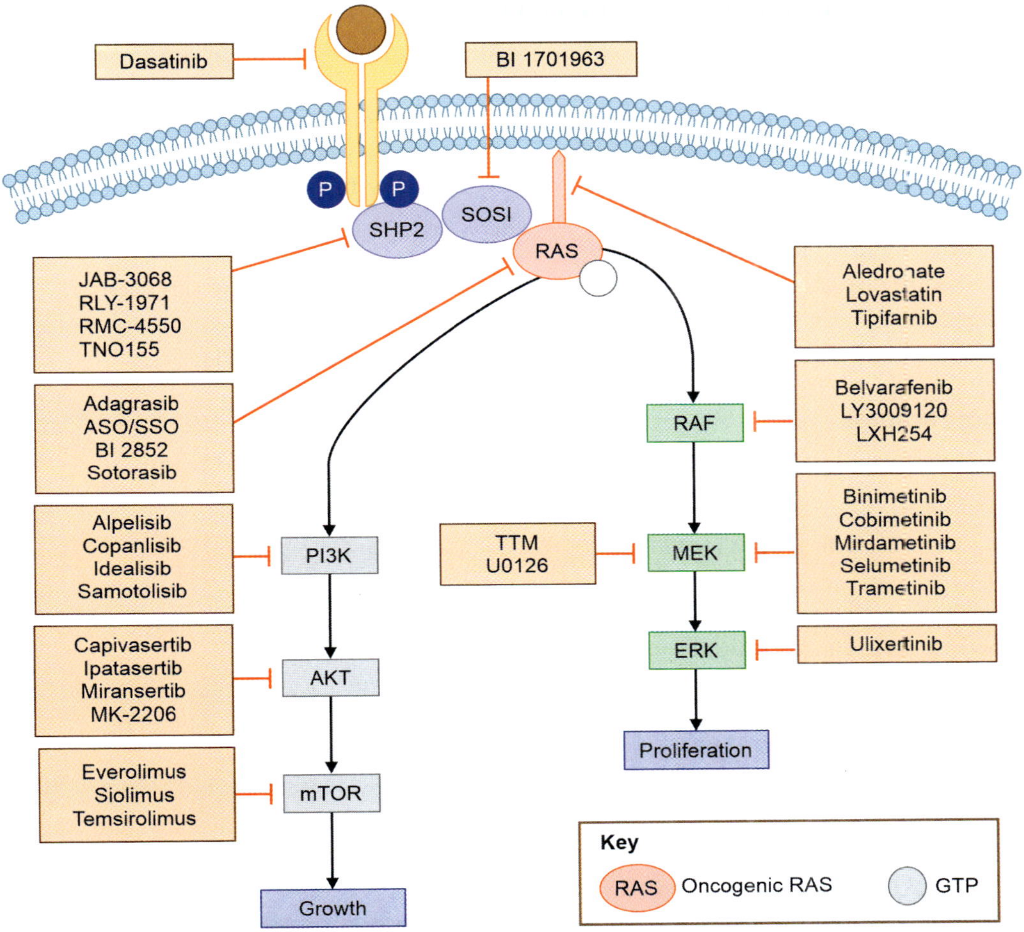

Fig. 13.23: Treating RASopathies. There are varied classes of drugs that target **RAS activation** and components of **the MAPK or the PI3K/AKT pathway**. Drugs that inhibit RAS activation include those that target RAS directly (e.g. **sotorasib**), inhibit RAS membrane localization (e.g. **tipifarnib**), prevent the activity of SHP2 (e.g. **RMC-4550**), inhibit the interaction of RAS with its exchange factor SOS1 (e.g. **BI 1701963**), or block the kinase activity of receptor tyrosine kinases (e.g. **dasatinib**). (Blue font indicates preclinical tool compounds; black font indicates a drug in clinical development). Several have been FDA approved for the treatment of cancer, including sotorasib, trametinib and copanlisib, among others, and could potentially be used for the treatment of RASopathies. TTM, tetrathiomolybate.

NEUROFIBROMATOSIS (NF)

Encompasses three distinct disorders (NF1, NF2, and schwannomatosis), characterized by ↑propensity toward tumor development, particularly of the nerve sheath:

- In 1882, Friedrich von Recklinghausen published a monograph describing NF1 and pointed out that the skin tumors were derived from peripheral nerves.
- 90% of cases are NF1
- 1 in 2500–3300 births.

1. NF1 (VON RECKLINGHAUSEN'S DISEASE)

- AD disorder caused by mutations in **neurofibromin** (NF1), a tumor suppressor gene on chromosome 17.
  - Neurofibromin is a cytoplasmic protein that negatively regulates Ras activation
  - **Mast cells** are increased in neurofibromas and may be involved in the development and growth of these tumors by producing several growth factors, such as histamine and tumor necrosis factor-α (TNF-α)
  - Almost 100% **manifest** by 5 years
  - 50% are due to sporadic mutations and mosaic/segmental disease can occur.
- Diagnostic criteria for NF-1 **(Box 13.6)**
- Clinical manifestations by age of presentation are listed in **Table 13.11**.

Clinical Features

These are depicted in **Fig. 13.24** and the varied manifestations are listed below.

BOX 13.6: Diagnostic criteria for NF1 (2021)

Must have ≥2 of the following:
- Six café au lait macules >0.5 cm (prepubertal) or >1.5 cm (postpubertal) (must be bilateral)
- Intertriginous freckling (axilla/groin) (must be bilateral)
- One plexiform neurofibroma or ≥2 dermal neurofibromas of any type
- ≥2 Lisch nodules or ≥2 choroidal abnormalities
- Optic nerve glioma
- Pathognomonic skeletal dysplasia (tibial or sphenoid wing dysplasia) or pseudoarthrosis of a long bone
- A heterozygous pathogenic NF1 variant

*Underlined portions are indicative of additions/changes in the updated NIH criteria (2021)

TABLE 13.11: Manifestations of NF1 according to the age of presentation

Average age of onset	Cutaneous	Ocular	Neurologic	Skeletal
Infancy to early childhood	• Café au lait macules • Plexiform neurofibromas	• Attention deficit	• Learning disabilities • Autism • Macrocephaly hyperactivity disorder	• Tibial dysplasia • Sphenoid wing dysplasia
Prepubertal	• Intertriginous freckling	• Optic gliomas	• Brainstem gliomas • Meningiomas	• Scoliosis
Adolescence	• Dermal or subcutaneous neurofibromas	• Lisch nodules		
Adulthood	• Malignant peripheral nerve sheath tumors			

1. ***Skin***

- **Neurofibroma:** Soft papule on trunk or limbs that invaginates upon finger pressure **("*button-holing*")**
  - Variant: Blue-red macules and pseudoatrophic macules
  - Females-areola (often missed site).

  Plexiform neurofibroma: May have an overlying CALM and/or hypertrichosis; "*bag of worms*" feel (seen in~25% of patients)
  - *Most commonly trigeminal or upper cervical* nerves and usually noticeable within the first 2 years of life.
  - Malignant peripheral nerve sheath tumor (MPNST, 3–15%): Rapid enlargement or pain of plexiform neurofibroma (10% risk), most common cutaneous malignancy in NF.
- **CALM** (typically ≥6 in number, ***1st to appear***, appear in 100% cases by **4 years** of age or less, in 82% by the first year).
  - Café au lait spots are present in **10–20% of normal individuals** (usually <6) and about 35% of patients with McCune-Albright syndrome **(Fig. 13.25)**. CALMs are also seen in Watson syndrome, Noonan syndrome, TSC, ring chromosome disorders and some other rare genetic disorders.
  - Children younger than 2.5 years old with ≥6 CALMS should be genetically tested for NF1 and SPRED1 genes due to high probability of testing positive and benefiting from early guidance.
- **Axillary freckling** (Crowe's sign): **70%** of patients, almost pathognomic—may be seen over an underlying plexiform neurofibroma, and if these extend to the midline of the spine it may indicate that the tumor involves the spinal cord.
- Pruritus—mast cells.

2. ***Eye***

- **Lisch nodules** (**pigmented iris hamartomas, >90%** of patients by **20** years of age), asymptomatic, not in segmental or bilateral acoustic NF.
- Choroid nevus and glaucoma.

3. ***Bone***

- *Sphenoid wing dysplasia*: Pulsating exophthalmos may be noted, though often asymptomatic.
- Macrocephaly, kyphoscoliosis, congenital tibial pseudarthroses.
- Additional skeletal abnormalities: Thoracic cage asymmetry, generalized *osteoporosis*, and pathologic fractures.
- Short stature and macrocephaly.

4. ***CNS***

- Learning disability, ADHD, and autism
- Seizures
- Hydrocephalus
- *Optic glioma* (can → blindness; seen with precocious puberty), astrocytomas, meningiomas, vestibular/acoustic schwannoma/neuroma, and ependymoma.
- Unidentified bright objects (UBO) on MRI (50–75%)

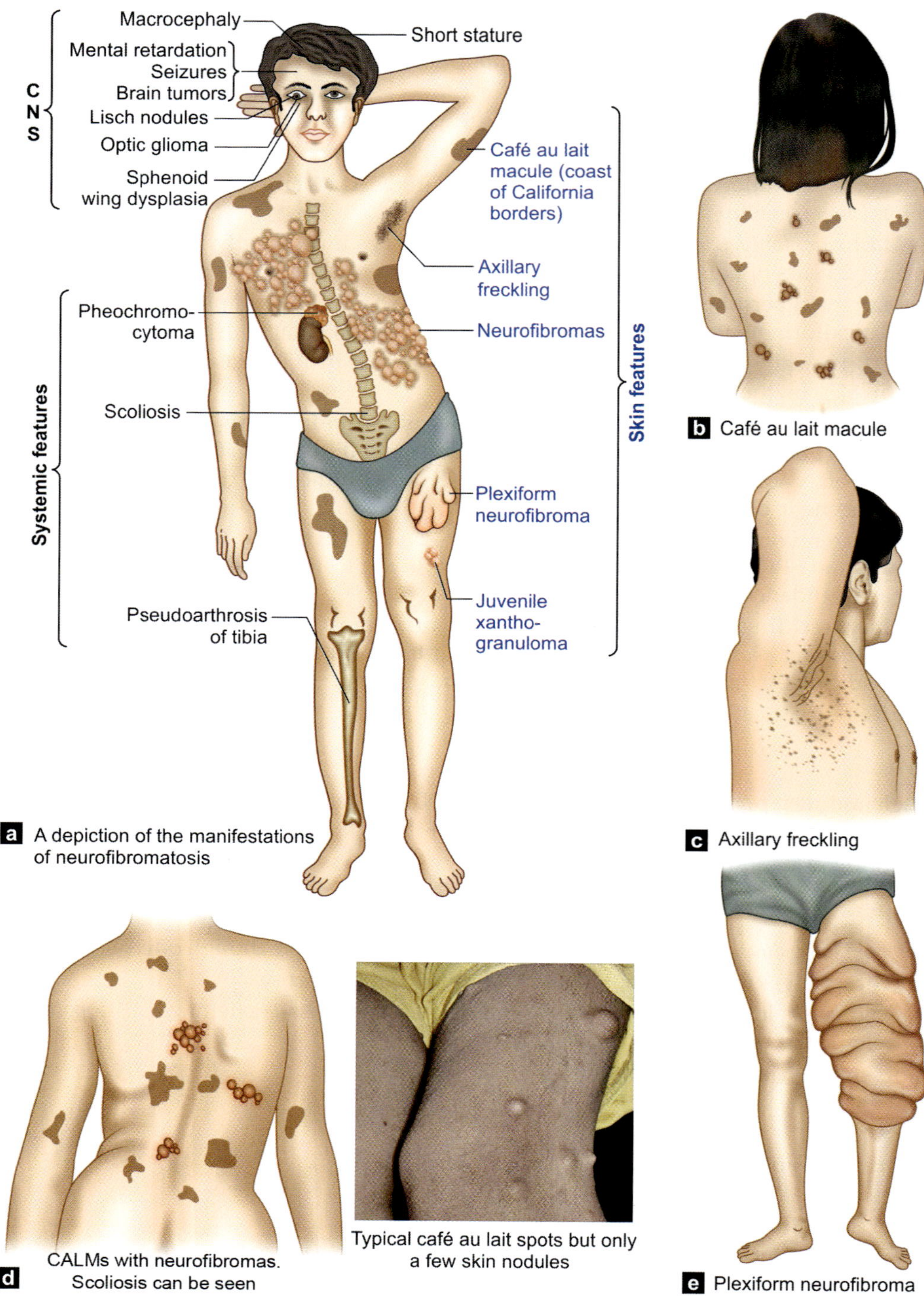

a A depiction of the manifestations of neurofibromatosis

b Café au lait macule

c Axillary freckling

d CALMs with neurofibromas. Scoliosis can be seen

Typical café au lait spots but only a few skin nodules

e Plexiform neurofibroma

Fig. 13.24: Varied manifestations of neurofibromatosis

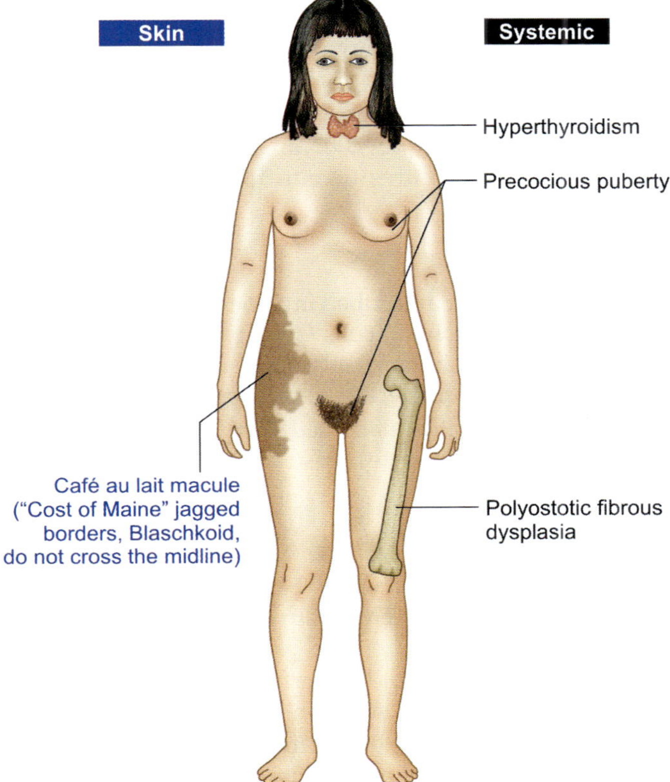

Fig. 13.25: Artistic depiction of McCune-Albright syndrome

5. *Miscellaneous*

Severity of cutaneous involvement gives no reliable indication of the extent of the disease in other organs.

- **Tumors**
  - **Most common** solitary **intracranial tumor is an <u>optic nerve glioma (10–15%)</u>**; astrocytomas and schwannomas also occur. <u>Maximum risk</u> for optic pathway tumors in <u>first 6 years</u>.
  - Sarcomatous change in NF (neurofibrosarcoma), rhabdomyosarcoma. Malignant peripheral nerve sheath tumors (MPNSTs) are highly aggressive-enlargement or pain should suggest the possibility of malignant change, although rapid enlargement may also occur secondary to intralesional hemorrhage.
  - Pheochromocytoma <u>(1%)</u>, Wilms' tumor, and chronic myelogenous leukemia.
  - <u>Breast cancer-5 fold risk</u> in women <50 years of age.
- **Hypertension** may develop as a result of a pheochromocytoma or renal vascular stenosis secondary to fibromuscular dysplasia.
- **Vascular:** Vascular dysplasia with cerebral, GI, and renal involvement; secondary infarction, renovascular hypertension.

6. *Associations and Variants*

- Strong **triple association** between NF1, juvenile xanthogranulomas, and juvenile chronic myelogenous leukemia
- Of note, **Watson syndrome** = NF1 features + pulmonary stenosis
- Legius syndrome (SPRED1 mutation) = In 2007, an important disorder that closely resembles NF1 was described. The cardinal features are **multiple CALMs, macrocephaly and axillary freckling**.

Pathology

- Cutaneous neurofibromas-well-circumscribed but unencapsulated dermal collection of small nerve fibers + loosely arranged spindle cells (scanty pale cytoplasm and elongated wavy nuclei) composed of fibroblasts, Schwann cells, and perineural cells in a collagenous stroma + varying amounts of mucin and scattered mast cells.
- In both café au lait spots and clinically unaffected skin, *giant pigment granules* are occasionally found in epidermal cells and melanocytes. Also seen in McCune–Albright syndrome, and never in normal skin.

Investigations (Table 13.12)

- Examine patient and all family members.
- Neurophysiological assessment, a skeletal survey, audiography and slit-lamp ocular examination.
- Magnetic resonance imaging (MRI) should be performed in children who have macrocephaly or who demonstrate focal neurological signs or symptoms.
- Annual blood pressure measurements, head circumference measurements, assessment of potential scoliosis, presence of painful lumps consistent with MPNSTs and eye examination.
- In the **UK**, screening is only suggested if *neurological* or *ophthalmological anomalies observed*.
- In the **USA**, all infants are screened routinely with cranial MRI scanning.

TABLE 13.12: Investigative protocol for NF1

Tests	**Rationale/Comments**
Baseline **ophthalmologic** examination	First at 5–6 years then every 2–3 years
Baseline **magnetic resonance imaging**	Optional
BP	Always check blood pressure; if elevated in *child*, consider renal artery stenosis (do renal arteriography); if elevated in adult, consider pheochromocytoma (24-hour urine collection for catecholamine)
CBC (complete blood count)	Multiple juvenile xanthogranuloma (JXG) may be associated with non-lymphocytic leukemia in a child with café au lait spots. If these xanthogranulomas are present, obtain a CBC, but recognize that the likelihood of finding evidence of leukemia is small
Serial **head circumference** measurements	Risk of hydrocephalus and the frequency of macrocephaly without hydrocephalus
Prenatal diagnosis	With such varied expression and complications, the decision to undergo prenatal diagnosis is far from clear. Prenatal diagnosis is also not an option for the approximately 50% of cases who represent new mutations

- Women screen for breast cancer with clinical examination/imaging (beginning by age 40 years).
- Genetic testing: MLPA (multiple ligation-dependent probe amplification), NGS array, CGH (comparative genomic hybridization).

Prognosis

- Majority have a benign course and long-term follow-up information on cohorts of NF1 patients has shown a reduced life expectancy related to the development of malignancy and other complications, such as hypertension due to renal artery stenosis or phaeochromocytoma.
- **Poor prognosis:** Extensive involvement of the *urinary* or *gastrointestinal tract* or the *central nervous system*.
- Pregnancy—unexplained hypertension frequently occurs and can cause rapid progression of existing lesions and the development of new ones, due to ↑hormonal influence.

Treatment

- Genetic counseling: 50% of the children are likely to be affected and the disease may be severe. First degree relatives (e.g. siblings and offspring) who have no stigmata of the disease are unlikely to carry the gene and the risk for their off spring is small but not absent, as gonadal mosaicism has been observed.

  Drugs that act on the membrane receptors, such as tyrosine kinase inhibitors in the mTOR pathway or MEK inhibitors are being tried. In April 2020, the FDA approved **selumetinib** (an oral selective inhibitor of MAPK kinase 1 and 2 (MEK 1/2) for pediatric patients, 2 years of age and older, with NF1 who have symptomatic, inoperable plexiform neurofibromas (PN).
- Regular follow-up with pediatrician, internist, ophthalmologist, neurologist, dermatologist.
- Referral to orthopedist, audiologist, psychiatrist, surgeon, neurosurgeon, oncologist if symptomatic.

2. NEUROFIBROMATOSIS, SEGMENTAL

This condition is characterized by café au lait spots, cutaneous neurofibromas and sometimes visceral neurofibromas, limited to a circumscribed body segment. The condition probably represents a somatic mosaicism of the *NF1* gene.

3. NF2 (BILATERAL ACOUSTIC SCHWANNOMAS)

- AD disorder caused by mutations in SCH gene (encodes schwannomin/merlin; tumor suppressor gene) on chromosome 22.
- Symptoms appear later than NF1 (usually in second to third decade).
- Cutaneous findings: Neurofibromas (less common than NF1)—more commonly *subcutaneous* type with overlying pigment/hair rather than intradermal (seen mainly in NF1), CALM (usually ≤2 lesions).
- Neurological findings: **Bilateral vestibular schwannomas (acoustic neuromas)** are diagnostic; may cause deafness, tinnitus, unsteadiness, headache (patients should not swim alone), meningiomas, astrocytomas, and ependymomas.
- Ocular findings: Juvenile posterior subcapsular lenticular opacity/cataract.
- Poor prognosis with worsening hearing, vision, ambulation; CNS tumors are most common cause of death.

As surgery can lead to morbidity **bevacizumab** is considered the first-line drug treatment for fast-growing NF2. Lately anlotinib has been tried in a case with recurrence after gamma knife (Zhao R, 2023).

4. TUBEROUS SCLEROSIS COMPLEX (TSC)

History

Rayer—described the fibrovascular papules.

It was described by Bourneville, a French neurologist and by John James Pringle.

Bourneville—reported the intellectual impairment, hemiplegia and epilepsy.

Sherlock coined the now outdated term 'epiloia' (epilepsy, low intelligence and adenoma sebaceum).

Inheritance: AD disorder caused by mutations in hamartin on 9q34 (TSC1) or tuberin (TSC2) (tumor suppressor genes) on 16p13.

Tuberin and hamartin form a complex that inhibits signal transduction of downstream effectors of mTOR (mammalian target of rapamycin) → abnormal regulation of cellular differentiation, proliferation, and migration of affected cell types with the formation of multiple hamartomas.

- Up to 66% may be spontaneous mutations.

Clinical Features

A depiction of the manifestations is given in **Fig. 13.26** and is detailed below.

1. *Skin*

- Cutaneous features are seen in up to 90% of affected patients, and may be the presenting symptom **(Table 13.13)**.
- Cutaneous findings: Adenoma sebaceum (facial angiofibromas), hypopigmented "ash-leaf" macules (confetti pattern pretibially; first cutaneous finding), Shagreen patch (connective tissue nevus), periungual fibromas ("Koenen tumors"), and CALMs.
- Angiofibromas (*at least 3 angifibroma should be +.*): Firm discrete red-brown telangiectatic papules in nasolabial furrows, cheeks and chin. Dermal fibrosis with stellate fibroblasts, atrophic sebaceous glands, dilated capillaries, and loss of elastin. Collagen synthesis is *increased* in the angiofibroma, although total collagen content is *decreased*, suggesting that there may be *an increased turnover of collagen*.
- Shagreen patch: Thickenend, slightly elevated skin-colored plaque in lumosacral reagion (connective tissue nevus). Broad sclerotic collagen bundles and reduced elastin.

TABLE 13.13: Cutaneous manifestations of TSC by age of presentation

Average age of onset	Cutaneous	Other
Infancy to early childhood	• Hypomelanotic macules • "Confetti"-like macules	• Cardiac rhabomyomas • Subependymal nodules • Seizures
Prepubertal	• Angiofibromas • Shagreen patch • Fibrous cephalic plaque • Dental pits	• Renal hamartomas
Adolescence	• Ungual **fibromas**	
Adulthood	• Intraoral fibromas	• Pulmonary lymphangioleiomyomatosis (females) • Renal cysts

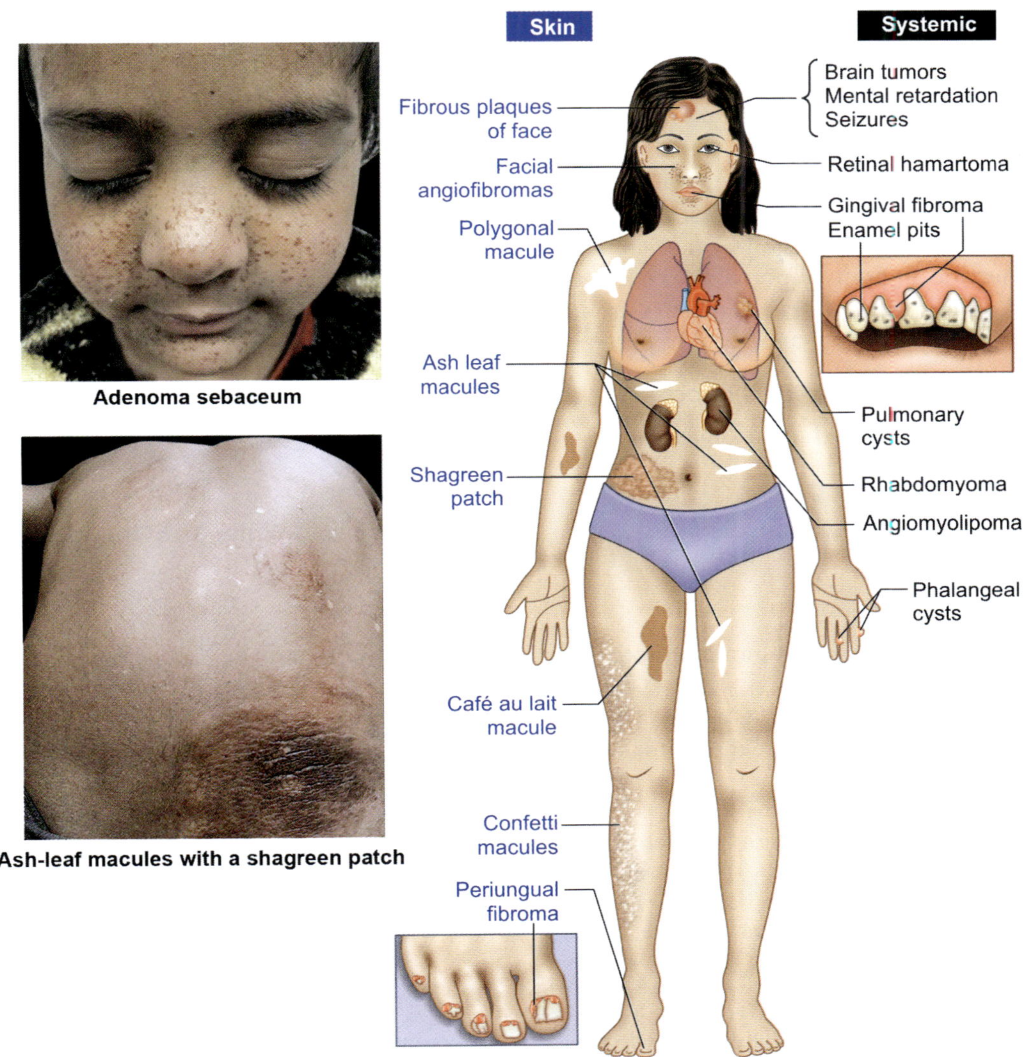

Fig. 13.26: A depiction of the varied manifestations of tuberous sclerosis complex

- Hypomelanotic macules: Ovoid/ash leaf-shaped, better seen under Wood's light, on trunk and limbs, earliest finding. Histology shows abnormal melanocytes, with ↓pigmentation due to decreased tyrosinase activity. Hypopigmented macules are seen in 2–3 per 1000 of apparently normal newborn babies as well.
- Molluscum pendulum necklace sign (soft pedunculated fibromas around neck).

2. *CNS*

Neurologic findings: **Cortical tubers**, subependymal nodules (may → hydrocephalus), subependymal giant cell astrocytomas, seizures/infantile spasms, hypsarrhythmia, intellectual impairment, and paraventricular calcification.

- Learning difficulties are present in 60–70% of cases:
  - Worse prognosis: Infantile spasms, a large number of cortical tubers, and early age of onset of seizures or intractable seizures.
  - MC cause of mortality → complications related to seizures.

3. *Renal Findings*

Renal cysts, angiomyolipomas, and renal cell carcinoma:
- Systemic mTOR inhibitors (i.e. *sirolimus* and *everolimus*) used for management of renal and hepatic angiomyolipomas and subependymal giant cell astrocytomas.
- Complications of renal disease (renal failure, catastrophic hemorrhage within a renal angiomyolipoma, and renal hypertension) = #2 cause of death.

4. *Ocular Findings (50% of cases)*

Retinal phakomas (hamartomas).

5. *Cardiac Findings*

Cardiac rhabdomyomas (50% of infants) → Wolff–Parkinson–White arrhythmia, resolve spontaneously.

6. *GI Findings*

Hepatic cysts, hepatic angiomyolipomas (usually asymptomatic), and GI polyps/hamartomas.

7. *Dental Findings*

Pits in enamel and gingival fibromas.

8. *Lung Findings*

- Pulmonary lymph angioleiomyomatosis and pulmonary cysts
- Pulmonary complications: Pneumothorax, chylothorax, hemoptysis, and pulmonary insufficiency.

9. *Radiological Findings*

Skull	• X-ray calcification in about 50% of patients in later childhood or adult life. • CT: Periventricular (subependymal) nodules, parenchymal hamartomas (cortical tubers), ventriculomegaly and, rarely, subependymal giant cell astrocytomas. • MRI is more sensitive in the detection of parenchymal lesions.
Hand and feet	Cyst-like lesions of the phalanges and irregular thickening of the cortex of the metatarsals and metacarpals.
Lungs	Irregular reticulation like interstitial fibrosis.
Kidneys	It is helpful in differentiating renal hamartomas from other lesions.

Prognosis

- Poor in severely affected infant: Three percent die in the first year, 28% under 10 years and 75% before the age of 25 years.
- **Death:** Epilepsy, intercurrent infection, others—tumor, cardiac failure or pulmonary fibrosis.
- Prognosis for the older child or young adult with cutaneous stigmata and epilepsy is unpredictable.

Diagnosis

- Prenatal diagnosis: Fetal echocardiogram revealing rhabdomyoma. DNA analysis if mutation known.
- Tests: Wood's light examination, transfontanel ultrasound, CT scan/MRI of brain, electro-encephalogram (EEG), fundoscopic examination, renal ultrasound, ECG and echo-cardiogram in infancy, HRCT chest and PFT, abdominal MRI.

  Approximately **60–70%** of TSC cases are thought to be the result of **new mutations**, but before genetic counseling of unaffected parents of an affected child, both parents should be fully investigated, including a full skin examination using the Wood's lamp, and possibly computed tomography (CT), renal ultrasound or intravenous pyelography, and expert ophthalmological examination. Almost **30%** of apparently unaffected parents have TSC.
- A definitive diagnosis of TSC requires two major features **(Box 13.7)**.

BOX 13.7: Diagnostic criteria for TSC

Major	Minor
• Facial angiofibromas (≥3) or forehead plaque	• Multiple randomly distributed pits in dental enamel
• Nontraumatic ungual or periungual fibroma (≥2)	• Hamartomatous rectal polyps
• Hypomelanotic macules (≥3)	• Bone cysts
• Shagreen patch (connective tissue naevus)	• Cerebral white matter migration lines
• Multiple retinal nodular hamartomas	• Gingival fibromas
• Cortical tuber	• Nonrenal hamartoma
• Subependymal nodule	• Retinal achromic patch
• Subependymal giant cell astrocytoma	• 'Confetti' skin lesions
• Cardiac rhabdomyoma, single or multiple	• Multiple renal cysts
• Lymphangiomyomatosis	
• Renal angiomyolipoma	

Definite TSC: Either 2 major features **or** 1 major feature with 2 minor features
Probable TSC: 1 major feature **and 1** minor feature
Possible TSC: Either 1 major feature **or** 2 or more minor features.

Treatment

- Cosmetic treatment—angiofibromas—PDL (wavelength 595 nm), which reduces redness. Papular/nodular lesions—carbon dioxide laser.
- Therapy: Topical rapamycin at 1–2% concentration may be of great benefit in treating cutaneous angiofibromas, systemic rapamycin may be useful in the therapy of visceral tumors and neurological complications including epilepsy **(Box 13.8)**. Various drugs that work on mTOR pathway have been tried in TSC.

Rationale of Therapy

Histologically, angiofibromas show increased dermal vascular and fibrotic components. These changes result from the tumor-inductive effects of fibroblast-like cells with biallelic mutations in TSC1 or TSC2, resulting in hyperactivation of mechanistic target of rapamycin (mTOR). Rapamycin treatment inhibits mTOR in these fibroblast-like tumor cells, but does not eliminate them even after prolonged oral therapy. Also mTOR-independent transforming growth factor (TGF)-β signaling also contributes to the proliferation of angiofibromas. Hence, using vitamin

BOX 13.8: Drugs tried in TSC

- Topical **sirolimus/rapamycin** (0.03–1%) have been used for angiofibromas.* (0.1% concentration represents the first choice)
- Topical **calcitriol** (0.0003%) recently tried.
- In April 2022, FDA approved sirolimus topical gel 0.2% for facial angiofibromas in adults and children > = 6 years of age.
- In April 2018, the FDA approved **everolimus** tablets for the adjunctive treatment of adult and pediatric patients aged 2 years and older with TSC-associated partial-onset seizures.
- Everolimus is also approved for two other manifestations of TSC: TSC-associated subependymal giant cell astrocytoma (SEGA) and TSC-associated renal angiomyolipoma.
- Metformin has been shown to have the potential to reduce the SEGA volume in younger patients. It also appeared to reduce seizures in patients with TS.
- **Vigabatrin** is the drug of choice for infants with TSC who have infantile spasms.

*__Sirolimus__, also known as rapamycin; 1 mg/mL solution or 1–2 mg tablet is crushed and compounded with an ointment.

D_3 to inhibit TGF-β signalling represents a novel approach to providing additional antifibrotic effects [Chen PL].

Follow-up

- Brain MRI every 1–3 years until age 25
- EEG if seizure activity or behavior change/cognitive decline
- Ophthalmologic examination annually if known eye lesions or visual symptoms
- ECG every 3–5 years in asymptomatic patients
- Echocardiography every 1–3 years in patients with cardiac rhabdomyomas until regression is documented
- Abdominal MRI every 1–3 years to evaluate for progression of angiomyolipomas and renal cysts
- Assess blood pressure and determine GFR at least annually
- High-resolution CT chest every 5–10 years in asymptomatic individuals at risk for lymphangioleiomyomatosis and every 2–3 years together with annual PFTs if known lung cysts.
- Dental examination at least every 6 months
- Annual dermatologic examination
- Offer genetic testing/counseling in patients of reproductive age.

PORPHYRIA

The porphyrias are a group of disorders caused by defects in the biosynthesis of haem. Their relevance to the skin arises from the phototoxic properties of the porphyrins, which accumulate in most porphyrias and cause photosensitivity.

The basic metabolic pathway is the formation of haem and various steps in this process. The defects of certain enzymes which cause the various types of porphyria are depicted in **Flowchart 13.2**.

- Eighty percent of hame is synthesized in erythroid cell precursors.
- Decarboxylation of uroporphyrinogen → coproporphyrinogen → protoporphyrinogen decreases water solubility, so that uroporphyrinogen is only excreted via the kidneys. Hydrophobic protoporphyrinogen and protoporphyrin are exclusively excreted into the bile.
- Physiological concentrations of porphyrins stay low because of the high efficiency of hame synthesis.

Classification

1. <u>Cutaneous disease</u> only:
   - Porphyria cutanea tarda (PCT)
   - Congenital erythropoietic porphyria (CEP).
   - Erythropoietic protoporphyria (EPP).

Flowchart 13.2: Hame synthesis pathway depicting the important defects in porphyria (ALA, aminolevulinic acid)

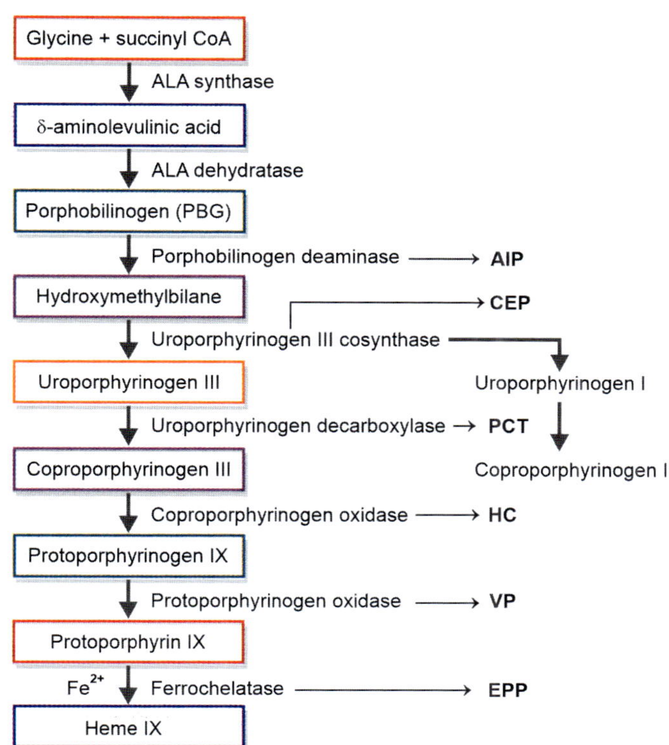

2. Cutaneous disease and acute attacks:
   - Hereditary coproporphyria (HCP).
   - Variegate porphyria (VP).
3. Acute attacks:
   - Acute intermittent porphyria (AIP)

All the cutaneous porphyrias, **except EPP**, present with **fragility** and **blistering** of exposed skin and are termed **'bullous porphyrias'**. Thus, they may be similar clinically and histopathologically.

The main absorption peak is at **408 nm ('Soret band')**, and this long wavelength of light leads to the phototoxic behavior by the porphyrin.

Site of the phototoxic reaction in the skin determines the clinical characteristics of the porphyria **(Fig. 13.27)**.

1. EPP, *lipophilic protoporphyrin* → localized to membranes/endothelial cell → upper dermal blood vessels causing **pain**.
2. PCT, the *water soluble uroporphyrin* → diffuses into surrounding tissues/upper dermis (causes blister under the basal lamina).
3. In VP, copro- and protoporphyrin accumulate but patients suffer from PCT-like upper dermal blisters rather than EPP-like acute pain (due to accumulation of uroporphyrin secondary to local photoinactivation of UROD by coproporphyrin).

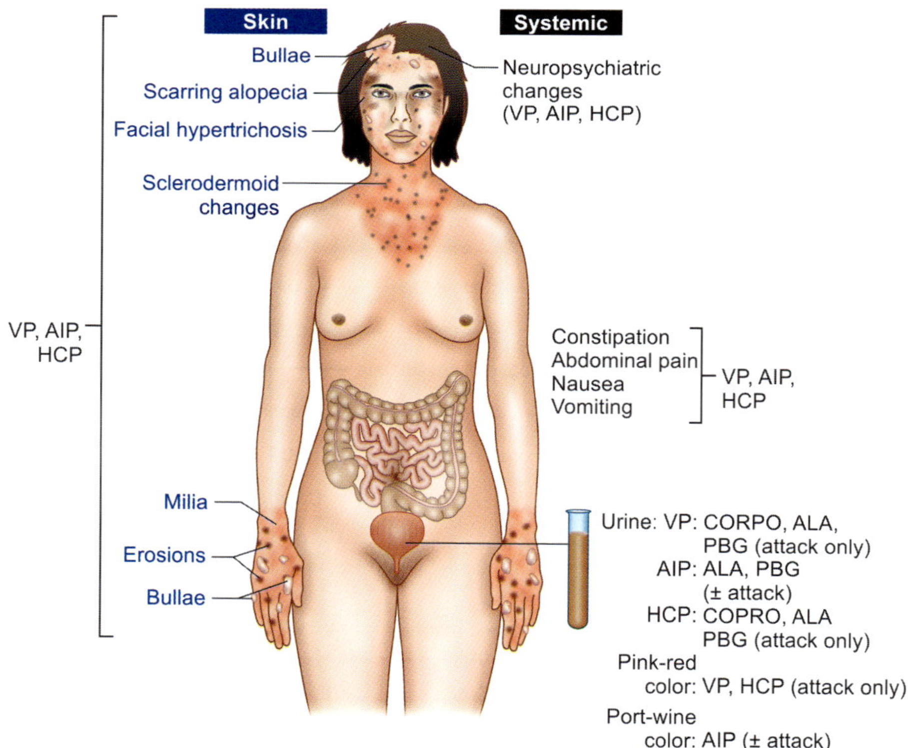

Fig. 13.27: A depiction of the clinical features of porpyhria

Histopathology

- Cutaneous porphyrias—Homogeneous material is seen within the vessel walls of the upper dermal and papillary vascular plexus (PAS + and diastase resistant).
- DIF-IgG in vascular distribution and dermal–epidermal basement membrane zone.

Principles of Treatment

- Preventing violet (Soret wavelength) light penetrating the epidermis.
- Sunscreen, sun avoidance behavior, sun protective clothing and hats.

Use sunscreens that are **opaque** or use large particle size **titanium dioxide** (pigmentary grade), **zinc oxide** and **iron oxide**.

- Dihydroxyacetone paint
- Car with clear window films (tinted).

PORPHYRIA CUTANEA TARDA

Most common porphyria

Defect: Due to ↓*hepatic uroporphyrinogen decarboxylase* (UROD) activity:

- 3 types (I: Sporadic, II: Familial, AD, III: UROD deficiency only localized to liver)
- Type I (sporadic/acquired) form most common (75%).

Clinical Features (Fig. 13.28)

- Age at presentation usually third to fourth decade of life.
- Skin findings include: Skin fragility, vesicles, bullae, erosions, milia, scarring, hyperpigmentation, and hypertrichosis in photodistributed areas (especially dorsal hands/forearms).
- Systemic: Hepatomegaly, cirrhosis and diabetes mellitus may be seen.
- Associations and triggers: Multifactorial disease with various associations/triggers (alcohol abuse, estrogen, iron and hemochromatosis, hepatitis C, and HIV).
- Common differential diagnosis:

a. **VP**

Skin: Identical to PCT can have acute attacks (also seen in acute intermittent porphyria and hereditary coproporphyria)
Gastrointestinal: Colicky abdominal pain, nausea, vomiting, constipation
Central nervous system: Peripheral neuropathy with pain, weakness, paralysis; confusional state, anxiety, depression, delerium, seizures, coma
Cardiovascular: Tachycardia, hypertension.

b. **Hereditary Coproporphyria**

Skin: Features like VP and PCT, acute attacks +
Central nervous system: Similar to AIP and VP;
Gastrointestinal: Similar to AIP and VP.

Histology

- Cell-poor **subepidermal bulla** with "festooning" of dermal papillae, **"caterpillar bodies"** (pink BMZ material in blister cavity and epidermis).
- DIF: IgG, IgM, fibrinogen, and C3 linearly along BMZ and in superficial dermal vessels (thickened deposits around vessels).

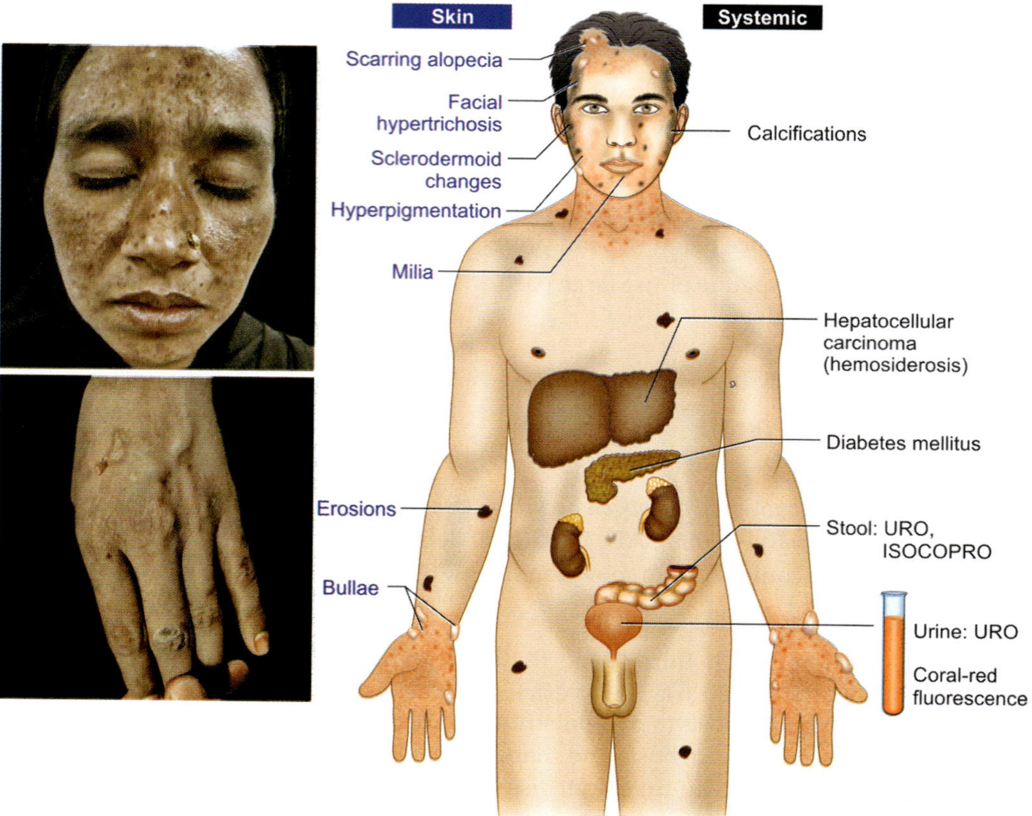

Fig. 13.28: PCT which inhibits increased skin fragility, with vesicles and bulla on the exposed sites which heal hyperpigmentation

Investigations

- Plasma fluorescence emission peak at 620 nm; ↑uroporphyrin III, ↑heptaporphyrin, ↑other porphyrins (including pentacarboxy porphyrin and coproporphyrin) in urine; ↑isocoproporphyrin, ↑heptacarboxylporphyrin III in stool.
- Complete blood count (CBC), liver function tests, iron level, hepatitis panel, liver scan.
- Differentiate VP from PCT as they can have identical cutaneous findings.
- Once you have a positive porphyrin screen, you must rule out a *seizure history*, and check the ratio of URO to COPRO in the urine. In PCT, 8:1; in VP, 1:1 or COPRO >URO.

Treatment

- Photoprotection.
- **Venesection** depletes iron stores and eliminates hepatic iron overload, thus restoring normal enzyme activity.
  - **500 mL** of blood is removed every week or every 2 weeks.
  - **Aim:** ↓transferrin saturation to 15%, hemoglobin to 11–12 g/dL and plasma ferritin to below 25 g/L.

Effect: Blistering usually resolves within 2–3 months, skin fragility within 6–9 months and porphyrin concentrations generally normalize within 13 months.

- **Low dose antimalarial**, HCQS 100 mg twice a week or chloroquine 250 mg twice a week.
- **Erythropoietin** mobilizes hepatic iron into hemoglobin and is the treatment of choice for PCT in renal failure where patients are too anemic for venesection and cannot excrete chloroquine.

  Ledipasvir/sofosbuvir (and likely other direct-acting antivirals) is an effective treatment for HCV in the presence of PCT and leads to clinical remission of PCT without additional phlebotomy or low-dose hydroxychloroquine treatment (Bonkovsky HL).
- Normal lifespan with clinical and biochemical remission achievable with treatment; premature death with hepatocellular carcinoma.

CONGENITAL ERYTHROPOIETIC PORPHYRIA (GUNTHER'S DISEASE)

Defect: AR deficiency of uroporphyrinogen/III cosynthetase (UROS) → overproduction of uroporphyrin I and coporphyrin I in erythrocytes, plasma, urine, and feces.

Also XLR mutation in GATA1 (transcription factor that regulates expression of UROS).

Clinical Features

First feature is child's mother noting brown discoloration of amniotic fluid at the onset of labor, or observing pink or brown porphyrin staining of nappies.

Cutaneous Features

- Photosensitivity with blistering, scarring, mutilating cutaneous deformity, *sclerodermatous changes*, hypertrichosis, dyschromia, and alopecia **(Fig. 13.29)**.
- Red urine noted during infancy due to porphyrins, which are excited by visible light at 400–410 nm (Soret band) and emit a red fluorescence.

Systemic

- Splenomegaly, cholelithiasis, hypersplenism and hemolytic anemia
- Pathologic fractures, osteopenia, vertebral compression, and contractures of fingers
- Conjunctivitis and corneal scarring
- A milder late-onset form, presenting at any age from the third decade onward, mimics PCT.

Investigations

- Erythrodontia → teeth fluoresce under Wood's lamp examination
- ↑urinary/erythrocyte uroporphyrin I;
- ↑urinary and fecal coproporphyrinogen I and uroporphyrinogen I.

Treatment

- Photoprotection
- Hypertransfusion with regular blood transfusions to maintain a polycythemia inhibits endogenous hemoglobin production and decreases porphyrin formation.

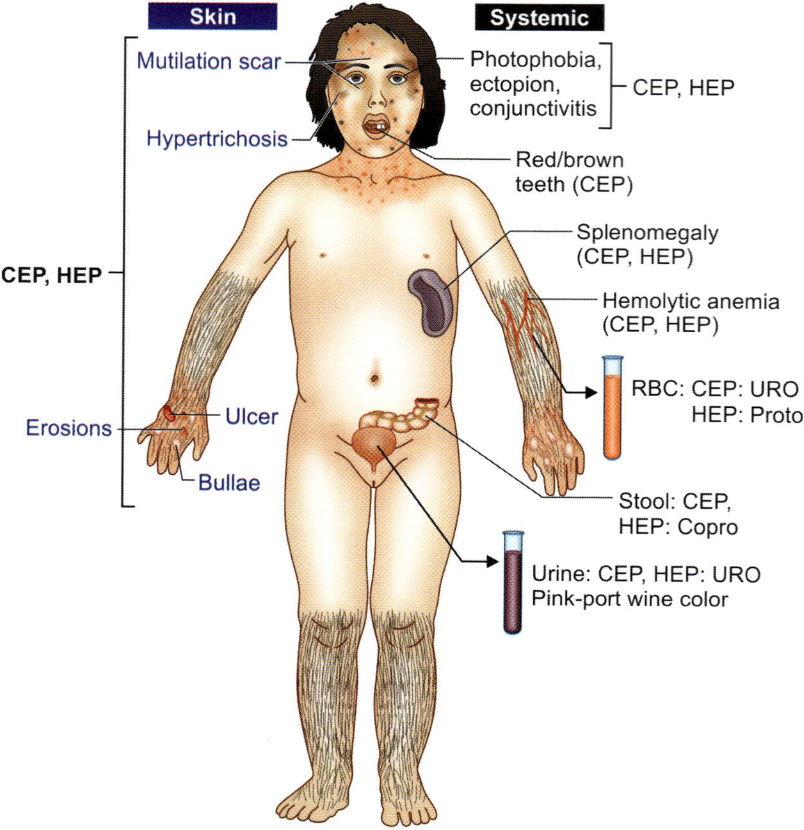

Fig. 13.29: Artistic depiction of CEP and HEP

- Allogeneic bone marrow transplantation (bone marrow or umbilical cord blood stem cells) from an HLA compatible donor has emerged as the treatment of choice in severe CEP.
- Genetic counselling: For parents of an affected child, the chance of each future offspring suffering from the disease is 25%.

ERYTHROPOIETIC PROTOPORPHYRIA

Most common form of porphyria seen in children, AD (rarely AR).

Defect: Caused by *ferrochelatase mutations*.

Clinical Features

Skin

- First year, babies usually present with crying in their prams in sunny weather, or crying for no obvious reason at night in the summer.
- Usually becomes symptomatic between 1 and 6 years of age.

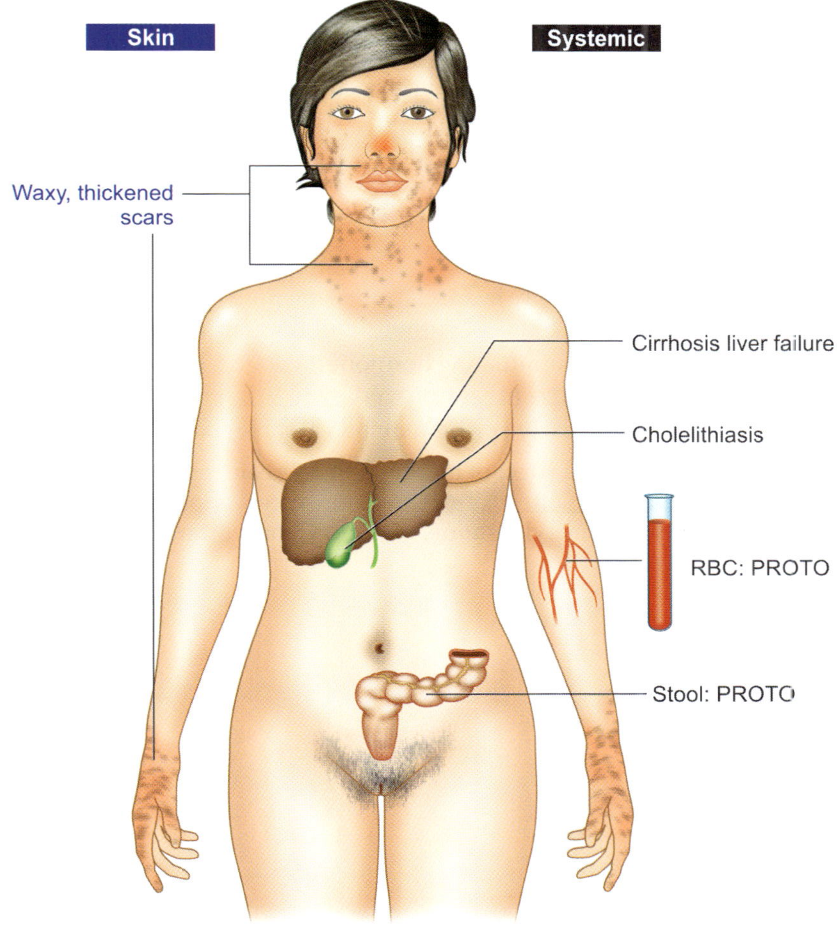

Fig. 13.30: A depiction of erythropoietic protoporphyria

- Early: Manifests as *burning/stinging/itching* 5–30 minutes post-sunlight exposure. The pain lasts for about 24 hours after outdoor exposure. The children learn to put ice on skin to relieve burning and stinging.
- Pruritic erythematous/edematous plaques that last 1–2 days post-sunlight exposure. Hypo-/hyperpigmentation, photo-onycholysis.
- Late: Shallow *linear pits* may develop on the face, alongwith a waxy, thickened scarring over nose, face, back of hands **(Fig. 13.30)**.

Systemic

- Hemolytic anemia and mild hypertriglyceridemia may be seen.
- Cholelithiasis; protoporphyrin accumulation in the liver may cause hepatotoxicity and progressive hepatic dysfunction.

Investigations

- Plasma porphyrin level and fluorescence spectrum
- Increased free protoporphyrin in red blood cells, stool
- CBC, liver function tests
- Liver/gallbladder scans if symptomatic.

Treatment

- Strict photoprotection.
- Oral β-carotene (around 180 mg daily in adults) or (90 mg daily in children) taken throughout the spring and summer (critical to take synthetic and not natural carotene.)
- **Afamelanotide**, the melanocyte stimulating hormone analogue, has shown promising results in initial trials in EPP patients (recently approved by FDA).
- Narrowband UVB used in the early spring may be valuable, particularly in milder cases.

Trials show a moderate positive effect of inorganic sunscreen application and subcutaneous implant of afamelanotide and no effect of organic sunscreen application, or oral treatment with beta-carotene, cysteine, N-acetylcysteine, vitamin C, or warfarin. [Heerfordt IM]

PALMOPLANTAR KERATODERMA

Palmoplantar keratodermas form a heterogeneous group of hereditary or acquired disorders defined by excessive epidermal thickening of the palms and soles.

A very useful way of classifying it is as syndromic and nonsyndromic PPK and is detailed in **Table 13.14**.

Definitions

1. **Diffuse keratodermas**, the whole of the palmar or plantar epidermis, usually including the centripalmar skin and the instep, is uniformly thickened **(Fig. 13.31a)**.
2. **Focal, areate or nummular keratoderma**, the areas of palmoplantar skin under most pressure are disproportionately thickened.
3. **Striate keratoderma** overlaps clinically with focal keratoderma, but the lesions are conspicuously longitudinal, particularly on the fingers, where keratoderma overlies flexor tendons.

TABLE 13.14: Classification of PPK

Diffuse	Nonsyndromic	• Epidermolytic palmoplantar keratoderma (EPPK) • Nonepidermolytic palmoplantar keratoderma (NEPPK) – Mal de Meleda – Type Gamborg–Nielsen – Type Nagashima – Type Bothnia – Type Kimonis • Loricrin keratoderma (LK)
	Syndromic	• Vohwinkel syndrome • Mitochondrial PPK with hearing impairment • Clouston syndrome • Papillon–Lefèvre syndrome • Olmsted syndrome (OLS)
Localized	Nonsyndromic	• Pachyonychia congenita (PC) **(Fig. 13.31b)** • Striate • Punctate palmoplantar keratoderma (PPPK) • Cole disease (CD)—punctate keratoderma with irregularly shaped hypopigmented macules • Spiny keratoderma (SK) • Marginal papular keratoderma (MPK)* • Transient aquagenic keratoderma (TAK)**
	Syndromic	• Carvajal-Huerta syndrome • Huriez syndrome • Howel-Evans syndrome • Richner-Hanhart syndrome • Tyrosinemia

*Marginal keratoderma (2 types—hereditary type (acrokeratoelastoidosis) and focal acral HK)

TAK = typically shows a subtle keratoderma appearing after a few minutes of immersion of their hands in water sweating. Characteristic sign might be that patients bring with them a vessel to immerse their hands in water ('hands in the bucket**' sign)

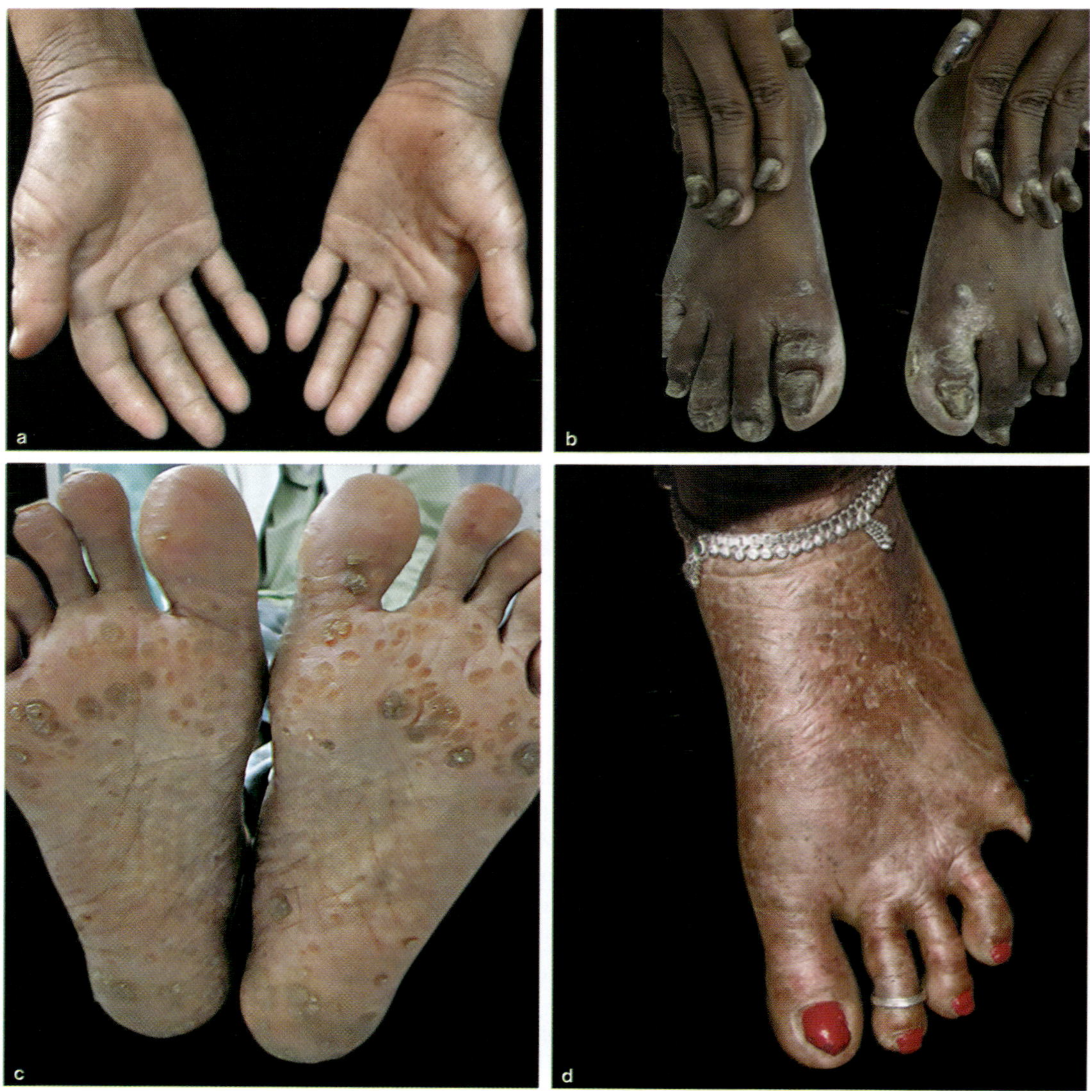

Fig. 13.31: (a) Diffuse keratoderma with extension beyond the palms; (b) Pachyonychia congenita in a child; (c) Punctate palmoplantar keratoderma; (d) Keratoderma with transgradiens and pseudoainhum

4. **Punctate**, papular or disseminated keratoderma consists of multiple scattered discrete round lesions **(Fig. 13.31c)**.
5. **Transgradient** keratoderma extends beyond palmoplantar skin, contiguously or as callosities on pressure points on the fingers or knuckles, or elsewhere **(Fig. 13.31a)**.
6. **Cicatrizing keratodermas** ('mutilating') are those in which constricting bands appear around digits. 'Pseudoainhum' can be found in many severe transgradient keratodermas **(Fig. 13.31d)** and the different types are listed in **Box 13.9**.

BOX 13.9: Inherited skin diseases and pseudoainhum

Keratodermas
- Vohwinkel syndrome (and Bart–Pumphrey syndrome)
- Clouston syndrome
- Mal de Meleda
- Papillon–Lefèvre syndrome
- Olmsted syndrome
- Loricrin keratoderma or KLICK (less common and severe than in Vohwinkel syndrome)

Generalized MeDOC
- Lamellar ichthyosis
- Erythrokeratoderma variabilis
  - Inherited epidermolysis bullosa
- Chronic epidermolysis bullosa
- Kindler syndrome

Others
- Tuberous sclerosis
- Erythropoietic protoporphyria

- The syndromic variants have been divided on the basis of the various organs involved and they are listed in **Box 13.10**. PPK can also be associated with other disorders including, *cancer* (Huriez syndrome), *ectodermal dysplasia*, *ichthyosis* and epidermolysis bullosa.

BOX 13.10: An overview of syndromic PPK

	Types, inheritance, gene
PPK with hearing impairment	• Vohwinkel syndrome AD, GJB2 • Bart–Pumphrey syndrome AD, GJB2 • PPK with deafness AD, GJB2
PPK with mucosal involvement	• Haim–Munk syndrome AR, CTSC • Papillon–Lefèvre syndrome AR, CTSC • Focal PPK and gingival keratosis AD, unknown • Howel–Evans syndrome AD, RHBDF2 (iRHOM2) • Multiple self-healing palmoplantar carcinoma
PPK with cardiomyopathy and woolly hair	• Naxos disease, AR, JUP • Carvajal syndrome, AR, DSP Carvajal syndrome with tooth agenesis AD DSP • Arrhythmogenic right ventricular dysplasia, with mild palmoplantar keratoderma and woolly hair, AR, DSC2
Others	• Tyrosinemia type II (Richner-Hanhart syndrome), AR, TAT • SAM syndrome AR DSG1/DSP • PPK with squamous cell carcinomas and 46, XX sex reversal/ true hermaphroditism, AR, RSPO1 • Aquagenic keratoderma, AR, AD

Clinical Overview

For the clinician and students, a description of PPK can be an onerous task. Thus we have detailed the main aspects of the commonly seen disorders in **Tables 13.15** and **13.16**. Most of them seem to overlap with other similar disorders, but some are unique.

One of the most common type is NEEPK in which the defect lies in *Aquaporins* which are a family of cell membrane proteins that allow the osmotic movement of water across the cell membrane. AQP5 is localized to the plasma membrane of the keratinocytes of the stratum granulosum. Nagashima PPK (NPPK) is an autosomal recessive disorder almost exclusively observed in Asia and caused by nonsense mutations in the SERPINB7 gene.

Variants: NEPPK type Nagashima, NEPPK type Bothnia, NEPPK type Kimonis, Mal de Meleda, type Gamborg-Nielsen Greither (Greither keratoderma is not considered as a clearly defined entity.)

An approach to the diagnosis of PPK is depicted in **Flowchart 13.3**.

TABLE 13.15: Overview of diffuse variant of PPK

Type	Gene/ inheritance	Onset	TG	Clinical/histopathology	R_x
Vörner Epidermolytic PPK **(EPPK)**	• KRT1 KRT9 • AD	0–3 years	X	• **Most common PPK** • **Disabling pain**: 'Tonotubular' PPK • Limited transgradient lesions • Epidermolytic change in suprabasal keratinocytes—**'tonotubules'** (ultrastructure may reveal the peculiar finding of whorls of keratins containing tubular structures)	Keratolytic Acitretin
Unna-Thost Nonepi-dermolytic PPK **(NEPPK)**	• KRT1 KRT6 AQp5 • AD	2–5 years	+/–	• **Second most common PPK** • **Hyperhidrosis** • Dermatophyte infections and pitted keratolysis • Histology with prominent orthokeratosis	• Keratolytic • Systemic acitretin (0.2–0.5 mg/kg) • Erythromycin • Tacrolimus
Mal de Meleda Nonepi-dermolytic PPK (NEPPK) **(Fig. 13.32)**	• SLURP-1 • AR	0–3 years	+	• Atopic dermatitis • PPK erythematous with fissures/ hyperhidrosis/maceration/**horrible odor**/ often infected	• Acitretin • Surgery
Mutilating PPK (Vohwinkel) (Fig. 13.33)	• GJB2 (Connexin 26) • AD	Child-hood		• **Starfish keratoses** on the knuckles/ feet/elbows/knees, linear keratoses on elbows/knees, sensorineural deafness (Connexin26) • Generalized ichthyosis (loricrin) • Alopecia, nail dystrophy (sporadic), hyperhidrosis • Mild to moderate sensorineural hearing loss • Progradiens +	• Isotretinoin • Inhibitors of VEGF receptor 2 • Acitretin • Surgical release of cicatricial bands

(Contd.)

TABLE 13.15: Overview of diffuse variant of PPK *(Contd.)*

Type	Gene/ inheritance	Onset	TG	Clinical/histopathology	R_x
Loricin Keratoderma	• LOR (+) • Loricrin ichthyosis	Child-hood		• **Honeycombed** palmar PPK, • **Pseudoainhum** (especially fifth finger –constriction bands → auto-amputation)	Isotretinoin
Papillon-Lefèvre syndrome (Fig. 13.34)	• CTSC (Cathepsin C) • AR	Birth to early infancy	+	• Bad odor (soles > palms) • **Pyogenic infections—periodontitis/ gingivitis** >premature loss of teeth • Psoriasiform lesions on elbows/knees • Diffuse or focal (friction-related), yellowish or reddish-yellow hyperkeratosis, hyperhidrosis • Severe periodontitis, premature loss of deciduous and permanent teeth, intracranial calcifications, mild mental retardation	Good response to retinoids, combination with antibiotics and dental care lessen the gingival inflammation and save the teeth
Naxos disease	• JUP • Plakoglobin • AR (orAD)	Infancy	X	• Diffuse keratoderma • **Woolly hair**; arrhythmias and **right ventricular cardiomyopathy** develop during adolescence	

TG, transgradience

Flowchart 13.3: Approach to the diagnosis of PPK

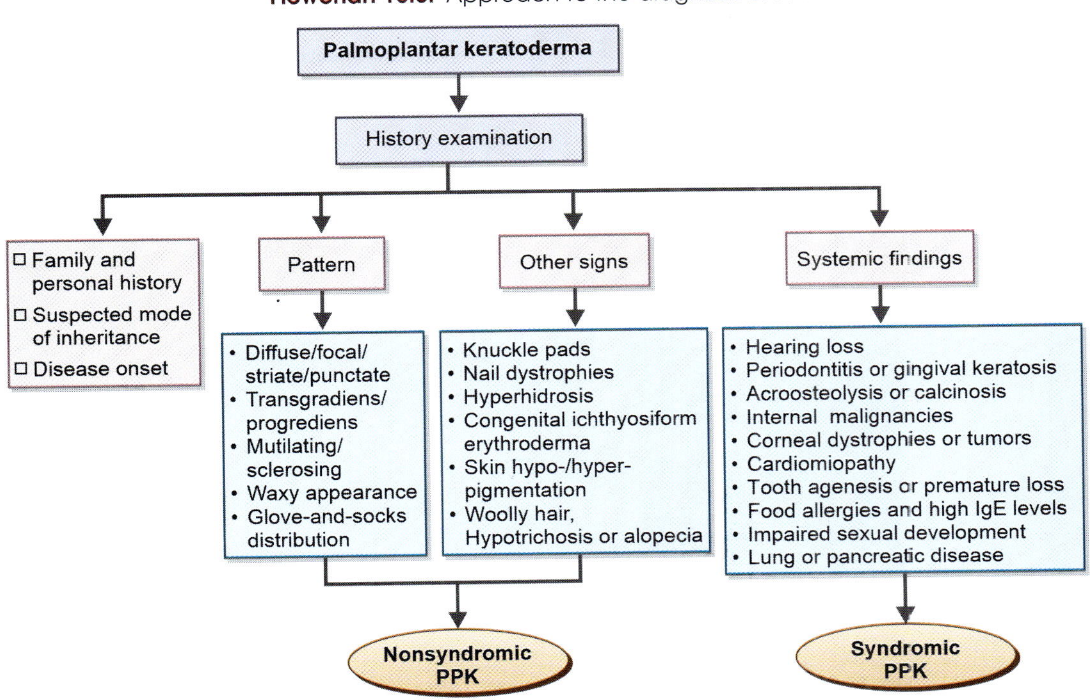

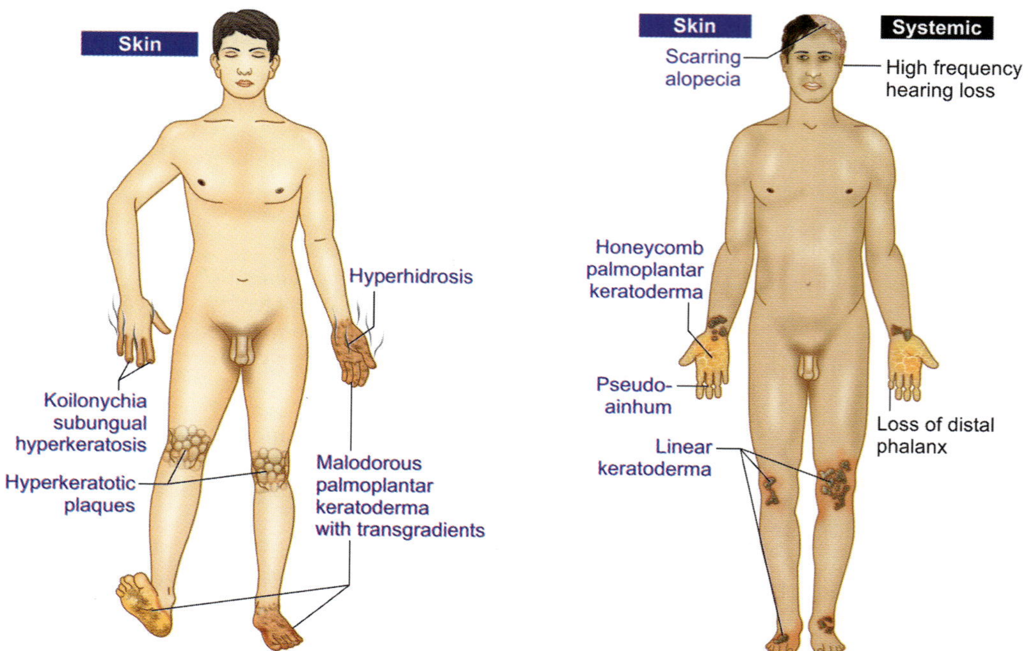

Figs 13.32 and 13.33: Overview of NEPPK (Mal de Meleda) and Vohwinkel (PPK)—both diffuse forms of PPK

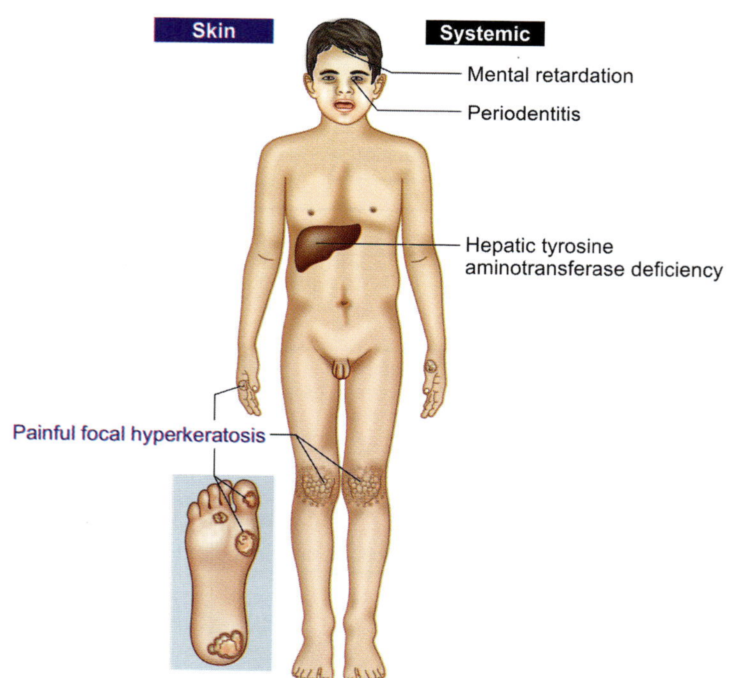

Fig. 13.34: A depiction of Papillon-Lefèvre syndrome (diffuse PPK)

Treatment

Treatment is not curative but the essentials of therapy are listed below:

- Daily bathing and professional foot and hand care is helpful for mechanical scale removal (e.g. with pumice stone) in some PPK types.
- Regular application of emollients (white petrolatum), keratolytics (urea, salicylic acid) and wet dressings may be used to control hyperkeratosis.
- Topical corticosteroids are useful to reduce inflammation, when present.
- Hyperhidrosis may respond to aluminum chloride containing products.
- Local infections should be treated by antifungal and antibacterial drugs.
- Iontophoresis and botulinum toxin have been reported to alleviate symptoms in PPK caused or exacerbated by water exposure.
- Acitretin can be used but not in epidermolytic PPK.
- Proper footwear is indicated for pain relief during everyday activity.
- EGFR Signaling Holds Promise for Treating Palmoplantar Keratodermas and has been tried for the treatment of pachyonychia congenita.

TABLE 13.16: Overview of localized variants of PPK

Type	Gene/ inheritance	Onset	TG	Clinical	Treatment
• Striate/focal type • Striate palmoplantar keratodermas (SPPK)	• DSG1-SPPK1 • DSP-SPPK2 • KRT1-SPPK3	4–10 years	X	• **Striate hyperkeratosis** on the flexure sites of fingers and palms, more diffuse and focal changes on the soles; triggered by manual work/mechanical stress • **Disadhesion of keratinocytes**	Acitretin Urea
Richner–Hanhart syndrome (tyrosinemia type II, oculo-cutaneously-rosinemia) **(Fig. 13.35)**	• TAT (tyrosine amino-transferase) • AR	• Infancy (ocular) • Early childhood to adole-scence (skin)	X	• **Focal painful PPK** on weight-bearing areas • **Eye:** Dendritic keratitis, corneal ulcers, and blindness (ocular findings prior to skin findings) • Hyperkeratosis of **elbows/knees** • Mental retardation	
Pachyonychia congenita (Fig. 13.36)	• KRT16 KRT6A KRT17 KRT6B AD	Infancy to early childhood	X	PC1: More severe NEPPK PC2: Steatocystoma multiplex and eruptive vellus hair cysts more common; natal teeth • **Three** clinical features are reported in more than 90% of patients across all mutation subtypes: **Toenail dystrophy**, **plantar keratoderma** and **plantar pain** which in patients older than 3 years are highly diagnostic for PC	EGFR inhibitor **erlotinib** or **lapati-nib**, a dual EGFR (Her1)/ Her2 × Her2 have been found to be useful.

(Contd.)

TABLE 13.16: Overview of localized variants of PPK *(Contd.)*

Type	Gene/ inheritance	Onset	TG	Clinical	Treatment
Howel–Evans syndrome (tylosis with esophageal cancer)	• RHBDF2/ IRHOM2 • AD	Childhood	X	• Thick yellow PPK on weight bearing areas (heels and balls of feet) starting in second decade • Significant risk for development of esophageal cancer in third to fifth decade	
Aquagenic acrokeratoderma (Fig. 13.37)	• AR, AD • CFTR	Late adolescence to adulthood	X	• Transient, symmetrical whitish or yellowish translucent hyperkeratotic papules and plaques on hands and rarely on feet after water exposure (hand-in-the-bucket sign) • Acral hyperhidrosis, pruritus, burning, tingling, pain or discomfort • Cystic fibrosis	Oral oxybutynin 5 mg/d

TG: Transgradient

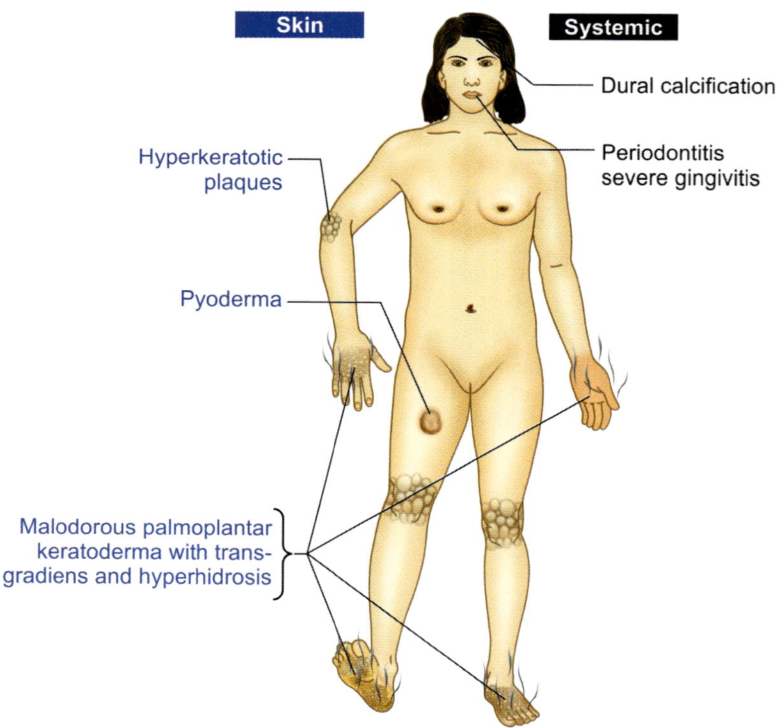

Fig. 13.35: Artistic depiction of Richner–Hanhart syndrome

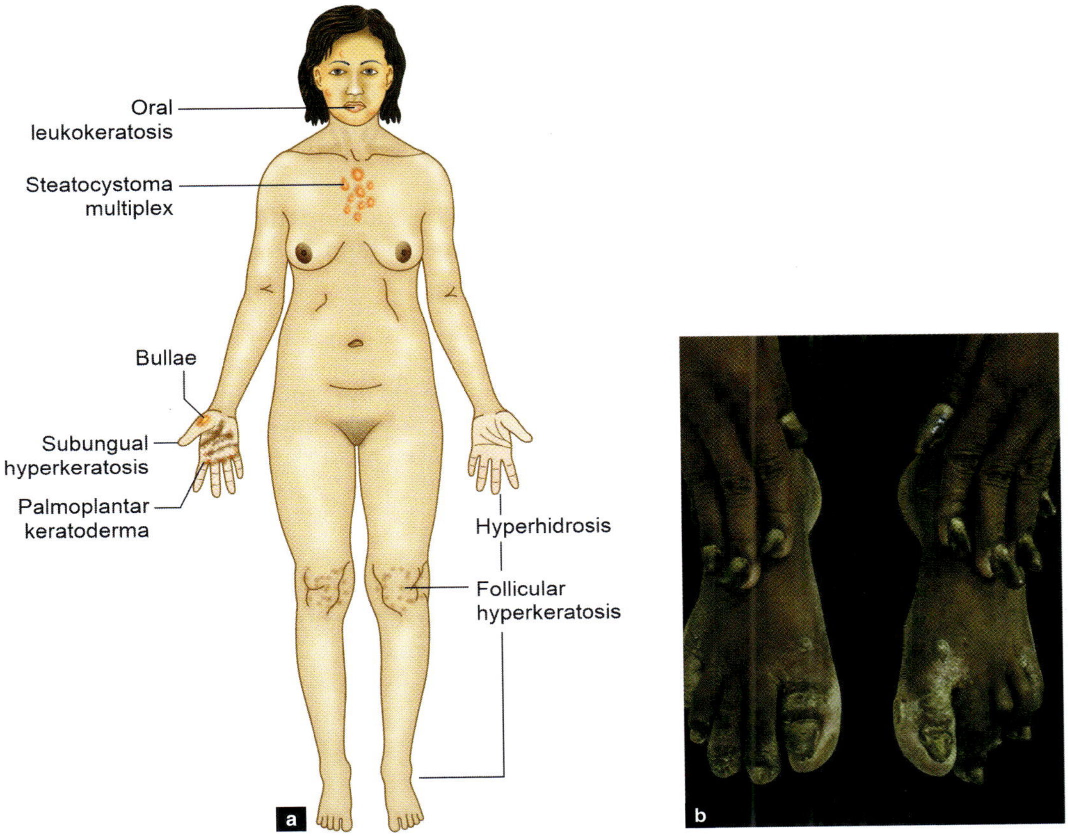

Oral leukokeratosis
Steatocystoma multiplex
Bullae
Subungual hyperkeratosis
Palmoplantar keratoderma
Hyperhidrosis
Follicular hyperkeratosis
a
b

Fig. 13.36: (a) Artistic depiction of pachyonychia congenita; (b) Pachyonychia congenita in a child

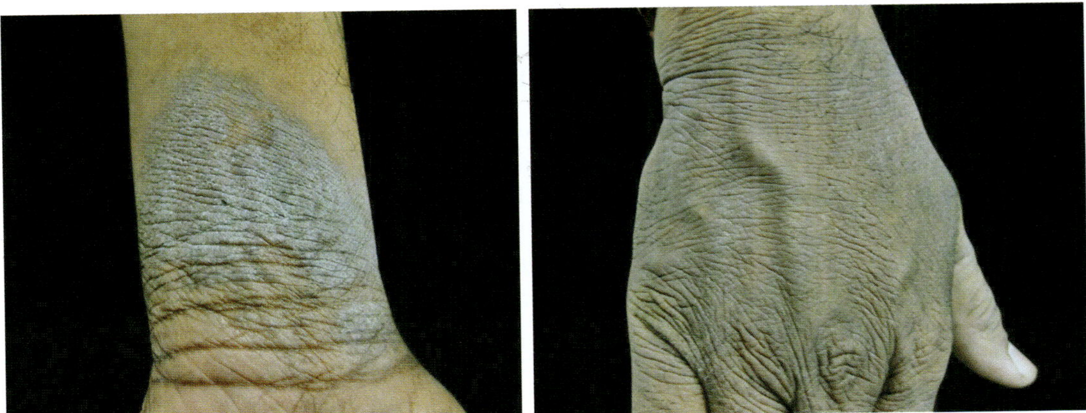

Fig. 13.37: Aquagenic acrokeratoderma in which transient whitening of skin is seen on immersion in water (atypical aquagenic keratoderma treated with oxybutynin chloride. An Brcs Dermatol. 2018 Mar;93(2):308–309)

PREMATURE AGING SYNDROME

These can be of 3 types:

1. **DNA repair defects:** Bloom syndrome, Werner syndrome and Xeroderma pigmentosum.
2. **Progeroid laminopathies:** Hutchinson–Gilford syndrome, mandibuloacral dysplasia.
3. **Elastic fiber defects:** Cutis laxa.
4. **Others:** Cockayne syndrome, trichothiodystrophy, Hallermann-Streiff syndrome, restrictive dermopathy, neonatal progeria syndrome (Wiedemann–Rautenstrauch syndrome).

PROGERIA

Hutchinson–Gilford Progeria Syndrome (HGPS)

Progeria is derived from the Greek word *geras*, meaning old age, and is the commonest of the progeria syndromes. It is a segmental aging syndrome as some of the other typical features of aging, such as cataracts, presbycusis, presbyopia, increased incidence of cancer and dementia do *not occur*.

Defect

- AD disorder caused by specific mutation (1824 C → T) in the **LMNA gene** (encodes lamin A)
- **Lamin A** protein contributes to the structure/function of the nuclear envelope
- Mutation introduces a splice site that results in the protein being abnormally *farnesylated*.
- With **abnormal farnesylation**, lamina cannot insert normally into the nuclear envelope.
- This results in genomic instability, decreased cell proliferation and premature cell senescence and death.

Clinical Features

A. **Cutaneous manifestations begin around 6–18 months (Fig. 13.38)**
   - Localized sclerodermatous changes of lower trunk/thigh.
   - Cyanosis around mouth or nasolabial folds.
   - Dyspigmentation.
   - Facial features: Enlarged head (**the head appears large for the face and scalp veins are prominent**, made more noticeable due to alopecia which may be partial or total, and which may also affect the eyebrows and eyelashes). The eyes tend to be prominent, the lips are thin and may have surrounding cyanosis, and earlobes may be absent. The facial appearance is reminiscent of a **"fledgling bird"**.
   - Also have failure to thrive.
   - Overtime, patients show signs of premature aging.
   - Other dermatologic manifestations: Lipodystrophy, onychodystrophy, and breast hypoplasia.

B. **Systemic**
   - Atherosclerosis and angina.
   - Bone density loss/osteoporosis (with susceptibility to fractures), coxa valga, and osteolysis of distal phalanges, **'horse-riding'** stance.
     - *A high-pitched voice* is characteristic.

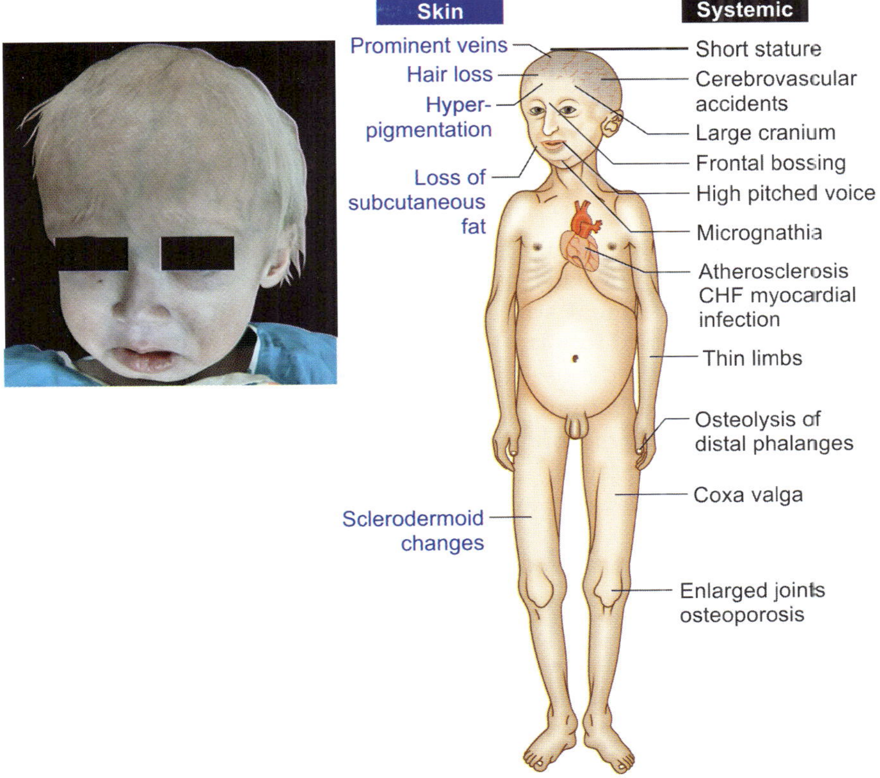

Fig. 13.38: A depiction of cutaneous features in progeria. The image on the left shows the face of a child with loss of hair, prominent veins, gray hair-visible signs of progeria (*Courtesy*: Dr Mala Bhalla, GMC, Chandigarh)

- Rapid and progressive features of *premature aging develop*—complications include cerebrovascular and cardiovascular events (CHF and MI), limited mobility and exercise tolerance, and poor growth.
- Complications of cardiovascular disease are the most common cause of mortality (mean age of death = 13 years) (range of 6–20 years).
- Death usually results from myocardial infarction, heart failure or stroke.

Pathology

Skin shows atrophy of epidermis and dermis, progressive hyalinization of dermal collagen and loss of subcutaneous fat.

Investigations

- 6–12-monthly growth, cardiovascular, neurological, musculoskeletal, dental, ear and eye assessments.
- Annual—lipids, electrocardiogram, echocardiogram, carotid duplex scanning, hip X-rays and bone densitometry scans.

Treatment

Management

1st Line: Infants and children may experience feeding difficulties and failure to thrive and require advice regarding nutrition. Measures to reduce the risk of atherosclerotic disease are important. Early input from physiotherapy and occupational therapy should be arranged to help reduce the complications of arthritis.

2nd Line: A clinical trial of a farnesyl transferase inhibitor, lonafarnib, improved weight gain, vascular stiffness, bone structure and audiological status in affected children. This drug Zokinvy™ received FDA approval in Nov 2020 and can help prolong the life span of patients.

A wide spectrum of treatment strategies, targeting several processes with different specificities, has been proposed to correct the defects in HGPS **(Fig. 13.39)**:

i. To directly "repair" the disease-causing mutation;
ii. To inhibit pre-mRNA aberrant splicing leading to progerin mRNA production;
iii. To decrease the toxicity of isoprenylated and methylated progerin;
iv. To induce progerin clearance;
v. To decrease the noxious downstream effects linked to progerin accumulation.

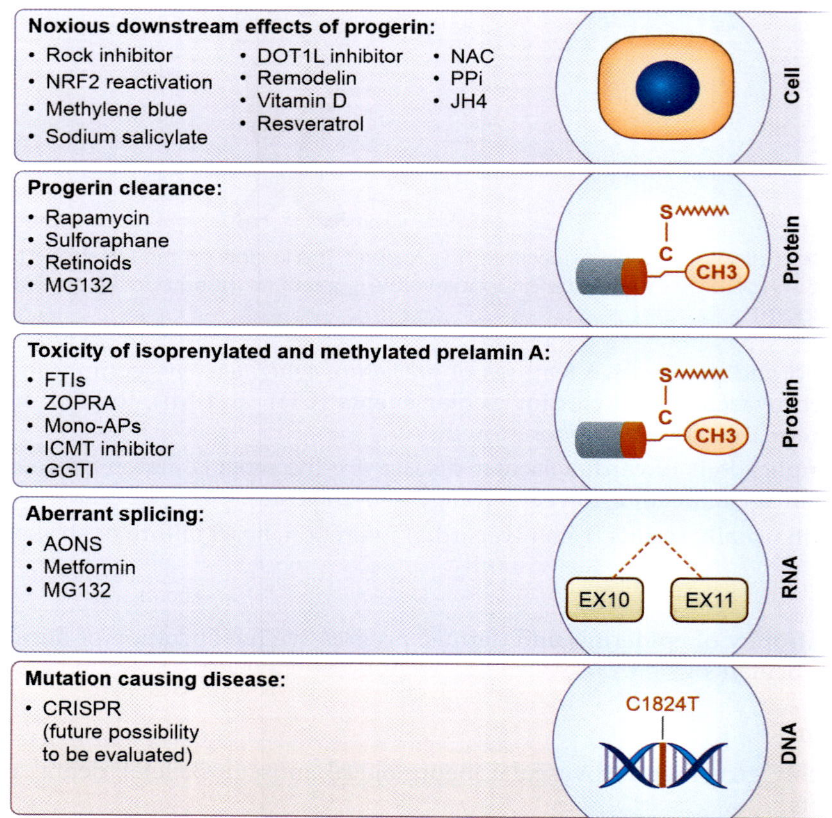

Fig. 13.39: Overview of various defects and the possible treatments in progeria (Harhari K, et al., 2018)

WERNER SYNDROME (PANGERIA)

Defect: AR disorder as a result of mutations in the **RECQL2**/WRN gene (encodes a DNA helicase that helps maintain genomic stability):

- Mutations in RECQL2/WRN →↑ expression of inhibitors of DNA synthesis and → telomere-driven replicative senescence → accelerated aging.
- Tissues of mesenchymal origin are preferentially affected compared with tissues of neural origin, thus they do not have neurological involvement such as Alzheimer or Parkinson diseases.

Clinical Features

- Children with Werner syndrome generally have normal growth and development **until puberty (Fig. 13.40)**.
- Symptoms/signs seen in second or third decade.
- **Cutaneous findings:** Premature canities, progressive alopecia, bird-like facial appearance, sclerodermatous/atrophic change acrally/facially, mottled pigmentation, telangiectases, hyperkeratotic ulcers over pressure points, leg ulcers, calcinosis cutis, and loss of subcutaneous fat.

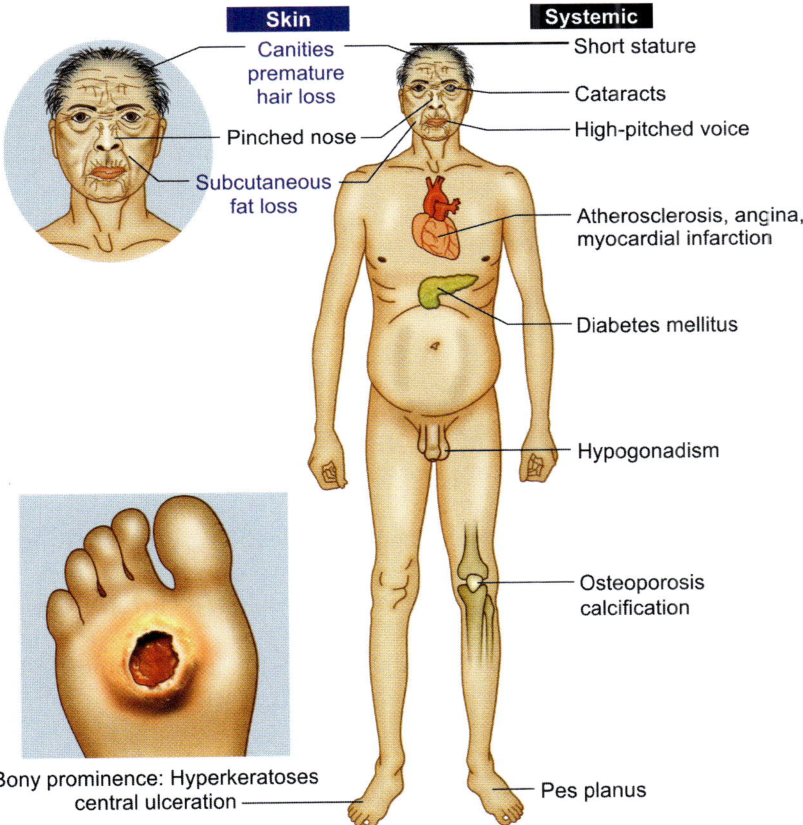

Fig. 13.40: A depiction of the clinical features of pangeria

- **Extracutaneous findings:** Short stature, muscle wasting, **atherosclerosis** (can cause CVA/MI), diabetes mellitus, hypogonadism, osteoporosis, arthritis, posterior subcapsular cataracts, DM2, and hypogonadism. A high pitched or hoarse voice **from thinning of the vocal cords and fixation of the epiglottis is characteristic**.
- ↑**Risk of malignancy:** Most frequent tumors are thyroid carcinomas (16.1%), carcinoma of breast or ovary, thyroid adenocarcinoma, fibrosarcoma, osteogenic sarcoma, meningioma, skin cancers, and hepatoma.
- Malignancy and cerebrovascular/cardiovascular events are main causes of mortality (mid-50s typically).

Differential Diagnosis

This includes progeria, Rothmund-Thomson syndrome, systemic sclerosis and Huriez syndrome.

Treatment

Abnormal cellular phenotype in Werner's syndrome might be amenable to treatment with mitogen-activated protein **(MAP) kinase inhibitors or rapamycin**.

BLOOM SYNDROME (CONGENITAL TELANGIECTATIC ERYTHEMA)

Defect: AR disorder due to mutations in BLM/**RECQL3** (DNA helicase) →↑rates of sister chromatid exchange and chromosomal instability. *Seen* more commonly in Ashkenazi Jews.

Clinical Features

- Presents early in life with prenatal and postnatal growth impairment (short stature; do not exceed 5 feet in height) **(Fig. 13.41)**.
- **Cutaneous manifestations:** Photosensitivity, telangiectatic erythema in a malar distribution, cheilitis, CALM, and hypopigmentation.
- Facies: Narrow face with prominent ears, malar hypoplasia, and prominent/bird-like nose. The limbs tend to be long with large hands and feet, and there may be reduced subcutaneous fat.
- **Systemic:**
  - Primary hypogonadism (men are sterile, women have decreased fertility).
    (Although the tubular elements of the testes function poorly, the androgen-secreting portions are spared, thus permitting normal puberty).
  - High-pitched voice.
  - Gastroesophageal reflux is also common and may lead to aspiration, contributing to the risk of chronic lung disease.
  - ↓**IgA** and **IgM** → bronchiectasis/chronic lung disease/recurrent respiratory and GI infections.
  - ↑Risk of **lymphoma and leukemia** (150–300-fold ↑risk), ↑risk of some solid tissue tumors (squamous cell carcinomas and adenocarcinomas [especially GI].

Prognosis

Cutaneous and immunologic findings improve with age, but ↑risk of mortality from malignancy (most common cause of death, especially leukemia) in the second to third decades; patients do not survive beyond 50 years.

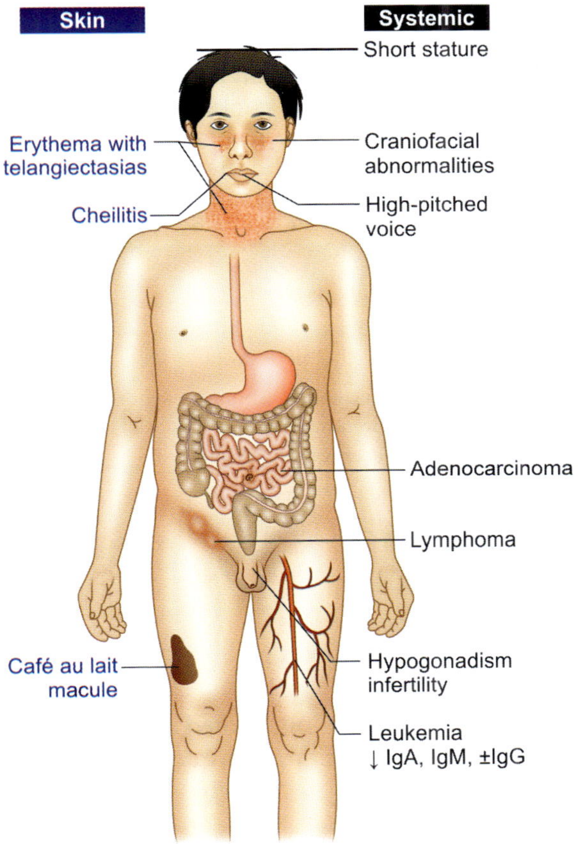

Fig. 13.41: A depiction of the clinical features of Bloom syndrome

Diagnosis

- A characteristic pattern of chromosomal breakage and rearrangement may be seen on chromosomal instability testing, which can be performed at specialized centers.
- Immunoglobulin levels.

Differential Diagnosis

- Cockayne syndrome
- Rothmund–Thomson syndrome
- Lupus erythematosus
- Erythropoietic protoporphyria.

Treatment

Referral to dermatologist—diagnosis, sun protection.

Referral to pediatric infectious disease specialist, hematologist/oncologist, endocrinologist, antibiotics, carcinoma surveillance, short stature management.

DNA REPAIR DISORDERS

The human genome is made up of about 3 billion DNA base pairs containing an estimated 30,000 protein-encoding genes. This DNA is continually being damaged by a variety of endogenous sources (such as reactive oxygen species) and exogenous sources (such as ultraviolet and ionizing radiation). There are multiple elaborate mechanisms to avoid this damage and defects in these DNA repair pathways result in a number of disorders **(Table 13.17)**.

TABLE 13.17: DNA repair disorders

Nucleotide excision repair	• **Xeroderma pigmentosum** • Cockayne syndrome • Trichothiodystrophy
Recombination Q helicase	• **Rothmund–Thomson syndrome** • **Bloom syndrome** • **Werner's syndrome**
Double strand break repair	Ataxia telangiectasia
Interstrand cross-link repair	Fanconi anemia
Mismatch repair	Muir–Torre syndrome

Note: Those in bold are important for examinees.

XERODERMA PIGMENTOSUM (XP)

The term xeroderma pigmentosum, means "pigmented dry skin".
In Indian and Middle Eastern areas, the incidence is quoted at one per 10,000–30,000.

Defect and Clinical Correlates

- AR disorder due to mutations in XPA to XPG genes (as well as variant XPV gene)—each gene encodes a protein important in the nucleotide excision repair pathway:
  The defect is in the nucleotide excision repair (NER) pathways and is of two types: **(Fig. 13.42)**
  a. Global genome nucleotide excision repair (GG-NER) in which damage to DNA not undergoing transcription is repaired.
  b. Transcription-coupled nucleotide excision repair (TC-NER) in which damage in transcribed regions of DNA is rapidly repaired.
- GG-NER can globally repair lesions in the genome, whereas TC-NER will only repair lesions on actively transcribed genes. The **subtypes** (7 complementation groups) of XP (XPA to XPG) correspond to the affected genes **either of nucleotide excision repair (NER) (XPA-XPG) or translesion synthesis (XPV)**.
  1. Steps unique to **GG-NER involve XPC and XPE**. Patients with defects in XPC and XPE show evidence of **freckling** but generally do **not** have an abnormal **sunburn reaction. However, they have highest increased risk of skin cancer**, which is thought to be at least partly attributable to the fact they do not have the adverse reaction to sun-light that would lead them to avoid sun exposure.

     Patients in the XPC complementation group have also recently been observed to have high sensitivity to ocular damage.

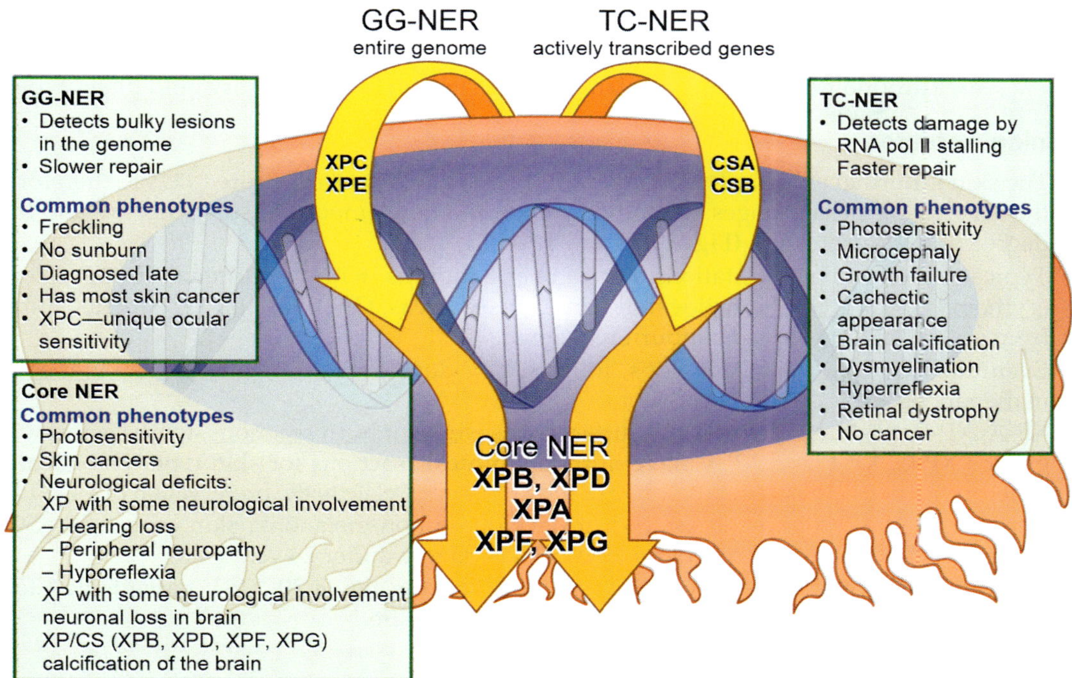

Fig. 13.42: Correlation of phenotypes with molecular deficits in xeroderma pigmentosum (XP). The two types of nucleotide excision repair (NER), global genome NER (GG-NER) and transcription-coupled NER (TC-NER), are shown. After initial recognition of the DNA damage, GG-NER and TC-NER both utilize a common pathway with core NER proteins for excision and repair

2. Steps unique to **TC-NER involve two genes** (CSA, CSB) involved in Cockayne syndrome (CS).
3. The core **NER proteins**, are utilized by both GG-NER and TC-NER, include **XPA, XPB, XPD, XPF and XPG**.
   Clinical features are of both GG-NER and TC-NER phenotypes, both skin cancer and neurological abnormalities.
4. XPV group have mutations in polymerase: Similarly to patients with XP who have mutations in proteins involved in the initial steps of GG-NER (XPC, XPE), patients in the XPV group do not present with abnormal sun-burn reactions and also show high susceptibility to developing skin cancer, albeit later in life.
5. A **summary** is given below:
   - Most common subtypes in the United States are XPA and XPC; XPA is most common subtype in Japan.
   - Broad range of neurological involvement in XP, including XP with some neurological features, XP with severe neurological features (which can be associated with mutations in XPA), and those with XP/CS complex common in Japan.
   - De Sanctis-Cacchione syndrome: Rare XP phenotype with severe neurologic deficits (severe mental retardation, deafness, at axia and paralysis). This term is no longer in general use as it is now appreciated that XP can be associated with neurological problems of widely varying severity.

- A subset of XPB and XPD mutations are known to cause trichothiodystrophy.
- A type of XPA group, ranging from 6 years to 79 years of age, originating from an area around north India, Pakistan and Afghanistan have only very mild phenotypes.

Clinical Features

- The skin is normal at birth. The changes in XP are the result of exposure to UVR, therefore, the severity of these changes is totally dependent on the amount of sun exposure and the degree of UVR protection **(Figs 13.43** and **13.44)**.
- Typical cutaneous manifestations appear *after* **6 months**, with development of persistent erythema, scaling, and ephelides on sun-exposed areas. Only **50%** of XP patients suffer from severe and prolonged sunburn reactions.
- Eventually poikiloderma develops, followed by development of numerous cutaneous malignancies.
- XP-A, XP-B, XP-D, XP-F and XP-G suffer from severe sunburn reactions, whereas those in groups **XP-C, XP-E and XP-V have normal sunburn** reactions for skin type. The normal sunburn reactions in approximately half of the XP patients relate to the preservation of TC-NER.
- Carcinoma: 10000-fold increased risk of developing non-melanoma skin cancer (NMSC) and a 2000-fold increased risk of melanoma skin cancer under 20 years old.
- XP-A to XP-G, generally develop skin cancer before the age of 20, XP-V patients develop their first skin cancers in the second or third decade of life.

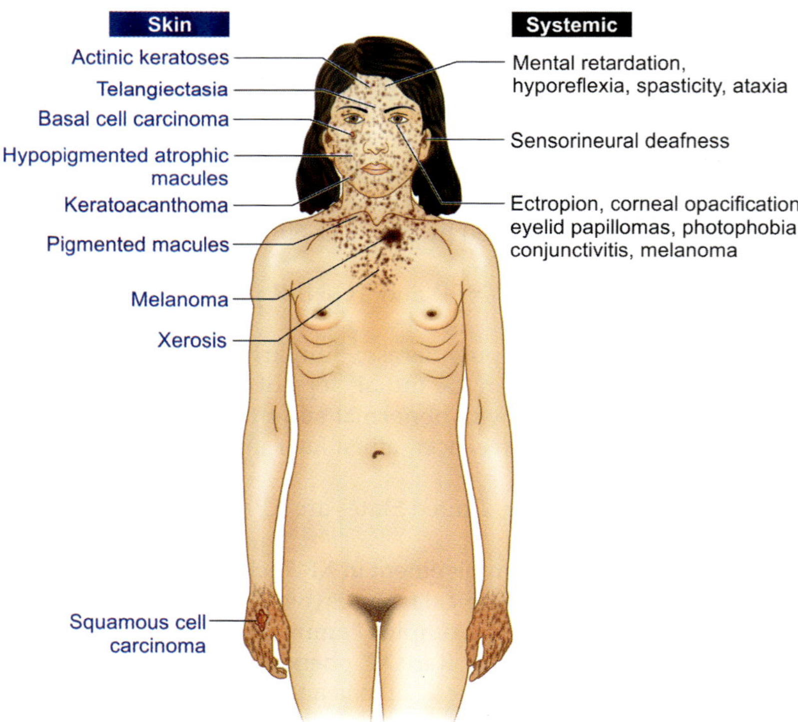

Fig. 13.43: A depiction of clinical features of xeroderma pigmentosum

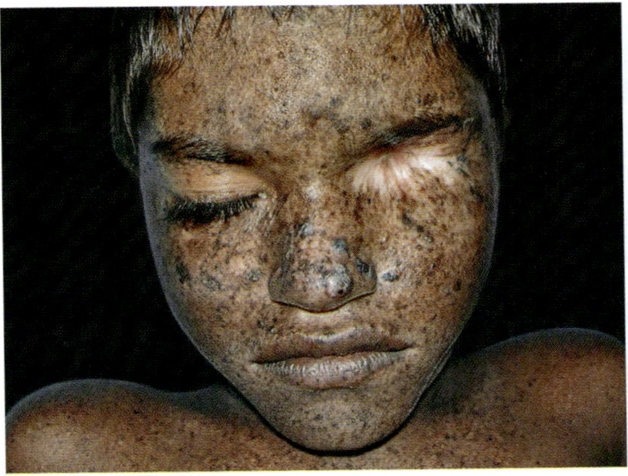
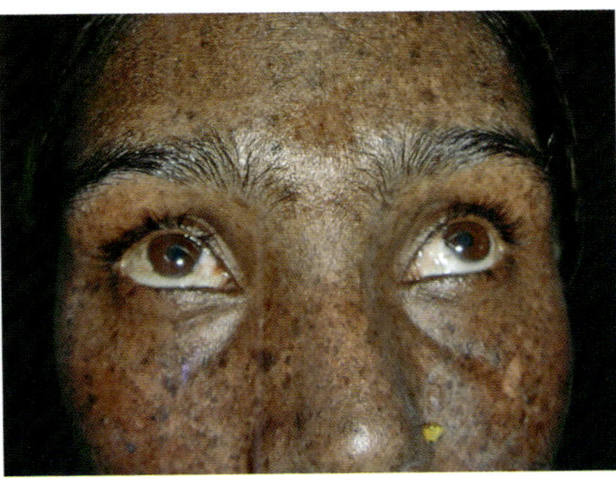

Fig. 13.44: A patient with XP showing freckles, lentigines, actinic keratosis, seborrheic keratosis, hypo-/hyperpigmentation, dry skin. If left untreated, NMSC often develops, with unfortunate sequelae as in the case on the left

- XP patients who have severe and exaggerated sunburn reactions generally have a lower frequency of skin cancer than those patients with sunburn reactions that are normal for skin type.
- Ophthalmologic complications: Photophobia, conjunctivitis, ectropion, and symblepharon.
- Neurodevelopmental complications, including developmental delay, intellectual impairment, sensorineural hearing loss, hyporeflexia, and/or ataxia occurs in 20–30% of XP patients (especially XPA and XPD groups) XPV patients have no neurologic complications.
- Severely affected individuals usually die as a result of complications from metastatic melanoma or invasive squamous cell carcinoma by ~20 years of age.

Disease Course and Prognosis

There is no cure for XP. The overall median age of death is reported as 32 years with skin cancer and neurodegeneration as the main causes of death. For those without neurological disease and rigorous UVR protection, the prognosis is good.

Treatment (Leung AK, 2022)

- Sun avoidance/limit outdoor activity to early morning, late afternoon and night;
- Photoprotect with physical block sunscreen, long-sleeve, long pants, frog skin clothing, wide-brimmed hat, UV-blocking glasses with side shields, long hairstyles.
- Dermatologic cancer screening every three months with weekly examination by informed parent.
- Removal of cutaneous neoplasms, cryotherapy, 5-fluorouracil, imiquimod.
- Oral isotretinoin, oral niacinamide, topical imiquimod and topical fluorouracil can be used for the prevention of skin malignancy (Leung AK, 2022).
  Topical Calcipotriol and Fluorouracil hs been used to prevent malignancies.
- Referral to ophthalmologist—corneal protection with methylcellulose drops, soft contact lens; corneal transplantation, regular cancer screening.
- Referral to neurologist if symptomatic.

Investigational therapies include the use of **T4 endonuclease-V liposome** lotion and **oral nicotinamide** to reduce the rate of actinic keratoses and nonmelanoma skin cancers and gene therapy for radical cure of this condition.

A summary of the various other agents that can be used in XP are listed below:

Target	Treatment
DNA repair defect	Liposomes of bacterial T4 endonuclease V or gene transfer,
Antibiotics	Gentamicin
Oral antioxidants	Coenzyme Q
Acetohexamide or glimepiride	Enhance viability after ultraviolet radiation
Caloric restriction	Enhances life span and attenuate neuron loss.
Nicotinamide (500 mg twice daily)	Promoted recovery of transcript expression after UVR exposure
Others	Oral isotretinoin, topical imiquimod, intralesional interferon-α, oral vismodegib (Hedgehog inhibitor), pembrolizumab

ROTHMUND-THOMSON SYNDROME (POIKILODERMA CONGENITALE)

Defect: AR disorder caused by mutations in **RECQL4** (DNA helicase that facilitates DNA replication and repair of UV damage).

Clinical Features (Fig. 13.45)

- Cutaneous manifestations (present in first year of life):
  - Erythema, edema on face, heals to leave behind red-brown reticulated areas
  - Photosensitivity with/without bullae.
  - **Poikiloderma** (hypo- and hyperpigmentation + atrophy + telangiectases) is subsequently noted at these sites.
  - Acral verrucous keratoses (may → SCC)
  - Photosensitivity (in 30%)
  - Alopecia of scalp/lashes/brows
  - Dystrophic nails
  - Musculoskeletal
- Short stature and skeletal dysplasia (e.g. **absence or hypoplasia of thumbs**, radius, and ulna). Triangular appearing face with frontal bossing/saddle nose/micrognathia; juvenile cataracts; dental anomalies; hypogonadism.
- Malignancy may lead to premature death:
  - **Osteosarcoma** (mean onset = 14 years of age) in ~30% patients.
  - Non-melanoma skin cancer (especially SCC)
  - Mean age at death = 34 years of age.

Differential diagnsosis: Dyskeratosis congenita, Kindler syndrome, progeria, Werner syndrome.

COCKAYNE SYNDROME (CS)

Defect: AR disorder due to defective *transcription-coupled NER* (nucleotide excision repair) = inability to resume RNA synthesis after UVR exposure (differs from XP, which has defective global genomic NER).

- Identical phenotypes may occur due to mutations in either of two genes:
  - CS-A (20%): Mutations in excision repair, cross complementing group 8 **(ERCC8)**

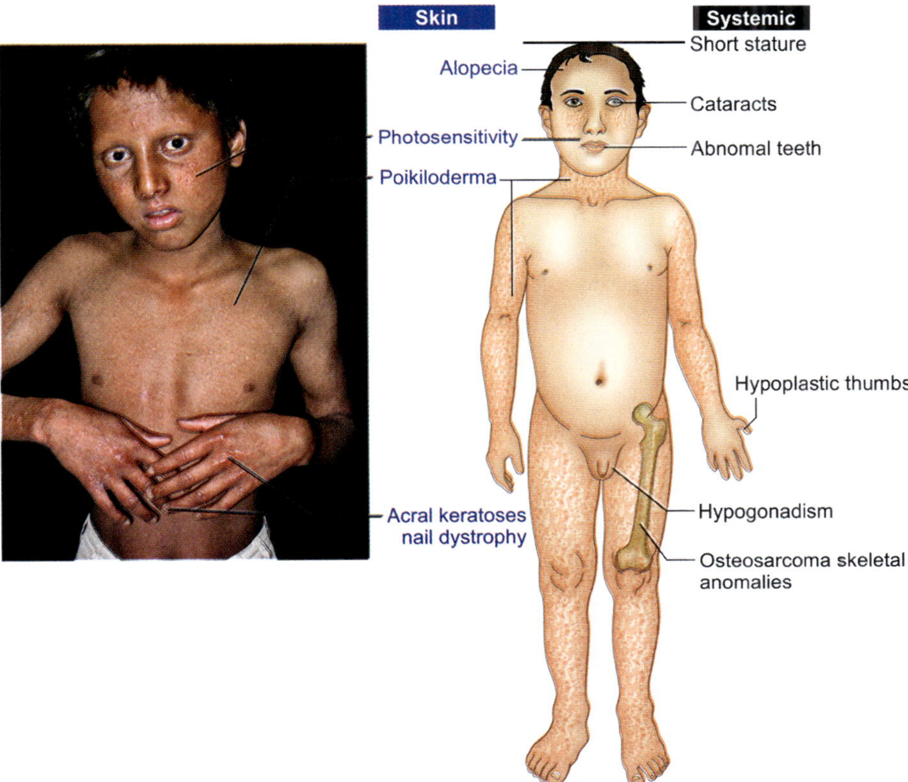

Fig. 13.45: Rothmund-Thomson syndrome—the marked erythema on the face with poikiloderma is a characteristic finding

- CS-B (80%): Mutations in **ERCC6**

  In general, CS-A is milder in clinical course than CS-B, but within each type, no clear genotype–phenotype correlation has been established.

  The age of onset and severity of disease are variable.

  1. CS I (classic CSI) presents during the first year of life.
  2. CS II (severe CS) presents at birth; early onset, progresses more rapidly, severe.
  3. CS III—late onset and milder.

Rare Variants

- Cerebro-oculo-facio-skeletal (COFS) syndrome is a very rare autosomal recessive disorder of DNA repair and constitutes the prenatal extreme form of CS.
- UV-sensitive syndrome (UVSS) is an autosomal recessive disorder of DNA repair characterized by sensitivity to UVR but without any increased risk of skin cancers or any evidence of neurological disease.

Clinical Features

- **Cutaneous manifestations: Photosensitivity**, with telangiectatic erythema **(Fig. 13.46)**.
  - Photosensitivity is present from birth and the abnormal growth and development becomes evident within the first few years of life.

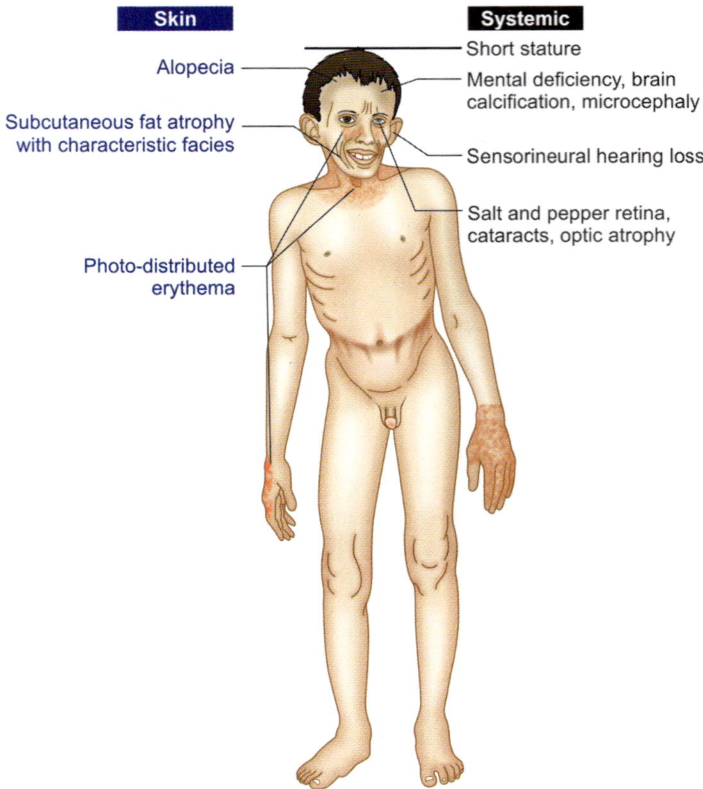

Fig. 13.46: A depiction of the salient features of Cockayne syndrome

- Typical **facies**: Pinched, narrow **"bird-like"** face (prognathism, enophthalmia, a prominent thin nose, large ears and loss of subcutaneous fat); growth failure and cachexia.
- The skin is **dry and thin**, and the hair is often sparse and is sometimes prematurely grey.
- Unlike XP, has **NO ↑risk of skin cancer and lacks pigmentary changes**.

- CNS: Basal ganglia calcification, progressive deterioration/demyelination of CNS/PNS with ataxia and spasticity, intellectual impairment, microcephaly, and progressive sensorineural hearing loss.
- Skeletal manifestations: Short stature + cachectic/thin body **("cachectic dwarfism")**, joint contractures, and kyphosis.
- Eye: Salt and pepper retinopathy, optic atrophy, cataracts, and nystagmus.
- Hypogonadism may be seen in affected males.
- Most patients *die* by *fourth decade* from progressive neurologic disease complications.

TRICHOTHIODYSTROPHY

AR, heterogeneous group of diseases with brittle hair and nails (reduced content of cysteine-rich proteins), ichthyosis, and **neurodevelopmental disability**.

Classified as photosensitive or nonphotosensitive:

- **TTD with photosensitivity (TTD-P):** Caused by mutations in three genes (ERCC2, ERCC3, and GTF2H5) encoding proteins (XPD, XPB, and TTDA), respectively, that function in the transcription repair protein IIH complex, which is involved in DNA transcription and excision repair.

- **TTD, nonphotosensitive (TTD-NP):** Results in about 10–20% of cases from mutations in the C7Orf11 gene or M-phase specific PLK1 interacting protein (MPLKIP), which is thought to regulate transcription efficiency; *lacks ichthyosis.*

Clinical Features (Fig. 13.47)

- Photosensitivity (unlike XP, has **NO increased skin cancer risk**).
- Ichthyosis: The ichthyosis, when present, often resembles mild CIE and requires minimal therapy.
- Brittle hair (short/sparse on scalp/brows/lashes with alternating light and dark bands on polarizing light microscopy **("tiger-tail" abnormality)**. Trichoschisis and trichorrhexis nodosa may be seen.
- Intellectual impairment and ataxia.
- Decreased fertility/hypogonadism.
- Short stature
- Other findings: Hypoplastic/dysplastic nails, palmoplantar keratoderma, keratosis pilaris, atopic dermatitis, cataracts, osteosclerosis, joint contractures, aged facial appearance, and hypogammaglobinemia with recurrent infections.

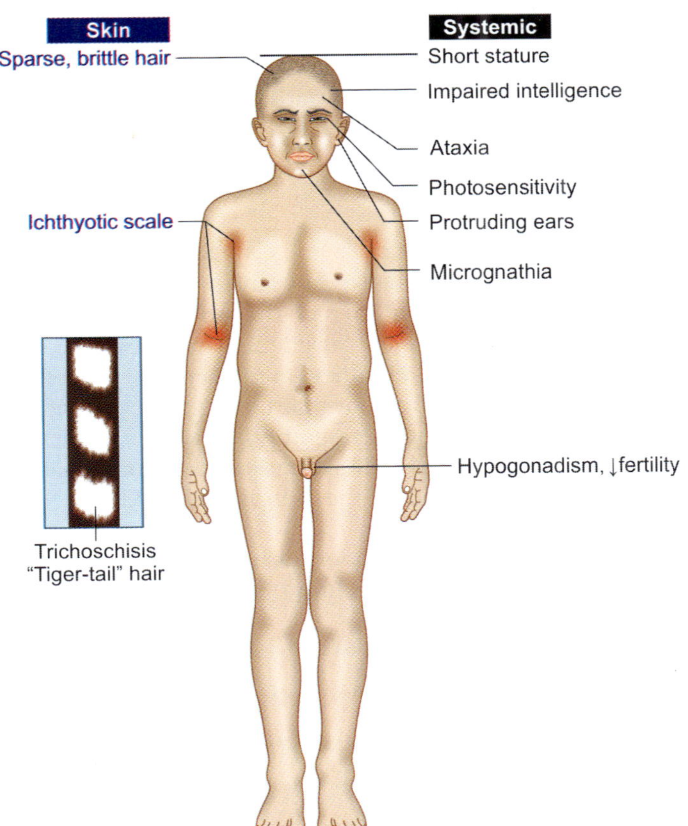

Fig. 13.47: A depiction of the salient features of trichothiodystrophy

DYSKERATOTIC–ACANTHOLYTIC DISORDERS

The following two disorders are important with abnormal keratinization (dyskeratosis) and loss of adhesion between keratinocytes (primary acantholysis).

DARIER DISEASE (DD)

Epidemiology

- Inherited acantholytic disorder
- Sex F = M
- Age peak at 6–20 years
- **Autosomal dominant** with *complete penetrance* but variable phenotypic expression.

Pathogenesis

- Due to mutation in **ATP2A2** gene on 12q24 chromosome.
- **ATP2A2** encodes **sarco-/endoplasmic reticulum Ca^{++} ATPase type 2 (SERCA 2) Transmembrane calcium pumps: 3 types**
  - SERCA2a—slow-twitch skeletal and cardiac muscle.
  - **SERCA2b—major isoform in epidermis**, other tissues too.
  - SERCA2c—more widely expressed.
- Normally epidermal keratinocyte differentiation and adhesion are dependent on high concentrations of Ca^{++}. Epidermal Ca^{++} increases from basal to superficial layers. Calcium-dependent signaling regulates transport of adhesion proteins to the cell membranes. Purinergic signals → ER calcium rapidly discharged into cytoplasm → cytoplasmic calcium increases → **TRPC1 (transient receptor potential cationic 1)** admits more extracellular calcium → increase in calcium flux.
- Defect
  - Reduced ER Ca^{++} and increased cytoplasmic Ca^{++} levels → upregulation of TRPC1 → increases cell proliferation and decreases apoptosis.
  - Reduced ER Ca^{++} interferes with correct protein folding and post-translational modification by molecular chaperones calreticulin and calnexin.
  - Impaired trafficking of desmoplakin adhesion molecule to the cell membrane.
  - Translocation of protein kinase C also impaired (regulates desmoplakin-intermediate filament association and desmosomes assembly).
  - Anti-apoptotic effect of upregulated TRPC1 may lead to abnormal keratosis (dyskeratosis).
- Why disease manifestation is limited to the skin is still unknown even though there is widespread expression of SERCA2.

  May be due to lack of compensation in epidermis by SERCA3.

  A summary of the pathogenesis is given in **Box 13.11**.

BOX 13.11: Overview of pathogenesis of Darier disease

TP2A2 (encodes SERCA2 = calcium ATPase of endoplasmic reticulum)

↓

Defective Ca^{2+} sequestration into ER

↓

Impaired synthesis and folding of cell adhesion proteins

↓

Keratinocyte acantholysis and apoptosis

Aggravating Factors

Friction, heat, sweating, sunlight, UVB.

Clinical Features (Fig. 13.48)

- Begins on sun-exposed areas usually, isolated nipple hyperkeratosis may occur as first manifestation.
- Discrete/confluent rough, *malodorous, greasy* skin-colored brownish papules.
- **Sites:**
  Seborrheic areas of trunk, face, scalp, temples, ears, neck and flexures—axillae, groin and perineum.
  Flexures: Papules may coalesce-irregular warty fissured plaques—vegetating malodorous plaques.
  Hands and feet: Acrokeratosis verruciformis on dorsa of hands. Plane wart-like papules.
  Palms and soles: Focal keratoses, palmar pits.
- **Nails:** May show earliest signs. Nail fragility, longitudinal splits, V-shaped nicking, nail dystrophy. Nails with multiple red and white bands resembling **'candy-canes'**, are **pathognomonic** for Darier disease.
- **Oral mucosa:** White umbilicated/cobble-stone papules (50%), most common on hard palate **(Fig. 13.48)**. Buccal lesions may simulate leukoplakia.
- **Eye:** Hyperkeratotic plaques, seborrheic debris at eyelid margin, chronic blepharitis.

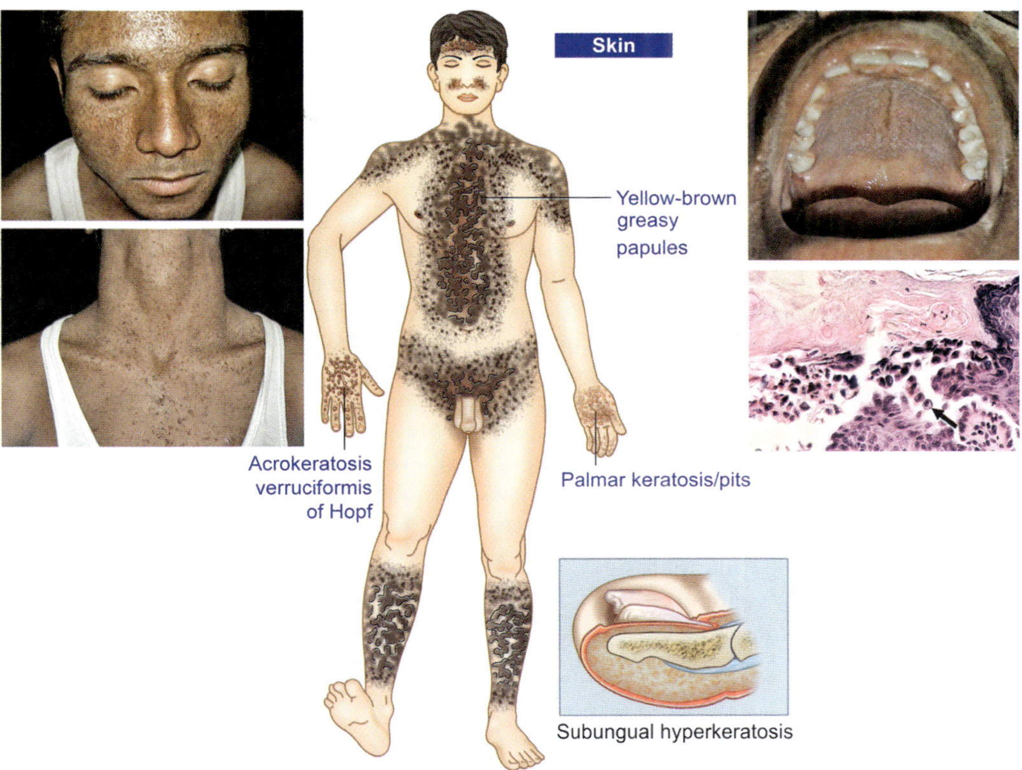

Fig. 13.48: A depiction of Darier disease with greasy papules on the seborrheic areas and papules on the palate. The histopathology shows "corps ronds" (black arrow)

Clinical Variants and other Features

- Isolated palmar/nail/nipple involvement
- Erosive/vesiculobullous—flexural
- Eroded hyperkeratotic plaques—distal limbs
- Comedonal
- Palmoplantar hemorrhagic macules
- Pigmented papular lesions similar to Grover's disease
- Guttate leukoderma in dark skinned
  - Segmental Darier/Type 1 (most common): Blaschkoid streaks of Darier lesions; postzygotic ATP2A2 mutation.
  - Type 2: Generalized Darier disease with focal areas of severe involvement; heterozygous germline mutation+ postzygotic loss of other allele.

Clinical Course

Chronic persistent/relapsing course.

Severity Scale

- Grade 0: Subclinical
- Grade I: Mild localized disease <10%
- Grade II: 10–30%
- Grade III: >30%

Complications

- Impetiginization including secondary infection with HSV/VZV viruses (Kaposi's varicelliform eruption is most concerning
- Eczematization
- Increased incidence of SCC and mammary Paget's disease (controversial)
- Neuropsychiatric diseases—depression, bipolar disorder, seizures, intellectual abnormalities due to high calcium pump expression in the brain (lithium treatment could exacerbate too). (Heart muscle also expresses SERCA but no cardiac manifestations reported).

Differential Diagnosis

- Seborrheic dermatitis
- Hailey-Hailey disease
- Dowling–Degos disease/Galli–Galli disease
- Acanthosis nigricans
- Confluent reticulate papillomatosis
- Pemphigus vulgaris/vegetans
- Plane warts/acrokeratosis of Hopf
- Grover's disease.

Investigations

- **Bedside tests: Tzanck smear**
  - Acantholytic cells
  - Dyskeratotic keratinocytes

- **HPE (Table 13.18)**
  - Compact hyperkeratosis
  - Suprabasal acantholysis and irregular acantholysis in all levels of the epidermis.
  - Dyskeratotic keratinocytes: *Corps ronds* (cells with small pyknotic nuclei, perinuclear halo and eosinophilic cytoplasm in granular layer) and grains (compressed cells with elongated nuclei in S. corneum and S. granulosum).

TABLE 13.18: Differential diagnosis of suprabasal bulla

	Pemphigus vulgaris*	Darier's disease*	Hailey–Hailey disease*
Types of lesions	Intraepithelial bullae	Suprabasal clefts	Intraepithelial bullae
Adjacent epithelium	Intact	Intact	Disintegrating
Involvement of adnexae	Yes	Yes	No
Corps ronds and grains	No	Yes	Rarely
Dermal inflammation	Mononuclears, eosinophils	Mononuclear	Mononuclear
DIF	Positive	Negative	Negative

*The lesions of Grover's disease may histologically mimic any of these and can only be distinguished by immunofluorescence.

Treatment

There is no curative treatment for Darier's disease; the various therapies are palliative and address the varied morphological presentations. An important aim should be to address the possibility of superinfection. Also there are certain trigger factors that should be addressed including heat, perspiration, exposure to the sun and superinfections (regular hygienic care). Being a genetic disorder the risk of transmitting the disease to progeny should be informed to the index patient. An evidence based treatment protocol is given in **Table 13.19**.

Naltrexone is a known Toll-like receptor 4 antagonist, which leads to decreased amounts of TNF-α, IL-6, and nitric oxide. These effects are involved in calcium homeostasis. Dose ranges from 3 mg to 12.5 mg; common side effects are vivid dreams and headache. While naltrexone and magnesium has been shown to be useful this may not be effective in severe cases [Bohemer D]. Recently Baricitinib has been tried in a singular case.

TABLE 13.19: Evidence-based treatment of Darier's disease

	Topical	Oral	Surgical and Cosmetic
1st line	• 0.05% isotretinoin • 0.1% adapalene • Tazarotene gel 0.05% combined with a topical corticosteroid	• Antibiotics are useful to treat superinfections of the skin • The antiviral drugs aciclovir or famciclovir may be administered in case of viral infections	
2nd line	• Tacrolimus 0.1% • Diclofenac sodium 3% gel	• **Acitretin** (30 mg daily) for 16 weeks • **Isotretinoin** (0.5 mg/kg) • **Alitretinoin** (30 mg daily)	
3rd line		• **Cyclosporine** as a bridge therapy • **Prednisolone**—short course • Low-dose **naltrexone** hydrochloride (1.5 to 3.0 mg per day)	• Fractional CO_2 • Erbium: YAG laser ablation • Botulinum (100 U) • Surgery

HAILEY-HAILEY DISEASE

AD. Family history (+), the disorder is not fully penetrant and in mild cases may never be diagnosed.

Pathogenesis

Defect in ATP2C1, a gene at chromosome 3q21-24 (encodes human secretory pathway Ca^{2+}/Mn^{2+} ATPase isoform 1 **(SPCA1)** → defective Ca^{2+} sequestration into Golgi apparatus → impaired processing of proteins involved in cell-cell adhesion → acantholysis.)

ATP2C1 is most highly expressed in the basal layer of epidermis.

Trigger: Heat, friction or infection.

Clinical Features

- Second and fourth decade, wider range of age of onset than Darier (teens—20 years mostly, but may arise later).
- Painful, pruritic and often malodorous lesions of flexures or other sites of friction. Lesions show fissuring and erosions **(Fig. 13.49a** and **b)**.
- Less occluded areas, such as truncal or neck lesions, are more likely to show *vesicopustules or flaccid bullae*, but may simply be crusted erosions resembling discoid eczema, or annular plaques with peripheral scales.
- No mucosal involvement (*helps differentiate from Darier*).
- Triggers: Heat, sweating, friction, infection, contact allergy, adhesive dressings or electrocardiogram electrodes, UV irradiation and scabies.

Grading

1. *Grade 0*: Subclinical—an obligate carrier in a family, with no apparent disease or nail lesions only.
2. *Grade I*: Mild disease—localized (e.g. perineal or axillary) and intermittent lesions responding to simple topical therapies.
3. *Grade II*: Moderate—chronic lesions at two or more body sites (e.g. axillary and groins) or locally severe and refractory to topical treatment.
4. *Grade III*: Severe—extensive or chronically disabling disease despite topical and systemic treatment.

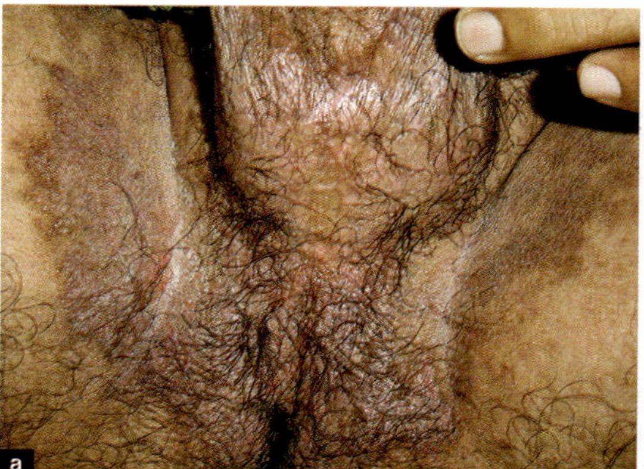

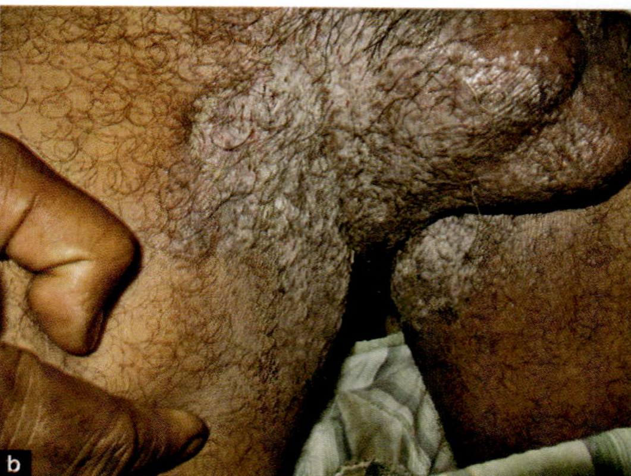

Fig. 13.49a abd b: Vegetative malodorous plaques with fissuring and erosions in Hailey–Hailey disease

Pathology

- Disorder of keratinocyte adhesion.
- Widespread partial loss of cohesion between suprabasal keratinocytes, or acantholysis, said to resemble a ***dilapidated brick wall*** **(Fig. 13.49c** and **d)**.
- Acantholytic clefts and bullae form suprabasally, and may contain floating clusters of loosely coherent cells. Adherens junctions may allow keratinocytes to continue to adhere and mild dyskeratosis may be present.
- Fewer dyskeratotic keratinocytes than Darier disease.

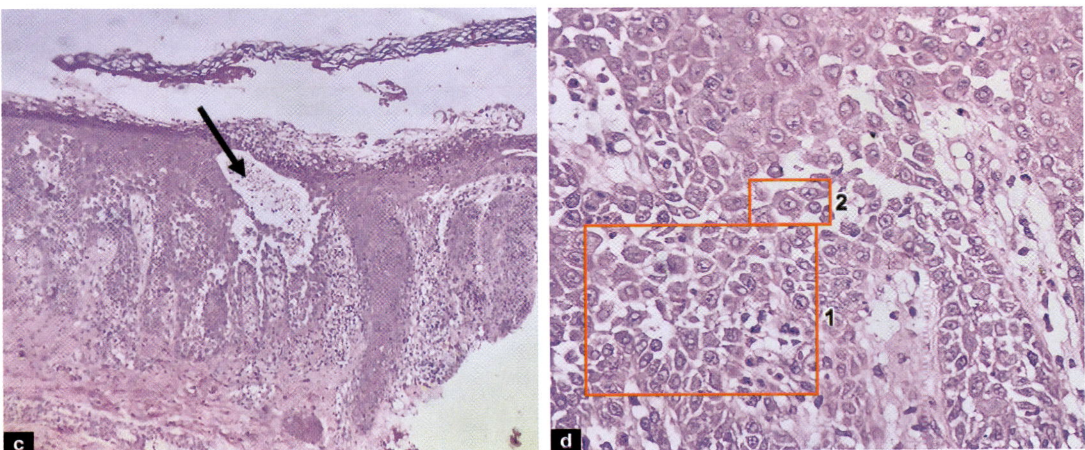

Fig. 13.49c and d: Skin biopsy shows suprabasal clefting with a pronounced intraepidermal bulla (c) and high power view (d) shows the dilapidated brick wall appearance (1) with partial loss of cohesion with numerous acantholytic cells (2) in Hailey–Hailey disease

Differential Diagnosis

- Pemphigus is distinguished from Hailey–Hailey disease by the presence of relatively intact epithelium in the adjacent epidermis (versus disintegrating 'dilapidated brick wall') and involvement of adnexal structures. DIF is (+) in pemphigus.
- Darier disease tends to show prominent suprabasal cleft formation with involvement of adnexae and is associated with numerous corps ronds and grains.

Treatment

While topical corticosteroids remain the first-line therapy, caution should be exercised. The combination of potent steroids in combination with gentamicin is a good choice. The results with Botulinum toxin are impressive but the cost is a deterrent. If considering a systemic agent, oral antibiotics have the largest volume of data to support their use in HHD, specially tetracyclines.

Newer agents tried include, dupilumab, adalimumab and PDT.

Of the procedural modalities, continuous wave CO_2 laser therapy has the most supportive data and could be considered as an alternative for patients failing to respond to first-line therapies **(Flowchart 13.4)**.

Flowchart 13.4: Treatment algorithm for Hailey-Hailey disease

1st line

- Emollients, topical antiseptics
- TCS—Combinations with topical antimicrobial agents seem to be more effective than TCS alone
- Avoidance of heat/sunlight
- Oral doxycycline (100 mg daily) for 3 months

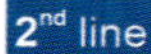

2nd line

- Tacrolimus 0.1%/calcitriol 3 μg/g ointment.
- Dapsone (100–200 mg/day)
- Cyclosporine (2.5 mg/kg/day) for 3 weeks and taper over 6 months
- Naltrexone low dose (12.5–50 mg daily)

3rd line

- Topical 5-FU cream/topical tacrolimus/topical tacalcitol
- Oral acitretin (0.25–0.50 mg/kg/day) or isotretinoin (0.5 mg/kg/d)
- Mtx (15 mg weekly)
- Surgical/physical therapies
- Botulinum toxin (50–500 IU per site)

EPIDERMOLYSIS BULLOSA

Introduction

- Epidermolysis bullosa (EB) is characterized by inherited fragility of skin and formation of blisters with seemingly mild trauma/friction.
- Some types affect only limited areas on the body.
- Others can be severe enough to cause mortality or complications.

Pathogenesis

Like any organ, the integrity of skin and its functions are dependent on the cohesion and cross-talk between the individual components.

Mutations

EB occurs due to mutation in the genes encoding several structural proteins, usually the ones present at the dermoepidermal junction (DEJ), and rarely those encoding desmogleins.

Based on the protein involved, its location in the skin and thus, the resultant level of split in the skin, EB is divided into **4 major types (Fig. 13.50)**:

- **EB simplex** (EBS, split at the level of basal cells, keratins 5 and 14 are involved)
- **Junctional EB** (JEB, split at the level of lamina lucida, usually laminin 5 and collagen 17 are involved)
- **Dystrophic EB** (DEB, split at the level of anchoring fibrils and sub-lamina densa, collagen 7 is involved)
- **Kindler EB** (defective kindling protein).

Classification

The recently proposed classification system is summarized in **Table 13.20** and many of the specific names have now been abandoned. The proposed system remains largely clinically

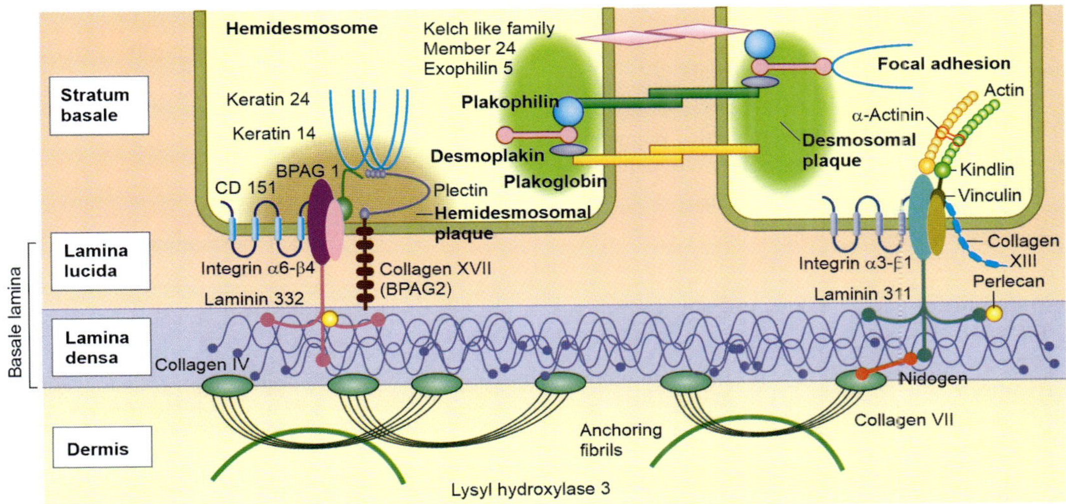

Fig. 13.50: An overview of the BMZ zone and stratum basale depicting various components that determine the variants of EB

oriented, and aims at a bedside diagnosis which can be supplemented later by the laboratory diagnosis, which in turn enables more accurate subclassification of these patients based on molecular findings.

The EB classification is complex because mutations in the same gene may be inherited in an autosomal dominant or recessive manner and may result in distinct clinical phenotypes (e.g. KRT5, KRT14, LAMB3, LAMA3, LAMC3, COL17A1 or COL7A1). On the other hand, in DEB and EBS, similar phenotypes may be either dominant or recessive, or may be caused by mutations in different genes (e.g. COL7A1, KRT5, KRT14, PLEC, DST, EXPH5 or KLHL24).

Unifying clinical and molecular aspects, the previously introduced 'onion skin' approach for subclassification of EB, can still be used **(Box 13.12)**. The concept of syndromic disorders has been proposed recently, and comprises those entities which are characterized by primary manifestations of other organs or systems such as the gastrointestinal or urogenital tract, myocardium, skeletal muscle.

BOX 13.12: "Onion skin" approach for EB classification

1. **First** the disease is classified into one of the **four main EB types**
   - **Junctional**
   - **Simplex**
   - **Dystrophic**
   - **Kindler**

   Then other information is added to classify the condition better:
2. **Phenotype, severity, and distribution are described**
3. **Mode of transmission, autosomal dominant or recessive**
4. **Site of cleavage ultrastructurally and associated findings**
5. **Protein involved**
6. **Gene involved**
7. **Mutation**

TABLE 13.20: Classification and inheritance pattern in EB (Has C, BJD 2020)

Type	Subtype	Inheritance	Defective antigen/protein
EB simplex (intraepidermal ectodermal dysplasia syndrome) • **Autosomal dominant EBS**	• Localized • Intermediate • Severe	AD	Keratin 5, keratin 14 (KRT5, KRT14)
	• With mottled pigmentation • Migratory circinate erythema		Keratin 5
	• Intermediate		Plectin
	• Intermediate with cardiomyopathy **(syndromic)**		Kelch-like member 24 (KLHL24)
• **Autosomal recessive EBS**	• Intermediate or severe	AR	K5, K14
	• Intermediate		Plectin (PLEC)
	• Localized or intermediate with BP230 deficiency		Bullous pemphigoid antigen 230 (BP230) (syn. BPAG1e or DST gene)
	• Localized or intermediate with exophilin-5 deficiency		Exophilin-5 (EXPH5)
	• Intermediate with muscular Dystrophy **(syndromic)**		Plectin (PLEC)

(Contd.)

TABLE 13.20: Classification and inheritance pattern in EB (Has C, BJD 2020) (*Contd.*)			
Type	**Subtype**	**Inheritance**	**Defective antigen/protein**
	• Severe with pyloric atresia **(syndromic)**		Plectin (PLEC)
	• Localized with nephropathy **(syndromic)**		CD151 (CD151 antigen)
Junctional EB (JEB, involves lamina lucida)	• Severe • Intermediate	AR	Laminin 332 (LAMA3/LAMB3/LAMC2 gene)
	• Intermediate		Laminin 332, type XVII collagen (BPAg2, COL17A1 gene)
	• Pyloric atresia **(syndromic)**		α6 β4 integrin (α6 β4 integrin, ITGA6/ITGB4 gene)
	• Localized		Laminin 332, type XVII collagen, integrin α6β4, integrin α3 subunit
	• Inversa		Laminin 332
	• Late onset		Type XVII collagen
	• LOC* syndrome		Laminin α3A
	• With interstitial lung disease and nephrotic syndrome **(syndromic)**		Integrin α3 subunit
Dystrophic EB (DEB, involves sub-lamina densa, dermolytic EB) (COL7A1 gene)	• Intermediate **(common)** • Localized **(common)** • Pruriginosa • Self-improving	AD	Type VII collagen (COL7A1 gene)
	• Severe **(common)** • Intermediate **(common)** • Inversa • Localized • Pruriginosa • Self-improving	AR	Type VII collagen
	• Dominant and recessive • DEB, severe	Compound heterozygosity	Type VII collagen
Kindler syndrome/ Kindler EB (photosensitivity and blistering at multiple levels)		AR	Kindlin 1 (fermitin family homolog 1) (FERMT1 or KIND1 gene)

LOC, laryngo-onycho-cutaneous

Clinical Features (Fine JD et al., 2014; Has C, et al., 2015)

Cardinal Features

- A fragile skin, milia, nail dystrophy or absence, scarring (usually atrophic), granulation tissue, palmoplantar keratoderma, dyspigmentation and alopecia characterize EB.
- The presence or absence of these findings may be age-dependent.

- As such, their absence cannot be reliably used for diagnosis during that window of time (i.e. early infancy) when classification and subclassification are most needed.
- In general, skin from patients with JEB and RDEB is much more fragile than that of EBS patients.
- An overview of the salient clinical features is given in **Box 13.13** and details are as follows.

BOX 13.13: Overview of salient clinical features of EB

- All EB simplex is autosomal dominant except for some rarer subtypes
- Hemidesmosomal and junctional EB are autosomal recessive
- Grouped blisters are most commonly seen in generalized, severe subtype of EB simplex
- Enamel hypoplasia is more characteristic of the junctional subtypes
- Exuberant granulation tissue in perioral/axillary/neck area is most characteristic of the generalized, severe subtype of junctional EB.
- Increased risk of squamous cell carcinomas in the generalized-severe type of recessive dystrophic EB.

1. EBS (Fig. 13.51)

- The most common type of EB: In most cases, EBS is inherited in an autosomal dominant manner; autosomal recessive inheritance is rare in Western countries but quite common in some regions in the world. Blistering is usually manifested at or shortly after birth. As a general rule, far less scarring, milia formation, and nail dystrophy are seen in EBS, as compared to JEB and DEB.

  New genes, KLHL24 and CD151, have been identified since the previous classification and extend the spectrum of EBS.

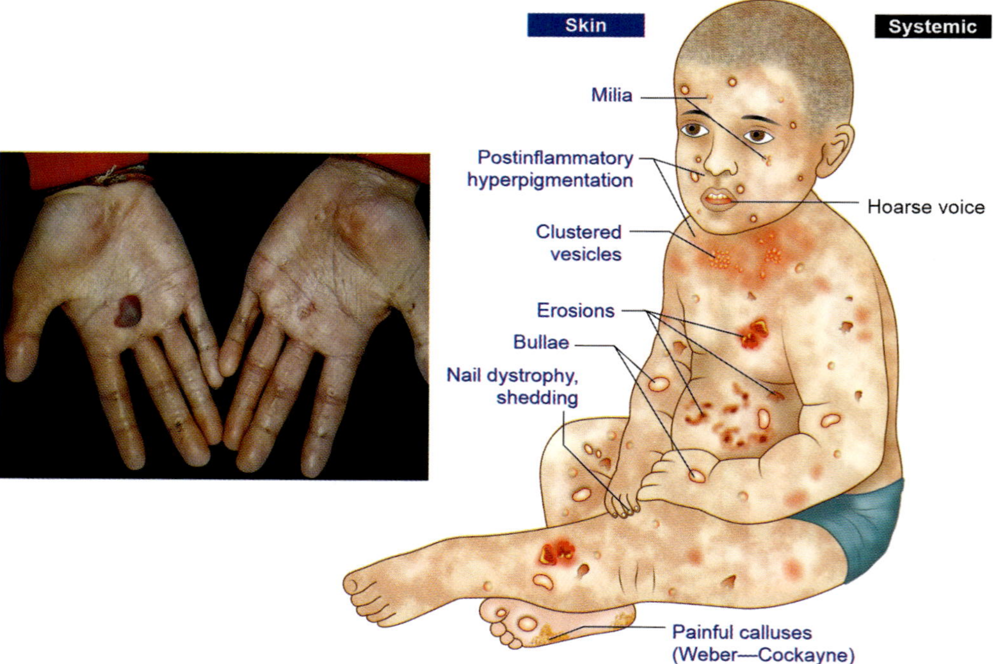

Fig. 13.51: Pictorial description of Dowling-Meara or generalized severe epidermolysis bullosa simplex (EBS), after the first months or year of life, grouped or herpetiform blistering and crusting on an inflammatory base are seen; Localized EB simplex (localized to palms and soles) is seen in the clinical image

- The most common subtype is **localized EBS** (formerly known as Weber–Cockayne disease).
- The usual distribution of blisters in these patients is on the palms, soles and oral cavity.
- EBS **generalized severe** (formerly known as EBS—Dowling Meara) is frequently associated with marked morbidity and features intact vesicles or small blisters in grouped or arcuate configuration.

  By late childhood, most patients develop palmoplantar keratoderma. The most notable complication in EBS is tracheolaryngeal compromise and a markedly increased risk of developing basal cell carcinoma.
- **EBS** generalized intermediate (earlier known as EBS-Koebner) is characterized by non-herpetiform blisters and erosions arising on any skin surface, but these usually tend to spare the palms and soles.

2. **JEB (Fig. 13.52):** There are two major JEB subtypes.

a. **JEB-generalized severe** (previously known as JEB-Herlitz) is present at birth.
   - Involves all skin surfaces
   - An essentially pathognomonic finding is exuberant granulation tissue, which usually arises within the first several months of life, and may involve the skin (periorificial;

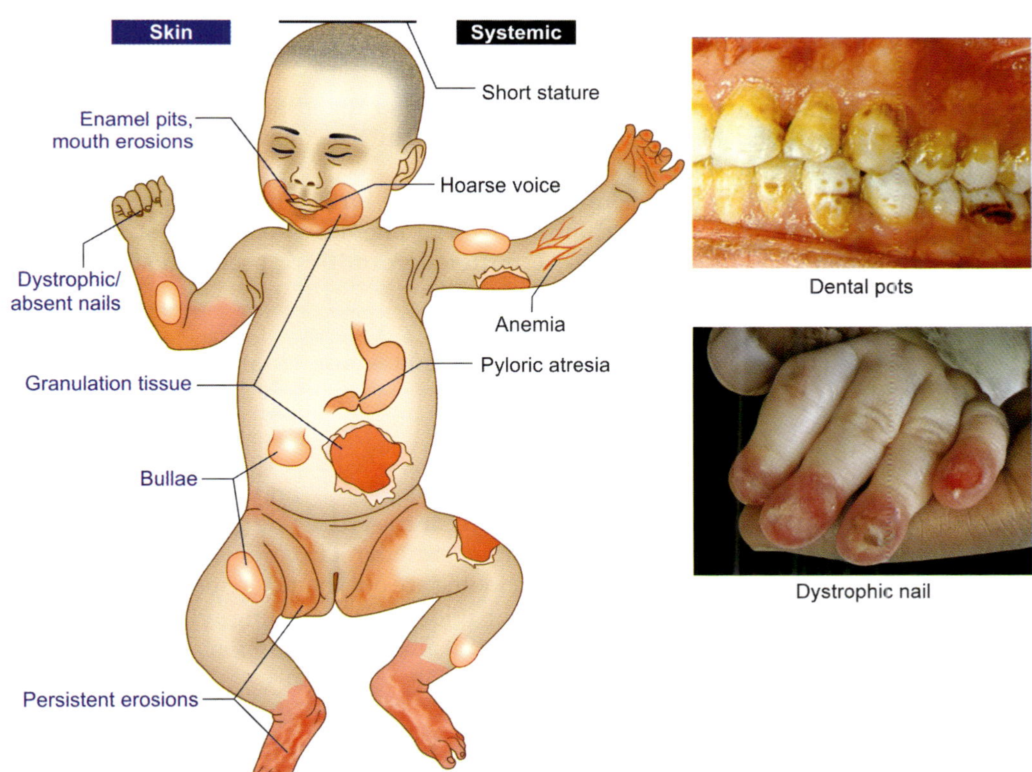

Fig. 13.52: Pictorial description of generalized severe junctional epidermolysis bullosa JEB or JEB-Herlitz where granulation tissue of the distal digits, face and ears are typical. Nail involvement is marked with dystrophic nails

axillary vaults; nape of the neck; lumbosacral spine; periungual and proximal nail folds) and the upper airway.

- Profound growth retardation, failure to thrive and multifactorial anemia are the norms in JEB-H.
- Esophagus (strictures), external eye (corneal blisters, erosions, and scarring; ectropion formation), upper airway (strictures and occlusion) and genitourinary tract are usually involved.
- The **highest** risk of infant **mortality** occurs in generalized severe JEB, and is most often the result of sepsis, failure to thrive, or tracheolaryngeal obstruction.

b. **Generalized intermediate JEB (previously known as non-Herlitz JEB) is:**
- Less severe than the generalized severe counterpart.
- Prominently has scarring alopecia of the scalp.
- Enamel hypoplasia is an extremely useful clinical feature to diagnose JEB.

3. DEB: DEB is characterized by a plane of skin cleavage just beneath the lamina densa and corresponds to the level of the anchoring fibrils, and is consequent to the defect in the gene encoding type VII collagen. The hallmark of DEB is that of scarring following blistering, both in the skin and in a variety of mucosae. Milia are also a specific finding in areas of healed blistering in DEB. DEB may be inherited as a dominant or recessive trait; generally, RDEB is more severe than dominant disease (DDEB) though there is a phenotypic overlap between types.

- **RDEB:** There are two main subtypes of RDEB generalized severe (formerly named Hallopeau-Siemens RDEB, **Fig. 13.53a**) and generalized intermediate RDEB (non-Hallopeau-Siemens RDEB).
  a. Generalized-severe RDEB—generalized blistering at birth, progressive scarring of the skin, corneal blisters or scarring, multi-factorial anemia, esophageal strictures, and debilitating hand and foot deformities (**"mitten deformities"**; pseudosyndactyly).
     - Severe ankyloglossia and microstomia.
     - Chronic renal failure.
     - These patients are at risk of developing metastatic cutaneous squamous cell carcinomas by age 40–45 years.
  b. Generalized-**Intermediate** RDEB—has similar but less severe cutaneous involvement.
- **DDEB**
  Localized dominant dystrophic epidermolysis bullosa (DDEB) and intermediate recessive DEB (RDEB) often display phenotypic overlap. In contrast to severe generalized RDEB and generalized severe JEB, however, failure to thrive, growth retardation, severe anemia, early infant mortality, and risk of squamous cell carcinoma are not characteristic features of DDEB.
  Skin: Bullae can be localized to extremities or widespread; healing with/without milia **(Fig. 13.53b)**, scars; mild oral disease; with/without albopapuloid lesions—hypopigmented scar-like papules increased on trunk
  Nails: Dystrophic to absent

4. **Kindler Epidermolysis Bullosa (earlier known as Kindler syndrome)** is characterized by generalized blistering, colitis, esophagitis, urethral strictures, ectropion, gingivitis and gingival hyperplasia, poikilodermatous pigmentation and photosensitivity. The genetic basis is represented by mutations in FERMT1 (syn. KIND1), encoding fermitin family homolog 1 (kindlin-1), an intracellular protein of focal adhesions.

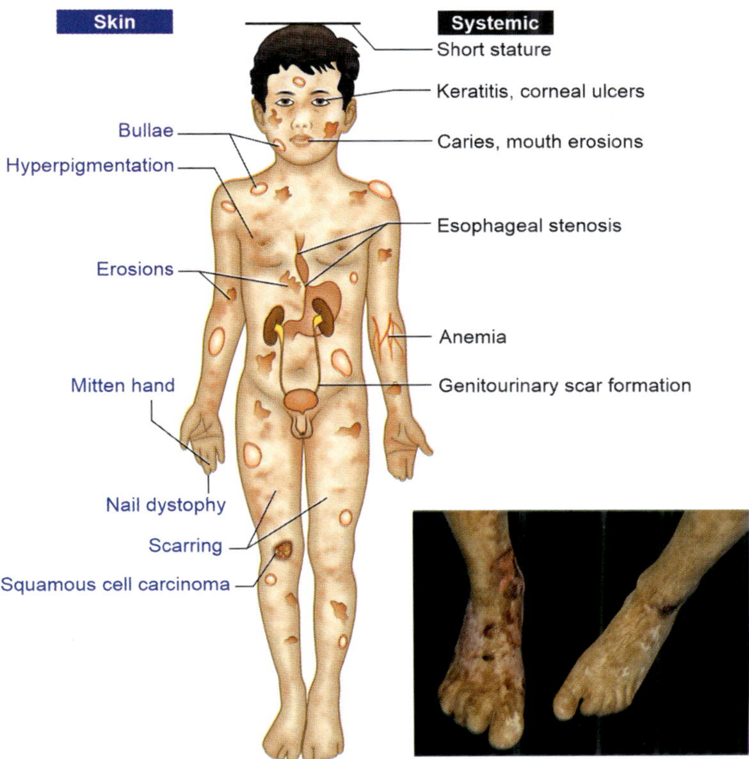

Fig. 13.53a: Pictorial description of generalized severe autosomal recessive dystroph c epidermolysis bullosa (RDEB). There is widespread skin fragility and ulceration in neonates which leads to scarring and joint contractures. This leads to loss of the distal digits, digital fusion and flexicn contractures. Severe scarring can ensue and cause contractures and pseudosyndactyly (clinical image)

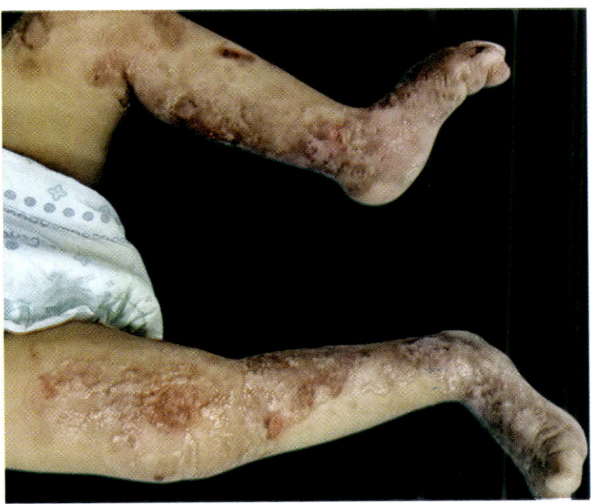

Fig. 13.53b: Dystrophic EB with extensive milia

DIAGNOSIS

Clinical

The incidence of blistering, erosions, scarring, milia formation, nail, hair, dental and mucosal involvement, granulation tissue formation, contractures and carcinomas varies in different types and subtypes.

Accordingly, the differential diagnoses in a patient can be narrowed down to a significant degree helping in reaching at the most probable diagnosis on clinical grounds. A clinical approach is immensely important in resource poor settings **(Table 13.21)**.

Disease Severity Assessment Scores

Severity scores named Birmingham EB severity score (BEBs), EB disease activity and scarring index (EBDASI) and iSCOREB have been developed.

Investigations (Has C, 2020)

- The diagnostic samples are the skin and the blood.
- Although genetic testing and electron microscopy are considered gold standards in diagnosing EB, investigations like immunohistochemistry (IHC) and immunofluorescence antigen mapping (IFM) have certain advantages in form of easier availability and lesser cost.
- In neonates, **IFM** should be the first diagnostic step as it delivers rapid results. In parallel, genetic testing should always be performed.
- In cases with characteristic clinical features, including localized dominant EBS or DEB, for which **IFM** will frequently not deliver a useful result, **genetic testing** by NGS (next-generation sequencing) or SS (Sanger sequencing) can deliver a final diagnosis.
- **TEM** (transmission electron microscope) is useful in a limited number of cases, and should be performed when IFM and genetic testing do not deliver conclusive results.

a. *Biopsy*

In order to make an accurate diagnosis, it is essential that a freshly induced blister is biopsied, from a clinically uninvolved area.

The area to be biopsied (upper arm, upper leg and flank) is gently rubbed firmly with a clean pencil eraser or index finger for 15–30 seconds.

This will induce a microsplit at the dermoepidermal junction (DEJ). Either a punch, shave or incisional biopsy is taken and the sample should be placed in the tubes of fixative provided for EM (glutaraldehyde), IFM (Mitchell's medium) and IHC (formalin).

1. **Electron microscopy:** EM still remains the gold standard for the diagnosis of EB. In addition, it permits the direct visualization and semiquantitative assessment of the specific structures. *Shave biopsy samples* are usually preferred since only shallow skin samples are required (punch biopsy technique may result in total separation of the dermis from the epidermis).
2. **Immunofluorescence antigen mapping:** IFM is a modified indirect immunofluorescence. The procedure consists of exposing the cryostat section of the skin biopsy to FITC labelled monoclonal antibodies directed against various antigenic proteins of the DEJ.

   The primary antibodies used are directed for **cytokeratin 14, laminin 332** (formerly known as laminin 5), **type VII collagen and type IV collagen**.

TABLE 13.21: Clinical diagnostic matrix: Columns represent the nine common subtypes of epidermolysis bullosa (EB) while rows represent the clinical features; –, +, ++ or not applicable (NA) represent typical scores agree by consensus

Clinical	EBs-L	EBs-GI	EBs-GS	JEB-GS	JEB-GI	DDEB	RDEB-GS	RDEB-GI	KS
Distribution of skin lesions excess grannulation tissue	Hand and feet –	Generalized/ limited –	Herpetiform/ generalized –	Generalized +	Generalized – or +	Generalized limited –	Generalized –	Generalized –	Generalized limited –
Scarring milia	– –	– –	– – or +	– –	– or + + or ++	+ or ++ + or ++	+ or ++ + or ++	+ or ++ –	– or +
Nail dystrophy	–	–	– or + or ++	+ or ++	– or + or ++	– or + or ++	– or + or ++	– or + or ++	– or +
Nail loss	–	–	–	+ or ++	– or + or ++	– or +	+ or ++	– or + or ++	– or +
Mucosal erosion	–	–	– or +	+ or ++	– or +	– or +	+ or ++	– or + or ++	–
Eye involvement	–	–	–	– or + or ++	– or + or ++	–	– or + or ++	– or + or ++	–
Hoarseness	–	–	–	+ or ++	– or +	–	– or +	– or +	–
Microstomia/ ankyloglossia	–	–	–	–	–	–	– or +	– or +	–
Poor dental enamel	– or NA	– or NA	– or NA	+ or NA	+ or NA	– or NA	– or NA	– or NA	– or NA
Keratoderma	– or +	– or NA	– or + or ++	–	–	–	–	–	– or +
Chronic wounds	–	–	–	– or +	– or +	– or +	– or + or ++	– or +	– or +
Syndactyly	–	–	–	–	–	–	+ or ++	– or +	– or +
Alopecta	–	–	–	–	+ or ++	–	– or +	– or +	–
Poikiloderma	–	–	–	–	–	–	–	–	+
Relative growth failure	–	–	–	+ or ++	– or +	–	+ or ++	– or +	– or +
Survival after 3 years	+ or NA	+ or NA	+ or NA	– or NA	+ or NA	+ or NA	+ or NA	+ or NA	+ or NA
Parents affected	+ or NA	+ or NA	– or + or NA	– or NA	– or NA	– or NA	– or NA	– or NA	– or NA
Total number of boxes ticked									

EBs, Eb simplex; L, localized; GI, generalized intermediate; GS, generalized severe; JEB, junctional EB, DEB, dystrophic EB; DDEB, dominant DEB; RDEB, recessive DEB; KS, Kindler syndrome.

Clinical and diagnostic matrix (CDM) as *Adapted from* Yenamandra et al., Br Journal of Dermatol, 2017; 176:1624–1632.

TABLE 13.22: Patterns of staining of various antibodies in the major subtypes of epidermolysis bullosa (EB) in IFM

	Type of EB		
Antibody	**EB simplex**	**Junctional EB**	**Dystrophic EB**
Type IV collagen	Normal, floor	Normal, floor	Normal, roof
Keratin 14	**Normal, clumping, holes, irregular staining, absent**	Normal	Normal
Laminin 332	Normal, floor	**Absent or weak, floor**	Normal, roof
Type VII collagen	Normal, floor	Normal, floor	**Absent or weak or normal, roof**

IFM is described based on the following parameters

- The level of separation is based on the location of the blister and staining of type IV collagen to the roof or floor of the blister. In cases where the level of separation cannot be ascertained, diagnosis is based on the pattern of staining of the various antibodies **(Table 13.22)**.
- The advantages are that it is an easy technique, gives rapid results, may indicate the candidate protein, may indicate the consequence of the genetic variant(s) on the protein level, has a prognostic value and may also help in the identification of areas of revertant mosaicism.

3. **Immunohistochemistry:** Immunohistochemistry involves the use of specific monoclonal antibodies against various proteins.
   - Laminin-5 is absent/reduced in JEB and type VII collagen is absent in DEB.

   Interpretation of staining pattern:

   The *bullous pemphigoid* 230 antigen is normally expressed in the intracellular and transmembrane portion of the hemidesmosome, *laminin* is present in lamina lucida and *collagen 4* is a component of lamina densa of the basement membrane.
   - EBS: Bullous pemphigoid, laminin and collagen IV antibodies will be located at the floor of the blister in the skin biopsy specimen.
   - JEB: Bullous pemphigoid antibodies will be seen at the roof of the blister and laminin and collagen IV will be at the floor of the blister. The staining pattern of laminin varies from partial to complete absence.
   - EBD: Bullous pemphigoid, laminin and collagen IV antibodies will be located on the roof of the blister.

b. *Blood Samples*

Genomic DNA isolated from peripheral blood leukocytes (ethylene diamine tetra-acetic acid treated), saliva or buccal smear from patients and their parents is analysed. These are used for genetic testing either by NGS (next-generation sequencing) or SS (Sanger sequencing).

c. *Prenatal Diagnosis*

Fetoscopy, chorionic villus biopsy, amniocentesis, pre-implantation genetic diagnosis are methods by which cellular DNA is extracted and the gene harboring mutation is amplified using polymerase chain reaction (PCR).

TREATMENT OF EB

Care of EB Patient *(Adapted from* Birmingham EB Care Tips)

Care of an EB patient primarily involves thoroughly educating the parents/caretakers.

The primary goals of EB care are:

- Protection of the skin against *trauma*
- Prevention of *infection*
- Maintaining the highest possible level of *nutrition*
- Minimizing *deformities*
- Sustaining a strong *support* system and a positive attitude.

Management of pain and pruritus can be achieved with antihistamines, non-steroidal anti-inflammatory drugs and opioids.

(A detailed management protocol is detailed in the first edition of this book).

Current Treatments under Consideration

These vary from targeting the inflammatory pathways to corrective gene editing. **Table 13.23** briefly summarizes the various treatment modalities currently under trial for EB.

TABLE 13.23: Current treatments under consideration for EB

Type of treatment modality	Mechanism of action
Use of genetically corrected cultured epidermal autograft, genetically-modified autologous human dermal fibroblasts	Gene therapy
Topical delivery of antisense oligonucleotide	Exon skipping, i.e. exclusion of mutated part from the mRNA
Mesenchymal stem cell (MSC) infusions from a related donor, allogeneic stem cell transplantation, fibroblast-based cell therapy for RDEB patients	Cell therapy
Gentamicin-topical/intraleasional/intravenous	PTC read-through
Oral apremilast, systemic losartan, topical diacerein, topical oleogel, topical sirolimus, 4-phenylbutyrate	Anti-inflammatory, antifibrotic, reduction of cellular stress and regulation of autophagy

Updates in Treatment

Dystrophic epidermolysis bullosa is caused by a defect in type VII collagen (C7). Type VII collagen is a major component of anchoring fibrils, which provide stability between the epidermis and dermis. Gene changes that alter the ability to form structurally sound C7 lead to increased separation of the epidermis and dermis/blisters.

In a recent phase III placebo-controlled trial (sponsored by Krystal Biotech), healing of paired wounds after introduction of a topical gene-based therapy versus placebo was evaluated. **Beremagene geperpavec** (B-VEC) is a topical investigational herpes simplex virus type 1 (HSV-1)-based gene therapy designed to restore C7 protein by delivering COL7A1 (Guide SV, 2022).

ECTODERMAL DYSPLASIA

Congenital defects in two or more ectodermal structures, one of which at least involves the **hair** (trichodysplasia), **teeth** (dental defects), **nails** (onychodysplasia) or **sweat glands** (dyshidrosis).

It is a **misnomer** because the ectoderm is hypoplastic, not dysplastic (if dysplasia is defined as cytologic atypia of epithelium).

- The term 'ectodermal dysplasia' did not appear in the literature until coined by Weech in 1929.
- Pinheiro and Freire-Maia gave classification of ED assigned conditions to groups using a '1234' system, depending on the presence of hair, nail, tooth or sweat gland abnormalities.
- EDs may also be divided into those with isolated involvement of hair, teeth and nails- **'pure' EDs**–whereas those with abnormalities of other structures and organs are referred to as **'ectodermal dysplasia syndromes'**.
- EDs has also been classified into **two broad categories: Group 1**, indicating defects in developmental regulation and epithelial-mesenchymal interaction, and **Group 2**, indicating defects in proteins of cytoskeleton or adhesion, which are involved in cell-cell communication as well as structural integrity.
- More than 170 conditions have been described under this category.

Epidemiology

- Affects first year of life, affect both sexes but females have less serious manifestation.
- Associated diseases, like atopic eczema, allergic asthma, rhinitis and food allergies.

Molecular Pathways that are Important in Ectodermal Dysplasias

- Hedgehog signaling pathway
- Wingless signaling pathway
- TNF-α signaling pathway
- **NF-κβ** signaling pathway defect-impair immune and stress responses, cell adhesion, and protection against apoptosis and inflammatory reactions, causing hypohidrotic ED.
- ED signaling pathway
- p63 signaling pathway
- Gap junctions-connexin pathway
- Axin pathway.
- Mutations in TP63-interfere with transcription factors and cause EDs associated with ectrodactyly, cleft palate, and ankyloblepharon.
- Wnt β catenin pathway is particularly associated with impaired hair and tooth formation.
- Mutations in epithelial structural proteins (cytokeratins) or adhesive molecules (desmosal components.

Genetics

- Autosomal recessive, autosomal dominant, X-linked and mitochondrial.
- X-linked—hypohidrotic—ectodermal dysplasia with immunodeficiency—rare
  Early age of onset, affects men only
  - Characteristic **clinical features** are:
    i. Hypohidrosis leads to heat intolerance.

ii. Delayed teeth eruption, conical teeth.
iii. Coarse, sparse hair with hypotrichosis or complete alopecia.
iv. Immunodeficiency complicated by frequent bacterial infections.

Associated Diseases

- IBD
- Rheumatoid arthritis
- Lymphoedema
- Osteopetrosis.

HYPOHIDROTIC ED (CHRIST–SIEMENS–TOURAINE SYNDROME)

- **Inheritance:** XLR, AD, AR
- Gene(s): EDA1, EDAR, EDARADD
- Most common of the ED

Clinical Features

Clinical triad: Sweating, hypotrichosis, and abnormal dentition.

- **Facial features: "Dysmorphic features" Frontal bossing**, **large nostrils**, wide/flat malar cheeks, **thick everted lower lip**, and prominent chin **(Fig. 13.54)**.
- **Hair:** Hypotrichosis with thin, light hair; eyelashes absent.
- **Skin:** Soft/smooth, thin wrinkled skin; darkening of skin under eyes; mild-onychodystrophy.

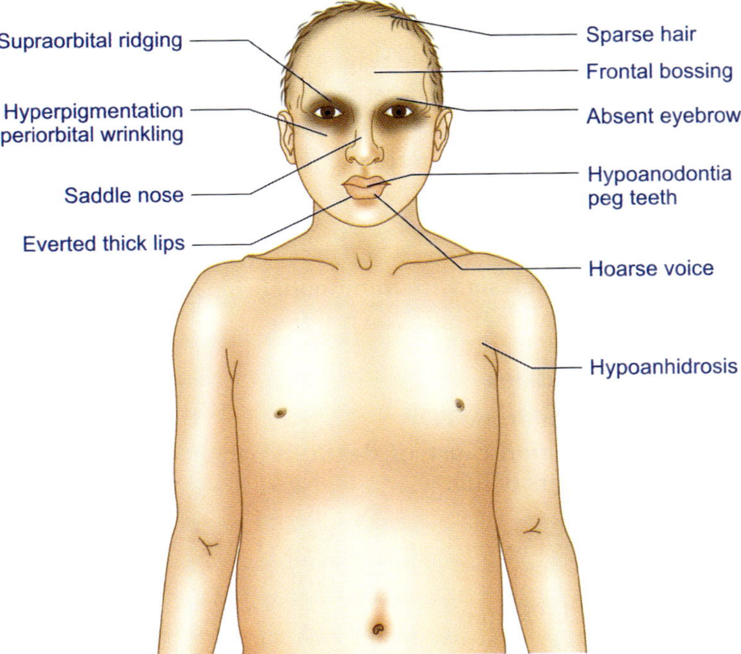

Fig. 13.54: Depiction of Christ–Siemens–Touraine syndrome

- **Teeth:** Dentition delayed; may have peg-shaped, conical or missing teeth.
- **Eccrine glands:** Risk for hyperthermia as a result of ↓perspiration; ↓lacrimation may be seen.
- May develop chronic sinus disease, pulmonary infections, and asthma.

The main clinical features are listed in **Box 13.14**.

BOX 13.14: Overview of clinical features of CST syndrome

Features	%
Smooth, dry skin	78
Sparse hair	89
Sparse eyebrows	100
Sparse body hair	62
Decreased sweating	85
Heat intolerance	50
Onychodysplasia	39
Dental anomalies	100

Clinical Variants

- Heat intolerance is subjective
- Hairs may be black or light colored, some have absent hairs
- Hypohidrotic ectodermal dysplasia with immunodeficiency is a result of mutations in IKBKG/NEMO (XLR) or NFKBIA (AD); susceptible to recurrent pyogenic or atypical mycobacterial infections.

Pathology

- Thin epidermis with flattening of the rete ridges
- Reduced hair follicles, sweat glands, sebaceous glands
- Apocrine glands may be absent, sparse or even normal
- Light and electron microscopy shows variable hair shaft defects including twisting, pili canaliculi and trichorrhexis nodosa.

Differential Diagnosis

- Other form of ectodermal dysplasia with immunodeficiency or deafness
- Sjögren syndrome with symptomatic sicca syndrome

Complications and Comorbidities

- There is **21%** mortality in anhidrotic ED.
- Heatstroke is the most **common cause of death** in patients with anhidrotic ectodermal dysplasia within the first years of life.
- Eczema
- Asthma and recurring wheezing
- Nasal crusting
- Recurring respiratory tract infections
- Feeding problems in infancy
- Recurrent fever in infancy.

Disease Course and Prognosis

- Early diagnosis is important to avoid life-threatening complications induced by hyperthermia and infections.
- Screening evaluation, regular monitoring and consideration of therapeutic intervention should begin in early childhood.
- DNA analysis: Fetoscopy (20 weeks)—skin biopsy showing absent pilo sebaceous units.

Management

- Avoidance of heat and physical over-exertion is an important preventive measure.
- Cooling the body with wet clothing and cool drink is advised.
- Orthodontic intervention is required for language development, restoring function and improving the appearance of the teeth
- HED with immunodeficiency requires immune-based therapies plus aggressive management of infections or hematopoietic stem cell transplantation.

Update

In **X-linked hypohidrotic ectodermal dysplasia** (XLHED), the genetic deficiency of the signaling molecule ectodysplasin A1 (EDA1) may be overcome before birth by administration of a recombinant replacement protein. This has been shown at least for the key problem of male subjects with XLHED, which is the near complete absence of sweat glands and perspiration which can lead to life-threatening hyperthermia. Prenatal treatment of six boys by injection of an EDA1 replacement protein into the amniotic fluid consistently induced the development of functional sweat glands. [Schneider H]

HIDROTIC ED (CLOUSTON DISEASE)

- Rare genodermatosis, normal sweating, involves skin, hair, nail only
- Inheritance: Autosomal dominant
- Gene: connexin gene (GJB6)
- Occur at early age and affects both sex equally.

Associated Diseases

- Photophobia
- Conjunctivitis
- Sensorineural deafness.
- Blepharitis
- Thickened skull bones

Clinical Features

- Three important features: **Nail dystrophy, alopecia and keratoderma**.
- **Skin:** Diffuse palmoplantar keratoderma with transgradiens. Hyperpigmentation over joints is common teeth and sweat glands *normal* (unlike hypohidrotic ED).
- **Hair:** Partial or total alopecia, sparse scalp hairs. Sparse and short hairs over eyelashes, eyebrows, axillary and pubic hairs.
- **Nail:** Thickened and whitish nails, triangular nails, distal onycholysis.
- **Eye:** Possible ophthalmologic (e.g. conjunctivitis, strabismus, and cataracts) and musculoskeletal (tufted distal phalanges) anomalies.
- **Musculoskeletal:** Tufting of terminal phalanges and thickened skull bones may occur.

Pathology

- Histological features from palm and sole shows orthohyperkeratosis
- Normal granular layer
- Increased number of desmosomes seen in stratum corneum.

Differential Diagnosis

- Pachyonychia congenita
- Pure hair and nail ectodermal dysplasia.

Disease Course and Severity

Normal life expectancy, despite increase in clinical features over times.

Investigations

- To confirm clinical diagnosis—gene mutation analysis for GJB6 gene (connexin 30) is mandatory
- Prenatal diagnosis—DNA analysis by fetoscopy (20 weeks)—skin biopsy showing absent pilosebaceous units.

Management

- Keratolytics and emollients
- Professional pedicures and manicures
- Alopecia–wig
- Topical tretinoin and minoxidil.

ECTODERMAL DYSPLASIAS DUE TO P63 MUTATION

AD mutation in p63 (critical transcription factor required for ectodermal, orofacial, and limb development).

Clinical Features

All syndromes may have wiry/sparse hair, dystrophic nails, ↓number of teeth/hypoplastic enamel, hypohidrosis, tearing, and short stature or poor weight gain.

Clinical Syndromes

- Rapp-Hodgkin syndrome: Clefting of lip/palate/uvula, hypoplasia of maxilla, small narrow nails, and small conical teeth.
- Ankyloblepharon-ectodermal dysplasia-cleft lip/palate **(AEC)** syndrome (Hay-Wells syndrome): Congenital fusion of eyelids (ankyloblepharon) associated with facial clefting or mid-face hypoplasia; diffuse collodion-like peeling/erythema seen at birth; scalp with chronic erosive dermatitis → frequent Staphylococcus infections.
- Ectrodactyly ectodermal dysplasia-cleft lip/palate **(EEC)** syndrome: Ectrodactyly (developmental anomaly of median ray of feet > hands → "lobster claw" deformity/missing digits), facial clefting, mild PPK, conductive hearing loss, and genitourinary anomalies.
- p63 mutations also underlie acrodermato-ungual-lacrimal-tooth **(ADULT)** syndrome, limb-mammary syndrome (LMS), and split hand-foot malformation (SHFM).

BIBLIOGRAPHY

Books

1. Genodermatoses: A Clinical Guide to Genetic Skin Disorders. Second Edition.
2. Rook's Textbook of Dermatology, 9th ed. Part 6, Chapter 80: Hamartoneoplastic Syndromes.
3. Rook's Textbook of Dermatology, 9th, ed.Part5, Chapter 60: Cutaneous Porphyrias.

Journals

1. Almeida HL, Jr. Rossi G, Karam OR, Rocha NM, Silva RM. Comparative scanning electron microscopy of bullous diseases. An Bras Dermatol 2014;89:347–50.
2. Boehmer D,. Variable response to low-dose naltrexone in patients with Darier disease: a case series. J Eur Acad Dermatol Venereol. 2019 May;33(5):950–953.
3. Bonkovsky HL, Ledipasvir/Sofosbuvir Is Effective as Sole Treatment of Porphyria Cutanea Tarda with Chronic Hepatitis C. Dig Dis Sci. 2023 Feb 22:1–9.
4. Chen PL The efficacy and safety of topical rapamycin-calcitriol for facial angiofibromas in patients with tuberous sclerosis complex: a prospective, double-blind, randomized clinical trial. Br J Dermatol. 2020 Oct;183(4):655–663.
5. Christiano AM, Pulkkinen L, McGrath JA, UittoJ. Mutation-based prenatal diagnosis of Herlitz junctional epidermolysis bullosa. Prenat Diagn 1997;17:343–54.
6. Dom GE. et al. Activity of Selumetinibin Neurofibromatosis Type 1-Related Plexiform Neurofibromas. N Engl J Med. 2016 Dec 29;375 (26):2550–60.
7. Duat-Rodriguez A, Hernandez-Martin A.[Update on the treatment of RAS opathies]. Rev Neurol. 2017 May17;64 (s03):S13–S17.
8. Eady RA, McGrath JA, McMillan JR. Ultrastructural clues to genetic disorders of skin: the dermal-epidermal junction. J Invest Dermatol 1994;103: 13S–8S.
9. El Hachem M, Zambruno G, Bourdon-Lanoy E, Ciasulli A, Buisson C, Hadj-Rabia S, et al. Multicent reconsensus recommendations for skin care ininherited epidermolysis bullosa. Orphanet J Rare Dis2014;9:76.
10. Fine JD, Bruckner-Tuderman L, Eady RA, Bauer EA, Bauer JW, Has C, et al. Inherited epidermolysis bullosa: updated recommendations on diagnosis and classification. J Am Acad Dermatol 2014;70: 1103–26.
11. Frew JW, Martin LK, NijstenT, Murrell DF. Quality of life evaluation in epidermolysis bullosa (EB) through the development of the QOLEB question naire: an EB-specific quality of life instrument. Br J Dermatol 2009;161:1323–30.
12. Frew JW, Murrell DF. Quality of life measurements in epidermolysis bullosa: tools for clinical research and patient care. Dermatol Clin 2010;28:185–90.
13. Goldschneider KR, Good J, Harrop E, Liossi C, Lynch-JordanA, Martinez AE, et al. Paincarefor patients with epidermolysis bullosa: best care practice guidelines. BMC Med2014;12:178.
14. Gordon LB, Association of Lonafarnib Treatment vs No Treatment With Mortality Rate in Patients With Hutchinson-Gilford Progeria Syndrome. JAMA. 2018 Apr 24;319(16):1687–1695.
15. Guide SV,. Trial of Beremagene Geperpavec (B-VEC) for Dystrophic Epidermolysis Bullosa. N Engl J Med. 2022 Dec 15;387(24):2211–2219.
16. Harhouri K, Frankel D, Bartoli C, Roll P. Sandre-Giovannoli A, Levy N. An overview of treatment strategies for Hutchison-Gilford progeria syndrome. Nucleus. 2018; 9(1): 246–257.
17. Has C, Kiritsi D. Therapies for inherited skin fragility disorders. Exp Dermatol 2015;24:325–31.
18. Heerfordt IM, Experimental and approved treatments for skin photosensitivity in individuals with erythropoietic protoporphyria or X-linked protoporphyria: A systematic review. Biomed Pharmacother. 2023 Feb;158:114132.
19. Hiremagalore R, Kubba A, Bansel S, Jerajani H. Immunofluorescence mapping in inherited epidermolysis bullosa: a study of 86 cases from India. Br J Dermatol2015;172:384–91.
20. HsuCK, Wang SP, LeeJY, McGrath JA.Treatment of hereditary epidermolysis bullosa: updates and future prospects. Am J Clin Dermatol 2014;15:1–6.

21. Leung AK, Barankin B, Lam JM, Leong KF, Hon KL. Xeroderma pigmentosum: an updated review. Drugs Context. 2022 Apr 25;11:2022-2-5.
22. Li Q, van de Wetering K, Uitto J. Pseudoxanthoma Elasticum as a Paradigm of Heritable Ectopic Mineralization Disorders: Pathomechanisms and Treatment Development. Am J Pathol. 2019 Feb;189(2):216–225.
23. Mazereeuw-Hautier J, Management of congenital ichthyoses: European guidelines of care, part two. Br J Dermatol. 2019 Mar;180 (3):484–495.
24. Mazereeuw-Hautier J. Management of congenital ichthyoses: European guidelines of care, part one. Br J Dermatol. 2019 Feb;180 (2):272–281.
25. McGrath JA, Eady RA. The role of immunohistochemistry in the diagnosis of the non-lethal forms of junctional epidermolysis bullosa. J Dermatol Sci1997;14:68–75.
26. McGrath JA. Recently Identified Forms of Epidermolysis Bullosa. Ann Dermatol 2015;27: 658–66.
27. Mellerio JE, Robertson SJ, Bernardis C, Diem A, Fine JD, George R, et al. Managementofcutaneous squamous cell carcinoma in patients with epidermolysis bullosa: best clinical practice guidelines. Br J Dermatol 2016;174:56–67.
28. Murauer EM, Koller U, Pellegrini G, De Luca M, Bauer JW. Advances in Gene/Cell Therapy in Epidermolysis Bullosa. Keio J Med 2015;64:21–5.
29. Murrell DF. Burden of disease scoring in epidermolysis bullosa. Br J Dermatol 2015;173: 1357–8.
30. Murrell DF. The pit falls of skin biopsies to diagnose epidermolysis bullosa. Pediatr Dermatol 2013;30:273–5.
31. Negosanti F, Tengattini V, GurioliC, NeriI. Facial angiofibromas treated by rapamycin 0.05% ointment and acombined laser therapy. J Cosmet Dermatol. 2018Oct;17 (5):762–5.
32. Pfendner EG. Next-generation sequencing: comprehensive genetic testing for epidermolysis bullosa. Br J Dermatol 2015;173:638–9.
33. Ralston SH, Gaston MS. Management of Osteogenesis Imperfecta. Front Endocrinol (Lausanne). 2020 Feb 11;10:924.
34. Rao R, Mellerio J, Bhogal BS, Groves R. Immunofluorescence antigen mapping for hereditary epidermolysis bullosa. Indian J Dermatol Venereol Leprol2012;78:692–7.
35. Schneider H. Ectodermal dysplasias: New perspectives on the treatment of so far immedicable genetic disorders. Front Genet. 2022 Sep 6;13:1000744.
36. Simpson JK, et al. Genotype-phenotype correlation in a large English cohort of patients with autosomal recessive ichthyosis. Br J Dermatol. 2020 Mar;182 (3):729–737.
37. Weon JL, Glass DA 2nd. Novel therapeutic approaches to xeroderma pigmentosum. Br J Dermatol. 2019 Aug;181(2):249–255.
38. Zhao R, Zou W, Zhao X. Treatment of neurofibromatosis type II with anlotinib: a case report and literature review. Anticancer Drugs. 2023 Jan 24. doi: 10.1097/CAD.0000000000001502.

Chapter 14

Hair Disorders

Surabhi Sinha, Kabir Sardana, Sweta Singh

INTRODUCTION

Hair disorders are conventionally divided into three main types: Nonscarring alopecia, scarring alopecia and hirsutism.

While androgenetic alopecia and telogen effluvium are commonly seen, we will not cover them here as they are of interest in clinical practice and are not asked in examinations.

ALOPECIA AREATA

Epidemiology

- Incidence—0.1–0.2% with a lifetime risk of 1.7% (6% in a child if a parent has AA)
- First episode usually below 40 years of age with peak in second to fourth decade of life.
- Children—peak between 1 and 5 years.
- Seen equally in both the sexes.
- 5% develop alopecia totalis (AT) and 1% develop alopecia universalis (AU).

Pathophysiology

A brief overview of the loss of immune privilege of the hair follicle is given in **Fig. 14.1a**, while detailed steps of pathogenesis are delineated in **Fig. 14.1b**.

A genome-wide association study (GWAS) on AA implicated both innate and adaptive immunity (Petukhova L, 2010). A genetic predisposition and risk factors increase the chances of developing AA in an individual.

Genetic Predisposition

- MHC class II alleles—HLA DQB1*0301 and HLA DRB1*1104.
- NKG2D/NKG2D ligands:
  - Natural killer group 2, member D (NKG2D) receptors are expressed by NK cells and CD8+ T cells—serve as recognition receptors for elimination of damaged or transformed cells.
  - NKG2D ligands belong to two families—MIC (MICA and MICB) and ULBP (ULBP1-ULBP6)—expressed by numerous target cells during infection/autoimmunity/inflammation. In the normal hair follicle, ULBP3 is turned off.

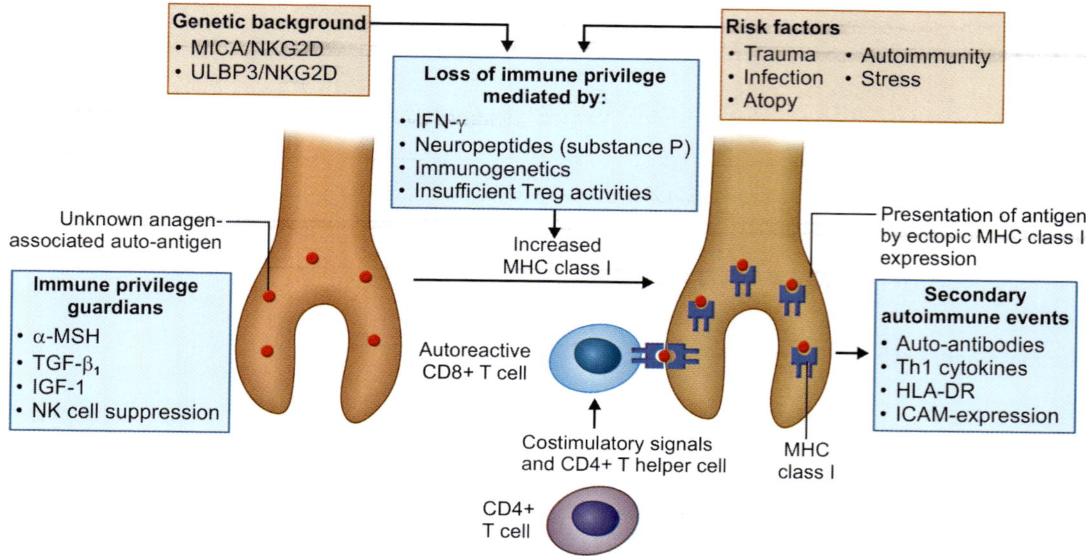

Fig. 14.1a: An overview of the steps of causation of alopecia areata from loss of immune privilege to activation of CD8+ T cells

- *MICA and ULBP3* gene cluster (code for the NKG2D-activating ligand that can trigger the NKG2D receptor, thus initiating an autoimmune response) are highly expressed in AA patients.
- It is now postulated that the characteristic T cell 'swarm of bees' infiltrate seen in alopecia areata is the result of T cells being attracted to the hair follicle by NKG2D-activating ligands.

- Positive family history: A family history of alopecia areata is more common in those with disease onset before the age of 30 years.

Risk Factors

- Trauma
- Atopy
- Psychologic stress
- Infection
- Autoimmunity
- Oxidative stress

Both genetic and risk factors when combined lead to the following steps:

Step 1: Collapse of hair follicle (HF) immune privilege (IP)

What preserves IP?

- The absence or low-expression of major histocompatibility complex (MHC) class I
- ↓ IFN regulatory factor-1
- ↑ upregulation of immunosuppressive or pro-apoptotic molecules (IP guardians)—TGF-β, α-melanocyte-stimulating hormone (MSH), IGF-1, absence of MHC class II cells or Langerhans cells.
- The sparse distribution of T cell and natural killer (NK) cells
- Absence of lymphatics

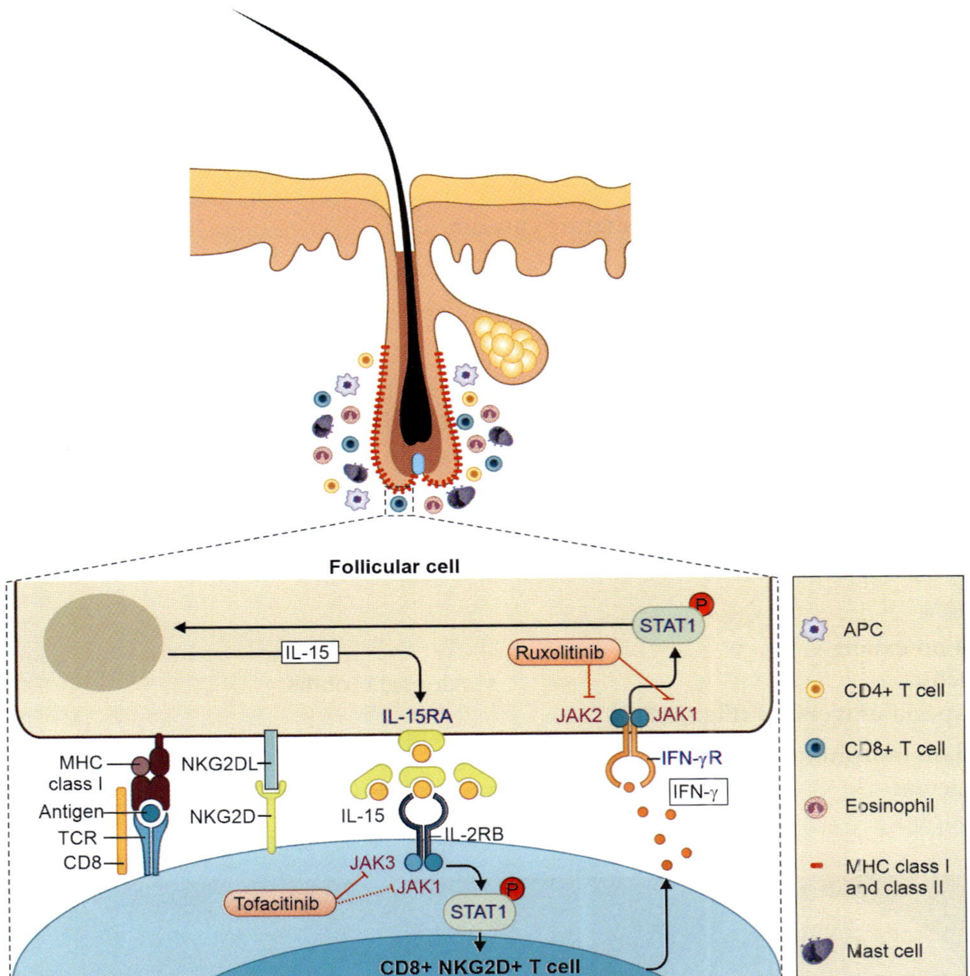

- Loss of immune privilege leads to exposure of hair follicle antigens to lymphocytes
- CD8+ NKG2D+ T cells infiltrate the dermis and localize to the hair follicle bulb and interact with follicular epithelial cells through major histocompatibility complex (MHC) class I—peptide complexes with NKG2DL
- Activated CD8+ T cells release IFN-γ which bind to follicular epithelial cell
- Signals JAK1 and JAK2 which lead to production of IL-15, a mediator of CD8+ T cell induction
- This in an autocrine loop activates CD8+ T cell surface, via JAK1 and JAK3, to enhance the production of IFN-γ amplifying the feedback loop
- Ruxolitinib and tofacitinib are small molecule JAK inhibitors that interfere with this feedback loop
- Ruxolitinib inhibits JAK1 and JAK2 while tofacitinib inhibits JAK3 more strongly than JAK1

Fig. 14.1b: A depiction of the interaction of hair follicle, APCs and CD8+ T cells in AA

Step 2: Exposure of autoantigens of hair follicle

- HF immune privilege collapse is the most important factor in the causation of AA.
- Normally, sequestered HF autoantigens are now presented via ectopic MHC I/β2-microglobulin expression to infiltrating autoreactive CD8+ T cells. This is an absolute requirement for autoimmune AA to develop.

- Interferon-γ (IFN)-producing immune cells and MHC class I upregulation
- Leads to presentation of hair follicle autoantigens to T lymphocytes

Step 3: Local IFN-γ-IL-15-JAK axis activation

- Activation of JAK pathway
- CD8+ T cell autoreactivity
- Hair bulb damage
- Induces HF dystrophy and premature catagen.

Clinical Features

- Circumscribed smooth hairless patch of skin
- Erythema +/–
- **Exclamation mark hair:** Presence of short easily extractable broken hair at the margins of the patch with broad distal ends and narrowed proximally.
- Scalp is the most common and, usually, the first site affected.
- Can involve the beard, eyebrows and eyelashes also.
- Sparing of white hair—'Canities Subita'.
- Regrowth can be depigmented to hypopigmented.

Variants

Based on extent

- Patchy
- Alopecia universalis **(Fig. 14.2a)**
- Alopecia totalis

Based on morphology

- Reticular
- Sisaipho
- Ophiasis **(Fig. 14.2b)**

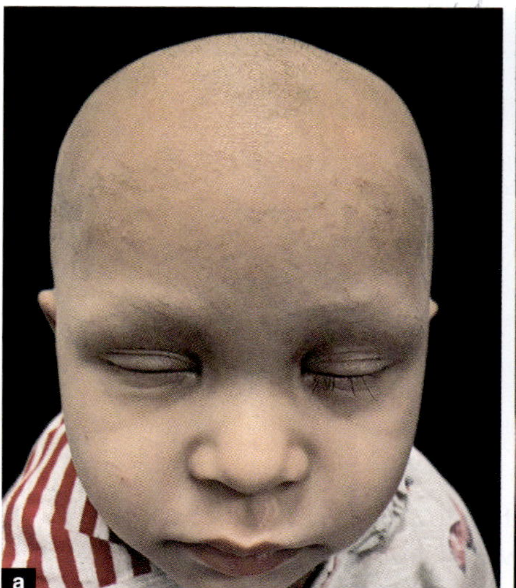

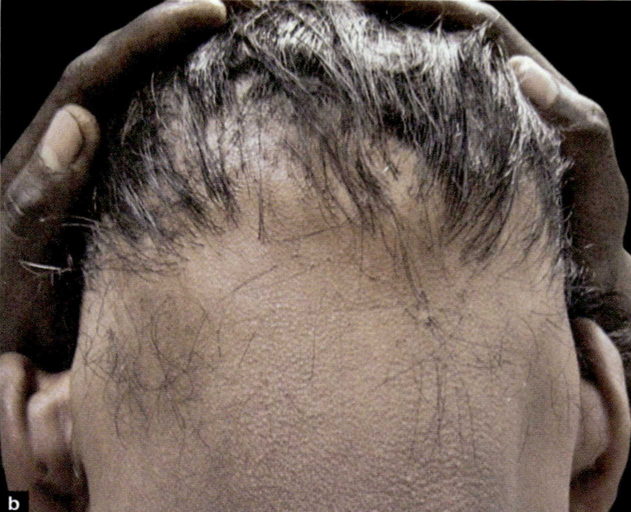

Fig. 14.2: (a) A child with alopecia universalis; (b) Ophiasis pattern of alopecia areata

Unusual variants
- Linear
- Perinevoid
- Acute diffuse and total (rapid progressive AA but favorable prognosis)
- Diffuse (overall reduced density without patches of hair loss)

Nail involvement: Seen in 10–66% of the cases.
- Geometric pitting and trachyonychia.
- Presence of red lunulae indicate acute disease.

Scoring System

Severity of Alopecia Tool Score (SALT Score)

Scalp is divided into four areas, namely vertex—40% (0.4) of scalp surface area; right profile of scalp—18% (0.18) of scalp surface area; left profile of scalp—18% (0.18) of scalp surface area; posterior aspect of scalp—24% (0.24) of scalp surface area.

Percentage of hairloss in any of these areas is percentage hair loss multiplied by percentage surface area of the scalp in that area.

SALT score is the sum of percentage of hair loss in all above mentioned areas.

Differential Diagnosis

See **Table 14.1**.

TABLE 14.1: Differential diagnosis of AA

Disease	Differentiation from AA
T. capitis	Presence of scaling and erythema, easy pluckability, itching
Trichotillomania	• Artificial shapes of the patches of hair loss • Broken hair has a bristle like texture, broken at varying lengths • Only accessible areas are involved
Cicatricial alopecia	Loss of follicular orifices, visible epidermal atrophy
Congenital triangular alopecia	Appears by 2 years of age, distinct triangular or oval shape, non-progressive

Prognosis

One of the most useful studies to predict response and progression is the seminal study by Ikeda et al. who studied the natural history of AA among 1989 patients in Kyoto, Japan. She noted that:
- 40% of patients develop a solitary patch of AA that regrows spontaneously within 6 months.
- 27% develop additional patches, but still achieve a complete and persistent remission at 1 year.
- Chronic AA, defined as AA that continues beyond 1 year, tends to develop additional areas of AA and has persistent hair loss for many years. Many never achieve complete remission. Among those with chronic AA, 30% ultimately develop alopecia totalis (AT) and 15% alopecia universalis (AU).

A summary of the results of Ikeda and the consequent prognostic factors are listed in **Table 14.2**.

TABLE 14.2: Prognosis of AA (based on the Ikeda study)

Clinical type	Spontaneous growth	Risk of chronic AA/AT, AU
Solitary stable patch		
• AA ≤6 months duration	87%	13%, 6%
• AA ≥6 months but ≤12 months	35%	65%, 30%
• AA ≥12 months duration	0%	100%, 45%
Multiple patches within 6 months of initial presentation	65%	35%, 15%
Age		
• 0–6 years at **initial presentation**	0%	100%, 45%
• 6–12 years at **initial presentation**	60%	40%, 18%

Poor prognostic factors in AA are:
- **Onset of disease**—onset before the age of 12 and in particular before the age of 6 years.
- **Duration**—more than 1 year
- **Extent/type**—development of multiple discrete patches, extensive hair loss involving >50% of the scalp, ophiasis pattern of alopecia, AT or AU.
- **Associated disorders**—nail disease, trisomy 21, atopy
- **Famliy history**—AA or other organ-specific autoimmune disease.

Investigations*

Trichoscopy (Fig. 14.3)
- Yellow dots, black dots, broken hairs, tapering hair/exclamation hair, and short vellus hairs.
- Yellow dots are not specific for AA as they are also seen in AGA.
- Presence of black dots, broken hair (cadaverized hair), and tapering hair suggest active disease and are most specific for AA.
- No pathognomonic marker on trichoscopy.

Histopathology

Active disease: In the acute stage, terminal hairs are surrounded by lymphocytes ('swarm of bees'). The inflammatory infiltrate is composed mainly of activated T lymphocytes, with a preponderance of CD4 cells, and an admixture of macrophages, Langerhans cells and cells expressing NK cell markers. Hair follicles do not progress beyond anagen III–IV stage.

Subacute phase: Decreased anagen and increased catagen and telogen hairs are characteristic.

Chronic phase: In chronic cases, follicular miniaturization with variable inflammatory infiltrate is seen in papillary dermis. The terminal to vellus hair ratio is decreased to 1:1 in contrast to 7:1 in normal population.

Additional investigations (*only if indicated*)
- KOH mount
- Fungal culture
- Syphilis serology
- Lupus serology

*AA is the second leading cause of psychiatric referrals by dermatologists (after psoriasis)—DLQI should be measured and psychiatric opinion sought, especially in AT/AU.

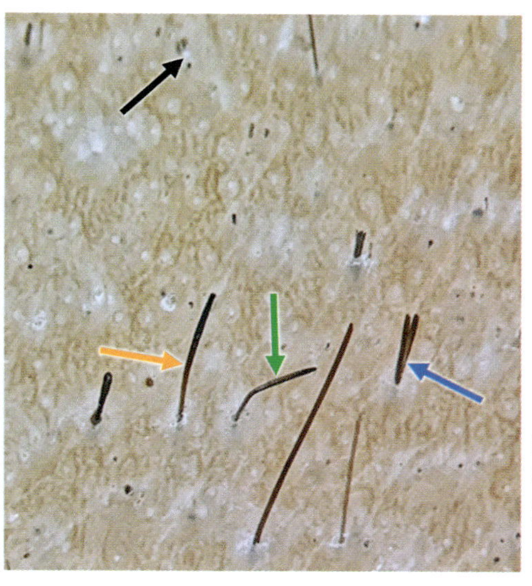

Active hair loss	Longstanding inactive disease	Hair regrowth
Black dots Micro-exclamation mark hairs Broken hairs Monilethrix-like hairs Trichorrhexis nodosa	Yellow dots Vellus hairs Follicular opening may not be visible	Upright regrowing hairs Pigtail hairs (oval or circular Vellus hairs

Fig. 14.3a: Trichoscopy of AA showing black dots (**black** arrow), broken hair or fractured hair shaft (**blue** arrow), exclamation mark hair (**orange** arrow) and coudability hair (**green** arrow). The accompanying box shows the markers for different stages of activity of the disease

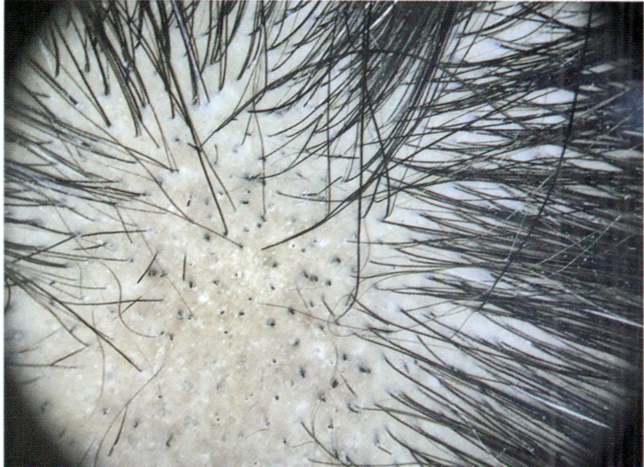

Fig. 14.3B: Trichoscopy of AA with black dots and exclamation mark hair (*Courtesy*: Dr Deepak Jakhar, MD)

Treatment (Flowcharts 14.1 and 14.2)

The various agents are listed below, but the kind of intervention would depend on the severity, prognostic factors, progression and age of the patient. As a general rule, for localized disease of duration <12 months, topical agents would suffice, but for the rest, systemic therapies are needed. There is as yet no disease modifying agent known for AA.

It would be reasonable to segregate acute AA and chronic AA, and reserve JAKi for patients with chronic AA defined by an episode duration of **≥12 months**. Of the cases with chronic AA, without systemic treatment 55% will have persistent multifocal relapsing and remitting disease, 30% will ultimately develop alopecia totalis (AT) and 15% will develop alopecia universalis (AU). Here it must be noted that the treatment of AT or AU, will need long term maintenance therapy and do not respond to treatment as well as patchy AA. This is especially true when the episode duration exceeds 7–10 years. JAK inhibitor would be ideal for chronic multifocal AA.

1. **Steroids (topical or intralesional)**
   - High-potency steroid, such as clobetasol propionate 0.05% as gel, foam, or solution
   - I/L steroids can be used 2.5–10 mg/mL at 4–6 weekly intervals.
2. **Oral steroids:** Systemic therapy is a possible option in case of acute rapidly progressing alopecia areata and in localized but very active cases. Systemic steroids are not a good option in alopecia totalis/universalis as response is poor. Response varies from 11% to 88%, with relapse rates of 28–100%.
3. **Immunosuppressive agents (ISA):** The various drugs tried include cyclosporine (CyS A), methotrexate, and azathioprine and these are used in combination with steroids.

   Cyclosporine is not useful in the severe variants of the diseases as it requires high doses (6 mg/kg/day), results are not consistent, and the safety profile is a concern.

   Methotrexate (15 mg/week) and azathioprine are safer and better drugs.

   Azathioprine is commonly started at a low dose (0.5–1 mg/kg daily) to minimise the risk of GI upset and gradually titrated every 4–6 weeks up to 2–3 mg/kg according to patient response and tolerance.
4. **Topical immunotherapy:** The two agents that are used are squaric acid dibutylester (SADBE) and 2,3-diphenylcyclopropenone (DPCP) and the efficacy ranges from 22 to 77%. No significant difference exists between these and they should be used only in stable disease.

Flowchart 14.1: Algorithmic approach to management of AA

Alopecia areata
Age
Age <10 years
Minoxidil 5% solution +/– Topical corticosteroid or Short contact anthralin
Age >10 years
Extent of scalp involvement
<50% Involvement
Intralesional corticosteroids +/– Minoxidil 5% solution +/– Topical corticosteroid +/– Short contact anthralin
>50% Involvement
Scalp prosthesis should be considered in patients with >50% scalp involvement
Topical immunotherapy DPCP/SADBE/DNCB
Response
Poor
Minoxidil 5% solution +/– Topical corticosteroid or Short contact anthralin or PUVA
Good
Continue topical immunotherapy

Flowchart 14.2: Treatment of AA

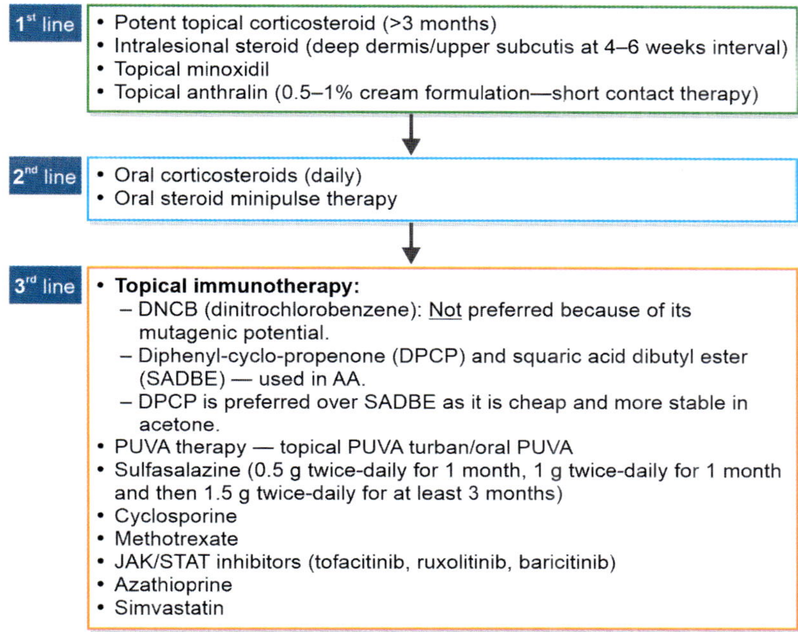

5. **Anthralin:** The efficacy ranges from 25 to 75%. It is applied onto the affected areas and washed off until mild dermatitis appears.
6. **Phototherapy/excimer laser:** Phototherapy and excimer laser are second-line options in both pediatric and adult patients with localized alopecia areata. Treatments that have shown efficacy in alopecia areata are PUVA therapy, PUVA-turban therapy, narrow-band UVB, and excimer laser. Even though the efficacy of this type of treatment is variable, when available, it may be a good option as an alternative or adjuvant therapy.
7. **JAK inhibitors**
   - **Tofacitinib** (JAK3/1 inhibitor)—Tofacitinib blocks STAT phosphorylation induced by IL- 15 (affects the IL-15/INF-γ pathway) and also inhibits the release of IFN-γ, IL-2, IL-4, IL-7 (as can be seen in **Fig. 14.1b**) (5–10 mg BD).
   - **Ruxolitinib** (JAK 1/2 inhibitor)—other than the effects of JAK-STAT pathway inhibition, ruxolitinib has been shown to have anti-inflammatory effects, which are thought to be due to interruption of the IL-17 signalling axis (15–20 mg BD).
   - **Baricitinib** (JAK 1/2 inhibitor). Seen to be effective in very severe treatment refractory AA. **Recently approved for severe AA by FDA (June 2022)**.
   - **Ritlecitinib** a JAK3 inhibitor drug and **Ifidancitinib** a potent and selective next-generation JAK1/3 inhibitor drug are novel drugs in this group.
   - Topical JAK inhibitors—not yet available commercially, have been tried in some studies. (Topical preparations of tofacitinib 2% or ruxolitinib 0.6% ointment or liposomal cream did not show efficacy in a study where they were utilized for 6 months or less, but some studies have shown improvement.)

An overview of the existing JAK inhibitors is given below **(Box 14.1)**.

BOX 14.1: Overview of JAK inhibitors in AA

		Dosage	Duration	Response	Relapse
Oral	Tofacitinib	5 mg BID	3 months	64%	100%
		10 mg BID*	6–18 months	66%	85%
	Ruxolitinib	20 mg BID	3–6 months	75%	33%
	Baricitinib#	2–4 mg QD	9 months	20–38%	—

*A recent black box warning has been released regarding tofacitinib in rheumatoid arthritis, reporting an increase of pulmonary thromboembolism in doses of 10 mg twice daily.
#Only Baricitinib has controlled trials supporting its efficacy in AA.

TRICHOTILLOMANIA

It is a type of obsessive-compulsive disorder and is diagnosed by the criteria given below in **Box 14.2**. [Compulsive hair rubbing (trichoteiromania) and hair cutting (trichotemnomania)—fall in the same category].

BOX 14.2: DSM-V criteria for trichotillomania (TTM)

A. Recurrent pulling out of one's hair, resulting in hair loss.
B. Repeated attempts to decrease or stop hair pulling.
C. The hair pulling causes clinically significant distress or impairment in social, occupational, or other important areas of functioning.
D. The hair pulling or hair loss is not attributable to another medical condition (e.g. a dermatological condition).
E. The hair pulling is not better explained by the symptoms of another mental disorder (e.g. attempts to improve a perceived defect or flaw in appearance in body dysmorphic disorder).

Clinical Features (Figs 14.4 and 14.5)

- Young children
  - As a 'habit tic'

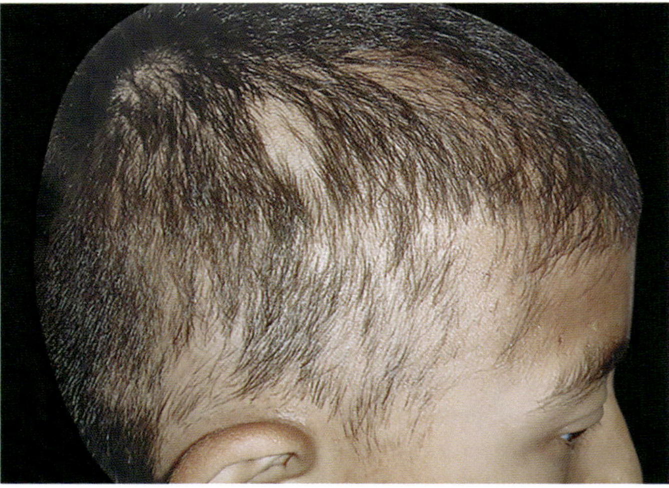

Fig. 14.4: A boy with TTM showing asymmetrical areas of hair loss with short hair of unequal length

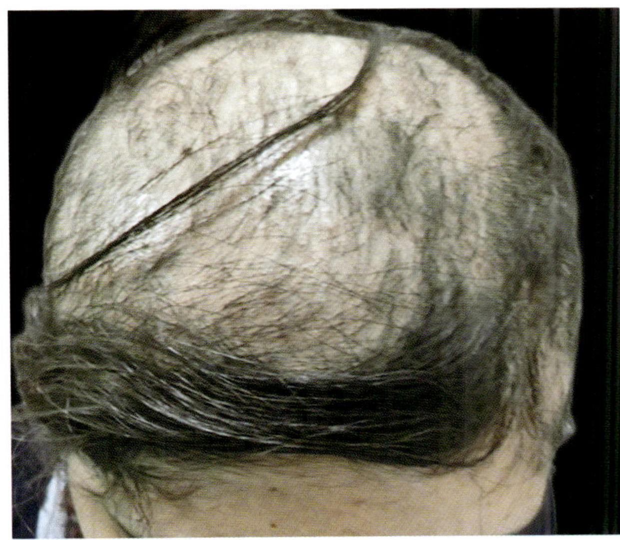

Fig. 14.5: Friar Tuck sign seen in an adult female with trichotillomania

- Frontoparietal region
- Bizarre/angular patch of hair loss with varying lengths of broken-off hair
- Adults
  - More in females
  - May be associated with psychiatric disorder/OCD
  - Patch with a coarse stubble of hair left
  - One asymmetrical patch/whole scalp except margin **(Friar Tuck sign)**
  - Unusual for patch to be completely bald
- Other sites can be affected other than scalp
- Trichobezoar-hair ball may occur if trichophagia present.

Neurobiology of TTM

There are 3 subtypes of TTM described with unique clinical presentations: one subtype is the "sensory sensitive pullers" with highly focused pulling, but infrequent and low intensity urges to pull; "low awareness pullers" with automatic pulling and pulling due to emotional triggers; and "impulsive/perfectionist pullers" who pull to control unpleasant feelings and feel unable to resist their pulling. These have different anatomical changes in the brain (Grant JE, 2023).

Diagnosis

Trichoscopy (Fig. 14.6a)	• *Flame hair*—wavy cone-shaped residues. Correspond to pigment casts. Most characteristic feature of TTM. • V sign, Tulip hair, circular hair • Hair broken at varying lengths—most common finding, not specific • Hair dust/hair powder—complete damage to hair shaft by mechanical friction • 'Burnt matchstick'—dark bulbar proximal tip with linear stem

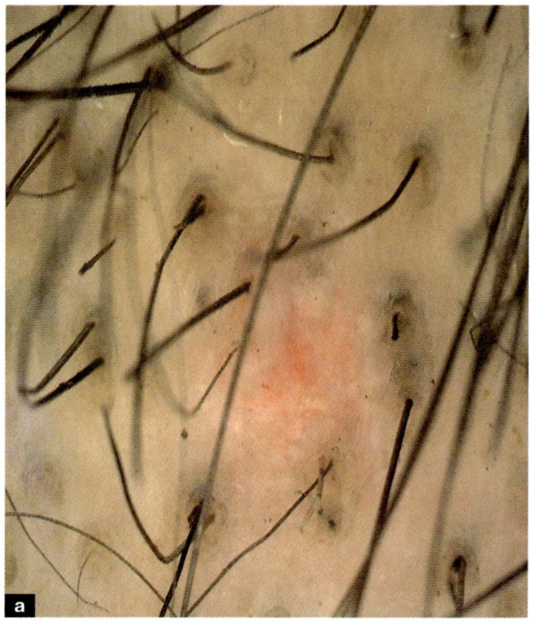

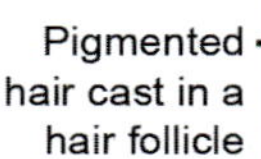

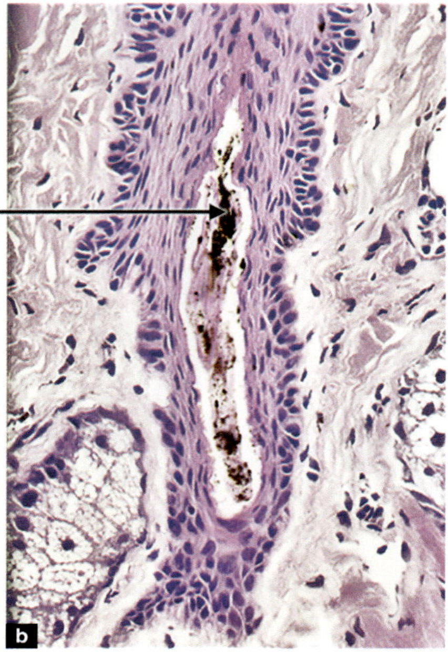

Fig. 14.6: (a) Hair shafts broken at different levels, hemorrhage, V sign and twisted hair shafts in a case of Trichotillomania (*Courtesy*: Ananta Khurana, MD); (b) Histopathology of TTM showing a pigmented hair cast within a hair follicle

	• Perifollicular hemorrhage • Black dots—broken stubs of hair on scalp surface • Trichoptilosis (split ends), microexclamation mark hair
HPE (Fig. 14.6b)	• Numerous *empty* canals—<u>*most consistent* feature of TTM</u> • Intrafollicular pigment casts (blobs of melanin) • Trichomalacia—deformed hair shafts and follicles • Many follicles in catagen, none in telogen • Clefts in the hair matrix, follicular epithelium separated from the connective tissue sheath, intraepithelial and perifollicular hemorrhages.

Differential Diagnosis

- Tinea capitis—scaly, easily pluckable hair, itching.
- Alopecia areata—complete loss of hair from patch, exclamation mark hair not firmly anchored (unlike broken hair of TTM).

Treatment

- Clomipramine—more effective than placebo
- SSRIs—no convincing benefit
- N-acetyl cysteine—better than placebo (Glutamate-modulating agent)
- Help groups, counselling, psychotherapy
- Novel Treatments-memantine, a glutamate modulator, 10–20 mg/d and onabotulinumtoxinA.

CICATRICIAL ALOPECIA

Pathogenesis

- Due to permanent hair follicle destruction, either due to disease of hair follicles themselves (primary) or by an external process (secondary).
- Stem cells in the *bulge area* are destroyed.
- Follicles disappear/are replaced by fibrous stelae.

Epidemiology

- LPP: Commonest cause in Europeans, F>M, 30–50 years
- CCCA: Commonest cause in Africans, F>M, 40s.
- CCLE: F>M, ↑ in Africans
- FFA: Exclusively in postmenopausal women, may occur earlier in association with LP pigmentosus
- Folliculitis decalvans (FD): F = M, >30 years
- Dissecting cellulitis: M >F, 20 years
- Folliculitis keloidalis: African men, >30 years
- Erosive pustular dermatosis: Fair skinned, M = F, 70 years

Associated Diseases

- 40% scalp LPP—cutaneous LP
- 30% scalp CCLE—cutaneous lesions of CCLE
- Dissecting cellulitis—follicular occlusion tetrad
- KPSD—KP elsewhere
- Follicular mucinosis—CTCL

Diagnosis

• **Dermoscopy**	• Loss of follicular ostia in all follicles • Some may have some characteristic features (*see* later)
• **HPE**	• Take early lesion • 2 biopsy samples (one for horizontal and one for vertical sections) • *Vertical sections*: Best for **scarring alopecia** → shows all levels of follicle • *Transverse horizontal sections*: Show all follicular units in specimen → best method for **non-scarring alopecia** • **If only one biopsy** → take 4 mm biopsy from clinically active area → horizontal sectioning (or the Hovert technique may be employed—vertical and horizontal sectioning of a single specimen) • Special stains: Acid orcein (elastin), PAS (mucin)
• **DIF**	• IgG, IgM, fibrinogen, C3

- Most common diagnosis is **non-specific cicatricial alopecia** (may be diagnosed as LPP/pseudopelade/another diagnosis later in the course of the disease).

Classification of Cicatricial Alopecia

It can be due to developmental defects **(Table 14.3)** or primary **(Table 14.4)** or secondary **(Table 14.5)** causes.

TABLE 14.3: Cicatricial alopecia due to developmental defects and hereditary disorders

- Aplasia cutis
- Facial hemiatrophy (Romberg syndrome)
- Epidermal nevi
- Hair follicle hamartomas
- Incontinentia pigmenti
- Focal dermal hypoplasia of Goltz
- Porokeratosis of Mibelli
- Ichthyosis
- Epidermolysis bullosa
- Polyostotic fibrous dysplasia
- Conradi-Hünermann syndrome (chondrodysplasia punctata)

TABLE 14.4: Classification of primary cicatricial alopecia

Lymphocytic	Chronic cutaneous LE (CCLE) Lichen planopilaris (LPP) • Classic LPP • Graham Little syndrome • Frontal fibrosing alopecia (FFA) Pseudopelade of Brocq Central centrifugal cicatricial alopecia (CCCA) Alopecia mucinosa Keratosis pilaris spinulosa decalvans (KPSD) Graft-versus-host disease
Neutrophilic	• Folliculitis decalvans (including tufted folliculitis) • Dissecting cellulitis/folliculitis
Mixed	• Acne keloidalis • Acne necrotica • Erosive pustular dermatosis
Non-specific*	Non-specific/end-stage cicatricial alopecia

*Non-specific scarring primary alopecia is defined as an *idiopathic* scarring alopecia with *inconclusive* clinical and histopathological findings, which is usually the *end stage* of a variety of inflammatory primary scarring alopecias, such as lichen planopilaris and folliculitis decalvans. But, this should *not* be labelled **as pseudopelade** which is a distinct entity.

TABLE 14.5: Classification of secondary cicatricial alopecia

Traumatic	Radiodermatitis, mechanical trauma, postoperative, burns, accidental, dermatitis artefacta, traction alopecia, hot comb alopecia
Sclerosing disorders	• Morphea • Scleroderma • Lichen sclerosus • Sclerodermoid PCT • Chronic GVHD

(Contd.)

TABLE 14.5: Classification of secondary cicatricial alopecia *(Contd.)*

Granulomatous	• Sarcoidosis • Necrobiosis lipoidica • Infectious granuloma
Infections	
• Bacterial	Folliculitis, carbuncle/furuncle
• Fungal	Kerion, favus, tinea capitis (rarely scarring)
• Viral	HZV, VZV, HIV
• Protozoal	Leishmaniasis
• Treponemal	Syphilis
• Mycobacterial	Tuberculosis
Neoplastic	
• Benign	Cylindroma, other adnexal tumors
• Malignant, primary	BCC, SCC, CTCL
• Malignant, secondary	Renal, breast, lung, GIT tumors, lymphoma, leukemia

FOLLICULAR LP

1. Classic (LPP) **(Fig. 14. 7)**
2. Frontal fibrosing alopecia (FFA) **(Fig. 14.8)**
3. Graham-Little syndrome (GLS)

Epidemiology

Commonest follicular LP—LPP.

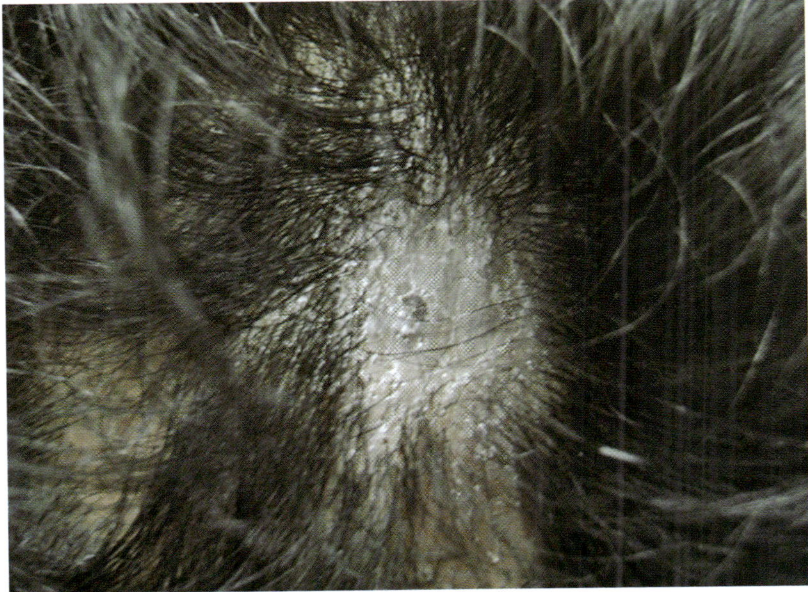

Fig. 14.7a: Lichen planopilaris with cicatricial alopecia

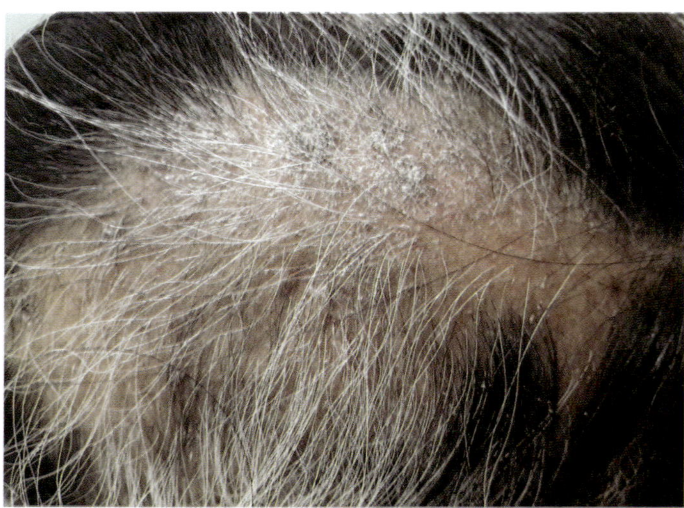

Fig. 14.7b: Lichen planopilaris with violaceous plaques with follicular plugging and perifollicular scaling seen with cicatricial alopecia

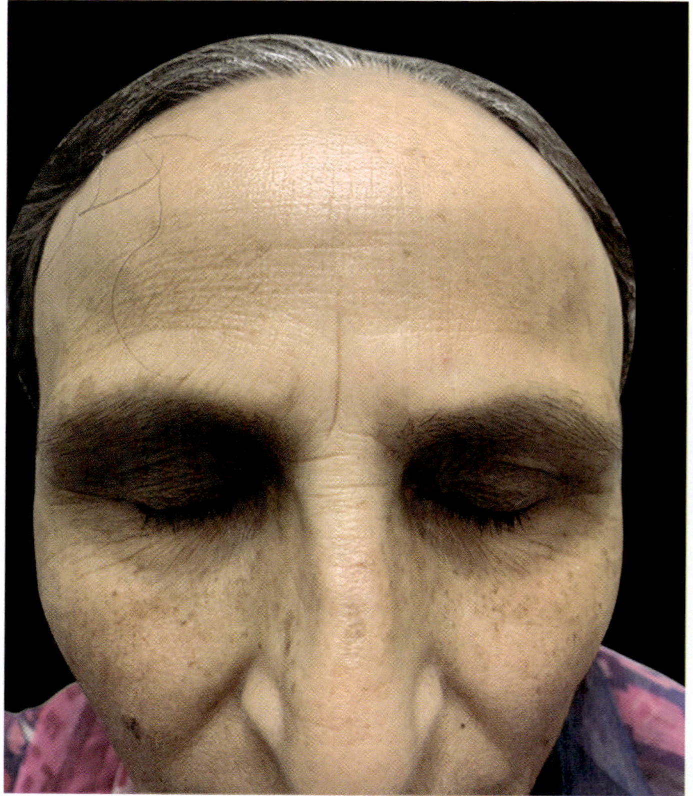

Fig. 14.8a: Frontal fibrosing alopecia (FFA) with cicatricial alopecia in the frontal scalp

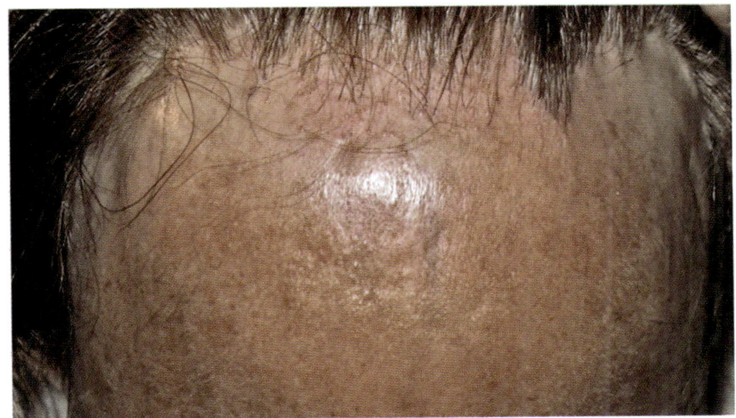

Fig. 14.8b: FFA showing a symmetric, cicatricial band of frontal hairline recession

Pathogenesis

Possibly PPAR-γ (peroxisome proliferator activated receptor γ)—decreased in LPP → aberrant lipid metabolism in the sebaceous gland → toxic build-up of lipids → inflammatory response → scarring.

Clinical Features

See **Table 14.6**. Also *see* **Table 14.7** for differentiating features of two commonly confused entities: LPP scalp *vs* CCLE scalp.

TABLE 14.6: Summary of types of follicular LP

	Classic LPP	FFA	GLS
Morphology	Violaceous papules, erythema, scaling → follicular plugging → smooth atrophic bald patches	• Recession of frontal hairline (recedes at 0.3–1.7 mm per month) in a straight line, loss of eyebrows • Diminished follicular markings • Some **perifollicular erythema**	Scalp—follicular plugging → atrophic bald patches; axillae and pubis—follicular plugging, non-cicatricial alopecia; keratosis pilaris elsewhere
Associated diseases	LP elsewhere, LP only on nails, bullous LP	LP of scalp may coexist, lichen planus pigmentosus +/–	LP may coexist
Sites	Scalp (also on axillae, inguinal folds, sacrum, limb flexures)	Frontal hairline, posterior hairline occasionally	Scalp, axillae, pubis
Age and sex	F>M, 30–50 years	Post-menopausal women exclusively	F>M, 30–70 years
Trichoscopy	• Tubular perifollicular scaling and casts • Elongated blood vessels • Diminished follicular ostia—white dots (impending perifollicular fibrosis) • 'Target' pattern (circular arrangement of melanin around the perifollicular area sparing the interfollicular area) of arrangement of blue-gray dots (melanin incontinence)	Same as LPP	Same as LPP

(Contd.)

TABLE 14.6: Summary of types of follicular LP *(Contd.)*

	Classic LPP	FFA	GLS
HPE	• Irregular acanthosis • Saw toothing of rete ridges • Liquefactive degeneration of basal layer • Lymphohistiocytic infiltrate abutting basal layer • Colloid bodies • Pigment laden macrophages • Hair follicles—periappendageal infiltrate, total destruction, fibrous stellae	Same as LPP	Same as LPP
DIF	Fibrin, IgM, C3—upper dermis in and/or BMZ	Same as LPP	Same as LPP
Treatment	Steroid (topical, I/L, systemic), methotrexate Anti-malarials, ciclosporin, thalidomide, pioglitazone (PPAR-γ agonist—results disappointing), tofacitinib, oral minoxidil	Disappointing. Steroids, anti-malarials, doxycycline, finasteride/ dutasteride, naltrexone	Disappointing. Steroids, anti-malarials, ciclosporin, thalidomide

TABLE 14.7: Lichen planopilaris versus CCLE scalp

	LPP scalp	CCLE scalp
Clinical features	Perifollicular erythema and scale of cicatricial alopecia more common cause	Dilated, plugged follicular ostia (Carpet tack sign), peripheral hyperpigmentation and central depigmentation, less common than LLP
Trichoscopy	• Tubular perifollicular scaling and cast **(Fig. 14.9a)** • Elongated blood vessels • Diminished follicular ostia • **White dots (impending perifollicular fibrosis)** • **No white areas** (due to lack of interfollicular involvement) • **'Target' pattern** (circular arrangement of melanin around the perifollicular area only) arrangement of the blue-gray dots (melanin incontinence)	• Branching/arborizing capillaries **(Fig. 14.9b and c)** • **White areas (due to tissue fibrosis in interfollicular area)—characteristic of CCLE (not seen in LPP)** • Keratin plugs • Reduced follicular ostia • White dots (impeding perifollicular fibrosis) • Blue-grey dots arranged in **'speckles' pattern** (involvement of interfollicular areas with sprinkling of melanin in these areas too)
Histopathology	• Infundibular **hyperkeratosis** • **Hypergranulosis** • **Saw-toothed rete ridges** • Band-like infiltrate of lymphocytes **(Fig. 14.9d)** • **Perifollicular inflammation ++** • Follicular horny plugs –ve • Dropping off of necrotic keratinocytes along the follicular basement membrane • Perifollicular <u>fibrosis</u> and <u>clefts</u> seen commonly • Dermal mucin if seen in LPP is <u>perifollicular</u> • Elastic fibers absent from scar • **No basement membrane thickening** usually • Interfollicular involvement in LPP occurs uncommonly	• **Thinning** of epidermis, • **Hypogranulosis**, • **No saw toothing** • Band-like infiltrate • Perifollicular inflammation not prominent • Follicular horny plugs ++ • Vacuolar changes +, necrotic keratinocytes at the DEJ • Perifollicular fibrosis and clefts not seen • Dermal mucin in CCLE is <u>increased</u> dermis • Elastic fibers absent • Basement membrane thickening is <u>prominent</u> and <u>striking</u> • Interfollicular involvement ±
DIF	**Fibrinogen, IgM, C3**—upper dermis and/or BMZ	Linear **IgG**, IgM, C3 in BMZ

Treatment

The general principle of treatment of **lymphocytic cicatricial alopecias** is given below:
1st line: Hydroxychloroquine 200 mg twice daily for 6–12 months, or doxycycline 100 mg twice daily for 6–12 months.
2nd line: Mycophenolate mofetil 0.5 g twice daily for first month, then 1 g twice daily for 5 months, or cyclosporine 3–5 mg/kg per day or 300 mg/day for 3–5 months or methotrexate (15 mg weekly for 6 months).
3rd line: Pioglitazone 15 mg daily or rosiglitazone 4 mg daily for 3–6 months, particularly for lichen planopilaris.
Intralesional: Injection of triamcinolone acetonide 10 mg/mL to inflamed, symptomatic sites.
Topical: Tacrolimus or steroids.

Update

Lichen planopilaris (LPP) which is a common subtype of primary lymphocytic cicatricial alopecia and it seems that follicular stem cells undergo epithelial-mesenchymal transition (EMT). Thus drugs that acts at this site would be useful and four of these drugs (pioglitazone, tofacitinib, barcitinib and apremilast) have been found to be useful and hold potential for treatment of LPP.

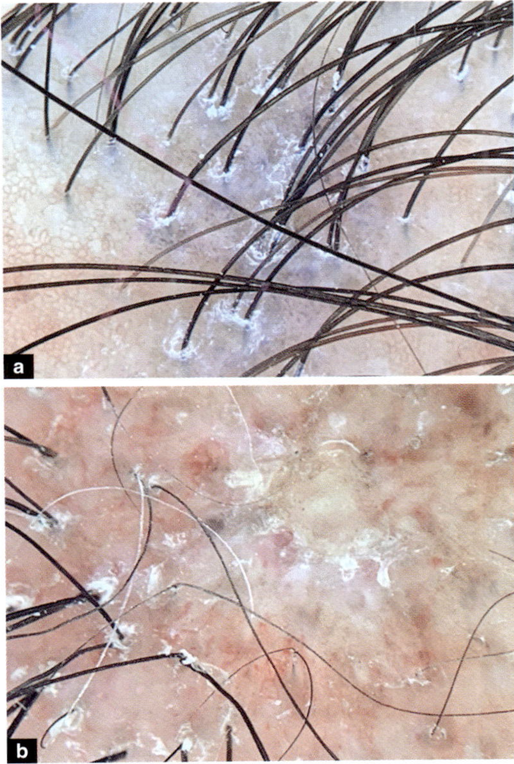

Fig. 14.9a and b: (a) Trichoscopy of LPP scalp (perifollicular scales and casts, blue-gray dots, diminished follicular ostia); (b) Trichoscopy of CCLE scalp (branching capillaries, white structureless areas, keratin plugs, reduced follicular ostia)

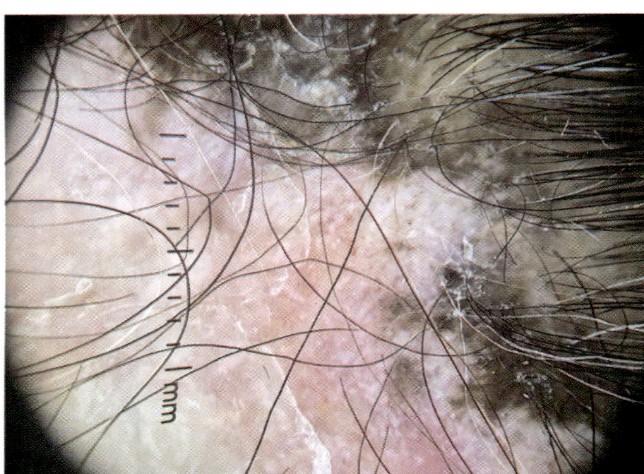

Fig. 14.9c: Trichoscopy of CCLE scalp showing atrophy with complete loss of follicular ostia, gray brown-to-blue colored blotches at the periphery and arborising blood vessels (*Courtesy*: Dr Deepak Jakhar, MD)

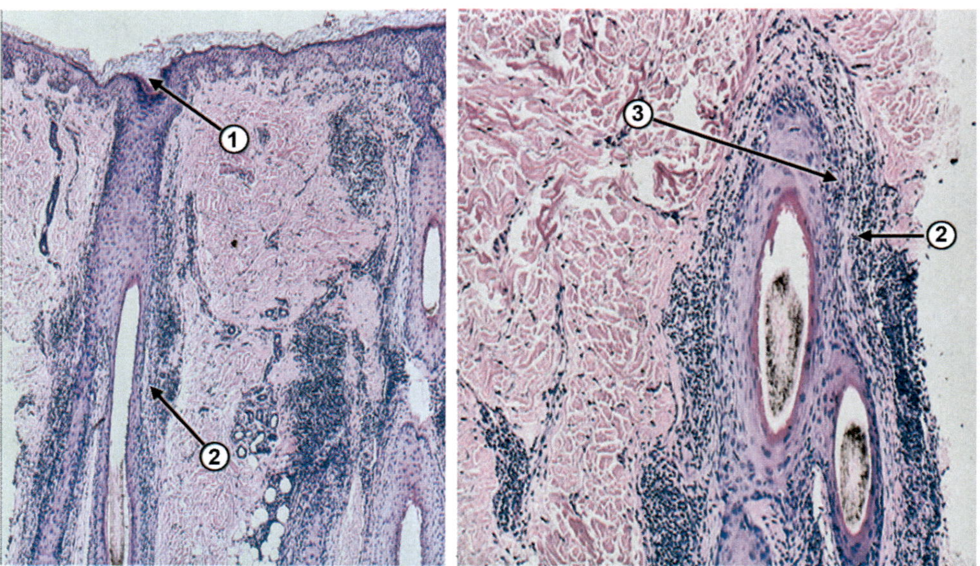

Fig. 14.9d: Histopathology of lichen planopilaris showing characteristic findings. (1) Follicular plugging; (2) Lymphocytic infiltrate; (3) Basal cell degeneration

FFA: Due to the common misdiagnosis, evaluating the response of individual therapeutic agents is difficult. Monotherapy is seldom used, and combination drug therapy is used. While activity markers have been suggested, the disease progression is variable and it is difficult to know whether the disease process has truly stabilized.

An algorithm is given in the figure below, usually aggressive treatment with 1/L steroids, topical tacrolimus and oral agents is the norm **(Flowchart 14.3)**. 5α-reductase inhibitors, intralesional steroids, and hydroxychloroquine have the highest level of evidence for treatment.

Flowchart 14.3: Treatment algorithm for FFA (HoA, et al., 2019)

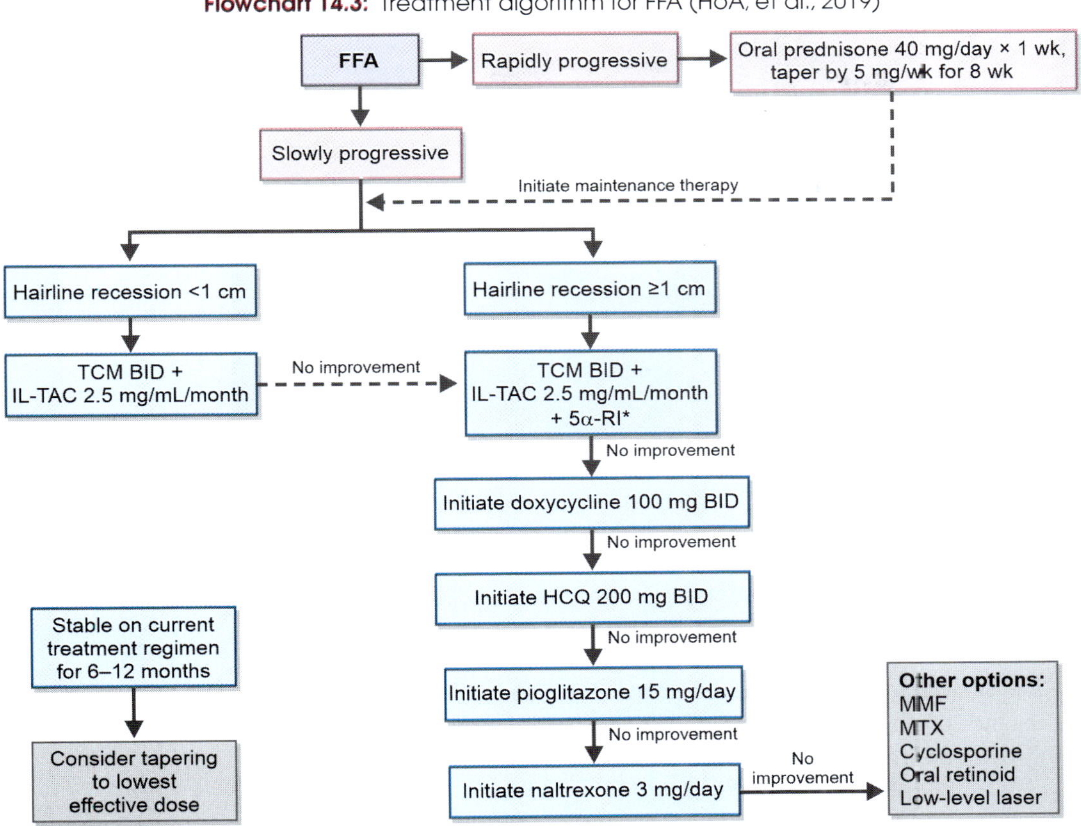

*Finasteride 5 mg/day (premenopausal) or dutasteride 0.5 mg/day (postmenopausal).
5α-RI = 5 alpha-reductase inhibitor; BID = Twice daily; HCQ = Hydroxychloroquine; IL-TAC = Intralesional triamcino-one acetonide; MMF = Mycophenolate mofetil; MTX = Methotrexate; TCM (tacrolimus 0.3% in cetaphil cleanser+ Clobetasol solution + Minoxidil 5% solution)

PSEUDOPELADE OF BROCQ

This is considered as a specific diagnosis because of its characteristic clinical appearance of islands of clumps of terminal hairs that persist in a background of severe sclerosis ('foot-prints in the snow'). **Pelade** is a French term for alopecia areata, so pseudopelade is supposed to resemble alopecia areata, but the latter is non-scarring.

Diagnostic Criteria (Braun-Falco, et al.)

Clinical Criteria

- Irregularly defined and confluent patches of alopecia **(Fig. 14.10)**
- Moderate atrophy (late stage)
- Mild perifollicular erythema (early stage)
- F:M = 3:1
- Long course more than 2 years
- Slow progression with spontaneous termination possible

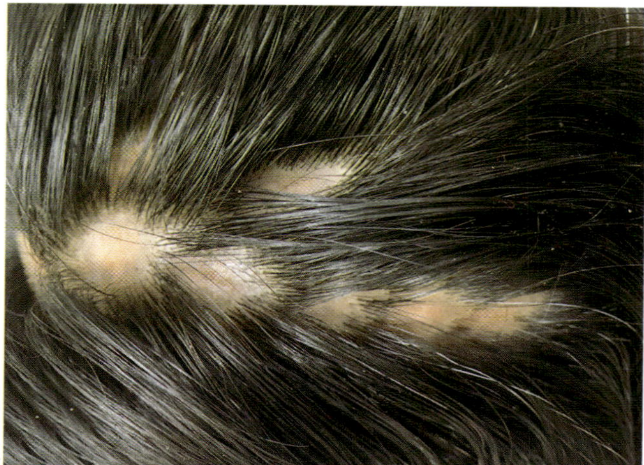

Fig. 14.10: A case of pseudopelade of Brocq with scarring alopecia and characteristic reticular elongation, visualized here as "footprints in the snow" pattern

HPE Criteria

- *Absence* of marked *inflammation*
- *Absence* of widespread *scarring* (Elastin stains)
- *Absence* of significant *follicular plugging*
- *Absence* or at least a decrease of *sebaceous glands*
- Presence of normal epidermis (only occasional atrophy)
- Fibrotic streams into the dermis

DIF

Negative (or only weak IgM on sun-exposed areas)

CENTRAL CENTRIFUGAL CICATRICIAL ALOPECIA (CCCA)

CCCA is a primary lymphocytic cicatricial alopecia of the central scalp which is not seen commonly in India and is restricted largely to Afro-Americans. An overview is given in **Box 14.3** and a clinical photograph shown in **Fig. 14.11**.

BOX 14.3: CCCA in a nutshell

Clinical features

- Slowly progressive scarring of vertex
- Islands of unaffected hairs within scar area **(Fig. 14.11)**
- Spreads symmetrically and centrifugally

Histopathology

- Premature disintegration of inner root sheath resulting in outward migration of the hair shaft through the ORS at the level of the isthmus
- Lamellar fibroplasias and variably dense lymphocytic inflammation surround the follicle at this level
- Follicular destruction and fibrous tract formation

Treatment options

- Potent topical and intralesional corticosteroid
- Hydroxychloroquine, isotretinoin
- Minoxidil
- Thalidomide, cyclosporine, mycofenolate mofetil

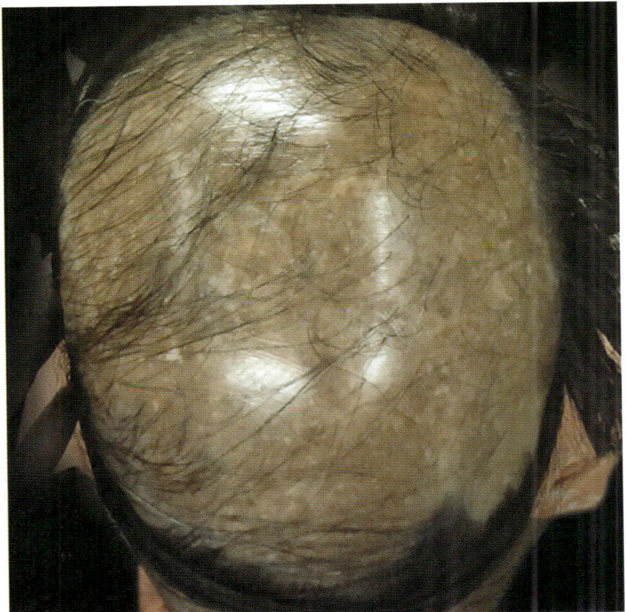

Fig. 14.11: Central centrifugal cicatricial alopecia

FOLLICULITIS DECALVANS

Folliculitis decalvans (FD) is the third most frequent primary cicatricial alopecia after lichen planopilaris and frontal fibrosing alopecia. It is a neutrophilic cicatricial alopecia that usually affects young patients, predominantly males. An onset before 25 years of age is associated with severe forms of FD.

Etiopathogenesis of this disease is not yet well known; however, the presence of *Staphylococcus aureus* in most cases and alteration of the patient's local immune response have been suggested as possible triggers.

It is characterized by discrete, crusted/inflammatory/papulopustules arising in crops on vertex of the scalp and is often colonized by *S. aureus*. An overview is given in **Box 14.4**.

BOX 14.4: Folliculitis decalvans at a glance

Clinical features (Fig. 14.12a)

- Destructive, suppurative folliculitis
- Caused by *Staphylococcus aureus*
- 70% of patients present with symptoms such as pruritus, burning sensation, or trychodynia
- Painful/pruritic erythematous pinpoint follicular pustules, papules with boggy swelling
- Crusting and scarring in the center
- Tufts of hair appear from dilated follicular opening giving 'Dolls hair' appearance **(Fig. 14.12b)**

Histopathology

- Perifollicular neutrophilic inflammation around the upper follicle
- Later develops into a more mixed inflammatory infiltrate of neutrophils, lymphocytes and plasma cells
- In burnt out stage, follicular and adventitial fibrosis is seen.

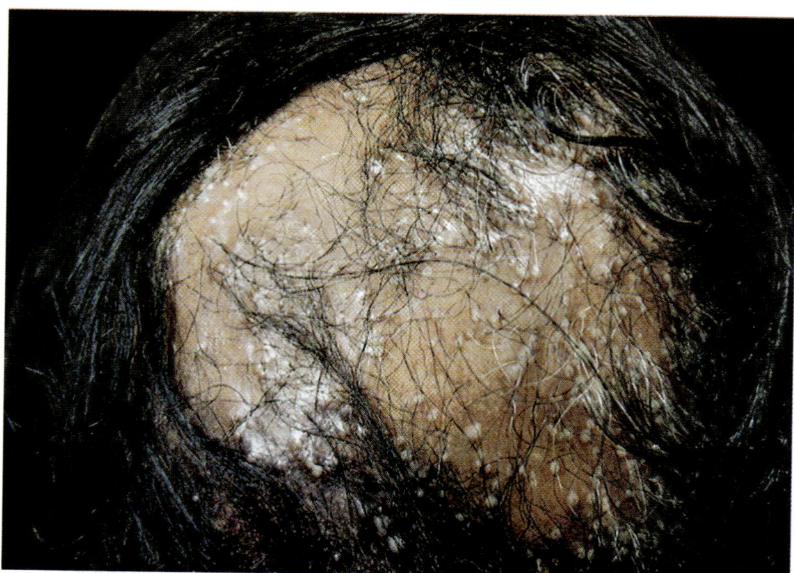

Fig. 14.12a: Multiple pustules associated with cicatricial alopecia in a case of folliculitis decalvans

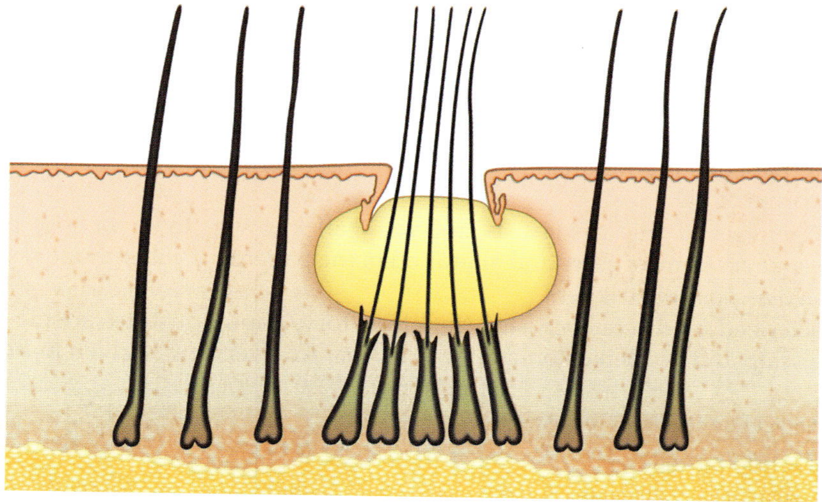

Fig. 14.12b: Tufted folliculitis: Multiple hair shafts emerge from a single dilated follicular opening (tuft consists of a central anagen hair surrounded by telogen hairs, each arising from independent follicles, converging toward a common dilated follicular infundilbulum)

Treatment

The aim is to intervene early so that the late stage of scarring does not ensue. The basis of treatment aims at tackling the inflammation and administering long-term antibiotics which can help to keep the *S. aureus* under control **(Table 14.8)**. In refractory cases adalimumab has been found to be useful and lately baricitinib has also been tried in FD.

TABLE 14.8: Evidence-based treatment of folliculitis decalvans

	Topical	Oral	Surgery/others
Acute therapy	• Intralesional steroids (triamcinolone) • Topical antibiotic + topical steroid • Dexamethasone (0.1 mg/kg/day 2 days/week)	• Clindamycin (300 mg twice daily) + Rifampicin (300 mg twice daily) (preferred regimen) × 10 weeks • Ciprofloxacin or levofloxacin (500 mg BD × 7 days) • Doxycycline (100 mg daily × 2 months)	
Maintenance	• Topical antibiotic + topical steroid • Intralesional steroids (triamcinolone) 1–2 monthly	• **Doxycycline** (100 mg two to three times/week)	
3rd line		• **Oral isotretinoin** (10–30 mg/day) • **Dapsone** (100 mg/day) • Anti-TNFα biologicals	• Surgery

HAIR SHAFT DISORDERS

Conditions with hair shaft defects are usually not amenable to treatment but can provide clues to other abnormalities. The diagnosis is based on light microscopy (LM) and trichoscopy. The disorders can be conveniently classified into those with increased fragility and those without increased fragility **(Box 14.5)**. The common disorders are depicted in **Fig. 14.13** and microscopy images of select disorders are shown in **Fig. 14.14**.

A summary of the hair shaft disorders is given in **Table 14.9**.

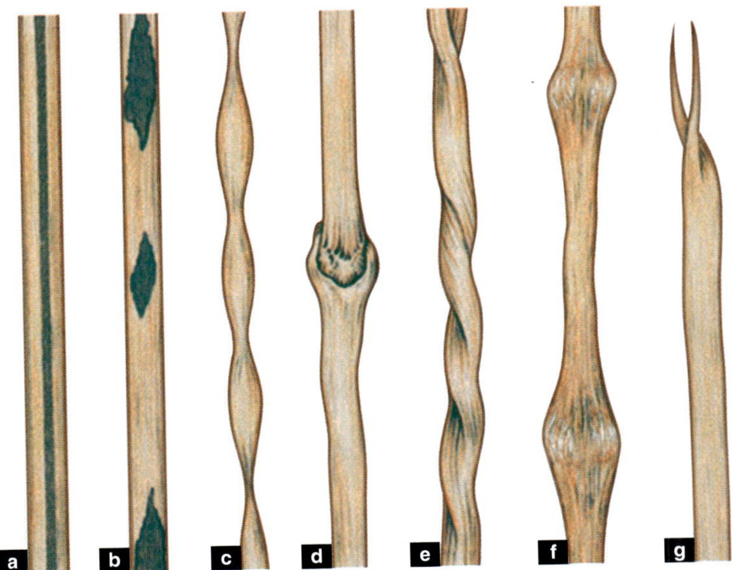

Fig. 14.13: A figurative depiction of the common hair shaft defects: (a) Normal hair; (b) Pili annulati; (c) Monilethrix; (d) Trichorrhexis invaginata; (e) Pili torti; (f) Trichorrhexis nodosa; (g) Trichoptilosis

BOX 14.5: Classification of hair shaft disorders

With increased fragility	Without increased fragility
Pili torti	Pili annulati
Monilethrix	Pili trianguli et canaliculi
Trichorrhexis invaginata	Trichonodosis
Trichorrhexis nodosa	Trichostasis spinulosa
Trichothiodystrophy	Trichoptilosis
Trichoschisis	Loose anagen hair
	Woolly hair

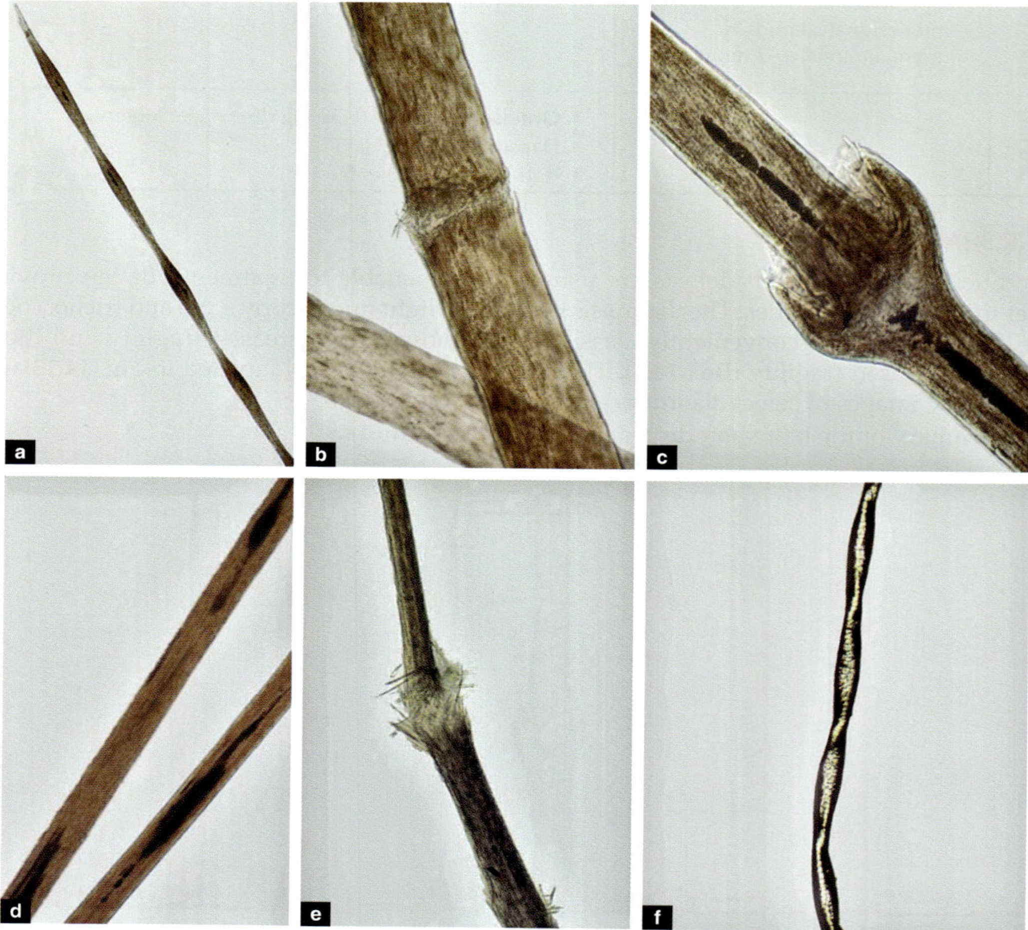

Fig. 14.14: (a) In monilethrix, the nodes correspond to the normal caliber of the hair and the defective portion resides in the constrictions; (b) Trichoschisis in a patient with trichothiodystrophy; (c) Netherton syndrome. The distal portion of this hair shaft (upper left) has sunken into the proximal portion (lower right) to create a node of trichorrhexis invaginata; (d) Pili annulati. Air-filled spaces within the shaft create dark areas when viewed with a light microscope; (e) Focal loss of the hair cuticle results in cortical fiber separation and the fragile 'nodes' of trichorrhexis nodosa; (f) Pili torti

TABLE 14.9: Summary of hair shaft disorders

Name	Etiology	Clinical features	Associations and syndromes	Management
1. Monilethrix (↑) **(Fig. 14.15)**	• AD: Mutations in **KRT81, KRT83, KRT86** • AR: **Dsg4**	• Presents with normal appearing hair at birth • Hypotrichosis • Beaded hair • Increased fragility • Improves with age, summers and puberty • Body hair and eye lashes can be involved	• Follicular papules in nape of the neck • Keratosis pilaris • Nail dystrophy **Pili torti—**hair shafts are twisted and flattened **Pseudomonilethrix**—due to trauma to hair shafts Presence of irregular nodes and irregular twisting without flattening	Minoxidil, oral retinoids
2. Woolly hair **(Fig. 14.16)**	• AD: **KRT71and KRT74** • AR: **LPAR6 and LIPH** (Noonan syndrome)	• Generalised/localized presence of curly and easily breakable hair • Hypopigmentation – elliptical cross-sections, axial twisting, +/– trichorrhexis nodosa	• Noonan syndrome • Ulerythema ophyrogenes • Naxos and Carvajal syndrome – **Naxos** disease (diffuse non-epidermolytic PPK, **RVH** and woolly hair): **Plakoglobin** mutations – **Carvajal syndrome** (striate epidermolytic PPK, **LVH**, woolly hair): **Desmoplakin** mutations	
3. Pili torti **(Fig. 14.14f)**	Inherited in an autosomal dominant manner but the exact genetic mutation has not been found Most misdiagnosed structural hair shaft defect	• Hair abnormal from birth, or normal at birth, and then during infancy becomes replaced by brittle and fragile hair • Brittle, **spangled hairs**, especially in the occipital and temporal regions. The spangled appearance is due to unequal reflection of light from the twisted surface • Hair are flattened and twisted on their longitudinal axes each twist may be 90°, 180°, or up to 360°	• **Menkes disease**—ATP7A mutation leading to a defect in copper transport across the Golgi apparatus, trichorrhexis nodosa; mental/psychomotor retardation, fractures, '**Cupid bow**' upper lip, *doughy skin*; *diffuse hypopigmentation* • **Björnstad syndrome**—pili torti with progressive sensory neural *deafness*—BSC1L gene mutation • **Crandall syndrome** = Björnstad syndrome + *hypogonadism* (mnemonic 'Crandall's = Cranberry balls') • **Netherton syndrome**: SPINK5 gene (encodes serine protease inhibitor LEKTI) • **Urea cycle defects** (citrullinemia, argininosuccinic aciduria) • **Acquired pili torti**: Anorexia nervosa and oral retinoids	

(Contd.)

TABLE 14.9: Summary of hair shaft disorders *(Contd.)*

Name	Etiology	Clinical features	Associations and syndromes	Management
4. Trichorrhexis nodosa (↑) **(Fig. 14.14e)**	**Congenital:** Argininosuccinic aciduria (AR, arginosuccinate lyase) or citrullinemia (AR, arginosuccinate synthetase) most commonly; also may see in Menkes, trichothiodystrophy, Netherton syndrome **Acquired** (three variants): 1. Proximal trichorrhexis nodosa: Arises in patients after years of hair straightening 2. Distal trichorrhexis nodosa: Due to acquired, cumulative, cuticular damage 3. Circumscribed trichorrhexis nodosa: Affects scalp, moustache, or beard	• **Most common** of all the structural hair abnormalities • Increased hair fragility • *'Nodes' of trichorrhexis nodosa represent foci of frayed cortical fibers that bulge out through a ruptured cuticle* • Characterized on light microscopic examination by a hair shaft fracture with adjacent fragments splaying out, <u>*resembling the ends of two brushes pushed against each other*</u> • Neonatal form more severe—failure to thrive, hepatomegaly, lethargy • Adult—onset form less severe but still have mental retardation and ataxia	• **Netherton syndrome—**ichthyosis linearis circumflexa, atopy and hair abnormality (trichorrhexis invaginata, trichorrhexis nodosa) • **Menkes disease** • **Trichohepatoenteric syndrome** • **Argininosuccinic aciduria** • **Trichothiodystrophy**	
5. Pili triangulata et canaliculi	Transmitted as AD as well as AR trait No specific genetic loci found	• Also known as **uncombable hair syndrome** • Light colored frizzy **hair stand up from the scalp** • Microscopy shows <u>*a triangular cross-section and longitudinal grooves*</u>	Skeletal dysplasias	

(Contd.)

TABLE 14.9: Summary of hair shaft disorders *(Contd.)*

Name	Etiology	Clinical features	Associations and syndromes	Management
6. Loose anagen hair syndrome **(Fig. 14.17)**	• Poor adhesion between the cuticle and the inner root sheath • AD inheritance • Underlying keratin defect • Classic presentation: Young girl with short blond hair that seldom needs to be cut	• Disease starts in early childhood • Scalp hair has easy pluckability • *Light colored hair* • Poor growth • Patchy alopecia • Anagen hairs can be **easily and painlessly pulled from the scalp** • Trichogram shows 'floppy sock appearance' in >70% of the examined hair	• Pili trianguli et canaliculi • Noonan phenotype	Improves with age Loom (≤0.02) Dose in HTC (Ped) 0.2 mg/kg in normotensive it has minimal hypotension Jerjon R, BJD
7. Trichothiodystrophy (↑)	• A decrease in the high **sulfur content** proteins of the hair shaft • Numerous genetic mutations have been described—C7ORF11 (non-photosensitive type) TTFIH, ERCC3, ERCC2, GTF2H5 (photosensitive trichothiodystrophy)	• Hypotrichosis affecting the scalp and body hair • Nail dystrophy • Progeroid facies • Microcephaly cataracts and microcornea • Short stature and joint contractures • Photosensitivity • Different variants of the syndrome have been described (A-H) • Polarized microscopy shows *tiger tail appearance. and transverse fractures (trichoschisis)*		
8. Pili annulati et pseudoannulati	• Inherited as an AD trait • Presence of air-filled cavities within the hair shaft	• Presence of alternating dark and light bands under microscope • Pili pseudoannulati results from reflection of the light over flattened or twisted surfaces of the hair shaft, and is considered as a normal variant	Do NOT need polarized light to see (*vs* trichothiodystrophy)	

(↑) Increased fragility.

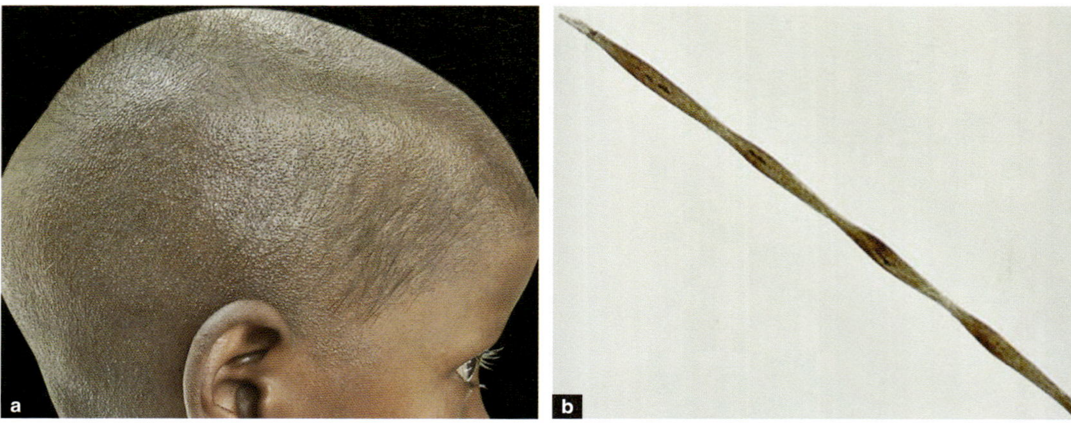

Fig. 14.15: In monilethrix, the nodes correspond to the normal caliber of the hair and the defective portion resides in the constrictions

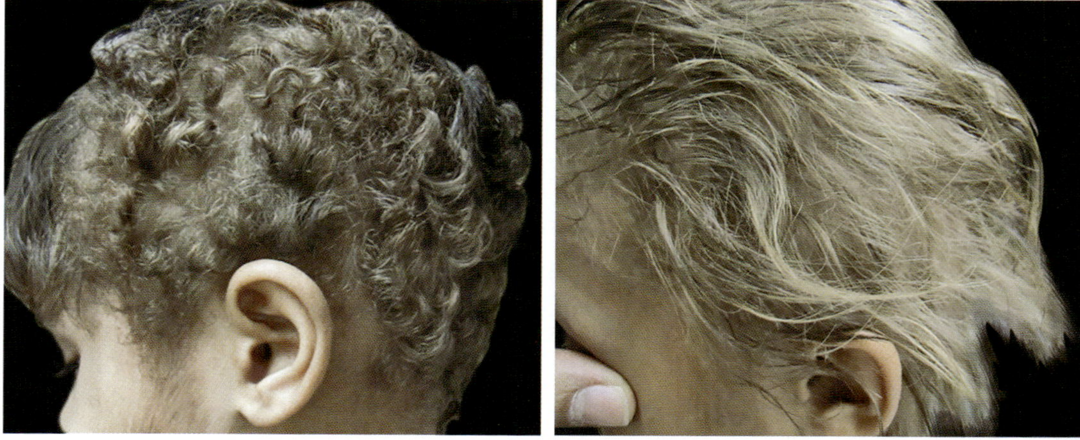

Fig. 14.16: Woolly hair nevus

Fig. 14.17: Loose anagen hair syndrome

Acknowledgments

The authors thank **Dr Sidharth Tandon**, MD, for his work on this chapter in the previous edition of this book.

BIBLIOGRAPHY

Books

1. Dermatology (Bolognia). 4th ed. Elsevier Chapter 6. Alopecias.
2. Hair Loss Disorders, Restoration and Management 2nd ed. 2018 CBS Kabir Sardana.
3. Rook's Textbook of Dermatology, 9th ed. Wiley Blackwell. Chapter 89. Acquired Disorders of Hair.

Journals

1. Ankad BS, Beergouder SL, Moodalgiri VM. Lichen planopilaris versus discoid lupus erythematosus: A trichoscopic perspective. Int J Trichology. 2013;5(4):204–7.

2. Bokhari L, Sinclair R. Treatment of alopecia universalis with topical Janus kinase inhibitors—a double blind, placebo, and active controlled pilot study. Int J Dermatol. 2018 Dec;57(12):1464–70.
3. Divito SJ, Kupper TS. Inhibiting Janus kinases to treat alopecia areata. Nat Med 2014; 20:989.
4. Gilhar A, Paus R, Kalish RS. Lymphocytes, neuropeptides, and genes involved in alopecia areata. J Clin Invest 2007;117:2019–27.
5. Grant JE,. Neurobiology of subtypes of trichotillomania and skin picking disorder. CNS Spectr. 2023 Feb;28(1):98–103.
6. Ho A, Shapiro J. Medical therapy for frontal fibrosing alopecia: A review and clinical approach. J Am Acad Dermatol. 2019 Aug;81(2):568–80. doi: 10.1016/j.jaad.2019.03.079. Epub 2019.
7. Ikeda T. A new classification of alopecia areata. Dermatology 1965;131:421–45.
8. Nambudiri, et al. Clinicopathologic lessons in distinguishing cicatricial alopecia: 7 Cases of lichen planopilarism is diagnosed as discoid lupus. J Am Acad Dermatol 2014;71:e135–e138.
9. Petukhova L, Duvic M, Hordinsky M, et al. Genome-wide association study in alopecia areata implicates both innate and adaptive immunity. Nature. 2010 Jul;466(7302):113–7. DOI: 10.1038/nature09114.
10. Rajabi F, Drake LA, Senna MM, Rezaei N. Alopecia areata: A review of disease pathogenesis. Br J Dermatol 2018;179:1033–48.
11. Strazzulla LC, Wang EHC, Avila L, Lo Sicco K, Brinster N, Christiano AM, Shapiro J. Alopecia areata: An appraisal of new treatment approaches and overview of current therapies. J Am Acad Dermatol. 2018 Jan;78(1):15–24.

Chapter

15

Hemangioma and Vascular Malformations

Seema Rani, Kabir Sardana, Snigdha Saxena

The classification proposed by the International Society for the Study of Vascular Anomalies (ISSVA) adopted in 2014 and modified in 2018, divides vascular anomalies into tumors (including infantile hemangiomas and congenital hemangiomas) and malformations **(Tables 15.1 and 15.2)**. This is based on the distinction between proliferative lesions (tumors) and lesions due to a congenital anomaly of vascular morphogenesis (vascular malformations). **Table 15.3** lists the differences between hemangiomas and vascular malformations.

TABLE 15.1: ISSVA classification for vascular tumors

Benign	Locally aggressive or borderline	Malignant
• Infantile hemangioma • Congenital hemangioma (RICH, PICH, NICH) • Tufted angioma • Spindle-cell hemangioma • Epithelioid hemangioma • Pyogenic granuloma (lobular capillary hemangioma)	• Kaposiform hemangioendothelioma • Retiform hemangioendothelioma • Composite hemangioendothelioma • Pseudomyogenic hemangioendothelioma • Polymorphous hemangioendothelioma • Dabska tumor • Kaposi sarcoma	• Angiosarcoma • Epithelioid hemangio-endothelioma

RICH, rapidly involuting congenital hemangioma; PICH, partially involuting congenital hemangioma, NICH, non-involuting congenital hemangioma.

HEMANGIOMA

INFANTILE HEMANGIOMAS

- Infantile hemangiomas are common, benign, vascular tumors of infancy.
- Proliferation in the first few months of life followed by slow spontaneous involution over a matter of years.
- **Risk factors:** Amniocentesis, *in vitro* fertilization, breech presentation, being first born and low birth weight (<2500 g).

TABLE 15.2: ISSVA classification for vascular malformations

Simple	Combined	Anomalies of major named vessels (truncal VM)	Associated with other anomalies
• **Capillary (CM)** – Nevus simplex/salmon patch ("'stork bite') – Cutaneous and/or mucosal CM ('port-wine' stain) ▪ Nonsyndromic CM ▪ CM with CNS and/or ocular anomalies ▪ CM with bone and/or soft tissues overgrowth – Reticulate CM – CM of CM-AVM – Cutis marmorata telangiectatica congenita – Telangiectasia ▪ Hereditary hemorrhagic telangiectasia • **Lymphatic (LM)** – Common (cystic) LM ▪ Macrocystic/microcystic/mixed – Generalized lymphatic anomaly (GLA) ▪ Kaposiform lymphangiomatosis – Primary lymphedema • **Venous (VM)** – Common VM – Blue rubber bleb nevus (Bean) syndrome – Glomuvenous malformation (GVM) – Verrucous VM (verrucous hemangioma) • **Arteriovenous malformations (AVM)** – Sporadic – In HHT – In CM-AVM • **Arteriovenous fistula (AVF)** – Sporadic – In HHT – In CM-AVM	• Capillary-venous malformation (CVM) • Capillary-lymphatic malformation (CLM) • Capillary-arteriovenous malformation (CAVM) • Lymphatic-venous malformation (LVM) • Capillary-lymphatic-venous malformation (CLVM) • Capillary-lymphatic-arteriovenous malformation (CLAVM) • Capillary-venous-arteriovenous malformation (CVAVM)	• **Affect** – Lymphatics – Veins – Arteries • **Anomalies of** – Origin – Course – Number – Length – Diameter – Valves – Communication (AVF) – Persistence (of embryonal vessel)	• **Klippel–Trénaunay sydnrome** (CM + VM +/– LM + limb overgrowth) • **Parkes Weber syndrome** (CM + AVF + limb overgrowth) • **Sturge–Weber syndrome** (Facial + Leptomeningeal CM + Eye anomalies +/– Bone and/or soft tissue overgrowth) • **Servelle–Martorell syndrome** (Limb VM + Bone undergrowth) • **Maffucci syndrome** (VM +/– Spindle-cell hemangioma + Enchondroma) • **CLOVES syndrome** (LM + VM + CM +/– AVM + Lipomatous overgrowth) • **Proteus syndrome** (CM, VM and/or LM + Asymmetrical somatic overgrowth) • **Bannayan–Riley–Ruvalcaba syndrome** (AVM + VM + Macrocephaly, lipomatous overgrowth) • **CLAPO syndrome** (Lower lip CM + Face and neck LM + Asymmetry and partial/generalized overgrowth)

TABLE 15.3: Differences between hemangiomas and vascular malformations

Hemangioma	Vascular malformation
Usually appears in early life	Usually present at birth
Has a growth cycle with proliferative and involuting/involuted phases	Continues to grow proportional to the growth rate of the body, no involution
'Self-limited' tumor with endothelial cell proliferation	'Self-perpetuating' embryologic tissue with malformed vessels
No recurrence	May recur due to persistence of mesenchymal cells (angioblasts), triggered by trauma, pregnancy, surgery
GLUT1 positive (infantile hemangioma)	GLUT1 negative
HPE—intralesional nerve bundles often absent, mast cells increased (proliferating > involuting), elastin stain often –ve	HPE—intralesional nerve bundles often present, mast cells less, elastic stain often +ve in AVM

- **Classification (based on morphology):**
  - Superficial (most common, 50–60%)
  - Deep
  - Mixed (superficial and deep)
  - Reticular, abortive or minimal growth

  These can exist in different patterns:
  - Focal
  - Segmental
  - Multifocal
  - Indeterminate

Etiopathogenesis

- **Placental hypothesis:**
  - Endothelial cells are characterized by the surface marker **GLUT1**, an erythrocyte type glucose transporter protein, which is expressed by infantile hemangiomas during all phases of their development (proliferating, involuting, involuted) as well as by the placenta.
  - It has been proposed that this placental phenotype may be the result of embolization of placental endothelial cells to the fetal circulation.
- **Endothelial cell origin**
  - Hemangiomas may be derived from endothelial progenitor cells or multipotent stem cells.
  - Vascular endothelial growth factor (VEGF) signalling and other pathways that affect vascular development (e.g. [$VEGF_2$>$VEGF_1$], dual-specificity phosphatase-5 [DUSP5]) have been identified in hemangioma tissue. Mutations in the integrin-like receptor tumor endothelial marker 8, and $VEGFR_2$ have been identified in hemangioma.
  - Familial hemangiomas have been linked to chromosome 5q.

Pathology

Proliferating: Endothelial cell hyperplasia, lobule formation, mast cells, prominent basement membrane.

Involuting: Fibrofatty tissue replacement, decreased mast cells (when fully involuted).

Clinical Features

- A faint telangiectatic patch or an area of pallor or as a flat pink mark which rapidly becomes red and raised.
- Two phases:
  1. **Proliferation:** The maximum rate of proliferation occurs within the **first 2 months** and is complete in 85% of patients by **6 months of age**.
  2. **Involution** gradually over several years (e.g. 30% completed by 3 years of age and 50% by 5 years).

  The maximum rate of involution occurs between **12 months to 24 months** of age.
- Most infantile hemangiomas reach **80%** of their final size by **3 months of age** and in untreated lesions, involution is complete at a median age of **3 years**.
- **Superficial** types of infantile hemangioma show their most rapid growth between 5.5 and 7.5 weeks of age.
- **Deep hemangiomas**, often present later and continue to grow for longer than superficial hemangiomas, develop in the lower dermis and subcutis and tend to appear blue or purple without any overlying skin changes.
- During the proliferative phase, infantile hemangiomas are firm. With involution, they become softer.
- Superficial hemangiomas develop islands of greying within the redness, with some flattening of the surface.
- Permanent changes—most frequently telangiectases, atrophy and residual bulk in the form of fibrofatty tissue have been reported in up to 69% of untreated hemangiomas.

Clinical Variants

1. Segmental infantile hemangioma:
   - **Segmental infantile hemangioma** of the face and of the lumbosacral region may be associated with underlying structural anomalies.
     a. **Face: PHACES syndrome** (*P*osterior fossa malformations, *H*emangiomas, *A*rterial anomalies, *C*ardiac anomalies, *E*ye abnormalities and *S*ternal pit/*S*upraumbilical raphe), seen in up to **30%** of large segmental facial hemangioma **(Fig. 15.1)**.
     The risk of PHACES syndrome in an infant presenting with a large segmental IH of the head or neck is approximately 30% **(Fig. 15.2)**.
     b. **Beard,** bilateral are mostly associated with <u>airways</u> hemangiomas.
     c. **Large IHs on the lower body—risk of**
     LUMBAR association: *L*ower body/lumbosacral **IH** and lipomas; *U*rogenital anomalies and ulceration; *M*yelopathy (spinal dysraphism); *B*ony deformities; *A*norectal and *A*rterial anomalies; *R*enal anomalies.
     SACRAL association: *S*pinal dysraphism, *A*no-genital anomalies, *C*utaneous anomalies, *R*enal and urological anomalies, *L*umbosacral IH.
     PELVIS association: *P*erineal IH, *E*xternal genitalia malformations, *L*ipomyelomeningocele, *V*esicorenal abnormalities, *I*mperforate anus, *S*kin tag **(Fig. 15.3)**.
2. **Multifocal hemangiomas** may range in number from a few to hundreds, and are usually small, some have symptomatic visceral lesions, with **liver involvement** being the most common **(Fig. 15.3)**.
3. **Hepatic hemangioma:** Hepatic hemangioma (HH) may occur with or without cutaneous infantile hemangioma. Many HH are asymptomatic, and those that become symptomatic usually do so within the first 3 months of life.

   The differential diagnoses of hemangioma is given in **Table 15.4**.

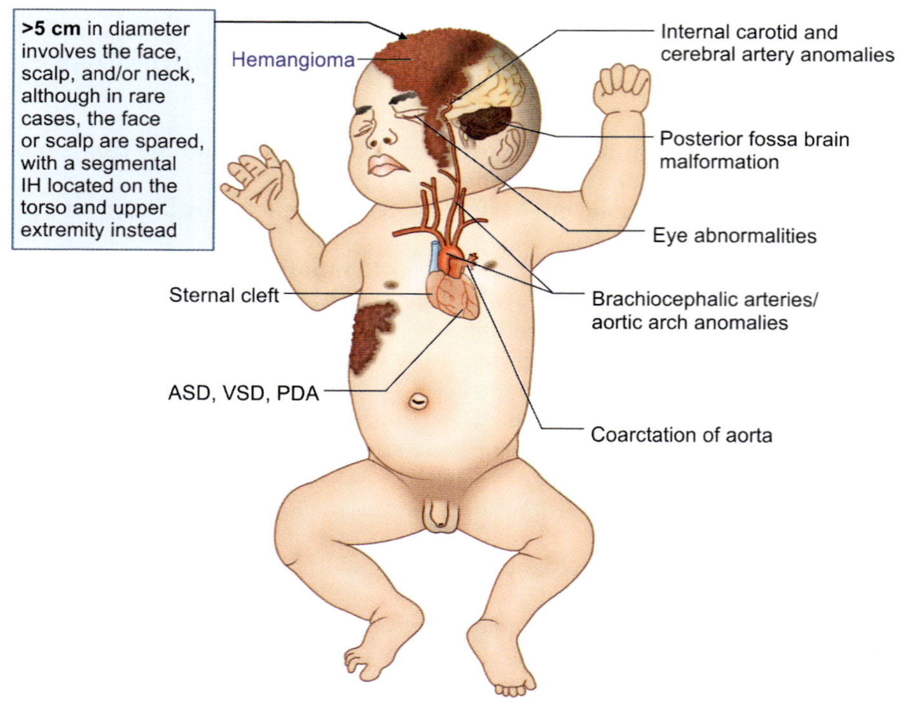

Fig. 15.1: A depiction of PHACES syndrome

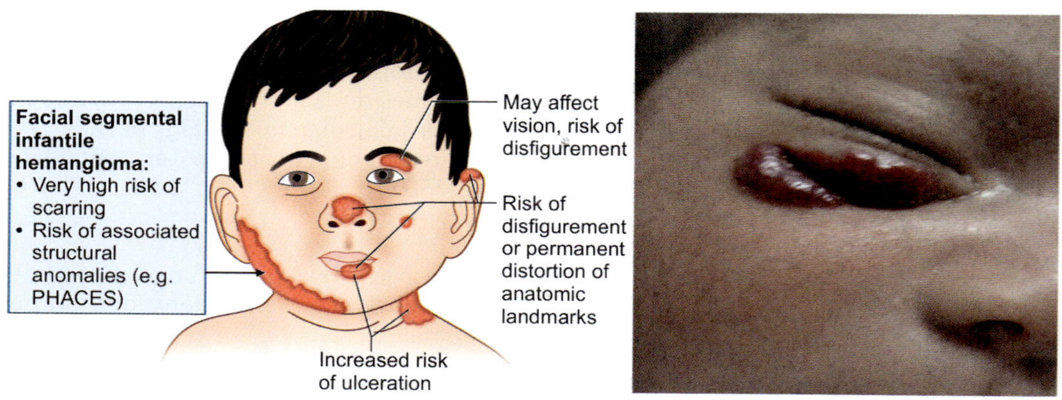

Fig. 15.2: High-risk hemangioma on face and neck

TABLE 15.4: Differential diagnoses of hemangioma

- Congenital hemangiomas (RICH, PICH, NICH)
- Port-wine stain
- Tufted angioma
- Kaposiform hemangioendothelioma
- Pyogenic granuloma
- Other vascular malformations—arteriovenous, venous and lymphatic

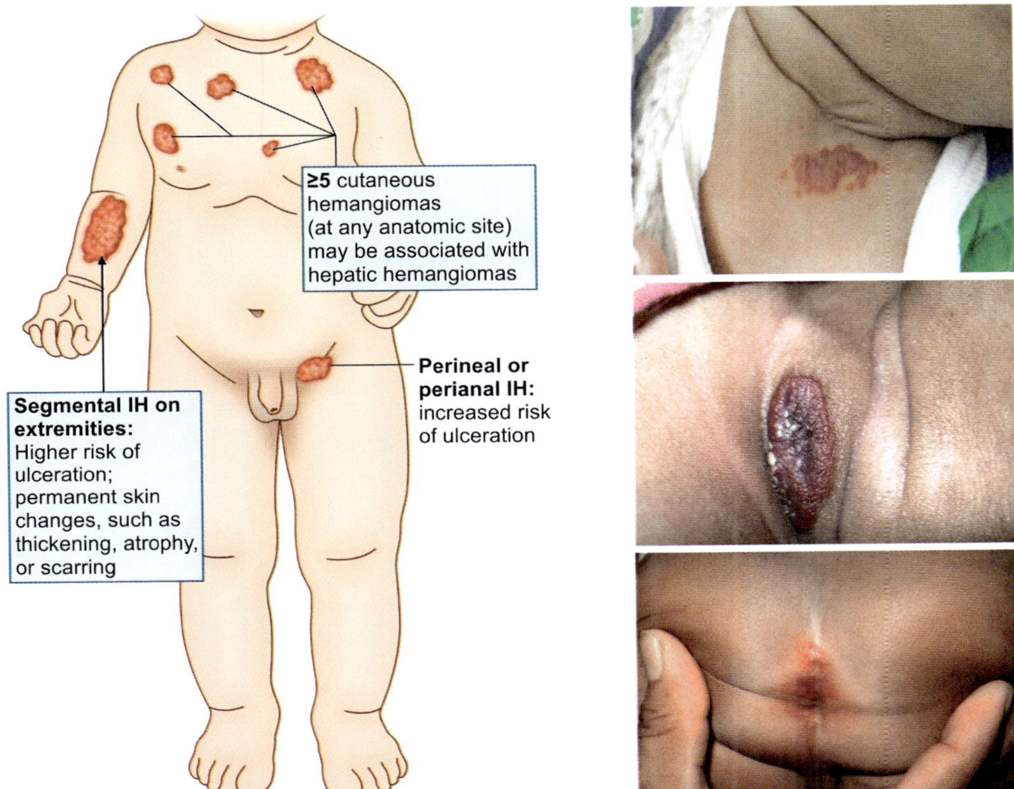

Fig. 15.3: High-risk hemangioma on trunk, extremities, and perineal area

Complications and Comorbidities

There are five major indications for consideration of early treatment or need for further evaluation of IHs:

1. Life-threatening complications
2. Functional impairment or risk
3. Ulceration or risk
4. Evaluation to identify important associated structural anomalies
5. Risk of leaving permanent scarring or distortion of anatomic landmarks.

1. **Ulceration**
   - **Occurs in 20% of cases**, associated with bleeding, infection and almost always results in scarring, being more common at the site of friction or moisture, in hemangiomas of larger size, segmental morphology, location on neck, anogenital areas, lips **(Fig. 15.4)**.
   - **Whitish discoloration** of an IH in an infant <3 months of age may signal impending ulceration.
2. **Disfigurement:** This risk is greatest in IHs with a prominent and thick superficial (strawberry) component, especially when there is a steep step-off (i.e. ledge effect) from affected to surrounding normal skin.

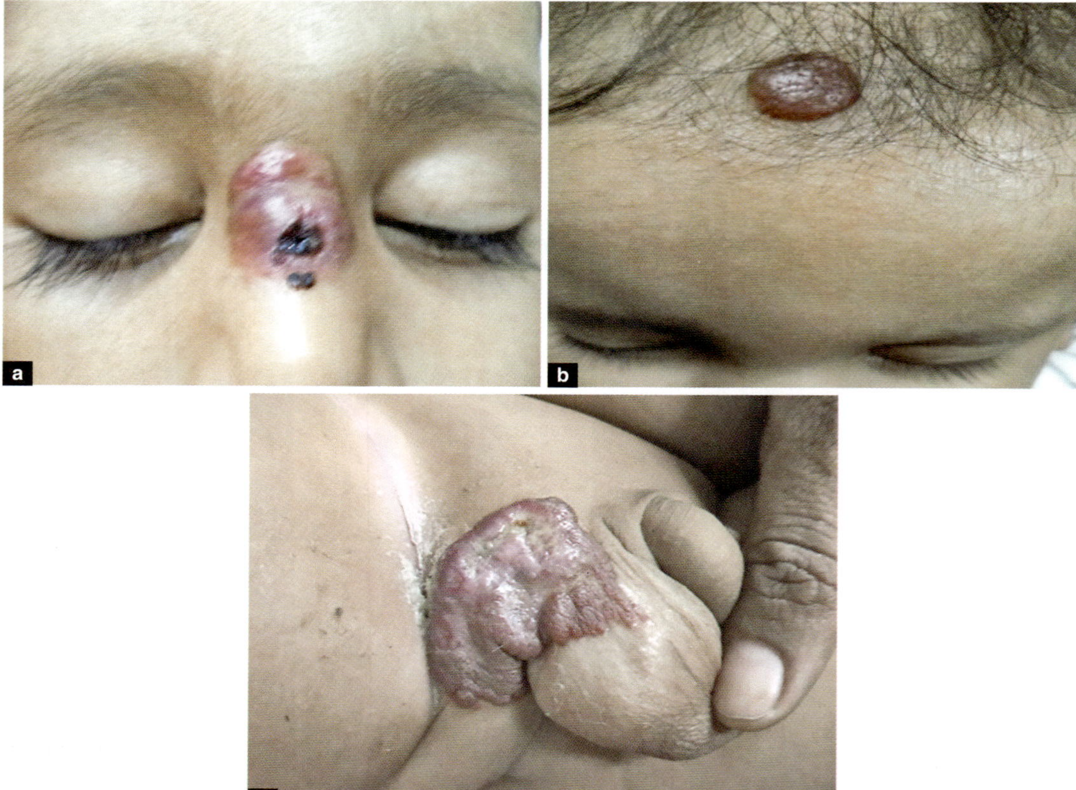

Fig. 15.4: (a and b) Midline superficial infantile hemangioma with ulceration; (c) Segmental infantile hemangioma in area of moisture and friction associated with ulceration

Depends on the location, morphological subtype and size.

- Periocular—**astigmatism**, due to pressure on globe; **amblyopia**, if it obstructs the visual axis; and **strabismus**, if it affects orbital musculature.
- IH on nasal tip (**Pinocchio** or **Cyrano nose**), columella, or lip (especially if it crosses the vermilion border)—facial distortion.
- IH on breast (in girls)—may affect underlying breast bud and cause breast hypoplasia.

3. **Functional impairment**
   - Periocular infantile hemangiomas, which may cause **astigmatism, visual axis obstruction and strabismus, amblyopia and the risk of permanent visual loss.**
   - Hemangiomas involving the airway and the nose can endanger **breathing, and those on the lip may interfere with feeding.**
   - **Segmental hemangioma**—*see* above.

Disease Course and Prognosis

- **Follow a predictable course**—appearing shortly after birth, usually achieving 80% of their growth by 3 months, and completion of growth by about 9 months.

- **Prognosis is excellent** for small hemangiomas, also for large one, if there is no functional impairement or not on aesthetically important sites.
- It is important to identify high risk IH (listed in **Box 15.1**).

BOX 15.1: High-risk IHs

Life-threatening	Beard area: Obstructive airway hemangiomas ≥5 cutaneous IH: Liver hemangiomas, cardiac failure, hypothyroidism
Functional impairment	Periocular IH (>1 cm): Astigmatism, anisometropia, proptosis, amblyopia IH involving lip or oral cavity: Feeding impairment
Ulceration	Segmental IH on lips, columella, superior helix of ear, gluteal cleft and/or perineum, perianal skin, and other intertriginous areas
Associated structural anomalies	Segmental IH of face or scalp: PHACES syndrome Segmental IH of lumbosacral and/or perineal area: LUMBAR/SACRAL/PELVIS associations
Disfigurement	Segmental IH, especially of face and scalp • Facial IH (measurements refer to size during infancy): Nasal tip or lip (any size) or any facial location ≥2 cm (>1 cm if ≤3 months of age) • Scalp IH >2 cm • Neck, trunk, or extremity IH >2 cm, especially in growth phase or if abrupt transition from normal to affected skin (i.e. ledge effect); thick superficial IH (e.g. ≥2 mm thickness) • Breast IH (female infants)

Investigations

Immunostaining for **GLUT1** is positive in the proliferating, involuting and involuted phases, shows high sensitivity and specificity, and is useful for the diagnosis of infantile hemangiomas if the clinical diagnosis is difficult.

The other investigations are listed in **Table 15.5**.

Management

Active non-intervention is advised for small and uncomplicated hemangiomas. Systemic therapy is indicated under certain situations **(Box 15.2** and **Figs 15.2** and **15.3)**. Here it must be noted that while most rapid proliferation occurs in the first 2 months and regression by 2 years,

TABLE 15.5: Investigations in a case of hemangioma*

1. **Segmental hemangioma**	Face	• Head and neck magnetic resonance angiography (MRA) • Ophthalmological examination
	Beard	ENT opinion
	Lumbosacral and perineal region	Infants <3 months, spinal ultrasound may be useful for the initial assessment, but spinal MRI with contrast is advisable
2. **Ultrasound**—to distinguish between hemangiomas and other soft tissue masses or vascular malformations		
3. **Thyroid function tests**—liver, parotid or PHACES syndrome		

*Clinicians should not perform imaging unless the diagnosis of IH is uncertain, there are 5 or more cutaneous IHs, or associated anatomic abnormalities are suspected.

BOX 15.2: Indications for systemic therapy

- **Threatened vital functions**
  - Vision
  - Airway
- **Potential for disfigurement**
  - Nasal tip/columella
  - Lip
  - Large/rapidly growing lesion on face
- **Severe/recalcitrant ulceration**
- **High-output cardiac failure**

TABLE 15.6: Treatment of hemangioma

Topical	• Steroids/IL steroids* • Timolol maleate (0.5% eyedrops) • Topical imiquimod • Topical becaplermin (0.01% gel)
Systemic and surgical modalities	• Propranolol • Steroids • Vincristine • Recombinant interferon-α (2a and 2b) • Laser-PDL • Surgery

*Focal, bulky IHs during proliferation or in certain critical anatomic locations (e.g. the lip)

there is also a sesne of **"self awareness"** which is a fundamental issue, which in children is obvious at the age of 18 months and at 2 years of age children begin to express embarassment. By 3 years of age to 4 years this self awareness is estabilished. Also by the time the child is 5–6 years the childs sense of self image is ingrained. Thus the treatment should be done before the age of 3 years so that the childs "self image" is not affected. In case this is not possible, then effective therapy should be finished by the time of formal schooling, about 6 years.

Treatment of hemangiomas is summarized in **Table 15.6**.

Topical

Although it must be noted that there are no reports of comparison with placebo and that the degree of improvement is smaller compared with systemically administrated drugs, topical medication can be an option for the treatment of infantile hemangioma with no risk of complications if drugs with milder adverse effects are selected.

- Steroids
- Timolol maleate (0.5% eyedrops up to three times a day) in non-ulcerated, non-mucosal lesions appears to be safe.
- Topical imiquimod.
- Topical becaplermin (0.01% gel) (human platelet derived growth factor—for ulcerated hemangiomas).

Systemic

- **Propranolol: FDA approved for treatment of problematic infantile hemangiomas. Usual dose is 2 mg/kg, divided into two or three oral doses,** side effects—hypotension, bradycardia, hypoglycemia. A baseline cardiac assessment (including examination, electrocardiography, and in some cases, echocardiography), often requiring a referral to a pediatric cardiologist, prior to propranolol therapy. Clinicians should evaluate patients for and educate caregivers about potential adverse effects of propranolol, including sleep disturbances, bronchial irritation, and clinically symptomatic bradycardia and hypotension. Clinicians may prescribe oral prednisolone or prednisone to treat IHs, if there are contraindications or an inadequate response to oral propranolol.

A detailed protocol is given in **Table 15.7**.

TABLE 15.7: Use of propranolol in hemangioma

Before starting propranolol	• History and examination including HR, BP and oxygen saturation • Echocardiography and ECG in selected patients (echo for PHACES) • Baseline glucose is only required in selected cases • Clinicians should counsel that propranolol be administered with or after feeding and that doses be held at times of diminished oral intake or vomiting to reduce the risk of hypoglycemia
Dose	• 5 mg/5 mL • Starting dose 1 mg/kg/day • Maintenance dose for **uncomplicated patients**—2 mg/kg/day • Minimum time interval between dose increases—24 hours, (HR and BP monitored). With 30 minutes between observations, total length of observation—2–4 hours • Glucose to be checked only in patients at risk of hypoglycemia (preterm, low weight, faltering growth, neonates, history of hypoglycemia) • PHACES syndrome—**0.5 mg/kg/day**, under observation of a cardiologist/neurologists, after MRI-MRA
During treatment with propranolol	• Maximum dose for **non-responders** is 3 mg/kg/day • Routine follow-up for a patient on a stable treatment dose, without complications, should be at intervals of 2–3 months • BP and HR do not need to be monitored between appointments, if the infant is well • Night terrors or restless sleep is the main limiting factor with propanolol. The dose can be split twice daily and as the levels peak about 3–4 hours, the drug can be given at 7 AM and 5 PM, so that the effect of the dose wears off by the time child sleeps. Another option is to give atenolol that does not cross the blood brain barrier.
Review	4–6 weeks after starting treatment, then 3–4 monthly
Treatment stopping	A. Temporary cessation required, if: • Significantly reduced oral intake (due to risk of hypoglycemia) • Wheezing requiring treatment B. End of treatment: In many cases, treatment can be stopped at one year of age, and the majority of IH patients do not need treatment beyond 17 months of age. It is safe to stop propranolol abruptly (rather than weaning patients off treatment gradually) during or at the end of therapy

Other Drugs

- Atenolol (selective β-1 blocker)
- Vincristine
- Recombinant interferon-α (2a and 2b)
- Laser-PDL
- Surgery

Treatment for Ulceration

The various agents tried include, propranolol, topical antibiotics, dressings and laser therapy.

CONGENITAL HEMANGIOMA

Congenital hemangiomas are benign vascular tumors that proliferate *in utero*, and do not show further proliferation postnatally.

- GLUT1 negative, equal in M:F.
- Seen as early as 12 weeks of gestation by prenatal ultrasound studies.
  - RICH (rapidly involuting congenital hemangioma): Pink-red to bluish-red, often large vascular tumor with characteristic pale halo. Can be associated with transient coagulopathy due to localized intravascular coagulation, high-output cardiac failure. Regress within 1–2 years.
  - NICH (non-involuting congenital hemangioma): Grows proportionally or expands slowly.
  - Intermediate type partial involution, and referred to as partially involuting congenital hemangioma (PICH).

Treatment

- RICH—embolization or excision may need to be considered for RICHs that are ulcerated, bleeding or causing hemodynamic instability. β blockers not useful.
- NICH—surgery.

VASCULAR MALFORMATIONS

Vascular malformations are subcategorized depending on the predominant anomalous channels and flow characteristics:

- **Slow-flow—**may be capillary (port-wine stain)—red, macular.
- **Venous** (cavernous hemangioma)—blue, compressible, fill with dependency.
- **Lymphatic** (microcystic lymphangioma or macrocystic cystic hygroma)—vesicles or large cyst.
- **Fast-flow—**arterial anomalies, arteriovenous shunting (AVM).

CAPILLARY MALFORMATION (PORT-WINE STAIN, NEVUS FLAMMEUS)

- Sporadic, affecting 0.1–2% of newborns.
- Unknown pathogenesis; mutations in **GNAQ** reported—both for non-syndromic PWSs and Sturge–Weber syndrome.

Clinical Features

- Red-purple vascular macule or patch present at birth **(Fig. 15.5)**.
- Often located on the face, but may be found anywhere on the body, on the nape (stork bite), facial lesions often fade by early childhood.
- Usually an isolated cutaneous finding, but may be seen in several syndromes (Sturge–Weber syndrome, Klippel-Trénaunay syndrome, Parkes-Weber syndrome, Proteus syndrome, PTEN hamartoma syndromes, Cobb syndrome, Beckwith-Wiedemann syndrome, phakomatosis pigmentovascularis, and capillary malformation-arteriovenous malformation [CM-AVM]).

Histology

- On histology, dilated venules in dermis with normal number of vessels and *no endothelial proliferation* (is a malformation rather than true neoplasm).
  In adults, fibrosis around the vessels and vascular dilation can be seen.

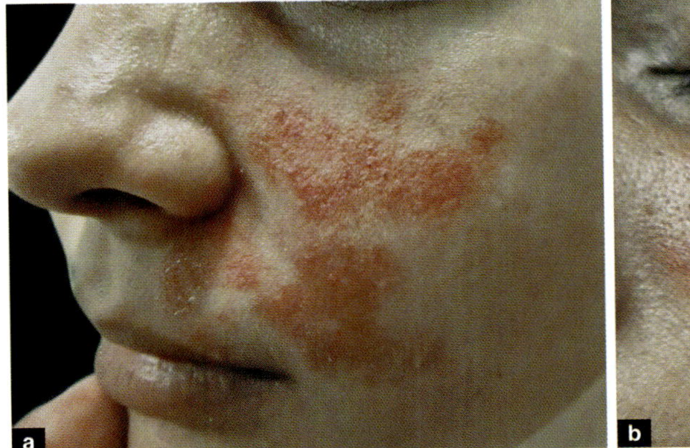

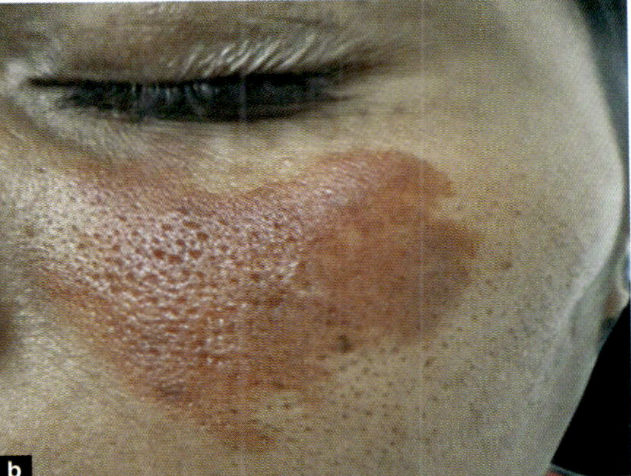

Fig. 15.5: Port-wine stain over face

Approach to Management (Flowchart 15.1)

Treatment

- Pulsed dye laser = First-line therapy
    a. Site—pulsed dye laser treatment for CM is likely more effective in the face and neck.
    b. The recurrence rate may increase with time after treatment.
    c. Laser therapy before the age of 1 year may be effective, and the earliest possible initiation of treatment is recommended.
    d. Topical agents, timolol, imiquimod, and rapamycin (RPM) have been tried in combination with PDL. Topical imiquimod and RPM have shown better results.

Ideal Wavelength (Li D)

Various wavelengths used include but are not limited to pulsed dye laser (PDL) in 585–600 nm, long-pulse 755-nm alexandrite, and 1064-nm Nd:YAG lasers. The varied parameters that are important include, epidermal melanin content, epidermal thickness, dermal blood content, blood vessel depth, and diameter on laser energy deposition.

a. In lightly pigmented skin with small and shallow target blood vessels the ideal device is with a 580–610 nm, in the visible band which is seen in most PDL.
b. If the epidermal pigment increases or size or depth of vessels increase 940 nm is ideal
c. With marked epidermal pigment the optimal wavelength changes to 1005 nm
   Thus 940 nm is ideal wavelength in PWS treatment to meet the need in most widely morphological structure. Lasers with wavelengths in the 580–610, 940, and 1005 nm regions are effective for treating PWS because of their high optical selectivity in blood over the epidermis.

- Lesions do not fade spontaneously; ↑↑ in size proportionately to the child's growth; may become gradually darker and hypertrophic over time.
- Management of limb overgrowths
    a. If leg-length inequality is insignificant, shoe lift is recommended.
    b. As significant inequality causes gait disturbance complicated with scoliosis, surgical treatment aimed to arrest epiphyseal growth is performed in the growth period.
    c. Shortening of the femur or tibia may be performed as an additional treatment.
    d. Bone elongation of the intact side is considered effective for the correction of leg-length inequality.

1. Sturge-Weber Syndrome (SWS) (Encephalotrigeminal Angiomatosis)

- Due to somatic mosaic mutations in the **GNAQ** gene.
- Capillary malformation in V1 (ophthalmic branch of trigeminal nerve) and V2 (>V3) distribution.

Clinical Features

- Only **10%** with a V1 capillary malformation will have SWS **(Flowchart 15.1)**.
- Unilateral > bilateral
- Soft tissue/skeletal hypertrophy under malformation:
    - Ipsilateral leptomeningeal capillary malformation (angiomatosis) of the brain and eye.
    - Neurologic complications include **seizures** (usually develop in **first** year of life), developmental delay, intellectual disability, and focal neurologic deficits.
- Head CT = **Cortical calcifications** that resemble **tram-track lines**.
    - Ophthalmologic complications affect 60% (the most common is **glaucoma**).
    - Clinical course depends on extent of leptomeningeal involvement.

Flowchart 15.1: Approach to capillary malformations

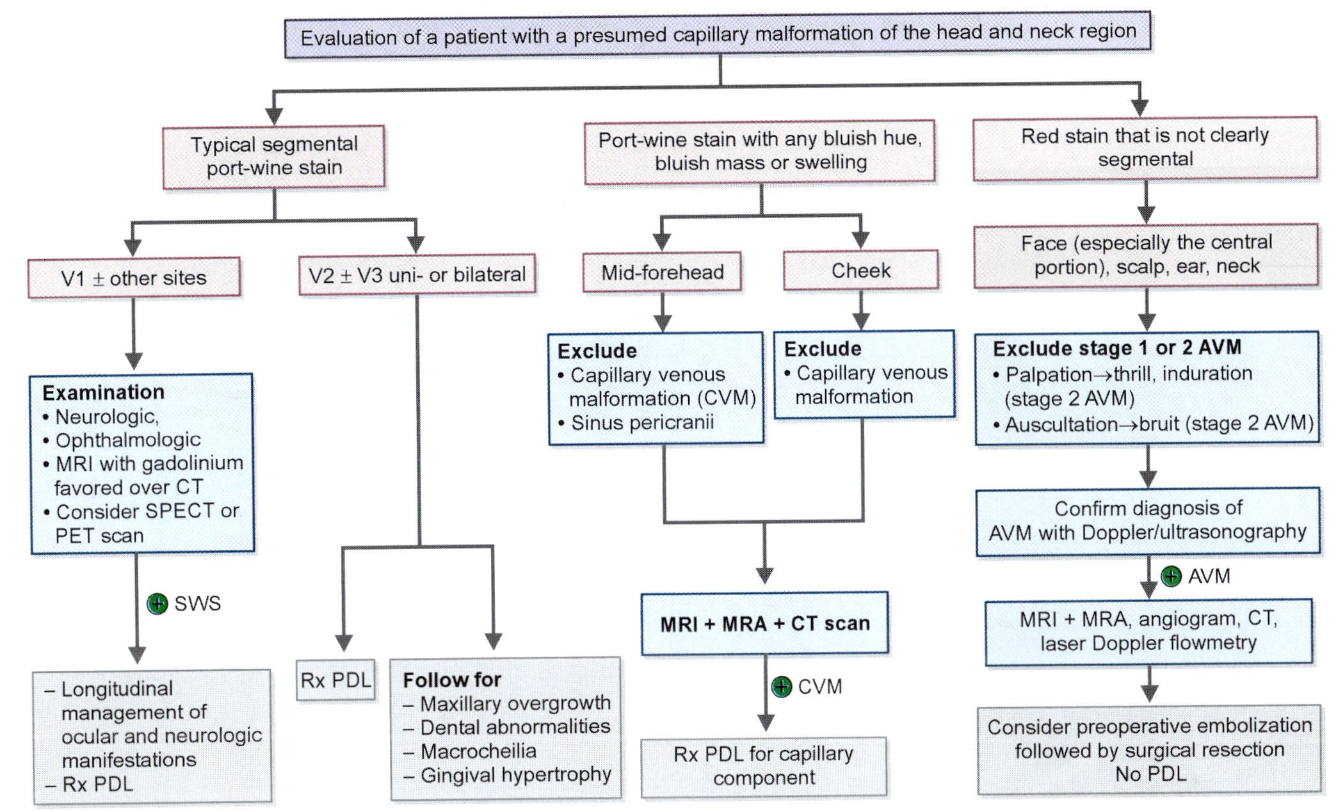

Rx, treatment

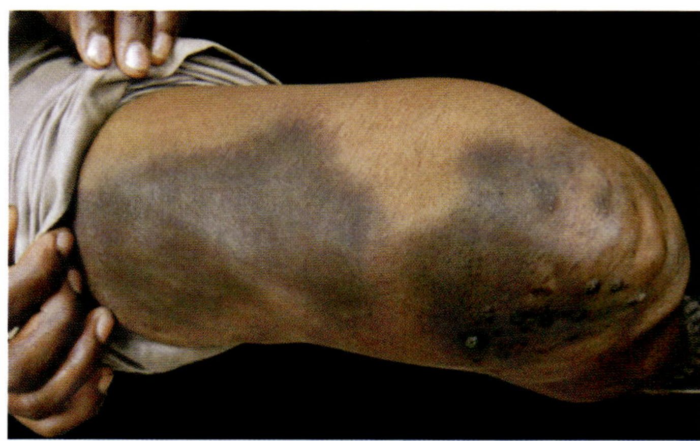

Fig. 15.6: Klippel–Trénaunay syndrome

– Bilateral facial capillary malformations involving V1 distribution = Worst prognosis (↑ risk of seizures and more profound developmental delay).

2. Klippel–Trénaunay Syndrome (Fig. 15.6)

Sporadic, somatic PIK3CA mutations in some.

Klippel-Trénaunay syndrome is characterized by three features:

i. **Capillary malformation (port-wine stain) of the skin (98%)**
ii. **Soft tissue and bone overgrowth and hypertrophy (67%)**
iii. **Varicose veins (72%), with or without deep venous and lymphatic abnormalities.**

It can be diagnosed if only 2 of the 3 features are present; **63%** cases have all three features, whereas **37%** have 2 out of 3 features.

- Involves the lower limbs, followed by the arms, the trunk and rarely the head and neck.
- Parkes-Weber syndrome has the above, plus arteriovenous fistulas, caused by somatic mutations in RASA1.

Pathology

- Ectatic capillaries, superficial dilated dermal venules, lymphatic hypoplasia corresponding to capillary, nodular growth within port-wine stain and lymphatic malformations, respectively.
- Atypical varicose veins are persistent embryonic veins of long, tortuous and without valves superficial venous system.
- Deep venous systems are abnormal in 25% cases of KTS, includes aneurysm, duplications, hypoplasia, aplasia and external compression from anomalous vessels or fibrotic bands.

Clinical Features

- **Capillary malformation:** PWS, pink or reddish may become purple with age with linear border, 10% are nodular. Does not cross the midline. May be deep and involve underlying structure.
- **Venous abnormalities:** Dilated tortuous veins skin ulcers and scarring, if deep venous system involved.
- **Hypertrophy:** Increase in limb girth and/or length, bony and soft tissue enlargement, may have hand and feet abnormalities (macrodactyly, syndactyly, ectodactyly, clinodactyly and camptodactyly).

Differential Diagnosis

- Proteus syndrome
- Maffucci syndrome
- Bannayan–Riley–Ruvalcaba syndrome

Investigations

- Duplex ultrasound
- MRI scan
- Lymphoscintigraphy

Complications and Comorbidities

- **Skin:** Stasis dermatitis
  - Ulcers and secondary infections
- **Veins:** Thrombosis and thrombophlebitis
  - Hemorrhage
  - Pulmonary emboli
- **Hypertrophy**
  - Vertebral scoliosis
  - Gait problems
  - Impaired functions
  - Premature onset of degenerative joint diseases
- **Rare complications (depending upon the site and depth of the lesions)**
  - Genitourinary, gastrointestinal hemorrhage
  - Hemothorax
  - Pulmonary emboli secondary to venous thrombosis
  - Heart failure
  - Central nervous system involvement—hemimegalencephaly, hydrocephalus, atrophy, epilepsy.

Disease Course and Prognosis

Risk of thrombosis and venous complication increase with age.

Management

Medical-compression garments: Orthotics and orthopedic-length heel inserts (for small difference in limb) osteotomy, epiphysiodesis, epiphyseal stapling (for larger differences).

- Avoidance of anticoagulants and oral contraceptives (in female)
- **Laser:** Pulse dye for PWS
  Endovenous laser for varicosities
- **Surgery:** Sclerotherapy, venous stripping, ligation and excision for venous malformation and varicosities.

3. Phakomatosis Pigmentovascularis

('twin spotting' in which a PWS coexists with aberrant Mongolian spots (dermal melanocytosis, also caused by mosaic GNAQ mutations; type 2 PPV) or a nevus spilus (type 3 PPV); a nevus anemicus may also be present.)

Type 1: Nevus flammeus + Epidermal nevus

Type 2: Nevus flammeus + Dermal melanocytosis ± Nevus anemicus **(most common)**
Type 3: Nevus flammeus + Nevus spilus ± Nevus anemicus
Type 4: Nevus flammeus + Dermal melanocytosis + Nevus spilus ± Nevus anemicus
Type 5: Cutis marmorata telangiectatica congenita + Dermal melanocytosis (associated findings can include ocular abnormalities, choroidal melanoma and hemihypertrophy of the limbs, visual vascular anomalies).

4. Proteus Syndrome

Previously was thought to be due to PTEN mutations, but now known to be due to AKT1 somatic activating mutation → asymmetric progressive overgrowth **(Fig. 15.7)**.

Clinical Features

1. Skin:

- Cerebriform connective tissue nevi (plantar collagenoma): Pathognomonic, if present **(Fig. 15.7)**.
- Capillary/venous/lymphatic malformations.
- Epidermal nevi

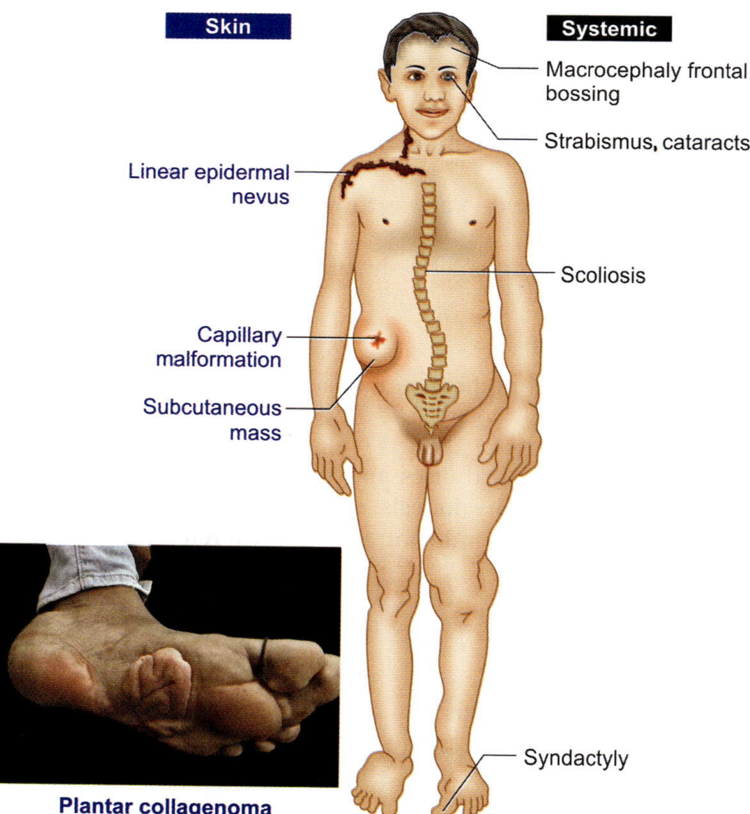

Fig. 15.7: Proteus syndrome

- Lipomas
- CALM
- Focal atrophy/dermal hypoplasia
- Varicosities
- Partial lipohypoplasia

2. **CNS:** Hemimegalencephaly and impaired intelligence
3. **Ophthalmologic:** Nystagmus, strabismus, cataracts, and myopia
4. **Musculoskeletal**
   - *Typical facies:* Dolichocephaly, down-slanting palpebral fissures, depressed nasal bridge, anteverted nares, and open mouth position at rest.
   - *Overgrowth of one or more of the following (involves soft tissue and bone)*: Extremities, digits, cranium (hemifacial macrosomia), vertebrae, and external auditory meatus.
   - Hyperostoses
   - Scoliosis
5. **Others**
   - Bilateral ovarian cystadenoma and parotid monomorphic adenoma
   - Organomegaly
6. **Lung**
   - Cystic lung malformations
   - Pulmonary emphysema
   - Restrictive lung disease
   - Recurrent pneumonia
7. Risk of venous thrombosis and pulmonary embolism.

5. Megalencephaly-capillary Malformation Syndrome

- Reticulated port-wine stains
- Asymmetric somatic growth
- CNS and neurological abnormalities

PIK3CA gene mutation (same as CLOVES [congenital lipomatous (fatty) overgrowth, vascular malformations, epidermal nevi and scoliosis/skeletal/spinal anomalies] syndrome).

VENOUS MALFORMATIONS

- Sporadic, but 50% of sporadic VMs have **TIE2 (aka TEK)** mutations.
  i. **Classical**—soft, compressible bluish nodules that fill with dependency; may be focal, segmental, or widespread, and often extend into underlying muscles and bones **(Fig. 15.8)**.
  ii. **Familial** cutaneous and mucosal venous malformation syndrome (VMCM): Widespread VMs of skin, mucosa and visceral organs due to TIE2 (aka TEK) mutations; has significant overlap with blue rubber bleb syndrome.
- Present at birth, but may become more apparent in childhood.
- Erythematous to violaceous, soft, compressible nodule or plaque without warmth, vascular thrill, or pulsations +/– radiating veins.

Histology

Dilated vascular spaces with single-layer endothelial wall that is surrounded by fibrous tissue; involves deep dermis or subcutaneous fat.

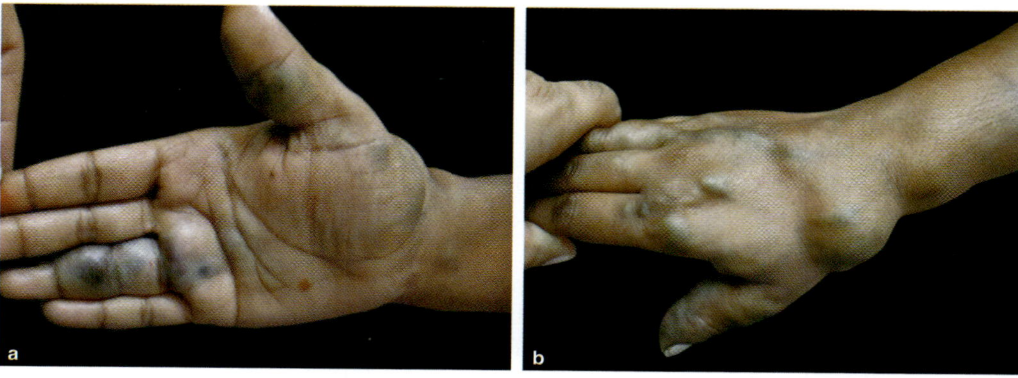

Fig. 15.8: Soft compressible bluish nodules of venous malformations

Imaging

Ultrasound shows slow-flow lesion; MRI is best imaging modality to determine extent; on plain films, calcification can be seen 2° to phleboliths.

Fibrinogen may be ↓ and D-dimer may be ↑.

Management

The essential therapy revolves around sclerotherapy in which various agents have been used including bleomycin, polidoconal, electrotherapy and cyanoacrylate glue embolisation.

An approach to management is given in **Flowchart 15.2**.

1. Blue Rubber Bleb Nevus (Bean) Syndrome

- Presents at birth to early childhood with venous malformations
- Multiple blue-violaceous **compressible** papules and nodules
- **Hyperhidrosis** overlying lesions; with compression, an **empty wrinkled sac** is noted that quickly fills with release of pressure) **(Fig. 15.9)**.
- Venous malformations involve the trunk/extremities, mucosa, GI tract (especially small intestine), liver, and CNS. GI bleeding, resulting in anemia, intussusception.
- ↑ size with age.

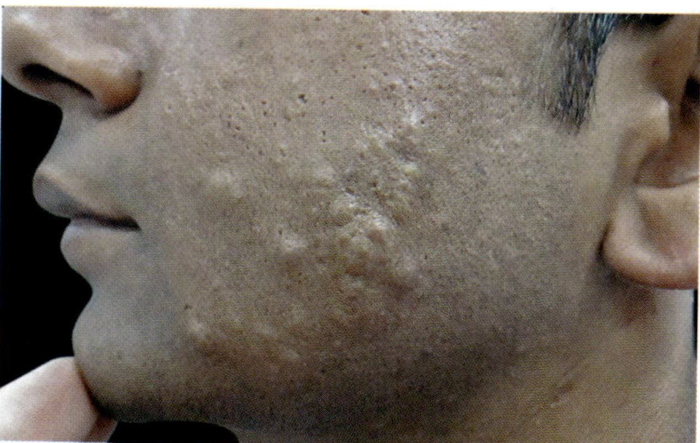

Fig. 15.9: Blue rubber bleb nevus

Flowchart 15.2: An approach to the evaluation and management of venous malformations (VMs)

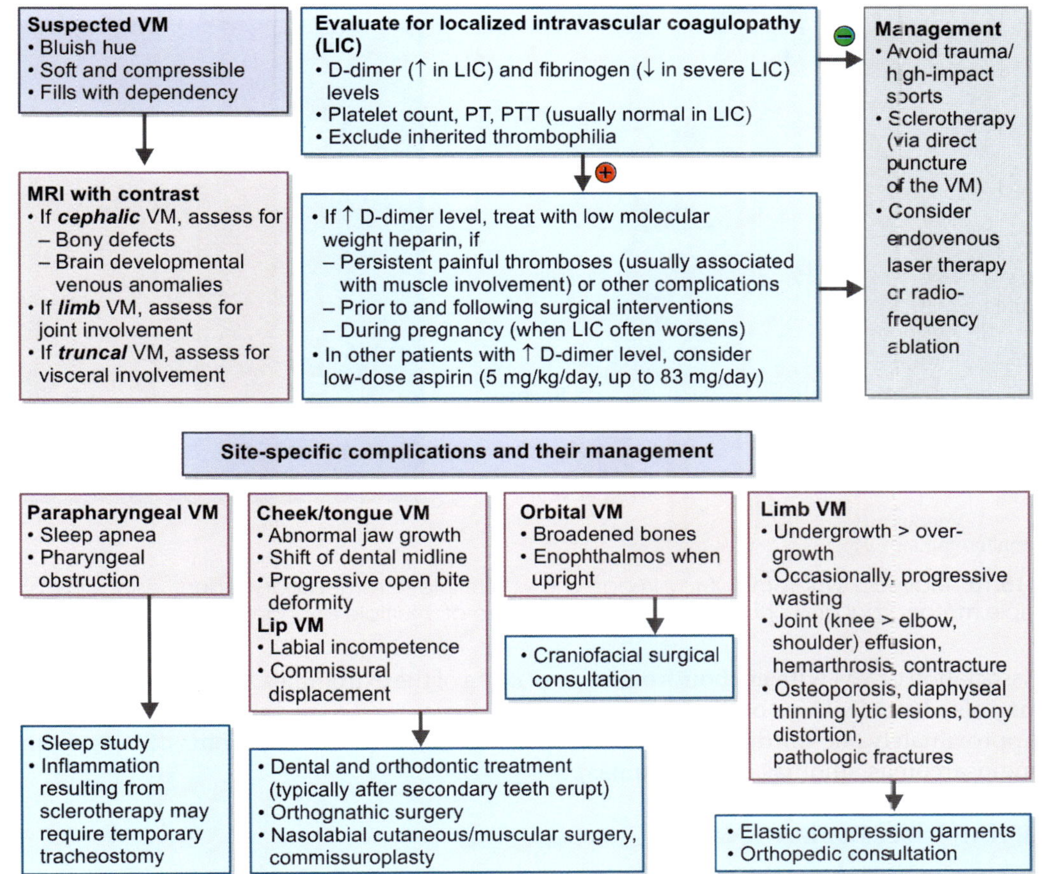

2. Glomulovenous Malformations (GVM; Previously Termed 'Glomangiomas')

Variant of venous malformation (is not a neoplasm → no longer referred to as 'glomangioma') where ectatic vessels are lined by a small number of glomus cells.

- Glomus cells are modified smooth muscle cells of Sucquet-Hoyer canal origin.
- AD inheritance, due to loss of function mutations in **glomulin (GLMN) gene**.

Clinical Features

- Presents in infancy or childhood.
- Multiple lesions (soft, partially compressible blue nodules > confluent plaques); favors lower extremities; usually asymptomatic (pain is more common with glomus tumors).

Histology: Large, dilated vessels surrounded by a small number of glomus cells.

3. Maffucci Syndrome

- Sporadic, parathyroid hormone/parathyroid hormone-related protein (PTH/PTHrP) type I receptor.

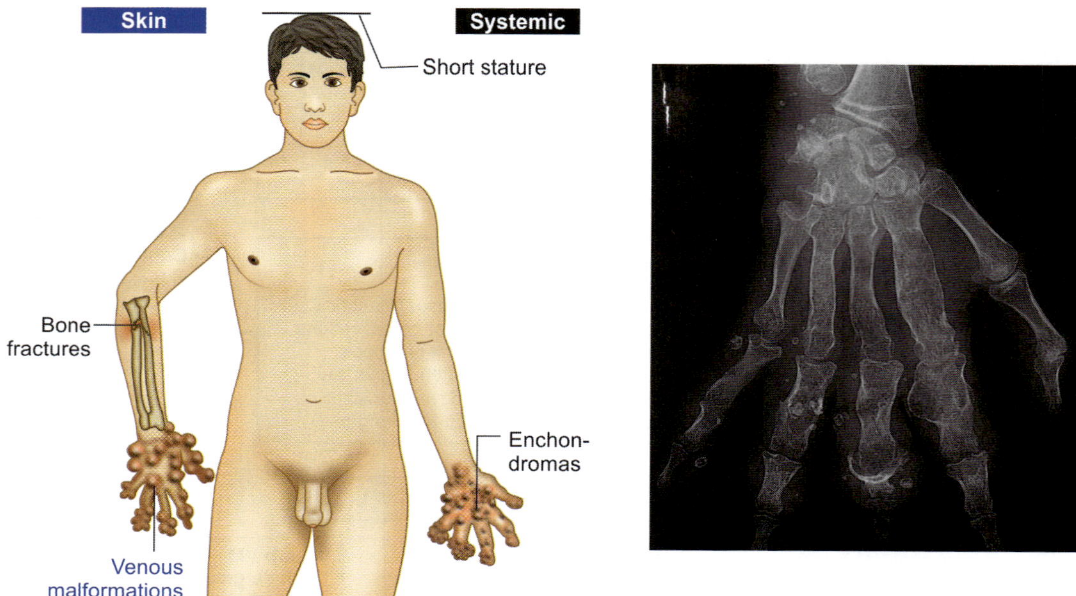

Fig. 15.10: Maffucci syndrome: X-ray image shows multiple intramedullary lucent lesions involving multiple metacarpal and phalanges bones suggestive of multiple enchondromas

- Association of VM with **enchondromas**, most often of the extremities; **(Fig. 15.10)** skin lesions may also have features of a spindle cell hemangioma.
- Approximately one-third of patients develop malignancies (chondrosarcomas, fibrosarcomas, angiosarcomas, gliomas and teratomas).

LYMPHATIC MALFORMATIONS

Lymphatic malformations (*LMs*) are due to excessive aberrant lymphatic channels, whereas *lymphedema* results from hypoplasia or disruption of the lymphatics.

Lymphangioma Circumscriptum (Microcystic LM)

- Lymphatic malformations account for 4% of all vascular malformations. Most common type of lymphatic malformation.
- Results from an error in the embryonic development of the lymphatic system, grows only by expansion/distension, not proliferation.

Etiopathogenesis

Somatic mutation restricted to cells of the lesion.

Clinical Features

- Manifest at birth or during infancy, as localized subcutaneous swelling or **frogspawn** (groups of watery or hemorrhagic vesicles or lymph blisters) on the skin **(Fig. 15.11)**.
- Site: Can occur anywhere on skin, favorable sites are axillary folds, shoulders, flanks, proximal parts of the limbs and perineum. In mouth (buccal mucosa, lips, tongue and oral floor).

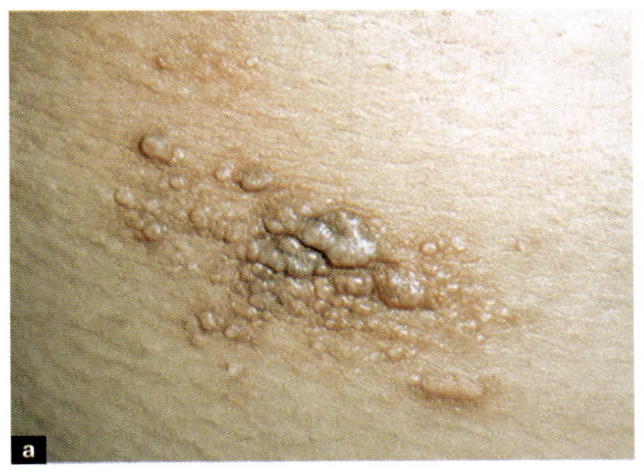

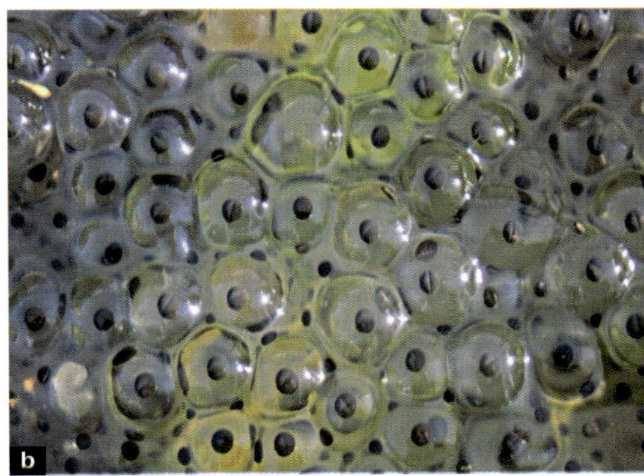

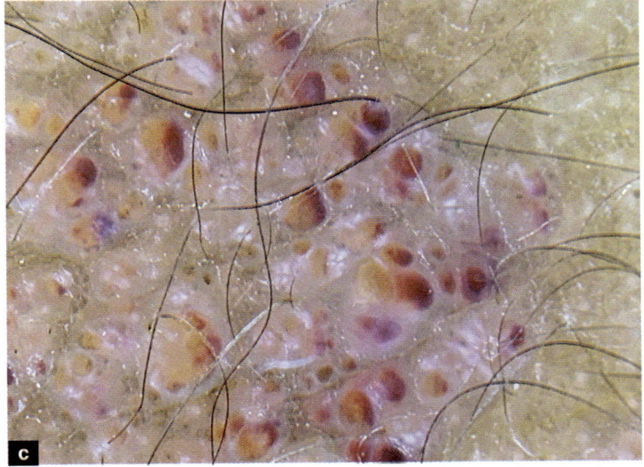

Fig. 15.11: Lymphangioma circumscriptum, plaque with surface showing scattered or hemorrhagic vesicles of variable sizes which resemble frogspawn (b), (c) dermoscopy of LC showing multiple well-circumscribed rounded yellowish and reddish lacunae surrounded by pale septae and few lacunae contain blood, characteristically accumulated in the bottom like a "hypopyon" (half-and-half lacuna) (*Courtesy*: Surabhi Sinha, MD)

- Surface of the lymphangiomas may appear warty and the lesions may be mistaken for viral warts.
- Additional features include swelling, hemorrhage and leakage of lymph from superficial vesicles and local cellulitis.
- Lymphedema will be a presenting feature, if there is connection to underlying normally draining lymphatic pathways.

Differential Diagnosis

- Vascular malformation
- Hamartomas
- Tumors
- HPV

Complications

- Frequent discharge of lymph fluid (lymphorrhea)
- Ulceration and infection
- Erysipelas-like reactions
- Squamous cell carcinoma

Prognosis

Excellent, if no lymphangiomatosis.

Investigations

- Biopsy will reveal angulated channels, which stain for **CD31** and **D240**.
- Ultrasonography, demonstrate fluid-filled lesions.
- MRI to know the extent of growth of lymphangioma.

Management

First line

- Conservative, compression garment for truncal lesions
- Sclerotherapy
- Bleomycin
- Dithermy or laser

Second line: Sildenafil.

Third line: Sirolimus, mTOR inhibitors (if there is mutation in the AKT/PIK3/mTOR pathway).

Macrocystic LM ('Cystic Hygroma')

- Associated with fetal aneuploidy, including **Turner syndrome** and **Down syndrome**; also associated with Noonan syndrome and achondroplasia.
- Presents as a large, soft, bluish, and sometimes translucent tumor, with normal overlying skin
  - Transilluminates with light
  - Head, neck, and axilla/chest most common locations, favoring left side.
- Sudden size ↑ may herald infection or intralesional hemorrhage.

LYMPHEDEMA

Primary Lymphedema

Most often affects the extremities (lower > upper), with occasional genital, cephalic, or generalized involvement; may be associated with pulmonary or GI lymphangiectasia.

Congenital Lymphedema

- Present at birth or develops during infancy; variants include *Milroy disease* (mutations in the gene encoding vascular endothelial growth factor receptor 3) and *Turner* and *Noonan syndromes*.
- *Milroy disease:* AD inheritance; due to loss-of-function mutations in FLT4 gene (encodes VEGFR3, which is required for lymphatic development)
  - Presents at birth (or soon after) and persists for life

- Painless pitting edema of bilateral lower extremities
- Over time, involved area becomes firm and fibrotic
- Associated features: Hydrocele, prominent veins, and upslanting toenails.

Lymphedema Praecox

Presents around puberty; variants include ***Meige disease*** **and** ***lymphedema—distichiasis syndrome***.

Lymphedema—distichiasis syndrome: Is a form of hereditary lymphedema but has peripubertal—onset (10–30 years); AD inheritance; FOXC2 mutation; lower-limb lymphedema + distichiasis (extra eyelashes ranging from a single hair to a full set).

ARTERIOVENOUS MALFORMATIONS (AVMs)

While the majority of AVMs are sporadic, recent studies have begun to elucidate the genetic basis of these lesions with the identification of somatic variants in genes associated with the RAS/MAPK signalling pathway. Most of these studies have focused on cerebral AVMs, and a meta-analysis revealed that a KRAS PV is present in 55% of these lesions. Rarest but most dangerous type of vascular malformation **(Fig. 15.12)**:

- Developmental anomaly arising early in embryogenesis → abnormal communication between an artery and vein causing high-flow (*fast-flow*) shunting of blood from the arterial circulation to the venous circulation (AV shunting).
- Erythematous to violaceous patches/nodules/tumors that are *warm* to touch and have palpable *thrill* or pulsation; most commonly cephalic (70%).

Divided into four stages based on clinical severity:

Stage 1—dormant: Red, warm and macular (mimicking a PWS) or slightly infiltrated.

Stage 2—expansion: Warm mass with thrill/throbbing and dilated draining veins.

Stage 3—destruction: Pain, necrosis, and ulceration; ± lytic bone lesions.

Stage 4—cardiac decompensation: High-output cardiac failure.

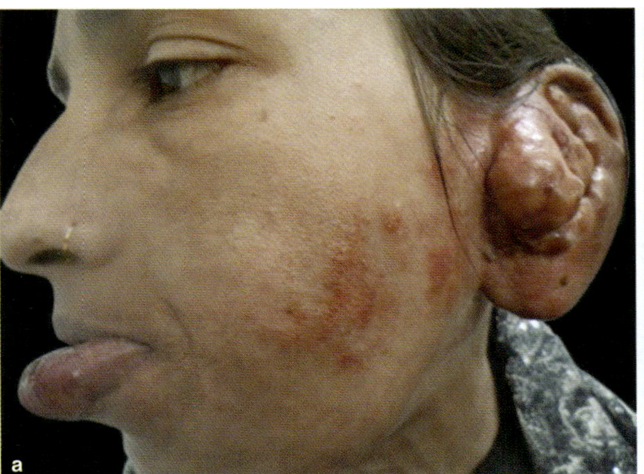

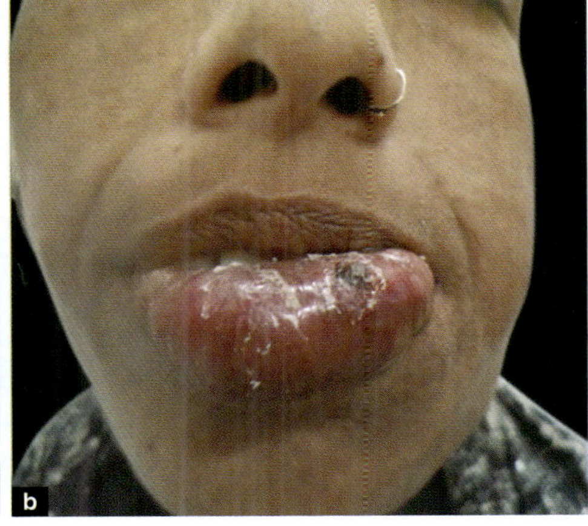

Fig. 15.12: Arteriovenous malformation over face in a segmental distribution

A recent study has noted high prevalence of pathogenic somatic variants, predominantly in MAP2K1 and KRAS, in extracranial arteriovenous malformations.

MAP2K1-usually focal

KRAS-severe, diffuse.

Investigations

MRI and ultrasound studies confirm diagnosis and assess disease extent.

Histology

On histology, circumscribed, unencapsulated, and thick-walled arterioles with direct connection to veins (thin-walled), and abundant superficial capillaries.

Treatment

- **Embolization** + **excision** is the treatment of choice for symptomatic lesions.
- Amputation may be required as a result of aggressive growth.
- Consumptive coagulopathy may develop in larger AVM.
- Vascular surgeon or an intervention radiologist are better suited to treat such cases.

Other AVM

1. **Acroangiodermatitis** (pseudo-Kaposi sarcoma) can occur in association with a lower extremity AVM.
2. **Metameric AVMs**
   - *Cobb syndrome*: Cutaneous (may mimic a CM or angiokeratoma) in dermatomal distribution + intraspinal/vertebral.
   - *Bonnet-Dechaume-Blanc* (*Wyburn-Mason*) *syndrome*: Cutaneous facial + Orbit/eye and/or brain.
   - *Parkes-Weber syndrome*: Characterized by capillary malformations, venous malformations, lymphatic malformations, and multiple fast-flow arteriovenous malformations/shunts (differentiates it from Klippel–Trénaunay syndrome, which only has slow-flow malformations).
     - Typically affects the lower extremities.
     - Soft tissue and bony hypertrophy.

OTHER VASCULAR DISORDERS

Angiokeratoma

- Well-defined benign vascular lesion not true angioma, comprising superficial vascular ectasia and overlying acanthosis or hyperkeratosis
- **Five** variants:
  i. Solitary or multiple angiokeratomas **(Fig. 15.13)**
  ii. Angiokeratomas of the scrotum and vulva (Angiokeratoma of Fordyce) **(Fig. 15.14)**
  iii. Angiokeratoma corporis diffusum (Fabry disease)
  iv. Angiokeratoma of Mibelli—acral skin
  v. Angiokeratoma circumscriptum

Table 15.8 shows important differentiating features among types of angiokeratoma.

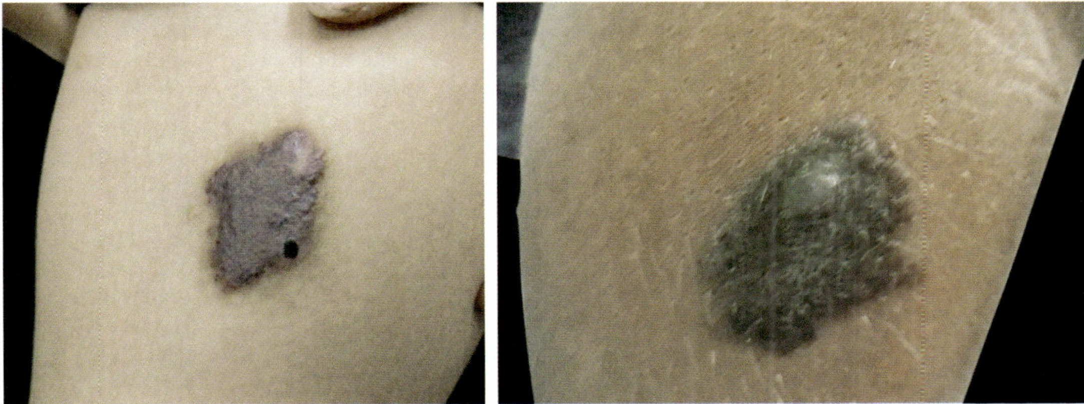

Fig. 15.13: Solitary angiokeratoma over extremity, bluish-red papules coalesce to form plaques

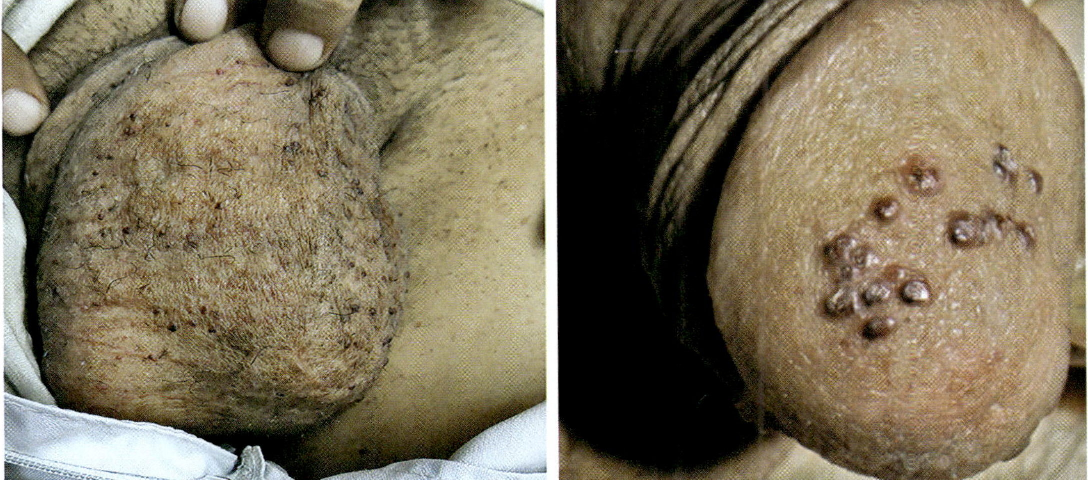

Fig. 15.14: Angiokeratoma of Fordyce on the scrotum and penis

Pathology

- Hyperkeratotic, acanthotic epidermis
- Marked dilation of papillary dermal vessels
- Elongated rete ridges enclosing partially or completely vascular channels
- In Fabry disease, vacuoles can be detected within endothelial cells and pericytes, glycolipid deposits can be demonstrated in PAS stain.

Clinical Features

- Red/blue or purple in color, sometimes with a slightly rough surface.
- May appear black, if thrombosed or traumatized or bled.
- Lesions may vary from papules to plaques.

TABLE 15.8: Types of angiokeratoma

Solitary or multiple angiokeratomas	Angiokeratoma of Fordyce	Angiokeratoma corporis diffusum	Angiokeratoma of Mibelli	Angiokeratoma circumscriptum
Small, warty, black papules	• The lesions are red-purple to black in color, may be single or multiple • Association with local venous hypertension varicocele, hernia, prostatitis, bladder or epididymal tumors, lymphogranuloma venereum (LGV)	• Development of multiple, often clustered angiokeratomas, usually in a bathing trunk distribution results from a deficiency of the lysosomal enzyme α-galactosidase A • Association with heart and renal failure, stroke, cornea verticillata, deafness	Associated with chilblains and acrocyanosis chilblains, or frostbite	• Plaque of multiple discrete papules or confluent hyperkeratotic papules and nodules • Association with Cobb syndrome, vascular malformation
Site—can occur anywhere, most commonly on the lower extremity	Scrotum, vulva	Trunk	Dorsal and lateral aspects of the fingers and toes, rarely on elbows and knees (AD)	Trunk, arms or legs and are unilateral
10–40 years, both sex	• Second or third decade • Mainly in old age (>60)	• Begin to appear during late childhood (5–12) or adolescence • X-linked recessive	• Seen in 10–15 years of age • Familial predisposition (AD)	Develop during infancy or childhood female predominance

Differential Diagnosis

- Malignant melanoma
- Cherry angioma

Complications and Comorbidities

Trauma can lead to bleeding and/or thrombosis.

Disease Course and Prognosis

- Benign and generally resolve spontaneously.
- No investigation required for single lesion, but for multiple lesions, Fabry disease should be considered and genetic counselling needed.

Management

- Excison for single lesion
- Hyfrecation
- Curettage

- Cryotherapy
- **Laser:** KTP laser or 800 nm diode laser give good cosmetic results, others—argon, carbon dioxide, erbium.
  Intralesional injection of Triamcinolone acetonide.

BIBLIOGRAPHY

Books

1. Anita N Haggstrom and Maria C Garzan. Infantile Hemangiomas. In: Bolognia JL, Jorizzo JL, Schayjer JV (eds). Dermatology (3rd ed.) London: Elsevier; 2002:1691–707.
2. El Sissy FN, Somatic mutational landscape of extracranial arteriovenous malformations and phenotypic correlations. J Eur Acad Dermatol Venereol. 2022 Jun;36(6):905–912.
3. O Dile Enjolras. Vascular Malformations. In: Bolognia JL, Jorizzo JL, Schaffer JV. eds. Dermatology (3rd ed). London: Elsevier; 2012:1711–27.
4. Peter S. Mortimer and kristiana Gorden. Disorder of the lymphatic vessels. In: Editors. Rook's Textbook of Dermatology (9th ed). UK Blackwell; 2016:2878–81.
5. Portia C. Goldsmith. Dermatoses Resulting from disorders of the veins and arteries. In: Rooks Textbook of Dermatology (9th ed). UK:Blackwell; 2016:2787–826.
6. Rook's Textbook of Dermatology—Part 10, Chapter 117: Dermatoses and Haemangiomas of Infancy.

Journals

1. ISSVA Classification of Vascular Anomalies ©2018 International Society for the Study of Vascular Anomalies Available at "issva.org/classification" Accessed [31.12.2020].
2. Krowchuk DP; subcommittee on the management of infantile hemangiomas. Clinical practice guideline for the management of infantile hemangiomas. pediatrics. 2019 jan;143(1):e20183475.
3. Li D. Wavelength optimization for the laser treatment of port wine stains. Lasers Med Sci. 2022 Jun;37(4):2165–2178.

Chapter

16

Hidradenitis Suppurativa

Surabhi Sinha, Kabir Sardana, Bhawuk Dhir

Hidradenitis suppurativa is a chronic inflammatory disease involving the follicles with a relapsing and debilitating course and characterized by deep-seated painful nodules. Other names for this condition include acne inversa, apocrine acne, pyoderma fistulans significa, etc.

EPIDEMIOLOGY

- Average age of patients is 24.2 years (peak 20 years).
- Disease onset-after puberty.
- F>M (3.3:1)
  - Women—axillary and genitofemoral lesions **(Fig. 16.1)**
  - Men—perineal and perianal disease

PREDISPOSING FACTORS

- **Hormonal influences:** Supported by a female preponderance, perimenstrual disease aggravation and improvement during pregnancy.
- **Smoking:** Higher risk of disease and more severe disease in smokers. (Role of nicotine in pathogenesis)
- **Obesity:** Major predisposing factors for HS. An increase of 1 kg/m^2 body mass index (BMI) is associated with a mean increase of 0.84 Sartorius HS severity score units.
  - Increased friction and maceration in skin folds
  - Proinflammatory cytokine release from visceral fat
  - Insulin resistance
- **Medications:** Lithium and sirolimus—exacerbate the disease.
- **Immune factors:**
  - Innate immune mechanisms are altered in HS (TLR and AMP down regulated)
  - Increased production of oxygen-free radicals is seen.
  - Upregulation in the levels of TNF-α, IL-1β and IL-10 (IL-23/Th17 pathway activated)
  - Down regulation of IL-2, IL-4, IL-5 and IFN-γ.

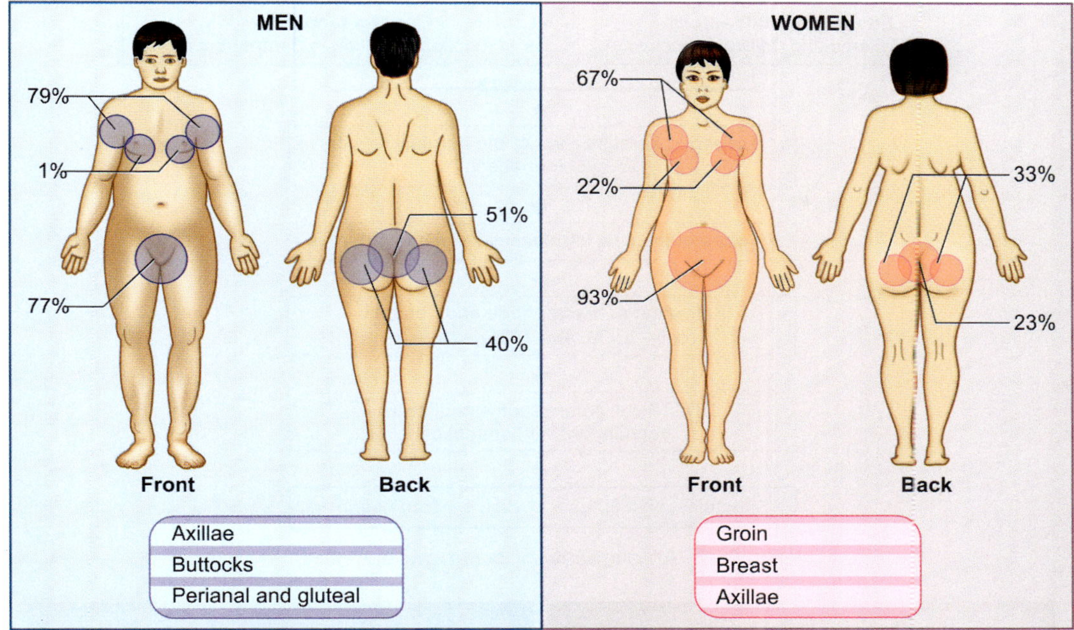

Fig. 16.1: Distribution of HS lesions in men and women

- **Genetics:** Family history +ve in one third patients
  - Loss of function mutation in genes encoding γ-secretase complex [presenilin (PSEN1/PSEN2), presenilin enhancer-2, nicastrin]
  - **γ-secretase deficiency** → Defective **NOTCH** signalling pathway → defective HF and epidermal differentiation, impaired anti-inflammatory regulator T-cell activity, and activation of TLR-induced proinflammatory responses.
- **Bacterial colonization**—overzealous immune response to commensal flora within hair follicles triggers the initial follicular inflammation.

PATHOGENESIS

Figure 16.2 shows an overview of the pathogenesis.

CLINICAL FEATURES

Key elements for diagnosis of HS:

1. **Characteristic lesions:** Deep seated nodules, painful abscesses, bridged scars, pseudo-comedones or multiheaded comedones **(Fig. 16.3)**.
2. **Characteristic sites:** Axillae, groins, perineum, buttocks, inframammary and intermammary areas **(Fig. 16.1)**.
3. **Chronicity and recurrence**
   - The lesion starts as a rounded abscess. Scarring is bridge or rope like. Mean duration of a single lesion is about 7–15 days following which it ruptures.
   - Scarring can be atrophic or hypertrophic.
   - Polyporous, paired and grouped comedones are seen. Closed comedones are never seen.
   - Other lesions include follicular papules and pustules along with pyogenic granulomas.

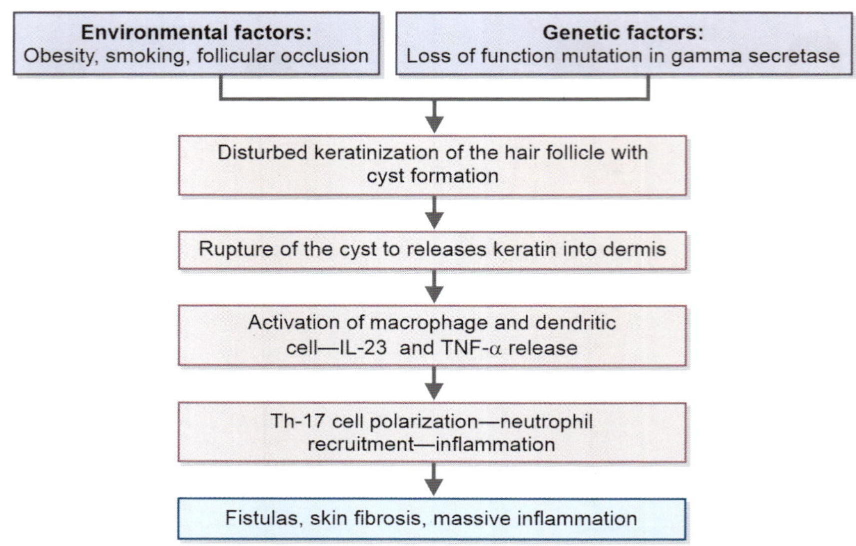

Fig. 16.2: An overview of pathogenesis of HS

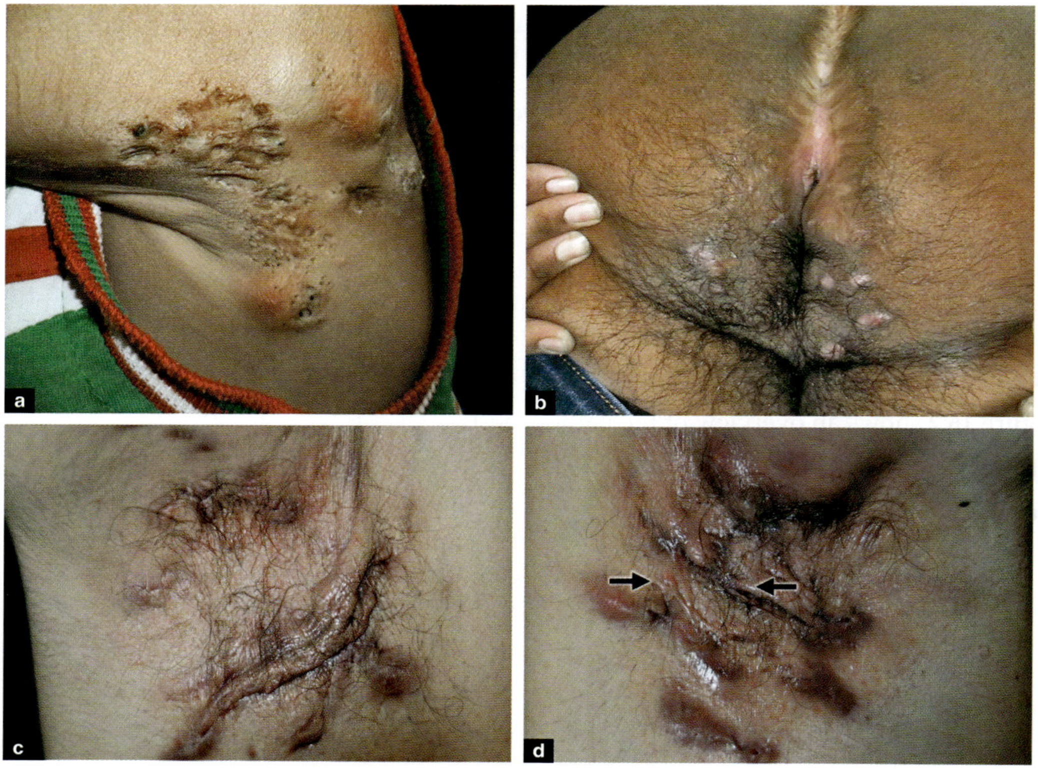

Fig. 16.3: (a) Multiporous comedones, nodules and cysts in the axillary folds; (b) Sinus and nodules in the perianal area; (c) Bridged scars with nodules; (d) Sinus and nodules in the axillae

CLINICAL VARIANTS

1. Classical type—**<u>Classic 'axillary-mammary'</u>** (48%)
2. Follicular type—associated with involvement of ears, back, legs and chest. Severe acne and positive family history, male predominance (part of follicular occlusion tetrad)
3. Gluteal involvement—seen in males.

DIAGNOSIS (all three must be present—Ingram JR et al., 2009)

1. Typical lesions—inflamed nodules, open comedones, sinus tracts, bridging scars
2. Predominantly flexural location—axillary, groins, perineum, infra or intermammary areas
3. Chronicity: ≥2 lesions in last 6 months/lifetime history of ≥5 lesions.

DIFFERENTIAL DIAGNOSIS

Table 16.1 represents a list of common differential diagnosis.

INVESTIGATIONS

Box 16.1 shows a list of relevant investigations.

TABLE 16.1: Differential diagnosis of HS

Disease	Similarity	Dissimilarity
Crohn disease	Perianal and genital fistulae, abscesses, scars	'Knife-cut' ulcers; fistulae communicate with the gastrointestinal tract; often concurrent with gastrointestinal Crohn disease; no comedones
Intergluteal pilonidal disease	Sinus tract formation; swollen, inflamed, and painful lesions; can occur in patients with hidradenitis suppurativa	Localization, recurrence is limited to the intergluteal area
Furuncles and carbuncles	Painful nodules and abscesses	Lack of chronicity
Tuberculosis (lupus vulgaris)	Chronic inflammation and scarring	Absence of polyporous comedones, fistulae and sinuses
Lymphogranuloma venereum	Localization in the genital and inguinal folds	Bacterial etiology: *Chlamydia trachomatis* (serotype L1–L3)

BOX 16.1: Investigations in HS

- WBC count, erythrocyte sedimentation rate
- Serum iron levels (reduced in HS)
- Serum protein abnormalities on serum electrophoresis
- Complete blood counts, and blood cultures (febrile or toxic patients)
- Blood sugar and lipid profile
- Purulent drainage should be sent for bacterial cultures and sensitivities (only if required)
- Deep-tissue culture for bacterial and fungal organisms (if suspected)
- USG or MRI

Severity Scoring

1. **Hurley staging system (Table 16.2)**
   Limitations of Hurley system
   - Not a quantitative staging
   - Fixed/static
   - Cannot assess treatment efficacy
2. Modified Sartorious score—takes into account the treatment response.
3. Hidradenitis suppurativa clinical response (HiSCR) score.
   - Defined as a **>50% reduction** in inflammatory nodule count without concomitant increase in number of draining fistulae
   - Recommended by HS ALLIANCE, Canadian, European, and Brazilian guidelines for assessment of treatment response
4. HS physician's global assessment (PGA) system.

COMPLICATIONS

- Superinfection
- Lymphedema with scrotal elephantiasis
- Fistulae
- Squamous cell carcinoma—most commonly on gluteal skin of males
- Amyloidosis
- Bacterial osteomyelitis
- Inflammatory eye disease—bilateral interstitial keratitis, uveitis, Mooren-type ulcerations, scleritis
- Profound psychosocial impact—social embarrassment, sexual dysfunction, higher suicide rates
- Degree of quality-of-life impairment (DLQI) **more severe** for HS *vs* other dermatological diseases (alopecia, psoriatic arthritis, and chronic urticaria).

COURSE AND PROGNOSIS

Mean duration of disease is 18.8 years, chronicity is the hallmark.
It is rarely seen in age group above 50 years.

TREATMENT

The treatment of HS involves general advice **(Box 16.2)** and specific interventions depending on the severity of the disorder. Each intervention is initiated for 12 weeks before proceeding to the next level. In case of antibiotics, it advisable to give a break in therapy to avoid resistance. Pain relief is required in severe cases. While **Table 16.3** lists an evidence-based treatment outline

TABLE 16.2: Hurley staging system

Stage	Abscesses	Sinus tracts	Cicatrization
I (mild)	Single or multiple	–	–
II (moderate)	Recurrent (separated)	+ (separated)	+
III (severe)	+++	Multiple, interconnected	++, diffuse

BOX 16.2: General advice for HS

- Advise wearing loose clothing to avoid friction with skin
- Washing with chlorhexidine, zinc pyrithione, or other anti-bacterial washes
- Recommend smoking cessation
- Recommend weight loss
- Eradication of *S. aureus* carriage with topical mupirocin in nose, axillae, perianal area
- Screen for CVS risk factors, depression and anxiety

TABLE 16.3: Evidence-based treatment of HS

		Mild	Moderate	Severe
1st line	Medical	• Clindamycin gel (1%) • Resorcinol (15%)	• Doxycycline/ minocycline (50–100 mg) BD/ lymecycline 408 mg	• Clindamycin + Rifampicin × 10 weeks[1] • Adalimumab × 12 weeks[3]
	Surgical	Intralesional triamcinolone (3–5 mg)	Excision, carbon dioxide laser evaporation, drainage of abscesses	
2nd line	Medical		Clindamycin + Rifampicin × 10 weeks[1]	Prednisone (40–60 mg) daily for 3–4 days then taper Or Cyclosporine (3–5 mg/kg) daily
	Surgical		Local procedures for sinus tracts[2]	
3rd line	Medical		• Adalimumab × 12 weeks[3] • Dapsone (25–200 mg) daily • Acitretin (0.5 mg/kg) daily	—
	Surgical		—	• Wide excision for larger affected areas • Radical wide excision

[1]Clindamycin (300 mg) BD + Rifampicin (300 mg) BD daily. [2]Deroofing of sinus tracts, sinus tract excision, STEEP surgery, carbon dioxide laser evaporation of diseased tissue. [3]Loading doses at week 0 (160 mg SC), week 2 (80 mg SC), Maintenance (40 mg SC) weekly.

for HS, salient agents are detailed below. Here it must be noted that the cardinal feature of HS is the presence of "tunneled comedones" which can only be cured by surgery. The other complications of HS are bridged lesions, epithelialized sinuses, cysts and, in extreme cases, fistulae in internal organs. The role of medical therapy here is merely adjunctive.

1. **Antibiotics:** Apart from the combination of rifampicin and clindamycin, other agents tried include moxifloxacin and metronidazole but are associated with adverse effects including gastrointestinal symptoms, vaginal candidiasis and tendinitis. Ertapenem is a broad-spectrum antibiotic that has demonstrated efficacy in treating HS. The dose used is 1 g of intravenous ertapenem for an average of 59 days. This might be used to achieve rapid improvement prior to surgery or other maintenance therapies, but can otherwise be considered for patients who are refractory to or contraindicated for other treatments.
2. **Surgical intervention in HS—basic principles:**
   - Option for unresponsive lesions with extensive scarring

- Recurrence is very common, if the lesions are merely drained.
- Roof of the sinus tract is excised, floor is left intact. The principle of treatment is to enable marsupialization (deroofing), in which the roof of the tunnel is laid open and the wall of the tunnel is ablated. Subsequent healing is best achieved by secondary intention.
- Excision of all hair bearing in the affected region provides much higher benefits compared to excision of just the inflamed lesions.
- Alcohol intake seen to be associated with post-surgery recurrence.
- For severe disease, wide excision with grafting is the only potentially curative treatment.

3. **Biologics in HS—basic principles (Fig. 16.4)**
   - Consider in moderate-to-severe HS who are unresponsive to, or intolerant of, antibiotic therapy.
   - Adalimumab should be considered as first-choice biologic agent in moderate/severe HS after failure of conventional treatments (*First FDA-approved therapy for HS*—in October 2018, in ages 12 and above). Adalimumab efficacy might be related to mTORC1 signaling, which is important for innate and adaptive immunity and Th17 differentiation. However, dose is higher than that for psoriasis.
   - Ixekizumab and secukinumab are being trialed.
   - Ustekinumab (a monoclonal antibody against IL-12/IL-23) and anakinra have also been tried.

Recently 2 randomized, placebo-controlled, phase III trials have shown that in moderate to severe hidradenitis suppurativa, secukinumab 300 mg every 2 weeks had a greater hidradenitis suppurativa clinical response compared with those receiving placebo (Kimball AB, 2023).

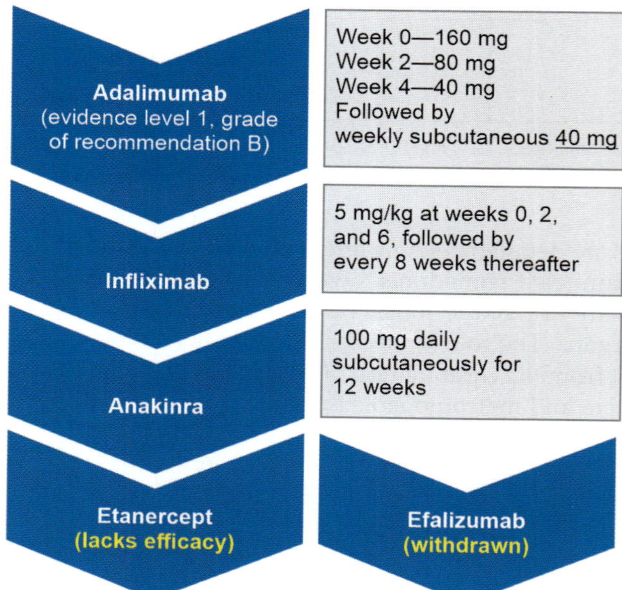

Fig. 16.4: Biologics in HS

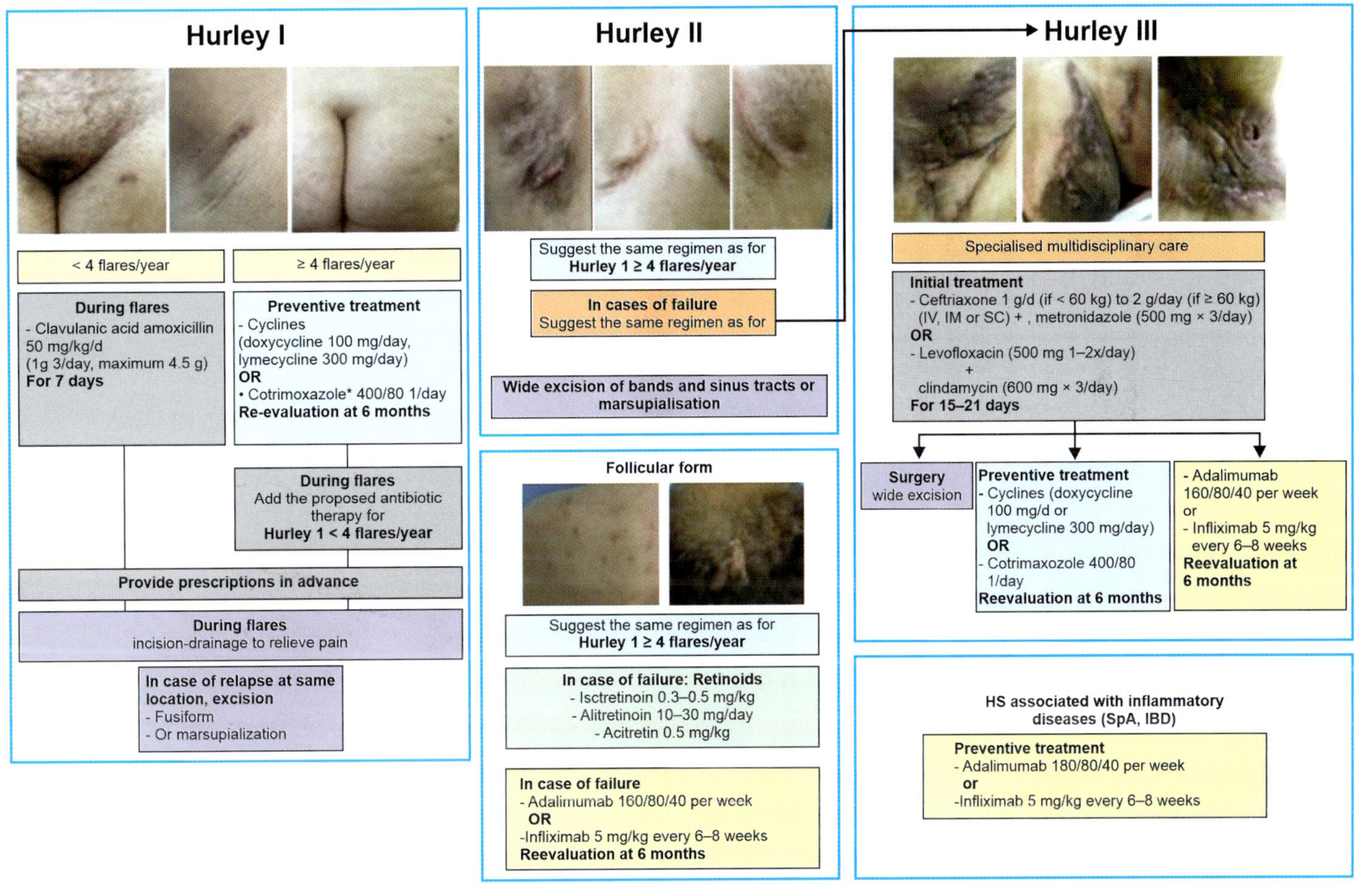

Fig. 16.5: Algorithm based approach to management of HS

4. **Other agents:** Various other agents have been tried including hormonal therapy (OCP/ spironolactone), retinoids, dapsone, metformin, finasteride, apremilast, IFX-1 (monoclonal antibody against C5a) and INCB054707 (JAK inhibitor) **(Fig. 16.5)**.

BIBLIOGRAPHY

Books

1. Fitzpatrick's Dermatology 9th Edition, Chapter 84: Hidradenitis Suppurativa.
2. Rook's Textbook of Dermatology, 9th ed. Chapter 92: Hidradenitis Suppurativa.
3. Textbook of Dermatology and Sexually Transmitted Diseases with HIV Infections, 1st edn. CBS 2019.

Journals

1. Goldburg SR, Strober BE, Payette MJ. Hidradenitis suppurativa: Current and emerging treatments. J Am Acad Dermatol. 2020 May;82(5):1061–82.
2. Hendricks A et al. A Comparison of International Management Guidelines for Hidradenitis Suppurativa. Dermatology 2019.
3. Ingram JR, Collier F, Brown D, Burton T, Burton J, Chin MF, Desai N, Goodacre TEE, Piguet V, Pink AE, Exton LS, Mohd Mustapa MF. British Association of Dermatologists guidelines for the management of hidradenitis suppurativa (acne inversa) 2018. Br J Dermatol. 2019 May; 180 (5): 1009–17.
4. Kimball AB,. Secukinumab in moderate-to-severe hidradenitis suppurativa (SUNSHINE and SUNRISE): week 16 and week 52 results of two identical, multicentre, randomised, placebo-controlled, double-blind phase 3 trials. Lancet. 2023 Mar 4;401(10378):747–761.
5. Von der Werth JM, Jemec GB. Morbidity in patients with hidradenitis suppurativa. Br J Dermatol. 2001;144(4):809–13.

Chapter 17

Infections

Kabir Sardana, Surabhi Sinha, Snigdha Saxena

BACTERIAL AND MYCOBACTERIAL INFECTIONS

ACTINOMYCOSIS

Agent: *Actinomyces israelii*

- Gram-positive, **non-acid-fast**, **anaerobic/microaerophilic** filamentous bacteria.
- When an adequate bacteriologic evaluation is performed, most, if not all, actinomycotic infections are **polymicrobial** in nature.
- The mixture of aerobic and anaerobic organisms involved in actinomycosis is not purely accidental but is synergistic. These companion bacteria strengthen the low invasive power of actinomycetes and cause treatment failures.
- *Aggregatibacter* (*previously Actinobacillus*) *actinomycetemcomitans* (a gram-negative bacillus) is the most common, followed by *Peptostreptococcus, Prevotella, Fusobacterium, Bacteroides, Staphylococcus*, *Streptococcus* and *Enterobacteriaceae*.

Three clinical presentations that should prompt consideration of this unique infection are:

1. The combination of **chronicity**, progression across tissue boundaries, and **mass**-like features, which mimic malignancy (with which it is often confused);
2. The development of a **sinus tract**, which may spontaneously resolve and recur; and
3. **A refractory or relapsing** infection after a short course of therapy, because cure of established actinomycosis requires prolonged treatment.

Pathogenesis

Actinomycetes are part of the normal flora of mouth, GI and GU tracts → infection usually arises after trauma (dental procedures or surgical interventions). A pivotal step in the pathogenesis of actinomycosis is disruption of the mucosal barrier.

- Oral and cervicofacial disease: Associated with dental procedures, trauma, oral surgery, head and neck radiotherapy, or oncologic surgical procedures.
- Pulmonary infections: Aspiration of oral secretions.

- Abdominal infection: Gastrointestinal surgery, diverticulitis, appendicitis, or foreign bodies (e.g. fish bones).
- Pelvic infection—after prolonged IUD use.

Clinical Features

Subacute or chronic granulomatous lesions with suppurating abscesses.

Types

1. **Cervicofacial** (most common, accounts for 70%): **"Lumpy jaw disease"**, red-brown nodules with fistulous abscesses draining characteristic yellow sulfur granules (= clumps of bacteria); associated with poor dental hygiene and dental procedures **(Fig. 17.1)**.
   - Most common location is **perimandibular** region. Periapical infection or trauma is often, but not always, the inciting event. The classic lesion is usually located at the angle of the jaw. The overlying skin often develops a bluish or purplish red hue. Involvement of the muscles of mastication frequently occurs, resulting in trismus.
   - Other causes are infected osteoradionecrosis, a site of complication of radiation therapy used in the treatment of head and neck cancer, and bisphosphonate-associated osteonecrosis.
2. **Pulmonary/thoracic:** As a result of aspiration, leading to pulmonary cavities at base of lungs.
   - Presents as mass lesion or pneumonia with or without pleural involvement. Pleural thickening, effusion, or empyema is present in more than 50% cases.
3. **GI:** As a result of trauma or inflammatory disease, presents with granulomatous lesions in bowel wall.
   - Appendicitis, especially with perforation, is the most common predisposing event and is associated with 65% of the cases of actinomycosis originating in the abdomen. As a result, the right iliac fossa is the most frequent primary site of abdominal disease and right-sided abdominal infection is more common than left.

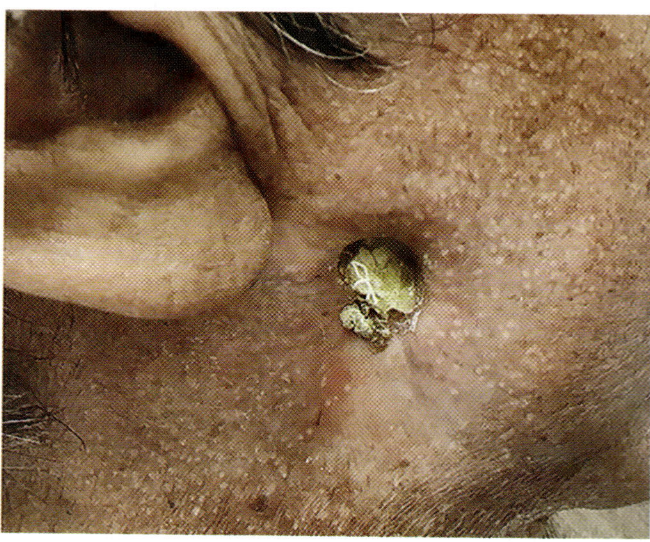

Fig. 17.1: Actinomycosis (cervicofacial)

4. **Pelvic disease**—the only type more common in females, associated with IUD use >8 years.
5. **Other sites:** Meningitis, endocarditis, mediastinal involvement, bone, skin, disseminated disease.

Primary cutaneous actinomycosis: Rare, chronic, usually follows trauma. Present with chronic nodules/masses/abscesses with fistulae or sinuses.

[**Note:** Actinomycotic mycetoma is caused by **aerobic** actinomycetes (*Nocardia*, *Streptomyces*, *Actinomadura*) (*see* under "*Mycetoma*")].

Diagnosis

- Clinical suspicion
- X-ray, CT, PET (to demonstrate hypermetabolism), MRI
- Fine-needle aspiration or biopsy and CT-or ultrasound guided aspirations or biopsies
- **Gram stain** of the tissue/crushed granule specimen (usually **more sensitive** than **culture**, especially if the patient has received prior antibiotics)
- **Culture:** 50% sensitivity only, less sensitive than Gram/HPE, anaerobic culture for >3 weeks, add metronidazole to suppress fast-growing anaerobes. "Molar tooth" appearance of colonies on blood/chocolate agar.
- **Histology**
  - Dense granulomatous and suppurative inflammation with "sulfur granules" with basophilic center (gram-positive branching filaments of *Actinomyces*) and eosinophilic rim (***Splendore–Hoeppli* phenomenon**) **(Fig. 17.2)**.

    This phenomenon is *not specific* for actinomycosis and can also be seen in *other* chronic infections, such as schistosomiasis, orbital pythiosis, cutaneous larva migrans, sporotrichosis, basidiobolomycosis, aspergillosis, blastomycosis, *Malassezia* folliculitis, mycetoma, botryomycosis, nocardiosis, and some noninfectious entities.
- **Sulfur granules**
  - Conglomeration of micro-organisms that forms only *in vivo*.
  - Visible with the unaided eye (up to 1–2 mm)—yellowish to brownish spherical particles made of filamentous actinomycete microcolonies, various concomitant bacteria and surrounding tissue reaction material, especially polymorphs and polysaccharides.

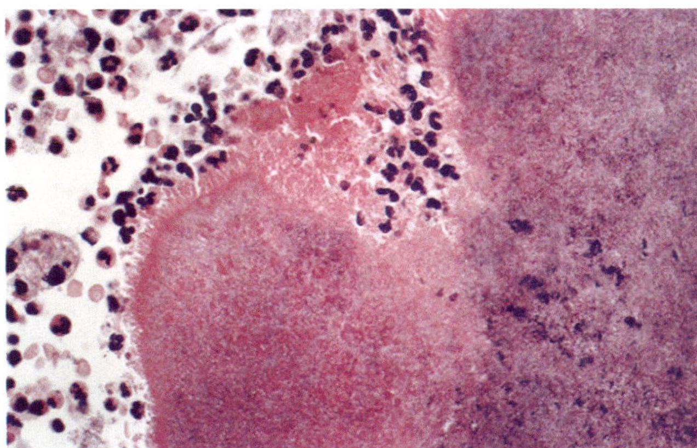

Fig. 17.2: A histology section in actinomycosis showing the "sulfur granule" and the tissue reaction that represents the Splendore–Hoeppli phenomenon

- Hematoxylin and eosin staining of tissue suffices to demonstrate the granules, but a special stain (e.g. gram, silver) is needed to show that the granule is composed of *branching* bacteria and not fungi (eumycetoma) or cocci/bacilli (botryomycosis).
- If branching bacteria are seen on staining of the granule and the infection did not originate in subcutaneous tissue (a characteristic of mycetoma) or tonsillar tissue, then the diagnosis of actinomycosis is established.

- **Differential diagnosis of grains**
  - *Nocardia*—on Gram's stain, the branching gram-positive bacilli are indistinguishable from *Actinomyces*, but they may be stained by a *modified Fite (acid-fast) stain*, whereas *Actinomyces* cannot. Ideal stain is methenamine silver **(Fig. 17.3a)**.
  - *Fungi* of mycetoma show *branching hyphae* on periodic acid-Schiff (PAS) or Gomori methenamine silver stain **(Fig. 17.3b)**.
  - Botryomycosis caused by *Staphylococcus, Streptococcus, Escherichia, Pseudomonas*, and *Proteus*, which are easily distinguished from the agents of actinomycosis by the presence of cocci or non-branching bacilli **(Fig. 17.3c)**.
  - *Actinomycosis*—sulfur granules of intertwined bacteria are seen as, radiating mycelial filaments, often with *opaque clubs at their tips* **(Fig. 17.3d)**.

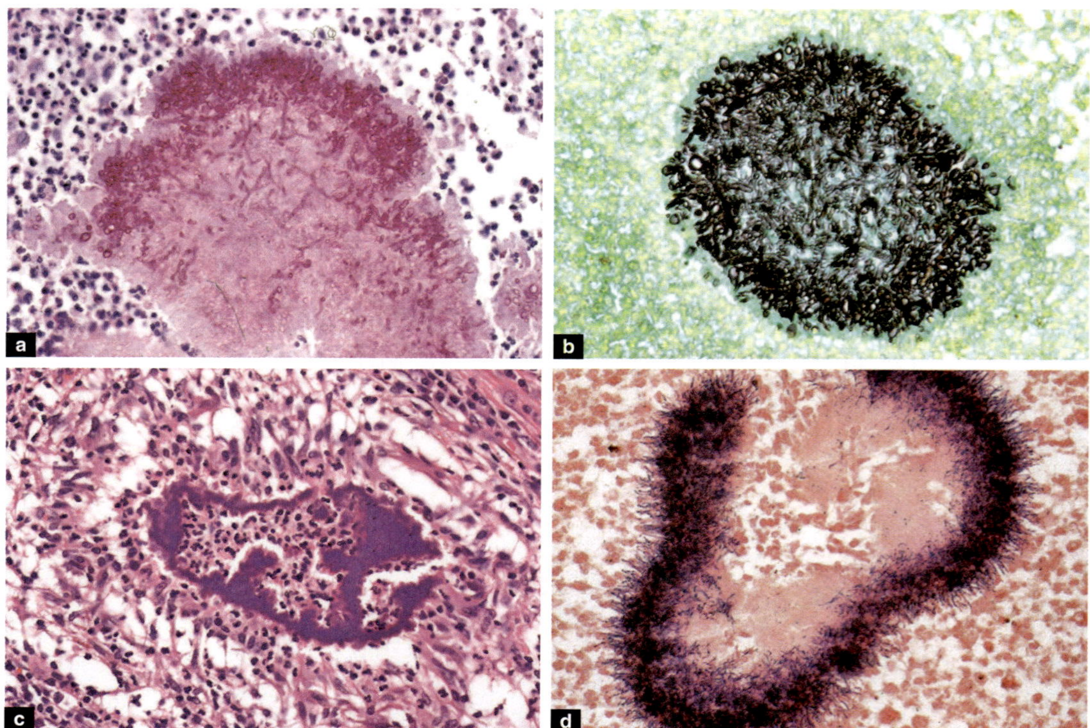

Fig. 17.3: Diseases with presence of grains: (a) *Nocardia*; (b) Eumycetoma; (c) Botryomycosis; (d) Actinomycosis: Gram-positive bacteria with club-shaped ends are present at the periphery of the granule

Treatment

- Principle—antibiotics at high doses and for a prolonged period of time.
- Drug of choice—**Penicillin-G** (18–24 million units of penicillin IV for 2–6 weeks, followed by oral therapy with penicillin or amoxicillin for 6–12 months).
- An overview of the therapeutic agents is listed in **Table 17.1**.
- Surgical debridement may be needed in some cases.

TABLE 17.1: Therapeutic agents used for actinomycosis

Group 1: Extensive successful clinical experience	
1. Penicillin (3–4 million units IV q4h) or amoxicillin (500 mg PO q6h)	
2. Erythromycin (500–1000 mg IV q6h or 500 mg PO q6h)	
3. Tetracycline (500 mg PO q6h)	
4. Doxycycline (100 mg IV q12h or 100 mg PO q12h)	
5. Minocycline (100 mg IV q12h or 100 mg PO q12h)	
6. Clindamycin (900 mg IV q8h or 300–450 mg PO q6h)	
Group 2: Anecdotal successful clinical experience	
1. Ceftriaxone‡	3. Imipenem-cilastatin
2. Ceftizoxime	4. Piperacillin-tazobactam
Group 3: Agents predicted to be efficacious based on *in vitro* activity	
1. Moxifloxacin	4. Quinupristin-dalfopristin
2. Vancomycin	5. Ertapenem‡
3. Linezolid	6. Azithromycin‡
Group 4: Agents that should be avoided	
1. Metronidazole	4. Dicloxacillin
2. Aminoglycosides	5. Cephalexin
3. Oxacillin	

‡parenteral therapy

NOCARDIOSIS

Agent: *Nocardia brasiliensis* (#1 cause of actinomycotic mycetoma), *N. asteroides* (#1 cause of pulmonary/systemic nocardiosis), other *Nocardia* spp.

- It is a gram-positive, weakly acid-fast (to 1% H_2SO_4), aerobic filamentous bacteria.
- Microscopically, *Nocardia* appear as gram-positive, beaded, weakly acid-fast, branching rods **(Fig. 17.4)**.
- Ubiquitous in soil (explains why foot is the most common site of actinomycotic mycetoma!)
- Mycetomas due to *Nocardia* spp, most often caused by *N. brasiliensis*, primarily affect immunocompetent hosts in tropical countries.
- They are differentiated from *Actinomycetes* by certain characteristics **(Box 17.1)**.

Fig. 17.4: Beaded gram-positive organisms of *Nocardia*

BOX 17.1: Differentiation between Actinomycetes and Nocardia

Anaerobic filamentous Actinomycetes can be distinguished from aerobic, filamentous bacteria such as *Nocardia* species in the following ways:

- Nocardiae are aerobes
- Nocardiae contain mycolic acids in their walls and are therefore partially acid-fast
- Nocardiae—aseptate hyphae branching at right angles (*Actinomyces*—aseptate broader hyphae branching at acute angles)
- Nocardiae—smaller grains of 1 mm (*Actinomyces*-1–2 mm hard yellow sulfur granules)
- Nocardiae are resistant to penicillin (drug of choice for *Actinomyces*)

Clinical Features

The classic sporotrichoid pattern is shown in **Fig. 17.5** and the four major forms of disease are depicted in **Table 17.2**.

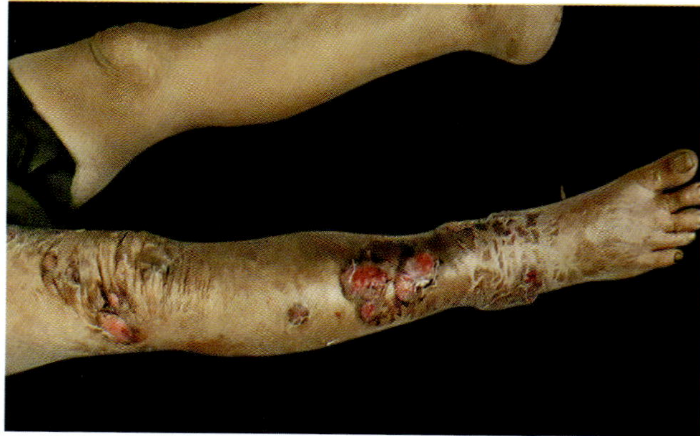

Fig. 17.5: Unilateral sporotrichoid lymphocutaneous nocardiosis in a patient with panhypopituitarism who was on oral steroids

TABLE 17.2: Cutaneous diseases caused by *Nocardia*	
Primary	
Actinomycotic mycetoma	Half of all cases of actinomycotic mycetoma are due to *Nocardia** **Traumatic inoculation** causes a painless nodule that enlarges, suppurates, and drains via the sinus tracts Purulent discharge contains sulfur granules The foot is the usual site of involvement May involve underlying muscle and bone
Lymphocutaneous	Occurs days to weeks after trauma Appears as a crusted pustule or abscess resistant to antibiotics Ascending lymphatic streaks, a **sporotrichoid** pattern of papulonodules, and tender palpable lymph nodes may be seen **(Fig. 17.5)**
Superficial cutaneous	Traumatic implantation of foreign objects (including soil and gravel) into the skin The diagnosis is based on a high index of suspicion, lack of response to routine antibiotic treatment, and laboratory results
Secondary	
Pulmonary/systemic	Subcutaneous abscesses of the **chest wall** Pustules, nodules, and cutaneous fistulae Almost universally fatal, if left untreated Most commonly caused by *Nocardia asteroides*

*In Mexico and Central and South America, *N. brasiliensis* is the etiology of 90% of actinomycotic mycetomas, whereas in the United States, most mycetomas are caused by true fungi (eumycotic).

Investigations

- Cerebral imaging, if indicated
- The microbiology laboratory should be informed of suspected nocardiosis because it may not be detected by routine laboratory methods. Respiratory secretions, skin biopsies, or aspirates from deep collections are the most useful diagnostic specimens and are typically positive on Gram's stain.
- Smear: Branching, beaded, filamentous bacteria, similar to those seen in smears taken from cultures, may be demonstrated within the abscesses on Gram's staining. "Sulfur granules" (bacterial macrocolonies) similar to those seen in actinomycosis may be found in nocardial mycetomas but *Nocardia* species usually stain acid fast in tissue sections if a method such as that of Fite-Faraco is used, whereas *Actinomyces* species do not.
- Species identification may be predictive of antimicrobial susceptibility.

Histology

Intense neutrophilic infiltrate + sulfur granules (only seen in actinomycotic mycetoma form); branching filaments are Gram positive, AFB+ (Fite > Ziehl–Neelsen), and GMS+.

Treatment

Sulfonamides (cotrimoxazole: Treatment of choice) +/– other antibiotics +/– surgical drainage.

- High risk patients: Amikacin + Panem + TMP/SMX
- Renal impaired patients: TMP/SMX, linezolid, carbapenem, ceftriaxone (avoid amikacin) (ideal drug based on antimicrobial spectrum)

CORYNEBACTERIAL CUTANEOUS INFECTIONS

ERYTHRASMA

Cause

C. minutissimum.

Epidemiology

- More in diabetics
- Although clinically most common on groin and axillae, Wood's lamp evidence suggests maximum in toe clefts.

Predisposing Factors

- Warm humid climate
- Diabetes mellitus

Clinical Features (Fig. 17.6)

- Sites—groin, axillae, submammary, intergluteal
- Sharply marginated irregular red smooth patches → brown scaly later

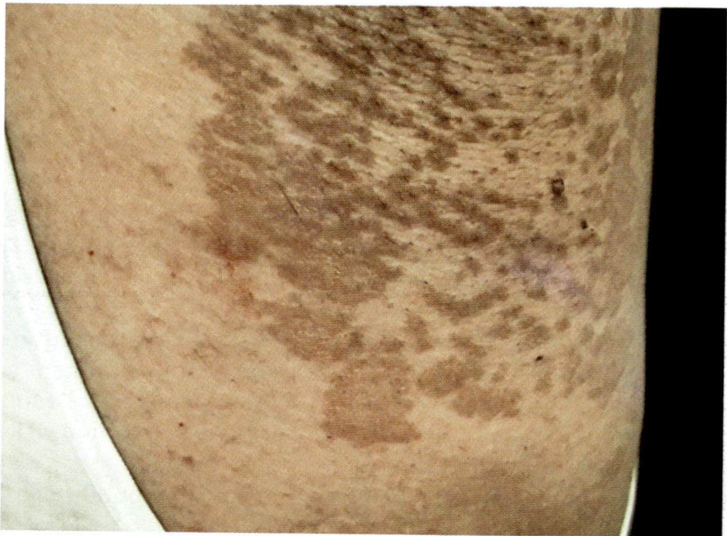

Fig. 17.6: Erythematous 'relatively' non-itchy lesion of erythrasma

Diagnosis

- **Bedside tests**
  - Wood's lamp—*coral-red/pink fluorescence* (coproporphyrin III by coryneforms).

Differential Diagnosis (Box 17.2)

- Pityriasis versicolor—occurs on upper trunk, smaller lesions, not erythematous.
- Tinea cruris—inflammations +, active raised border, satellite lesions absent.

BOX 17.2: Differential diagnoses of erythrasma

- Pityriasis versicolor
- Candidiasis
- Tinea cruris
- Acanthosis nigricans

- Candidiasis—satellite lesions, pustules.
- Acanthosis nigricans (may also fluorescence due to coryneform growth)—velvety, rugose skin.

Treatment (Fig. 17.7)

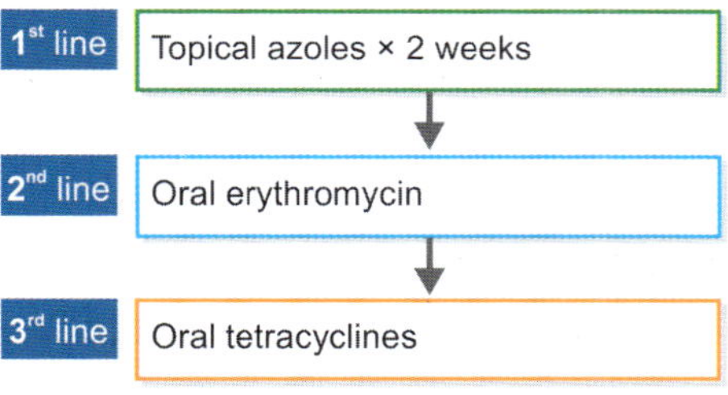

Fig. 17.7: Treatment of erythrasma

TRICHOMYCOSIS AXILLARIS/TRICHOMYCOSIS NODOSA

Cause

- *C. tenuis*, many other aerobic corynebacteria too
- Chemical environment changes responsible for different colors (not due to different strains)

Clinical Features (Fig. 17.8)

- Yellow/black/red adherent concretions on axillary and pubic hair shafts
- Axillary sweat—may be yellow/black/red
- Yellow—most common

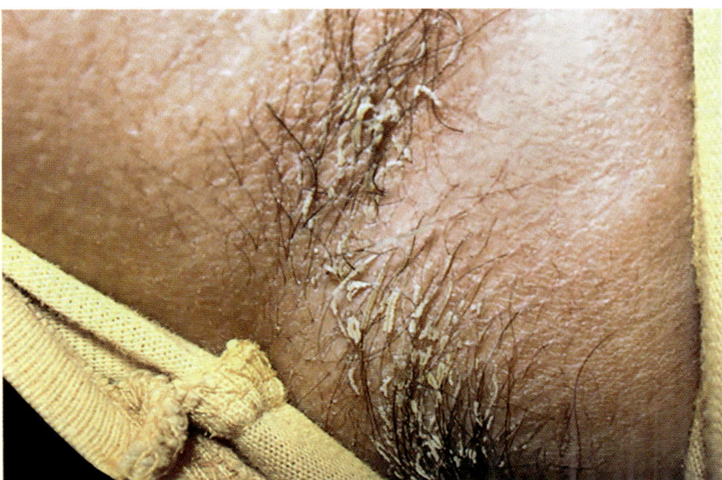

Fig. 17.8: Yellowish concretions on the axillary hair in a case of trichomycosis axillaris

Diagnosis

- **Bedside tests**
  - KOH mount
  - Gram stain
  - Culture—in blood agar

Differential Diagnosis

- Pediculosis pubis—matting of pubic hair, no concretions, lice can be visualized by dermoscopy.
- Piedra—scalp and beard more common, KOH mount shows hyphae.

Treatment (Fig 17.9)

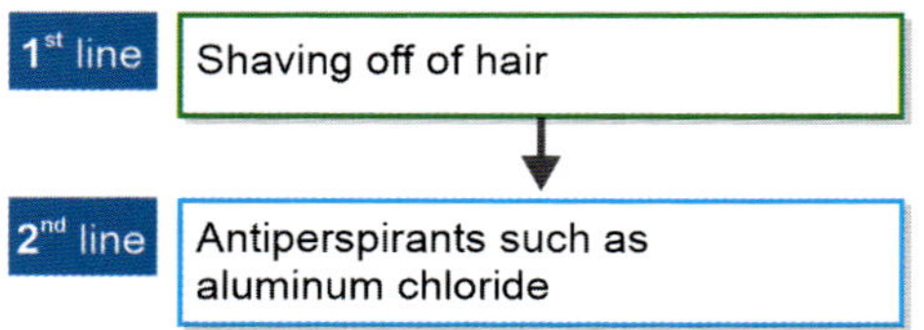

Fig. 17.9: Treatment of trichomycosis axillaris

PITTED KERATOLYSIS

Cause

Corynebacterium spp, *Actinomyces keratolytica*, *Dermatophilus congolensis*, *Kytococcus sedentarius*, etc.

Predisposing Factors

- Warm humid climate
- Hyperhidrosis

Clinical Features

- Sites on soles—pressure-bearing/friction areas **(Fig. 17.10)**
- Conspicuous, discrete, shallow, circular, punched out superficial erosions, coalescing at places to form irregular erosions.

Diagnosis

- **Bedside tests**
  - Gram stained smears
  - Culture on brain heart infusion agar

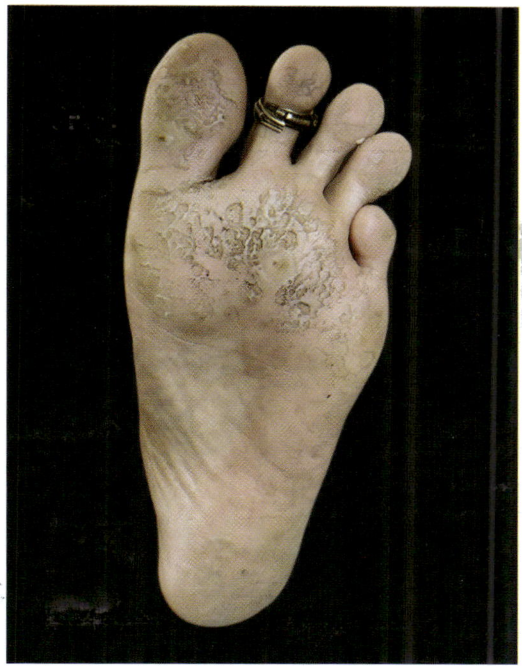

Fig. 17.10: Multiple pits associated with a foul odor and hyperhidrosis in pitted keratolysis

Treatment (Fig 17.11)

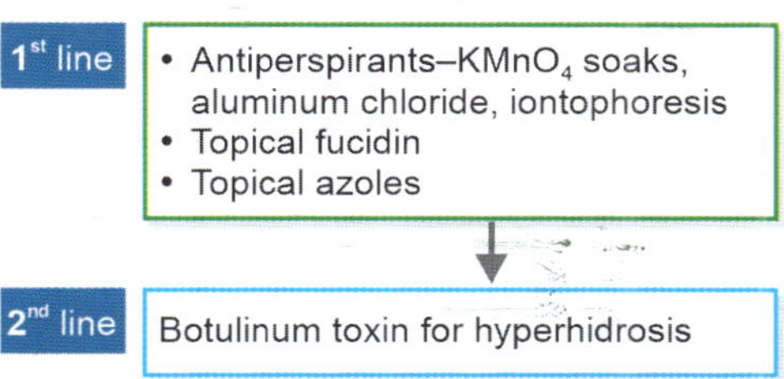

Fig. 17.11: Treatment of pitted keratolysis

CUTANEOUS TB

The genus *Mycobacterium* contains more than 140 species, of which around 25 are pathogenic in humans. **Table 17.3** lists the species causing human disease, the most important of which are *M. tuberculosis* and *M. leprae*. **Table 17.4** gives the classification of cutaneous TB.

TABLE 17.3: Classification of mycobacterial species causing human disease

I. *Mycobacterium tuberculosis* complex

M. tuberculosis
M. bovis
M. africanum
M. microti
M. canetti

II. Slowly growing nontuberculous mycobacteria

Photochromogens (pigment production only in light)
M. kansasii
M. marinum
M. simiae
M. asiaticum

Scotochromogens (pigment production in dark or light)
M. gordonae
M. scrofulaceum
M. szulgai

Nonchromogens (no pigment production)
M. avium complex
- *M. avium*
- *M. intracellulare*
- *M. chimaera*

M. terrae complex
M. ulcerans
M. xenopi
M. malmoense
M. haemophilum

III. Rapidly growing nontuberculous mycobacteria (no pigment though may be late-pigmenting, colonies in 5 days)

M. fortuitum complex
- *M. fortuitum*
- *M. peregrinum*
- *M. porcinum*

M. chelonae
M. abscessus
- *M. abscessus* subspecies *abscessus*
- *M. abscessus* subspecies *bolletii*
- *M. abscessus* subspecies *massiliense*

M. smegmatis
M. mucogenicum

IV. Non-culturable

M. leprae
M. lepromatis

TABLE 17.4: Classification of cutaneous tuberculosis

Host immunity	Method of inoculation	Disease
Multibacillary forms		
• Naive host	Direct inoculation	Tuberculous chancre
• Low	Contiguous spread	Scrofuloderma
• Low	Autoinoculation	Orificial tuberculosis
• Low	Hematogenous spread	Acute miliary/cutaneous
• Low	Hematogenous spread	Tuberculous gumma
Paucibacillary forms		
• High	Direct inoculation	Tuberculosis verrucosa cutis/warty tuberculosis
• High	Hematogenous spread (majority)/ direct inoculation (few)	Lupus vulgaris
• High	?Hematogenous spread	Tuberculids

A 2nd classification has been followed which divides them into two types:

- **Exogenous** (TB Chancre, TBVC)
- **Endogenous** (Scrofuloderma, Lupus Vulgaris, Orificial TB, Miliary TB, TB Gumma and Tuberculide).

A large Indian study has shown that the most common type remains lupus vulgaris followed by scrofuloderma and lichen scrofulosorum. Almost 41% had systemic involvement in lymph nodes (50%), lungs (35%), bone (10%), and abdomen (6%) (Singal A, 2022).

Investigations

While ideally isolation of AFB is suggested this is rarely possible in cutaneous TB. Other tests that are useful are the tuberculin skin test (TST/PPD) or IFN-γ release assays (e.g. QuantiFERON-TB Gold [In-Tube]) or PCR of the tissue biopsy. The advantage of the interferon relese is that it is not influenced by BCG vaccination. The most commonly used test remains histopathology.

Histopathology

The reaction to the bacterium depends on:

- The <u>size</u> of the inoculum
- The <u>immune state</u> of the patient
- The <u>virulence</u> of the organism

In general, the cellular response is characterized by epithelioid macrophages, Langhans' giant cells, and caseous necrosis, with perivascular lymphocytes in the surrounding tissue (tuberculous granuloma).

The presence of large numbers of bacilli in a lesion implies a non-immune or anergic state, such as in tuberculous chancre or orificial lesions.

Caseation is an indication of hypersensitivity and is not a toxic effect of the organisms; it is clear that it is not always beneficial to the host because it is invariably associated with destruction of surrounding tissue.

Three types of HPE pictures are described in cutaneous TB:

1. Well formed granulomas without caseous necrosis
   - Lupus vulgaris
   - Lichen scrofulosorum
2. Granulomas with caseous necrosis
   - TBVC
   - Acute miliary TB
   - Papulonecrotic tuberculid
   - Primary tubercular chancre
   - TB cutis orificialis
3. Poorly formed granulomas with intense caseous necrosis
   - Scrofuloderma
   - TB gumma/metastatic abscess

Differential Diagnosis (Table 17.5)

1. **Sarcoidosis:** Sarcoid can be distinguished by the lack of caseation, but often this is not particularly helpful since necrosis is seen in only a minority of cases of tuberculosis. Necrosis when present in sarcoidosis is rather more *fibrinoid* than caseating. More helpful is the lack of a surrounding lymphocytic infiltrate and fewer giant cells in sarcoidosis and a more discrete arrangement of the granulomata (the sarcoidal naked granuloma).

TABLE 17.5: Differential diagnosis of cutaneous TB

1. Sarcoidosis	5. Late secondary and tertiary syphilis
2. Leprosy	6. Acne agminata
3. Deep fungal infections	7. Foreign body reactions
4. Leishmaniasis	

2. In less granulomatous forms of cutaneous tuberculosis, a distinction from **leprosy** must be made. The *perineural* distribution of the inflammation is a pointer towards leprosy.
3. **Deep fungal infections** and **leishmaniasis** may also be confused with tuberculosis and recognition of the organism is vital.
4. Granulomatous late secondary and tertiary syphilis is distinguished by the vascular changes and numerous *plasma cells.*
5. Caseation necrosis is typical of acne **agminata** and may also be seen in **foreign body reactions** to beryllium and zirconium. It may also be a feature of Wegener's granulomatosis, although this would be distinctly unusual in cutaneous lesions.

TUBERCULOUS CHANCRE

Epidemiology

Age: Children (usually unvaccinated and exposed to infected caregiver), healthcare/laboratory workers.

Sex: No predominance.

Predisposing Factors

Low socioeconomic status, overcrowding.

Course of Infection and Clinical Course (Flowchart 17.1)

Flowchart 17.1: Pathogenesis of TB chancre

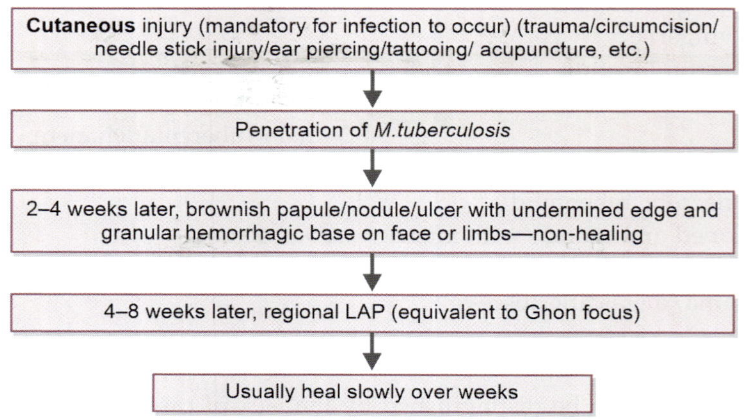

Clinical Variants

- Mucosal
- Paronychia-like changes on fingernails.

HPE

A neutrophilic abscess with numerous bacilli, associated with necrosis leading to ulceration. This is gradually surrounded by histiocytes; after 6 weeks, giant cells (derived by fusion of epithelioid cells) are seen. Central necrosis remains prominent, but diminishes, along with the number of bacilli, as the granulomatous element increases.

Differential Diagnosis (Box 17.3)

BOX 17.3: Differential diagnosis of tuberculous chancre

- Non-tuberculous mycobacterial ulcers (*M. ulcerans, M. marinum*)
- Actinomycosis
- Cutaneous leishmaniasis
- Sporotrichoid pattern—sporotrichosis, cat scratch disease, tularemia
- Cutaneous malignancy

Associated diseases: Other forms of cutaneous TB may develop at the site:

- Lupus vulgaris
- TBVC
- Scrofuloderma
- Rarely, systemic TB

Complications

Disseminated tuberculosis (rare).

Diagnosis

Mainly clinical.

- **Tuberculin skin test:** Initially negative, later becomes positive (once immunity develops).
- **HPE:**
  - Early—acute neutrophilic inflammation with necrosis with numerous acid-fast bacilli (AFB).
  - After 3–6 weeks—organized granulomas with caseation with disappearance of bacilli.
- **Rapid test:** Xpert® MTB/RIF-simultaneously test for pulmonary tuberculosis and rifampicin resistance (as an indicator of MDR TB), endorsed by WHO in 2010.

LUPUS VULGARIS

Epidemiology

- Hematogenous spread from tubercular focus (on face)/direct inoculation or after BCG vaccination (on extremities) in previously sensitized individual.
- **Most common form** of cutaneous TB in adults.
- Sex: Females > males.

Course of Infection and Clinical Course (Flowchart 17.2)

Most common sites in India-buttocks, trunk.
"Apple jelly"—applies to the feel on probing as the color is actually greyish.

Clinical Variants

1. **Plaque**—hyperkeratotic irregular or serpiginous edge, one edge may heal with scarring while other may continue to extend **(Fig. 17.12)**.

Flowchart 17.2: Clinical evolution of lupus vulgaris

Small reddish-brown soft flat plaque (apple jelly nodules)
↓
Grows to become elevated and infiltrated, extends peripherally
↓
One edge may heal with atrophic scarring while other may continue to extend

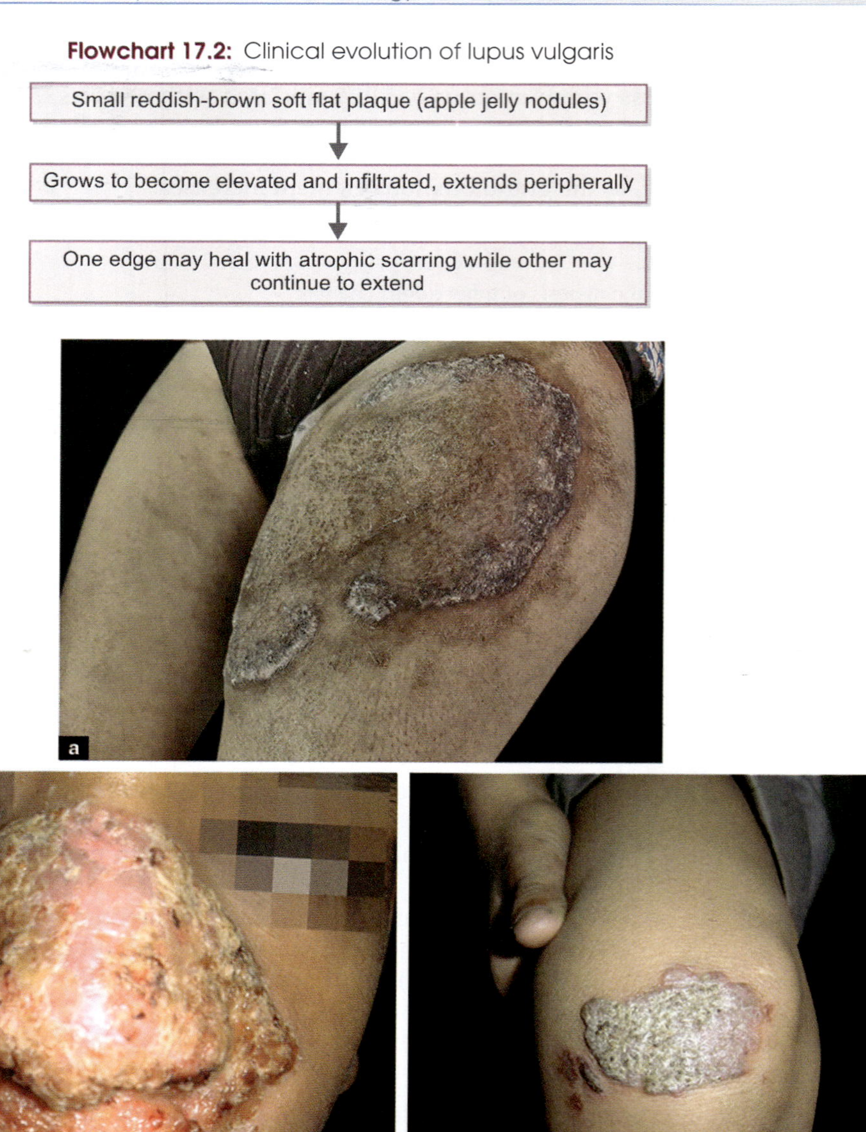

Fig. 17.12: (a and b) Plaque form of lupus vulgaris; (c) Large plaque of lupus vulgaris with hypertrophy and areas of ulceration on the nose in a child

2. **Ulcerative and mutilating**—ulceration and scarring predominate. Involve deep tissue and cartilage and cause mutilation **(Fig. 17.13)**.

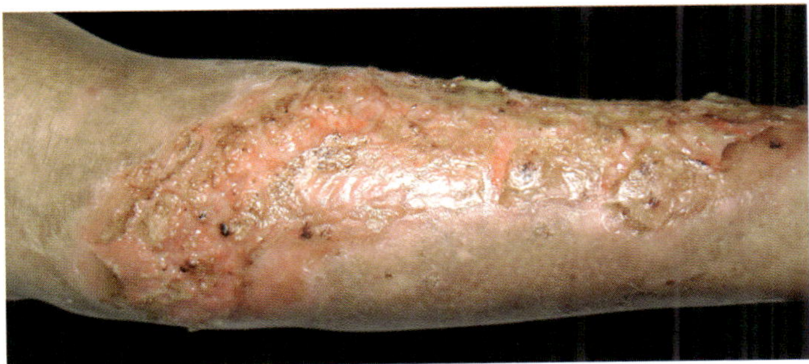

Fig. 17.13: Ulcerative variant of lupus vulgaris

3. **Vegetating**—marked infiltration, ulceration and necrosis with very little scarring. Mucosae and cartilage destroyed gradually causing extensive disfigurement.
4. **Tumor-like**—hypertrophic soft tumor-like nodules.
5. **Papular and nodular**—disseminated lupus-true "miliary lupus". In immunosuppressed individuals or in children after an episode of measles.

Rare Variants

1. Lupus vulgaris postexanthematicus (a form of papular nodular LV)
   - After a transient impairment of immunity, especially measles
   - Multiple disseminated lesions simultaneously due to hematogeneous spread from a latent focus
   - TST may be –ve but later +ve after general condition improves
   - Clinical and HPE—typical LV (versus acute miliary TB)
2. Annular LV
3. Giant LV

HPE (Fig. 17.14)

- Varied
- Granuloma in the ***superficial dermis***, consisting of tubercles, some of which coalesce, with *scanty or absent* central caseation surrounded by epithelioid histiocytes and multinucleate giant cells.
- *Peripheral lymphocytes* are also usually prominent.
- Epidermis may be ulcerated (in which case there is usually a more mixed inflammatory infiltrate), atrophic or acanthotic.

Differential Diagnosis (Box 17.4)

BOX 17.4: Differential diagnosis of lupus vulgaris

- Leprosy
- Sarcoidosis
- DLE
- Deep mycosis
- Lupoid leishmaniasis
- Non-tuberculous mycobacterial lymphadenitis and skin infection (*M. avium complex, M. scrofulaceum*)

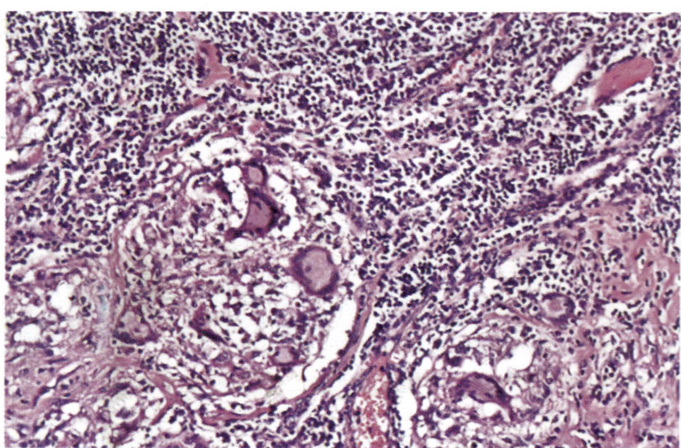

Fig. 17 .14: Lupus vulgaris: Tuberculoid granulomas that are often concentrated in the upper dermis, particularly around follicular units, although they can also extend into the subcutis. The granuloma contains epithelioid macrophages, including multinucleated giant cells (some of the Langhans' type), surrounded by lymphocytes and plasma cells, caseation is frequently absent or slight, zones of fibrosis can be seen in long-standing lesions

Complications

- Scarring
- Contractures
- Tissue destruction and mutilation
- Relapse of lupus vulgaris in scar
- Malignancy—SCC in 0.5–20% after 25–30 years.

Diagnosis

See **Box 17.5** for important tests done in a case of lupus vulgaris.

BOX 17.5: Diagnosis of lupus vulgaris

Mainly clinical
- **Tuberculin skin test:** Positive
- **HPE:**
  - Epidermis—atrophic/acanthotic
  - Superficial tuberculoid granulomas with absent/scanty caseation and surrounded by epithelioid histiocytes and MNGCs and lymphocytic cuff
  - AFB +/–

SCROFULODERMA

Epidemiology

- Worldwide, it is the commonest form of cutaneous TB.
- **Age:** Children (commonest form of cutaneous TB in children and adolescents)
- **Sex:** Males > females

Predisposing Factors

Low socioeconomic status, overcrowding, HIV infection.

Course of Infection and Clinical Course (Flowchart 17.3)

- Most common sources—cervical, epitrochlear, retroauricular, tubercular lymphadenitis.
- Most common sites—face and neck (worldwide), buttocks (India).

Flowchart 17.3: Clinical evolution of scrofuloderma

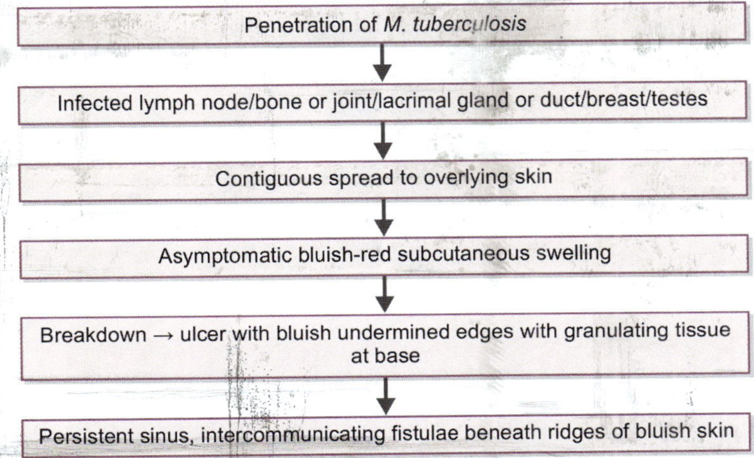

Clinical Variants (Fig. 17.15)

There is a nodular swelling or ulceration resulting from direct extension of underlying bone or lymph node TB **(Fig. 17.16)**.

HPE

- Ulcerated dermal abscess with an ill-defined histiocytic component **(Fig. 17.17)**.
- Peripheral granuloma with marked caseation necrosis, in which bacilli may be numerous, can be seen in the deeper tissues.

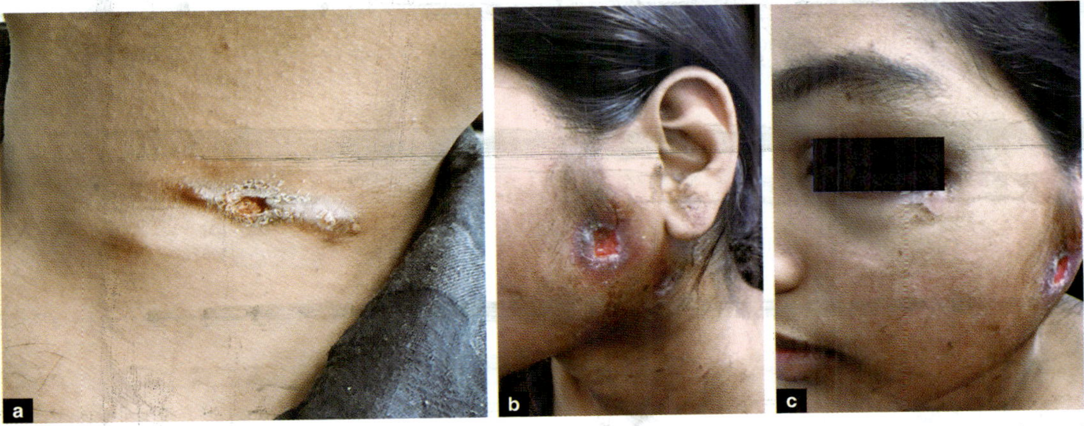

Fig. 17.15: Various presentations of scrofuloderma affecting the cervical lymph nodes, neck and face

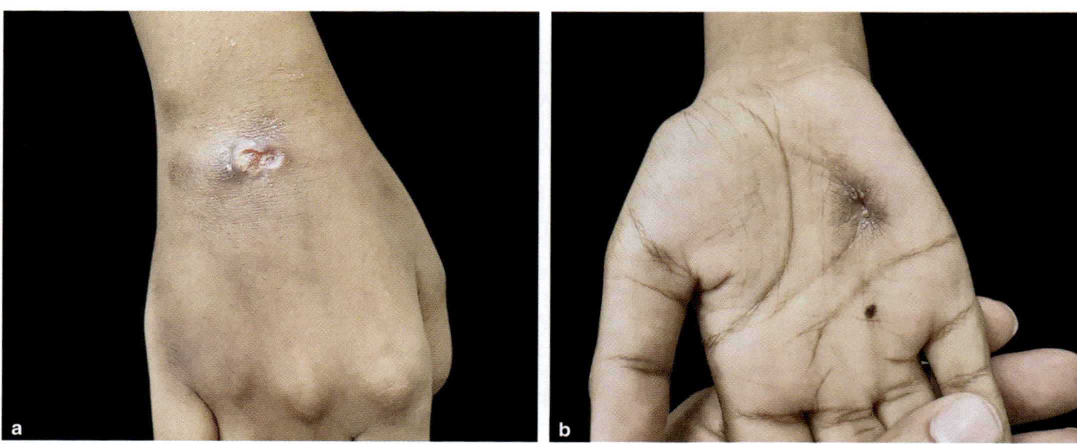

Fig. 17.16: Scrofuloderma involving dorsum of hand and palm

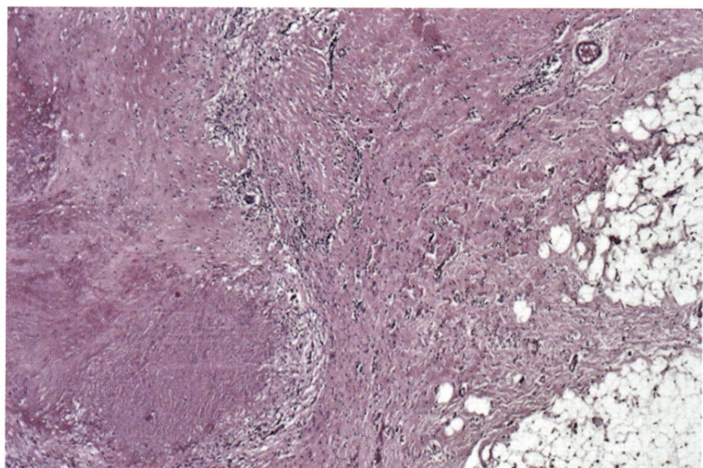

Fig. 17.17: Scrofuloderma features a zone of caseous necrosis, surrounded by epithelioid macrophages, multinucleated giant cells of Langhans' type, and plasma cells which may not be consistently seen

Differential Diagnosis (Box 17.6)

BOX 17.6: Differential diagnosis of scrofuloderma

- Nontuberculous mycobacterial lymphadenitis and skin infection (*M. avium complex, M. scrofulaceum*)
- Actinomycosis
- Bacterial abscess
- Sporotrichoid pattern—sporotrichosis
- Hidradenitis suppurativa

Complications

Persistent discharging sinus.

Diagnosis (Box 17.7)

BOX 17.7: Diagnosis of scrofuloderma

- Mainly clinical
  - **Tuberculin skin test:** Positive
  - **FNAC:** AFB ++ (may be 1st line of investigation)
  - **HPE** (taken from edge of ulcer or sinus)
- Ulcerated epidermis and dermis
- Dermal abscess—with marked caseation necrosis, ill-defined histiocytic component
- AFB ++

WARTY TUBERCULOSIS (TUBERCULOSIS VERRUCOSA CUTIS: TBVC)

Epidemiology

- Previously sensitized healthcare/laboratory workers (anatomist's warts/verruca necrogenica).
- Through autoinoculation with sputum in patient with active tuberculosis.

Course of Infection and Clinical Course (Flowchart 17.14)

Sites—knees, ankles, buttocks, fingers (exposed to trauma and sputum).

Flowchart 17.4: Clinical evolution of TBVC

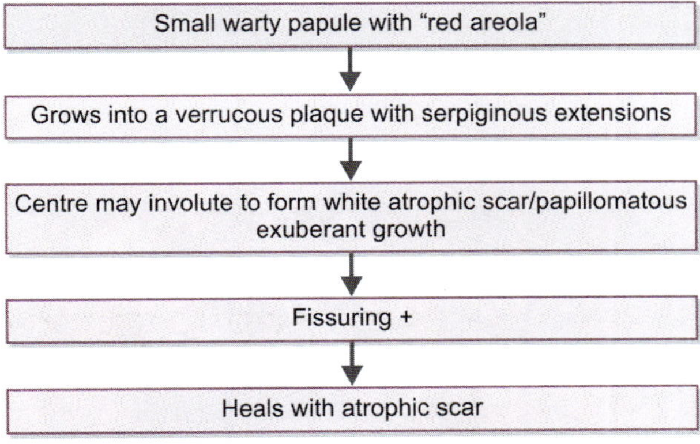

Clinical Variants (Fig. 17.18)

- Destructive papillomatous
- Sclerotic
- Tumor-like

HPE (Fig. 17.19)

- Acanthotic papillomatosis with marked hyperkeratosis.
- Dermal infiltrate consists mainly of neutrophils and lymphocytes, and abscesses may sometimes be present.
- Granulomas are present in the deeper dermis and caseation is occasionally a feature.

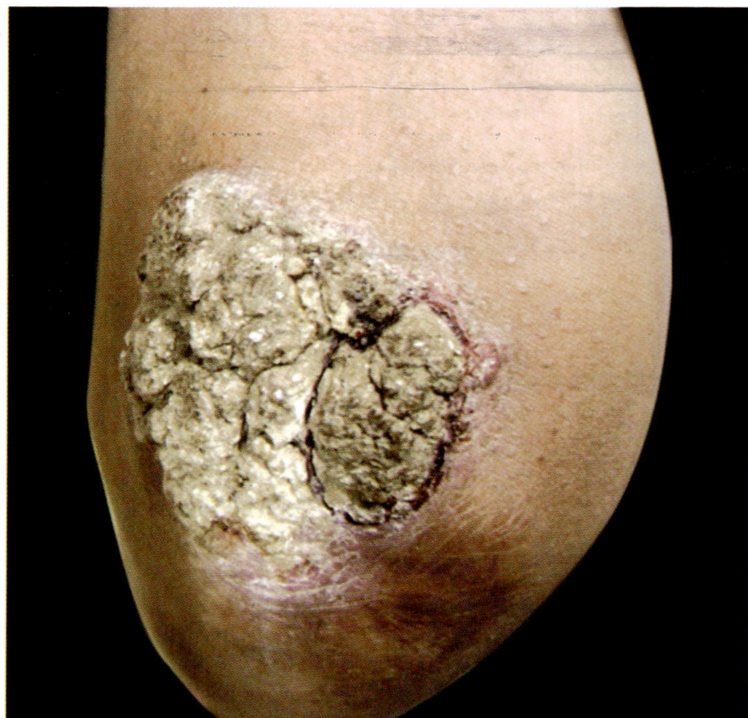

Fig. 17.18: Chronic verrucous growth with fissuring in a case of TBVC

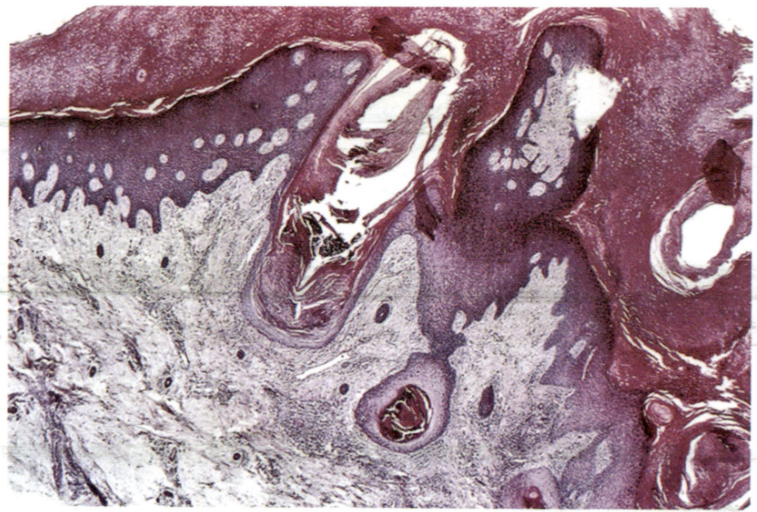

Fig. 17.19: Tuberculosis verrucosa cutis: Hyperkeratosis, papillomatosis, and acanthosis. The inflammatory infiltrate varies from a mixture of neutrophils (which form usually intraepidermal or dermal abscess), lymphocytes, and granulomatous elements. Sometimes there is a tuberculoid granulomatous infiltrate, uncommonly with caseous necrosis

Differential Diagnosis (Box 17.8)

BOX 17.8: Differential diagnosis of TBVC

- Warts (fingers, sole)
- Keratoses
- Chromoblastomycosis, blastomycosis
- Actinomycosis
- Non-tuberculous mycobacterial ulcers (*M. ulcerans*, *M. marinum*)
- Cutaneous leishmaniasis
- Hypertrophic lichen planus, lichen simplex chronicus
- Lupus vulgaris

Associated Diseases

Look for active TB elsewhere.

Diagnosis (Box 17.9)

BOX 17.9: Diagnosis of TBVC

- Mainly clinical
  - **Tuberculin skin test:** Positive
  - **HPE:**
    - Marked pseudoepitheliomatous hyperplasia
    - Superficial abscess—mixed infiltrate
    - AFB—+/–

TUBERCULIDS

The etiopathogenesis is depicted in **Flowchart 17.5**.

Flowchart 17.5: Pathogenesis of tuberculids

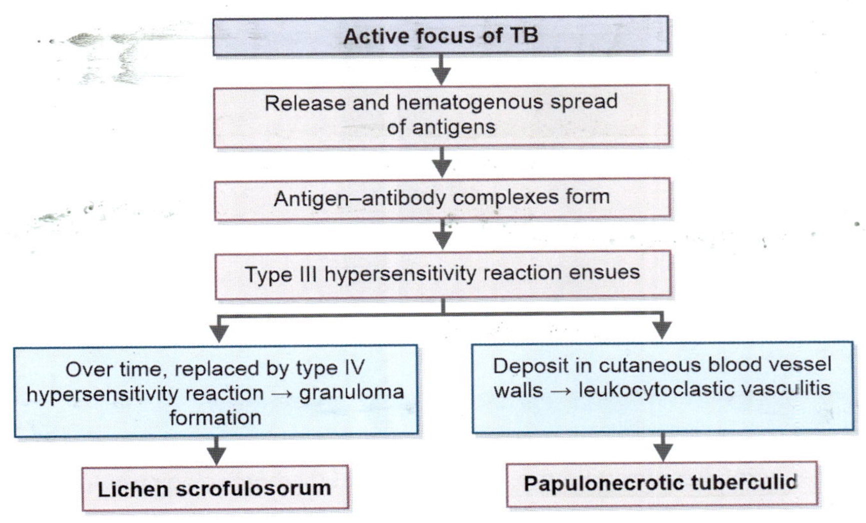

Diagnostic Criteria

1. Tuberculoid histopathology
2. Strongly positive Mantoux reaction
3. Smear negative for AFB
4. Culture negative for *M. tuberculosis*
5. Resolution of lesions with ATT.

Lichen Scrofulosorum

Epidemiology

- Mostly in children and adolescents
- Second most common cutaneous TB in children in India.

Predisposing Factors

- Overcrowding, poor SE condition.
- Patients typically show a strong positive reaction to PPD, often measuring 18 mm or larger, and the site may ulcerate. Prior vaccination with BCG does not prevent this condition from developing.
- 73% of patients have an associated focus of tuberculosis elsewhere (cervical, hilar and mediastinal lymph nodes—65%). Other foci include the lung, bone or intracranial sites.

Clinical Features

- Sites—chest, abdomen, back, proximal limbs, +/– face (centripetal distribution).
- Skin-colored/reddish-brown papules topped with crust/tiny pustule/perifollicular papules which can occasionally arrange in a annular configuration **(Figs 17.20** and **21)**.
- Clears without scarring within 4 weeks of ATT.

Clinical Types/Variants

- Lichenoid
- Psoriasiform/PR-like
- Granuloma annulare-like

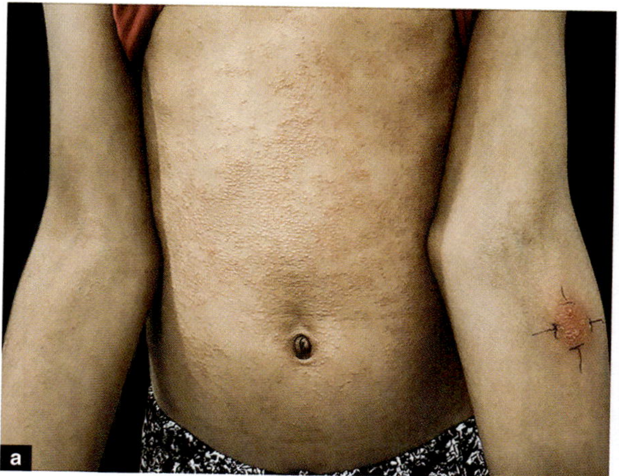

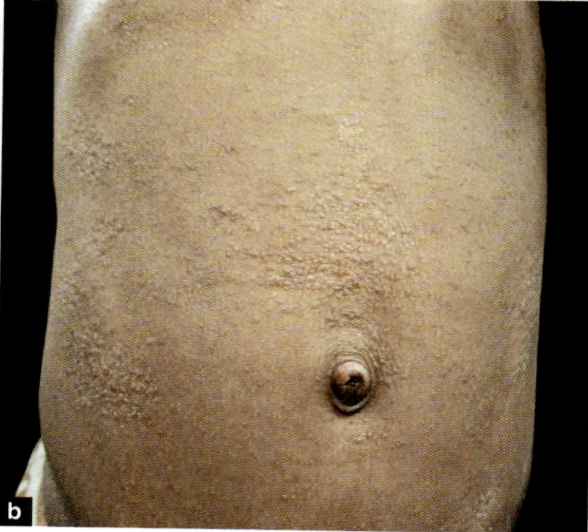

Fig. 17.20: Lichen scrofulosorum, note the prominent follicular morphology with a strongly positive Mantoux test

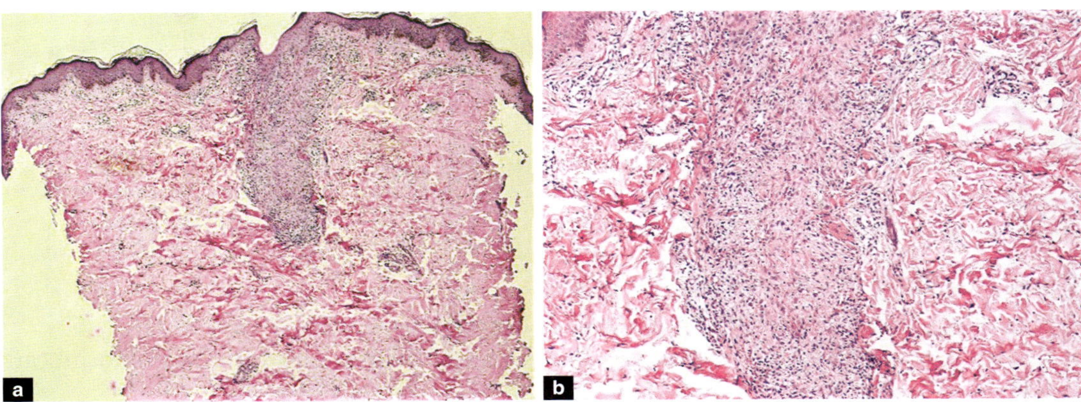

Fig. 17.21: Perifollicular non-caseating granuloma composed of epithelioid cells, lymphocytes and multinucleated giant cells (4X,10X) (*Courtesy*: Dr Geeti Khullar)

Differential Diagnosis

The important differential diagnoses are given in **Box 17.10** (for details *see* also Chapter 12: Follicular Disorders).

BOX 17.10: Differential diagnosis of lichen scrofulosorum

- Lichen nitidus
- Keratosis pilaris
- Secondary syphilis
- Drug eruptions
- Lichen spinulosus
- Papular/lichenoid sarcoidosis
- Pityriasis rosea

HPE (Fig. 17.21)

In lichen scrofulosorum, a granulomatous infiltrate in which Langhans' giant cells are conspicuous is centered around hair follicles and eccrine units.

Diagnosis

- **Mantoux reaction:** Strongly positive
- **HPE:**
  - Noncaseating epithelioid cell superficial dermal granulomas surrounding follicles and sweat glands
  - AFB-ve
  - Culture negative
- **PCR skin biopsy:** May be positive.

Treatment

First line	Second line	Third line
ATT	—	—

Papulonecrotic Tuberculid

Epidemiology

Young adults and sometimes children.

Predisposing Factors

Overcrowding, poor SEC.
38–75% of patients have a associated foci of TB.

Clinical Features of Classic Lesion

- Sites—legs, arms, elbows, knees, hands, feet (may favor perniotic areas)
- Recurrent crops of symmetrical red papules → crust/ulcerate → heal with varioliform scars **(Fig. 17.22)**.

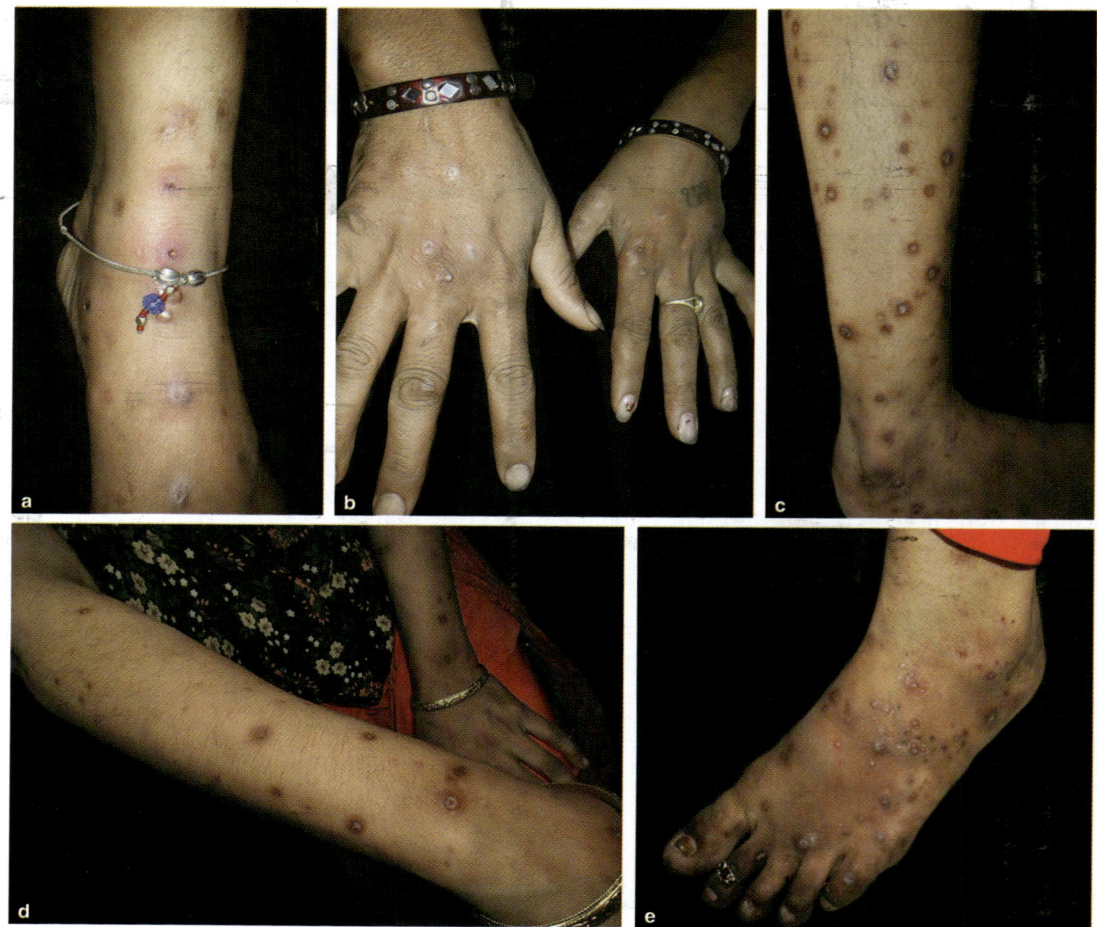

Fig. 17.22: Bilateral symmetrical, papules and nodules with central crusting in a case with papulonecrotic tuberculid. The papules may become pustular, ulcerate or develop crusts and often heal with depressed, varioliform scars

Clinical Types/Variants

- Isolated genital lesions
- Verrucous

Differential Diagnosis (Table 17.6)

TABLE 17.6: Differential diagnosis of hyperkeratotic and/or ulcerated papules on extremities

	Papulo-necrotic tuberculid	PLEVA	Papular urticaria	Cutaneous small vessel vasculitis (CSVV)	Prurigo nodularis	Acquired perforating dermatosis	Perforating granuloma annulare
Sites	Legs, arms, elbows, knees, hands, feet, perniotic areas	Trunk, flexors of proximal limbs	Exposed parts of limbs, especially lower legs	Stasis prone areas especially ankles and lower legs, sparing toe web spaces	Extensors of limbs, neck, shoulders, back, buttocks	Extensors of limbs, trunk	Acral areas mainly
Classical lesion	Recurrent crops, B/L red ulcerated/ crusted papules, atrophic varioliform scars	Crops of edematous pink papules → vesicles → hemorr-hagic necrosis → varioliform scars	Clusters of very itchy urticarial wheals with central hemorrhagic puncta → firm pruritic papules with tiny vesicles on top	Simultaneous crop of palpable purpura papules → nodules, vesicles, plaques +/– ulceration and PIH	Papule/ plaque/ nodule which is hyperkerato-tic/eroded	Dome-shaped keratotic papule with central crust	Papules with yellowish centers with TEE of clear viscous fluid that form a crust
Associated findings	Active focus of TB else-where	Constitutional symptoms +/–	History of exposure to fleas/bedbugs/ other arthro-pod bites	Pedal edema, livedo reticularis (in cPAN), urticaria (in UV)	Atopy, chronic kidney disease, diabetes, many other disorders may be associated	Chronic kidney disease (+/– hemo-dialysis), diabetes mellitus	?diabetes mellitus, autoimmune thryroiditis
Histopatho-logy	Lymphohistio-cytic vasculitis causing thrombosis of vessels and central tissue necrosis	Edematous epidermis, deep dense wedge-shaped lymphocytic infiltrate, endothelial proliferation, necrotic keratinocytes, intraepidermal and perivas-cular extra-vasation of RBCs	Mixed perivascular infiltrate with many eosino-phils, with prominent papillary dermal edema	Findings of leukocyto-clastic vasculitis	Thick com-pact ortho-keratosis, pseudoepi-theliomatous hyperplasia, hairy palm sign*, fibrosis of papillary dermis, vertically arranged collagen fibers	Cup-shaped invagination of epidermis plugged with necrotic inflammatory debris. TEE of collagen fibers	Superficial necrobiotic area surrounded by palisading histiocytes situated beneath a perforation, TEE of necrobiotic material

PLEVA—pityriasis lichenoides et varioliformis acuta, TB—tuberculosis, PIH—post-inflammatory hyperpigmentation, cPAN—cutaneous polyarteritis nodosa, UV—urticarial vasculitis, TEE—transepidermal elimination

*Hairy palm sign—thick compact cornified layer (like volar skin of palms) with folliculosebaceous units (like non-volar skin)

Clinical Course

May clear within 4 weeks of ATT.

HPE

Histologically, the lesions show variable combinations of vasculitis with necrosis, a moderate to intense lymphohistiocytic infiltrate, and granulomatous inflammation.

- Papulonecrotic tuberculid, when fully developed, shows cutaneous infarction comprising a necrotic epidermis with ulceration and an underlying V-shaped zone of dermal coagulative necrosis accompanied by a dense chronic inflammatory cell infiltrate with scattered giant cells.
- Necrosis of hair follicles may occur.
- On occasion, a histiocytic palisade has been described, resulting in features reminiscent of granuloma annulare.
- Neutrophils are generally inconspicuous.
- Vasculitis may be present.

Complications

Varioliform scarring and hyperpigmentation.

Diagnosis

- **Mantoux reaction:** Strongly positive
- **HPE:**
  - Lymphohistiocytic vasculitis with thrombosis of small dermal blood vessels, wedge-shaped infarct with central coagulation necrosis surrounded by inflammation
  - Culture negative
- **PCR skin biopsy:** *M. tuberculosis* DNA can be detected fairly frequently by PCR [Rook's]
- **IGRA (interferon release assay):** May be positive.

Treatment

First line	Second line	Third line
ATT	—	—

ERYTHEMA INDURATUM OF BAZIN

Epidemiology

- Past (more common) or active focus of tuberculosis
- Young and middle-aged women
- Lobular panniculitis with vasculitis

Predisposing Factors

More persistent if preexisting erythrocyanotic (perniotic) features.

Clinical Features of Classic Lesion

Usually asymptomatic (sometimes painful) nodules/subcutaneous plaques on posterior lower legs—indurated, scaly → may ulcerate centrally → ragged, irregular, shallow ulcers with bluish edges → heals with atrophic hyperpigmented scars **(Fig. 17.23)**.

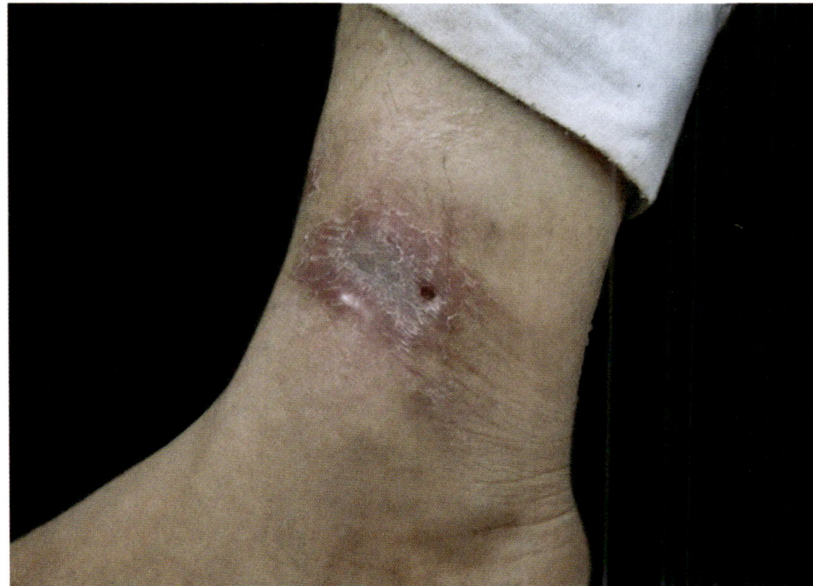

Fig. 17.23: Erythema induratum

Clinical Types/Variants

Nodular tuberculid and subcutaneous nodules along great saphenous vein-granulomatous phlebitis/superficial thrombophlebitic tuberculid.

Differential Diagnosis (Box 17.11)

BOX 17.11: Differential diagnosis of erythema induratum of Bazin

- Erythema nodosum (painful, anterior, no ulceration, joint swellings, elsewhere on body, other causes, septal panniculitis without vasculitis)
- Panniculitis due to other causes inlcuding erythema nodosum leprosum
- Polyarteritis nodosa
- Lupus profundus
- Subcutaneous sarcoidosis
- CTCL
- Perniosis
- Nodular vasculitis

Clinical Course

- Recurrent crops
- Slow response to ATT (around 6 months)—slower response if associated erythrocyanotic features.

HPE

- Erythema induratum has a less histiocytic infiltrate and is indistinguishable from nodular vasculitis.

- The presence of both primary vasculitic changes and granulomatous inflammation suggests that type III and type IV hypersensitivity reactions are important in the latter condition.

Complications

Hyperpigmented scars.

Diagnosis

- **Mantoux reaction:** Strongly positive
- **HPE:**
  - Lobular/septolobular granulomatous panniculitis with neutrophilic vasculitis
  - Areas of coagulative and caseous necrosis
  - Culture negative
- **PCR skin biopsy:** May be positive.
- **IGRA (interferon release assay):** May be positive.

Treatment

Response is slow (1–6 months)

First line	Second line	Third line
ATT	—	—

TREATMENT OF CUTANEOUS TB

As sometimes a definitive diagnosis cannot be made as there is failure to demonstrate bacilli even in definite cases of tuberculosis occasionally, it may be a diagnosis of exclusion, which is confirmed by a therapeutic trial of anti-tuberculous drugs of 6 weeks (Sehgal VN, 2008).

Standard Recommended Regime (Table 17.7)

- All drug sensitive TB cases are treated with 2 HRZE/4 HRE as FDCs in weight bands.
- **MDR TB:** Multidrug-resistant TB is caused by an organism that is resistant to at least isoniazid and rifampin, the two most potent TB drugs. Rifampicin resistant TB (RR–TB) is treated similarly.
- **Pre-XDR TB:** MDR–TB or RR–TB PLUS resistance to any fluoroquinolone.
- **XDR–TB:** MDR–TB or RR–TB PLUS resistance any fluoroquinolone PLUS at least one additional group A drug (group A drugs are the most potent second–line drugs for drug resistant TB and include levofloxacin, moxifloxacin, bedaquiline and linezolid.

TABLE 17.7: ATT regimen*

Drug	Dose	Duration
1. Isoniazid	5 mg/kg	6 months
2. Rifampicin	10 mg/kg	6 months
3. Pyrazinamide	25 mg/kg	First 2 months
4. Ethambutol	15 mg/kg	6 months

*All on empty stomach once daily as FDCs as per weight band.

MANAGEMENT OF CUTANEOUS ADVERSE EFFECTS OF ATT

In a recent study from India, maculopapular rash was the most common adverse effect due to ATT, most frequently caused by ethambutol. Among different types of SCAR, ATT drugs more frequently cause DRESS rather than SJS/TEN or AGEP compared with other causative drugs of SCAR.

Though rechallenge is usually discouraged in the management of SCAR due to the possible serious risks, previously prescribed ATT drugs have occasionally been re-administered in cases of ATT-related DRESS. Recommendations by the GOI and the Philadelphia TB Control Programme are given below:

ICMR and Central TB Division, DGHS, Ministry of Health and Family Welfare Recommendations (2016)

- ATT-induced rash/urticaria (all ATT)–desensitization with the ATT drugs and substitution with second line drugs if it fails.
- Allergic dermatitis and erythroderma (FQ most common)–continue drugs till substitution is possible.
- SJS/TEN (H, R, E, FQ)–immediate drug withdrawal, no rechallenge.

The Philadelphia Tuberculosis Control Program gave the following Recommendations (1998):

Adverse effect	Features	Drugs	Management
Mild flushing	Type 1: ± itching	R, Z	Antihistamine drugs
	Type 2: + hot flash/ palpitations/headache	H with tyramine	Avoid cheese, red wine, tuna fish (contains tyramine)
Moderate-severe cutaneous hypersensitivity reaction	Hives ± fever	H<R<Z<E<S	Discontinue ATT R/o viral infection (EBV, HSV) **Rechallenge** each drug every 4 days.

Drug Rechallenge Protocol

Drug	Challenge doses	
	Day 1 (mg)	Day 2 (mg)
H	50	300
R	75	300
Z	250	1000
E	100	500
S	125	500

- If a reaction occurs during drug rechallenge and the causative drug cannot be discontinued, drug desensitization will be necessary.
- Consideration should be given to desensitizing patients under monitored conditions for severe reactions.
- The patient should be receiving >2 other TB medications before undergoing drug desensitization.

The most common desensitization protocol is as follows:

a. Initiate the day 1 dose as indicated in **Table 17.1**.
b. If a reaction occurs after day 1 of drug rechallenge, begin desensitization with 1/10th of the day 1 dose.
c. Double each dose and administer twice daily until the recommended daily dose has been achieved.
d. Administer the recommended daily dose for 3 days, then switch to once daily dosing (e.g. INH 150 mg bid × 3 days, then 300 mg/day).
e. If a reaction develops during desensitization, decrease the dose to the highest dose (the previous dose) that did not cause a reaction and begin increasing the doses in smaller increments.

Based on the table above, begin rechallenge with H on day 1 (give 1/10th dose if initial reaction was severe). If no reaction, increase dose on day 2. In case of no reaction after 2nd dose, continue H 300 mg/day. Continue to add a new drug every 4 days in the given order.

If Day 2 dose is less than normal recommended dose/kg increase to appropriate dose on day 3. (e.g. ethambutol for 70 kg: Day 1–100 mg, Day 2–500 mg, Day 3–1000 mg).

However, desensitization should not be attempted with severe skin reactions or those involving the mouth or mucous membranes (e.g. exfoliative dermatitis and Stevens–Johnson syndrome).

ATYPICAL MYCOBACTERIAL INFECTIONS

Also known as nontuberculous mycobacteria (NTM)/mycobacteria other than TB (MOTT).

- Found naturally in the environment (water and soil).
- Transferred via dust, skin injuries, droplets, and occasionally cause opportunistic infections. Not known to spread via human-to-human transmission.
- Almost all NTM can cause cutaneous disease, which is the most common extrapulmonary organ involved.
- Run a more benign course than *M. tuberculosis*. Only *M. marinum* and *M. ulcerans* produce a characteristic clinical picture.
- Much less responsive to ATT drugs.

Rapidly growing mycobacteria (RGM) are associated more with cosmetic and surgical procedures, while slow growing mycobacteria (SGM) are limited to traumatic injuries.

Approach to Diagnosis

Apart from clinical suspicion, both mycobacterial tissue culture and histopathology with special stains for AFB are recommended to increase diagnostic yield.

- Histopathology shows granulomatous and suppurative inflammation with variable pseudoepitheliomatous hyperplasia, ulceration, microabscesses, necrosis, and fibrosis. In immunosuppressed patients, the infiltrate tends to be more diffuse, with increased neutrophils and decreased granulomatous inflammation.

  In case of *M. abscessus/chelonae*-neutrophilc abscesses, and epitheliod granulomas with vaculoes are suggestive.

  Special stains to detect AFB, such as Fite or Ziehl–Neelsen, should be performed, but have low sensitivity (e.g. 34–51% positive in tissue culture-confirmed cases). AFB are more readily seen with immunosuppression.

- Tissue culture submitted specifically for mycobacterial detection is recommended. RGM and *M. marinum* grow best at 28–30°C, *M. ulcerans* grows at 25–33°C, and most other slowly growing mycobacteria grow at 35–37°C. Therefore, skin specimens for mycobacteria are typically incubated at both 28–30°C and 35–37°C. Most cultures are incubated for 6 weeks, with growth typically in 2–3 weeks. *M. ulcerans* may require 8–12 weeks.

An overview of the various types of NTM is listed in **Table 17.8**.

TABLE 17.8: Atypical mycobacterial infections

Organism	Epidemiology	Site of lesions	Clinical lesions	Associated findings	Differential diagnosis	Treatment**
M. marinum (**swimming pool granuloma** or Fish fancier's finger) (slow growers)	Occupational/ recreational exposure to saltwater/ freshwater	Dominant hands of fish fanciers; elbows, knees, feet of swimmers	• Single or occasional "ascending" multiple sporotrichoid lesions • Violaceous papules → nodule or verrucous plaques on an extremity, → progressing subsequently to shallow ulceration → scarring in 1–2 years • Clinical involvement of regional nodes is uncommon	Complications—tenosynovitis/ osteomyelitis/ septic arthritis	Sporotrichosis, blastomycosis, Coccidioido-mycosis, other NTM	• Rifampicin + Ethambutol + Azithromycin/ clarithro-mycin + Amikacin **Resistant** to Isoniazid and pyrazinamide • Treat with **two active agents** for 2 months after resolution of symptoms, typically 3–4 months in total • **Surgical debridement** for disease involving closed spaces of hand and in recalcitrant cases. • Local heat application as *M. marinum* grows at low temperatures.
M. kansasii (slow growers)	Occupational exposure to dust/lung diseases, HIV, **immuno-compromised, on immuno-suppressants**	Distal extremities	• Sporotrchoid papules/ pustules coalescing into granulo-matous or verrucous plaques/ nodules → ulcers • In immuno-suppressed, cellulitis and abscesses.	**Mostly pulmo-nary** disease in COPD or cystic fibrosis patients, cutaneous disease only in immunocom-promised	Sporotrichosis, cutaneous TB, other NTM	• Rifampicin + Ethambutol + Isoniazid or Azithromycin/ Clarithromycin • Continue for minimum of 12 months after culture conversion

(Contd.)

TABLE 17.8: Atypical mycobacterial infections *(Contd.)*

Organism	Epidemiology	Site of lesions	Clinical lesions	Associated findings	Differential diagnosis	Treatment**
*M. ulcerans** (**Buruli ulcer**) (slow growers)	• Endemic to Buruli, Uganda. Very common in some African communities. Maximum cases in children (F>M) 5–15 years old living in marshy/ swampy areas. • Globally, *M. ulcerans* is now the third most prevalent mycobacterial species, after *M. tuberculosis* and *M. leprae*, in immunocompetent individuals.	Extremities, usually lower	Single indolent subcutaneous nodule → painless necrotic ulcer with undermined scalloped edges ("buruli ulcer") → extends rapidly leading to local complications (fat and muscle necrosis, severe scarring). Clinical involvement of regional nodes is uncommon.	Complications—osteomyelitis, fat and muscle necrosis, disabling scarring	Ulcerated cutaneous TB, blastomycosis and other deep mycoses, pyoderma gangrenosum, necrotizing cellulitis/ fasciitis, panniculitis	• Most antimycobacterial agents ineffective • Rifampicin + Streptomycin/ clarithromycin × 2 months (WHO) • Surgical debridement combined with skin grafting • Postsurgical antimycobacterial treatment to prevent relapse/ metastasis of infection.
M. avium, M. intracellulare (MAC) (slow growers)	MAC infection seen mostly in HIV positive patients	Neck in cervical lymphadenitis cases, anywhere in disseminated cases. Follows trauma, injections or surgery.	**Cervical lymphadenitis** → fistula/sinus In immunocompromised patients–disseminated MAC lesions (nodules, abscesses, ulcers), sporotrichoid +/–	Cutaneous involvement rare, mostly causes cervical lymphadenitis in children	Scrofuloderma, lepromatous leprosy, lupus vulgaris	• Rifampicin + Ethambutol + Azithromycin/ clarithromycin + consider intravenous amikacin for up to 3 months or nebulised amikacin • Antibiotic treatment continued for a minimum of 12 months after culture conversion
M. hemophilum (slow growers)	HIV, immunocompromised, on immunosuppressants	Extremities, usually joints	Erythematous/ violaceous papules or nodules painful ulcers or abscesses. Classically, an AFB smear positive, draining	Synovitis, less frequently pulmonary or disseminated infections	*M. marinum*, MAC infections, bacterial ulcerations, Kaposi sarcoma	• Susceptible to Amikacin, clarithromycin, ciprofloxacin, rifampin, and rifabutin • All isolates resistant to ethambutol

(Contd.)

TABLE 17.8: Atypical mycobacterial infections *(Contd.)*

Organism	Epidemiology	Site of lesions	Clinical lesions	Associated findings	Differential diagnosis	Treatment**
			skin lesion that has no growth on ordinary (routine) AFB media in immunosuppressed patients (especially organ transplant recipients).			
M. scrofulaceum (slow growers)	Children 1–3 years	Neck in cervical lympadenitis (unilateral)	Unilateral cervical lympadenitis ulcer → fistula Submandibular/submaxillary lymphadenopathy	Lung/other organ involvement very rare	Scrofuloderma, mumps, mononucleosis, Hodgkin's lymphoma	• Susceptible to amikacin, clarithromycin, ciprofloxacin, rifampin, and rifabutin • All isolates resistant to ethambutol
M. fortuitum, *M. chelonae* *M. abscessus* (rapid growers or RGM)#	Both in immunocompetent and immunocompromised, mostly post-traumatic or postoperative	Follows a puncture wound (such as occurs after stepping on a nail) or surgical procedure, acupuncture, mesotherapy, dermal filler injection or surgery	Immunocompetent–dark red nodule → local abscess Immunocompromised—disseminated erythematous nodules, cellulitis, ulcers, sinuses, abscesses, cause usually single-site rather than multiple-site infections.	Endocarditis, meningitis, osteomyelitis, keratitis, catheter-related infections	Other NTM, sporotrichosis, bacterial ulcers and cellulitis	**Box 17.12** lists the antibiotic treatment of RGM. • Surgery for extensive disease/abscess/recalcitrant cases • Removal of foreign bodies like breast implants/percutaneous catheters is essential

*Surgical management is the mainstay for *M. ulcerans*.
**Based on BTS 2017/ATS 2020 guidelines. Daily doses for severe infections and thrice weekly dosing for mild-moderate cases.
#HPE of rapid growers—"dimorphic inflammatory response"— simultaneous PMN microabscesses with granuloma with foreign-body giant cells.

BOX 17.12: Antibiotic treatment of RGM

- Recommended duration is 4 months for mild disease and 6 months for severe disease.
- At least 2 antibiotics should be used.
- *M. abscessus* complex-Amikacin + Imipenem/ cefoxitin + Tigecycline (macrolide resistant) OR Azithromycin/ Clarithromycin (macrolide susceptible).
- *M. abscessus* may have inducible macrolide resistance.
- *M. chelonae*-susceptible to macrolides but cefoxitin resistant. Azithromycin/ clarithromycin + doxycycline + tobramycin.
- *M. fortuitum*-susceptible to multiple oral antibiotics. Amikacin + minocycline + quinolone.

We are detailing the principles that determine treatment of common causes and a summary of treatment is detailed in **Table 17.9**.

Principles of Treatment

M. marinum

Antibiotic therapy with two or more agents is recommended for 3–4 months, or 1–2 months beyond clinical resolution. **Monotherapy** can be considered for **limited infection**. Routine susceptibility testing is not required for *M. marinum*, except in cases of treatment failure. Isolates are typically susceptible to macrolides, sulfonamides, rifampin, ethambutol, and amikacin, and are susceptible or intermediate in susceptibility to tetracyclines. Treatment failure is usually related to deep structure involvement, rather than a particular antibiotic.

Tetracyclines tended to be prescribed more for **superficial infection**, while rifampin, rifabutin, and ethambutol are prescribed more for **deep infection**. Clarithromycin is equally prescribed in **superficial and deep infections**. Duration of therapy is significantly longer for patients with deep infections (median 7.5 *vs* 4 months), and 48% of patients need surgery, which was significantlyassociated with deep structure infection.

Due to **rifampicin's** excellent bone-penetrating ability, combination therapy with rifampicin plus ethambutol or minocycline for previously untreated patients for 6 months, or at least 2 months beyond clinical improvement is advised. For relapse, **triple therapy** with clarithromycin, minocycline, and ethambutol is advised and for deep structure infections surgical excision/debridement.

Rapidly Growing Mycobacteria

Treatment of RGM infections is not standardized. Species identification and *in vitro* susceptibility testing should be performed to guide treatment. Antibiotic therapy with at least **two antibiotics** with *in vitro* susceptibility is recommended for a minimum of **4 months**.

M. chelonae isolates have in vitro susceptibility or intermediate susceptibility to tobramycin (100%), clarithromycin (100%), linezolid (90%), imipenem (60%), amikacin (50%), doxycycline (25%), and ciprofloxacin (20%). Isolates are uniformly resistant to cefoxitin.

M. fortuitum isolates display in vitro susceptibility to amikacin (100%), ciprofloxacin and ofloxacin (100%), sulfonamides (100%), cefoxitin (50%), imipenem (100%), clarithromycin (80%), and doxycycline (50%).

M. abscessus is often the most challenging to treat due to broad antibiotic resistance. *M. abscessus* subsp. abscessus and subsp. bolletii possess an erm (41) gene, which confers macrolide resistance. Surgery has an adjunctive role. Foreign material (e.g. breast implant) at the site of infection should be removed.

M. ulcerans

While initially surgery was the ideal treatment the recurrence rates were high (16–28%) and now antibiotic therapy has lead to very good results (recurrence rates of 0–2%). The World Health Organization (WHO) recommends combination antibiotic therapy for 8 weeks as first-line treatment for all stages of disease. In 2004, oral rifampicin and intramuscular streptomycin were recommended. Recent oral alternatives, such as rifampicin in combination with clarithromycin or moxifloxacin, show similar efficacy.

Treatment of NTM

Tables 17.9 and **17.10** give the treatment and suggested dosages for extrapulmonary NTM infections.

TABLE 17.9: Treatment of extrapulmonary nontuberculous mycobacterial diseases (Wi YM, Infect Chemother, 2019)

Species	Suggested regimens
Mycobacterium abscessus complex	**Macrolide resistant** **Initial:** Amikacin + cefoxitin/imipenem + tigecycline **Maintenance or mild:** 3–5 of the following antibiotics: Clofazimine, linezolid, minocycline, moxifloxacin, cotrimoxazole **Macrolide susceptible:** **Initial:** Amikacin + Cefoxitin/Imipenem + Azithromycin/Clarithromycin **Maintenance or mild:** Azithromycin/Clarithromycin + 2–4 of the following—clofazimine, linezolid, minocycline, moxifloxacin, cotrimoxazole.
Mycobacterium chelonae	**Initial:** Azithromycin/clarithromycin + tobramycin ± imipenem **Maintenance or mild:** Azithromycin/clarithromycin + doxycycline or clofazimine or linezolid
Mycobacterium fortuitum	**Initial:** Amikacin + quinolone + minocycline **Maintenance or mild:** Quinolone + minocycline
Mycobacterium marinum	**Initial:** Amikacin + azithromycin/clarithromycin + rifampin + ethambutol **Maintenance or mild:** Azithromycin/clarithromycin + rifampin + ethambutol
Mycobacterium ulcerans	**Initial:** Rifampicin + streptomycin **Maintenance or mild:** Rifampicin + clarithromycin or moxifloxacin
Mycobacterium avium complex	**Macrolide susceptible:** **Initial:** Amikacin/streptomycin + rifampin + ethambutol + azithromycin/clarithromycin **Maintenance or mild:** Rifampin + ethambutol + azithromycin/clarithromycin

TABLE 17.10: Doses of oral and parenteral drugs in NTM

Drug (oral)	Daily dosing
Azithromycin	250–500 mg/day
Ciprofloxacin	500–750 mg BD
Clarithromycin	500 mg BD
Clofazimine	100–200 mg/day
Doxycycline	100 mg BD
Ethambutol	15 mg/kg
Isoniazid	5 mg/kg
Linezolid	600 mg OD–BD
Moxifloxacin	400 mg/day
Rifabutin	150–300 mg/day
Rifampicin	10 mg/kg
Cotrimoxazole	800 mg/160 mg BD
Drug (parenteral)	**Daily dosing**
Amikacin	10–15 mg/kg
Cefoxitin	2–4 g BD–TDS
Imipenem	500–1000 mg BD–TDS
Streptomycin	10–15 mg/kg
Tigecycline	25–50 mg OD–BD

FUNGAL INFECTIONS

INTRODUCTION

Fungal infections have been grouped according to their clinical presentation, subdividing them into superficial, subcutaneous, systemic, and opportunistic mycoses and an updated classification is given in **Tables 17.11** and **17.12**.

TABLE 17.11: Superficial cutaneous mycoses

Disease	Causative agent
• Tinea (pityriasis) versicolor, seborrheic dermatitis, including dandruff and *Malassezia* folliculitis	*Malassezia* spp (a lipophilic yeast)
• Tinea nigra	*Exophiala werneckii*
• White piedra	*Trichosporon asahii*
• Black piedra	*Piedraia hortae*
• Dermatophytosis, ring-worm of the scalp, glabrous skin, and nails	Dematophytes (*Microsporum, Trichophyton, Epidermophyton*)
• Candidiasis of skin, mucous membranes, and nails	*Candida albicans* and related species
• Dermatomycosis	Nondermatophyte molds, *Hendersonula toruloidea, Scytalidium hyalinum, Scopulariopsis brevicaulis*

TABLE 17.12: Subcutaneous and systemic mycoses

Disease	Causative agent
Subcutaneous mycoses	
Sporotrichosis	*Sporothrix complex*
Chromoblastomycosis	*Fonsecaea, Phialophora, Cladosporium*
Phaeohyphomycosis	*Cladosporium, Exophiala, Wangiella, Bipolaris, Exserohilum, Curvularia*
Eumycetoma	*Madurella, Fusarium, Scedosporium* spp
Subcutaneous zygomycosis (entomophthoromycosis)	*Basidiobolus ranarum* *Conidiobolus coronatus*
Subcutaneous zygomycosis (mucormycosis)	*Rhizopus, Mucor, Rhizomucor, Mycocladus, Saksenaea*
Lobomycosis	*Lacazia loboi*
Dimorphic systemic mycoses	
Histoplasmosis	*Histoplasma capsulatum* var *capsulatum*, *Histoplasma capsulatum* var *duboisii*
Coccidioidomycosis	*Coccidioides immitis, Coccidioides posadasii*
Blastomycosis	*Blastomyces dermatitidis*
Paracoccidioidomycosis	*Paracoccidioides brasiliensis*
Opportunistic systemic mycoses	
Candidiasis	*Candida albicans* and related spp
Cryptococcosis	*Cryptococcus neoformans* (var *neoformans*, var *gattii*)
Aspergillosis	*Aspergillus fumigatus*, other spp
Pseudallescheriasis	*Scedosporium* (*Pseudallescheria boydii*)
Zygomycosis (mucormycosis)	*Rhizopus, Mucor, Rhizomucor, Mycocladus*
Fusariosis	*Fusarium* spp
Penicilliosis	*Penicillium marneffei*
Trichosporonosis	*Trichosporon* spp
Hyalohyphomycosis	*Penicillium, Paecilomyces, Beauveria, Fusarium, Scopulariopsis*
Phaeohyphomycosis	*Cladosporium, Exophiala, Wangiella, Bipolaris*

SUPERFICIAL MYCOSES

PITYRIASIS VERSICOLOR

Epidemiology

- Caused by different species of Malassezia—*M. globosa*—most common. *M. sympodialis* (most commonly found on normal skin) and *M. furfur* too may cause.
- Age—late teens
- Sex—equally prone
- Hypopigmented forms (P. versicolor alba)—more common in skin type III and higher
- Associated with—Cushing syndrome, malnutrition.

Predisposing Factors

- Oil application on skin
- Humid warm climates

Clinical Features

- Sharply demarcated, slightly erythematous macules with fine furfuraceous scaling on large confluent areas.
- Scaling more apparent on scraping with fingernail **(Scratch sign/Besnier sign/coup d'ongle sign)**.
- Upper trunk.

Clinical Variants

- Facial and scalp involvement in tropics.
- Pale ochre (in darker skins) to medium brown (lighter skins) color. Could be due to *Malassezia* metabolites.
  (Azelaic acid: A dicarboxylic acid that inhibits tyrosinase, Malassezin: An aryl hydrocarbon receptor agonist that induces apoptosis in melanocytes).

Complications

Pulmonary and systemic infection due to *Malassezia* in infants on long-term IV lipid therapy.

Differential Diagnosis (Box 17.13)

BOX 17.13: Differential diagnosis of pityriasis versicolor

- Pityriasis alba
- Dermatophytic infections
- Vitiligo
- Erythrasma
- Pityriasis rosea
- Seborrheic dermatitis
- Progressive macular hypomelanosis
- Hypopigmented MF

Diagnosis (Box 17.14)

BOX 17.14: Diagnosis of pityriasis versicolor

- KOH—coarse mycelium, fragmented to short filaments with spherical thick-walled yeasts. Mycelium is diagnostic. (spaghetti and meatball appearance)
- Wood's lamp—pale yellow fluorescence.
- Dermoscopy:
  - Hyperchromic
- Fine whitish scaling.
- Pigmented network composed of brown stripes/diffuse brownish pigmentation.
  - Achromic
- Fairly demarcated white area.
- Fine scales in the skin furrows.

Treatment (Fig. 17.24)

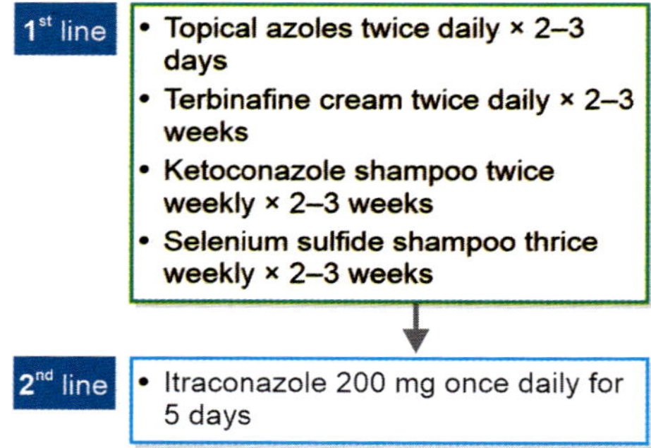

Fig. 17.24: Treatment of pityriasis versicolor

DERMATOPHYTOSES

Dermatophytes live as parasites in tissue containing keratin. They can be divided into:

1. **Anthropophilic: Found in humans**
2. **Zoophilic: Found in animals**
3. **Geophilic: Found in soil.**

The clinical presentation is determined by the nature of the dermatophyte, by the tissue it invades, and by the degree of host response. Dermatophytes invade keratin only, and the inflammation they cause is due to metabolic products of the fungus or delayed hypersensitivity.

The most common cause of superficial fungal infections is ***Trichophyton rubrum***. In India though, *Trichophyton mentagrophytes/interdigitale* spp is now the commonest cause of superficial dermatophytosis, as confirmed by molecular studies; even though taxonomy keeps changing and now this species has been renamed as *Trichophyton indotineae*.

Notably the first case of Terbinafine resistance with SQLE mutations and the first case of proven azole resistance with mutations in Erg 1,3,11 and efflux transporters has been reported from Delhi, RML Hospital (Singh A, 2018).

Most cases of the present dermatophyte species either need updosed terbinafine 250 mg BD or Itraconazole.

Even though tinea corporis and its atypical variants are common in India; in the examinations, tinea capitis and onychomycosis are the focus of examiners.

TINEA CAPITIS

Epidemiology

- *M. canis*—increasing in Europe
- *T. tonsurans*—most prevalent in UK, increasing in USA
- *T. violaceum*—commonest cause in India

Causative Organisms

- *Trichophyton* species—special predilection for hair shaft.
- *Epidermophyton* spp, *T. concentricum*, *T. interdigitale*—never infect hair shaft.
- *Trichophyton tonsurans* and *Microsporum canis* are the most common causes.
- A depiction of the involvement of the hair shaft is given in **Fig. 17.25** with the species listed below
  - **Endothrix:** *T. rubrum*, *T. tonsurans*, *T. schoenleinii*, *T. yaoundei*; *T. violaceum*, *T. gourvilli*, and *T. soudanense*
  - **Ectothrix** (arthrospores around hair shaft):
    a. **Fluorescent** (Wood lamp—due to pteridine): *M. canis*, *M. audouinii*, *M. gypseum*, *M. ferrugineum*, *M. distortum*, and *T. schoenleinii*.
    b. **Nonfluorescent:** *T. mentagrophytes*, *T. rubrum*, *M. manum*, *T. megninii*, *T. gypseum*, and *T. verrucosum*.

Pathogenesis

- Spores of fungi are seen in the air in close proximity to patients.
- The hair acts like a trapping device.
- First, there is invasion of the **stratum corneum** of the scalp → after approximately 3 weeks → clinical evidence of hair shaft infection → infection spread to other follicles, then for a period of variable duration the infection persists but does not spread further.

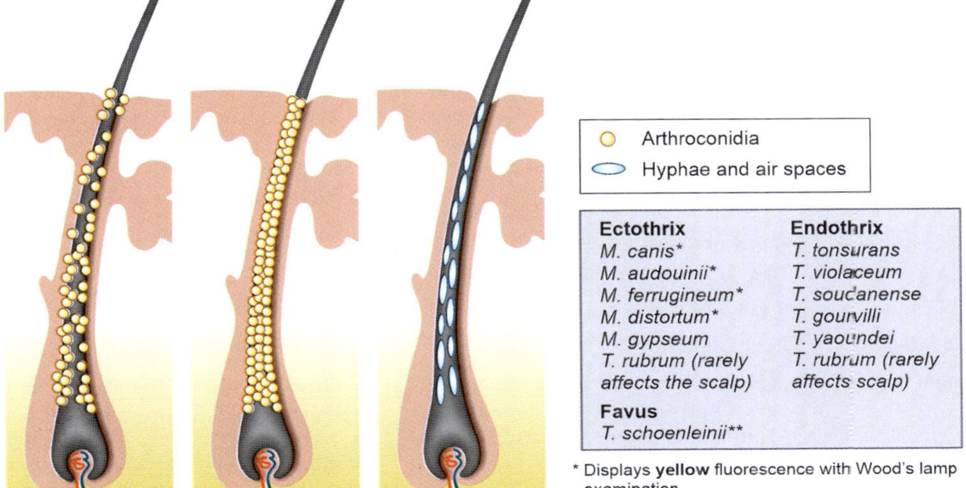

Fig. 17.25: An overview of the types of tinea capitis based on invasion of the hair shaft and the causative organism

Ectothrix: Hair shaft is invaded mid-follicle. The intrapilary hyphae continue to grow inwards towards the bulb of the hair and secondary, extrapilary hyphae burst out and grow in a tortuous manner over the surface of the hair shaft and produce a mass of small arthroconidia (2–3 µm diameter).

Endothrix: Intrapilary hyphae fragment into arthroconidia up to 8 µm in diameter, which are entirely contained within and completely fill the hair shaft. Hair thus affected is especially fragile, and breaks off close to the scalp surface.

Clinical Features

The clinical features are listed in **Table 17.13** and depicted in **Fig. 17.26**.

TABLE 17.13: Clinical features and types of hair shaft invasion

	Ectothrix	Endothrix	Favus	Kerion
Causative organisms	Small spored— *M. canis,* *M. ferugineum,* *M. audouinii,* *M. equinum* Large spored— *M. gypseum,* *M. fulvum*	*T. tonsurans,* *T. soudanense,* *T. yaoundei*	*T. schoenleinii*	*T. verrucosum,* *T. mentagrophytes*
Clinical features	• Circular patches with **gray** (d/t coating of arthrospores) broken-off hair, fine scaling, sharp margins **(Fig. 17.26a)** • Trichoscopy shows **zigzag and morse code hair**	• **Black dots** (swollen hair shafts) d/t hair breakage at surface • Multiple patches, minimal scaling • Commonly angular outlines instead of circular **(Fig. 17.26b)** • Trichoscopy shows **comma hair and corkscrew hair**	• Endemic in South Africa and Ethiopia • May run through generations, no tendency to resolve • Yellow cup-shaped crust **"Scutula"** around affected hair—pierced centrally by the hair • Adjacent crusts become confluent–mass of yellow crusting **(Fig. 17.26d)**	• Most severely inflammatory, usually zoophilic • Large boggy endematous swelling studded with pustules, crusting, matting of hair, lymphadenopathy • May have bacterial superinfection, usually only fungal **(Fig. 17.26c)**
Wood's lamp	Green fluorescence	None	Pale blue/green-gray	—
Treatment	• Griseofulvin/ itraconazole > Terbinafine • Griseofulvin (10–20 mg/kg × 6 weeks) • Itraconazole (2–4 mg/kg × 6 weeks)	• Terbinafine × 1 month (5–8 mg/kg per day)	• Griseofulvin • Itraconazole • Terbinafine • Removal of crusts • Cutting of hair around the alopecia patches • Antifungal shampoo	• Careful removal of crusts with wet compresses • Treat coexisting bacterial infection, if present • NSAIDs

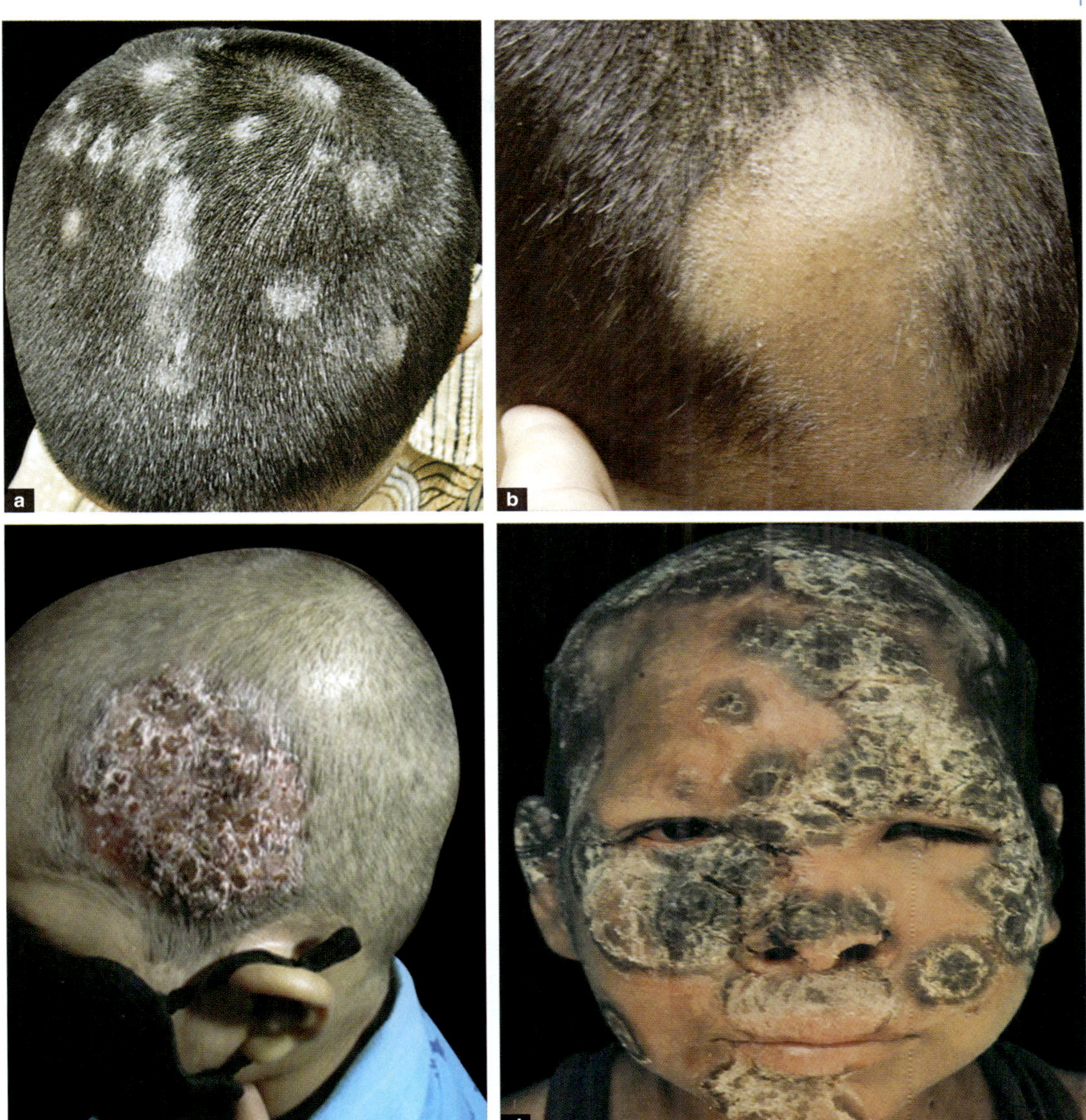

Fig. 17.26: (a) A case of gray patch tinea capitis. There is patchy circular alopecia and fine scaling. Fine scales represent the fungal arthrospores; (b) "Black dot" tinea capitis, which was initially misdiagnosed as a case of alopecia areata; (c) Inflamed, boggy, tender areas of alopecia in a case of kerion; (d) Tinea favosa

Associated Features

- Cervical lymphadenopathy: Palpable cervical lymphadenopathy is a frequent finding in patients with tinea capitis, particularly when clinical signs of inflammation are present.
- Dermatophytid reactions: Autoeczematization reactions (id reactions) are secondary dermatitic eruptions that occur in association with a localized inflammatory skin disorder.

Dermatophytid reactions often follow the onset of antifungal therapy, but may also precede treatment. Patients develop a widespread pruritic eczematous eruption characterized by erythematous, scaly papules.

- Other: Infrequently, erythema nodosum occurs in association with kerion

Differential Diagnosis (Box 17.15)

BOX 17.15: Differential diagnosis of tinea capitis

- Alopecia areata—exclamation mark hair, smooth nonscaly surface.
- Seborrheic dermatitis coexisting with alopecia areata—more confusing, but scaling and hair loss do not coexist in these cases.
- Trichotillomania
- Traumatic alopecia
- Impetigo of scalp
- Cicatricial alopecia

Diagnosis (Box 17.16)

BOX 17.16: Diagnosis of tinea capitis

- **Bedside tests**
  - KOH hair shaft
  - Wood's lamp
- **Trichoscopy:** Comma hairs, corkscrew hairs, morse code-like hairs, zigzag hairs
- **Culture:** Scales inoculated in SDA medium.

1. **Bedside tests:**
   - KOH hair shaft
   - Wood's lamp
     - Ectothrix—bright green
     - Endothrix—no fluorescence (except *T. schoenleinii*—pale blue/dull green)
2. **Trichoscopy:** Dhaille et al. (2019) found culture positivity in 53% and a typical trichoscopic finding in 94%. They found that even a single typical trichoscopic finding is highly predictive for tinea capitis.

   Typical trichoscopic findings include **(Fig. 17.27)**:

   - At low magnification (30×)—**comma hairs**—C-shaped short hair shafts due to bending and breakage of hair shafts filled with hyphae. More frequent with *Trichophyton* (endothrix) (Dhaille et al., 2019).
   - **Corkscrew hairs**—broken-coiled hairs seen at higher magnification (120–150×)—translucent, easily deformable hairs. These hairs are different from the surrounding ones, have no horizontal white bands, and look weakened and transparent, showing unusual bends; they are likely the result of a massive fungal invasion involving the entire length of the hair shaft. More with *Trichophyton*.
   - **Morse code-like hairs**—with multiple white bands across the hair shaft. These white bands are related to localized areas of fungal infection (large density of hyphae and arthroconidia). Highly specific for *Microsporum* (ectothrix).

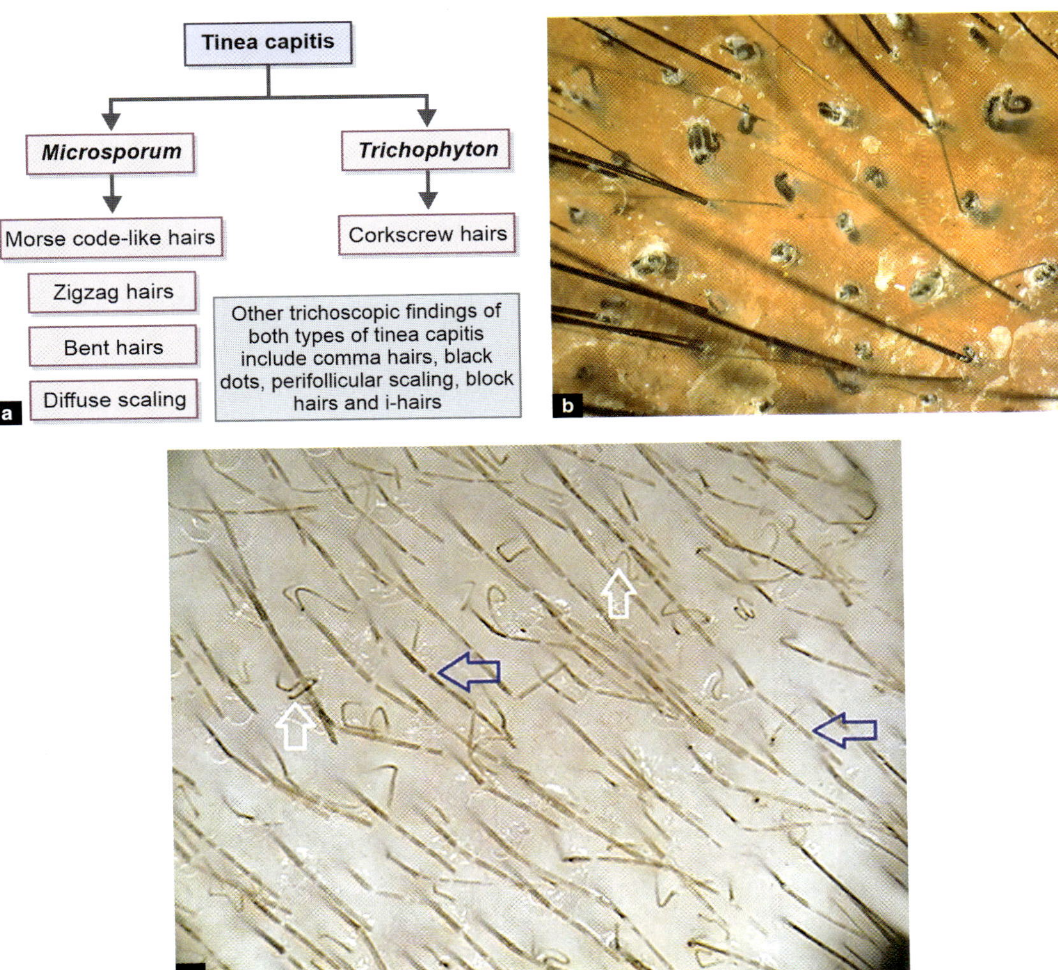

Fig. 17.27: (a) Overview of the Trichoscopic findings of t. capitis (Waskiel-Burnat, A, et al., 2020). Trichoscopy of tinea capitis: A systematic review (Dermatol Ther 2020); (b) Trichoscopic image of tinea capitis with numerous comma hair and corkscrew hair (*Courtesy*: Dr Ananta Khurana, Dr RML Hospital, New Delhi); (c) Trichoscopy of tinea capitis with the presence of morse code-like hairs (blue arrows) and corkscrew hairs (white arrows) (×20) (Waskiel-Burnat A, et al., 2020)

- **Zigzag hairs**—with numerous bands at sharp angles (also in other diseases associated with focal weakening of the hair shaft, such as alopecia areata and trichorrhexis nodosa). More common with *Microsporum*.
- White sheaths—more with *Microsporum*.

3. **Culture:** Scales inoculated in SDA medium.

Treatment (Table 17.14)

- A recent meta-analysis confirmed that for *Microsporum*, griseofulvin was most efficacious in terms of both mycological and complete cure while for *Trichophyton*, terbinafine was the

TABLE 17.14: Therapy of tinea capitis

Drug	Dosage	Duration
Griseofulvin (microsize) Available in 250 or 500 mg tablets or 125 mg/5 mL oral suspension	• 10–20 mg/kg/day, single or divided doses • Max daily 1 g	• 4–8 weeks • May need up to 12 weeks, if not cleared
Griseofulvin (ultramicrosize) Available in 125 and 250 mg (tablets)	• 10–15 mg/kg/day • Maximum dose is 750 mg/day	Same as above
Terbinafine 250 mg (tablet)	• <20 kg: 62.5 mg daily • 20–40 kg: 125 mg daily • >40 kg: 250 mg daily	2–4 weeks, up to 8 weeks for *Microsporum* infections
Terbinafine (granules) (oral granules sprinkled into non-acid foods such as pudding) 125 mg in a packet 187.5 mg in packet	• 125 mg daily for body weight less than 25 kg • 187.5 mg daily for body weight 25–35 kg • 250 mg daily for body weight greater than 35 kg	6 weeks
Itraconazole 100 mg capsule	• <20 kg: 5 mg/kg daily • 20–40 kg: 100 mg daily • >40 kg: 200 mg daily	2–6 weeks
Fluconazole 50, 100, 200 mg tablets or oral powder for suspension	• 5–6 mg/kg/day—three to six weeks. • Pulse dose of 6 mg/kg once weekly for 6 to 12 weeks	3–6 weeks

Except for *griseofulvin* and *terbinafine granules*, none of the rest is approved for use in T. capitis by USFDA.

most efficacious in terms of both mycological and complete cure (Gupta AK, et al., 2020). Itraconazole is more active against *Trichophyton* than *Microsporum*.

- **Trichoscopy** can be used as a guide to initiate treatment—Finding zigzag hairs and barcode hairs points to ectothrix infection **(*M. canis*)**, it is recommended to start treatment with **griseofulvin**. On the other hand, finding comma hairs and corkscrew hairs points to endothrix infection **(*T. violaceum*)**, and it is recommended to start treatment with **terbinafine** (Genedy RM, et al., 2020).
- Shampoos with antifungal properties (e.g. selenium sulfide 1 or 2.5%, ciclopirox 1%, or ketoconazole 2% shampoo) at least twice weekly can be used to decrease shedding of fungal spores.
- Clean combs, brushes, and hats to prevent reinfection (with household bleach).
- Sometimes pets may be the source.

TINEA PEDIS

Epidemiology

- Most common dermatophytosis in the developed world
- Males > females
- Adults > children

Predisposing Factors

- Wearing shoes for long durations
- Shared bathrooms and washing facilities

Causative Organisms

- Anthropophilic organisms
- ***T. rubrum* > *T. interdigitale* > *E. floccosum***
- Some may have Gram-negative bacteria too.

Clinical types of Tinea Pedis

- Interdigital tinea pedis: Can be caused by any of the three species
- Chronic hyperkeratotic (moccasin foot): *T. rubrum*
- Vesicobullous type: *T. interdigitale* (zoophilic strains)
- Ulcerative type: *T. interdigitale* (zoophilic strains)

Differential Diagnosis (Box 17.17)

BOX 17.17: Differential diagnosis of tinea pedis

- **Interdigital:** Erosio interdigitalis blastomycetica, erythrasma, bacterial coinfection
- **Hyperkeratotic:** Dyshidrosis, psoriasis, contact dermatitis, atopic dermatitis, hereditary or acquired keratodermas.
- **Vesiculobullous:** Dyshidrosis, contact dermatitis, pustular psoriasis, bacterid, palmoplantar pustulosis, bacterial pyodermas, scabies.

Diagnosis (Box 17.18)

BOX 17.18: Diagnosis of tinea pedis

- **Bedside tests**
  - KOH skin scraping
  - Wood's lamp
- **Culture:** Scales inoculated in SDA medium

Treatment

An overview of the types of tinea pedis and its treatment is depicted in Tables 17.15 and 17.16 respectively.

TABLE 17.15: Types and therapy of tinea pedis

	Interdigital type	Dry type	Wet/vesicobullous type
Causative organism	*T. rubrum, T. interdigitale, E. floccosum*	*T. rubrum* > *E. floccosum*	*T. interdigitale* > *E. floccosum*
Clinical features	Maceration and fissuring of lateral toe clefts	Hyperkeratotic pink lesions covered with fine silvery scales, "moccasin foot"—very extensive	Vesicles, pustules, rupturing leaving behind collarettes of scale, very inflammatory, may have associated with eruption
Sites	Interdigital spaces of lateral toes, may spread to under-surface of toes	Soles, sides, heels	Toe clefts, sole
Nail involvement		Very common (less with *E. floccosum*)	Common (less with *E. floccosum*)
Chronicity		Very chronic, resistant to treatment	Recurrent in summers, not chronic

(Contd.)

TABLE 17.15: Therapy of tinea pedis *(contd.)*

	Interdigital type	Dry type	Wet/vesicobullous type
D/D	• *Neoscytalidium* spp • *Fusarium* spp • Erythrasma • Candidiasis • Macerated soft corns	• *Neoscytalidium* spp. • Juvenile plantar dermatosis • Psoriasis • Contact dermatitis	• Pustular psoriasis • Diabetic bulla
Treatment	• Topical imidazole twice daily × 4 weeks • Topical terbinafine twice daily × 1 week	• Terbinafine 250 mg once daily × 2 weeks • Itraconazole 200 mg twice daily × 2 weeks	• Terbinafine 250 mg once daily × 2 weeks • Itraconazole 200 mg twice daily × 2 weeks

TABLE 17.16: Treatment of tinea pedis/mannum—drugs and dosages

	Griseofulvin	Fluconazole	Terbinafine	Itraconazole	Ketoconazole
Tinea pedis/ mannum	750–1000 mg/day (microsize) or 500–750 mg/day (ultramicrosize) × 6–12 weeks	150–200 mg/week × 4–6 weeks	250 mg daily × 2 weeks	200–400 mg/day 1–2 weeks	Not recommended
Tinea pedis/ mannum (children)	15–20 mg/kg/day (microsize suspension) × 4 weeks	6 mg/kg/week × 4–6 weeks	125 mg (<20–40 kg or 250 mg (>40 kg) × 2 weeks	3–5 mg/kg/day (maximum 200 mg) × 1 week	Not recommended

*In India, terbinafine is increasingly showing non-responsiveness lately.

ONYCHOMYCOSIS

For details *see* Chapter 22: Nail Disorders.

SUBCUTANEOUS MYCOSES

Subcutaneous mycoses belong to a group of infections acquired from ubiquitous saprophyte fungi that affect the skin and subcutaneous tissue. Inoculation is caused by traumatic implantation, and this infection has a subacute or chronic evolution. The fungal disease remains localized to the inoculation area, with slow peripheral growth. Lymphatic or hematologic dissemination is infrequent.

SPOROTRICHOSIS

Causative Organisms

- *Sporothrix schenckii* causes a **benign** chronic subcutaneous mycosis.
- *Sporothrix brasiliensis* is highly **virulent**.
- *Sporothrix globosa* mainly causes **fixed** cutaneous lesions.
- *S. brasiliensis* is the prevalent species related to cat-transmitted sporotrichosis.

Epidemiology

- Common in tropics and subtropics
- America (North, South and Central), sub-Saharan Africa, India, Egypt, Japan and Australia.

- Endemic—in Brazil
- Age—any age
- Sex—no gender predilection

Predisposing Factors

- Occupational exposure to the fungus in-mine workers, forestry workers, gardeners, florists, packing factory workers using straws.
- Different clinical variants in immunocompromised and HIV/AIDS patients.

Pathogenesis

- Fungus grows on decaying vegetable matter.
- Inoculated into the dermis directly or into subcutaneous tissue through a penetrating injury, or by a minor puncture wounds by thorn or splinter.
- Incubation period—8–30 days (can be variable).
- *S. shenckii* remains localized in subcutaneous tissue, rarely may locally spread into subcutaneous lymphatics or in blood-stream after pulmonary infection. This leads to mixed granulomatous reaction with neutrophil foci.
- T cell immunity is important in limiting the disease. The presence of ergosterol peroxide, cell wall compounds, and exoantigens have been described as virulence factors linked to activation of **Th1** or **Th2** responses. In the **early** phase of the disease, the **Th1** response is predominant, with **Th2** presence beginning in the **fifth** week, suggesting humoral immunity in advanced stages.
- Present in tissue as **cigar shaped** or oval yeasts (3–5 mm), or it may be surrounded by thick, radiate, eosinophilic substance forming **asteroid bodies**.

Clinical Features

It has three different clinical presentations: **Lymphangiitis, fixed,** and **disseminated. Extracutaneous disease** includes osteoarticular, which is the most common, pulmonary, mucosal, or systemic.

A. **Lymphangitic sporotrichosis**—most common type. Nodule or pustule follows the implantation of spores in wound, later may form ulcers.
   - Usual site—exposed parts, e.g. upper limbs **(Fig. 17.28)**.
   - Chronic—new papules or nodules appears along the tender lymphatic cords and ulcerate with thin purulent discharge. Regional lymphadenopathy may be present.

B. **Fixed**—less common, fungi remain localized at the site of inoculation **(Fig. 17.29)**.
   - Presentation—as acneiform, nodular, ulcerated or extensive verrucous type.

C. **Systemic type**
   - Mostly in cases with defect in host defense, e.g. AIDS cases.
   - Probably due to inhalation, presents as pulmonary symptoms/focal/wide-spread disseminated disease involving skin joints and meninges.
   - Pulmonary involvement: Presents as a productive cough with or without hemoptysis, fever, and weight loss.

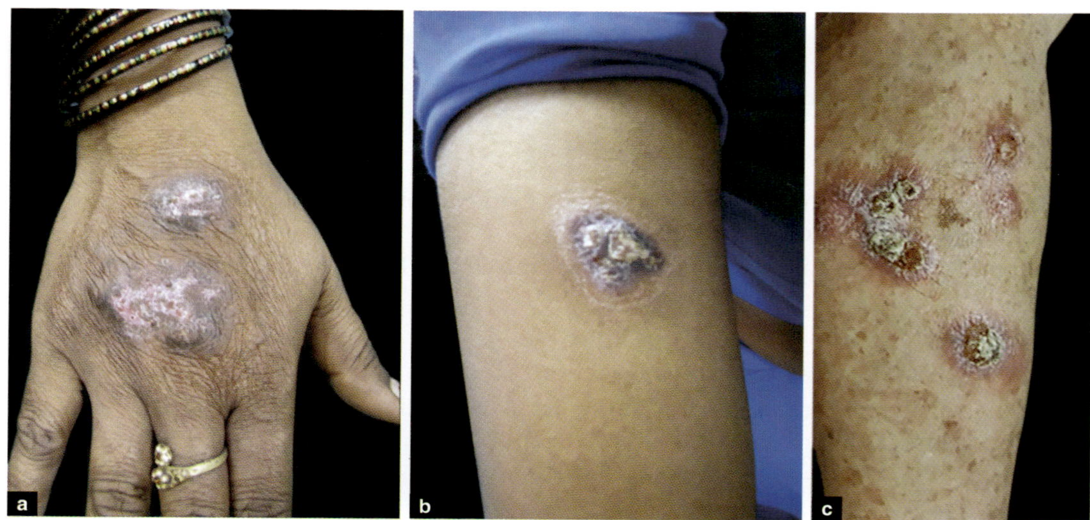

Fig. 17.28: Sporotrichosis: A sporotrichoid distribution can be discerned in these images

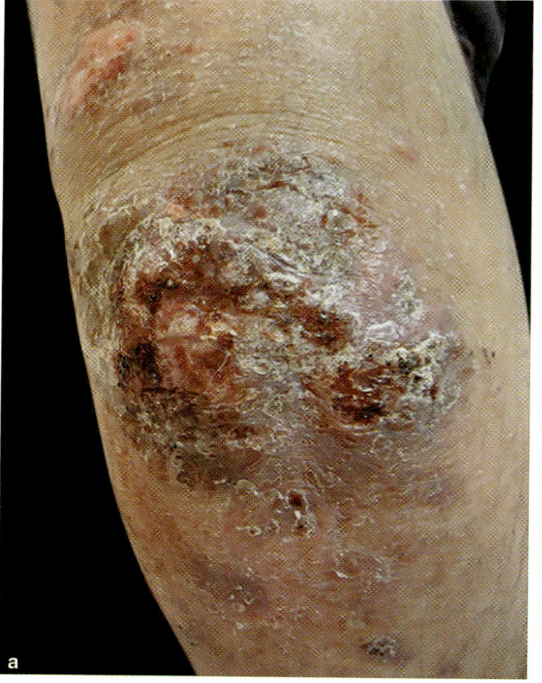

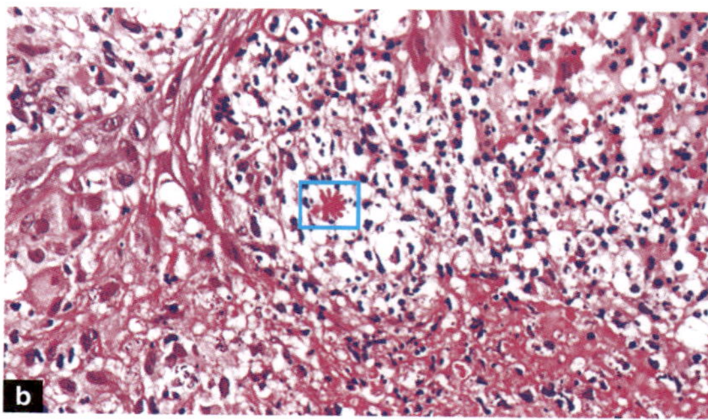

Fig. 17.29: (a) Sporotrichosis: Fixed variant (*Courtesy*: Dr Roberto Arenas, México City); (b) Sporotrichosis showing asteroid bodies within dermal abscesses

Differential Diagnosis

- **Sporotrichoid mimickers** *'mnemonic'*: No SALT—*Nocardia*, sporotrichosis, atypical mycobacteria, leishmaniasis, tularemia (a detailed list is given in **Table 17.17**).
- **Fixed type:** Lupus vulgaris, SCC, leishmaniasis, fish tank granuloma.

TABLE 17.17: Infectious and noninfectious causes of nodular lymphangiitis

Infectious	Non-infectious
Fungi • *Sporothrix schenckii* • *Blastomyces dermatitidis* • *Coccidioides immitis* • *Histoplasma capsulatum* • *Cryptococcus neoformans* • *Scedosporium apiospermum* • *Fusarium* sp • *Scopulariopsis blochii* *Bacteria* • *Nocardia* sp • *Pseudomonas* (*Burkholderia*) *pseudomallei* • *Francisella tularensis* • *Staphylococcus aureus* • *Streptococcus pyogenes* • *Bacillus anthracis* • *Erysilopethrix rhusiopathiae* *Mycobacterium* sp • NTM *Protozoa* • *Leishmania* sp *Viruses* • *Cowpox virus* (*Vaccinia virus*) • *Herpes simplex*	• Pyogenic granuloma • Sarcoidosis • Cutaneous PAN • Keratoacanthomas • BCC • SCC • T cell lymphoma • Langerhans' cell histiocytosis

An algorithmic approach to nodular lymphangiitis based on the smear characteristics is given in **Flowchart 17.6**.

Diagnosis

- **Samples**—smears, exudates and biopsy.
- **Culture on Sabouraud's agar:** The gold *standard* for diagnosis is the isolation of the fungus in Sabouraud agar. Culture is positve in 1 week in 90% of cases. In the remaining 10% it may take up to 4 weeks to achieve a positive result on Sabouraud agar culture. The colony is characterized by pigmented, membranous, radiated growth and the characteristic *microscopic features* of sympodial conidia resembling *daisy flowers*.
- **Microscopy:** They are diagnosed by demonstrating dimorphism, or conversion to the yeast phase. Oval to pyriform hyaline conidia produce along the sides of the hyphae.
- **HPE:** A hyperplastic epidermis, with or without ulceration, is seen with characteristic "sporotrichoid" suppurative granuloma seen in more than 80% of cases.

  The **sporotrichoid granuloma**—central microabscess with neutrophils and necrosis, with lymphocytes and macrophages, surrounded by plasma cells, fibroblasts, and blood vessels. **Asteroid bodies** may be observed in the centre of the granuloma in approximately 20% of cases, but they are not pathognomonic of the disease **(Fig. 17.29b)**. The asteroid body is thought to be a resistance mechanism of the yeast. It is surrounded by an eosinophilic radiating matrix **(Splendore-Hoeppli phenomenon)** composed of IgM and IgG antibodies that protect it from phagocytes.
- Intradermal sporotrichin skin test and molecular tests.

Flowchart 17.6: Algorithm for diagnostic approach in nodular lymphangiitis

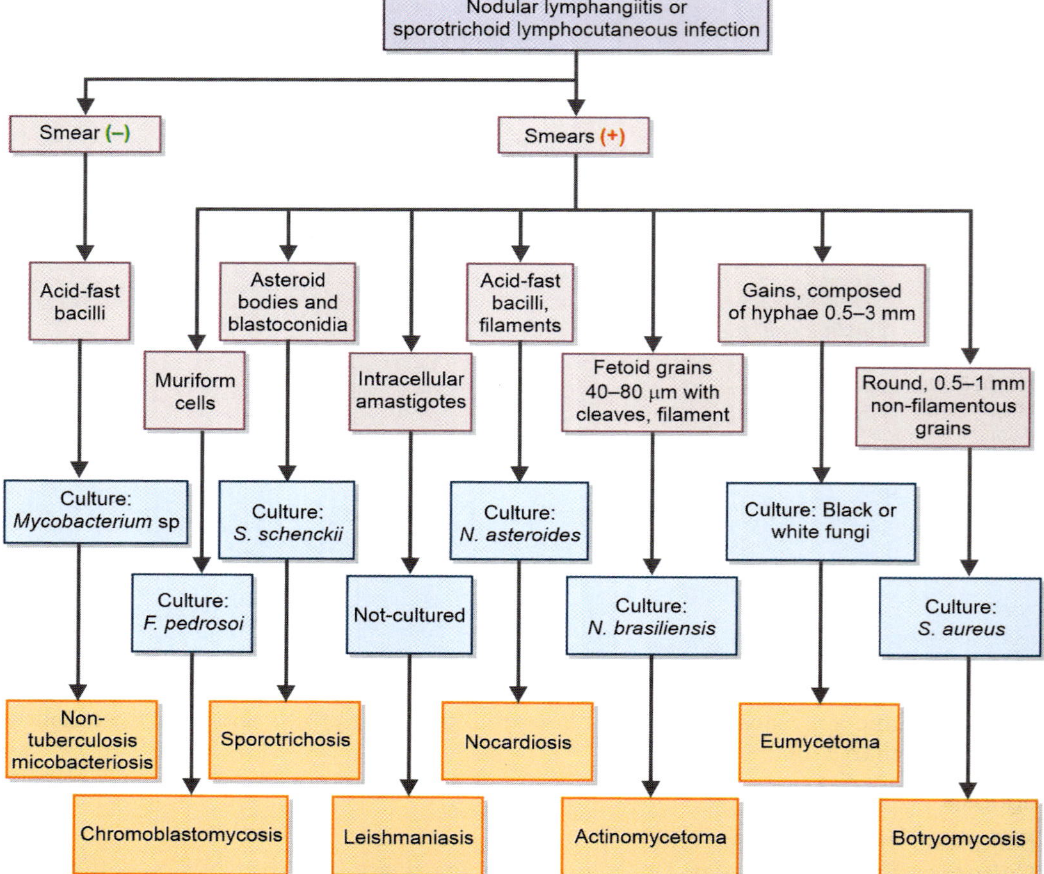

Treatment

Treatment includes localized physical therapies, saturated solution of potassium iodide (SSKI), azoles, terbinafine, and amphotericin B.

Thermotherapy

The rationale for heat therapy is the inhibition of fungal growth and enhanced killing by neutrophils; skin temperature should be maintained above 42°C for 30 minutes twice a day.

SSKI

It is used in cutaneous forms, especially fixed cases. It is known to have a immunomodulatory action, it suppresses the production of toxic intermediates from oxygen by the polymorphonuclear leukocytes and therefore, exert its anti-inflammatory effect. The dose is 5 drops TDS and increased as tolerated to 30 drops three times daily (47 mg/drop-SSKI). Dose is increased by 5 drops/week. In a study from India the initial response was seen in 2 weeks and treatment was curative in 76.8% patients and lesions healed in 2–9 months (average 5.2

months) (Sharam R, 2021). Treatment is continued for 3–4 weeks after clinical cure. Side effects include gastric intolerance, edema, rash, and erythema nodosum. Thyroid suppression (Wolff-Chaikoff effect) or thyrotoxicosis (Jod-Basedow effect) must be avoided, detected, and treated.

Antifungal Drugs

- *Sporothrix brasiliensis* is the major pathogen involved in feline-to-human sporotrichosis in and displays more virulent genotypes than the closely related species *S. schenckii*.
- Terbinafine has been demonstrated to be highly active *in vitro*, followed by ketoconazole and posaconazole.
  1. Terbinafine (*S. schenckii*)—250–500 mg for 3 or 4 months.
  2. Itraconazole: It should be initiated at a loading dose of 200 mg three times daily for 3 days, followed by 100–400 mg daily, depending on disease severity. It may be administered continuously or intermittently (pulse). Itrconazole is less effective against S. brasiliensis and this is due to the resistance mechanisms developed by this species, due to overexpression of efflux pumps. Of the other azoles posaconazole is effective against disseminated sporotrichosis in murine models.
  3. Fluconazole has been therapeutically effective in pregnant patients with sporotrichosis.
  4. Amphotericin B: Extracutaneous, immunosuppression and disseminated disease. Median doses of amphotericin B used in a large study was 750 mg and 4500 mg for deoxycholate and lipid complex formulations, respectively. Survival analysis showed an association between cure and the absence of bone, upper airway, and central nervous system involvemen. Sporothrix brasiliensis was the (Rodrigues AM, 2022).

MYCETOMA

- Also known as: Madura foot, maduramycosis.
- Chronic, localized infection of subcutaneous tissue characterized by single or multiple discharging sinuses. It could be due to fungi or actinomycetes.
- Causative organisms are listed in **Table 17.18**.

Epidemiology

- First described by Dr John Gill in 1842 in Madurai, India.
- Confined to tropical and subtropical climates ('Mycetoma belt').

TABLE 17.18: Common causative organisms of mycetoma

Dark grain eumycetoma	Pale grain eumycetoma	Actinomycotic mycetoma
Madurella mycetomatis	*Pseudallescheria boydii* **(*Scedosporium apiospermum*)**	***Nocardia brasiliensis*** (pale grains) ***Actinomadura madurae*** ***Actinomadura mexicana***
Madurella grisea	*Fusarium* spp.	*White* **(*Actinomadura syzygii* *Actinomadura bangladeshensis*)**
Curvularia geniculata	*Acremonium falciforme*	***Actinomadura pelletieri*** (pink-red grains)
Exophiala jeanselmei	*Aspergillus nidulans*	*Streptomyces* spp (yellow-brown grains)
Phialophora verrucosa		

MC in India—*Madurella mycetomatis, Nocardia brasiliensis* (Species in bold are commonly implicated).

- Most frequent organisms causing **actinomycetoma**: *Streptomyces somaliensis, Actinomadura madurae, A. pelletieri, Nocardia brasiliensis* and *N. asteroides*. The actinomycetoma-causative agents have a wide spatial geographical distribution worldwide. In parts of Latin America, notably Mexico, *Nocardia brasiliensis* is the most common causative agent reported while in Africa, *Streptomyces somaliensis, Actinomadura madurae* and *Actinomadura pelletieri* are frequently reported.
- Most common pathogens reported in **eumycetoma**: *M. mycetomatis, M. grisea, Pseudoallescheria boydii* (*anamorph Scedosporium apiospermum*) and *Leptosphaeria senegalensis*.
- By mapping mycetoma causative agents, an association with **Acacia trees** was found.

Predisposing Factors

Working in fields barefeet, malnutrition, cuts or injury on exposed parts of body.

Pathogenesis

- Inoculation of organism in the subcutaneous tissue by penetrating injury/thorn.
- Persistence of organism depends on its ability to evade host defense mechanisms, such as:
  - Formation of cell clusters or grains.
  - In actinomycetes, it forms a protective matrix.
  - In fungi, cell wall thickening due to intrahyphal growth and increase linkage to adjacent cell walls, deposition of melanin in cell wall and surrounding matrix.
  - The black colour of *M. mycetomatis* grains is due to the fungi ability to produce two types of melanin: Pyomelanin and dihydroxynaphthalene (DHN)-melanin. DHN melanin has the following protective effects:
    - It reduces the *in vitro* efficacy of itraconazole and ketoconazole by hindering the accessibility of these drugs to the fungal mycelia. *In vitro* studies have shown that the melanin pigments produced by *M. mycetomatis*, increases the MIC for itraconazole by 32 times and ketoconazole by 64 times, whereas the MIC for amphotericin B, posaconazole, and voriconazole were not affected.
    - Acts as a scavenger for free radicals produced by host.
    - Fungi were seen to increase the production of DHN-melanin when challenged with itraconazole, possibly conferring additional protection against the drug.

Clinical Features

In a study of patients in India, the average time to presentation with disease from history of probable inciting trauma was 3 years for *N. brasiliensis*, 7 years for *A. madurae*, and 9 years for *T. grisea* [Maiti et al].

Characteristic features of eumycetoma **(Fig. 17.30)** and actinomycetoma **(Fig. 17.31)** closely resemble each other and their differentiation is required for proper management. A comparison of the types of mycetoma is detailed in **Table 17.19**.

In spite of significant similarity, **actinomycetoma** tends to be **more aggressive** and **destructive, rapidly proliferating, inflammatory** and invades bone faster than eumycetoma.

Early Stage

- Starts as firm painless nodule at the site of inoculation which gradually progress to form papules or pustules and in-turn forms multiple discharging sinuses on skin surface.

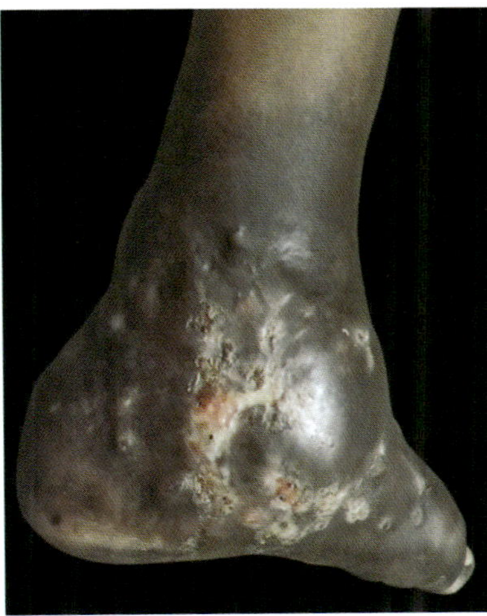

Fig. 17.30: Eumycotic mycetoma of the foot: Black grains popping out from a nodule are seen. Old nodules have become fibrosed. Hyperpigmentation is seen (*Courtesy*: Dr R Madhu)

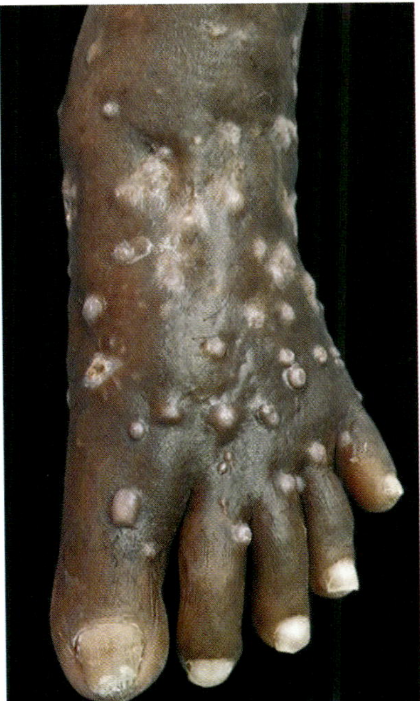

Fig. 17.31: Actinomycotic mycetoma of the foot: Swelling with multiple nodules and sinuses seen (*Courtesy*: Dr R Madhu)

- Later on, the area becomes hard and swollen.
- Involvement of underlying bone and joints can lead to periostitis, osteomyelitis and arthritis.
- Pain is hardly felt at this stage and has only been reported in 15% of patients. This absence of pain has been attributed to production of anesthetic substances by the organism.

TABLE 17.19: A comparison of the types of mycetoma

Characteristics	Eumycetoma	Actinomycetoma
Site	Usually hands, feet and other parts of arms and legs	Feet and hands, also chest, abdomen and head
Course	*Slow*	Rapid
Morphology	Well encapsulated with a clear margin	Diffuse, no clear margin
Sinus (number, morphology)	*Few, proliferative, protuberant*	Many, depressed, flat
Fistula	*Few*	Many
Bone	Delayed invasion and rare Cavities: *Fewer* but larger with clear margins on X-rays Dot in circle	Rapid Numerous, small with unclear margins Dot in circle
Lymphatic spread	Rarely	Frequent, sporotrichoid Nocardial infections are known
Veins proximal to lesion	Dilated	No
Grains/hyphae	Larger (0.5–2 mm) Coarser Melanin (+) Septate hyphae (4–5 μm thick)	Smaller (20–100 μm) Finer Melanin (–) Fine, branching filaments (<1 μm)
Color of grains	Different colors, but mostly white or black; coarse texture	Different colors but not black; fine texture
Stain	Modified AFB (–) Masson-Fontana silver/GMS (+) PAS staining (+) B and B staining (–)	Weakly positive (Nocardia) (–) (–) (+)
Treatment	Treatment—respond less well to drug therapy (mostly azoles, amphotericin B). Usually need debridement/surgical excision/amputation (last resort) with antifungals × 6 months pre-and post-surgery	Respond better to drugs—long course. Cotrimoxazole and aminoglycosides-mainstay. +/– rifampicin

B and B stain—Brown and Brenn stain

Late Phase of Mycetoma

- **Triad:** Classical **painless subcutaneous mass, multiple sinuses, and discharge containing grains (Fig. 17.32)**.
- Vital structures, such as tendons and nerves, are usually well preserved until late in the disease course due to adequate supply of blood in mycetoma.
- Regional lymph nodes may enlarge as a result of superimposed bacterial infection.

Differential Diagnosis

A tabular summary of the common grains is given in **Table 17.20**.

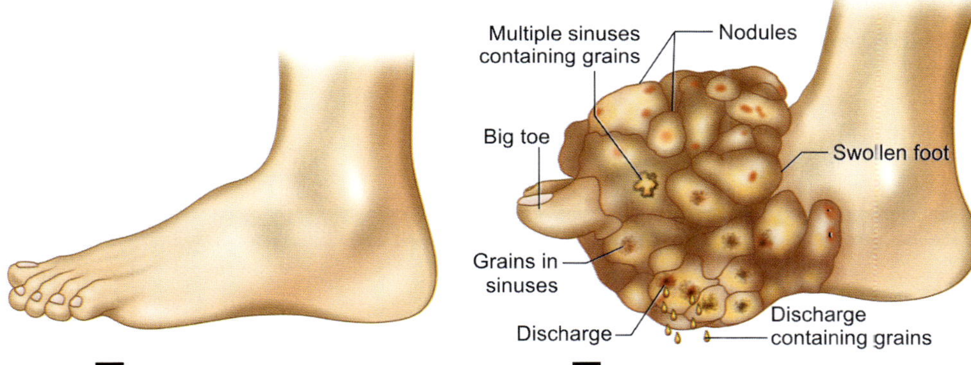

Fig. 17.32: Schematic diagram showing: (a) A normal foot and (b) foot disfigured by the destructive nature of mycetoma due to delay in instituting clinical management

TABLE 17.20: Characteristics of different grains according to stains (also *see* Fig. 17.3)

Stain	Botryomycosis	Actinomycetoma	Eumycetoma	Actinomycosis
Hematoxylin and eosin	Eosinophilic periphery and basophilic center	Basophilic mass of microfilaments	Basophilic or eosinophilic vesicles and filaments	Basophilic mass of microfilaments
Grocott-Gomori methenamine silver	Negative	Positive	Positive	Positive
Periodic acid–Schiff	Positive (bright)	Negative	Positive	Positive
Gram	Gram-positive or gram-negative clusters of bacteria	Gram-positive mass of filaments	Gram-negative	Gram-positive
Ziehl-Neelsen	Negative	Partially positive (*Nocardia* spp)	Negative	Negative

Investigations (Box 17.19)

- **Direct microscopy of grains (Table 17.21):** Grains are commonly obtained by *deep surgical biopsies* under aseptic conditions to avoid contamination. Grains obtained from open sinuses are commonly not viable and often contaminated.
  i. The grains can be directly examined under light microscope using 10% potassium hydroxide (KOH), Gram's stain and modified ZN stain:
    – Actinomycetoma causative organisms are gram-positive, while eumycetoma causative organisms are Gram-negative. *M. mycetomatis* have a light to drak brown color, *A. madura* stain violet and *A. pelletieri* are violet stained and have a fractured outline.
    – On inspection, actinomycetes are recognized by the production of 0.5 to 1 µm—wide filaments and fungi by 2 to 5 µm—wide hyphae.
    – The ZN staining technique is superior in discriminating between actinomycotic agents; *Nocardia* spp. are ZN positive (modified ZN with 1% H_2SO_4), whereas *A. madurae* and *S. somaliensis* are ZN negative.

BOX 17.19: Investigations in mycetoma

- **Direct microscopy of grains**
- **Imaging**
  - X-ray
  - Ultrasound
  - CT/MRI (dot in circle)
- **Tissue biopsy**
  - Culture
  - HPE
  - PCR

TABLE 17.21: Direct microscopy of grains of eumycetoma and actinomycetoma

	Eumycetoma	Actinomycetoma
Gram stain	Gram-negative	Gram-positive
Feature of organism	2–5 μm thick wide, septate hyphae ***Madurella mycetomatis*:** Large granules (up to 1–2 mm or more) with interlacing hyphae embedded in interstitial brownish matrix; hyphae at periphery arranged radially with numerous chlamydospores ***Scedosporium apiospermum*** (formerly Pseudallescheria boydii): Eosinophilic, lighter in the center; numerous vesicles or swollen hyphae; peripheral eosinophilic fringe	0.5–1 μm thin filaments ***Actinomadura madurae*:** Large (1–5 mm) and multilobulate; peripherally basophilic and centrally eosinophilic or pale-stained; filaments grow from the peripheral zone ***Streptomyces somaliensis*:** Large 0.5–2 mm or more) with dense thin filaments; often homogenously stained; transverse fracture lines ***Actinomyces israelii*:** Small grains (approximately 1 mm); central purple zone; loose clumps of filaments; Gram-positive delicate branching filaments breaking up into bacillary and coccal forms; Gram-negative amorphous matrix

ii. **Gross examination of Grains**
   - Color: Black—fungal, red/pale—actinomycetes. Eumycetoma causative organisms produce black or pale grains **(Fig. 17.33)**, and rarely yellow, and actinomycotic mycetoma commonly is caused by organisms that produce yellow, white, or red grains.
   - Size: *Madurella mycetomatis* and *A. madurae* have *large grains*, whereas *Nocardia brasiliensis*, *N. cavae*, and *N. asteroids* grains are *small* in size.
   - Consistency—most grains are soft, but *Streptomyces somaliensis* and *M. mycetomatis* are quite hard.

- **Culture:** Differentiation of the various dematiaceous fungi on the basis of morphology is sometimes difficult and time consuming, and culture usually takes about 3 weeks to give an accurate result. If extruded grains are used, most experts suggest rinsing these in 70% alcohol or with antibiotic-containing saline solutions to decrease bacterial contamination.
- **HPE (Figs 17.34 and 17.35):** Pseudoepitheliomatous hyperplasia, chronic inflammatory reaction leading to formation of focal neutrophilic abscesses with giant cells and fibrosis. Grains are formed by the compact colonies of organisms. Homogeneous eosinophilic material around the grain in a star-shaped manner **(Splendore–Hoeppli reaction)** can be seen in actinomycetomas.

- Special stains for eumycetoma—Gomori methamine silver or PAS stains. The host tissue reaction against the mycetoma causative organisms is distinctive. For actinomycetoma—Gram's stain and modified ZN stain. A approach to diagnosis of actinomycotic mycetoma is given in the **Fig. 17.35**.

- **Serology:** ELISA—low sensitivity.

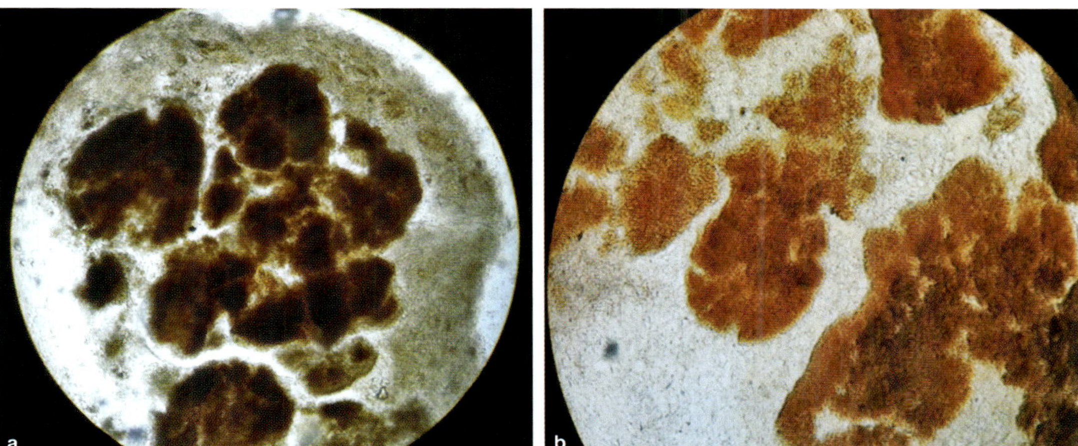

Fig. 17.33: (a) Low power view of potassium hydroxide (KOH) mount of discharge from a eumycetoma nodule: Multiple black grains are seen; (b) High-power view of the KOH mount showing eumycotic black grains with hyphae and chlamydospores in the periphery of the grains (*Courtesy*: Dr R Madhu)

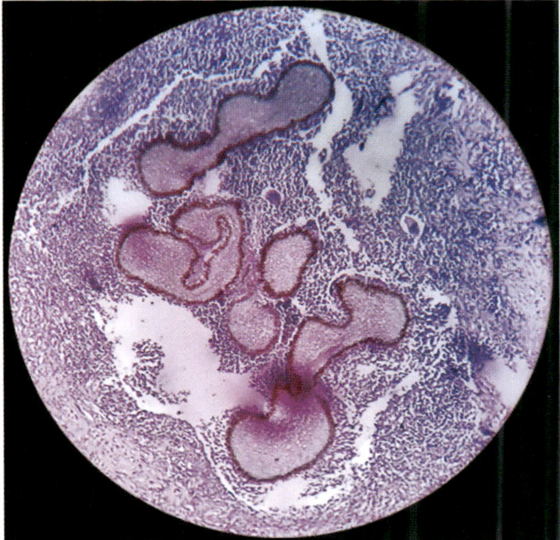

Fig. 17.34a: Low power view of histopathology (H&E) of eumycetoma showing multiple grains of *Madurella mycetomatis* seen as large rounded, oval or trilobed brown-colored grains with radiating hyphae and chlamydospores in the periphery, present within suppurative granulomatous reaction. Multiple vesicles are seen in the center of the grain (*Courtesy*: Dr R Madhu)

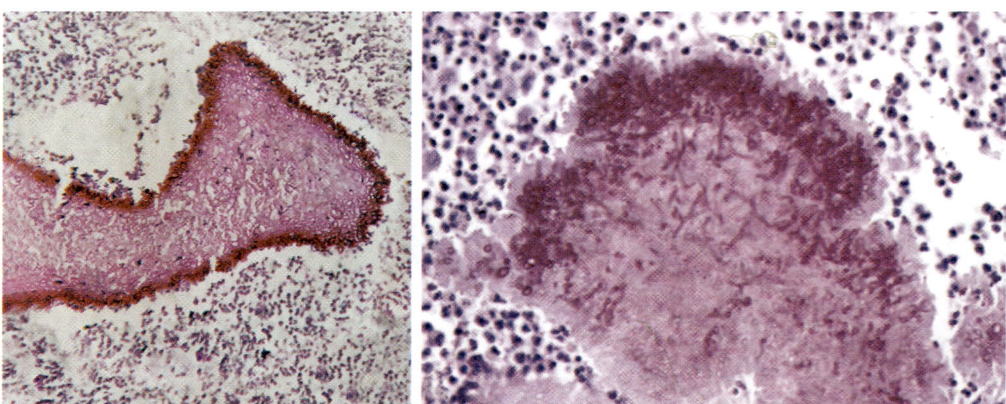

Fig. 17.34b: High power view of histopathology (H&E) of *Madurella mycetomatis*. Brown septate, radially arranged hyphae seen in the periphery (cortex) are slightly more swollen towards the edges. Hyphae are present in a haphazard manner in the medulla of the grain (*Courtesy*: Dr R Madhu)

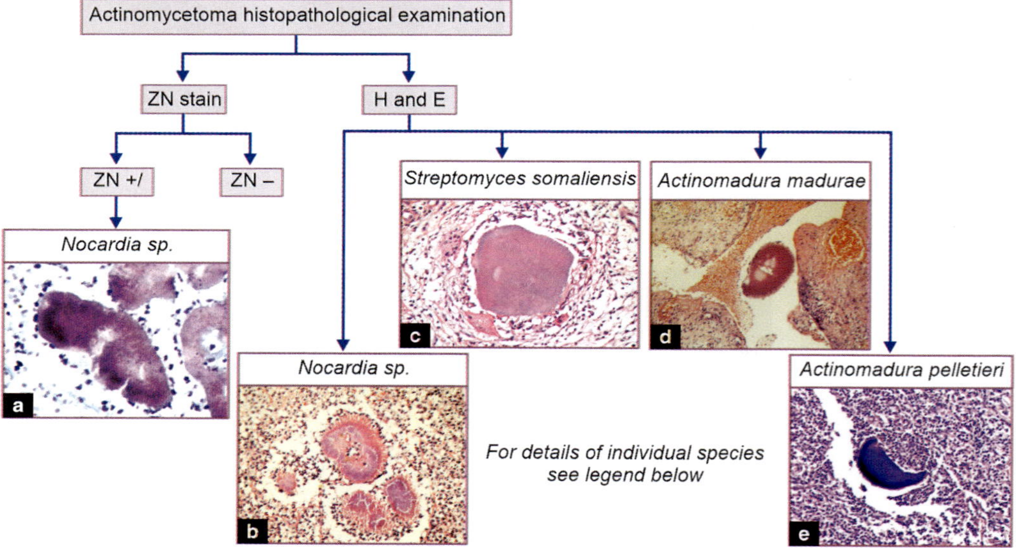

Fig. 17.35: Approach to diagnosis of grains of actinomycotic mycetoma

Histopathological appearance of individual species is given below:

(a) Histopathological appearance of Nocardia spp. grains shown to be positive by ZN staining; (b) Nocardia grains are small and rounded in shape about 40–70 µm in the smaller diameter and 70–100 µm in the larger diameter. The grains of Nocardia spp. stain bluish with routine H&E staining they have eosinophilic rays (finger-like) at the periphery; (c) The grains of Streptomyces are multilobulated measure about 250–600 µm in diameter, they have a smooth outline and as result of sectioning, they may show longitudinal cracks. Inside the grain, the filaments are fine (measuring 0.5–2 µm in diameter) and closely packaged and embedded in a cement matrix; (d) *Actinomadura*: The large grains have a characteristic variegated pattern. The periphery of the grain is opaque, homogenous and deep purple when stained with H&E, while the centre is less dense. Additionally, the periphery of the grains shows an immunoglobulin-rich eosinophilic material. *A. madurae* have a more deeply stained purple fringe; (e) *A. pelletieri* are smaller than *A. madurae* grains and measure about 60–150 m in diameter. They stain with a characteristic deep violet colour when using H&E staining. They are small in size and round to oval but semicircular, and sickle-like shapes have been observed.

- **Molecular-based identification methods** are more accurate.
- **Recent advances:** PCR on biopsy sample.
- **Radiographic studies**
  - X-ray can reveal bony involvement such as periosteal erosion secondary to invasion, osteoporosis, and changes consistent with osteomyelitis, including lytic lesions. Eumycetoma were found to produce single or multiple thick-walled cavities, without acoustic enhancement, with grains represented as distinct hyperreflective echoes. Actinomycetoma produced similar results, except grains produced fine echoes that were found at the bottom of the cavities.
  - Magnetic resonance imaging (MRI) and computed tomography (CT)—computed tomography appears to be more sensitive for detecting early changes consistent with bone involvement. A **dot-in-circle** sign has been described as a potentially specific diagnostic finding seen with **MRI**.

    [The dots are tiny hypointense foci (believed to be grains) within spherical, high-intensity lesions (the circle) surrounded by low-intensity matrix on T2-weighted imaging, which represent granulomas scattered in areas of fibrosis. An MRI grading system has been developed by the Mycetoma Research Centre (Khartoum, Sudan) for use in the diagnosis and management of mycetoma (El Shamy ME)]

Treatment

Treatment of mycetoma is still based on expert opinion in the absence of WHO treatment guidelines.

Actinomycetoma

Principle: The basic principle of the regimen was to combine an aminoglycoside with TMP/SMX. But there is a need to use MIC data to use better regimens which are more effective and safer than the use of Aminoglycosides.

In case of resistance or intolerance to cotrimoxazole or amikacin, amoxicillin-clavulanic acid can be used as an alternative to cotrimoxazole and netilmicin to amikacin. Alternative drugs that can be used in case of intolerance to TMP/SMX include: Minocycline, Amoxy/Clavulanate, Linezolid, the last of which should be given as a salvage therapy.

- **Welsh regime:**

  Initial—15 mg/kg IM of amikacin in 2 doses + sulfamethoxazole (35 mg/kg/day) and trimethoprim (7 mg/kg/day) in 3 divided doses for **21 days** with **15-day intervals.**

  (Most require one or two cycles; none required more than four cycles)

  Maintenance phase: Trimethoprim and sulfamethoxazole (7 mg/kg/day and 35 mg/kg/day, respectively) administered for 2 weeks after the last cycle.
- **Modified Welsh regime:**

  Initial—15 mg/kg/day of **amikacin** in divided doses + sulfamethoxazole-trimethoprim tablets (35 mg/kg/day + 7 mg/kg/day) + **rifampicin** capsule (10 mg/kg/day) for **21 days** (1–3 cycles of 15 days intervals).

  Maintenance: Sulfamethoxazole-trimethoprim tablets (35 mg/kg/day + 7 mg/kg/day) + **rifampicin** capsule (10 mg/kg/day) for 3 months in the maintenance phase.
- **Modified two-step regime (Raman et al. 2007):**

  Initial—**gentamicin** (80 mg twice daily, IV), and cotrimoxazole (two tablets of 960 mg twice daily) for **4 weeks** in the intensive phase.

  Maintenance: **Doxycycline** (100 mg orally, twice daily) and **cotrimoxazole** (two tablets of 960 mg twice daily) which are given until 5–6 months after complete healing of all sinuses.

The initial modifications were based on adding either doxycycline or rifampicin. **The newer regimens** use linezolid and penems (Sardana K, 2018). The 2 weeks interval of amikacin in the 5 weeks cycle is used for renal and audiometric monitoring. Other regimens are listed in **Table 17.22**.

Eumycetoma

- At present, the recommended treatment for eumycetoma is itraconazole 200–400 mg/day for 6–9 months followed by wide local excision, if the lesion is not fully cured by the drug. Postoperatively, itraconazole is continued until the patient is clinically, radiologically, ultrasonically, and cytologically cured.
- A patient is deemed clinically cured when the skin becomes normal, the mass disappears, the sinuses heal, and the organisms are eliminated from the tissue. Radiological examination is essential for follow-up of patients on medical treatment and to assure cure. It usually shows reappearance of normal bone pattern and the disappearance of the soft-tissue mass.
- Voriconazole and posaconazole have been assessed in a very limited number of patients with promising results. Isavuconazole and fosravuconazole were reported to have excellent *in vitro* activity.
- Because of its susceptibility pattern, mycetoma secondary to the *S. apiospermum* complex should be treated with voriconazole.
- *In vitro*, terbinafine has limited activity against *M. mycetomatis* compared with that observed with itraconazole, ketoconazole, or posaconazole.

The present treatments regimens are depicted in **Table 17.23**.

TABLE 17.22: Alternative treatments for actinomycetoma

Drug	Dose	Cure	Country
Oral TMP/SMX	(800 mg/160 mg) once daily for a minimum of 1 yr	60–90%	Sudan, Mexico and Senegal
Parenteral streptomycin + oral TMP/SMX	Streptomycin (14 mg/kg once daily) + TMP/SMX (800 mg/160 mg once daily)	63%	Sudan
Parenteral gentamicin	80 mg twice daily (for 4 weeks) then doxycycline (200 mg once daily) and TMP/SMX (800 mg/160 mg twice daily) given throughout therapy	66%	India
Parenteral amikacin + oral TMP/SMX	Parenteral amikacin (15 mg/kg once daily for 3 weeks cycle, up to 4 weeks) plus oral TMP/SMX (800 mg/160 mg once daily)	95%	Mexico
Parenteral imipenem, amikacin, oral TMP/SMX	Parenteral imipenem (1.5 g once daily) plus amikacin (15 mg/kg once daily) for 3 weeks cycle repeated every 6 months and oral TMP/SMX (800 mg/160 mg once daily)	40%	Mexico
Linezolid	600 mg twice daily for 2 months	Case report	USA
Rifampicin + TMP/SMX	Rifampicin (600 mg once daily) and TMP/SMX (800 mg/160 mg twice daily) for 10 months	Case report	India
Amoxicillin/clavulanic acid	Dose of 875/125 mg twice daily	71%	Mexico

SMX, sulfamethoxazole; TMP, trimethoprim, TMP/SMX → should always be part of the regimen as resistance to it is rare.

TABLE 17.23: Eumycetoma treatment

Drug	Dose	Cure	Country
Ketoconazole	200–400 mg once daily for 1 year + surgery	40–70%	Sudan and India
Terbinafine	500 mg twice daily for 24–48 weeks	25%	Senegal
Posaconazole	800 mg once daily for 24 months	80%	Argentina

CHROMOBLASTOMYCOSIS

- Also known as chromomycosis/verrucous dermatitis.
- Chronic fungal infection of skin and subcutaneous tissue.
- Causative organisms: ***Fonsecaea pedrosoi* (most common)**, *Rhinocladiella*, *Phialophora verrucosa*, and *Cladophialophora carrionii*.

Epidemiology

- Common in tropics with medium to heavy rainfall.
- Common in adult male farmers.

Predisposing Factors

Injury prone work like farming/gardening.

Pathogenesis

- Inoculation of fungi into subcutaneous tissue due to penetrating injury, puncture, wound.
- This leads to a foreign body granuloma formation along with foci of microabscess with presence of chestnut or golden brown-colored fungi in giant cells **(Medlar bodies) ("copper pennies")**.
- **Muriform or sclerotic cells** are thick-walled, single or multicelled clusters produed by fungi dividing in multiple planes **(Fig. 17.36)**.
- An imbalance between protective type 1 T-helper cell and less efficient type 2 T-helper cell responses has been noted. The humoral immune response involves IgM and IgA. Transforming growth factor-β has a double effect that induces fibrosis and immunosuppression in affected skin. Antimelanin antibodies are produced during human infection.

Clinical Features

- Presents as slowly progressive warty papules, which form a hypertrophic plaque with central scarring and active flat margin **(Fig. 17.37a)**.
- Plaque proceeds **centrifugally** and develops an irregular verrucous or papillomatous surface.
- Later on, it forms hyperkeratotic thick plaque with secondary ulceration, **satellite lesions**.
- Usually painless except with secondary bacterial infection.
- Lymphatic and hematogenous spread is exceptional.
  Multiple clinical types have been described (**Table 17.24**).

***Clinical course*:** Slowly progressive, nonfatal.

***Complications*:** Secondary bacterial infection due to chronic lymphatic stasis.

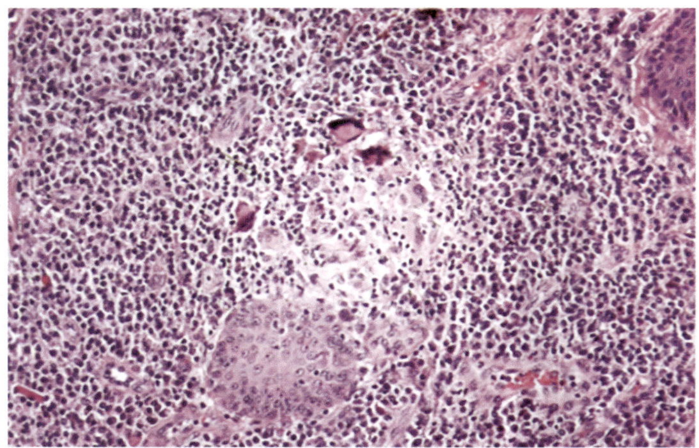

Fig. 17.38a: Suppurative granuloma within an abscess in chromoblastomycosis

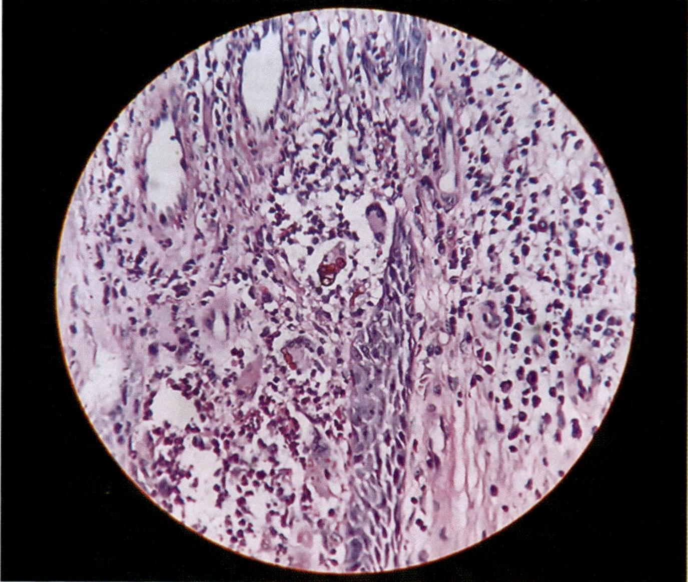

Fig. 17.38b: Sclerotic bodies seen in histopathological tissue section in H&E (x 400)

plasma cells, neutrophils, eosinophils, macrophages, and multi-nucleated giant cells. Fibrosis is present in older cases. Fumagoid cells are found alone or in clusters, both within and outside multi-nucleated giant cells, and can be identified with hematoxylin and eosin **(Fig. 17.38)**. **Box 17.20** lists recent developments in the diagnosis of subcutaneous mycoses.

Treatment

Treatment consists of long periods of anti-fungal drugs, often combined with physical treatments like surgery, cryotherapy, and thermotherapy. Studies report highly variable clinical and mycological cure rates, ranging from 15 to 80%.

BOX 17.20: Whats new? (Hay R, et al., 2019)

- WHO has formally recognized mycetoma and chromoblastomycosis as fungal neglected tropical diseases (NTDs), together with other unspecified deep mycoses viz. sporotrichosis.
- In basic healthcare settings, direct microscopy combined with clinical signs have been reported to be the most useful diagnostic indicators to prompt referral for treatment. Also, there is a key role of semi-invasive sampling methods such as biopsy for diagnosis as compared to swabs or impression smears.
- Recent developments in diagnosis of mycetoma include molecular methods to identify new etiologic agents, isothermal amplification techniques, adaptation of MALDI-ToF to fungal identification and finding of novel infection-related antigens.
- In chromoblastomycosis diagnostics also there is an upcoming role of molecular and MALDI ToF analyses.
- Though there have been major advances in identifying specific antigens, diagnosis of sporotrichosis is the most problematic with poor sensitivity across most widely available laboratory tests except fungal culture.

Drugs

Analysis of minimum inhibitory concentrations showed that the best drugs were—posaconazole, terbinafine, itraconazole and voriconazole.

In *drug combination* studies, terbinafine-voriconazole and itraconazole-caspofungin showed 100% of synergism for *Fonsecaea pedrosoi*, *Exophiala jeanselmei* and *Phialophora verrucosa*

1. Itraconazole (200–400 mg/day) and terbinafine (500–1000 mg/day) × 6–12 months.
   - The oral drugs can be given for 3 months before surgical excision and then for an additional 6–9 months.
   - Combination of itraconazole and fluorocytosine has only been evaluated in a small number of patients but has proven very effective even in severe forms of subcutaneous mycoses.
2. Pulse therapy with itraconazole (400 mg/day for 7 days/month).
3. Combination of an azole (itraconazole) and an allylamine (terbinafine) seems to be helpful in recalcitrant cases.
4. Combination of antifungal drugs with immunoadjuvant compounds such as glucan and imiquimod have been investigated in recent years.

PHAEOHYPHOMYCOSIS

- Also known as phaeomycotic subcutaneous cyst.
- **Causative organisms** (brown pigmented dematiaceous fungi):
  - *Exophiala jeanselmei*
  - *Alternaria* spp
  - *Cladophialophora bantiana*
  - *Exserohilum* spp
  - *Exophiala dermatitidis*
  - *Phialophora* spp
  - *Bipolaris* spp

Epidemiology

- Common in tropical climate
- Rare infection

Predisposing Factors

Immunocompromised state, e.g. on steroid therapy.

Pathogenesis

- Fungi is inoculated in subcutaneous tissue through penetrating injury.
- It leads to formation of *subcutaneous cyst*—well-organized wall with surrounding fibrosis, mixed cellular infiltrate with multinucleated giant cells, lymphocytes, macrophages and neutrophils.

Clinical Features

Well-defined, painless, single cystic lesion **(Fig. 17.39)** on trunk or limbs.

Clinical Course

No spontaneous healing.

Diagnosis

KOH: Hyphae are pigmented/brown, and also stain (+) with Fontana–Masson **(Fig. 17.40)**.

HPE: Single subcutaneous cyst with well-organized wall with surrounding fibrosis, mixed cellular infiltrate with multinucleated giant cells, lymphocytes, macrophages and neutrophils. Fungi can be seen in the cyst **(Fig. 17.41)**.

Treatment

First line	Second line
Excision	Post-excision oral itraconazole

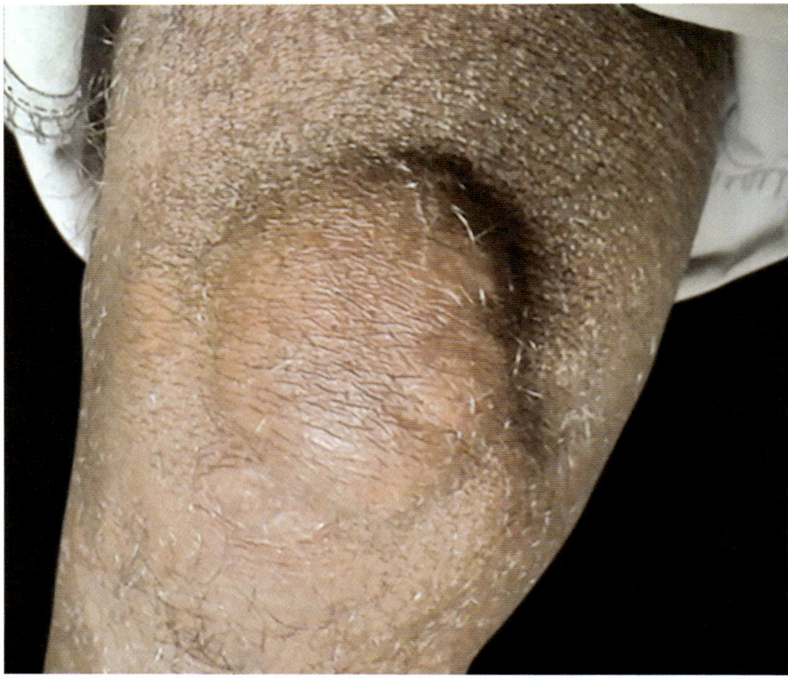

Fig. 17.39: Phaeohyphomycotic cyst in an immunocompetent male (*Courtesy*: Dr R Madhu)

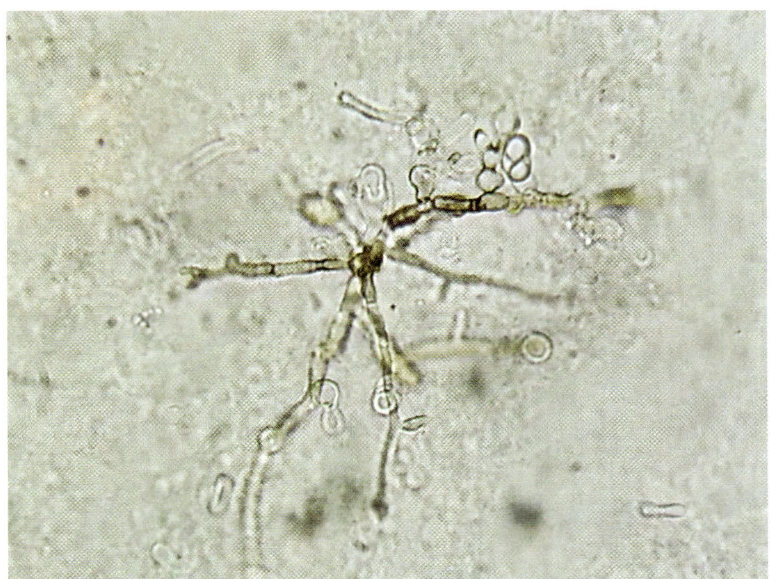

Fig. 17.40: High power view of KOH mount of phaeohyphomycosis showing brown-colored, septate moniliform hyphae and thin-walled yeast cells (*Courtesy*: Dr R Madhu)

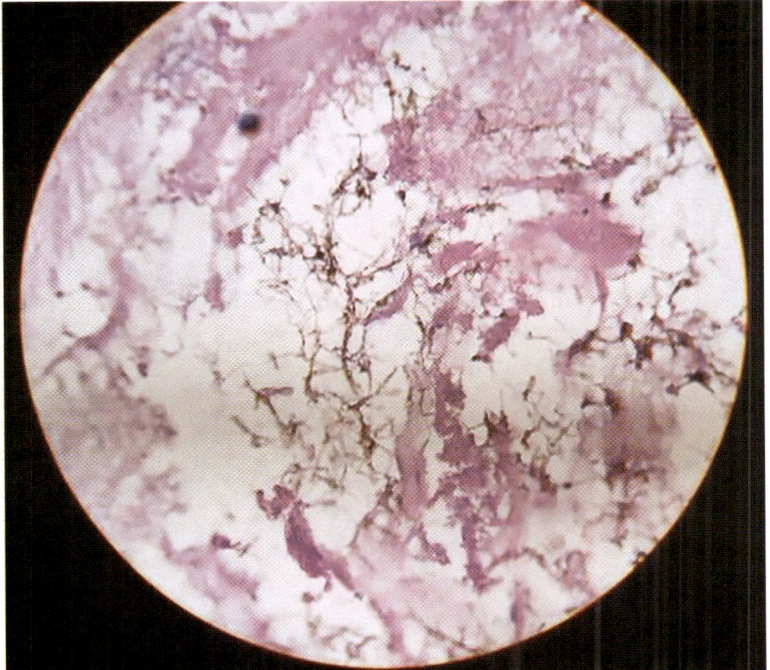

Fig. 17.41: Low power view of histopathology in H&E of phaeohyphomycosis showing pigmented (brown), septate moniliform hyphae (*Courtesy*: Dr R Madhu)

LOBOMYCOSIS

- Also known as Lobo disease/keloidal blastomycosis
- Causative organism: *Lacazia loboi*

Epidemiology

- Rare disease
- First reported in Amazon valley.

Predisposing Factors

Probably through contact of injured skin with infected water.

Clinical Features

- Usually present on exposed part of body.
- Present as elevated, crusted, keloidal/fungoid plaques.
- Autoinoculation may lead to spread of fungi.

Differential Diagnosis

Disease	Similarity	Dissimilarity
Chromoblastomycosis	Keloidal plaques	Muriform or sclerotic cells

Clinical Course

Slowly progressive, remains localized.

Complications

Squamous cell carcinoma in chronic lesions.

Diagnosis

- **HPE (H and E stain)**—diffuse lymphocytic infiltrate with macrophages and giant cells. Fungal cells, 5–10 µm in diameter, aligned in short chains of 3–8 oval or round, joined by short tubular structures, are present in giant cells.
- **Culture**—never been isolated *in vitro*.

Treatment

First line
Excision

RHINOSPORIDIOSIS

- **Causative organism:** *Rhinosporidium seeberi*.
- Organism has never been isolated *in vitro*.
- *Not a fungus*
- Taxonomical position is now changed to aquatic member of Protista.

Epidemiology

- Endemic in India and Sri Lanka
- More in adult males

Clinical Features of Classic Lesion

- Most common site—*mucous membrane of the nose*, the nasopharynx or soft palate (in ¾ cases) followed by conjunctiva or the lacrimal sac involvement (1/4 cases).
- Pedunculated or sessile growth **(Fig. 17.42)**.
- Presents as pink or red lobulated and cauliflower-like growth with small white spots on surface which represents the mature sporangia of fungus.
- It is not contagious.

Differential Diagnosis (Table 17.25)

TABLE 17.25: Differential diagnosis of rhinosporidiosis

Disease
Condylomata
Hemorrhoides
Genital warts

Clinical Course

Rarely spontaneous resolution.

Complications

Obstruction to breathing in nasal lesions.
In ocular lesions—conjunctivitis, photophobia or eversion of eyelids.

Diagnosis

Microscopy—single, thick-walled and spherical organism packed with numerous rounded endospores of 6–7 μm size in diameter when fully differentiated **(Fig. 17.43)**.

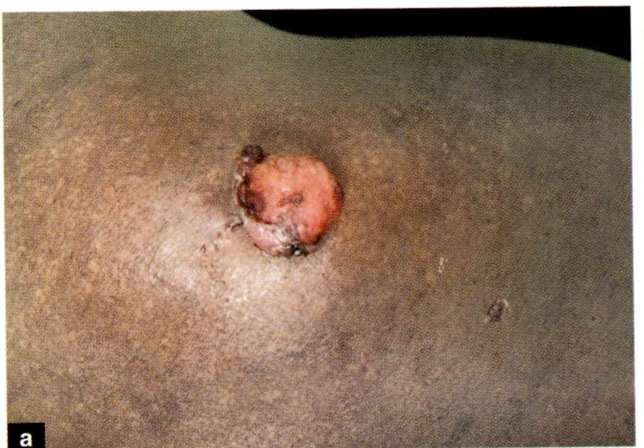
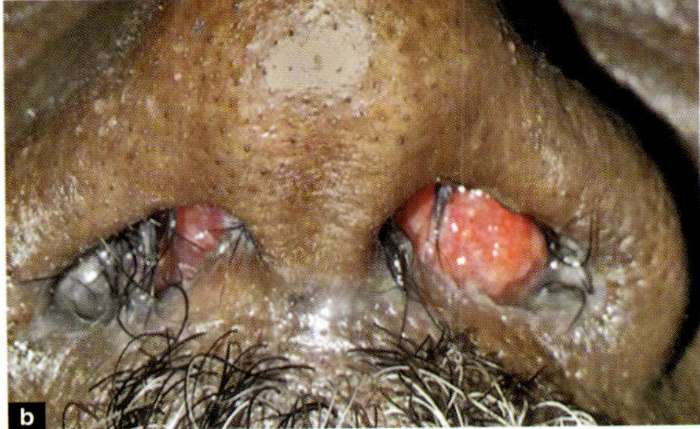

Fig. 17.42: (a) Cutaneous rhinosporidiosis—sessile fleshy mass seen; (b) Nasal rhinosporidiosis— fleshy polyps seen in both nostrils (*Courtesy*: Dr R Madhu)

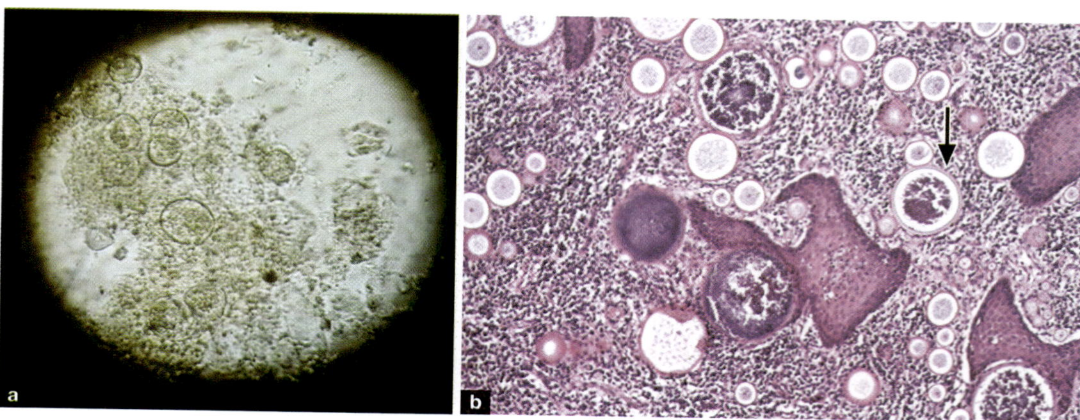

Fig. 17.43: (a) Low power view of KOH mount of rhinosporidiosis showing sporangia; (b) Low power view of histopathology (H&E) showing sporangia with endospores in different stages of maturation (*Courtesy*: Dr R Madhu); Cysts contain spores with a thick hyaline eosinophilic wall

HPE—large thick-walled sporangia with 1000+ endospores, accompanied by a mixed inflammatory infiltrate.

Treatment

Surgical removal.

VIRAL INFECTIONS

MOLLUSCUM CONTAGIOSUM (MC)

Epidemiology

Cause: MCV-1 (majority of infections), MCV-2 (HIV, adults), rarely MCV-3, 4. It is the only poxvirus (after smallpox eradication) that specifically afflicts humans.

Incidence: Two peaks—2–5 years and young adulthood (sexual transmission).

Predisposing Factors

- Atopic dermatitis (?due to TCS/TCI use)
- Widespread, atypical, giant, mucosal MC—in HIV, idiopathic CD4 lymphocytopenia, sarcoidosis, hematological malignancy, hyper-IgE syndrome, DOCK8 deficiency, immunosuppressive treatment.

Clinical Features

Shiny pearly-white hemispherical umbilicated papules with central core **(Fig. 17.44)**.

Clinical Course

- Individual lesions—2 months.
- Mostly self-limiting within 6–9 months.

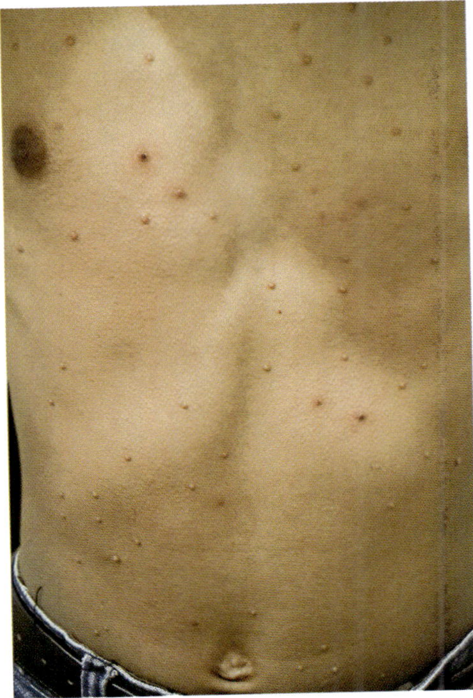

Fig. 17.44: Molluscum contagiosum. Some of the lesions show inflammation—a sign which precedes resolution and is known as the "beginning of the end" (BOTE) sign

Complications

- Eczematization around MC (especially in AD).
- Conjunctivitis/superficial punctate keratitis (near eyelid).
- Depressed scars/anetoderma-like lesions (after healing).

Differential Diagnosis (Table 17.26)

TABLE 17.26: Differential diagnosis of molluscum contagiosum

Disease	Similarity with MC	Dissimilarity with MC
Histoplasmosis, cryptococcosis, penicilliosis (HIV, immunosuppressed)	Central umbilication	Systemic features, microscopy
Pyogenic granuloma	Red like an inflamed MC	Bleeding on manipulation
Keratoacanthoma	Hemispherical dome-shaped nodule	Central keratin plug, larger
Plane warts (if many small lesions)	Papules	No central umbilication
Milia	White papule	Smaller, no central umbilication

Diagnosis

- **Bedside tests: Tzanck smear**—intracytoplasmic **molluscum bodies (Henderson–Paterson bodies):** The largest known inclusion bodies (30–35 μm), they are virus-transformed keratinocytes, appearing as ovoid, deeply basophilic bodies with a hyaline, homogeneous structure surrounded by a membrane, filled with eosinophilic granular inclusion bodies that contain MC virions and displace the nuclei to the periphery.
- **HPE:** Lobular hyperplasia of epidermis into dermis → cup-shaped lesions → keratinocytes of s. basale and s. spinosum become enlarged and transformed into—**Henderson–Paterson molluscum bodies** containing eosinophilic granular inclusion bodies **(Fig. 17.45)**.

  The virions increase in size as they progress up towards the *S. granulosum* → compress the nuclei to the periphery and change the staining to basophilic.
- **PCR** is now available for detection and typing but is currently used only in research settings.

Treatment

For treatment please *see* **Fig. 17.46**.

PITYRIASIS ROSEA (PR)

Epidemiology

- **Age:** 10–35 years (peak in adolescence)
- **Sex:** Slightly more in females

Predisposing Factors

None

Pathogenesis

- Herpesvirus-like particles have been found in 71% (15/21) PR lesions in a study. Viral DNA of human **herpesvirus 6 and 7 (HHV-6 and HHV-7)** has been reported in peripheral

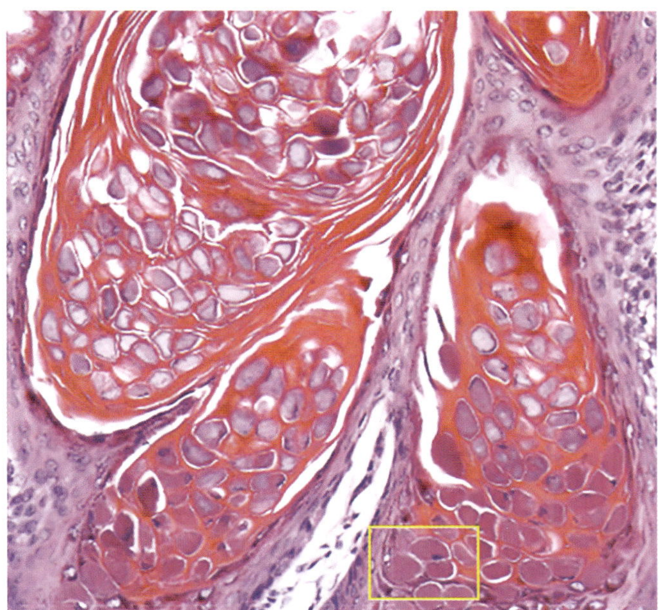

Fig. 17.45: The histology of molluscum contagiosum shows a lobulated, hyperplastic epidermis with the keratinocytes containing very large intracytoplasmic inclusions, which compress the nucleus against the cell membrane. These inclusion bodies are eosinophilic initially but acquires a basophilic tone when they are known as Henderson-Paterson or molluscum body

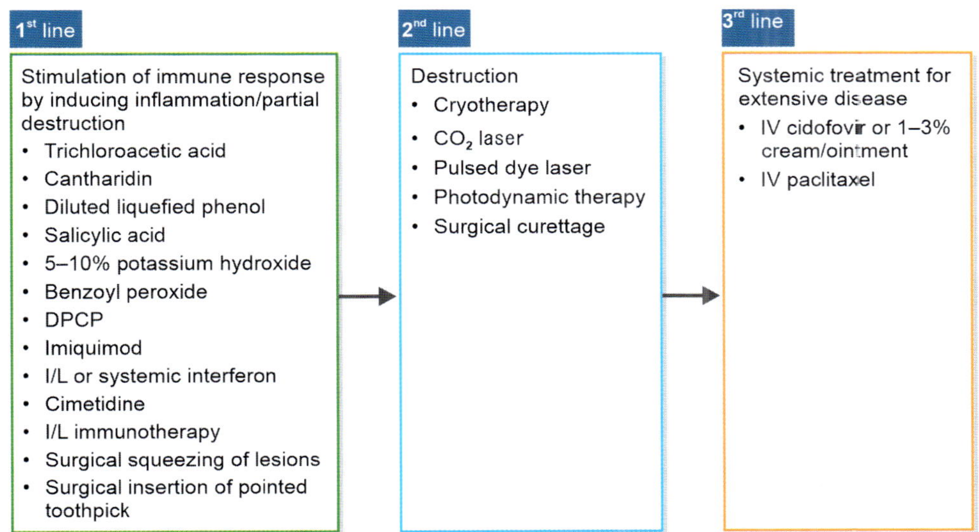

Fig. 17.46: Treatment of molluscum contagiosum (I/L: Interlesional)

blood mononuclear cells and in lesional and unaffected skin of patients. HHV-7 is detected more frequently than HHV-6. However, unaffected individuals may also have evidence of presence of HHV-6 and HHV-7; hence the causal relationship is still debatable.

- Possible association with HHV-8 and H1N1 also proposed.
- Certain drugs may also lead to a PR-like eruption **(Box 17.21)**.

BOX 17.21: Drugs causing pityriasis rosea-like eruption

ACE inhibitors, β-blockers, clonidine	Nortriptyline	Metronidazole
Adalimumab, rituximab	Griseofulvin, terbinafine	Omeprazole
Aspirin	Imatinib	Penicillin
Allopurinol	Isotretinoin	D-penicillamine
Barbiturates, lamotrigine	Ketotifen, levamisole	Vaccines—BCG, DT, hepatitis B, pneumococcal

Clinical Features

- Herald patch appears on arm/thigh/trunk—sharply defined, erythematous, round/oval patch covered with fine scales, 2–5 cm.
- Interval of 5–15 days before general eruption.
- General eruption begins to appear in crops over 7–10 days on trunk and proximal limbs—discrete oval dull-pink macules with marginal "collarette" of scales (attached at the periphery and free in the centre). Face and scalp involvement rare except in children. Palms and soles spared usually.
- Lesions are aligned with their long axes along lines of cleavage in a 'Christmas tree or fir tree' pattern.
- Hyperpigmented folliculocentric lesions may occur in darker skins.
- Oral lesions—red patches with a few erosions, punctate hemorrhages, bullae.
- Slight to moderate pruritus.
- Slight constitutional symptoms may occasionally accompany—fever, malaise, lymphadenopathy.

Clinical Types/Variants

Clinical variants of PR are numerous and are listed in **Table 17.27**.

TABLE 17.27: Clinical types of PR

Based on herald patch	Based on location of lesions	Based on morphology of lesions	Based on course of lesions
• No herald patch • Only herald patch • Multiple herald patches • Atypical location of herald patch	• Scalp only • Trunk only • Limbs-girdle only (pityriasis circinata et marginata of Vidal) • Flexures only • Extremities only • Acral only • Blaschkoid • Unilateral	• Purpuric • Urticaria • Erythema multiforme like • Papular • Follicular • Vesicular • Giant • Hypopigmented • Limited	• Relapsing • Recurrent • Persistent • Relapsing and persistent

Clinical Course

- Fades in 3–6 weeks (up to 3 months)
- Temporary hypo- or hyperpigmentation may occur in some
- 2%—recurrent PR

Complications

If it occurs in first trimester of pregnancy → higher risk of spontaneous abortion/preterm delivery/infant with hypotonia or hyporeactivity.

Differential Diagnosis

Differential diagnosis of PR are listed in **Table 17.28**.

TABLE 17.28: Differential diagnosis of pityriasis rosea (PR)

Disease	Differentiating features
Secondary syphilis	More systemic symptoms, peripheral lymphadenopathy, no herald patch, palms and soles affected, plasma cells on histology
Drug-induced eruption	No herald patch, severe pruritus, tendency to become very inflamed or lichenoid, resolution slower, eosinophil count high
Guttate psoriasis	Persistent lesions, smaller lesions, thicker silvery scales, scales attached in center and free peripherally (reverse of collarette), no fir tree appearance
Pityriasis lichenoides	Persistent lesions, polymorphic lesions, hemorrhagic crusts, adherent scales
Seborrheic dermatitis	Persistent lesions, no herald patch, mostly on upper midline of trunk, duller in color, thicker greasy scales
Tinea corporis (D/D of herald patch)	More erythematous and edematous, raised edges, marginal vesiculation may occur, scraping from edge KOH +ve

Diagnosis

Mostly clinical.

HPE: Spongiosis, patchy parakeratosis, acanthosis, psoriasiform hyperplasia and mononuclear cell infiltrate with exocytosis of lymphocytes to form subcorneal pustules.

Treatment

Figure 17.47 lists the treatment options. However, usually no treatment is required as it is a self-limiting disease

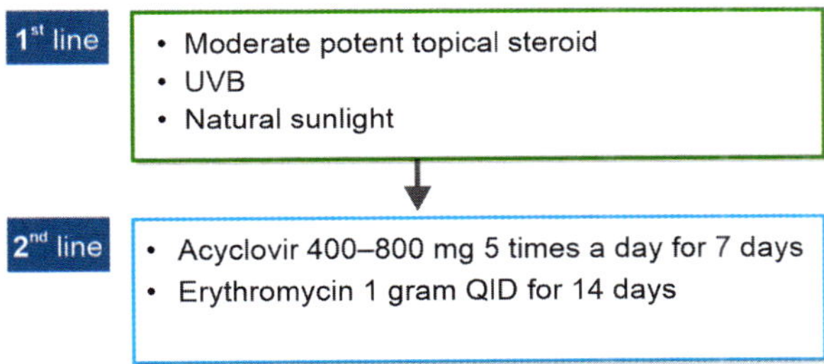

Fig. 17.47: Treatment of pityriasis rosea

HERPES ZOSTER (HZ)

Epidemiology

Zoster (= girdle)

Age: Incidence increases >50 years age.

Sex: Slightly more in females.

Predisposing Factors

Immunosuppression: HZ precipitated by—trauma/pressure to nerve roots, stem cell and organ transplantation, neoplastic deposits, surgery, radiotherapy, even trivial trauma.

Course of Infection and Clinical Course

- Pain +/– pruritus → unilateral (rarely bilateral) dermatomal skin eruption (grouped papules → vesicles → pustules) (after 1.4 days in trigeminal zoster and 3.2 days in thoracic zoster) **(Fig. 17.48)**.
- Mucous membranes within affected dermatome (s)—vesicles and erosions
- Regional tender lymphadenopathy
- "Zoster sine eruption"—pain is not followed by skin eruption.
- **Thoracic** > cervical > trigeminal (ophthalmic) > lumbosacral

Clinical Types/Variants

- **Disseminated zoster**—defined as more than **20 vesicles** outside the area of the primary and adjacent dermatomes—in 10% immunocompromised patients with HIV infection, immunosuppressed, lymphomas, bone marrow transplants, anti-TNF-α therapy.

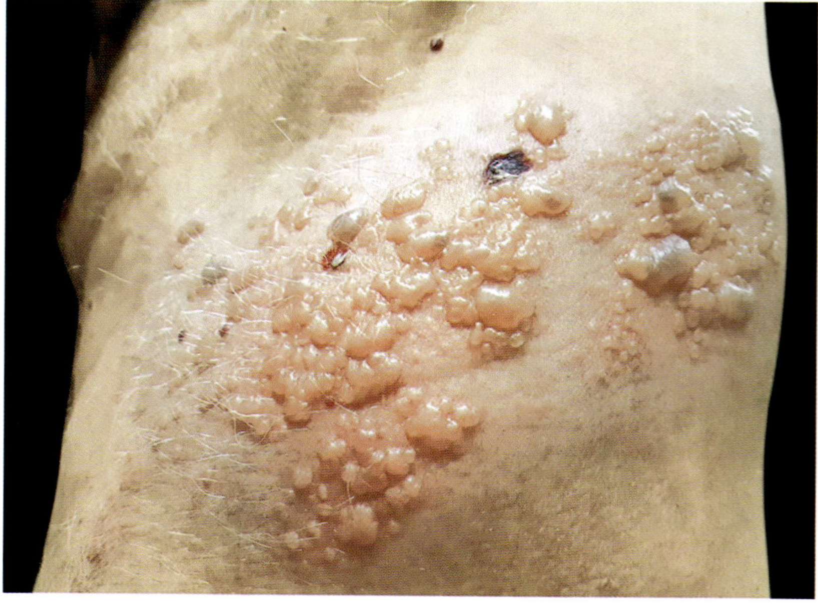

Fig. 17.48: Herpes zoster (thoracic)

- **Zoster in pregnancy**—not associated with intrauterine infection of fetus.
- **Zoster in infancy**—may follow material varicella, with the baby having developed varicella *in utero*.
- **Trigeminal nerve zoster:**
  - Most commonly involved division is **ophthalmic division** and the eye is involved in 2/3rd cases, especially if **Hutchinson sign** is positive (vesicles on the tip or side of the nose indicating nasociliary nerve involvement). Conjunctivitis and conjunctival congestion may occur.
  - Maxillary division—vesicles on uvula and tonsillar fossae.
  - Mandibular division—anterior part of tongue, floor of mouth, buccal mucous membrane.
- **Facial nerve zoster (HZ oticus) (Ramsay–Hunt syndrome):** Vesicles on pinna and external auditory meatus, tympanic membrane, tonsillar fossae and adjacent soft palate, anterior 2/3rd of tongue (sensory fibers). Ear pain, loss of taste in anterior 2/3rd of tongue, facial palsy [accounts for 10% facial palsy (motor fibers involvement)].

Differential Diagnosis of HZ (Table 17.29)

TABLE 17.29: Differential diagnosis of herpes zoster

Disease	Differentiating features
Zosteriform HSV	Size of vesicles uniform in a cluster, later recurrences more frequent, PCR
Paederus dermatitis	Predilection for exposed areas, presence of kissing lesions, similar cases in a given area, seasonal incidence, identification of the insect

Clinical Course

- Recovery within 2–3 weeks in young patients and 3–4 weeks in elderly patients.
- Recurrent HZ—same or different dermatome.

Complications

- **Postherpetic neuralgia (PHN)**—most common. Persistence or recurrence of pain for more than 1 month (3 months according to some authors). More likely if prolonged dermatomal pain before onset of eruption, severe acute pain, prolonged rash, immunodeficiency.
- Two main forms—continuous burning pain with hyperaesthesia [tricyclic antidepressants (TCAs) more effective] and spasmodic shooting pain (gabapentin and pregabalin more effective).
- Allodynia—most distressing symptom, in 90%.
- Secondary bacterial infection, necrosis and extensive scarring in elderly and malnourished.
- **Disseminated zoster**—defined as more than 20 vesicles outside the area of the primary and adjacent dermatomes. May also spread systemically and cause pneumonia, hepatitis, encephalitis.
- Motor involvement—complete paralysis of facial muscles, ocular muscle palsy, fecal or urinary incontinence.
- Scar sarcoidosis, granuloma annulare, fungal granulomas at site of healed HZ.
- Ocular complication in HZ ophthalmicus—scleritis, keratitis, uveitis, ocular muscle palsies, proptosis, ulceration and necrosis of the eyelid. Retinal vascular occlusion and acute retinal necrosis syndrome is rare.
- Guillain-Barré syndrome—may occasionally follow HZ.

Diagnosis

Mainly clinical.

HPE: Posterior nerve roots and ganglia show inflammatory infiltrate. Destruction of nerve fibers in mid and lower dermis.

Treatment of HZV

Treatment is needed both for the acute episode and for the ensuing postherpetic neuralgia as well. **Figure 17.49** depicts the treatment for HZ and PHN.

Patients with recurrent zoster should also be treated with similar dose and duration of antiviral therapy of initial episode.

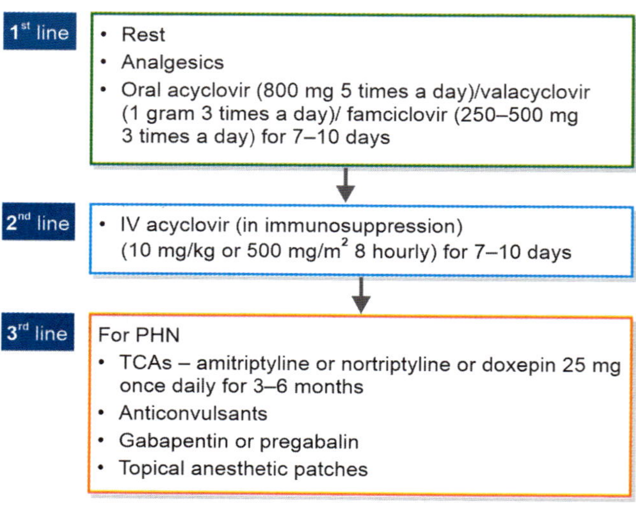

Fig. 17.49: Treatment of herpes zoster

HAND, FOOT AND MOUTH DISEASE (HFMD)

Epidemiology

Age: Children below 10 years.
Seasonal occurrence—summer, spring, autumn.

Predisposing Factors

None

Cause and Pathogenesis

Most outbreaks due to **coxsackievirus (CV)—A16, CV-A6 and enterovirus 71**. Many other coxsackieviruses may cause it.

Clinical Features

- Incubation period—1 week.
- Constitutional symptom—fever, malaise.

- Painful stomatitis, oral blisters breakdown into ulcers.
- Oval vesicles on palms > soles (children > adults)—most commonly on sides or backs of digits especially around the nails—fade in 2–3 days.
- 2–4 weeks later, nail changes may occur—Beau's lines, onycholysis, **onychomadesis**.

Differential Diagnosis (Table 17.30)

TABLE 17.30: Differential diagnosis of HFMD

Disease	Dissimilarity with HFMD
Herpes simplex gingivostomatitis	Primary herpes simplex would be more severe, involve gingivae (keratinized epithelium), limited lip involvement in recurrent lesions
Stevens-Johnson syndrome	Targetoid lesions on skin, history of drug intake, peeling off of skin at areas, rest of mucosal surfaces involved
Herpangina	Predominantly oral involvement only-vesicles with vivid red areolae on pharynx, tonsils, uvula and soft palate (nonkeratinized epithelium only), shallow ulcers
Chickenpox	More widespread, characteristic "dew drop on rose petal" appearance

Clinical Course

Fades in 1 week.

Complications

- Severe cases—high fever, myocarditis, pneumonitis, meningitis, encephalitis, Guillain-Barré syndrome, flaccid paralysis (mostly associated with enterovirus 71).
- Mortality rates up to 5% in enterovirus 71 outbreaks.

Diagnosis

Mostly clinical.

HPE: Spongiosis, intraepidermal vesicles, mononuclear cells invading the epidermis, necrosis of individual keratinocytes.

Antigen detection: PCR—skin vesicle fluid, blood, rectal swab, oral lesional swab, CSF samples.

Treatment

Symptomatic treatment only.

GIANOTTI-CROSTI SYNDROME (GCS) (Papular Acrodermatitis of Childhood)

Epidemiology

Age: 6 months to 12 years old children.

Cause and Pathogenesis

Early cases—most were associated with hepatitis B infection.

Now a number of viral and bacterial causes and immunizations are reported to cause GCS:

- **Viruses: HBV** (most common in Europe), **EBV** (most common in USA), HAV, HSV, CMV, HHV-6, coxsackie viruses A16, B4 and B5, echovirus 7 and 9, rotavirus, molluscum contagiosum, parvovirus B_{19}, mumps, influenza and parainfluenza virus, HIV.

- Bacteria: *Mycoplasma, Streptococcus, Bartonella, Borrelia burgdorferi*.
- Vaccines: Polio, MMR, diphtheria, pertussis, tetanus, influenza, H1N1 influenza, hepatitis B>A.

Clinical Features

- Dull-red flat-topped **papules** on thighs and buttocks → extensor aspect of arms, legs → face (mostly acral and face) **(Fig. 17.50)**.
- May be vesicular.
- Hepatitis B associated—non-itchy, others may be itchy.
- Slight constitutional symptoms may occasionally accompany—fever, malaise, lymphadenopathy.

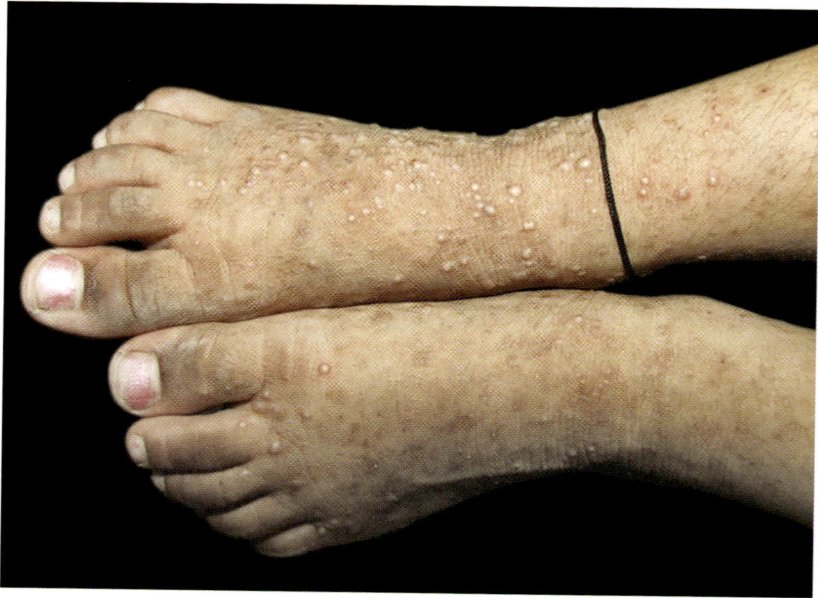

Fig. 17.50: Gianotti–Crosti syndrome

Differential Diagnosis (Table 17.31)

TABLE 17.31: Differential diagnosis of GCS

Disease	Dissimilarity with GCS
Scabies	Excoriated papules predominantly in genitalia and interdigital web spaces, family history, burrows
Lichen planus	Violaceous papules, flexor aspect of wrist and ankle joints, oral involvement, older individuals
Lichenoid drug eruption	Lesions more psoriasiform, history of drug intake
Erythema multiforme	History of drug intake or viral infection, target lesions with central crust/necrosis, more on palms and soles

Clinical Course

- Fades in 2–8 weeks.
- Recurrence may occur with infection/immunization.

Complications

No complications except liver sequelae in hepatitis B associated cases. Assess liver function tests.

Diagnosis

Mostly clinical. Look for triggering infections.

HPE: Spongiosis, patchy parakeratosis, epidermal vesicles, mild dermal edema, and lymphocytic infiltrate.

Treatment

Symptomatic treatment only. **Figure 17.51** lists the treatment options.

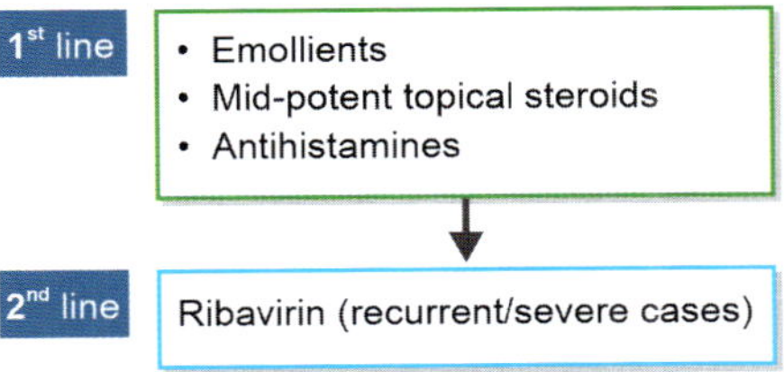

Fig. 17.51: Treatment of GCS

CUTANEOUS WARTS

Epidemiology

Age: Increases during school years, peak at adolescence and early adulthood.

Pathogenesis

Most often, warts developed within 3–4 months, although lesions occasionally grew as early as 6 weeks or as long as 2 years after inoculation.

- **HPV genome:** The HPV genome is divided functionally into three regions. A noncoding upstream regulatory region contributes to the control of DNA replication and transcription of eight to nine ORFs that are divided into early (E1–E7) and late (L1 and L2) regions. The functions of the ORFs (open reading frames) are listed below:
  - **E1** is involved in viral plasmid replication.
  - **E2** product is an important modulator of viral transcription and also plays a role in viral replication.
  - **E4** proteins form filamentous cytoplasmic networks and share the same cellular distribution as cytokeratin intermediate filaments, with which they may interact.
  - **E5** protein is located in the cellular membrane and prevents the acidification of endosomes, it stimulates the transforming activity of the epidermal growth factor receptor and contributes to the oncogenicity of HPV.
  - **E6** and **E7** of oncogenic HPV types have major transforming properties through the binding of various cellular factors and key tumor suppressor proteins. Both E6 and E7 bind to the p53 tumor suppressor gene product and abrogate its activity by accelerating its degradation.

Viral capsid proteins **L1** and **L2** are expressed and allow for the viral genome to be packaged. At the most apical layer of cells, the virus is released into the extracellular environment along with shedding skin cells in a nonlytic manner so as to avoid detection by immune cells.

1. **Viral invasion:** The virus replicative cycle is tightly dependent on epithelial differentiation. It begins with the entry of particles into the stratum germinativum (basale) because viral DNA is detected in the nuclei of the basal cells which requires a minor breach. As the basal cells differentiate and progress to the surface of the epithelium, HPV DNA replicates and is transcribed, and viral particles are assembled in the nucleus. Ultimately, complete virions are released, probably still tightly associated with the remnants of the shed dead keratinocyte shell **(Fig. 17.52a)**.
2. **Immune response:** Most times, a combination of innate and adaptive immunity eliminates infection **(Fig. 17.52b)**. Effector T cells targeting early viral proteins (notably E2, E6 and E7) can attack the virus-infected cells. Helper T cells that recognize L1 facilitate the induction of nAbs (natural antibodies) that can prevent virus transmission and reinfection of the host. However, with HPV persistence, lesion progression can be driven by de-repressed expression of E6 and E7.

E6 and/or **E7** interfere with recognition by intrinsic immune receptors cyclic GMP–AMP synthase-stimulator of interferon genes protein (cGAS–STING) and Toll-like receptor 9 (TLR9),

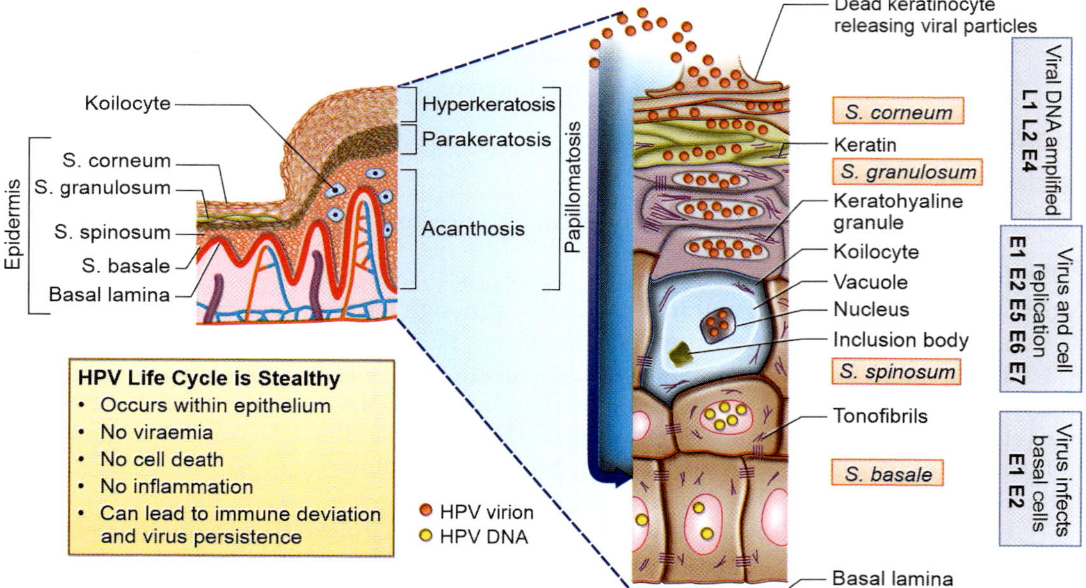

Fig. 17.52a: Pathogenesis of HPV infection: Abrasion of skin leads to denudation of epithelial cells, providing access to the basal keratinocytes. The virus, via the minor capsid protein L2, leads to infection. In the basal proliferating layers of the epithelium, the virus and cell replicate together and the DNA copy number is maintained at around 50–100 copies/cell. The early viral proteins E6 and E7 are key to stimulating the continued proliferation. Terminal differentiation of infected cells in the upper epithelial layers activates the expression of E4 and then L1 and L2 to package very high copy numbers of the viral genome. The virions are released as E4 leads to disintegration of cytokeratin filaments. The time taken between infection and the generation of infectious virus is 3 weeks

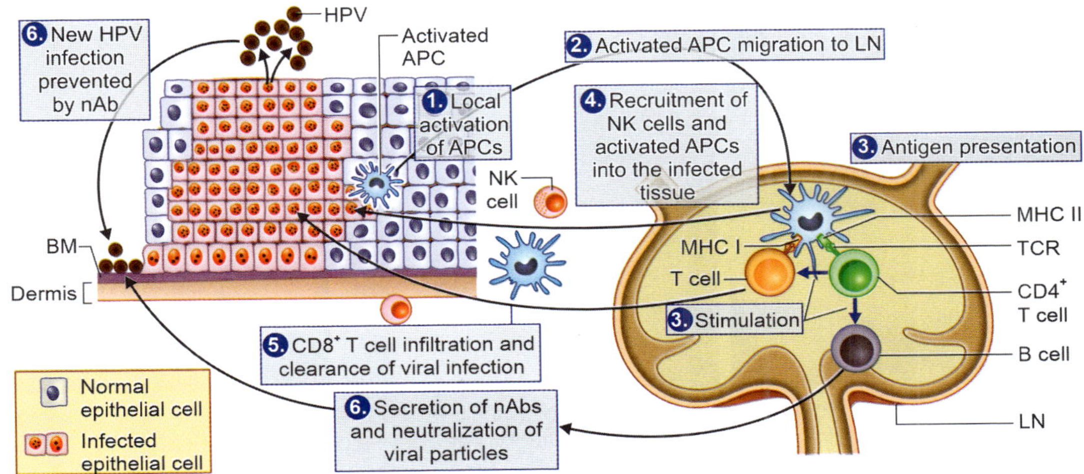

Fig. 17.52b: Immune response against HPV: The first step is the detection of virus by the APC **(1)**, this is followed by activaton of the host immune response in the LN **(2)**. The activated APCs stimulate various viral-antigen-specific CD4 + T cells that can either help activation of CD8 + T cells or help B cells to produce Abs that are, directed against capsid proteins **(3)**. There is then secretion of nonspecific effectors, interferons and the attraction of more APCs to further drive activation of adaptive immunity **(4)**. This inflammatory state provides the signals to attract the effector CD8 + T cells, which can target the virus-infected cells in the basal layers of the epithelium and are critical to clearance of the virus infection **(5)**. Only the viral particles, and not the HPV-infected cells, can be targeted by Abs, which are thus unable to cure infection but can stop further infections **(6)**

including through interferon regulatory factor 1 (IRF1) or IRF3 inhibition, and thereby block innate signalling of the viral genome presence while suppression of interferon-κ (IFNκ), CXC-chemokine ligand 14 (CXCL14) and CC-chemokine ligand 20 (CCL20) production prevents the recruitment of APCs to the site of infection. Such events compromise and/or delay the induction of an adaptive immune response, facilitating viral persistence and increased risk of cancer. E6 and E7 overexpression also compromises cellular DNA repair and induces extra centrosomes.

Clinical Types (Fig. 17.53)

Table 17.32 lists the various types of warts and the HPV types causing them. The natural history of cutaneous warts is poorly characterized. Spontaneous regression is seen in 30% warts by 3 months and in almost 70% warts by 2 years. In a given patient two-thirds of the warts that resolve spontaneously do so within 2 months and when warts resolve it is often synchronous.

Recurrence and recalcitrance is more likely to occur in the following groups:

- Long duration >2 years
- Involvement of palms and soles
- Beard area (shaving)
- Large number of warts
- Immunocompromised state
- Periungual (nail biters)

Differential Diagnosis

Table 17.33 lists the various clinical appearance of cutaneous warts and their differential diagnoses.

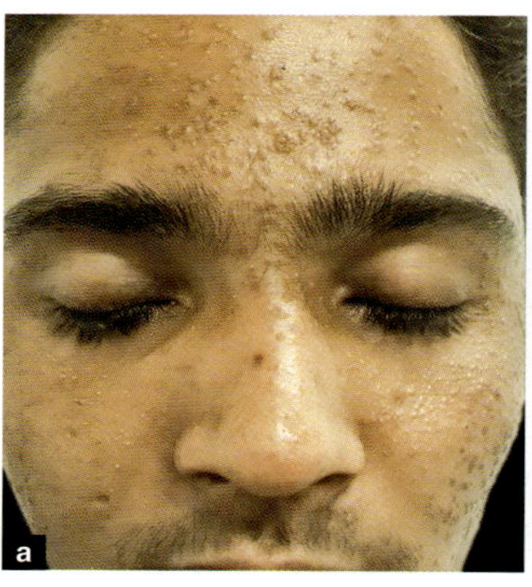
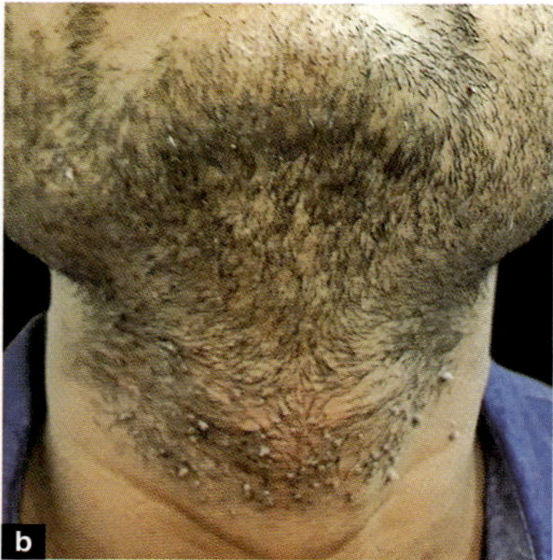
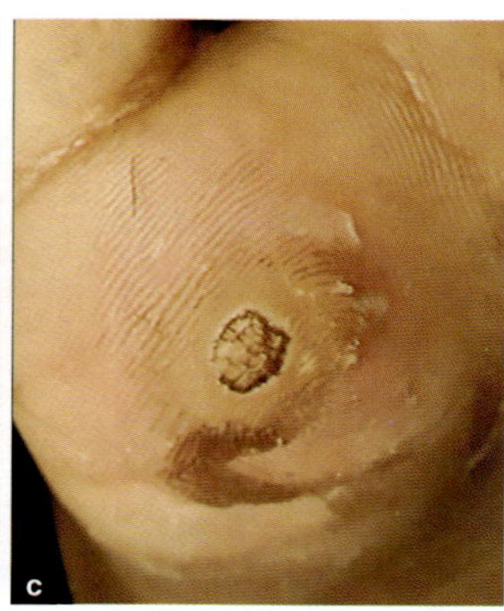

Fig. 17.53: (a) Verruca plana; (b) Filiform warts; (c) A plantar wart on treatment with 12% salicylic acid. Note the reversion of skin markings on the wart, which precedes resolution of the lesion

TABLE 17.32: Types of warts and HPV types causing them

Type of warts	HPV types most frequently detected
1. Common and plantar	1,2,4-Common (HPV 1,2 disseminate while HPV 27 and 57 do not) 1,2-Plantar
2. Plane	3, 10
3. Butcher's warts	7
4. Digital SCC and Bowen disease	16
5. Condylomata acuminata	6, 11
6. Respiratory and conjunctival papillomas	6, 11
7. Buschke–Löwenstein tumor	6, 11
8. High grade intraepithelial neoplasia	16
9. Heck disease (focal epithelial hyperplasia)	13, 32

TABLE 17.33: Clinical features and differential diagnosis of cutaneous warts

	Site	Clinical appearance	Differential diagnosis
Common	Anywhere, mostly on hands, fingers, knees, Koebner's +/–	Rough horny papules	VEN, Bowen disease, actinic keratosis
Plantar	Beneath pressure points, heel	Mosaic—superficial, painless, persistent, closely compressed small warts myrmecia—deeper, painful	Corn, callus
Plane	Face, dorsum of hands, shins, Koebner's +/–	Smooth, flat/slightly elevated	Lichen planus, acrokeratosis verruciformis
Filiform/ digitate	Face, neck, scalp in males mostly	Finger-like projections	Acrochordons
Pigmented	Palms and soles in Japanese	Pigmented warts	Seborrheic keratosis

VEN— verrucous epidermal nevus

Diagnosis

- Mostly clinical.
- Dermoscopy: Red/black dots (thrombosed capillaries) with a surrounding whitish halo (frog-spawn appearance).
- Investigations may be needed in atypical cases. **Table 17.34** gives the investigations in a case of cutaneous warts.
- In a wart or condyloma, viral replication is associated with excessive proliferation of all of the epidermal layers except the basal layer. This process produces acanthosis, parakeratosis, and hyperkeratosis. A deepening of the rete ridges, where normally present, produces the typical papillomatous cytoarchitecture. Some infected cells undergo the characteristic transformation of koilocytosis. *Koilocytes* (from the Greek *koilos*, "cavity") are large, usually polygonal, squamous cells with a shrunken nucleus lodged inside a large cytoplasmic vacuole.

TABLE 17.34: Investigations in a case of cutaneous warts

- **Histology:** Acanthosis, hyperkeratosis, characteristic koilocytes, papillomatosis, basophilic nuclear inclusion bodies (virus particles on EM), and eosinophilic cytoplasmic inclusion bodies (clumped keratohyaline granules) **(Fig. 17.54)**.
- Immunohistochemistry
- DNA *in situ* hybridization
- PCR for HPV DNA

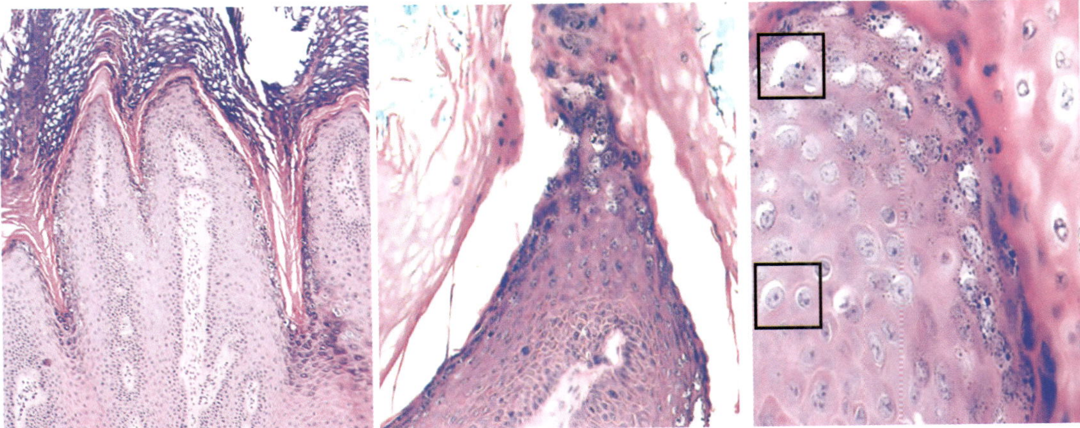

Fig. 17.54: Histopathology of cutaneous wart: Hyperkeratosis with acanthosis is seen with papillomatosis and HPV-induced cytopathic changes affecting keratinocytes in the granular layer. The koilocytes have typically halo-like bright cytoplasm and clumped keratohyalin granules

Treatment

A list of treatment options is listed in **Table 17.35** and a morphology-based treatment algorithm is given in **Table 17.36**.

Salient points about treatment of cutaneous warts:

- **Destructive modalities**
  - Cryotherapy and salicylic acid appear to be both effective and safe with no significant difference between them.

TABLE 17.35: A list of treatment modalities in nongenital cutaneous warts

Destructive	Antimitotic agents	Virucidal agents	Immunological therapy	Alternative treatment
• Salicylic acid 12–40% • Cryotherapy • Silver nitrate • Phenol • Cantharidin • Trichloroacetic acid • Hyperthermia • Lasers • Photodynamic therapy • Cautery-electrical	• Bleomycin • Retinoids • Vitamin D analogues • 5-Fluorouracil • Dithranol • Podophyllin/ podophyllotoxin	• Cidofovir • Formaldehyde • Glutaraldehyde	• Topical imiquimod • Contact immunotherapy • Intralesional vaccines–MMR, BCG, Mw • Intralesional anti-gens–*Candida*, PPD • Zinc • Levamisole • H_2 receptor antagonists • Autoimplantation	• Hypnotherapy • Homeopathic treatment • Acupuncture

TABLE 17.36: Treatment of cutaneous warts according to morphology

Type of wart	Recommendation (Zhu et al., 2022)
• Common warts-refractory, recurrent	• Cryotherapy (1B) • 5FU, Bleomycin, Cidofovir (2B) • Thermotherapy (2C)
• Flat warts	• 10% 5-ALA-PDT (1B) • CO_2 laser, PDL, YAG laser (2C) • Bleomycin (1B) • I/L *Candida albicans* antigen (1B)
• Plantar warts	• Cryotherapy (2B) • Long pulsed Nd:YAG laser (1B) • CO_2 laser (1B) • Bleomycin (1B)
• EDV	• 5-FU, imiquimod (2D) • Retinoic acid (oral/topical) (2D) • E/C, cryotherapy (2D) • Surgery (precancerous, cancerous) (2D) • Guidance on sunprotection (1D)
• <18 years with warts	• I/L *Candida albicaus* antigen (2C) • 5-ALA-PDT + E/C (2C) • 5% imiquimod (1B) • Monochloroacetic acid (MCA) (1B)
Pregnancy	• TCA (1A) • Cryotherapy (2C) • Surgery (2C)

– Increased efficacy of aggressive cryotherapy over gentle cryotherapy.
– Difficult to do in multiple/facial/children warts.
– More permanent adverse effects—dyspigmentation, scarring.

- **Antimitotic agents**
  - **Bleomycin** is cheap and effective in periungual and palmoplantar warts.
    - Intralesional injection and topical instillation of bleomycin with multiple puncture or microneedling methods are equally effective (patient comfort is more with the latter).
    - More effective than 5-FU and *Candida* antigen.
  - **5-FU** has moderate efficacy (less effective than bleomycin).
- **Retinoids**—recent systematic review concluded that oral acitretin plus *Candida* Ag was the highest-ranked in achieving a complete recovery among retinoids.
  - Topical retinoids were not inferior to systemic retinoids (some papers differ).
  - Topical retinoids may be effective in plane warts.
  - Combination of retinoids with immunotherapy is more effective than individual treatment.
- **Intralesional immunotherapy**
  - First line for >5 in number and >1 cm warts, multiple distant lesions, difficult-to-treat sites
  - Second line for recalcitrant warts
  - Avoid in immunosuppression, pregnancy, hypersensitivity.
  - Rationale: Proteins from various infectious agents are used as antigens to induce an immune response that is subsequently also directed against HPVs. The antigens are injected directly into the wart; in case of multiple warts, treating one will frequently suffice.
  - HPV vaccine-intralesional better efficacy than intramuscular.
    - Most HPV vaccines target the L1 antigen and induce a robust L1-specific CD8 + T cell response, but basal keratinocytes harbouring HPV do not detectably express L1 and thus presumably escape this response. The activity of T helper cells is important to achieve a robust response. Hence the vaccines do not necessarily eradicate existing infecton by HPV.
    - The fact that this treatment has been demonstrated to work best in prepubertal children may be explained by the influence of sex hormones on the expression of HPV proteins in infected cells. After the onset of puberty, class 1 MHC (major histocompatibility complex) molecules in HPV-infected cells disappear, and this likely results in a weaker vaccine-induced cytotoxic T-cell response against HPVs.
  - PPD and MMR—most effective specially in adults (Mohammed YF, 2021).

    MMR—the most effective in reducing the recurrence rate at the primary site after 3–6 sessions of treatment and is also effective in perianal warts [Sharma S]. A particularly useful study has compared it with cryotherapy and found MMR to be more effective in most warts except common warts. Injection of MMR vaccine was done intralesionally with a dose of 50 IU (0.5 mL) by an insulin syringe. Injections were repeated into the same wart (the largest wart) every 2 weeks for all patients until complete resolution or for a maximum of three sessions (Abd El-Magiud EM, 2020).

    It would seem that the exposure of the population to the vaccine previously is a determinant to the ultimate response though a recent study found that BCG has the best results (Shaker ESE, et al., 2021).
  - Combining intralesional immunotherapy with destructive methods might enhance the efficacy, shorten the treatment duration, and reduce the side effects.

- **Topical immunotherapy**
  - Imiquimod—moderate efficacy, main advantage is its use in immunosuppression
- **Systemic immunotherapy**
  - Not strongly proven role.

EPIDERMODYSPLASIA VERRUCIFORMIS (EV) (Treeman Syndrome)

Epidemiology

- Congenital EV—very rare, inherited (mostly AR).
- Acquired EV—in organ and bone marrow transplant recipients, on long-term immunosuppression, primary immunodeficiencies, HIV/AIDS.

Predisposing Factors

- Genetic—mutations on **EVER1** and **EVER2** on chromosome **17** in many cases.
- UV radiation-considered a prerequisite for development of malignancy.

Cause

- βHPV types—at least 20 types—HPV types 5, 8, 9, 12, 14, 15, 17, 19–25.
- HPV-5 and HPV-8—main types associated with malignancy.

Clinical Features

- Three types of lesions **(Fig. 17.55)**:
  - Plane wart-like lesions on face and neck, backs of hand and feet, develop in childhood.
  - Scaly macules similar to pityriasis versicolor—erythematous/hypopigmented/hyperpigmented—on trunk and limbs.
  - Erythematous/hyperpigmented plaques similar to seborrheic keratoses—on trunk and limbs.

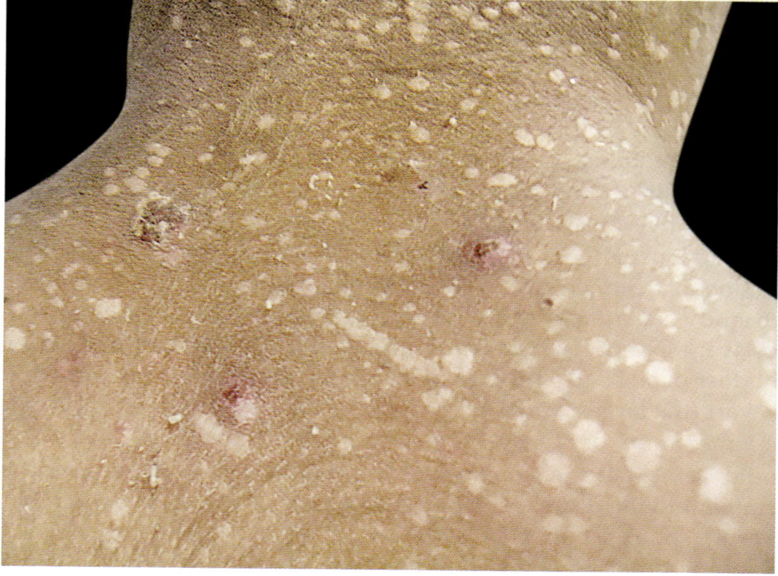

Fig. 17.55: Epidermodysplasia verruciformis

Differential Diagnosis (Table 17.37)

TABLE 17.37: Differential diagnosis of EDV

Disease	Differentiating features
Acrokeratosis verruciformis	Elbows and knees are a preferred site, palms show diffuse thickening and breaks in dermatoglyphic pattern and tiny keratoses, no vacuolation on HPE
Lichen planus	Purplish papules, pruritus, oral lesions, HPE diagnostic

Clinical Course

- Persistent
- Malignant transformation possible in approximately two-thirds of patients.
- May regress in pregnancy.

Complications

Malignancy on exposed lesions—SCC in 20–30% (HPV-5, HPV-8).

Diagnosis

Mainly clinical.
- PCR for → HPV DNA in skin biopsy.

HPE
- Hyperkeratosis and acanthosis
- Large cells with blue-grey cytoplasm in the upper dermis
- Extensive vacuolation/ballooning in perinuclear area of keratinocytes (much more than in plane warts).

Treatment (Fig. 17.56)

Photoprotection—essential to prevent the development of actinic keratoses and non-melanoma skin cancer.

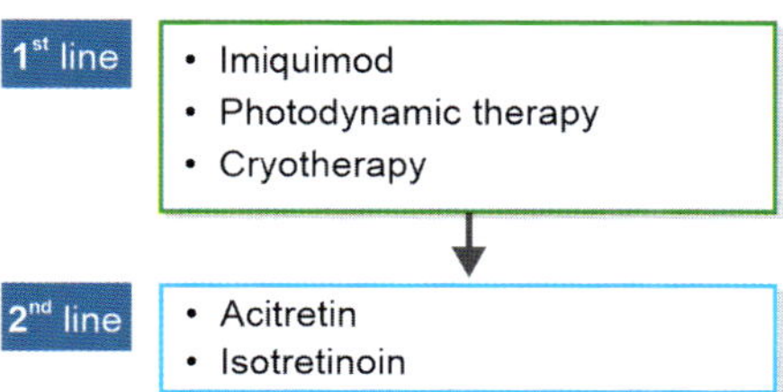

Fig. 17.56: Treatment of EDV

DENGUE (FLAVIVIRUS) AND CHIKUNGUNYA (TOGAVIRUS) FEVERS

Chikungunya ("Bending Up") Fever

Vector: *Aedes aegyptii, Aedes albopictus* (*vertical transmission also*).

Clinical Features

Dermatological (seen in up to 50%) **(Table 17.38)**.

TABLE 17.38: Dermatological manifestation of chikungunya fever		
Type of eruption	**Characteristics**	**Sites involed**
Generalized macular erythema	Within 24–48 hours of onset of fever	Upper limbs, face, trunk (most pronounced), neck, ear lobes
Maculopapular rash (vesicular/ pigmented in infants)	**Most common (within 2–3 days), severe pruritus**	
Xerosis, desquamation of palms and soles	During subsidence phase	
Hypermelanosis (postinflammatory) (around 2 weeks later)	After subsidence phase: • **Centrofacial/melasma-like** • Periorbital • Freckle-like • Diffuse face and extremity pigmentation • Flagellate/irregular • Pigmentation of existing acne • Addisonial palmar pigmentation	1. **Nose (most common (persists for 3–6 months—*Chik sign*)** 2. Face 3. Trunk 4. Neck 5. Palms
Oral lesions	Aphthae, erosions, cheilitis, hard palate pigmentation	
Nail lesions	Red/black lunulae, periungual ulcers, subungual hemorrhages, melanonychia (diffuse/longitudinal)	
Penoscrotal and perianal ulcers, oral ulcers (aphthae-like lesion)		Oral cavity, genitalia, axillae, perineum
Petechial/purpuric		
Localized erythema and swelling of the pinnae (mimicking the Milian's ear sign of erysipelas)		Pinna
Scar erythema over pre-existing scars (mimicking scar phenomenon of sarcoidosis)		Scars and striae

Non-dermatological

- High grade fever
- **Severe arthralgias and arthritis** (small joint)—hands, wrists, ankles (sometimes larger joints too)—may persist, 50% have for >1 year
- Conjunctival injection and conjunctivitis, photophobia
- Lymphadenopathy
- May lead to flare of psoriasis/other pre-existing dermatosis.

Diagnosis

- RT-PCR-fastest
- IgM antibody by ELISA

Dengue ("Break Bone") Fever

Vector: *Aedes aegypti*

Clinical Features

- Fluctuating fever
- Nausea, vomiting
- Headache, retrobulbar pain
- Severe back pain
- Rash (50%)—on 3rd/4th day of fever—fades around 7th day when fever subsides:
  - Transient flushing erythema of face—typically within the first 24–48 hours.
  - Second rash—3–6 days after the onset of fever and it is characterized by asymptomatic maculopapular or morbilliform eruption.
  - Generalized confluent erythema with petechiae and rounded islands of sparing—**"white islands in a sea of red"**.
  - Pruritus less common.
  - Start on legs/chest and trunk.
  - May pass through a petechial phase on limbs.
  - May be missed in dark skins.
  - Oropharyngeal/conjunctival mucosa—30%.
- **Chikungunya versus dengue:** Chikungunya patients have more joint pains and more typical postures, shorter fever, more flushing erythema, more conjunctival injection, more severe rash, less bleeding manifestations.

Diagnosis

- **NS-1 antigen for serotype 1 (most common)**
- RT-PCR—fastest
- IgM antibody by ELISA.

CUTANEOUS LEISHMANIASIS AND POST-KALA-AZAR DERMAL LEISHMANIASIS (PKDL)

Leishmaniasis is an infection by the protozoan parasites of the genus Leishmania and causes three primary clinical syndromes: **Visceral leishmaniasis (VL), cutaneous leishmaniasis (CL),** and **mucosal leishmaniasis (ML)**. A more detailed classification is given in **Table 17.39** though we will focus primarily on PKDL in this section.

- *Leishmania* organisms are transmitted by the bites of female sandflies of the *Lutzomyia* and *Phlebotomus* genera. Sand fly saliva and inoculum size influence human infection **(Fig. 17.57)**.

TABLE 17.39: Classification of cutaneous and visceral leishmaniasis

Type of leishmaniasis	Organism	Main lesion	Vector
OLD WORLD			
Cutaneous leishmaniasis	• *Leishmania donovani donovani* (viscerotropic) • *L. donovani infantum* (viscerotropic) • *L. major* • *L. tropica* • *L. aethiopica*	Kala-azar and PKDL Kala-azar and PKDL Self-healing rural sores → scars Self-healing urban sores Self-healing nodule	***Phlebotomus argentipes*** *and other* spp.
Leishmaniasis recidivans (chronic/ lupoid)	*L. tropica* (Iran, Afghanistan)	Chronic lupus vulgaris—like lesion, destructive, may ulcerate/ concentric rings	
Diffuse cutaneous leishmaniasis	*L. aethiopica*	Chronic relapsing disorder, nodules over large areas, no ulceration, no visceral involvement	
Mucocutaneous leishmaniasis	*L. aethiopica*	Chronic destructive	
Visceral leishmaniasis	*L. donovani*		*Phlebotomus argentipes*
PKDL	*L. donovani*		*Phlebotomus argentipes*
NEW WORLD	• *L. brasiliensis* • *L. mexicana*		***Lutzomyia longipalpis*** and other spp.
Cutaneous leishmaniasis	• *L.b. brasiliensis* • *L.b. peruviana* • *L.b. panamensis* • *L.b. guyanensis* • *L.m. mexicana* • *L.m. amazonensis*	Self-healing Self-healing Self-healing, Self-healing, lymphatic nodules Self-healing, chronic destructive Chiclero ear Self-healing	
Mucocutaneous leishmaniasis	• *L.b. brasiliensis, L.b. panamensis, L.b. guyanensis*	Persistent, destructive, Espundia	
Diffuse cutaneous leishmaniasis	• *L.m. amazonensis*	Chronic and relapsing, disfiguring	

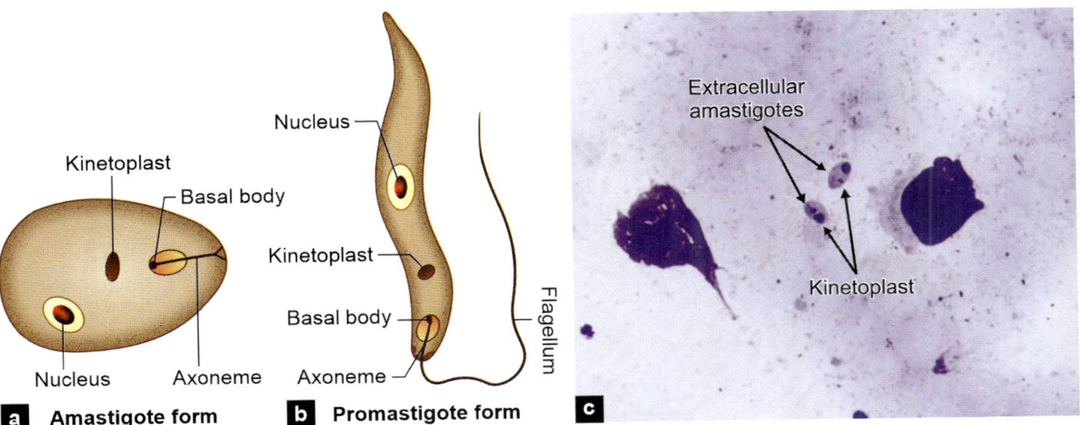

Fig. 17.57: (a) Diagrammatic representation of the amastigote form of *L. donovani*; (b) Diagrammmatic representation of the promastigote (in gut of sandfly) form of *L. donovani*; (c) Amastigotes, 3–4 μm in width and 4–5 μm in length are seen

- Leishmania parasites exist as flagellated promastigotes in sand flies and transform into oval amastigotes after tissue infection in mammalian hosts.
- **Life cycle: Figure 17.58** depicts life cycle of *Leishmania donovani*.
- Leishmaniasis is an intracellular infection, and as such adequate control requires a robust cell-mediated immune response. Parasite and host factors influence the tropism of infection **(Fig. 17.59)**.

Pathogenesis and Immunology

Leishmaniasis can be thought of as a polar disorder similar to other intracellular infections such as leprosy **(Fig. 17.59)**. On one end of the spectrum are **polyparasitic** infections (e.g. diffuse CL or VL) characterized by a predominantly Th2-type immune response with relative anergy, akin to lepromatous leprosy. Heavily parasitized macrophages are abundant, and diagnosis is readily made by smear or in the biopsy tissue **(Fig. 17.60)**. Peripheral blood mononuclear cells neither proliferate nor produce interferon-γ (IFN-γ) nor interleukin-2 (IL-2) in response to leishmanial antigens *in vitro* and cutaneous delayed-type hypersensitivity (DTH) reactions are absent. The **oligoparasitic** end of the spectrum includes ML and latent VL infection. Amastigotes are sparse, and a mononuclear cell infiltrate predominates in a Th1-type immune response, analogous to tuberculoid leprosy.

Why some species spread systemically causing visceral disease and others remain relatively confined to the skin is not fully understood. The A2 gene family, found as a functional gene among species that cause VL, is likely important in visceralization, protecting the parasite from heat shock and oxidative stress.

Diagnosis

There are three ways to approach the diagnosis of all suspected *Leishmania* infections: Clinical, parasitologic, and immunologic.

- Clinical diagnosis combines epidemiology with clinical manifestations and serves as a useful guide but is rarely adequate in and of itself due to the cost and toxicity of available

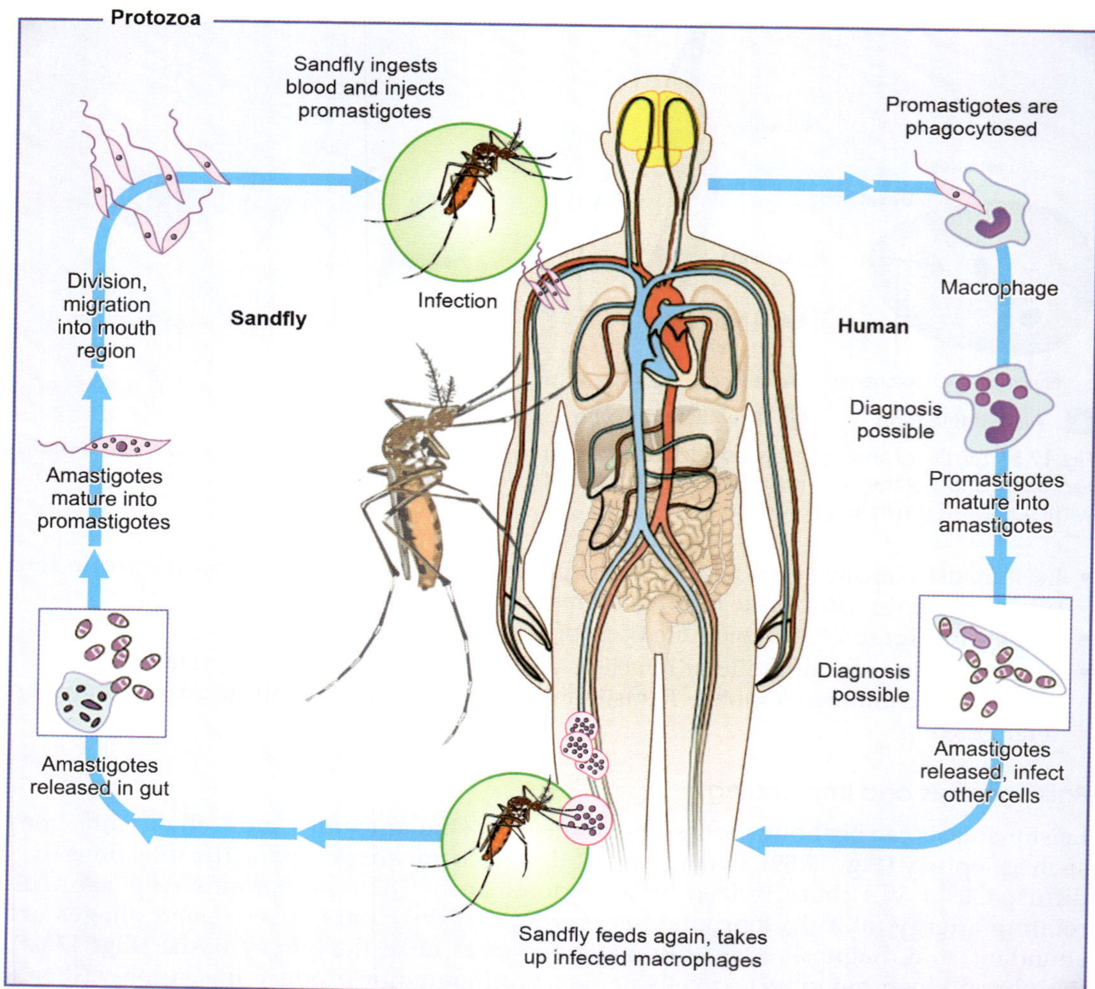

Fig. 17.58: Life cycle of *Leishmania donovani*

therapies as well as the prognostic importance of species identification, particularly in CL.

- Parasitologic diagnosis is confirmed by visualizing amastigotes in a tissue biopsy specimen or smear **(Fig. 17.60)**, visualizing promastigotes in culture, or amplifying *Leishmania*—specific nucleic acids by polymerase chain reaction (PCR).
- Immunologic diagnosis is an adjunct in most cases, with various antibody tests, cytokine release assays, and the Leishmanin (Montenegro) skin test. The leishmanin skin test and cytokine release assays such as the interferon gamma (INF-γ) release assay (IGRA), evaluate for cell-mediated immune responses, but neither the skin test nor cytokine release assays are standardized or commercially available.

The choice of the optimal diagnostic test or procedure depends on the parasite burden of the leishmaniasis syndrome **(Fig. 17.59)**.

Spectrum of Disease

Cutaneous

ML, DL, LR | LCL | DCL

Visceral

Latent VL infection | Subclinical VL | VL, PKDL

Parasite Burden

Oligoparasitic | Polyparasitic

Diagnostic Tests

PCR, LST, IGRA | Culture/species | Histology serology

Immune Response

Th1 Cell-mediated | Antibody Th2

Fig. 17.59: A depiction of the spectrum of Leishmania infection and disease. DCL, diffuse cutaneous leishmaniasis; DL, disseminated leishmaniasis; IGRA, interferon-γ release assay; LCL, localized cutaneous leishmaniasis; LR, leishmaniasis recidivans; LST, Leishmanin skin test; ML, mucosal leishmaniasis; PCR, polymerase chain reaction; PKDL, post-kala-azar dermal leishmaniasis; Th1, Th1-predominant

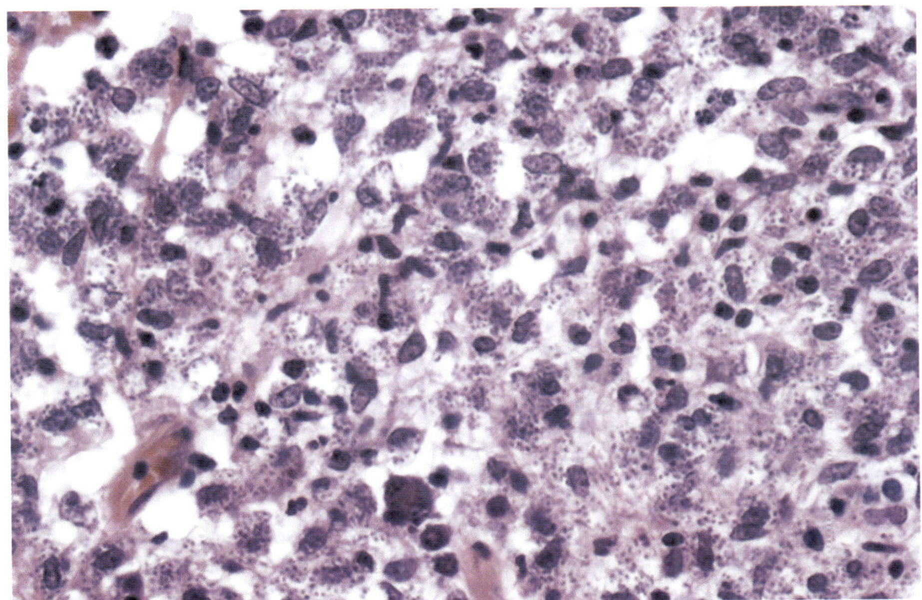

Fig. 17.60: Tissue biopsy reveals histiocytes with LD bodies in most of the cells in the polyparasitic variant of leishmaniasis, in cutaneous leishmaniasis this density of LD bodies is not seen

Treatment of Cutaneous Leishmaniasis

***Uncomplicated versus complicated infection*:** The approach to management of cutaneous leishmaniasis (CL) begins with establishing the **clinical severity** of infection and 2 types are described **simple** and **complex** CL as given in **Table 17.40.**

TABLE 17.40: Clinical characteristics of cutaneous *leishmaniasis* (CL) that may determine management*

Simple CL	Complex CL
Caused by a *Leishmania species* unlikely to be associated with mucosal leishmaniasis (ML)	Caused by a *Leishmania* species that can be associated with increased risk for ML, particularly *Viannia* spp. in the "mucosal belt" of Bolivia, Peru, and Brazil
No mucosal involvement noted	Local subcutaneous nodules
Absence of characteristics of complex CL	Large regional adenopathy
Only a single or a few skin lesions	>4 skin lesions of substantial size (e.g. >1 cm)
Small lesion size (diameter <1 cm)	Large individual skin lesion (diameter ≥5 cm)
Location of lesion feasible for local treatment	Size or location of lesion such that local treatment is not feasible
Nonexposed skin (i.e. not cosmetically important)	Lesion on face, including ears, eyelids, or lips; fingers, toes, or other joints; or genitalia
Immunocompetent host	Immunocompromised host (especially with respect to cell-mediated immunity)
Lesion(s) resolving without prior therapy	Clinical failure of local therapy Unusual syndromes; leishmaniasis recidivans, diffuse CL, or disseminated CL
Management options: Simple CL	**Management options: Complex CL**
Watchful waiting (wound care) Local therapy • Cryotherapy • Thermotherapy • Topical paromomycin • Intralesional SbV or pentamidine • Photodynamic therapy Systemic therapy—azoles	Systemic therapy • Miltefosine • SbV • Liposomal amphotericin B • Amphotericin B deoxycholate • Pentamidine Adjuvant immunomodulatory therapies, including imiquimod, pentoxifylline, CpG DNA

*Clin. Infect. Dis. 2016–63;e202–e264.

Whom to Treat?

- The objective of CL treatment is clinical cure not parasitological cure. Many CL infections eventually resolve clinically without treatment, and not all patients who undergo treatment demonstrate elimination of parasitic infection.
- Clinical observation (in the absence of treatment) is reasonable for immunocompetent patients with uncomplicated lesions that are healing spontaneously and whose infection is either known to be caused by a *Leishmania* species not associated with increased risk for ML **or** whose species is unknown but whose infection was acquired outside of areas with *Leishmania* species associated with increased risk for ML.

- **Local therapy** is reasonable for patients with uncomplicated CL who are not already healing spontaneously and/or who would like to pursue therapeutic intervention. Local therapy is appropriate for management of Old World CL as well as for treatment of New World CL caused by species unlikely to cause disseminated infection.
- **Systemic therapy** is warranted for patients with complicated CL, for immunocompromised patients, for patients with spontaneously healing or recently healed lesions whose infection is known to be caused by a *Leishmania* species associated with increased risk for ML, and for patients with healing lesions whose species is unknown but whose infection was acquired within an area with *Leishmania* species associated with increased risk for ML. Systemic therapy is also warranted for patients with less common syndromes including leishmaniasis recidivans, diffuse cutaneous leishmaniasis, and disseminated cutaneous leishmaniasis.

An overview of the medical treatment of cutaneous leishmaniasis is given in **Table 17.41**. Other options include cryotherapy, heat therapy and 15% paromomycin and 0.5% gentamicin cream.

TABLE 17.41: Treatment options for cutaneous leishmaniasis

Cutaneous leishmaniasis (CL)	There is no generally applicable treatment of choice; choice should be individualized		For cases of CL associated with increased risk for ML, the choices include miltefosine, amphotericin B formulations, and pentavalent antimonials.
IV/IM	**Amphotericin B deoxycholate**	0.5–1.0 mg/kg per dose daily or every other day for cumulative total of ~ 15–30 mg/kg	
	Sodium stibogluconate	20 mg Sb/kg/day for 20 days	Dilute dose in D5W (~ 50–100 mL) for IV, ~ 10–30-minute infusion. Use of an in-line filter is recommended
	Liposomal amphotericin B	3 mg/kg/day on days 1–5 and 10 or on days 1–7 (total 18–21 mg/kg)	Off label
Oral	**Fluconazole**	Adults: 200 mg daily for 6 weeks	Off label
	Ketoconazole	Adults: 600 mg daily for 28 days	Off label
	Miltefosine	FDA-approved regimen: If 30–44 kg, 50 mg bid for 28 days; if ≥ 45 kg, 50 mg tid for 28 days	Target dose is ~ 2.5 mg/kg/day, but doses >150 mg/day have not been studied. GI side effects may limit higher doses
Intralesional alternatives	**Sodium stibogluconate**	Various regimens, e.g. 0.2–5 mL per session every 3–7 days (or up to every 3 weeks) +/– cryotherapy for 5–8 sessions or until healing. 5 sites/lesion with a 25–27G needle intradermally for 0.1 mL/cm^2 until blanched	

POST-KALA-AZAR DERMAL LEISHMANIASIS

Post-kala-azar dermal leishmaniasis (PKDL) occurs almost exclusively in patients with visceral leishmaniasis caused by *L. donovani*; it is rare in cases caused by *L. infantum*. However, there are marked differences in the rate of developing PKDL even in areas where *L. donovani* is the causative parasite.

Epidemiology

- Bihar (90%) > Jharkhand > West Bengal > Uttar Pradesh (incidence of visceral leishmaniasis; VL).
- Highest number of PKDL patients in Northern Bihar.
- 10–20%—no history of VL (but are usually natives of the endemic states).
- **"Para-kala-azar dermal leishmaniasis"**—concomitant VL + PKDL—seen in Sudan, sporadic in India.
- **Association between VL and PKDL:** It is widely believed that as the immunity improves, the visceral disease (kala-azar) improves and there is a decrease in the parasite load. This is associated with the emergence of signs of PKDL. Based on this concept, three types of presentations have been described:
  - **Classic:** In these cases, there is a gradual transition from VL to PKDL.
  - **Intermediate stage:** In this, the patients have a disseminated disease as demonstrated by the presence of parasites in lymph nodes or in bone marrow aspirates. These patients with PKDL and concomitant VL may be more appropriately referred to as cases of **para-kala-azar** dermal leishmaniasis and they have an intermediate position between VL and PKDL.
  - PKDL may also occur <u>without</u> a previous history of VL (4–29%).

The differences between the African and Indian PKDL are listed in **Table 17.42**.

TABLE 17.42: Indian PKDL versus African PKDL

Features	Africa	India
Clinical		
PKDL can develop in the absence of *previous VL*	Yes	Yes
PKDL can develop while therapy is on for *VL*	Yes	**No**
PKDL can develop with visceral disease	Yes	Yes
Site	Face > trunk > arms > legs	Face > trunk > arms > legs
Morphology	PN > MP > microP > M	Erythema, induration M, P, N
Lymphadenopathy	Yes	Rare
Epidemiology		
Frequency of PKDL following VL	>20% (up to 50–60%)	5–10%
Interval between VL and PKDL	0–6 mo, children	2–7 y, young adults
Diagnosis		
Smear (+)	20–30%	20–40%
PCR	83%	94%
LST (+)[#]	16–65%	0–67%
Spontaneous cure	The rule	Not reported

*M, macular; MicroP, micropapular; MP, maculopapular; N, nodular; PN, papulonodular.

[#]LST: leishmanin skin test

Pathogenesis/Immunology

PKDL occurs after treatment for visceral leishmaniasis in a proportion of patients, and is considered to be triggered immunologically. In visceral leishmaniasis, the predominant immune response is a Th2 response, whereas in **PKDL**, Th2-type response in the skin with alternative macrophage activation despite a Th1 response predominating in the viscera is noted. Increased **interleukin-10 (IL-10) is seen which** inhibits the nitric oxide (NO)-mediated killing of the parasites.

Predictive Factors

- **Suboptimal therapy of VL:** Inadequate treatment for VL (e.g. treatment with a low dose of medicine or for a short duration).

  In a prospective cohort of 1700 patients treated for VL with 3 different regimes—single dose AmBisome (10 mg/kg), AmBisome (5 mg/kg) + Oral miltefosine and Intramuscular Paromomycin (11 mg/kg) + Oral miltefosine—least relapses of VL (median onset—6 months after VL treatment) but highest risk of PKDL (median onset—2 years after VL treatment) were seen with Paromomycin + Miltefosine, while the reverse was seen with the two AmBisome regimes (Goyal V, 2020). In another study, the mean interval reported was 21 months, 36 months and 48 months when VL was treated with miltefosine, sodium stibogluconate, and amphotericin deoxycholate, respectively. (Mondal D, 2019)
- **Host genetic predisposition:** In Sudan, genetic studies have shown decreased expression of the **interferon-gamma receptor gene** in patients with PKDL; this was not found in patients with visceral leishmaniasis.
- Environmental factors such as ultraviolet light exposure or water arsenic levels
- Young age (generally 5–17 years)
- Malnutrition
- HIV infection and antiretroviral treatment
- Persistence of parasites

Favourable outcomes for patients with PKDL are predicted by a positive leishmanin skin test (LST) or when levels of interferon-γ are higher than levels of IL-10.

Clinical Features

In Sudan, three grades of PKDL severity have been described; this clinical grading has also been adapted for case management in Ethiopia and South Sudan. The grades are:

- **Grade 1**—scattered maculopapular or nodular rash on the face, with or without lesions on the upper chest or arms.
- **Grade 2**—dense maculopapular or nodular rash covering most of the face and extending to the chest, back, upper arms and legs, with only scattered lesions on the forearms and legs.
- **Grade 3**—dense maculopapular or nodular rash covering most of the body, including the hands and feet; the mucosa of the lips and palate may be involved.

Most patients in the **Indian** subcontinent have a polymorphic presentation comprising macular, papular or nodular lesions, with a predilection for the area around the chin and mouth ("muzzle area"). This presentation can be subdivided into different forms:

- Monomorphic (macular or nodular) **(Fig. 17.61a** to **c)**.
- Polymorphic or mixed (both macules and indurated lesions, such as nodules are present) **(Fig. 17.61d)**.

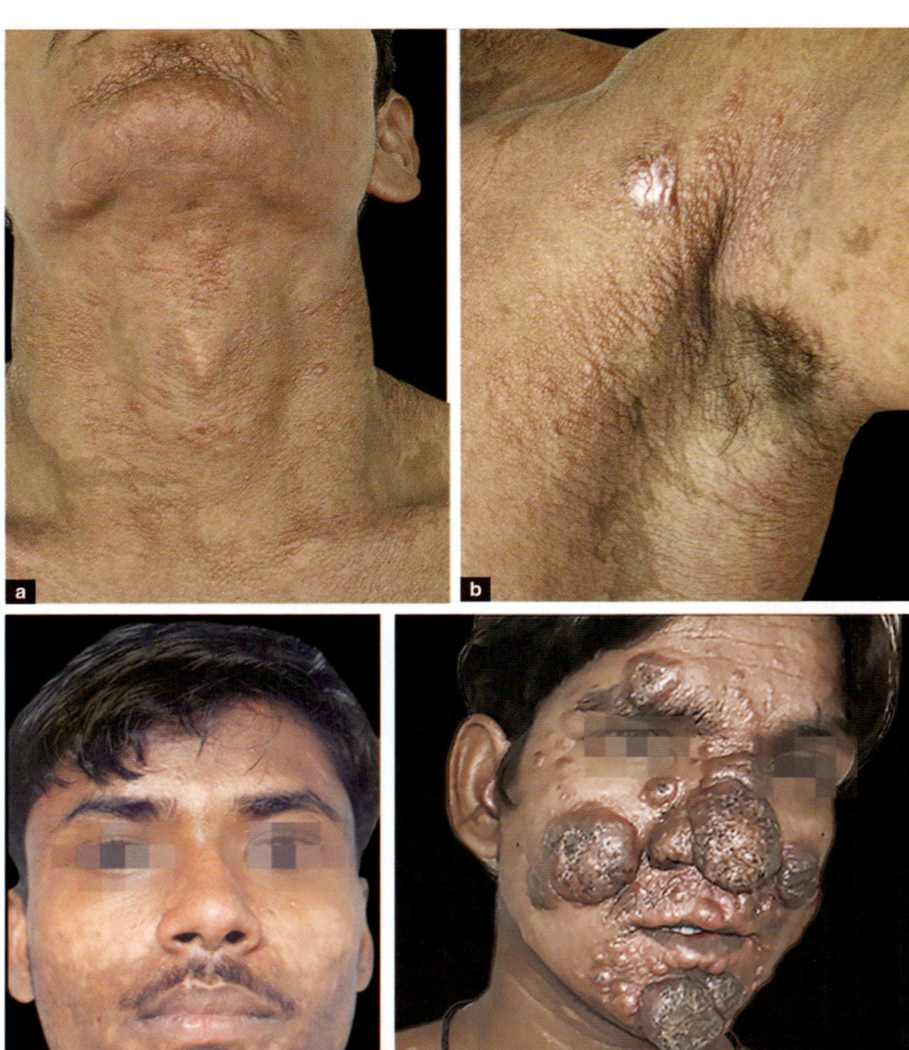

Fig. 17.61: (a and b) Monomorphic papular variant of PKDL on the face and shoulder. (c) Macular lesions pronounced in the muzzle area of the face. (d) Polymorphic PKDL with hypopigmented macules on trunk, and papules and nodules on face

- Hypopigmented macules—initial lesion in most cases (due to local effect on melanocyte)/(kala-azar hyperpigmentation due to effect on adrenal suppression).
- Mucosal—infiltrated nodules in oral cavity and lips and angle of mouth
- Genital—papules and nodules on glans, prepuce, shaft of penis
- Rare presentations (e.g. erythrodermic, xanthomatous, keloidal, measles-like, photosensitivity, verrucous, papillomatous, fibroid, spontaneous ulceration).

Differential Diagnosis

A summary of the common differentials are listed in **Table 17.43**. Macular PKDI should be most importantly differentiated from Borderline leprosy **(Table 17.44)**.

Similarity of PKDL and Leprosy

- Similar endemic area.
- Epithelioid cell granulomas of PKDL similar to tuberculoid granulomas of BT leprosy.
- Parasites may not be visible in both.
- Dermal nerve involvement possible in both.
- N-ramp (in lysosomal compartment of macrophages) affects replication of both parasites.

TABLE 17.43: Differential diagnosis of PKDL in Asia (most important causes)

Macular rash	Papulonodular
Leprosy	Leprosy
Chronic arsenic poisoning	Neurofibromatosis
Pityriasis vesicolor	Secondary syphilis
Vitiligo	
Pityriasis alba	

TABLE 17.44: Differentiating features of PKDL and borderline leprosy

	PKDL	Borderline leprosy
Sites	Ear lobes *spared, centrofacial* involvement	Ear lobes preferentially involved, centrofacial area spared
rK39 antigen (on plasma, on slit skin smear)	+ve (95–100% sensitive, 95–100% specific)	–ve
Histopathology	Superficial infiltrate Peripheral limits of infiltrate have fairly sharp margins LD bodies +ve, especially just beneath the epidermis	Infiltrate around neurovascular bundle Peripheral limits of infiltrate are infiltrative *M. leprae* +ve intracellularly in macrophages

Diagnosis

The investigations in a case of PKDL are listed in **Table 17.45**.

TABLE 17.45: Tests for the diagnosis of PKDL

- Slit skin smear or sample obtained from tissue biopsy–to identify Leishman-Donovan bodies or amastigotes (Gold standard due to high specificity)
- Serological tests–direct agglutination test (DAT), enzyme-linked immunosorbent assay (ELISA) and the rK39 rapid diagnostic ELISA. rKE-16 is another recombinant antigen (obtained from *L. donovani*) that has been used in some studies.
- Leishmanin skin test (LST)
- Histopathology
- DNA amplification methods: PCR, LAMP (loop-mediated isothermal amplification), qPCR
- Serum ADA levels
- Serum IL-10 levels

PKDL should be suspected in patients in endemic areas who present with a skin rash combined with previous or concomitant visceral leishmaniasis. The diagnosis can be made using clinical criteria or by identifying the parasite, or both.

There are 2 algorithms for diagnosis of a suspected PKDL case: The 1st is recommended by the **GOI** and 2nd is proposed by **WHO (Flowcharts 17.7** and **17.8)**.

1. **Slit skin smear:** Slit skin smears or samples obtained by biopsy can be used to identify parasites to confirm the diagnosis of PKDL. Studies in India and Sudan have found that smears are more likely to show amastigotes, if they are taken from nodular lesions rather than papular lesions; samples are least likely to show amastigotes, if taken from macular lesions.
2. **Serological tests:** Serological tests **(Table 17.46)** such as the direct agglutination test (DAT), enzyme-linked immunosorbent assay (ELISA) and the rK39 rapid diagnostic ELISA are usually positive but are of limited value because a positive result may be caused by antibodies persisting after a past episode of visceral leishmaniasis too. Nevertheless, serology can be helpful when other diseases (e.g. leprosy) are considered in the differential diagnosis, or if a history of visceral leishmaniasis is uncertain. A summary of the various antigens against which antibodies are detected are listed in **Table 17.46.**
   a. **rK39 rapid dipstick test (point of care test—POCT)**
      - Immunochromatographic test.
      - Detects circulating IgG against recombinant K39 protein antigen.
      - Can be done on slit skin smear or plasma.
      - Sensitivity 100%, specificity 100% even on SSS (from nodular lesions).

Flowchart 17.7: NVBDCP (Government of India) protocol for diagnosis of PKDL

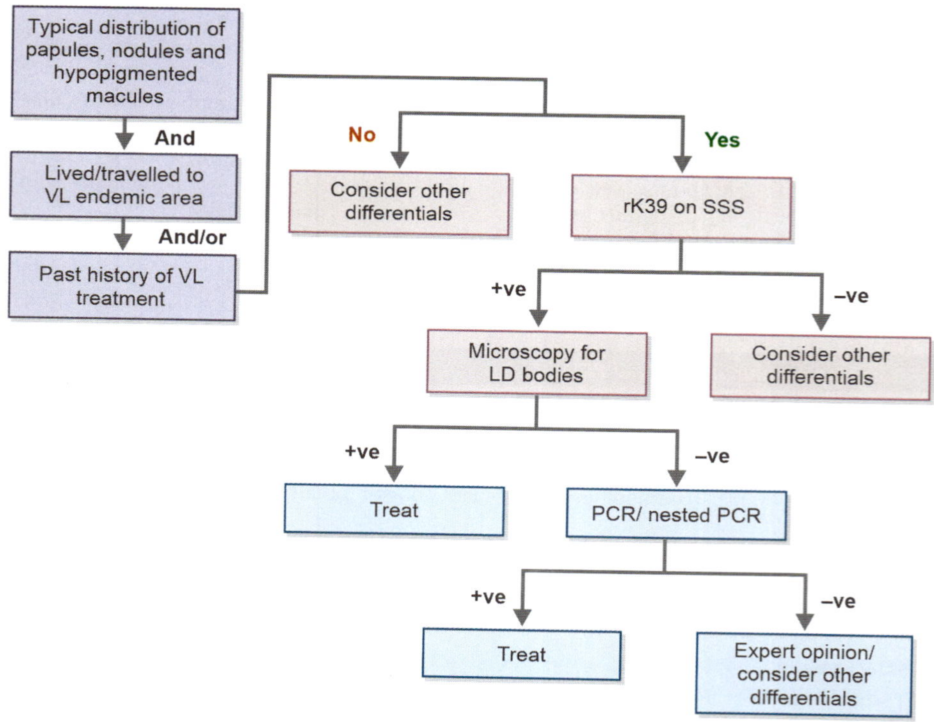

Flowchart 17.8: WHO algorithm for diagnosing and treating PKDL

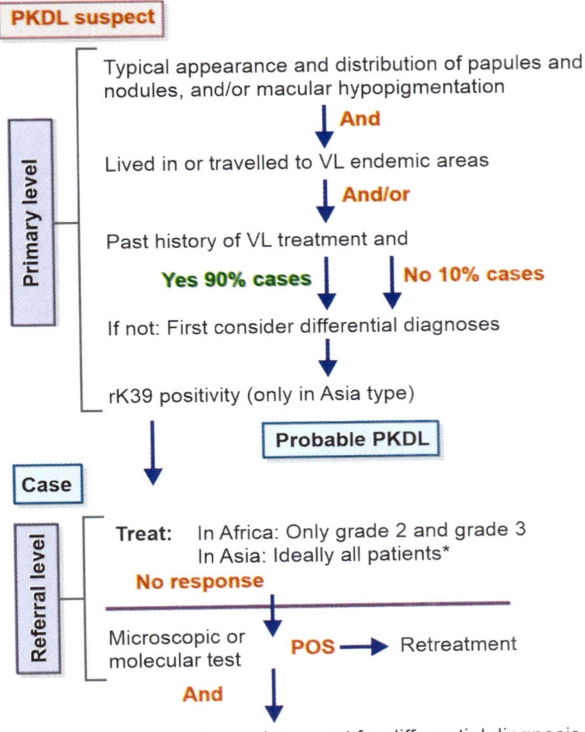

*As soon as an effective and safe regimen is identified

TABLE 17.46: Antigens used in ELISA for detection of antileishmanial antibody in sera of patients with PKDL

Antigen	Sensitivity (%)	Specificity (%)
CLA	86–100	90–100
SLA	83	90–100
MP	100	96.7
rK39*	94.5–100	93.7–100
GBP	93–100	83
GRP78	78	90
C-ELISA (D2)	100	100

*Used in India as a strip test.

- Positive when both T and C lines red, results available in 5 minutes.
- It can be used as strong evidence for past VL in both Africa and the Indian subcontinent. However, this test is more sensitive in the Indian subcontinent than in Africa; therefore, if negative, it rules out past disease in the Indian subcontinent but not in Africa.

b. **Direct agglutination test (DAT):** It has high sensitivity and specificity. Can be carried out on whole blood or serum. Uses freeze dried whole promastigotes as antigen.

3. **Leishmanin skin test**
4. **HPE**
   - Superficial (upper dermal) mixed chronic infiltrate of histiocytes, mainly lymphocytes and a few plasma cells with macrophages interspersed seen in macules while the entire dermis is involved in nodules.
   - 3 patterns seen (Ramesh & Ramam, 2020):
     - macules—mild superficial infiltrate
     - papules—dense upper dermal infiltrate
     - nodules—diffuse dermal infiltrate. Prominent follicular plugging with dense plasma cell—rich lymphohistiocytic dermal infiltrate with abrupt cut-off in lower dermis—very characteristic of PKDL even without LDBs. Grenz zone usually present.
   - **LD bodies +ve in macrophages or extracellularly**, especially just beneath the epidermis. Can confirm the diagnosis. *Histoplasma capsulatum* is the closest differential by histological appearance. Rates of positivity—macules (7–33%), papules (36–69%) and nodules (61–100%). Mucosal lesions more likely to demonstrate LDBs so they must be biopsied if present.
   - **HPE differences in Sudan:** Biopsy samples of PKDL in India show a diffuse dermal infiltrate of macrophages, lymphocytes and plasma cells; in PKDL, biopsy samples from Sudan, epithelioid cells are seen but plasma cells are scanty or absent. The inflammatory cells are mainly CD3+ cells; IL-10 is prominent in the lesions; interferon-γ and tumor necrosis factor alpha (TNF α) are found uniformly; and IL-4 is present in varying amounts. Diminished expression of interferon-gamma receptor 1 and TNF-R1 receptors during PKDL may interfere with an effective host response.
5. **DNA amplification methods:** Indicate live parasite → active infection, can work as test of cure
   - PCR, nested PCR, qPCR. Target most commonly used is the multi-copy kDNA as it has very high sensitivity.
   - LAMP (loop-mediated isothermal amplification)—does not need high temperatures unlike PCR, more suited for development as POCT.
6. **Serum ADA levels:** Increased, decrease during treatment.
7. **Serum IL-10 levels:** Proportionate to *L. donovani* load.

A comparison of the various tests is given in **Table 17.47**.

Treatment (Box 17.22)

There is limited evidence about the efficacy of PKDL treatment, and the outcome may depend on the severity of the condition and the duration of symptoms before treatment. Evaluating the efficacy of treatment for macular lesions clinically is not straight-forward because repigmentation of lesions may take place long after the goal of parasite clearance has been reached.

Treatment of PKDL implemented as a disease-control intervention is justified, only if the treatment is safe, effective, acceptable to the patient, and if it is not likely to lead to the development of resistant strains when monotherapy is used. Consideration should be given to preventing the development of resistant strains when monotherapy lasting longer than 4 weeks is prescribed.

A combination regimen is now used where MIL and LAmB combination for 45 days (3 injections of LAmB, 5 mg/kg body weight, and 100 mg/day MIL) and patients treated with combination therapy demonstrated a rapid decline in parasite load and achieved 100% cure, with no reports of relapse. Those treated with MIL monotherapy attained clinical cure with a gradual decrease in parasite load; however, 25% relapsed within 18 months of follow-up.

TABLE 17.47: Comparison of diagnostic methods between macular and nonmacular (polymorphic) PKDL

Features	Nonmacular type (polymorphic)*	Macular
Histology	Specific	Non-specific
Cellular infiltration	Dense in superficial and mid-dermis	Scattered in perivascular areas/superficial dermis
LDB	Present	Not seen commonly
Overall sensitivity	Up to 85%	Low positivity
IHC	100%	72%
ELISA	100%	90%
rK39 strip test	94–100%	73%
DAT		
Amastigote	100%	90–98%
Promastigote	90–100%	0–80%
PCR	100%	90–100%

DAT, direct agglutination test; H&E, hematoxylin and eosin; IHC, immunohistochemistry; LDB, Leishman–Donovan bodies; PCR, polymerase chain reaction

*Papules, nodules, erythema and induration/combination of one or more.

(Modified from *Indian J Med Res* 2006; 123:295–231).

BOX 17.22: Treatment of PKDL in Bangladesh, India and Nepal (based on WHO Technical Report Series 949)

1. **Miltefosine:** In India the dose is given as 25 kg >100 mg, <25 kg 50 mg
   - 150 mg orally per day for 12 weeks for patients weighing >50 kg,
   - 100 mg orally per day for 12 weeks for patients weighing 25–50 kg;
   - 50 mg orally per day for 12 weeks for patients weighing <25 kg; (grade of recommendation A).
2. **Amphotericin B deoxycholate:** 1 mg/kg per day by infusion, up to 60–80 doses delivered over 4 months; (grade of recommendation C).
3. **Liposomal amphotericin B:** 5 mg/kg per day by infusion two times per week for 3 weeks for a total dose of 30 mg/kg; (grade of recommendation A).

- Pregnant women should **not** be treated with miltefosine. Women of reproductive age and their partners should be counselled appropriately about the need to use effective contraception during the 12-week course of miltefosine treatment and for 4–6 months after completing treatment.
- Sodium stibogluconate should **not** be used to treat patients coinfected with HIV, pregnant women, or patients with underlying cardiac disease or renal disease.
- Clinical and parasitologic end points in PKDL are poorly defined, although PCR may have an emerging role in future trials.

Though cure is difficult to define, a proposed definition is given in **Box 17.23**. In addition, the role of PKDL as a reservoir for VL should be kept in mind as both nodular and macular PKDL can be infectious to sandflies. Active PKDL case detection and prompt treatment should be instituted and maintained as an integral part of VL control and elimination programs (Lancet, 2018).

BOX 17.23: Definitions of cure of PKDL

Clinical cure: Demonstrated by clinical cure of papular and nodular lesions, and complete resolution of macular lesion or repigmentation of macular lesions at 12-month follow-up visit.

Parasitological cure: At the end of treatment and at subsequent follow-up visits, parasites should no longer be present.

1. *Miltefosine*

- Hexadecylphosphocholine
- Preferred drug since it is an oral drug
- MOA:
  - Anti-leishmanial action—inhibition of synthesis of phosphatidylcholine (inhibits synthesis of glycerophospholipids)—present in cell membrane of parasites.
  - Anti-cancer action induces apoptosis in various cell lines, interferes with mitogenic signal transduction pathways **(miltefosine lacks bone marrow toxicity unlike other anti-cancer drugs; instead stimulates growth of hematopoietic stem cells)**.
- Dosage (available as capsules), *see* **Box 17.21** (any dosage above 150 mg has GI side effects)
- Contraindications:
  - <2 years
  - Pregnant and lactating females
  - Women in reproductive age group who refuse contraception during and for at least 5 months after treatment completion (due to long primary elimination t½ of 170 hours or 7 days and terminal elimination t½ of 30.9 days.
- Adverse reactions:
  - Nausea, vomiting, diarrhea—most common, up to 20%.
  - Teratogenicity (hence contraception essential and depot preparations of IUCD preferred)
  - Probably impaired male fertility
  - Hypersensitivity, SJS/TEN
  - Keratitis, scleritis
  - Few—LFT/KFT derangement—monitoring essential
- Resistance: Miltefosine was FDA approved for VL, CL and ML in 2014. It has been used for PKDL since 2006. However, relapses have been reported with miltefosine monotherapy—15% at 18 months (Ramesh V, 2015). Also, due to high chances of gastrointestinal side effects, compliance may be compromised leading to higher chances of development of resistance (Pijpers J, 2019). Lab confirmed cases of miltefosine resistance have been reported.

A study has shown that a a combination of Miltefosine + LAMB is better than miltefosine alone and thus in difficult cases a combination of MIL and LAMB combination for 45 days (3 injections of LAmB, 5 mg/kg body weight, and 100 mg/day MIL) is advisable (Ramesh V, et al., 2020).

2. *Amphotericin B*

- MOA: Similar to that in fungi (binds to ergosterol in cell membrane leading to formation of pores)
- Indications:
  - Failed first line treatment
  - Adverse effects of other first line drugs
  - Pregnant and lactating females
  - <2 years of age
  - LFT/KFT deranged significantly
- Contraindications:
  - Significant liver disease/kidney disease
  - Heart disease

- Monitoring required for:
  - Hypokalemia
  - Hypomagnesemia
  - Hypoglycemia
  - KFT derangement
  - Hypersensitivity reactions
- Dosage:
  - Amphotericin B deoxycholate IV **1 mg/kg/day (20 days on, 15 days off)** for up to **4 months**.
  - Liposomal amphotericin B (**5 mg/kg** per dose) 2/week × 3 weeks (a total of **30** mg/kg). A short-course treatment of 3 mg/kg given for 5 doses (a total of 15 mg/kg) has also been tried successfully.

3. *Antimonial Compounds*

- Sodium antimony gluconate (SAG) contains 100 mg/mL of antimony
- MOA:
  - Interferes with phosphorylation of ADP and GDP (dose dependent—thus higher dose needed in PKDL for enough drug to reach dermis)
  - Anti-inflammatory too (hence used in leprosy reactions occasionally)
- Contraindications: Tuberculosis
- Dosage: 20 mg/kg body weight (up to 850 mg/day) for 120 days (IM or slow IV in evening)
- Adverse effects:
  - Nausea, headache, lethargy
  - Myalgias
- Monitoring required for:
  - Heart function (ECG)
  - LFT/KFT.
- Resistance
  - Drug resistance due to reduced biological reduction of Sb^{5+} to Sb^{3+}, decreased internalization of drug, increased level of the target enzyme trypanothione reductase.

4. *Paromomycin*

- An aminoglycoside antibiotic with antileishmanial properties.
- *MOA*:
  - inhibition of leishmanial cyt C enzyme
  - inhibition of translocation and recycling of ribosomes
- *Dosage*: 11 mg/kg I/M × 45 days
- *Adverse effects*: Reversible ototoxicity, reversible nephrotoxicity, hypokalemia
- *Use*: Monotherapy has a very low cure rate, but its combination with SSG is effective and safe.

5. *Update*

Triclabendazole (TCBZ) is a benzimidazole used to treat fasciolosis in adults and children. It presents a lower toxicity profile than amphotericin B (AmpB) and is administered orally, making it an attractive candidate for treating other parasitoses and has been studied in combination with Amphotericin B and has shown synergy and can be a potential drug for PKDL (Borges BS, et al., 2023).

SCABIES

Epidemiology

- Causative agent: *Sarcoptes scabiei var hominis* **(Fig. 17.62)**
- **Name:** Greek *sarx* = meat; *koptein* = twisted. *Latin* scaber = rough, not clean.
- Scabies—added to list of **neglected tropical diseases by WHO**.

Transmission

- Unlike ectoparasitic fleas and flies, scabies mites cannot jump or fly, but they can crawl at a rate of 2.5 cm/min on warm, moist skin.
- They can survive for 24–36 hours at room temperature and average humidity and remain capable of infesting humans.
- Scabies is most easily transmitted by skin-to-skin contact, as with sex partners, children playing.
- Animal scabies are facultative ectoparasites and cannot complete their life cycle in humans.

Predisposing Factors

Overcrowding, low socioeconomic status.

Pathogenesis

- Mite—attracted to human host by heat and nitrogen waste.
- Average number of mites/patient—**12** and about **10–15** fertile mites are transmitted from one patient to another host. Females live for about **2–3 months**.

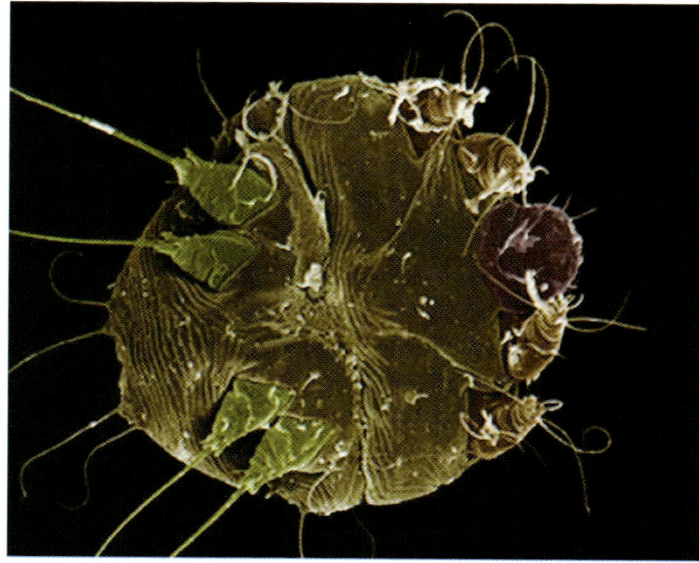

Fig. 17.62: Scanning electron micrograph of the scabies mite (*Sarcoptes scabiei*)

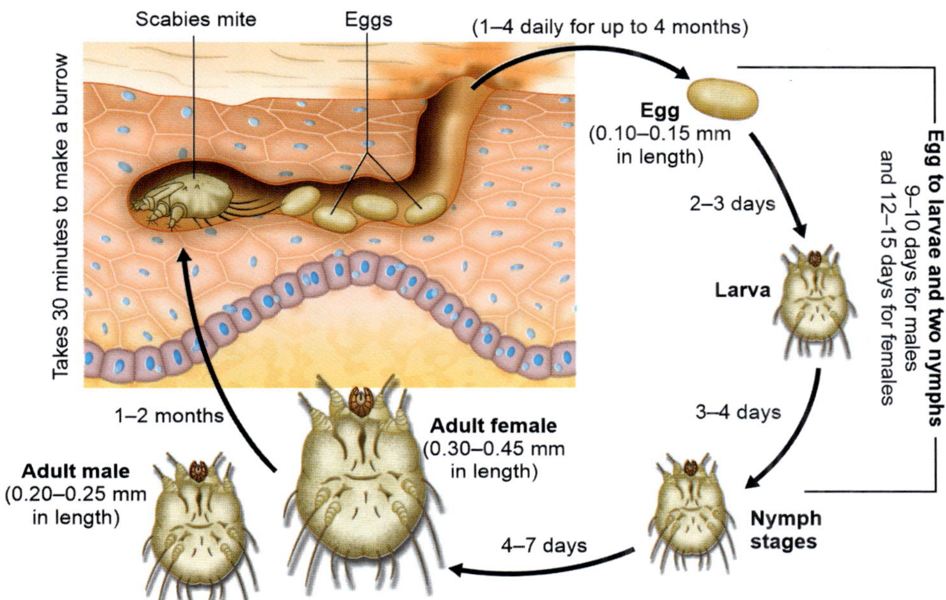

Fig. 17.63: Life cycle of *Sarcoptes scabiei*

- <u>Less</u> at areas with high density of pilosebaceous units (seborrheic areas).
- Life cycle—Egg → adult—**14–15** days **(Fig. 17.63)**.
- **IP**—from infection to symptoms is **3–6 weeks** for initial infection **and 1–3 days** in case of reinfection.
- Immediate hypersensitivity to mite/products—itching
- Delayed type hypersensitivity—leads to symptoms after **3–6** weeks, T cell pseudolymphoma on HPE.

Clinical Features of Classic Lesion

- **Nocturnal itching**
  Itching occurs due to:
  - Activation of TLR-3, 4, 7 expressed on sensory neurons
  - Mite feces proteases activate protease—activated receptors
  - Activation of pruritus receptors through direct action on keratinocytes
- **Burrows:** <u>Pathognomonic lesions</u>
  - Slightly raised brownish serpiginous/linear papule **(Fig. 17.64)**
  - As thin as human hair, 2–3 mm

  (The burrow is dotted with fecal lithes (pellets) or scybala, and terminates in raised papules hiding ovipositing females)
- **Other lesions:** Excoriated papules, vesicles (infants), pustules, nodules, excoriation marks—present in a <u>**circle of Hebra**</u> distribution **(Fig. 17.64)**.

Clinical Types/Variants

Table 17.48 details the clinical types of scabies.

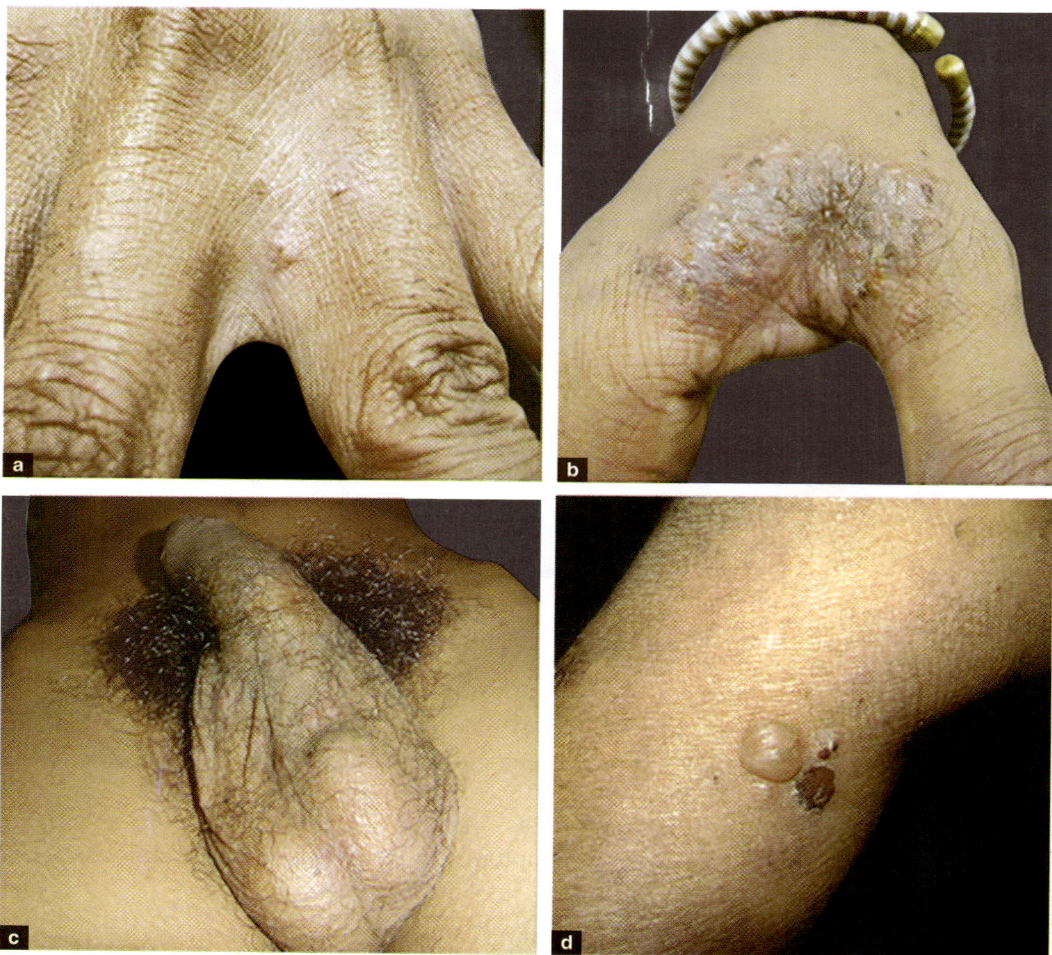

Fig. 17.64: (a) Interdigital papules and burrow seen in scabies; (b) Secondarily infected and impetiginized burrow; (c) Nodules of scabies; (d) Bullous lesions in scabies

TABLE 17.48: Clinical types/variants of scabies	
1. Crusted (Norwegian) scabies	• <u>No/mild pruritus</u> • Thick crusted plaques, subungual hyperkeratosis, nail dystrophy, palmoplantar keratoderma, erythroderma, generalized lymphadenopathy • Seen in debilitated bedridden patients, syringomyelia, tabes dorsalis, Down syndrome, stroke, malignancies, leprosy, HIV, SLE, mental retardation • Initial misdiagnosis (e.g. eczema, prurigo, drug-related eruptions, psoriasis) is seen in 43% of cases
2. Infantile scabies	• Atypical sites (face, palms/soles) • Vesicular lesions

(Contd.)

TABLE 17.48: Clinical types/variants of scabies (Contd.)	
3. Animal scabies	• Sarcoptic mange • Mite from animal can be transmitted to humans but cannot complete its life cycle.
4. Atypical sites	• Scalp (infants, children, elderly, HIV/AIDS, crusted scabies; differential diagnosis seborrheic dermatitis) • Palms and soles (infants; differential diagnosis infantile acropustulosis)
5. Atypical presentations	Mimic bullous pemphigoid, urticaria, chronic lymphocytic leukemia, B cell lymphoma with monoclonal infiltrate, CD 30+ lymphoid proliferations, necrotizing vasculitis, lupus erythematosus
6. Scabies galeuse/chancre galeuse	• A syphilitic chancre may occasionally develop in a lesion of scabies. • Initial lesion of scabies may be the route of entry of *Treponema pallidum*.

Complications

- Impetiginization
- Eczematization
- Psychosocial impact
- Poststreptococcal glomerulonephritis (PSGN) **(Australian aboriginal communities**—highest rate of PSGN in the world due to scabies super-infection**)**
- Induction of bullous pemphigoid (rare).

Diagnosis

The diagnosis is mostly clinical but investigations may sometimes be needed to differentiate from close mimickers and are detailed in **Table 17.49**.

TABLE 17.49: Diagnosis of scabies	
• **Bedside tests** [visualization of mite with/without fecal pellets (scybala) and eggs-confirmatory]	• Drop of mineral oil/10% KOH—scrape entire lesion with blade, transfer to slide, put cover slip, examine under microscope **(Fig. 17.65)** • Shave biopsy—examine under microscope. • **Burrow ink test/Parker ink test**—rub underside of cartridge pen nib on papule, wipe off excess, ink tracks down burrow, dark zigzag line visible • Adhesive tape—pulled off and adhered on to slide—seen under light microscope
• Dermoscopy	• **Jet with contrail (40×)** (= mite with eggs and scybala) • **Circumflex-accent like image (similar to the French letter)—Ô (on 10×)** (= head and 2 pairs of front legs of the mite)—91% sensitive, 86% specific
• Serum IgE	• Elevated in many studies • Indicative of type I hypersensitivity
• Histopathology (rarely required) **(Fig. 17.66)**	• May show the mite and its parts but in most cases, nonspecific features such as spongiosis, papillary edema,superficial and deep perivascular inflammatory infiltrate, eosinophils • Nodular scabies: Pseudolymphoma like picture on HPE with plasma cells, lymphocytes,histiocytes, eosinophils

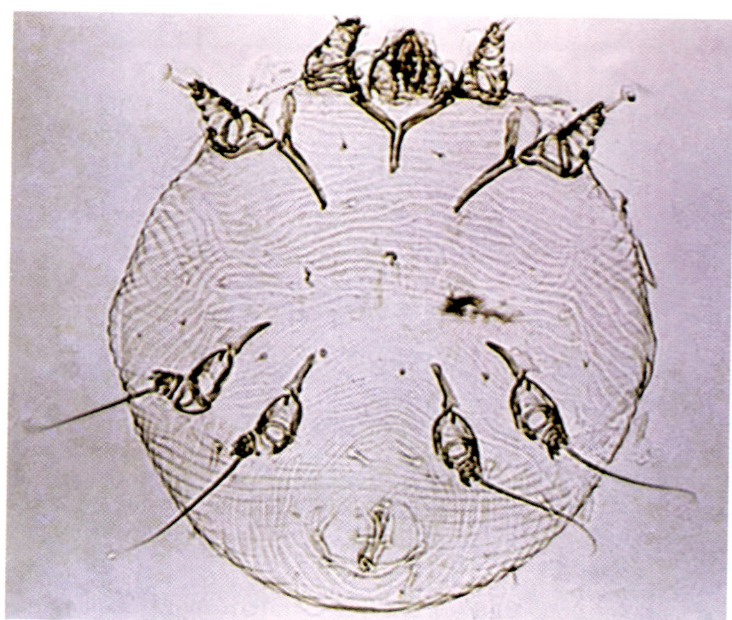

Fig. 17.65: A KOH mount of scabies mite

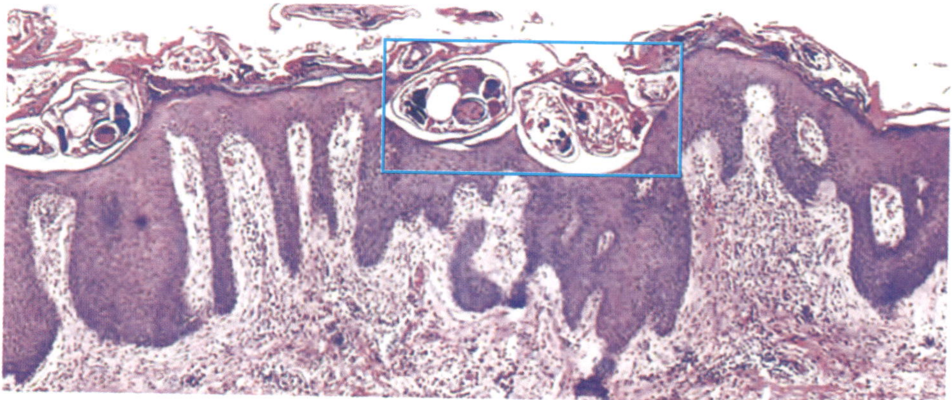

Fig. 17.66: Presence of scabies mites, scybala and eggs within the stratum corneum

Treatment

While the treatment modalities are listed in **Table 17.50**, resistance has developed in certain parts of the world. For **crusted scabies**, Currie and McCarthy have recommended both 5% topical permethrin every 2–3 days for 1–2 weeks and oral ivermectin, 200 μg/kg/dose, taken with food and administered as three doses (days 1, 2, and 8), five doses (days 1, 2, 8, 9, and 15), or seven doses, depending on the severity of the infection **(Table 17.51)**. In refractory institutional and community outbreaks, combined therapy with topical permethrin and oral ivermectin for all symptomatic cases with classic or crusted scabies and a single oral dose of ivermectin, 200 μg/kg, for all exposed, asymptomatic residents, visitors, and staff is advised.

TABLE 17.50: List of topical and systemic anti-scabietic agents

Name	Strength	MOA	Application	Side effects	Precautions	Safety in infants	Pregnancy/ lactation	Safety in CNS disease patients
Lindane/ GBHC (FDA approved)	1% lotion	Blockage of GABA gated Cl channels → hyperexcitation of CNS → Causes convulsions death	Apply overnight—wash off after 6–8 hours. Repeat after 1 week	Headache, vertigo, convulsions Aplastic anemia	Excessive excoriations on skin → Higher systemic absorption → higher CNS s/e, Black box warning (carcinogenic)	Approved for children > 2 years who have failed first line treatment	Cat C/ avoid	Avoid
Malathion (organophosphate insecticide)	0.5% lotion	Irreversibly binds to acetylcholinesterase → death	Apply to dry skin × 24 hours. Repeat after 1 week	Irritation, conjunctivitis	—	Avoid	Cat C/ avoid	Avoid
Precipitated sulfur	5%, 10% in petrolatum	Scabicidal, keratolytic	3 applications at night after bath every 24 hours	Messy, smelly, stains burning sensation	—	Safe	Cat C/safe	Safe
Crotamiton (FDA approved)	10% cream/ lotion	Unknown, also an anti-pruritic	2 applications at night, after bath for 24 hours	Irritation, pruritus, methemoglobinemia (children)	—	Not approved	Cat C/safe	Safe
Benzyl benzoate (from Balsam of Peru)	25% emulsion (12.5% for children)	Inhibits respiration	3 applications at night after bath for 24 hours	ICD, ACD, skin irritation	Avoid alcohol for 2 days due to disulfiram-like reaction	Safe	Cat C/safe	Safe
Permethrin (pyrethroid insecticide)* (FDA approved)	5% cream/ lotion	Irreversibly binds to sodium channels → delayed repolarization → flaccid paralysis → death	Apply overnight—wash off after 8–12 hr. Repeat after 1 week	Irritation, contact dermatitis (rare)	—	>2 months	Cat B/safe	Safe
Ivermectin (from soil actinomycete *Streptomyces avermitilis*)#	1% cream and tablet 200 µg/kg	Binds to glutamated Chloride channels → flaccid paralysis → death	Apply overnight—wash off after 8–12 hours. Repeat after 1 week take orally with food for better bioavailability	Lethargy, hypotension, asthenia, headache, myalgias, arthralgias, rash, eosinophilia	Does not cross BBB, 3 weekly doses in crusted scabies	Avoid in children <5 years/ <15 kg	Cat C/ avoid	Avoid
Spinosad (FDA approved 2021)	0.9% suspension	Neuronal hyperexcitation → paralysis	Single applicaton – wash after 6 hours	Irritation, dry skin	—	>4 years	Safe	Safe

* Permethrin—acaricidal, larvicidal; #Ivermectin—only acaricidal, not ovicidal; s/e—side effect

TABLE 17.51: Treatment of scabies according to clinical type	
Classic scabies	Topical _permethrin_ and oral _ivermectin_ are the most common first-line treatment in the United States, United Kingdom, and Australia
Crusted scabies	Combination treatment with _permethrin_ and oral _ivermectin_ is considered the preferred first-line treatment for crusted scabies. CDC: • Topical 5% _permethrin_ or topical 5% benzoyl benzoate applied _daily for 7 days, then twice weekly until cure_, and • Oral _ivermectin_ (200 µg/kg/dose) given on days _1, 2, 8, 9, and 15_. Patients with severe infestations may require longer courses of oral _ivermectin_, with two additional doses (given on days 22 and 29).
Endemic scabies	Mass drug administration of oral _ivermectin_
Nodular scabies	Once to twice daily application of a potent topical steroid for 2 to 3 weeks or intralesional injection of a corticosteroid such as _triamcinolone_ acetonide (5 to 10 mg/mL).
Special population	**Children**—given its high efficacy and safety, _permethrin_ is preferred therapy. <2 months-topical sulfur Treatment with oral _ivermectin_ is not recommended for children who weight <15 kg **Pregnant women:** _Permethrin_ is considered safe for use in pregnant and lactating women and is a preferred treatment, second-line treatments for pregnant women include topical sulfur and benzyl benzoate.
Treatment failure	Therapy is likely successful, if active lesions resolve and nocturnal pruritus ceases by one week after treatment. Of note, some pruritus often persists for 2 to 4 weeks after successful treatment.

There is no need to treat pets as in animal scabies the mites are genetically distinct and cannot live on other hosts. Avoid contact with clothes/towels used for more than 3 days.

General measures including treatment of all contact cases and tumble drying of all clothes of index cases at >50° C is important. A recent paper has examined if current treatment strategies for scabies also cover the opportunistic bacteria, seen in scabies cases and **abametapir and mānuka oil** have antimicrobial properties against common scabies-associated bacteria, specifically *Staphylococcus aureus, Streptococcus pyogenes, Streptococcus dysgalactiae subsp. equisimilis* and *Acinetobacter baumannii*. The current scabicide ivermectin offers some antimicrobial activity and is capable of inhibiting the growth aforementioned bacteria. This is relevant as the commonest secondary infection is impetigo (Taylor S., 2022).

Common causes of pruritus >4 weeks include:

1. Treatment-related skin irritation or contact dermatitis.
2. Treatment failure may result from poor adherence to the treatment regimen, resistance, or reinfestation.
3. Other causes of persistent pruritus include delusional infestation (also called delusional parasitosis) and unrelated skin disease.

The **treatment of individual type of scabies is listed in Table 17.51**.

PEDICULOSIS

Epidemiology

Causative Agent

- ***Pediculus humanus***—*P. humanus capitis* (head louse) and *P. humanus humanus* (body/clothing louse)
- ***Pthirus pubis*** (pubic/crab louse)
- Wingless dorsoventrally flattened **blood sucking (solenophages) obligate ectoparasites** (suborder Anoplura of order Phthiraptera)
- Highly host-specific
- Highly territory-specific

PEDICULOSIS CAPITIS

Epidemiology

- **Age:** Children > adults, 3–11 years.
- **Sex:** F > M, length of hair (as lice favor dark areas—areas of higher hair density) more head-to-head contact in girls.
- Pomade use, curliness, increased combing in black Americans decreases incidence, but hair oils not seen to reduce incidence in Indian subcontinent.

Predisposing Factors

- Poverty, poor hygiene, overcrowding → more head-to-head contact.
- Role of fomites—doubtful, better to disinfect.

Pathogenesis

Life cycle

- Adult females—3–4 mm long (male slightly smaller).
- Egg hatch in 8–10 days, 3 nymphal/instar stages **(Figs 17.67** and **17.68)**. First 2 instar stages—immobile → cannot transmit. Only adult and 3rd instar stage responsible for transmission.
- Total lifespan—*40 days*.
- Male dies after copulation.

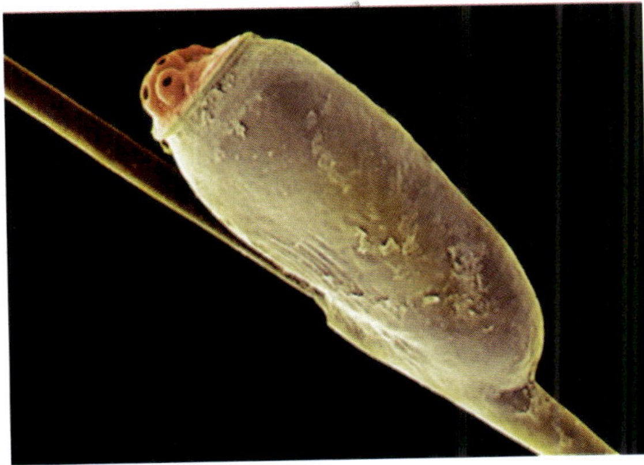

Fig. 17.67: Scanning electron micrograph of an egg of *P. humanus capitis* with a operculum (cover) which has aeropyles

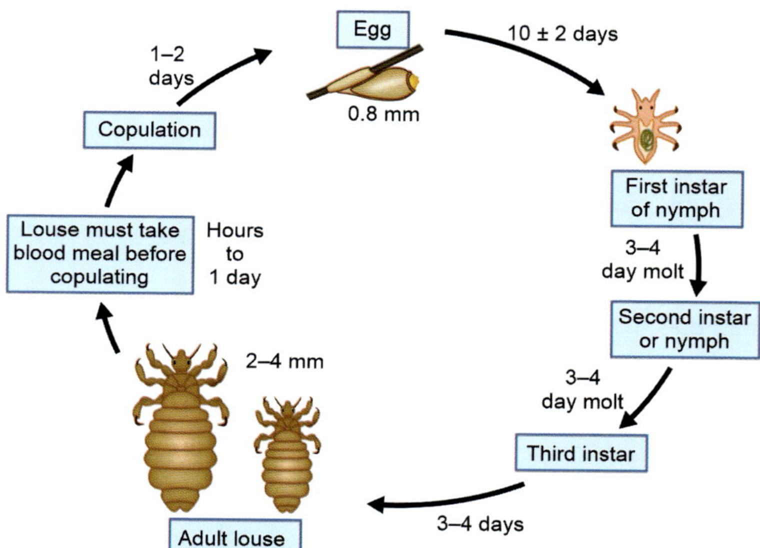

Fig. 17.68a: Life cycle of *Pediculus humanus capitis*

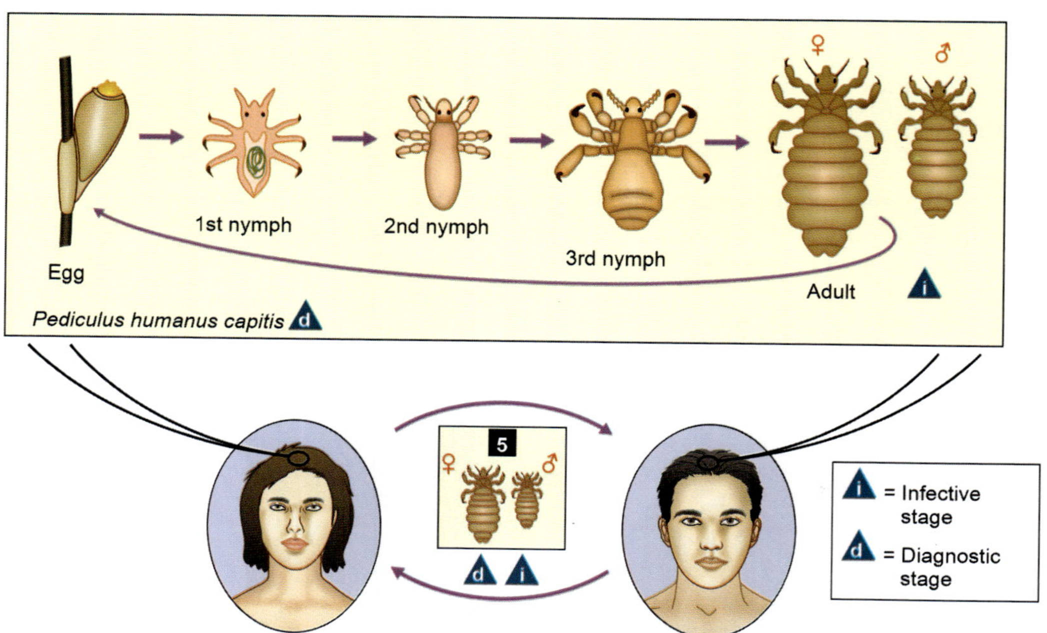

Fig. 17.68b: Diagnostic and infective stages in life cycle of *P. humanus capitis*

- Female lays 7 eggs a day—close to the scalp surface for optimum temperature for egg hatching, cemented by chitinous substance.
  Distance from scalp (eggs at 1–2 mm → nymph at 6–7 mm → thus if within 1 cm suggestive of active infestation).

- Females can live on their hosts for up to 3 months, lay up to 300 eggs/nits in a lifetime and die within 24 hours when separated from hosts. Speed of lice—up to 23 cm/day.

  In general only fertilized females creep up to the surface of the hair, while male and larvae stay mostly close to the surface of the scalp, since they need repeated blood meals (every 2–3 hours) **(Fig. 17.69)**. The fertilized females do not stay very long on the surface of the hair, but creep quickly back to the scalp in order to ingest again blood and to lay eggs. In case they are in contact with the hair of another person they transmit to this person.

Clinical Features

- Many—asymptomatic
- Typical—scalp pruritus **(Fig. 17.70)**
- Secondary bacterial infection +/−
- Pruritic papules, excoriations—nape of neck, behind ears (**lice maximum in occipital and parietal regions) (Fig. 17.71)**
- Matting—**"plica polonica"**

Complications

Not known to transmit any human pathogen (though some bacteria have been detected in the lice—significance unknown).

Diagnosis

- **Bedside tests**
  - Visualization of adult lice and nymphs—evidence of active infestation. Only eggs and nits is not proof that infection is active.

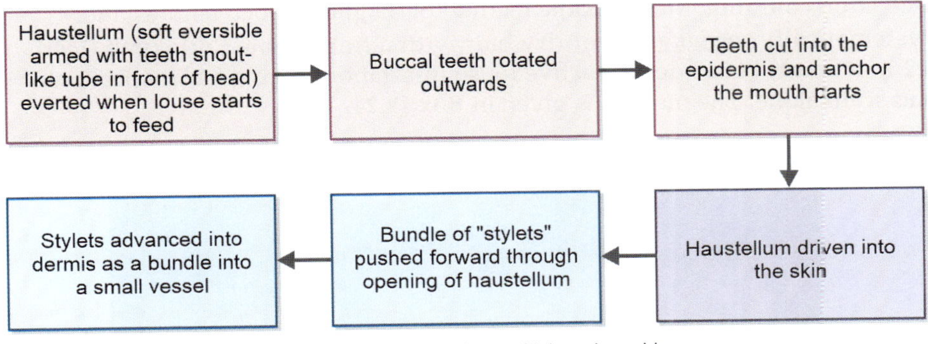

Fig. 17.69: Mechanism of blood sucking

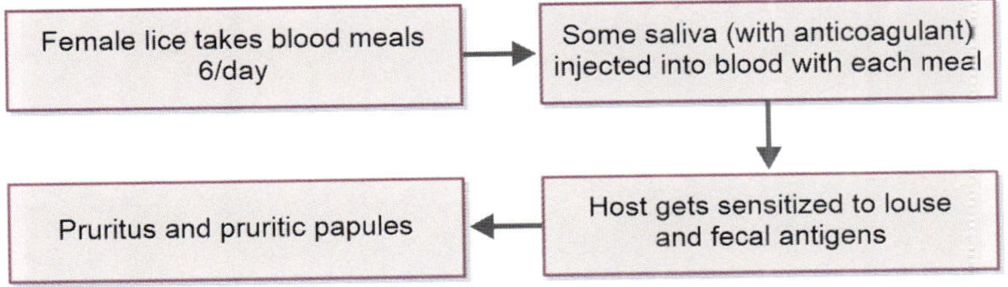

Fig. 17.70: Pathogenesis of symptoms of itching

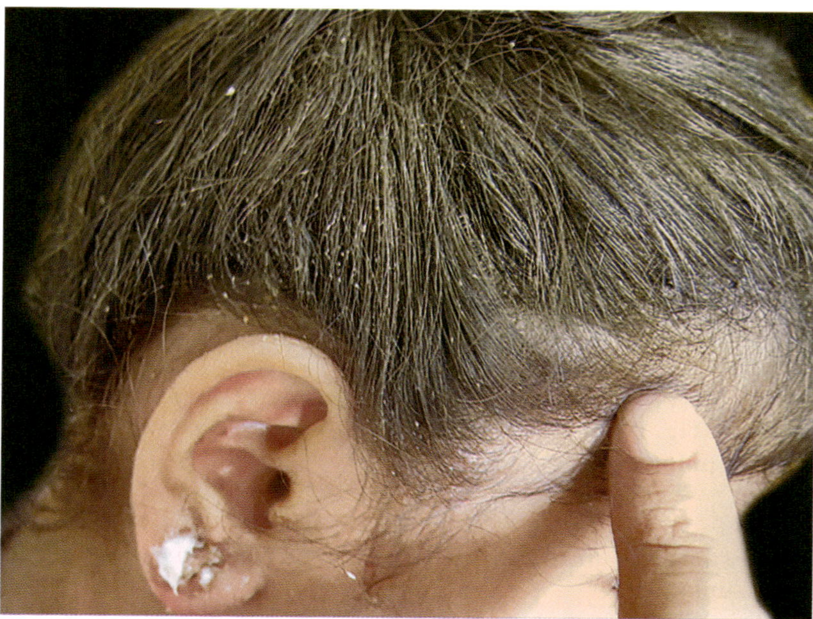

Fig. 17.71: A child with nits, the concomitant itching leads to scatching and secondary infection

- Adult lice are flattened dorsoventrally and are 1 mm (pubic lice) to 3 mm (head and body lice) in length, have three pairs of legs ending in powerful claws that can grip hair shafts, and exhibit a reddish-brown hue after blood feeding **(Fig. 17.72)**.
- **Detection combing:** Most reliable method of diagnosing active infestation. Systematically combing wet or dry hair with a fine-toothed nit comb (teeth of comb 0.2 mm apart) better detects active louse infestation than visual inspection of the hair and scalp alone. The method is given in **Box 17.24**.

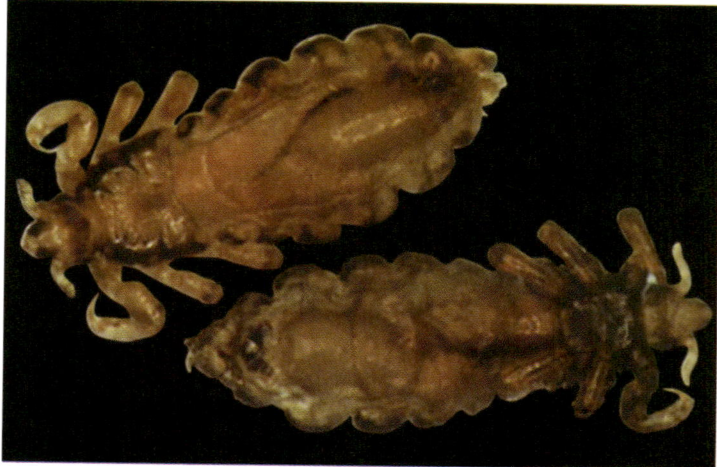

Fig. 17.72: Image of *Pediculus humanus capitis*

BOX 17.24: Combing method to detect lice

- A lubricant such as a hair conditioner is applied to the hair
- Hair is brushed or combed to remove tangles
- Fine-toothed comb is inserted near the crown until it gently touches the scalp, after which it is drawn firmly down and examined for lice after each stroke
- Combed systematically at least twice

- **Dermoscopy**
  - **To differentiate eggs** from pseudonits—peripilar keratin casts (remnants of IRS), debris, dried globules of cheap hair lacquer, dandruff or pityriasis sicca, white or black piedra, monilethrix, pseudomonilethrix, pili torti, Psocids or booklice.

Hair casts may be idiopathic (primary hair casts) or may occur in association with a scalp condition such as seborrheic dermatitis or psoriasis.

i. Eggs—attached to only a *part* of the hair shaft, piedra/casts—circumferentially *envelope* the hair haft, hair casts *slide* easily along the hair shaft.
ii. Eggs with nymph—appear opaque white, while empty nits—appear translucent flat.
iii. Egg with nymph—oval, flesh-colored, have a lid/operculum capping the free end which is opened by the hatching louse nymph **(*see* Fig. 17.68)**. Empty egg case/nit—white, easier to see.
iv. Nits also should be distinguished from white and black piedra, fungal infections most commonly found in tropical areas that present with white to beige (white piedra) or brown to black (black piedra) concretions on hair shafts.
   - White piedra: The nodules of white piedra tend to be *soft and loosely adhered* to the hair shaft. Sites: Face, axillae, and genitals more often than scalp hair.
   - Black piedra: *Hard and firmly attached*. Sites—scalp and facial hair.

Treatment

General Measures

- Furniture should be vacuumed.
- Boil/disinfect with insecticidal powder—hair combs/curlers, etc.
- Bedsheets laundered at >60°C.
- Fomites that cannot be laundered should be placed in a bag for >3 days (as lice cannot survive off host for >55 hours).
- Treat all family contacts within 1 week.
- Avoid sharing of hats/hair care items.
- *Prefer lotions* and *liquids* to shampoos due to short contact time and low concentrations in the latter → may contribute to resistance.
- Aqueous base preferable to alcoholic base— less irritation, no exacerbation of asthma, not flammable.
- Do not use sprays in asthma patients.
- Administer topical/oral treatment on 2–3 occasions at gap of 7–10 days.
- Patients with nits but no detectable nymphs or adult lice likely do not have active infection, if nits are specially found **>6.5 mm** from the scalp. These patients do not require treatment.

- Removal of all viable nits by carefully combing wet hair.
- Olive oil and petroleum jelly are preferred hair-wetting agents, and plastic combs are preferred over metal combs.

Medical Therapy

- Two topical or systemic treatments with pediculicides, 7–10 days apart.
- Single oral dose of **ivermectin**, **400**/μg/kg of body weight repeated at 7 days, established higher louse-free rates by day 15.
- In **2012**, the FDA approved the use of **topical 0.5% ivermectin** lotion for head lice infestations after two multisite, randomized, double-blind studies comparing single applications of 0.5% ivermectin lotion with vehicle control that demonstrated significantly greater louse-free days at 1, 7, and 14 days in the ivermectin group than in the vehicle control group.
- **Permethrin**

  Locations without prevalent pyrethroid resistance—*Permethrin* is commonly prescribed and the mode of application is detailed below.

  - Dry hair should be ensured before applying the pediculicide
  - Keep it for 20 minutes
  - 2nd treatment on day 9
  - Prescription-strength permethrin (5%) is also available but is not more effective than the over-the-counter preparation
  - S/E: May cause breathing difficulties in patients with ragweed allergy, and permethrin use is not recommended in patients who are allergic to chrysanthemums
  - Age: Pyrethrins can be used for patients >2 years of age

  Locations with prevalent pyrethroid resistance—*malathion, benzyl alcohol, spinosad*, and topical *ivermectin* are appropriate treatments.
- Combination therapy with topical permethrin and trimethoprim-sulfamethoxazole may be more effective than treatment with permethrin alone. The mechanism of action of trimethoprim-sulfamethoxazole may involve the death of symbiotic bacteria in the louse gut that produce B vitamins necessary for louse survival.

The ranked order of therapeutic effectiveness from most to least effective agent is 0.5% malathion, undiluted natural pyrethrins with piperonyl butoxide, 1% permethrin, diluted natural pyrethrins with piperonyl butoxide, and 1% lindane. Unfortunately, the ideal pediculicide with 100% killing activity against lice and nits does not exist. **Table 17.52** presents the most commonly used pediculicides for lice infestations. Drug resistance is increasing against the safest pediculicides (the pyrethrins and synthetic pyrethroids), and even against lindane and malathion which as of today remain the only effective ovicidal insecticide with 95% efficacy against viable nits.

Update

Abametapir 0.74% is a drug that chelates heavy metal cations and inhibits metalloproteinases critical to louse ova development, hatching, and adult survival. It has been found to have a direct ovicidal activity inhibiting 100% of treated louse eggs from hatching and a 10 min application is effective and is a newly FDA-approved, single-application treatment for head lice in patients aged 6 months and older.

TABLE 17.52: Common pediculocidal agents

Agent	Application/Efficacy	Comments
1% Permethrin creme rinse	• Apply for **20 minutes** → rinse • 2-week residual activity • Drug resistance reported	Infants and children age 6 months and younger; safety in pregnancy uncertain
Ivermectin, 200–400 µg/kg tablet	• Excellent but not ovicidal • Single PO dose, second dose in 7–10 days recommended	<15 kg
0.9% Spinosad suspension	• Apply to hair for 10 minutes • Repeat after 9 days • No reports of resistance; not ovicidal	Infants and children age under 4 years; presumed safe in pregnancy based on animal studies
0.5% Ivermectin lotion	• No resistance • Single 10-min application → rinse • Not ovicidal but nymphs die when they emerge from nits	CI: Infants and children age 6 months and younger; safety in pregnancy uncertain
0.5% Malathion lotion, 1% malathion shampoo	• 95% ovicidal • Rapid (5-minutes) killing • Good residual activity	CI: Infants and children <6 months of age; Avoid pregnancy; breastfeeding
1% Lindane lotion and shampoo	• Apply overnight or wash after 8 hours • 95% ovicidal • No residual activity, increasing drug resistance	CI: Pre-existing seizure disorder; infants and children <6 months of age; Avoid pregnancy; breastfeeding
Benzyl alcohol 5% lotion	• Non-neurotoxic • Kills lice by asphyxiation • Apply for 10 minutes → rinse • Repeat after 9 days	<6 months
Dimethicone 4% lotion	• Coats cuticles of lice → seals the spiracles → suffocation • Apply for 10 mins → rinse • Repeat after 8–10 days	<2 years
Cotrimoxazole tablet	• Kills symbiotic bacteria • Twice daily × 10 days	Resolve for cases not responding to topical pediculicides

Physical Methods

- **Bug busting:** Shampooing → apply conditioner in large amounts (lice cannot move on wet hair) → fine-toothed comb **(Wet combing)** repeat every 4 days for 2 weeks—so that freshly hatched eggs and nymphs removed too.
- **Hot air therapy—"louse buster"**—air at 58–60°C.
- **Dimethicone lotion**—blocks outer respiratory tract and water excretion → death.
- **Coconut-derived emulsion shampoo**
- **Benzyl alcohol 5% solution**—obstruction of respiratory spiracles

- CETAPHIL™ liquid cleanser
- Cyclomethicone + isopropyl myristate
- **Occlusives**—oils, margarine, petroleum jelly (most effective)

  (However, lice are difficult to suffocate, and a small study of such products concluded that they are not effective. Gasoline and kerosene are highly flammable and should not be used for pediculosis capitis.)

PEDICULOSIS CORPORIS

Predisposing Factors

- Poor socioeconomic condition
- ***Pediculosis vestimenti***—clothes not changed/washed regularly
- Homeless vagabonds, refugee-camp population—*"**Vagabonds' disease/Morbus errorum**"*
- Their preferred temperature ranges between 31° and 33°C. Thus, they leave persons with very high fevers. They are found more often in moderate climates than in the tropics. Temperatures higher than 50°C kill these lice and their eggs within about 30 min. At 90–100°C they die within one minute.
- Starving is tolerated only for short periods at higher temperatures, but they survive deep temperatures for a while or cold water.

Complications

- Transmission of:
  - Epidemic typhus (*Rickettsia prowazekii*)
  - Relapsing fever (*Borrelia recurrentis*)
  - Trench fever (*Bartonella quintana*)

Pathogenesis

- Natural habitat—clothing. Only visits the skin to feed.
- Eggs and lice cemented onto clothing fibers—especially seams **(Fig. 17.73)**.

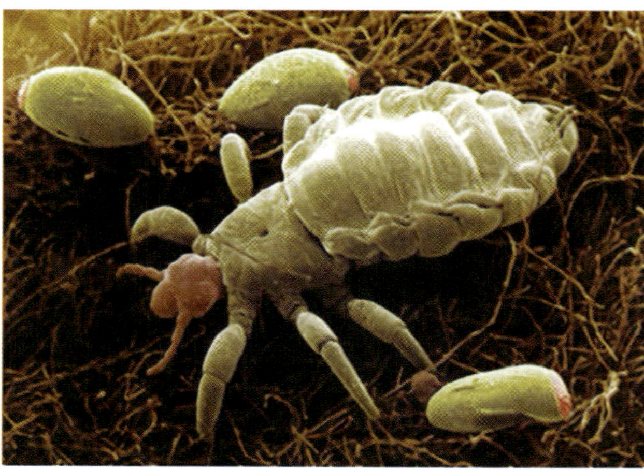

Fig. 17.73: Scanning electron micrograph of a female body louse (*Pediculus humanus corporis*) with eggs glued to the tissue

- Female adults live for 30–40 days and produce during this time up to 300 eggs (about 5–15 eggs per day). The larvae hatch after about **7 days** and it takes another **8–15 days** and three moults until the adults are developed, so that a body louse population spreads very quickly inside a dwelling.

Clinical Features

- Pruritus
- Excoriations
- Secondary bacterial infection
- Postinflammatory hyperpigmentation
- The diagnosis of an infestation with body lice can be done easily by examination of clothes for attached lice and eggs as well as for feces which appear as dense glued particles.

Treatment

- Bed linen and clothes—decontaminate—should suffice usually.
- Ironing clothing with particular attention to the seams will also kill lice on fabrics.
- Wash body with soap → followed by two applications of
  - Malathion (8 hours) to pyrethrins, pyrethroids (24 hours).

    or
  - Ivermectin (3 doses of 12 mg each) at 7 day intervals—especially in patients living in shelters or institutions.

PEDICULOSIS PUBIS (Phthiriasis Pubis)

Epidemiology

Usually sexually transmitted.

Pathogenesis

- Crab louse—morphologically very different **(Fig. 17.74)**
- Eggs—light brown, cemented to pubic hair

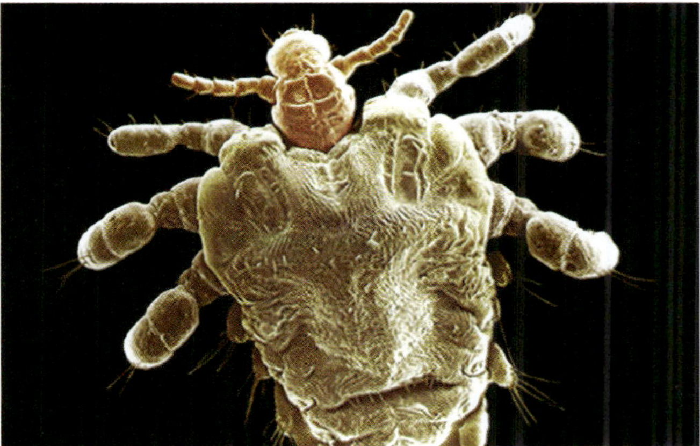

Fig. 17.74: Scanning electron micrograph of an adult female *Phthirus pubis.* Note the compressed body, where no separation between thorax (breast) and abdomen (hindbody)

- Can colonize axillary hair, eyebrows, eyelashes, beard hair, areolar hair, hair on trunk and limbs
- Mainly sedentary, becomes active at night
- Has difficulty moving when taken from its host (c.f. head and body lice)
- The average life span for *Phthirus pubis* is 17 days for females and 22 days for males.
- Incubation period is 7–8 days, and the life cycle from egg to adult is 22–27 days.

Clinical Features

- Pruritus is marked and the louse may be visualized sticking to the hair **(Fig. 17.75)**
- Louse feces—rust-colored specks on skin and hair
- Underclothes—altered blood
- **Maculae cerulea**—blue-gray macules on skin—due to subcutaneous tissue staining due to heme pigments altered by louse saliva and digestion
- Examine other body areas

Diagnosis

Dermoscopy/endodermoscopy: Adult *Pthirus pubis* identification:

- 1.5–2 mm long, slightly smaller than the body louse and head louse.
- Almost round body.
- Another distinguishing feature is that the posterior 2 pairs of legs of a crab louse are much thicker than the front legs and have large claws much like the pincers of a crab.
- Eggs with nymphs—convex lower border, empty nits are flat at the bottom.
- Alive and moving lice can be seen on digital dermoscopy in real-time projection on the monitor.

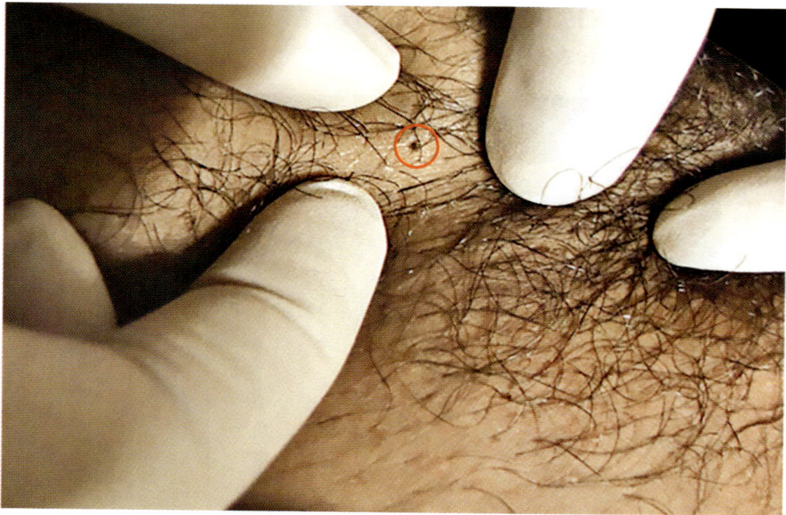

Fig. 17.75: Pediculosis pubis, note the louse which looks like a pigmented speck, patients complain of a creeping sensation that helps localize the louse

Differential Diagnosis

- **Trichomycosis axillaris:** Trichomycosis axillaris is a superficial bacterial infection in which tan concretions composed of corynebacteria occur on hair shafts. Corynebacteria are evident on Gram's stain.
- **White piedra:** White piedra, a fungal infection of the hair shaft characterized by white or tan, adherent nodules, can be mistaken for nits. Fungal hyphae can be seen on a potassium hydroxide (KOH) preparation.
- **Scabies:** Scabies can present with pruritus and excoriations in the pubic area. However, scabies mites are not visible with the naked eye, and nits are absent.

Treatment

- Permethrin 1%—repeat after 7–10 days. Since the typical incubation period for louse eggs is _6–8 days_, at least one week should elapse prior to retreatment. Reapply the drug after 9–10 days to kill any lice that have hatched from eggs that survived the initial treatment.
- Petrolatum jelly twice daily for 8–10 days.
- Oral ivermectin: Ivermectin should **not** be used in pregnant or lactating women; in addition, there are not adequate safety data for ivermectin in children weighing less than 15 kg.
- Examine and treat sexual contacts.
- Remove nits with fingernails, a nit comb, or tweezers.
- All general measures—as described earlier.

THERAPY OF PEDICULOSIS PALPEBRARUM

Manual removal, rather than topical pediculicide application, is the preferred first-line treatment.

Manual removal: Manual removal involves twice-daily application of petroleum jelly or an occlusive ophthalmic ointment to the eyelid margins followed by dislodging the lice and nits with fingernails or a nit comb. This regimen is repeated for 8–10 days.

Alternative therapies:

- **Oral therapy:** Oral _ivermectin_ (two doses of 200 μg/kg by mouth given one week apart) was effective in a case series of four patients.
- **Topical therapy:** Topical treatments have been reported as successful in small numbers of patients. These include _pilocarpine_ gel, _fluorescein_ 20% drops, yellow mercuric oxide ointment, _permethrin_ 1% créme rinse.
- **Eyelash removal:** Removal of the eyelashes is an infrequently employed alternative therapy.

Acknowledgements

The authors thank **Sidharth Tandon**, MD, and **Neha Meena**, MD, for their work on this chapter in the previous edition of this book.

BIBLIOGRAPHY

Books

1. Agents of actinomycosis.Thomas ARusso.Chapter 256 in. Mandell, Douglas, and Bennett's Principles and Practice of Infectious Diseases, 8th Edition.
2. Algorithm for diagnosis and treatment of PKDL (under NVBDCP Accelerated Plan for Kala-azar 2017).

3. Diagnosis and Management of Skin Disorders: An Evidence-Based Approach, 1/e Kabir Sardana Lippincott Williams and Wilkins 2012.
4. Leishmaniasis In. Mandell Douglas and Bennett's Principles and Practice of Infectious Diseases, 9th Edition.
5. Mancini AJ, Shani-Adir A, Sidbury R. Other viral diseases. Dermatology. BologniaJL,Schaffer JV, Cerroni L, Eds. 4th edn. Elsevier1434–35.
6. Mandell, Douglas, and Bennett's Principles and Practice of Infectious Diseases, 8th Edition https://expertconsult. inkling.com/read/mandell-douglas-bennetts-infectious-diseases-8/chapter-294/lice-pediculosis-Accessed on22/1/19.
7. Mckees Pathology of the Skin. https://expertconsult.inkling.com/read/mckees-pathology-of-the-skin-calonje-brenn-lazar-mckee-4th/chapter-18/bacterial-infections-Accessed on23/3/21.
8. NVBDCP Guidelines for treatment of Post-kala-azar dermal leishmaniasis (based on WHO Technical Report Series 949).
9. Post-kala-azar dermal leishmaniasis: Amanual for case management and control Kolkata, India, 2–3 July 2012 report of a WHO consultative meeting.
10. WHO Technical Report Series 949. "Control of the Leishmaniases." 2010. http://whqlibdoc.who. int/trs/WHO_TRS_949_eng.pdf (Accessed on October 25,2012).

Journals

1. Abd El-Magiud EM. Intralesional injection of measles, mumps, and rubella vaccine versus cryotherapy in treatment of warts: A randomized controlled trial. Dermatol Ther. 2020 Mar;33(2):e13257.
2. Agarwal R, Singh G, Ghosh A, Verma KK, Pandey M, XessI. Chromoblastomycosis in India: Review of 169 cases. PLoSNegl Trop Dis 2017; 11(8):e0005534.
3. Ahmed AA, van de Sande W, Fahal AH. Mycetoma laboratory diagnosis: Review article. PLoS Negl Trop Dis. 2017;11(8):e0005638.
4. Aithal S, Kuruvila S, Ganguly S. Zoster iform herpes simplex and herpes zoster: A clinical clue. Indian Dermatol Online J. 2013; 4(4):369.
5. Arora S, D'Souza P, Haroon MA, Ramesh V, Kaur O, Chandoke RK. PKDL mimicking leprosy relapse: A diagnostic dilemma. Int J Dermatol 2014;53:606–8.
6. Borges BS, Bueno GP, Tomiotto-Pellissier F, Figueiredo FB, Soares Medeiros LC. In vitro anti-Leishmania activity of triclabendazole and its synergic effect with amphotericin B. Front Cell Infect Microbiol. 2023 Jan 9;12:1044665.
7. Brahmachari PN. Post kala-azar infection of the skin by Leishmania donovani. Indian J Med Res 1942;30: 485–92.
8. Brito AC, Bittencourt MJS. Chromoblastomycosis: an etiological, epidemiological, clinical, diagnostic, and treatment update. An Bras Dermatol 2018;93(4):495–506.
9. Brown TJ, McCrary M, Tyring SK. Varicella-Zoster Virus (Herpes 3) J Am Acad Dermatol. 2002; 47: 972–97.
10. Cheung JP, Fung B, Wong SS, et al. Mycobacterium marinum infection of the hand and wrist. J Orthop Surg 2010; 18: 98–103.
11. Currie BJ, McCarthy JS: Permethrin and ivermectin for scabies. N Engl J Med. 2010;362:717–725.
12. Daley CL, Laccarino JM, Lange C, et al. Treatment of Nontuberculous Mycobacterial Pulmonary Disease: An Official ATS/ERS/ESCMID/IDSA Clinical Practice Guideline. Clin Infect Dis 2020;71:e1–e36.
13. Datta A, Podder I, Das A, et al. Therapeutic modalities in PKDL: A systematic review of the effectiveness and safety of the treatment options. Indian J Dermatol 2021;66:34–43.
14. DevoreCD,Schutze GE, Councilon School Health and Committee on Infectious Diseases, American Academy of Pediatrics. Headlice. Pediatrics 2015; 135:e1355.
15. Dhaille F, Dillies AS, Dessirier F, Reygagne P, Diouf M, Baltazard T, Lombart F, Hébert V, Chopinaud M, Verneuil L, Becquart C, Delaporte E, Lok C, Chaby G. A single typical trichoscopic feature is predictive of tinea capitis: a prospective multicentre study. Br J Dermatol. 2019 Nov;181(5):1046–1051.

16. Diagnosis and Treatment of Leishmaniasis: Clinical Practice Guidelines by the Infectious Diseases Society of America (IDSA) and theAmericanSociety of Tropical Medicine and Hygiene (ASTMH) (2016). http://cid.oxfordjournals.org/content/early/2016/11/03/cid.ciw670.full.pdf+html (Accessed on November 16,2016).
17. Drago F, Malaguti F, Ranieri E, Losi E, Rebora A. Human herpes virus-like particles in pityriasis rosea lesions: An electron microscopy study. J Cutan Pathol 2002;29(6):359–61.
18. Drake LA, Shear NH, Arlette JP, et al. Oral terbinafine in the treatment oftoenail onychomycosis: North American multicentertrial. J Am Acad Dermatol 1997;37:740.
19. El Shamy ME, Fahal AN, Shakir MY, et al. New MRI grading system for the diagnosis and management of mycetoma. Trans R Soc Trop Med Hyg. 2012;106:738–742.
20. Elsa Vásquez-del-Mercado, Roberto Arenas, Carmen Padilla-Desgarenes Sporotrichosis. Clinics in Dermatology 2012;30:437–43.
21. Escalonilla P, Esteban J, Soriano ML, et al. Cutaneous manifestations of infection by nontuberculous mycobacteria. ClinExpDermatol 1998;23:214.
22. Genedy RM, Sorour OA, Elokazy MAW. Trichoscopic signs of tinea capitis: a guide for selection of appropriate antifungal. Int J Dermatol. 2020 Nov 3. doi: 10.1111/ijd.15289.
23. González U, Pinart M, Rengifo-Pardo M, et al. Interventions for American cutaneous and mucocutaneous leishmaniasis. Cochrane Database Syst Rev 2009;CD004834.
24. Goyal V, Das VNR, Singh SN, Singh RS, Pandey K, et al. (2020) Long-term incidence of relapse and post-kala-azar dermal leishmaniasis after three different visceral leishmaniasis treatment regimens in Bihar, India. PLOS Neglected Tropical Diseases 14(7): e0008429.
25. Griffith, DE, Aksamit, T, Brown-Elliott BA, et al. An Official ATS/IDSA Statement: Diagnosis, Treatment, and Prevention of Nontuberculous Mycobacterial Diseases. Am J Resp Crit Care Med 2007;175(4), 367–416.
26. Gupta AK, Bamimore MA, Renaud HJ, Shear NH, Piguet V. A network meta-analysis on the efficacy and safety of monotherapies for tinea capitis, and an assessment of evidence quality. Pediatr Dermatol. 2020 Nov;37(6):1014-1022. doi: 10.1111/pde.14353. Epub 2020 Sep 8. PMID: 32897584.
27. Gupta AK, Ryder JE. How to improve cure rates for the management of onychomycosis. Dermatol Clin 2003;21:499–505.
28. Haworth CS, Banks J, Capstick T, et al. British Thoracic Society guidelines for the management of non-tuberculous mycobacterial pulmonary disease (NTM-PD). Thorax 2017;72:ii1–ii64.
29. Hay R, Denning DW, Bonifaz A, et al. The Diagnosis of Fungal Neglected Tropical Diseases (Fungal NTDs) and the Role of Investigation and Laboratory Tests: An Expert Consensus Report. Trop Med Infect Dis. 2019 Sep 24;4(4):122.
30. Hellwig AHDS, Heidrich D, Zanette RA, Scroferneker ML. In vitro susceptibility of chromoblastomycosis agents to antifungal drugs-asystematic review. J Glob Antimicrob Resist 2018 Sep25.
31. Heras-Mosteiro J, Monge-Maillo B, Pinart M, et al. Interventions for Old World cutaneous leishmaniasis. Cochrane Database Syst Rev2017; 12:CD005067.
32. https://tbcindia.gov.in/WriteReadData/Prevention%20and%20Management%20of%20Adverse%20Reaction/files/assets/common/downloads/publication.pdf
33. http://www.uphs.upenn.edu/tbpa/treatment/managingsideeffects.pdf
34. Jahnke C, Bauer E, Hengge UR, Feldmeier H. Accuracy of diagnosis of pediculosis capitis: visual inspection *vs* wetcombing. Arch Dermatol 2009; 145:309.
35. Kalter DC, Sperber J, Rosen T, Matarasso S. Treatment of pediculosis pubis. Clinical comparison of efficacy and tolerance of 1% lindane shampoo *vs* 1% permethrin cremerinse. Arch Dermatol 1987;123:1315.
36. Kumar P, Chatterjee M, Das NK. PKDL: Clinical features and differential diagnosis. Indian J Dermatol 2021;66:24–33.
37. Kumar R, Sharma MK, Jain SK, Yadav SK, Singhal AK. Cutaneous Manifestations of Chikungunya Fever: Observations from an Outbreak at a Tertiary Care Hospital in Southeast Rajasthan, India. Indian Dermatol Online J 2017;8(5):336–342.
38. Madke B, Khopkar U. Pediculosis capitis: An update. IJDVL 2012;78:429–438.
39. Maiti PK, Ray A, Bandyopadhyay S. Epidemiological aspects of mycetoma from a retrospective study of 264 cases in West Bengal. Trop Med Int Health. 2002;7:788–792.

40. Many C, Aunauilt V, Faugero B, et al. Controlof L. infantum infection is associated with CD8+ and IFN- and IL-5 producing CD4+ Ag-specific cells. Infect Immun. 1997;67:5559–66.
41. Mohammed YF, Comparative study of intralesional tuberculin protein purified derivative (PPD) and intralesional measles, mumps, rubella (MMR) vaccine for multiple resistant warts. J Cosmet Dermatol. 2021 Mar;20(3):868–874.
42. Mumcuoglu KY, Friger M, Ioffe-UspenskyI, et al. Louse comb versus direct visual examination for the diagnosis of headlouse infestations. Pediatr Dermatol 2001;18:9.
43. Newsom JH, Fiore JLJr, Hackett E. Treatment of infestation with Phthirus pubis: comparative efficacies of synergized pyrethrins and gamma-benzene hexachloride. Sex Transm Dis 1979; 6:203.
44. Nodular Lymphangiitis (Sporotrichoid Lympho-cutaneous Infections). Clues to Differential Diagnosis. J Fungi (Basel). 2018;4(2).
45. Pijpers J, den Boer ML, Essink DR, Ritmeijer K (2019). The safety and efficacy of miltefosine in the long-term treatment of post-kala-azar dermal leishmaniasis in South Asia-A review and meta-analysis. PLOS Neglected Tropical Diseases 13(2): e0007173.
46. Ramesh V, Ramam M. Histopathology of PKDL. Indian J Dermatol 2020;65:461–464.
47. Ramesh V, Singh R, Avishek K, Verma A, Deep DK, et al. (2015) Decline in Clinical Efficacy of Oral Miltefosine in Treatment of Post Kala-azar Dermal Leishmaniasis (PKDL) in India. PLOS Neglected Tropical Diseases 9(10): e0004093.
48. Ramesh V. Treatment of post-kala-azar dermal leishmaniasis. Int J Dermatol 1994;33:153–156.
49. Ramesh V, Dixit KK, Sharma N, Singh R, Salotra P. Assessing the Efficacy and Safety of Liposomal Amphotericin B and Miltefosine in Combination for Treatment of Post Kala-Azar Dermal Leishmaniasis. J Infect Dis. 2020 Feb 3;221(4):608–617.
50. Raman M, Bhat R, Garg T, Sharma VK, Ray R, Singh MK, et al. A modified two-step treatment for actinomycetoma. Indian J Dermatol Venereol Leprol 2007;73(4) 235–239.
51. Riyaz Najeeba, Riyaz A, Rahima, Abdul Latheef EN, Anitha PM, Aravindan KP, Nair Anupama S, Shameera P. Cutaneous manifestations of chikungunya during are centepidemic in Calicut, north Kerala, South India. Indian J Dermatol Venereol Leprol 2010;76:671.
52. Roberts LJ, Huffam SE, Walton SF, Currie BJ. Crusted scabies: clinical and immunological findings in seventy-eight patients and are view of the literature. J Infect 2005;50:375.
53. Rodrigues AM, Current Progress on Epidemiology, Diagnosis, and Treatment. Current Progress on Epidemiology, Diagnosis, and Treatment of Sporotrichosis and Their Future Trends. J Fungi (Basel). 2022 Jul 26;8(8):776.
54. Salavastru CM, Chosidow O, Boffa MJ, et al. European guideline for the management of scabies. J Eur Acad Dermatol Venereol 2017;31:1248.
55. Sardana K, Chugh S. Newer therapeutic modalities for Actinomycetoma by Nocardia species. Int J Dermatol. 2018 Sep;57(9):e64–e65.
56. Sarris I, Berendt AR, Athanasous N, et al. MRI of mycetoma of the foot: two cases demonstrating the dot-in-circle sign. Skeletal Radiol. 2003;32:179–183.
57. Scott GR, Chosidow O, IUSTI/WHO. European guideline for the management of pediculosis pubis, 2010. Int J STD AIDS 2011;22:304.
58. Sehgal VN, Sardana K, Sharma S. Inadequacy of clinical and/or laboratory criteria for the diagnosis of lupus vulgaris, re-infection cutaneous tuberculosis: fallout/implication of 6 weeks of anti-tubular therapy (ATT) as a precise diagnostic supplement to complete the scheduled regimen. J Dermatolog Treat. 2008;19(3):164–7.
59. Shaker ESE, Doghim NN, Hassan AM, Musafa SS, Fawzy MM. Immunotherapy in cutaneous warts: comparative clinical Study between MMR vaccine, tuberculin, and BCG Vaccine. J Cosmet Dermatol. 2021 Jan 6. doi: 10.1111/jocd.13921.
60. Sharma R, Mahajan VK, Singh Chauhan P, Mehta KS, Sharma A, Sharma J. The clinico-epidemiological characteristics and therapeutic experience of 152 patients with cutaneous sporotrichosis: a 10-year retrospective study from India. Int J Dermatol. 2021 Jan;60(1):99–106.
61. Sharma S, Agarwal S. Intralesional Immunotherapy with Measles Mumps Rubella Vaccine for the Treatment of Anogenital Warts: An Open-label Study. J Clin Aesthet Dermatol. 2020 Aug;13(8):40–44.
62. Singal A Clinicoepidemiological characteristics of cutaneous tuberculosis in 1458 Indian patients: a retrospective analytical study from a tertiary care center. Int J Dermatol. 2022 Aug;61(8):1012–1022.

63. Sigurgeirsson B, Olafsson JH, Steinsson JB, et al. Long-term effectiveness of treatment with terbinafine *vs* itraconazole in onychomycosis: a 5-year blinded prospective follow-up study. Arch Dermatol 2002;138:353.
64. Singh A, Masih A, Khurana A, Singh PK, Gupta M, Hagen F, Meis JF, Chowdhary A. High terbinafine resistance in Trichophyton interdigitale isolates in Delhi, India harbouring mutations in the squalene epoxidase gene. Mycoses. 2018 Jul;61(7):477–484.
65. Taylor S, Walther D, Fernando DD, Swe-Kay P, Fischer K. Investigating the Antibacterial Properties of Prospective Scabicides. Biomedicines. 2022 Dec 19;10(12):3287.
66. Thomas EA, John M, Kanish B. Mucocutaneous manifestations of Dengue fever. Indian J Dermatol. 2010;55(1):79–85.
67. Torres-Guerrero E, Isa-Isa R, Isa M, Arenas R. Chromoblastomycosis. Clinics in Dermatology (2012) 30,403–408.
68. Tosti A, Piraccini BM, Stinchi C, Colombo MD. Relapses of onychomycosis after successful treatment with systemic antifungals: athree-year follow-up. Dermatology 1998;197:162.
69. UrbinaF, DasA, SudyE. Clinical variants of pityriasis rosea. World J Clin Cases 2017;5(6):203–11.
70. van de Sande WW, Maghoub el S, Fahal AH, Goodfellow M, Welsh O, Zijlstra E. Themycetoma knowledge gap: identification of research priorities. PLoSNeglTropDis. 2014 Mar 27; 8(3):e2667.
71. VouldoukisI, BecherelPA,Riveros-Moreno V,et al. IL-10 and IL-4 inhibit intracellular killing of Leishmania infantum and L. major by human macrophages by decreasing nitric oxide generation. Eur J Immunol 1997;27:860–5.
72. Wallace RJ Jr, Brown BA, Onyi GO. Skin, soft tissue, and bone infections due to Mycobacterium chelonae importance of prior corticosteroid therapy,frequency of disseminated infections, and resistance to oral antimicrobials other than clarithromycin. J Infect Dis 1992;166:405.
73. Wallace RJJr, Bedsole G, Sumter G, et al. Activities of ciprofloxacin and ofloxacin against rapidly growing mycobacteria with demonstration of acquired resistance following single-drug therapy. Antimicrob Agents Chemother 1990;34:65.
74. Waskiel-Burnat, A., Rakowska, A., Sikora, M. et al. Trichoscopy of Tinea Capitis: A Systematic Review. Dermatol Ther (Heidelb) 10, 43–52 (2020).
75. Wi YM. Treatment of Extrapulmonary Nontuberculous Mycobacterial Diseases. Infect Chemother. 2019 Sep;51(3):245–255.
76. Woods GL, Washington JA 2nd. Mycobacteria other than Mycobacterium tuberculosis: review of microbiologic and clinical aspects. Rev Infect Dis 1987;9:275.
77. Zijlstra EE,vande Sande WWJ, Welsh O, MahgoubES, Goodfellow M, FahalAH. Mycetoma: a unique neglected tropical disease. Lancet Infect Dis.2016 Jan;16(1):100–112.

Chapter

18

Leprosy

Kabir Sardana, Ananta Khurana, Surabhi Sinha, Sweta Singh

HISTORY OF LEPROSY

Rudolf Virchow had discovered the lepra cell in the late 1850s and described 'brown bodies' within these. In 1871 or 1872, Hansen noted the tiny rods within these same cells in material obtained from nodules of leprosy patients and asserted that these represented bacteria and thus proposed leprosy as a bacterial disease for the first time. This was further confirmed with aniline dyes developed later by Albert Neisser.

Chemotherapy

- **Chaulmoogra oil:** It is believed that a Burmese King contracted leprosy and was directed by the gods to enter a forest and eat the fruit of the Kalaw (the Brazil Burmese name for Chaulmoogra), which cured his disease. In India, it was used by Mouat (1854), a British physician, as a topical agent.
- **Dapsone:** First used by Cochrane et al. (1949), who gave it intramuscular (IM). Lowe and Smith (1949) were the first to use dapsone orally. Dapsone resistance was first reported by Pettit and Rees in 1964.
- **Clofazimine:** First used by Browne in 1965.
- **Rifampicin:** First used by Opromolla (1963), initially given IM. Opromolla also recommended that rifamycin should not be used alone for fear of resultant resistance to the drug, a problem which was eventually observed by Jacobson and Hastings (1976).
- **Thalidomide:** First used by Sheskin (1965) in six ENL patients in Israel; the dose given was 100 mg orally three times daily leading to an improvement within 3 days.
- **MDT:** This was introduced based on the Malta trial which involved over 200 patients, 80 of whom had lepromatous leprosy. Patients in this trial received dapsone, rifampin, isoniazid and prothionamide for periods of up to 2 years. The results were exceptionally good, with the added bonus of only one relapse being reported within a 5-year period following the cessation of treatment (World Health Organization, 1982); and through 1988, there were no additional relapses reported.

Investigations

- Smear and its examination: Developed by Wade and Rodriguez in 1927 and described further by Wade in 1935. Modified by Cochrane in 1947 and standardized to a logarithmic scale by Ridley (1958).

- Mouse footpad inoculation: The successful inoculation with *M. leprae* was achieved by Shepard (1960). The footpad was chosen because of the coolness of this area (average 30°C at normal room temperature). Binford had suggested in 1956 that leprosy bacilli probably preferred to multiply in cooler sites and Brand (1959) demonstrated a relationship between leprosy-related deformities and the temperature of the body.
- Use of the armadillo: One armadillo can supply about one trillion lepra bacilli. The use of armadillo for leprosy research is in the following aspects:
  1. Screening new drugs
  2. Testing for the presence or absence of drug resistance
  3. Determining the generation time of the bacilli
- Other animals that can develop leprosy are: Rhesus monkey, sooty mangabey, and African green monkeys.

EPIDEMIOLOGY

World: During 2018, 184,212 leprosy patients were 'on treatment'; with prevalence rate (PR) of 0.24 per 10,000 population. In the same year 208,619 new cases were reported globally and the rate of detection of new cases was 2.74 per 100,000 population (WHO, 2019).

India: The total number of cases on record during 2018 were 85,302 while 120,334 new cases were detected by the end of 2018, with **a PR of 0.67 per 10,000**. The salient features are given in **Box 18.1**.

Age: The age of presentation ranges from 3 weeks to 70 years. There is a bimodal peak with the first peak at 10–14 years and a second peak at 30–60 years in high endemic areas. The latter is presumably because of superinfection/reinfection in elderly because of lowered immunity.

Sex: Male:female :: 2:1. However, interestingly when the disease is first introduced to an area or where the disease is dying out, the ratio is equal.

Mortality in leprosy: Lepromatous patients 3.5 times and non-lepromatous patients 2 times the general population.

Inactivation of disease: Majority of patients, particularly of the tuberculoid spectrum and indeterminate leprosy, tend to get cured spontaneously. An earlier study in India had shown that over a period of 20 years, the extent of spontaneous regression among children with tuberculoid leprosy was about 90%.

BOX 18.1: Data on leprosy (NLEP)

• New cases detected in 2017–18	1,20,334
• Annual new case detection rate (ANDCR)	10.17 per 100,000
• Leprosy cases by end of 2018	85,302
• Prevalence rate	0.67 per 10,000 population
• MB	49.57%
• Female	39.17%
• Child	8.7%
• Grade II deformity	3.34%
• Grade II disability rate	3.94/million population

Transmission of Leprosy

Incubation period: 2.9–5.3 years for tuberculoid leprosy and 9.3–11.6 years for lepromatous leprosy. Important aspects of the disease transmission are given in **Box 18.2**.

- **The most important route of transmission to,** as well as entry into, the human host is by respiratory route. The contact with *M. leprae* likely leads to a primary nasal infection. A protective mucosal immunity however overcomes the infection in most cases and is likely long lasting. In those in whom this immunity does not develop, spread occurs via the bloodstream and/or lymphatics lodging the lepra bacilli in nerves, skin and other sites.
- There is yet conflicting evidence on skin as a route of transmission of leprosy, with anecdotal reports on infection following tattooing and injuries. But there is now some clarity on the presence of bacilli in superficial skin structures (epidermis, hair follicles, sweat and sebaceous glands) which may probably act as exit points for *M. leprae*.
- Recently, environmental presence of *M. leprae* in soil and water of highly endemic regions has been brought to attention in studies from India and Indonesia. Further, it has been demonstrated that free-living pathogenic amoebae are capable of ingesting and supporting the viability of *M. leprae* expelled into the environment.

BOX 18.2: Salient aspects of leprosy and its transmission*

Reservoir load	• LL—load of organisms—**7 billion/g of tissue** • Non-lepromatous—**1 million/g of tissue**
Portal of exit	• **Nose**—10 thousand to 10 million/day (Shepard, 1960) • Milk—2 million/feed (Pedley, 1967) • Skin—contradictory past evidence, now being revisited
Viability of *M. leprae*	• 36 hours to 9 days—possibility of contaminated clothing and other fomites acting as sources of infection. Environmental reservoirs now demonstrated in hyperendemic regions
Minimal infective dose	• 3–40 solidly staining bacteria (McRae and Shepard, 1971)
Portal of entry	• Respiratory is the main route. Skin (tattoo and trauma) are less important
Transmission	• By contact: Depends on index case (Noordeen, 1978) relative risk: LL:TT = 9.5:3.7 • Respiratory route: Rees and McDougall (1977) showed transmission by aerosols • Bloodstream (through the lungs) • ?Breast milk

*Hastings, Leprosy, 2nd Edn.
? = Questionable

Natural Course of Disease

Figure 18.1 depicts the natural course after infection with *M. leprae*.

Microbiology

The salient features of the microbiology of *M. leprae* are listed in **Box 18.3**.

- The functional genome of *M. leprae* appears to be less than 40% of the size of the genome of *M. tuberculosis*. This is because *M. leprae* has undergone reductive evolution, whereby many genes and associated functions were lost through shrinkage of the genome and gene decay.

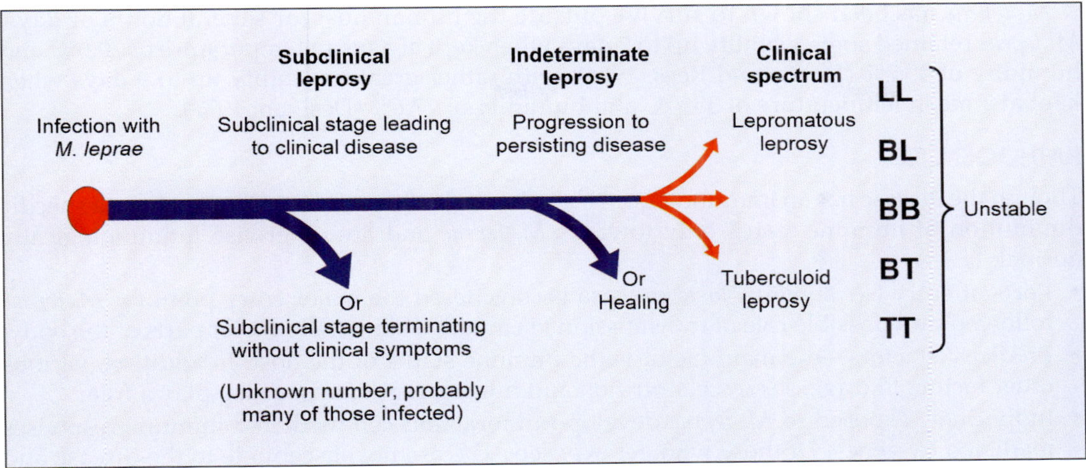

Fig. 18.1: The natural course after infection with *M. leprae*

BOX 18.3: Microbiology of *M. leprae**

Biological properties	• Doubling time **11–13 days** • Optimum temperature 27–30°C • Sensitive to dapsone (MIC 0.003 μg/mL), rifampin (0.3 g/mL) and clofazimine
Ultrastructural properties	• Rod-shaped bacilli, **1–8 μm long, 0.3 μm diameter** • Tends to form clumps or globi, surrounded by electron transparent zone—strongly acid-fast, but majority stain granular • Non-acid-fast after pyridine extraction
Biochemical properties	**Cell wall and capsule** • Phenolic glycolipid (PGL) with species-specific antigenic oligosaccharide L- alanine replaced by glycine in peptidoglycan **Proteins** • Range of proteins with species-specific antigenic determinants (65 kD, 36 kD, 35 kD, 28 kD, 18 kD, 12 kD) **Genome** • Low G + C content relative to other mycobacteria, species-specific repetitive element, species-specific sequences in genes encoding protein antigens and rRNA

*Jopling's Handbook of Leprosy, 6th Edn.

- Recently genotyping had revealed different subtypes of leprosy, by using the SNP **(SNP types 1, 2 and 3)** and rpoT gene polymorphisms. This genotyping may help in studying the sources and transmission chain in leprosy.

SNP type 4, which is prevalent in West Africa arose from SNP type 3. The evidence also suggests that *M. leprae* entered Asia by a Southern route and also by a Northern route that corresponded to the Silk Road.

A study from India (Lavania M, et al., 2009) using PCR amplification of rpoT gene and sequencing of amplicons showed the presence of two genotypes of *M. leprae*, 73.4% having three copies (ancient Indian type) and 26.6% containing 4 copies (considered to be Japanese and Korean) origin.

M. leprae has been shown to survive outside the human host for several hours or days. *M. leprae* retained some viability up to **7 days** when kept at a mean temperature of 20.6°C and humidity of 43.7% (Davey and Rees, 1974), with rather greater viability up to **9 days** when kept at a mean temperature of 35.7°C and humidity of 77.6% (Desikan, 1977).

PATHOGENESIS

Though the disease has an immunological basis, by itself, the patients of leprosy have a specific diminution of immune status only towards *M. leprae* and are otherwise immunologically normal.

- Ports of entry (*see* above): Nasal mucosa is considered the major entry point for *M. leprae* followed by a possible role of transmission via abraded skin in the cooler parts of the body.
- Predictive factors—the main factor is the immune status of the host. In addition, various other factors like age, sex, race, nutrition and intercurrent diseases may play a role.
- Individuals exposed to *M. leprae* develop humoral and cell-mediated immune responses mediated by genes. Of those who get exposed, 95% are not susceptible to the disease and only a relatively small percentage develop leprosy (Newell, 1966). The majority of those who are disease-free are lepromin positive, indicating a well-developed cell-mediated immunity. A small number among the resistant individuals are lepromin negative and the mechanism of resistance in this group is an enigma. The few who develop the disease can be divided into two groups: A lepromin negative group who eventually develop disseminated lepromatous leprosy and a lepromin positive group in whom the disease is localized **(Flowchart 18.1)**.
- **Genetic:** Genome-wide linkage analysis in multi-case families has defined susceptibility alleles in many components of the innate and adaptive immune response including the genes for toll-like receptors 2 and 4, NOD2, VDR, MICA, MRC1, several cytokines, lymphotoxin, the ubiquitin and proteasome-related enzymes—PARK2 and PACRG, in addition to the recognized linkage to HLA class II and tumor necrosis factor genes (A Alter).

Flowchart 18.1: Sequence of the natural course of infection with the role of relevant gene expression

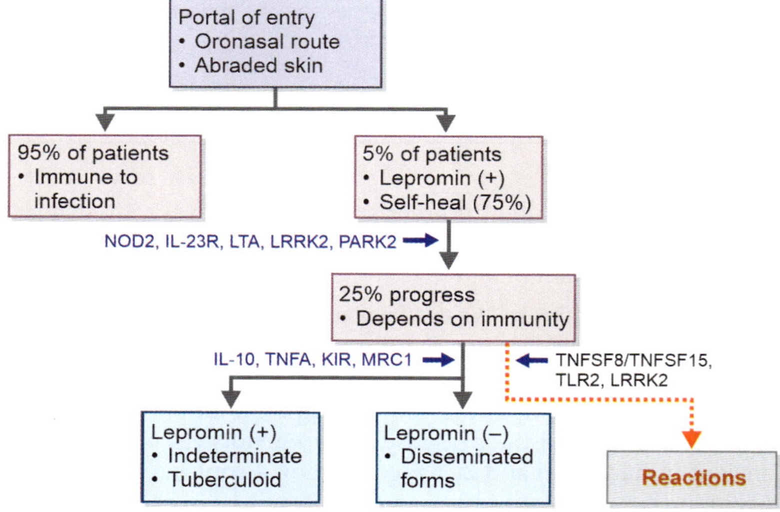

- HLA-DR2 and -DR3 are associated with tuberculoid disease and HLA-DQ1 with lepromatous leprosy.
- **Nerve involvement:** This is seen in almost all cases of leprosy. Involvement can be via naked axons in the epidermis or in the papillary layer of the superficial dermis following denudation of the epithelium. Another route is via endoneural blood vessels during bacteremia.

Stages of nerve involvement are shown in **Flowchart 18.2**.

Schwann cell is the target of *M. leprae*. Increased PGL1, an *M. leprae* 19 kDa lipoprotein, can mediate Schwann cell apoptosis acting as an agonist of TLR2. *M. leprae* specifically interacts with G-domain of the laminin-α_2 chain in the basal lamina of Schwann cells and the laminin receptor, α-dystroglycan (A Rambukkana).

After the initial inoculation, the bacilli may get into the cutaneous nerves at the site of entry, they may spread via the lymphatics or there may be a bacillemia (Khanolkar, 1955; Ridley, 1971; Ramu et al., 1985). Since the nerves offer a protected site, the bacilli lodging there as a result of the bacteremia escape elimination by the defense mechanisms of the body. This results in the pure neuritic type of leprosy seen in about 18% of cases (Noordeen, 1972).

M. leprae is capable of direct peripheral nerve damage even in the absence of inflammation or a cellular immune response. These mechanisms are likely to be especially responsible for peripheral nerve damage in multibacillary leprosy.

Flowchart 18.2: Stages of nerve involvement with their consequences

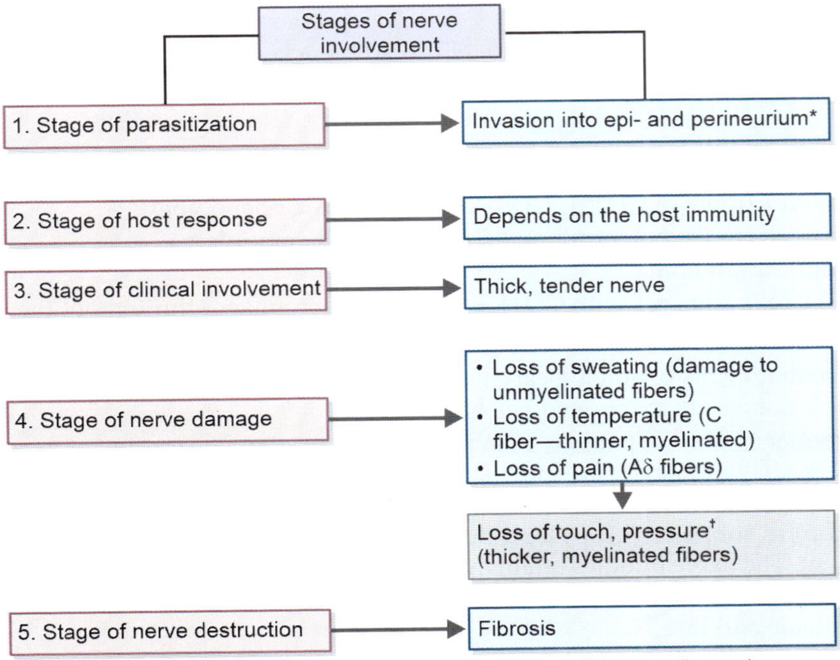

Stages of nerve involvement

- 1. Stage of parasitization → Invasion into epi- and perineurium*
- 2. Stage of host response → Depends on the host immunity
- 3. Stage of clinical involvement → Thick, tender nerve
- 4. Stage of nerve damage →
  - Loss of sweating (damage to unmyelinated fibers)
  - Loss of temperature (C fiber—thinner, myelinated)
  - Loss of pain (Aδ fibers)

  ↓ Loss of touch, pressure† (thicker, myelinated fibers)
- 5. Stage of nerve destruction → Fibrosis

**M. leprae* (lipoproteins, toll-like receptor, PGL1) bind to laminin-2 (on Schwann cell—axon).

†Stocking-glove pattern of sensory impairment (S-GPSI).

Pathology

The basic overview of the pathology of different stages in the disease spectrum is given below.

i. Inflammatory Cells

Macrophages, epithelioid cells, lymphocytes and plasma cells are the inflammatory cells existent in leprosy lesions; their presence and relative numbers varying across the spectrum. Whereas the collection of **epithelioid cells (TT, BT)** appears as a syncytium with no histologically recognizable cell borders, **macrophages (BL, LL)** have fairly well outlined cell structures and 'a fine network of reticular fibers' around these cells can be demonstrated using a reticulin stain.

Macrophages and **plasma cells** predominate in LL. Although the BB group has numerous epithelioid cells, macrophages also form a fairly significant proportion of the cells in this spectrum. A few epithelioid cells may be seen in some BL patients but never in LL.

Fairly large numbers of **lymphocytes** are found in the TT and BL types. They are a little less in BT and scanty in BB and LL.

ii. Nerves

- Perineural cell proliferation, thickening, and the inflammatory cell infiltration of the perineurium are minimal in TT, gradually increase along the spectrum and are seen at their **maximum in BL (giving the nerves an onion peel appearance)**.
- **TT-marked intraneural inflammation** and granuloma formation and even caseous necrosis in some instances.
- Endoneural granulomas are classic of leprosy.

iii. Bacterial Load

Varies from a near absence of *M. leprae* in TT to AFB-packed macrophages in LL.

iv. Type of T cells (on IHC)

- Tuberculoid granuloma
  - CD4+ T cells predominate; with CD8+ T cells only in the mantle surrounding the granuloma (more of CD28+, CD8+ cells—cytotoxic phenotype)
  - CD1a+ cells in the epidermis and periphery of the granuloma.
- Lepromatous granuloma
  - CD8+ T cells admixed with CD4+ T cells and macrophages throughout the granuloma.
  - CD8+T cells here are of the suppressor type (CD8+, CD28 –ve).

Some differentiating histopathological characteristics of specific spectral types and time points in the disease course are mentioned below.

- TTs (secondary TT) *vs* TTp (polar TT): In polar variety (TTp) the erosion of the epidermis is more marked; lymphocytes are more abundant; Langhans giant cells are less conspicuous; and tubercles are well-formed.
- Polar (LLp) *vs* subpolar (LLsp) lepromatous disease: LLsp there is a sizable lymphocytic component. The nerve bundles retain the multi-laminated perineurium as they downgrade from BL to LL.
- BB is unstable and rare.
- Histoid leprosy: Interlacing bands of spindle-shaped histiocytes arranged in criss-cross or whorled (storiform) fashion.

- **Resolving phase**
  a. Tuberculoid leprosy—slow disappearance of granuloma, no fibrosis; takes 1–3 years.
  b. Lepromatous lesions—pink granular cytoplasm of the foamy cells undergoes fatty degeneration; increased lymphocytic infiltration occurs; foamy giant cells; dermal collagen and elastic tissue are mostly destroyed; skin adnexa atrophy and disappear without any fibrosis, nerve bundles are replaced by fibrous tissue.
- **Relapse:** Relapse in lepromatous areas—new arrival of active macrophages and solid staining AFB. LLsp patients may relapse with lesions of BL, and BT and BL patients may relapse with BT. In the tuberculoid pole they can be mistaken for reactions. The return of epithelioid cell collections along with scattered macrophages containing AFB is diagnostic.

Diagnosis of Leprosy (WHO): The diagnosis of leprosy is based on the presence of at least 1 of the 3 cardinal signs:

1. Definite loss of sensation in a pale (hypopigmented) or reddish skin patch.
2. Thickened or enlarged peripheral nerve with loss of sensation and/or weakness of the muscles supplied by that nerve.
3. Presence of acid-fast bacilli in a slit-skin smear.

Slit-skin smears are positive only in MB leprosy (i.e. any positive slit-skin smear is classified as MB irrespective of the number of patches and/or nerve involvement).

CLASSIFICATION

There are five different methods of classifying the disease. In research institutions, the Ridley-Jopling classification is followed. However, in primary care centers, the WHO and NLEP classifications are followed. Others are Madrid classification and Indian classification.

1. Ridley-Jopling/immunological classification: It is based on a combination of clinical findings, bacteriological index (BI), immunological reactivity and the histological findings. This classification ranges from a spectrum of high-to-low resistance pattern.

The various types are TT (*typical* tuberculoid), BT (borderline tuberculoid), BB (borderline), BL (borderline lepromatous), LLsp (subpolar lepromatous) and, finally, LLp (polar *typical* lepromatous). The inter-relationship between the various types is shown in **Fig. 18.2**. TTp and LLp (polar) are clinically and immunologically stable. Thus, the disease cannot progress from these types. The other types (BT, BB and BL) are unstable and the immune response may change as indicated by the arrows and the spectrum may upgrade or downgrade silently or with reactional episodes. The 'reaction' is more common/prominent in the upgrading phenomenon.

Patients with BT may upgrade to TTs (TT—secondary) but LLsp patients do not downgrade to LLp *nor* do LLp patients upgrade to LLsp. Jopling states: "Borderline patients may upgrade to the tuberculoid type (TT) but form a subgroup—secondary tuberculoid or TTs, which, in contrast to its counterpart at the other end of the spectrum (subpolar LL or LLsp), appears to be immunologically stable. The various shifts which can occur with upgrading reactions across the leprosy spectrum are: LLsp → BL → BB → BT → TTs. The reverse holds good in downgrading reactions: BT → BB → BL → LLsp **(Fig. 18.2)**.

Evidence indicates that patients in the tuberculoid portion of the spectrum have a prominent Th1 and Th17 type of immune response to *M. leprae*, producing interleukin 2 (IL-2), interferon-γ (IFN-γ) and the Th17 cytokines—IL-17 and IL-22. At the other pole, lepromatous patients have a Th2-like pattern, with greater production of IL-4 and IL-10 and also show prominent presence of T regulatory cells contributing to immunological unresponsiveness or anergy characteristic of the lepromatous pole. An overview of the histological features of the major types of leprosy is given in **Table 18.1**.

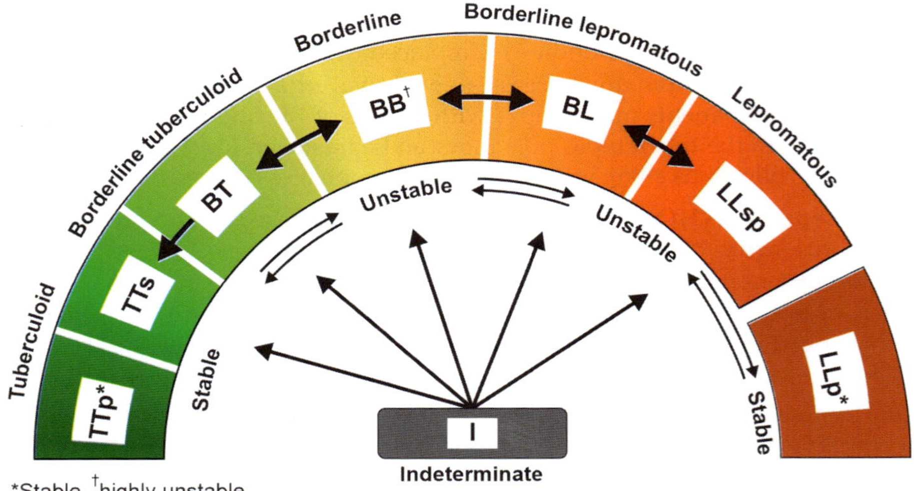

Fig. 18.2: Diagrammatic depiction of the relationship between various leprosy types according to the Ridley-Jopling classification

TABLE 18.1: Salient features of the histopathology of leprosy (derived from Hastings)

Types	Epidermis	Dermis	Nerve	AFB
Indeterminate	Normal	• Mononuclear cell infiltrates occupying less than a tenth of the dermis • Mast cells—around the neurovascular bundle is a significant finding	• Perineural cuffing along with infiltration of the peri- and endoneurium are diagnostic if seen	Can be seen in: Cutaneous nerve bundles, the sub-epidermal zone just beneath the basal layer, and the arrector pili muscles
TT	Atrophic	**Granuloma** • *Hugs* the epidermis • Composed of epithelioid cells, Langhans giant cells surrounded by a *dense collection of lymphocytes* • Skin adnexa *destroyed*	Nerves infiltrated and destroyed; remnants of nerve tissue in the granuloma	Very uncommon to see
BT	Atrophy and flattening of the rete ridges	**Granuloma** • Less compact than TT • Composed of epitheloid cells, Langhans giant cells • *Clear* subepidermal zone • Skin adnexal structures destroyed	• Nerves show intra- and perineural granuloma • Nerve fragments seen	AFB inside Schwann cells

(Contd.)

TABLE 18.1: Salient features of the histopathology of leprosy (derived from Hastings) *(Contd.)*

Types	Epidermis	Dermis	Nerve	AFB
BB	Epidermis is atrophic	**Granuloma** • Grenz zone (+) • Plump epithelioid cells, some macrophages and a sprinkling of lymphocytes • Interstitial edema • Giant cells (rare)	• Nerves are infiltrated by epithelioid cells and lymphocytes • Reactive proliferation of perineurial cells and edematous thickening of the perineurium	AFB in small numbers are detected in Schwann cells and in the macrophages
BL	Atrophic	• Grenz zone (+) • Many macrophages and numerous lymphocytes • A few epithelioid cells are present	• Nerve bundles show marked perineurial cell proliferation • Edema	Numerous bacilli inside macrophages, Schwann cells, endothelial cells and arrector pili muscles
LL	Atrophic	• Grenz zone—macrophages have granular cytoplasm to foamy cells • A few lymphocytes and plasma cells	• Nerves also show perineural collections of macrophages • Intraneural infiltration by inflammatory cells is insignificant	Acid-fast stain shows clumps of bacilli in Schwann cells and appendages

2. Indian: In addition to the Ridley–Jopling classification, there are two additional types unique to India—the indeterminate and neuritic types.

For the purpose of treatment, WHO and NLEP have given simpler classifications which are widely followed.

3. WHO (2018) classifies leprosy as PB or MB based on the following criteria:

i. Paucibacillary (PB) case: A case of leprosy with **1–5** skin lesions, without demonstrated presence of bacilli in a skin smear.
ii. Multibacillary (MB) case: A case of leprosy with more than 5 skin lesions; **or** with nerve involvement (pure neuritic, or any number of skin lesions and neural involvement); **or** with the demonstrated presence of bacilli in a slit-skin smear, irrespective of the number of skin lesions (WHO Guidelines, 2018).

4. NLEP classification criteria has minor differences from the WHO criteria and is given in **Table 18.2**.

TABLE 18.2: NLEP criteria for grouping PB and MB leprosy

S. No.	Characteristic	PB (Paucibacillary)	MB (Multibacillary)
1.	Skin lesions	1–5 lesions	6 and above
2.	Peripheral nerve involvement	No nerve/only one nerve with or without 1–5 lesions	More than one nerve irrespective of number of skin lesions
3.	Skin smear	Negative at all sites	Positive at any site

Note: If skin smear is positive irrespective of number of skin and nerve lesions, the disease is classified as MB leprosy but if skin smear is negative it is classified on the basis of the number of skin and nerve lesions.

CLINICAL FEATURES

- The commonest early lesion is an area of numbness of the skin or visible skin lesions in the form of a few hypopigmented macules of indeterminate leprosy.
- Early tuberculoid lesions are more or less well-defined macules or plaques of hypopigmented and often erythematous skin, and are usually anesthetic.
- Early lepromatous macules are hypopigmented and so vague that they are often missed, and thus the disease is not noticed until the skin becomes infiltrated.
- Neuritic pain may be the first symptom of leprosy with localized paresthesia, pain, or rarely hyperalgesia.
- Examine nerves carefully **(Fig. 18.3)** in all patients, irrespective of neurological complaints, to detect early involvement.
- Also test for sensory, motor and autonomic functions.

Sensory function
- First explain the procedure to the patient.
- Ask him to *close* his *eyes*.
- For touch sensation, use a ball point pen or Semmes-Weinstein monofilaments if available. Remember to only 'touch' and not brush against the skin.
- Ask the patient to point to where he felt the touch. If he cannot identify-it is anesthesia.
- If the patient feels it but cannot point to the exact point, it is called '*misreference*' (the normal reference for spatial differentiation on palms is within 1 cm, the face—2 cm, and up to 7 cm on the back and buttocks).
- Pain (pinprick) and temperature (test tubes containing hot and cold water) are tested next.
- Stocking-glove pattern of sensory impairment (S-GPSI) may be seen.
- Loss of hot and cold discrimination (mediated by type C fibers) occurs before loss of sensations of pain or light touch.

- Voluntary muscle tests (*see* page 633 in the section of nerve testing)
- Autonomic nerve damage: Signs of this include—dryness and fissuring, dusky cyanosis of hands, postural hypotension, hair loss, hypopigmentation, fingers do not wrinkle when immersed in water, more prone to burns.

Clinical Features of Nerve Damage

Ulnar: The ulnar nerve is usually damaged just proximal to the olecranon groove, leading to paresis or paralysis of the interossei, the hypothenar muscles and the two medial lumbrical muscles ('ulnar or minimal claw'). Rarely, it is damaged proximally which leads to weakness of the deep flexors of the little and ring fingers.

Median nerve: Low palsy commonly leads to weakness or paralysis of 3 muscles of the thenar eminence (opponens pollicis, abductor pollicis brevis, flexor pollicis brevis), and the two lateral lumbricals.

Common peroneal nerve: Damage commonly occurs proximal to where the nerve passes around the neck of the fibula, and in the popliteal fossa. This results in anesthesia of the lateral side of the leg and the dorsum of the foot and motor deficit of the peroneal muscles and the dorsiflexors of the foot. The earliest sign is difficulty in dorsiflexion or eversion of the foot (footdrop with a high stepping gait).

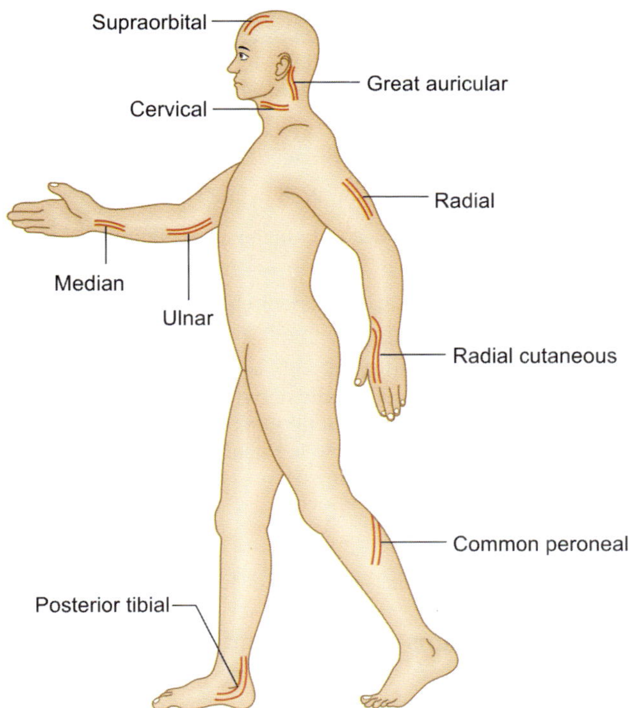

Fig. 18.3: Sites of predilection of peripheral nerves enlarged and palpable in leprosy

Posterior tibial nerve: Damaged proximal to where it passes around the medial malleoli. Damage results in anesthesia of the sole of the foot, and paralysis of the intrinsic musculature of the foot, leading to clawing of the toes, and collapse of arches.

Facial nerve: Temporal and zygomatic branches of the facial nerve are involved as they cross the zygoma. Their damage causes lagophthalmos. The lower lid is most affected. (For details of nerve testing, *see* section on deformity.)

Diagnosis of Clinical Types

Some important diagnostic points are listed in **Table 18.3** that can enable an accurate clinical diagnosis of leprosy type.

The following pointers can be used to determine the spectrum of disease:

1. Higher immunity (I, TT and BT): There are a few countable lesions which are asymmetrically distributed. Macules/plaques usually with well-defined and regular borders. Anesthesia, hair loss and hypo-/anhidrosis are seen and a few asymmetrical nerve enlargements are seen. As a corollary, AFB are scant and the lepromin test is positive.
2. Lower immunity (BL and LL): There is symmetrical distribution of numerous lesions that are hypo-/normoesthetic and are composed of macules/papules that have ill-defined borders. Numerous symmetrical nerve enlargement is seen. As a corollary, AFB are numerous and the lepromin test is negative.
3. Mid-immune (BB): Features of both the spectra are present and as it is immunologically unstable, and prone to reactions. The instability makes this the rarest type.

TABLE 18.3: Salient features that predict leprosy types

Number of skin lesions	The higher the resistance, the fewer the lesions (tuberculoid). With no resistance, skin lesions may be so numerous that they become confluent (lepromatous)
Distribution and symmetry	When few, leprosy lesions are not symmetrical; when numerous, they are more likely to be symmetrically placed
Definition and clarity	Abruptness of the margin; **Well** defined margins are seen in tuberculoid pole
Anesthesia	More the **lesional** anesthesia higher the immunity; this is seen in the tuberculoid pole
Loss of sweating and reduced hair growth	Occurs early in paucibacillary disease **(lesional)** and late in multibacillary disease **(diffuse)**
Peripheral nerve	• Tuberculoid leprosy, one or a few nerves is enlarged and there is commonly sensory, motor, autonomic nerve deficit • Lepromatous leprosy, all peripheral nerves are affected symmetrically, not appreciably enlarged and the neurological deficit appears slowly • Borderline disease, many nerves are thickened, usually asymmetrically, and nerve damage may be severe
Mucosal and systemic	More in multibacillary
Slit smear	BI calculation predicts spectrum of leprosy

It is also important to know the signs of activity of disease, in the form of

- Erythema/infiltration
- Extension or appearance of new lesions
- Extension/new appearance of anesthesia, paresis and paralysis
- Tenderness and pain in nerves
- High morphological index (MI)
- Occurrence of reaction

Clinical Types

1. *Indeterminate Leprosy*

This is described in the Indian classification and refers to a lesion appearing before the host mounts a definitive immunological response.

- Indeterminate leprosy is the first sign of disease in 20–80% of patients.
- The patient is usually a child.
- One or more hypopigmented faintly-erythematous, ill-defined, macules are seen. Infiltration, by definition, is absent **(Fig. 18.4)**.
- Normoesthetic lesions; no enlarged nerves.
- If lesions are inconclusive, and histology is not available, review after 3 months.
- Lepromin test (±)
- Slit smear for AFB (–)

2. *Tuberculoid (TT) Leprosy*

The primary lesion is a plaque. There are two types:

1. TTp: Refers to the stable type of TT that does not downgrade or upgrade.
2. TTs: Refers to a type of TT that has upgraded from BT.

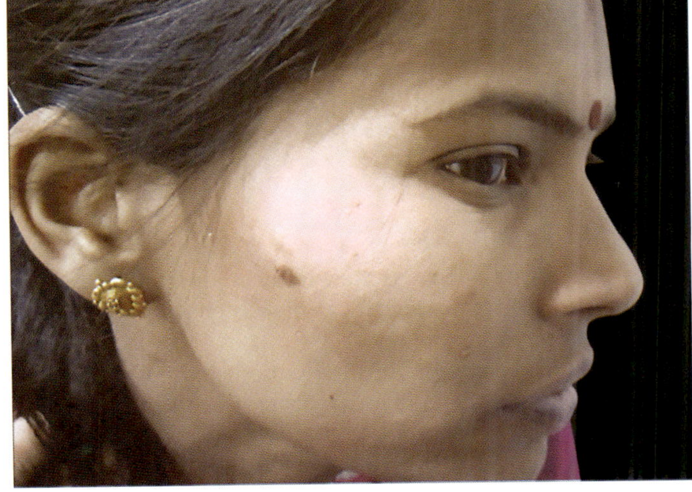

Fig. 18.4: Indeterminate Hansen: Ill-defined hypopigmented, normoesthetic macule is seen over the right cheek

Skin lesions

- Single or few in number, large (up to 10 cm in diameter) **(Fig. 18.5)**
- Asymmetrical, well-defined, anesthetic, hypopigmented, erythematous or copper colored annular lesions. (The shape is described as 'saucer right way-up').

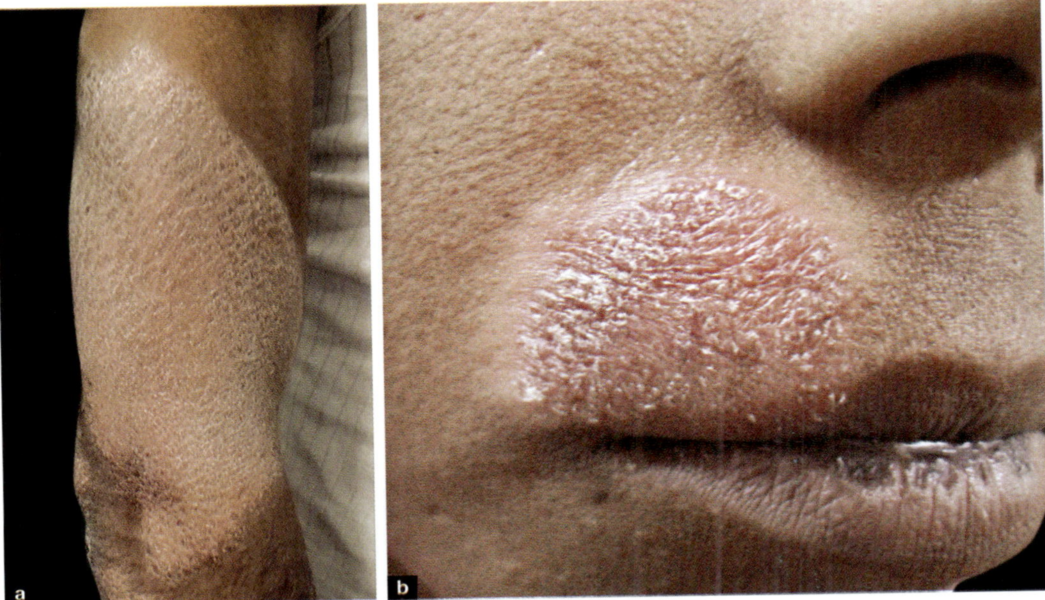

Fig. 18.5: (a) TT Hansen: Well-defined, hypopigmented, anesthetic, dry scaly, hairless plaque with sharply raised border seen over the right elbow; (b) A case of TTs Hansen in an untreated patient showing reaction

- The initial lesion may be hyperesthetic.
- Autonomic nerve damage: Dry and scaly, with complete loss of hair and sweating. (Loss of sweating is tested by exercising the patient in the sun.)

Nerve involvement

- Minimal or nil.
- There may be enlargement of one or at most two nerves in the area near a skin lesion.

3. *Borderline Leprosy* (*BT, BB and BL*)

The lesions may be plaques or macules and vary in number from a few in BT to numerous in BL. The slit smear is used for the final classification which may place the patient in a lower pole than clinically obvious.

Instability is a feature of this spectrum and the patient may downgrade to LLs or upgrade to TTs. Both these changes may be seen on treatment (adequate/inadequate) or without treatment. The downgrading may be silent or is uncommonly associated with reactions. In BT, the CMI defines the clinical features, while in BL, bacillary load is important for defining the clinical features.

Borderline tuberculoid (BT)

Skin

- Up to 10 or 20 or more lesions
- Large asymmetrical lesions that are well-to- ill-defined, with irregular borders and are hypoesthetic **(Fig. 18.6)**
- Margins show streaming and satellite lesions.
- Less scaling, erythema, induration and less elevation (than TT)
- Type I reactions can occur in either skin or nerves or both.

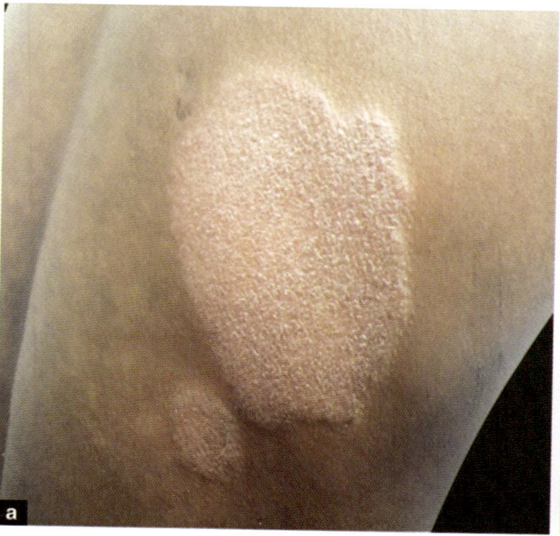

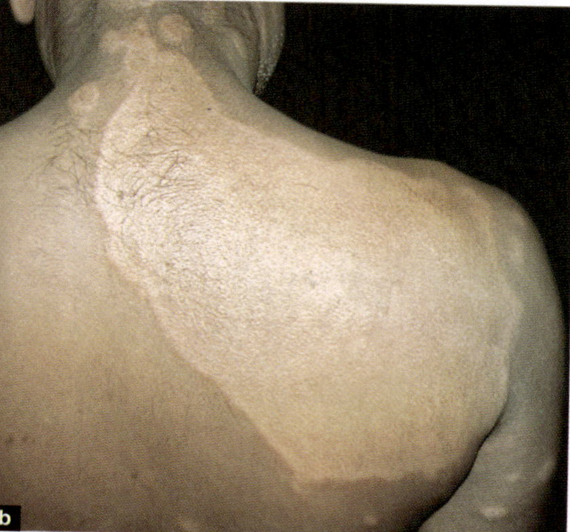

Fig. 18.6: BT Hansen: Well-defined large, hypopigmented to erythematous, hypoesthetic plaque with downward sloping edges seen over mid-outer back. Smaller satellite lesions are seen in the periphery of lesion indicating spread of the disease and lowered immune status

Nerve

- Widespread and asymmetrical nerve enlargement leading to widespread nerve damage is characteristic.

Borderline–Borderline (BB)

Because of its intrinsic instability, this is the rarest form of leprosy. The patients usually stabilize by up or downgrading with or without a clinical reaction.

Skin

- Asymmetrical well-demarcated, somewhat shiny lesions are seen.
- Admixture of TT and LL type. The lesions may be macules, plaques or papules or a combination of these types.
- Often, annular lesions are present with characteristic, punched-out or Swiss cheese appearance (the outer border is vague, inner border is clearly defined) **(Fig. 18.7)**. Thus, the border has a well-defined 'tuberculoid' interior margin but a poorly defined 'lepromatous' exterior margin. The presence of both these morphologies is also termed 'dimorphic' lesions.
- Geographic lesions: The shapes of lesions are characterized by streaming, irregular borders and satellites which represent an infiltration around immune areas.

Nerve: Widespread and asymmetrical nerve enlargement if downgraded from BT (multiple mononeuropathy); symmetrical nerve enlargement is seen if the patient has upgraded from BL (symmetrical polyneuritis).

Borderline-Lepromatous (BL)

In BL disease, there is a maximum damage as there is a high bacillary load with inherent immunological instability.

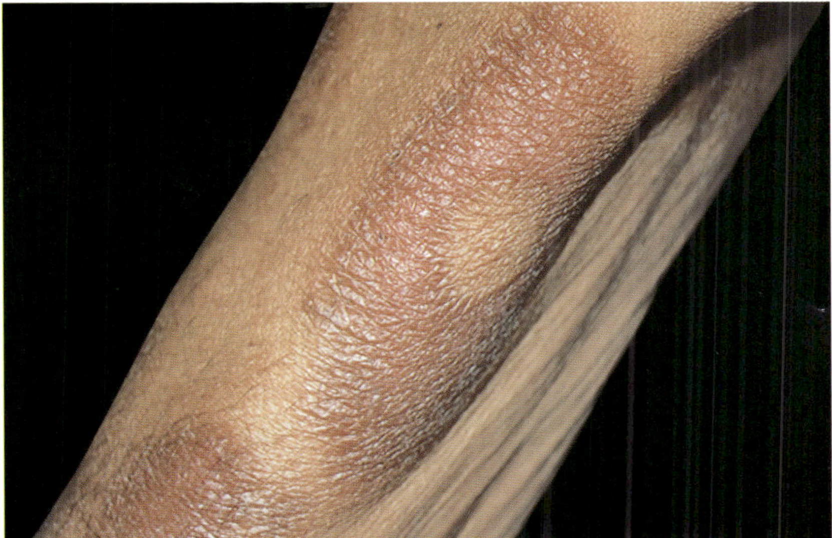

Fig. 18.7: BB Hansen: Well-defined large, irregularly shaped erythematous, slightly hypoesthetic punched out plaques with central raised edge and outwards sloping margins (punched-out or Swiss cheese lesion) seen over the right upper arm

Skin

- Variable in size, number and morphology.
- Symmetrical lesions are hypoesthetic.
- Symmetrical nerve involvement.
- Annular and plaque lesions, however numerous, are asymmetrical. The lepromatous-like nodules if numerous, are symmetrically arranged.
- Classically, the disease starts with macules. The signs of nerve damage (such as hypopigmentation, loss of hair, loss of sensation and decreased sweating and hair growth) start earlier than in LL. The earliest infiltration is in center of the macules.
- Papules and nodules: These lesions have a sloping margin and lie on normal looking skin **(Figs 18.8** and **18.9)**.

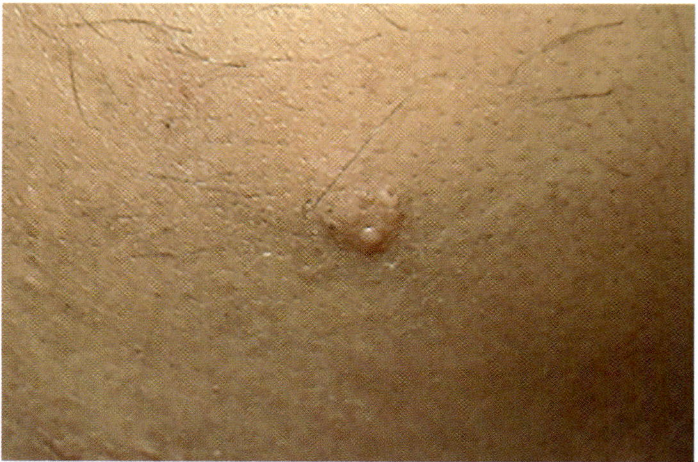

Fig. 18.8: Papule over a pre-existing macular lesion of leprosy

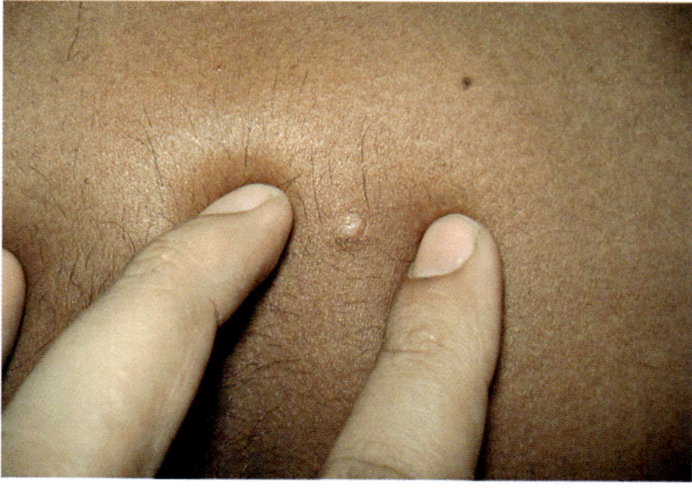

Fig. 18.9: Papule on apparently normal skin

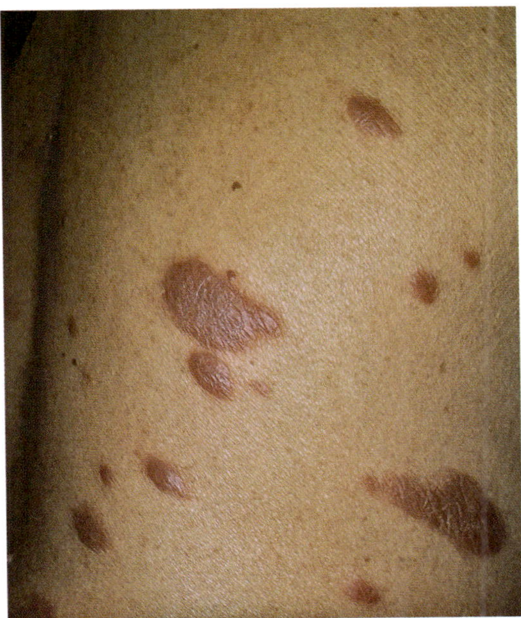

Fig. 18.10: A BL plaque is typically infiltrated in the center and gradually slopes away imperceptibly towards the periphery (the inverted saucer lesion of Molesworth) (*Jopling's Handbook of Leprosy, 6th Edition*)

- Classic lesion: Poorly marginated outer border (lepromatous-like) but a sharply marginated inner one (tuberculoid-like). As the center is raised and sloping towards the periphery the 'inverted saucer' appearance is seen **(Fig. 18.10)**.
- A case of BL can have lesions of BT leprosy as the majority of these patients have downgraded from BT Hansen's disease.

Nerves: Peripheral nerve involvement is symmetrical.

Prognosis: If the patients begin with a clinical diagnosis of BL and it is detected early, the prognosis is good. On the contrary, if the patient has downgraded from BT, then there will be nerve damage and further reactions are to be expected. Patients who downgrade to LLs can have additional type 2 reactions apart from type 1 reactions.

4. *Lepromatous Leprosy*

There are two types of LL:

1. LLp: This refers to the rare polar form of LL that arises *de novo* and is stable.
2. LLsp: This refers to the commoner subpolar type that arises after downgrading from BT/BB/BL.

Skin: There are numerous, symmetrically distributed, erythematous or copper-colored, shiny, macules, papules and nodules. Lesions are less on the warmer areas.

- Diffuse infiltration of skin leads to leonine facies, loss of eyebrows and eyelashes **(Fig. 18.11)** with infiltration of the earlobes **(Fig. 18.12)**. There occurs diffuse loss of sensation over the dorsum of the hands, feet, forearms, and lower legs.
- Macules: Ill-defined, slightly hypopigmented, shiny and moist appearing.

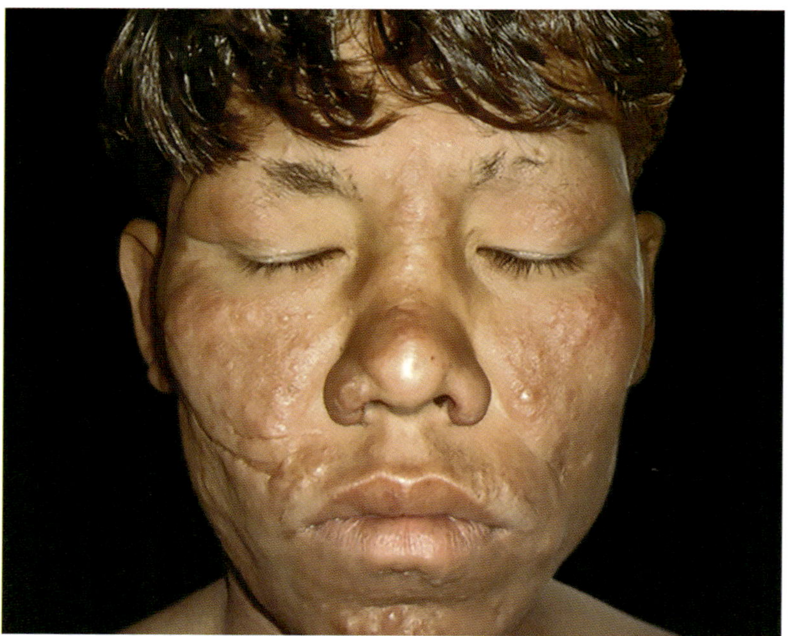

Fig. 18.11: Diffuse infiltration of the face in a case of lepromatous leprosy

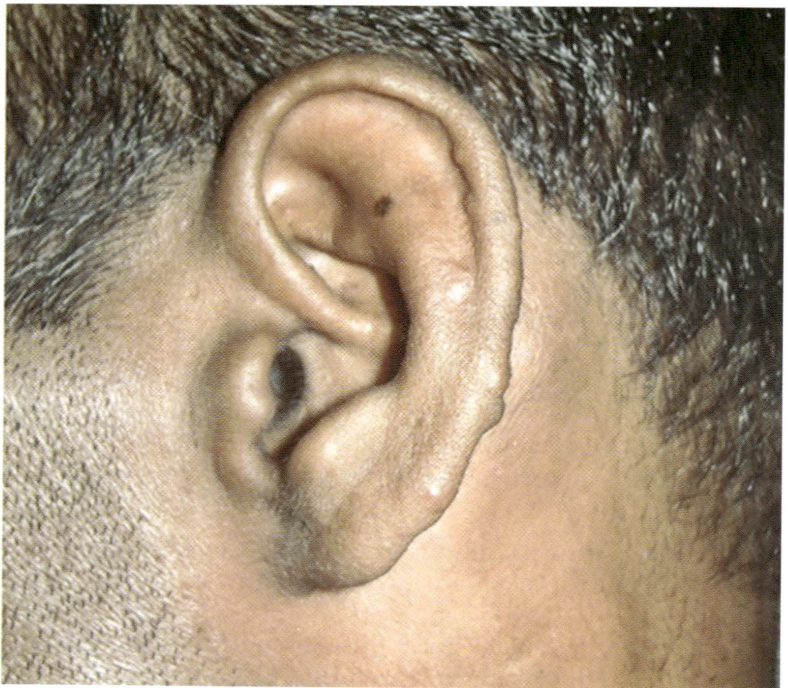

Fig. 18.12: Infiltration and papules on the ear

- The papules usually lie over infiltrated skin.
- Poorly defined nodules are the most common lesions; these are usually up to 2 cm in diameter and are symmetrically distributed.
- Rarely, in advanced lepromatous disease, hair is lost all over except the scalp with residual hair growing only in bands over the course of the arterial supply to the scalp, probably where it is warmer. This is called 'leprous alopecia.'

Nerve: Peripheral nerves at the sites of predilection first become firm, then enlarged and then hard; in a symmetrical manner. Muscular weakness, sometimes appears a little sooner, possibly because the muscles of the hands and feet are affected directly as well as also through the peripheral nerves.

Other organs affected

A detailed overview is given in **Table 18.4**.

As two important organs affected are the eye and the bone, the **Tables 18.5** and **18.6** detail the major findings in these two systems.

5. *Pure Neuritic Leprosy*

Wade (1952) was the first to recognize pure neuritic Hansen. A spectrum from TT to BL leprosy has been observed in the histopathology of nerves. A firm consistency and the lepromin response, if strong, indicates TT or BT leprosy. Ulnar, median and common peroneal are the commonly involved nerves.

TABLE 18.4: Systemic involvement in leprosy

UR tract mucosa (80%)	• A stuffy or blocked nose like coryza, often followed by epistaxis • **40%** of lepromatous patients lose their sense of smell
Eye	• Corneal anesthesia due directly to bacillary infiltration of corneal nerves, and later from damage to the ophthalmic division of the trigeminal nerve • Sclera may become erythematous • Anterior uveitis • Lagophthalmos
Hands and feet	• Swollen digits—joints become swollen and later angulated • Ground glass appearance, hairline fractures • Enlarged nutrient foramen (*earliest sign*), osteolysis
Testis	• The testes become small, soft to palpation, and insensitive • **Exocrine portion**—atrophy causes sterility • **Endocrine portion**—impotence, osteoporosis, gynecomastia • In the early stage, the patient remains sexually potent but his semen is devoid of spermatozoa and therefore he is sterile*
Liver	• Intercurrent hepatitis, caused by viral infection or drugs, hepatic amyloidosis • LL—miliary leproma, no cirrhosis, LFT dysfunction, no correlation with BI
Kidney	• Glomerulonephritis • Nephritis can occur without reaction and also in paucibacillary patients
LN	LL—cortex, medulla, never involve bronchial/mesenteric LN TT—epitrocheal LN

UR, upper respiratory

TABLE 18.5: Eye involvement in leprosy

How are they affected	• Due to involvement of the V and VII cranial nerves • Infiltration of the eyes and the surrounding tissues by the leprosy bacillus • Inflammation of the eyes secondary to the reactions • Complications of the eyes secondary to involvement of surrounding tissues
Cranial nerve	• **Vth nerve**—exposure conjunctivitis and keratitis • **VIIth nerve**—lagophthalmus, ectropion, exposure keratitis
Surrounding structures	Blockage of NLD → infection, conjunctivitis, corneal ulcers
Direct involvement	• Eyebrows: Madarosis • Eyelids: Nodules, conjunctiva, sclera nodules
Cornea	• Affected via the myelinated corneal nerves • **Lepromatous pearls**—clumps of globi packed within swollen macrophages • Superficial punctate keratitis • Avascular punctate keratitis most commonly found in the *superolateral aspect*; interstitial keratitis; pannus and perforation of cornea
Iris/ciliary body	• Iris pearls • Nodular lepromata • Acute and chronic plastic iridocyclitis

Cataract was found to be the most common cause of visual disability (although it is not directly caused by leprosy).

TABLE 18.6: Bone involvement in leprosy*

Why does it happen	• Repeated *trauma and disuse* • Impaired *blood supply* of bone due to endarteritis of nutrient vessels • *Osteoporosis* secondary to testicular atrophy, prolonged use of steroids and renal damage • Bacilli deposition • *Osteomyelitis* may complicate chronic ulceration of the overlying skin
Types	**Specific** • Lepra reactive = Terminal tuft dissolution, destruction of bone, sclerosis, subperiosteal bone erosion **Osteitis** • Enlarged nutrient foramen, pseudocyst, honeycomb appearance and sucked candy look **Nonspecific** • Bone erosion, absent phalanges, osteomyelitis, Charcot type joint **Osteoporosis**
Facies leprosa	• Atrophy of nasal spine—nasal collapse, with – atrophy of anterior alveolar process of maxilla—loss of central upper incisor 'flattening of cheeks and upper lip' • Described by Moller-Christensen

*Dharmendra, ed. Leprosy. Vol. 1. Bombay: Samant and Company, 1985.

6. *Rare or Uncharacteristic Presentations*

Tuberculoid type

1. **Tenosynovitis:** Seen in BT Hansen in type 1 reaction.
2. **Spontaneous ulceration:** Seen as a result of exaggerated hypersensitivity in type 1 reactions. Histopathology shows necrosis due to extreme cellular hypersensitivity in BT leprosy.

Lepromatous type

Four unusual types of lepromatous leprosy:

1. Localized lepromatous or borderline lepromatous disease (nodule or a localized area of nodules or papules).
2. Histoid leprosy by Wade: Pathologically characterized by appearance of spindle-shaped cells. Clinically, the lesions have very well-defined edges, are shiny and coppery red in color. The presented etiology cause is relapse after many years of apparently successful monotherapy with dapsone. The BI is 5+ to 6+; with elongated bacilli and may indicate a focal loss of immunity **(Fig. 18.13)**.
3. Acute exacerbation of leprosy: Seen mainly in very advanced lepromatous patients with nodular and plaque-like lesions. Clinically the lesions undergo ulceration, that mimic a

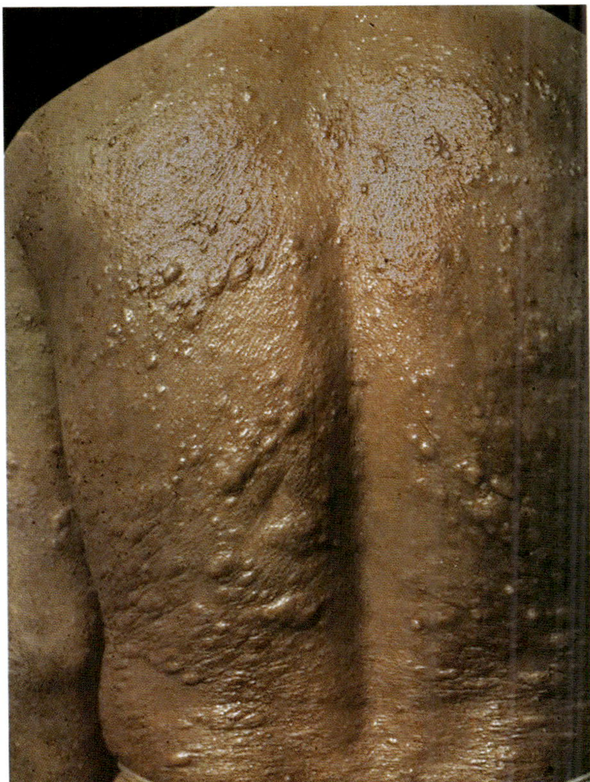

Fig. 18.13: Histoid Hansen: Multiple well-defined succulent, fleshy, skin-colored normoesthetic nodules scattered all over the back, both arms, forearms. There may be history of incomplete therapy or dapsone monotherapy in the past

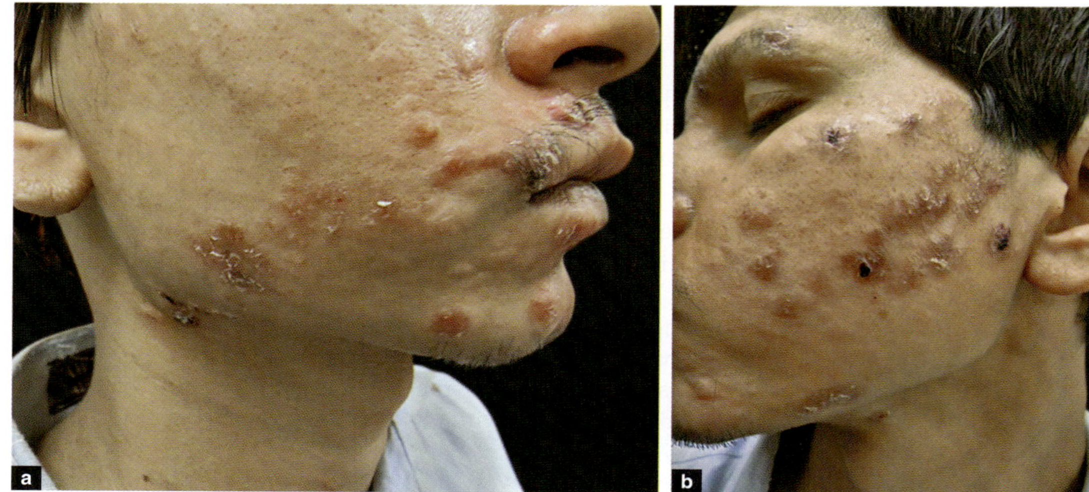

Fig. 18.14: Acute exacerbation in a patient with lepromatous leprosy

type 2 reaction, but there are no systemic features and there are intact bacilli on smears; while in ENL there are granular bacilli with neutrophils **(Fig. 18.14)**.

4. Lucio-Latapí leprosy and lazarine leprosy: Lucio-Latapí leprosy refers to the diffuse non-nodular type of leprosy described by Lucio and Alvarado in Mexico in 1852 and later by Latapí and Zamora in 1948. This form of leprosy has no specific lesions of leprosy on skin and has also been called the 'lepra bonita' (beautiful leprosy).

   The other name—lazarine leprosy, which is often alluded to in literature, is derived from the name of the Saint Lazaro Hospital (Hospital de San Lázaro) in Mexico City, where this form of leprosy was first described, in 1844. Lucio-Latapí leprosy refers to the diffuse infiltrative form; the terms "Lucio phenomenon, erythema necroticans, ENL necroticans, spotted leprosy (lepra manchada) and lazarine leprosy" describe the same entity and probably refer to the necrotic ulcerations seen in these patients. The cause is believed to be involvement of endothelial cells of the capillaries manifesting as hemorrhage and infarction of the overlying epidermis.

LEPROSY REACTIONS

These are immune-mediated events that occur during the otherwise indolent disease course.

Type 1 Lepra Reactions

Usually seen when the disease is upgrading, but can also be seen in the downgrading state.

Major cause of impairment of nerve function in leprosy and affect up to 30% of leprosy patients.

i. Upgrading (reversal reaction)
ii. Downgrading reaction
iii. Static reaction

- Mostly occur in borderline cases (BB, BT and BL) as they are immunologically unstable.
- Increased inflammation in established BT-BL skin lesions or new swollen lesions in BL and subpolar LL patients.

- Neuritis can be profound. Women commonly get extensive skin changes, especially in reactions associated with pregnancy.

Mechanism

Type IV hypersensitivity reaction.

Triggers and risk factors: Antigenic load (positive BI), pregnancy, intercurrent infections especially tuberculosis, vaccinations, psychological stress, extensive disease, established nerve function impairment at diagnosis, facial patches or *M. leprae*-specific IgM anti-PGL antibodies.

Th1 cellular immune response: IFN-γ and TNF-α combined with the effects of cytolytic CD4+ T cells produce tissue damage. Treg cells are also increased leading to localization of reaction (unlike ENL).

Clinical Features

Onset: Upgrading (reversal) reactions usually occur during the *first 6 months* of therapy in BT and BB patients while in BL reactions usually occur between *2 and 12 months* after treatment, in almost 50% of patients. Downgrading reactions occur spontaneously in untreated patients or in patients whose treatment has been interrupted. Untreated BT patients may suffer episodes of type 1 reaction in association with downgrading, presumably because the immunological balance is responding to an increasing antigenic stimulus. In this case, the reactions cease as the patient reaches BL, but are likely to recur during chemotherapy. Rarely they can occur up to 5 years after treatment where they have to be differentiated from a case of relapse of leprosy.

Systemic: Low-grade fever, malaise and anorexia. Sometimes, there is slight to severe edema of the hands, feet and face.

Types

- **Upgrading reaction (Fig. 18.15):** Some or all the existing leprosy lesions show signs of acute inflammation (pain, tenderness, erythema and edema). Necrosis and ulceration may occur in severe cases. The lesions desquamate as they subside. There may be severe neuritis. New lesions might appear occasionally in upgrading reactions. As the edema is profound, the existing lesion becomes more prominent.
- **Downgrading reaction:** The lesions worsen and the morphology progresses towards the lepromatous pole. The new skin lesions are lepromatous in appearance. Rapid onset of swelling of one or more nerves with pain and tenderness may be seen; edema of hands, feet or face may be present and nerve abscesses may form.

Type 2 Lepra Reactions

Seen most commonly in BL and LL patients. In most cases, the onset is after 6 months (within the first 2 years) of therapy or rarely they may occur *de novo*. Over 1/2 LL and 1/4th of BL patients will experience type 2 reactions.

Mechanism

It is a type 3 or immune complex-mediated lepra reaction and is triggered by infections, pregnancy, puberty, vaccinations, drugs and stress. It occurs when a large numbers of leprosy bacilli are killed and the proteins released from the dead bacilli provoke an allergic reaction (seen when the morphological index is under 5%). Since these proteins are present in the

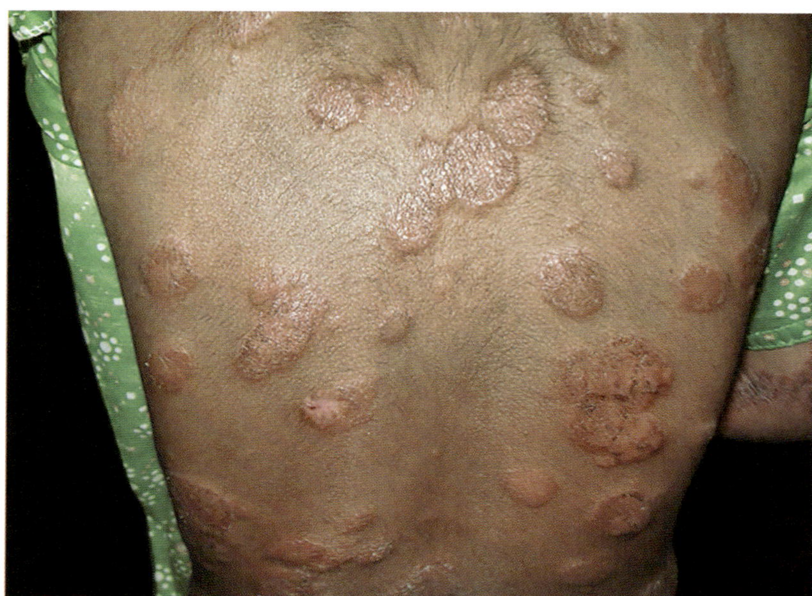

Fig. 18.15: Type I upgrading reaction. Painful, erythematous lesions which desquamate as the reaction subside

bloodstream, a type 2 reaction consequentially, is systemic in nature. Increased neutrophils lead to vasculitis, pustule formation, and ulceration. The **Th1** and **Th17** cell lines contribute to widespread tissue damage in the absence of the inhibitory Treg cells.

Clinical Features

- The classic lesions are tender, erythematous, evanescent nodules referred to as ENL.
- ENL may appear in any place where there has been a lepromatous infiltrate, even though this may not have been obvious clinically. Most common sites are the face and extensor surfaces of the limbs, but truncal lesions also commonly occur. Panniculitis may be seen.
- Atypical morphology: Targetoid, vesicular, pustular, ulcerative and necrotic lesions **(Fig. 18.16)**.
- Neuritis: Affected nerves are tender and a little enlarged.
- Systemic involvement: Conjunctivitis, keratitis, iritis, iridocyclitis, orchitis, hepatomegaly and lymphadenopathy. High-grade fever usually accompanies extensive crops.

Types

Three patterns of ENL have been described, which are as follows (Pocaterra L, et al., 2006):

1. *Acute episode* is defined as a single episode, lasting *less than 6 months*, which responds to steroid treatment; this accounts for only 6% of episodes.
2. *Recurrent ENL (32%)*: This is constituted by recurrent episodes (occurring 4 weeks or more apart) with intervening quiescent periods.
3. *Chronic ENL (62%)*: In this, the patient needs treatment for more than 6 months either continuously or with treatment-free period of 27 days or less. It is the most distressing type both for the patient and the clinician.

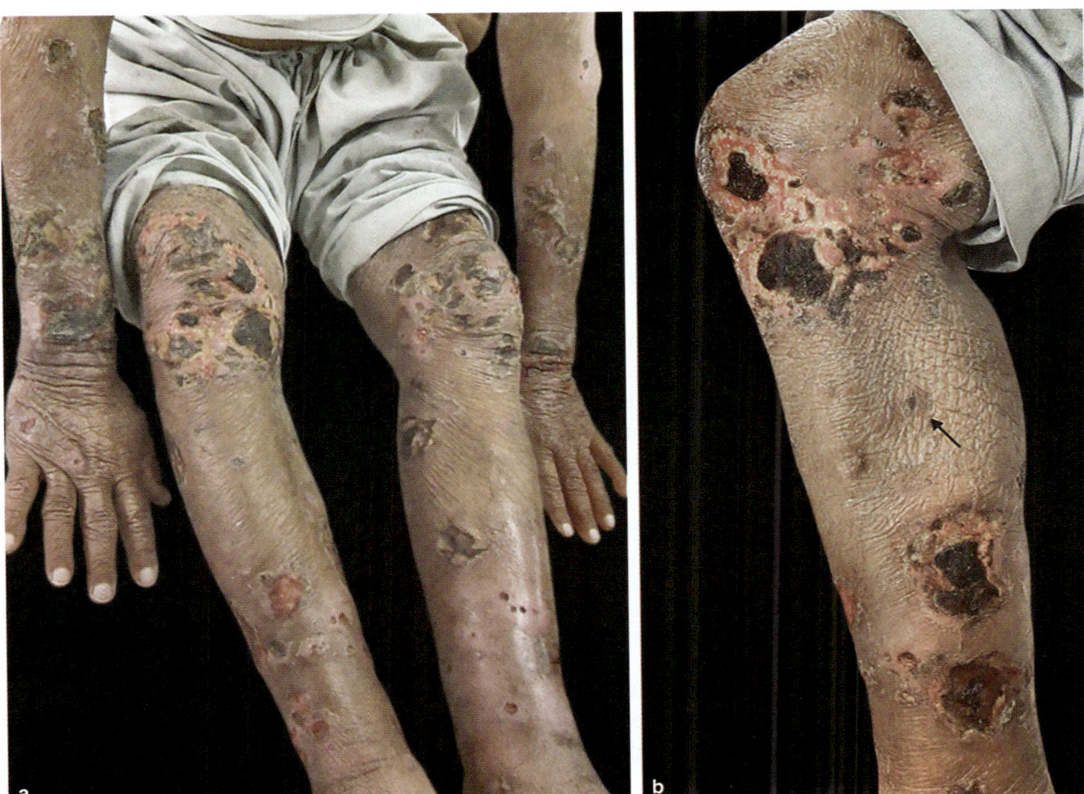

Fig. 18.16: Type II lepra reactions: Erythema nodosum leprosum (ENL) necroticans: (a) Multiple ulcers with central eschar present over both arms, forearms. Margins of the ulcers are punched-out with erythematous to yellowish pus exuding from the floor. Pedal and hand edema is seen; (b) A few ill-defined erythematous tender subcutaneous nodules are seen (black arrow) with and without necrotic centers

Grading of reaction: The older classification divides ENL into mild, moderate and severe varieties, but the latest recommendations grade them in two types:

1. A mild reaction is one that occurs in the skin only (as long as it does not occur over a major nerve or in the face); there may be mild fever and slight swelling (edema) of the limbs.
2. Severe reactions affect the nerves or eyes in addition to the skin and the signs include:
   - Pain or tenderness in the nerves
   - New loss of sensation
   - New muscle weakness
   - Reaction in a skin lesion lying over a major nerve
   - Reaction in a skin lesion on the face
   - Signs of inflammation in the eye
   - Severe edema (swelling) of the limbs
   - Involvement of other organs, such as testes, lymph nodes or joints
   - Ulceration of skin lesions

More recently, ENLIST scoring has been introduced for severity assessment of ENL.

INVESTIGATIONS

1. Slit-skin Smear

- *Whom to smear, and when*: All patients before commencing MDT, and all MB leprosy patients at end of therapy; post-treatment patients if suspected of relapse. Smears should be kept to a minimum (consistent with good practice) as there is nothing so demoralizing as having to examine large numbers of negative smears.
- *Sites to be smeared*: The *minimum* is 1 earlobe **plus** two active skin lesions in untreated patients, with the same sites used for follow-up smears. In patients suspected of relapse, new relapse lesions should also be smeared.
- Select the most active-looking lesion, but *not on the face*. 'Active' means raised and reddish in color. Take the smear in the most active area of the lesion (usually the **edge**).
- If there is no suitable skin lesion, take the second smear from the other earlobe, or from a site where active lesions were originally recorded or where a previous smear was positive.
- From previously untreated and suspected relapsed drug-resistant lepromatous patients, smears can be taken from six sites: Both earlobes and four representatives active skin sites. This is not recommended to avoid trauma and chance of spread of blood-borne infections.
- A particularly useful site for the detection of impending *relapses* in long treated lepromatous patients have been the *dorsa* of fingers.

How to make and stain a smear

Making the smear

- Take a new, clean, unscratched microscope slide. Using a slide marker, write the patient identification (ID) number at the bottom of the slide. This number must be on the request form.
- Clean the skin at the smear sites with a cotton wad drenched in alcohol. Let it dry.
- Light the spirit burner.
- Put a new blade (No. 15) on the scalpel handle. If you put the scalpel down, make sure the blade does not touch anything.
- Pinch the skin firmly between your thumb and forefinger; maintain pressure to press out the blood.
- Make an incision in the skin about **5 mm long and 2 mm deep**. Keep on pinching to make sure the cut remains bloodless. If bleeding, wipe the blood away with cotton wad.
- Turn the scalpel 90° and hold it at a right angle to the cut.
- Scrape inside the cut once or twice with the side of the scalpel, to collect tissue fluid and pulp. There should be *no blood* in the specimen, as this may interfere with staining and reading.
- Stop pinching the skin and absorb any bleeding with a wad of cotton.
- Spread the material scraped from the incision onto the slide, on the same side as the ID number. Spread it evenly with the flat of the scalpel, making a circle **8 mm** in diameter. Two smears can be made on each slide.

Fixing the smear: Heat fix over a flame. If hot plate is available, then heating for 5 min between 40–50°C is acceptable. The simplest way of avoiding heat-fixation is to fix the smears for 10 min in formalin fumes, which will also ensure that the bacilli are killed.

Staining the smear: AFB-mycolic acids confer resistance to decolorization by acids, including ethanol and hydrochloric acids, during staining procedures. Hence, the term 'acid-fast'. The smears are stained using the **hot Ziehl–Neelsen** method. Stain with 1% carbol fuchsin, which colors everything red. Washout the stain with 1% acid-alcohol, which removes the stain from everything except *M. leprae*. Counterstain the slide with 0.2% methylene blue. The leprosy bacilli will be seen as red rods on a blue background.

In 1915, Kinyoun published the **'cold staining'** variant, replacing the use of heat with the use of a higher concentration of carbol fuchsin in the primary stain.

Stain for human tissue on histopathology is **Fite-Faraco** method. Other stains are the fluorochromes.

Measurement of the bacteriological index (BI) and morphological index (MI)

BI: Report the BI for both smears on the slide. For smear-positive patients, either the average BI (total BI from different sites divided by number of sites) or the highest BI will be taken as the BI for that patient. The slides are examined by examining 25–100 fields, on a logarithmic scale ranging from 0–6 **(Box 18.4)**.

BOX 18.4: Bacteriological index (BI)

0	0 bacilli in 100 fields
1+	1–10 bacilli in 100 fields
2+	1–10 bacilli in 10 fields
3+	1–10 bacilli, on average, in each field
4+	10–100 bacilli, on average, in each field
5+	100–1000 bacilli, on average, in each field
6+	>1000 bacilli, on average, in each field

The BI falls at the rate of approximately 1 unit/year of effective treatment. The BI decreases across the spectrum from 5+/6+ in LL leprosy to 0–2+ in BT leprosy and 0 in TT leprosy. A BI of 6 indicates 10^9 bacilli/g of tissue, while tissues with a BI of 0 may have as many as 10^3 organisms/g.

MI: Regularly and irregularly stained bacteria are counted on preferably 200 red staining elements, lying singly. Only *individual* bacteria, the entire *outline* of which can be seen, and which are *not touching* or superimposed, are counted. Only bacteria showing *uniform* and *bright* staining down their length are called *regularly* stained; pale-staining organisms are counted as irregularly stained. Short organisms (length less than four times their width) are counted as irregularly stained.

Importance—it indicates the *viability* of bacilli, *infectiousness* of a patient and the patient's *response to treatment*; and in treated patients a positive MI will give early intimation of *relapse* and *resistance*. Theoretical *disadvantage* is that it may be an over estimate of viable bacilli as no one knows the interval between the biological death and regular stain of the bacilli.

In LL Hansen, there is *no fall of BI in the first 12 months*. The MI is 25–75% initially and should become zero in 6 weeks.

2. Nasal Smears

They are usually done for LL cases and rapidly become negative. Thus, these are an indication of the *response* to therapy. Not routinely recommended.

3. Lepromin Test

This is not done nowadays. Two antigens: Mitsuda and Dharmendra. Two reactions: Early (Fernandez) and late (Mistuda).

4. Histopathology (*See* Table 18.1)

An overview of pathology of the major types of leprosy is provided in **Table 18.7** and the nuances are given in the text that follows.

The pathology of leprosy reactions is given in **Table 18.8**.

- **Downgrading:** Without adequate, regular anti-leprosy therapy, many of the BT and BL lesions undergo a gradual downgrading shift. The process of downgrading is ordinarily insidious and silent.

TABLE 18.7: Comparison of the salient features of leprosy types (from Hastings)

	TT	BT	BB	BL	LL
Lepromin reaction	3+	1+			
Immunological stability	2+	+/–	–	+/–	2+
Type 1 reactions	–	1+	2+	1+	–
Type 2 reactions				1+	1+
Bacilli in granuloma	0	1–3+	3–4+	4–5+	5–6+
Epithelioid cells	1+	1+	1+	–	
Lymphocytes/erosion of epidermis	3+/1+	2+	1+	3+	+/–
Infiltration of subepidermis zone	1+	1+			
Nerve damage	2+	2+	1+	1+	+/–
Langhans giant cells	1+	2+			
Touton giant cells					1+
Globi				–	1+
Foam cells				1+	3+

TABLE 18.8: Overview of the histopathology of reactions*

	Dermis	Nerves/IHC	AFB
Type 1 borderline reactions			
Upgrading reactions	• Edema • Disorganized granuloma • Marked ↑ in *lymphocytes*, epithelioid cells	Nerves may undergo caseous necrosis Influx of CD4+ T cells ↑ CD28+ cells↑	AFB in the lesions of BL are considerably reduced or completely disappeared
Downgrading reactions	• Edema—↓in lymphocytes, paucity of cells, ↑*macrophages*		Appearance of increasing numbers of macrophages with AFB
ENL	• Dense infiltration of the superficial and/or deep dermis and/or subcutaneous tissue by neutrophils (seen in acute stage <12 hours) • Necrosis and ulceration of skin • Vasculitis (75% of cases)	CD28 –ve CD1a ↓	Reduction of bacterial load and most of the organisms present are broken and granular

*Lepr Rev. 2018; 89:256–271
Lepr Rev. 2017; 88:217–26

- **Acute exacerbations of disease:** Histologically, there are small localized areas of necrosis in the middle of a large sheet of macrophages eliciting a localized infiltration of neutrophils. Macrophages contain a relatively large load of AFB with many solid staining organisms which differentiate acute exacerbation from ENL.

5. Detection of DNA

The need for PCR tests for diagnosis of leprosy mainly lies in early leprosy, indeterminate, PB and pure neural leprosy. Further, the use of molecular-based techniques in finding mutations in drug-resistant determining region (DRDR) of *M. leprae* is also increasing.

6. Serology

The clinical utility of serological tests remains undetermined. While anti-PGL1 IgM or NDO-LID® may be useful in diagnosis of MB leprosy, serological methods are not sensitive enough to aid diagnosis of PB leprosy and the presence of anti-*M. leprae* antibodies is not predictive of disease.

NDO-LID® test, used for the rapid diagnosis of MB leprosy based on the complementary detection of antibodies against a novel protein—glycolipid conjugate. NDO-LID® is an immunochromatographic test that requires small amounts of serum or whole blood. Like the other serological tests for leprosy, it detects MB patients.

7. Immunodiagnostic Tests

These are based on the antigens to *M. leprae*, IFN-γ-induced protein 10 (IP-10), IFN-γ/IL-10 ratio, transcription profiles and cytokines released in reactions like, IL-2 receptors, TNF-γ, IL-6, IP-10, and IL-17F.

Lateral flow assays (LFAs) based on upconverting phosphor (UCP-LFAs) have been developed for the detection of IFN-γ, IP-10 (Th1), and IL-10 (Treg) as well as antibodies against the *M. leprae* specific PGL1.

TREATMENT

Rationale of Chemotherapy in Leprosy (Grosset JH)

In a patient with multibacillary (MB) leprosy, the maximal number of acid-fast bacilli (AFB) could be 10^{11-12} and out of this 1% (10^{10}) are viable. The proportion of *M. leprae* mutants resistant to dapsone, clofazimine or rifampin are given in **Table 18.9** and are diagrammatically represented in **Fig. 18.17**.

Thus, a patient with MB leprosy harbors, at most, $\mathbf{10^9}$ drug-susceptible organisms, $\mathbf{10^3}$ rifampin-resistant mutants and $\mathbf{10^4}$ dapsone or clofazimine mutants **(Fig. 18.17)**. As seen in **Table 18.9**, bacilli resistant to all 3 drugs are not possible.

Drug-resistant bacilli: For rifampin, a single dose of 600 mg kills more than 99% of the susceptible bacilli and it also kills the bacilli resistant to DDS/CLO. The time required for DDS+ CLO to kill the rifampin-resistant mutants is unknown, thus dapsone and clofazimine are advised during the whole course of therapy.

Drug susceptible bacilli: Rifampicin in the initial doses kills 99.999% of bacilli; thus, reducing the initial population of viable *M. leprae* in a MB patient from 10^{10} to 10^5. The objective is then

TABLE 18.9: Drug-resistant mutants in a normal strain of *M. leprae*

Drug(s)	Resistant mutant (%)	Total[a]
Rifampin (RMP)	1 per 10^7	10^3
Dapsone (DDS)	1 per 10^6	10^4
Clofazimine (CLO)	1 per 10^6	10^4
RMP + DDS	1 per 10^{13}	10^{-3}
RMP + CLO	1 per 10^{13}	10^{-3}
DDS + CLO	1 per 10^{12}	10^{-2}
RMP + DDS + CLO	1 per 10^{19}	10^{-9}

[a]In an MB patient harboring 10^{10} viable *M. leprae*.

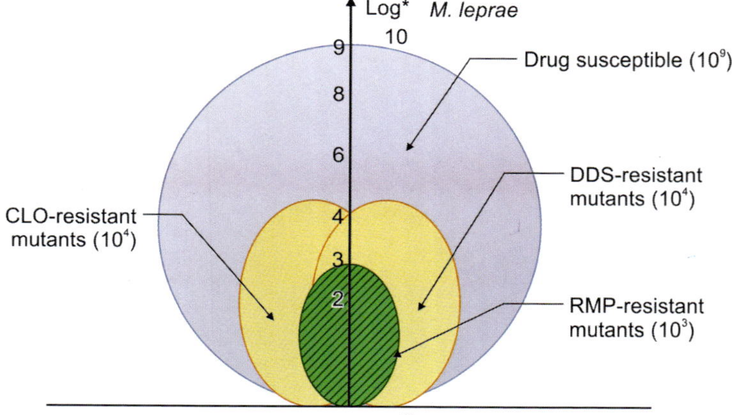

Fig. 18.17: Bacillary populations in multibacillary leprosy

to eliminate the remaining 10^5 viable drug-susceptible *M. leprae* in order to prevent relapse after stopping treatment.

After the initial rapid killing of bacilli, the proportion of *M. leprae* capable of multiplying in mice remained constant during the 2 years of treatment, suggesting that chemotherapy is mostly ineffective against the remaining organisms. These bacilli remain metabolically inactive or dormant and here the clearing mechanisms of the host can eliminate them progressively.

Conventional Drugs

An overview of the conventional drugs is given in **Tables 18.10** to **18.12**.

Newer Drugs

The newer drugs were primarily discovered for shortening the duration of MDT but now have importance as they are useful in drug-resistant **(Table 18.13)** leprosy which is increasingly being reported. It is clear that the three new drugs ofloxacin, minocycline and clarithromycin are individually and in combination much more active than dapsone and clofazimine. They are, therefore, natural candidates to replaced dapsone and clofazimine for improving leprosy chemotherapy.

1. *Fluoroquinolones*

OFLO: Acts by inhibiting the alpha subunit of the enzyme DNA gyrase, thereby interfering with bacterial DNA replication. Dose: **400** mg is bactericidal against *M. leprae*, although less

TABLE 18.10: Overview of dapsone

MIC	0.003 µg/mL, tissue levels about the same as plasma levels
Mode of action	Competitive inhibition with *para*-aminobenzoic acid for an enzyme (dihydropteroate synthetase) thereby blocking the synthesis of dihydrofolic acid
Resistance	Stepwise mutation (Hastings, 1977), rapid acetylators are not more likely to develop sulfone, resistant disease (Shepard et al., 1976)
Absorption metabolism	90% absorbed, equilibrium is set up between dapsone and its monoacetyl derivative (MADDS), secreted in the urine, T½ = 28 hours
Side effects	'DDS syndrome', agranulocytosis, hepatitis, peripheral neuropathies, methemoglobinemia, and hypoalbuminemia • **DDS syndrome:** 6 weeks after the start of therapy, erythroderma, skin rashes, generalized lymphadenopathy, hepatosplenomegaly, fever, and hepatitis. HLA-B * 13:01, which is present in Asian but not African populations, is a major risk factor for dapsone hypersensitivity • Methemoglobinemia—skin discoloration, cyanosis, headache, lightheadedness, weakness, syncope and palpitations • **Hemolytic anemia:** The reticulocyte count 2–5% range, usually with a mild drop in hemoglobin and hematocrit • **G6PD deficiency:** Start at 25 mg twice weekly, increase by 3–4 weeks to 50–100 mg daily • **Agranulocytosis:** 1:10000, fever, ulcerating pharyngitis (sore throat), pallor, or purpura • **Peripheral neuropathies:** Motor, ulnar /median, distal axonal degeneration, dose related, reversible • **Liver:** Toxic hepatitis or jaundice, reversible
Pregnancy	Safe
Dose	100 mg tablets, acedaposone 225 mg every 11 weeks

TABLE 18.11: Overview of rifampicin	
MIC	0.3 μg/mL
Mode of action	Inhibits DNA dependent RNA polymerase
Resistance	One step (Jacobson and Hastings, 1976)
Absorption	Rapidly absorbed if taken empty stomach
Metabolism	Stomach, peak conc. of 7 μg/mL in 2–4 hrs, t½ of 3 hours, excretion via GIT
Side effects	Toxicity appears to be uncommon after the first year of therapy Hepatotoxic: SGOT/SGPT—2–3 times—stop Flu-like syndrome: Chills, fever, headache, myalgia, bone pain rarely thrombocytopenia
Interaction	Reduces levels of dapsone and steroids
Dose	600 mg monthly

TABLE 18.12: Overview of clofazimine	
MIC	Unknown, multiplication of *M. leprae* is inhibited by feeding mice 0.0001 g% clofazimine in their diet
Mode of action	Unknown Postulated mechanism (acts on outer membrane): • Interaction with respiratory chain → redox cycling → oxidation of reduced clofazimine → ROS, H_2O_2 → interference with ATP production cell death • Interaction with membrane phospholipids—interference with K^+ transport → interference with ATP production → cell death
Resistance	Not common
Absorption metabolism	70% absorbed, t½ = 70 days, serum levels 0.5 μg/mL, 100 mg 3 weekly (exact half-life is difficult to determine because the drug seems to be excreted more rapidly from some tissues than others), excretion via sebum, sweat, feces and urine
Side effects	• Skin discoloration: Due to drug-induced reversible ceroid lipofuscinosis; blotchy; on stopping the color disappears in 6–12 months • Gastrointestinal tract: Mild crampy or burning mid-abdominal to epigastric pain occasionally associated with mild nausea and/or diarrhea (>100 mg), severe symptoms are uncommon during the first 6–12 months of therapy and less than 25% of patients develop any problem even on doses over 100 mg daily • Xerosis: Anticholinergic action
Pregnancy	Safe
Dose	50 mg daily, 300 mg monthly

than a single dose of RMP; **22** daily doses killed **99.99%** of the viable organisms (peak serum levels 2.9 μg/mL, serum half-life of 7 hours, excretion via kidneys).

Daily ofloxacin for 1 month is considered as capable as 2 years of dapsone plus clofazimine to kill the rifampin-resistant mutants.

Side effects: Nausea, diarrhea, and other gastrointestinal complaints, and a variety of central nervous system complaints including insomnia, headache, dizziness, nervousness and hallucinations. Serious problems are infrequent, and only occasionally require discontinuing the drug.

TABLE 18.13: Comparative bactericidal activities of a single dose of rifampin, the combinations of ofloxacin, clarithromycin and/or minocycline against *M. leprae*

Drug[a]	Killing activity
RMP	99.5%
MINO + CLARI	96%
OFLO + MINO + CLARI	98.4%
RMP + OFLO + MINO + CLARI	99.5%

[a]RMP, rifampin 10/kg; MINO, minocycline 25 mg/kg; CLARI, clarithromycin 100 mg/kg; OFLO, ofloxacin 150 mg/kg.

2. *Macrolides*

CLARI: The drug acts by linking to the 50S ribosomal subunit, thus inhibiting bacterial protein synthesis. Potent bactericidal activity but *less* than rifampicin.

Dose: 500 mg daily. Kills 99% of *M. leprae* by **28** days, and **99.9%** by **56** days (peak serum level 1 µg/mL, serum half-life of 6–7 hours). Tissue concentrations are higher than those in the serum. Active component—14-0H-CLARI.

Though some synergism between minocycline and clarithromycin was demonstrated in the mouse model, the combination of 100 mg minocycline and 500 mg clarithromycin was not more active in man than each component alone, perhaps because the potency of each individual drug was too strong.

Side effects: Gastrointestinal irritation, nausea, vomiting and diarrhea are the most common symptoms, but they do not usually require discontinuation of the drug.

3. *Minocycline*

MINO binds reversibly at the 30S unit of the ribosome, blocking the binding of aminoacyl transfer RNA to the messenger RNA-ribosomal complex, thereby inhibiting protein synthesis.

Dose: The standard dose is 100 mg daily, which yields a blood level of 2–4 µg/mL, well above the apparent minimal inhibitory concentration for *M. leprae* of 0.2 µg/mL. More than 99% and **99.9%** of the viable *M. leprae* are killed by **28** and **56** days of treatment.

Definite clinical improvement is seen in some patients as early as 14 days after beginning treatment, in all patients by 1 month, and on an average marked improvement occurs in all patients by 2 months.

Replacement of Drugs in WHO-MDT Pack

- Clofazimine: Based on clinical data, *ofloxacin* (400/mg/day) is used most commonly as a substitute for *clofazimine* (Ji B, et al., 1994) although others (including *moxifloxacin*) also appear to be effective in the treatment of leprosy (Pardiloo FE, et al., 2009).
- Dapsone or clofazimine: In addition to the fluoroquinolones, other alternative agents include *minocycline* (100/mg/day) in place of *dapsone* or *clofazimine*.
- Any drug: *Clarithromycin* (500/mg/day) in place of any of the three first-line agents, based on encouraging clinical results.

Special Situations

1. **MDT in tuberculosis:** Since WHO-MDT for leprosy is not the ideal treatment for tuberculosis, an appropriate anti-tubercular regimen should be added to the anti-leprosy MDT in patients

in whom the two diagnoses are confirmed. If daily RMP is part of the anti-tuberculosis treatment, there is no need to administer monthly RMP as part of the leprosy MDT. The remaining MDT drugs continue as per the treatment classification (PB/MB).

2. **MDT in pregnancy:** It is established that pregnancy exacerbates leprosy. Fortunately, MDT appears to be safe during pregnancy; no contraindications have been established currently. CLO is excreted through breast milk and can cause mild discoloration of the skin of the infant and has been reported as the cause of 3 deaths. DDS can cause hemolysis and arise in liver enzymes, while RMP can cause cleft palate and spina-bifida in rats. The use of newer drugs is not advised in pregnancy.
3. **Management of a defaulter:** The maximum time limit for completion for PB leprosy is 9 months while for MB leprosy the therapy must be completed in 18 months. A defaulter is an individual who fails to complete treatment within the maximum allowed time frame. Thus, whenever a PB patient has missed more than 3 months of treatment or an MB patient more than 6 months of treatment, they should be declared as defaulters from treatment. If the case was a PB case and on examination is now an MB case (more than five lesions), register the patient as a return from default, not as a new case and treat with a full course of MB-MDT (12 months) while if it remains PB, treat with a 6 month course of PB-MDT.
4. **Leprosy and human immunodeficiency virus infection:**
   - HIV has little effect on clinical type or histopathologic appearance of leprosy lesions. *M. leprae* may grow too slowly to affect the clinical form of leprosy in people with HIV infection in developing countries, because other complications of HIV infection may dominate.
   - ART therapy for HIV infection is believed to 'unmask' subclinical leprosy in these patients, and in addition, individuals with HIV and *M. leprae* coinfection frequently exhibit reversal reactions as a manifestation of immune reconstitution after anti-retroviral therapy (Sanghi S, et al., 2011).
5. **Leprosy in other immunocompromised hosts:**
   - In treating transplant recipients with leprosy, the potential for adverse medication interactions, particularly between rifampin and cyclosporine; for this reason, leprosy in this patient group may require the use of alternative anti-mycobacterial agents (e.g. minocycline, clarithromycin, ofloxacin).
   - A second population in whom leprosy has been reported are patients receiving TNF-blocking agents (e.g. infliximab, etanercept). These agents, which have been increasingly used in the treatment of autoimmune diseases, have been associated with the development or reactivation of infections typically contained by cell-mediated immunity (e.g. leprosy). Reversal reactions may develop on stopping the biological drugs—presumably because of a restoration of the host immunity.
6. **Non-responders to therapy:** There are four causes that should be systematically ruled out before considering any other possibility. These are as follows:
   - Misclassification of disease
   - Non-compliance
   - Side effects, interaction of drugs or GI upset leading to decreased absorption
   - Resistance.

There is confusion regarding relapse, reactivation, residual disease, resistance and reinfection **(Fig. 18.18)**. Reinfection is a theoretical possibility which can never be definitely confirmed but it is believed that if an elderly patient develops leprosy in an endemic area, it is most likely a case of reinfection.

DRUG-RESISTANT LEPROSY

A basic overview of the steps for diagnosing resistance is given in **Fig. 18.18**.

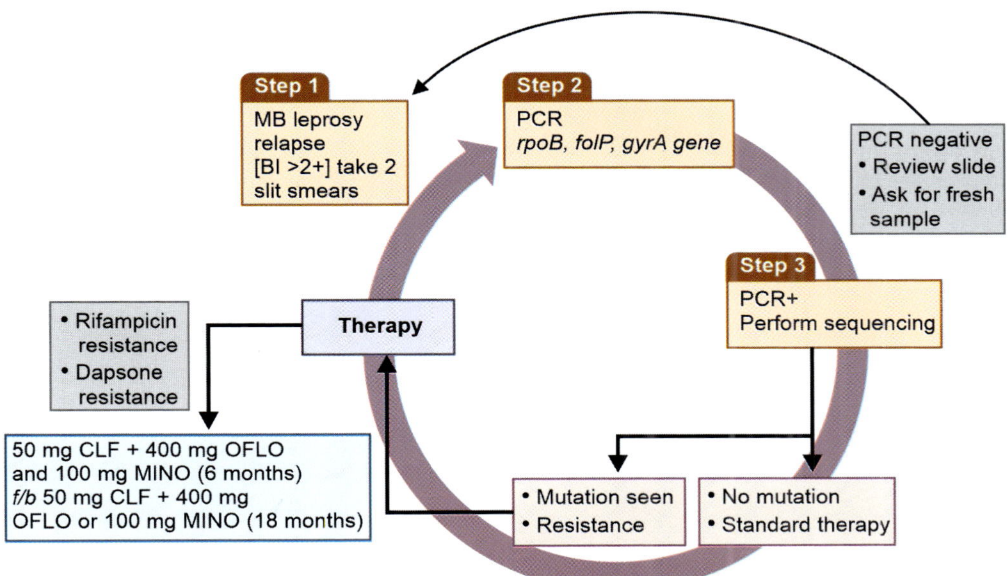

Fig. 18.18: An approach to diagnosis of resistance in leprosy

A summary of the present data on resistance and leprosy is given below.

- Studies (WHO) reported prevalence of rifampicin resistance to be 1.4% in new cases and 8% in *relapsed patients*.
- Patients who start MDT and are found to have resistance to rifampicin alone or in association with resistance to dapsone, shall *restart* a full course of second-line treatment, regardless of clinical outcomes with MDT.
- Cases with resistance to quinolones have also been detected. In India, the number of cases of quinolone resistance appears to equal the number of cases of dapsone resistance, highlighting the need to *limit the use of quinolones* to persons with clear indications. Because fluoroquinolones are active against TB, leprosy patients starting a second-line regimen should be investigated for signs and symptoms of TB, to ensure that persons with TB are treated with an appropriate regimen effective against both diseases, to avoid emergence of drug-resistant TB.
- Monitor with an electrocardiographic monitoring, due to the risk of QT interval prolongation and associated cardiac arrhythmia.

The GDG (Guidelines Development Group, WHO) recommends leprosy patients with rifampicin resistance be treated using at least two of the following second-line drugs: Clarithromycin, minocycline or a quinolone (ofloxacin, levofloxacin or moxifloxacin), plus clofazimine daily for 6 months, followed by clofazimine plus one of the second-line drugs daily for an additional 18 months **(Table 18.14)**.

TABLE 18.14: Treatment of resistant leprosy

Resistance type	Treatment	
	First 6 months (daily)	**Next 18 months (daily)**
Rifampicin resistance	Ofloxacin 400 mg* + Minocycline 100 mg + Clofazimine 50 mg Ofloxacin 400 mg* + Clarithromycin 500 mg + Clofazimine 50 mg	Ofloxacin 400 mg* OR Minocycline 100 mg + Clofazimine 50 mg
Rifampicin and ofloxacin resistance	Clarithromycin 500 mg + Minocycline 100 mg + Clofazimine 50 mg	Clarithromycin 500 mg OR Minocycline 100 mg + Clofazimine 50 mg

*Ofloxacin 400 mg can be replaced by levofloxacin 500 mg or moxifloxacin 400 mg.

TREATMENT OF REACTIONS

Type I Reaction

- The treatment largely depends on whether the reaction is limited to skin lesions (in which case nonsteroidal anti-inflammatory drugs would suffice) or involves nerves too (an indication for steroid treatment).
- Neural reaction may present as an acute neuritis or sudden nerve function impairment (NFI)—sensory/motor/both. Both manifestations may coexist or each may occur without the other.
- In patients with subpolar lepromatous and borderline lepromatous leprosy, and in some patients with borderline and borderline tuberculoid leprosy, reversal reactions may be low grade and management is based on clinical judgment and the patient's level of discomfort.
- Downgrading reactions often do not need steroids as neural involvement is uncommon.

The drug of choice (esp. in presence of definite neural involvement) remains prednisolone. Other drugs such as aspirin and chloroquine are at best used as adjuvants.

Principles of therapy in type I reaction associated with neurological impairment/neuritis

1. **Ideal drug:** Require high-dose corticosteroids for a prolonged duration to permit nerve function recovery.
2. **Duration:**
   - Treatment of early neuropathy in leprosy (TENLEP) trial, showed that a 20-week (5 months) steroid course is sufficient for restoring nerve function in 78% of patients (Wagenaar I, et al., 2017).
   - But duration of immunosuppression should be long enough to cover the period during which the antigen load is able to trigger the CMI response. Thus, ideal therapy should be for **3–6 months for BT, 6–9 months for BB and 18–24 months for BL leprosy**.
3. Most **responsive** patients are those with *recent paralysis* (less than 6 months), *BL leprosy and median nerve palsy*.
4. **Recovery:** The expected recovery of nerve function is variable and depends on the duration and severity of symptoms as well as the particular nerve involved:
   i. One study found neurologic improvement after corticosteroid treatment at 3 months in **30–84%** of patients. Patients who had the *shortest duration of symptoms* before the initiation of therapy and those who had *less severe symptoms* at presentation had the best prognosis (van Brakel WH, et al., 1996).
   ii. Another study found that the overall recovery rate for nerve function is **60–70%**, but may be higher in patients who have no nerve damage at diagnosis but develop acute neuropathy during MDT (Croft RP, et al., 2017).
   iii. Recovery is less in patients with pre-existing nerve function impairment or with chronic or recurrent reactions.
5. Thalidomide is not effective, and because of its ability to upregulate Th1 responses and its potential neurotoxicity, it is contraindicated in pure reversal reactions.
6. Anti-leprosy therapy is always continued.

Prednisolone

Regimen: WHO regimen/ILEP: This is a fixed duration regimen **(Box 18.5)**, while another schedule proposed by Naafs is given in **Table 18.15**.

- The regimen followed in tertiary centers is different and is often individualized.

BOX 18.5: ILEP regimen for type I reaction

PB case* Weeks of course	Daily dose of prednisolone (mg)
1–2	40
3–4	30
5–6	20
7–8	15
9–10	10
11–12	5

MB case[†] Weeks of course	Daily dose of prednisolone (mg)
1–4	40
5–8	30
9–12	20
13–16	15
17–20	10
21–24	5

*The total duration is 12 weeks.
[†]This course lasts 24 weeks.

TABLE 18.15: Steroid schedule (Naafs)

Paucibacillary		Multibacillary	
Dosage	**Time**	**Dosage**	**Time**
40 mg	2 weeks	30 mg	1 month
30 mg	2 weeks	25 mg	2 months
25 mg	1 month	20 mg	3 months
20 mg	2 months	15 mg	2 months
15 mg	1 month	10 mg	2 weeks
10 mg	2 weeks	5 mg	2 weeks
5 mg	2 weeks		
	Total: 6 months		**Total:** 9 months

Dose: Initial dose 40 mg/day (0.5–0.6 mg/kg/day), once a day. Hastings recommends a higher dose of 60–80 mg. If the improvement lasts only for 6–12 hours, then the dose may be divided to a twice daily regimen.

When to taper: The dose of prednisone should then be maintained until the skin changes have *completely resolved*, neuritic pain has *cleared* and neural function lost in the course of there active episode has *begun* to return.

How to taper: The dose can be reduced by 5 mg every 2 weeks over 2–3 months to 20–25 mg. Thereafter, the dose of prednisolone is reduced by 5 mg once monthly. The tapering is individualized and can be slower. The tapering can be faster if the reaction is mild. In cases where a chronic treatment is needed, an alternate day regimen can be given. Some may need long-term low-dose steroids.

Critical dose: 15–20 mg (0.30–0.35 mg/kg) is the critical dose of prednisolone to control an RR after the initial period. Consequentially, at this dose the therapy should be maintained for a longer time. Improvements can be appreciated after 3 months, which may continue for up to 6 months.

Other Drugs

Azathioprine, cyclosporine, chloroquine and non-steroidal anti-inflammatory drugs (NSAIDs) are best used as adjuvants in mild cases.

Surgical

This is indicated in the presence of nerve abscess, unresponsive nerve pain or nerve function impairment that does not respond to medical treatment. If required nerve decompression should be done within **2–3 months**.

Erythema Nodosum Leprosum/Type II Reaction

The therapy is similar to type I reaction. Though a mild self-limiting reaction does respond to aspirin and colchicine, most have chronic and recurrent reactions.

1. **Prednisolone:** The WHO protocol mandates a 12-week protocol. In practice though for most chronic cases a initial dose of 60 mg (1 mg/kg/day) which is tapered down gradually over 5 months.
2. **Combination of clofazimine and corticosteroids:** This is indicated in cases with severe ENL, who do not respond satisfactorily to treatment with corticosteroids or where the risk of toxicity with corticosteroids is high.
   Dose: Clofazimine should be used in a dose of 100 mg, three times a day, for a maximum of 12 weeks. The dose of clofazimine should then be tapered to 100 mg twice a day for 12 weeks and then 100 mg once a day for 12–24 weeks.
3. **Thalidomide**
   Initial dose: The starting dose is 100–200 mg at night, which can be increased to 100 mg three to four times a day. At a **TDS** dose, ENL is usually controlled *within 48 hours*. Tapering the dose of thalidomide should be started when there is 90% diminution of systemic symptoms or skin lesions. The tapering should be ideally completed in 4 weeks. A lower starting dose of thalidomide (50–100 mg/day) has also been seen to be effective in many ENL patients in clincal settings.
   - If patient is on steroids, first the steroid should be tapered till there is a flare of ENL, at which time thalidomide is initiated at a dose of 100 mg four times a day.
   - In case of *chronic ENL*, a maintenance dose of 100 mg is required. Attempts should then be made to discontinue it at least every 6 months, tapering the dose if the patient is on 100 mg or more daily. In case of partial effect, prednisone can be added (0.5–1.0 mg/kg) and after control has been achieved, prednisone can be tapered over the subsequent 6–8 weeks.
   - Thalidomide *failure* can occur specially in BB and BL cases in which concomitant steroids are invariably needed. Another scenario is when the reaction is in fact a reversal reaction or mixed reaction.
4. Other drugs tried include pentoxifylline, aspirin and indomethacin, colchicine, chloroquine, zinc, methotrexate and infliximab.

RELAPSE IN LEPROSY

Relapse

Relapse is defined as the reoccurrence of the disease at any time after the completion of a full course of treatment. It may be confused with a type 1 reaction and **Table 18.16** lists the salient differentiating features.

Criteria

- **Clinical criteria**
  1. Increase in the **size and extent** of lesions
  2. Appearance of **new lesions**

TABLE 18.16: Overview of difference between reversal reaction and relapse

Feature	Reversal reaction	Relapse
Duration from release from treatment (RFT)	Most occur _within 6 months_ of RFT; in recurrent reactions up to 2 years	Following complete subsidence _6 months to 3 years_ or more after RFT
Types of leprosy	BT, BB, BL, LLs	All types
Skin lesions	• Increased erythema, swelling, tenderness on pressure between fingers. There may be edema of feet, hands. Few new lesions of same morphology • Succulent consistency due to edema of lesions • Change in type from BL to BB, BB to BT • Ulceration seen in severe reactions	• Increase in extent and number of lesions. No tenderness. Fresh lesions rubbery in consistency • Edema of hands and feet—rare • Ulceration not seen • New lesions appear
Nerve lesions	• Acute painful neuritis often present Nerves exquisitely tender to touch Nerve abscess during subsidence of reaction • Sudden paralysis of muscles and increase and in extent of sensory loss	• Fresh nerve involvement • _No spontaneous pain_ • Tenderness on pressure • Sensory and motor deficit slow and creeping without treatment
Skin smears	Decrease in BI in reversal reaction in BL and BB types	Any degree of positivity for AFB in fresh lesions in patients rendered inactive signifies relapse
Lepromin	Reversal from BL to BB, and BB to BT evokes progressively positive Fernandez response	Lepromin response corresponds to the type of relapsed leprosy
Response to steroid treatment	There is complete subsidence of skin lesions in _2 to 4 weeks_ which remain subsided* This holds true for reaction in the nerve also in which the treatment should be prolonged	There may be response or only partial subsidence; lesions tend to reappear on stopping treatment. This holds true for the nerves also where progressive loss of function is encountered

*Hastings: 40 mg or more prednisone daily for 4 weeks. If the signs and symptoms clear it is probably a reversal (type I) reaction, but if they do not, relapse is more likely.

3. **Infiltration and erythema** in lesions which had completely subsided and remained subsided.
4. **Nerve involvement**, i.e. involvement (thickening and tenderness on pressure) of nerves which were previously unaffected or in which previous lesion had completely subsided. This fresh involvement is shown by tenderness on pressure and increase in sensory and motor deficit.

- **Bacteriological criteria:** Positivity at any site in skin smears for AFB at two examinations during the period of surveillance is diagnostic of relapse in a PB case. In patients who had high BI (5 to 6+) at the start of MDT, skin smears continue to be positive during surveillance while declining at 0.6 to 1 per one year. If there is an increase in BI by 2 over the previous smear at any site and it continues to be so at two examinations, relapse is diagnosed.
- **Histopathological criteria:** This includes the reappearance of granuloma in PB cases and increased macrophage infiltration with solid-staining bacilli and increasing BI in MB cases.
- **Therapeutic criteria:** If there is no subsidence or only a partial subsidence on steroid therapy with 1 mg/kg of body weight of prednisolone, the condition should be diagnosed as relapse **(Table 18.16)**.

Cause of Relapse

Relapse rate is very low—0.1% per year for PB and 0.06% per year for MB on an average. Latest studies also show a very low relapse rate, with respective values in PB and MB being 1.9% and 0.84%. Majority of relapses occur within 3–5 years of RFT. There is a close correlation of the risk of relapse with the bacterial load of the patient, as relapse occurs more among patients with a BI of 4 or more before MDT or with a BI of 3 or more at the end of MDT. Pure neuritic patients may relapse with lepromatous leprosy.

The main causes of relapse are:

i. Inadequate <u>therapy</u>: This may be result of miscategorization of the patient.
ii. <u>Irregularity</u> in ingesting self-administered clofazimine and dapsone, either due to irregular supply of clofazimine or irregular compliance by the patient. Such patients would be taking only the supervised doses of rifampicin monotherapy. There is a great danger of emergence of rifampicin resistance in them.
iii. **In MB:** *M. leprae* remain as <u>persisters</u> in certain locations like nerves, smooth muscles, lymph node, iris, bone marrow, liver. Persisters are physiologically dormant bacilli and can thus escape the action of drugs. These persisting organisms remain dormant multiplying at varying intervals after cessation of treatment and can produce disease.
iv. Patients with high bacteriological index (BI) initially have a greater risk of relapse than those who are negative or have low BI.
v. The risk of relapse rises with increase in <u>extent and number of skin</u> lesions and number of nerves involved in PB leprosy.
vi. HIV infection and relapse: Endogenous reactivation of leprosy due to HIV infection has been observed.
vii. Resistance can be a cause of relapse, but this is seen in only 3.6% of all cases.

In PB, relapses may occur in the following settings:

- Majority of PB cases are cured by 6 months but some need longer treatment and premature cessation of treatment can thus cause relapse.
- MB cases wrongly classified as PB.

Clinical Features (Refer to Table 18.16)

PB Leprosy

PB relapses: In PB, 50% of relapses occur within first **2.5 years** and 75% in **5 years**. If it is less than 3 years, a reaction is most likely, while if it is more than 3 years, a relapse becomes more likely.
Clinical: On relapsing, previously subsided skin lesions become active once more. This may occur in the form of increased erythema/infiltration or extension beyond original boundaries or appearance of satellite lesions. In macular lesions which relapse, there is usually an increase in the extent and infiltration of lesions.

Nerves: Relapses involving the nerve trunks may manifest as fresh nerve thickening and/or tenderness with/without increase in the extent of sensory loss and motor deficit. It is not uncommon to find relapses involving only nerves. This is evidently due to the 'high neural bacillation'.

Rx: If it is decided to treat someone as a case of relapse of PB leprosy, they are given a normal course of PB-MDT for the usual duration of 6 months, as they are responsive to MDT.

MB Leprosy

MB relapses: In MB, 50% of all cases of relapse occur within first **3 years** and 75% in **6 years**. An approach to diagnosis of relapse is given in **Flowchart 18.3**.

- The first manifestation of relapse in MB leprosy is the occurrence of bacteriological positivity in patients who had become bacteriologically negative or a BI higher than 2+ over the previous value in BI +ve patients.
- In patients with resolved infiltration, relapse occurs as localized areas of infiltration. The common sites are forehead, the lower part of the back, the dorsum of the hands and feet and the upper part of the buttocks.
- **Histoid leprosy:** A soft pink papule or nodule or several such lesions with or without a background of infiltration may be found at these sites. The papules may enlarge and become plaques of BL leprosy. Sometimes hypodermal nodules are the first manifestations of relapse. They feel like peas in size and consistency. The common sites are posterior aspects of arms and anterolateral aspects of thighs.
- Mucosal lesions: Papular or nodular lesions in the center of hard palate, inner aspects of lips or glans penis.
- Ocular lesions: Iris pearls or rarely leproma (in cases which have had lesions in iris).
- Peripheral nerve lesions: Like PB, here also fresh nerve thickening and tenderness on pressure can occur, with insidious loss of function. (Sometimes, nodular lesions may occur in the course of cutaneous and peripheral nerve trunks as manifestations of relapse.)
- Drug-resistant relapse: Seen primarily in those given monotherapies before.
- Change in spectral localization of leprosy may occur with a relapse, e.g. BT may relapse as BL and vice versa.

Thus, relapsed lesions may lie anywhere in the clinical spectrum of multibacillary leprosy. There has been a tendency to designate such relapses as reversal reaction even when signs of acute inflammation are absent. Likewise, relapses in the nerve are designated much too often as reversal reaction even in the absence of spontaneous pain and exquisite tenderness on touching the nerve. The silent neuritis due to relapse in the nerve in the absence of specific therapy will lead to disabilities.

Treatment

As PB cases usually relapse as PB, and MB cases as MB, in essence the treatment does not change except in case of resistance, which must ideally be tested for in every relapse case.

Flowchart 18.3: An algorithm to distinguish relapse, reactivation, reaction and resistance (RFT, release from treatment)

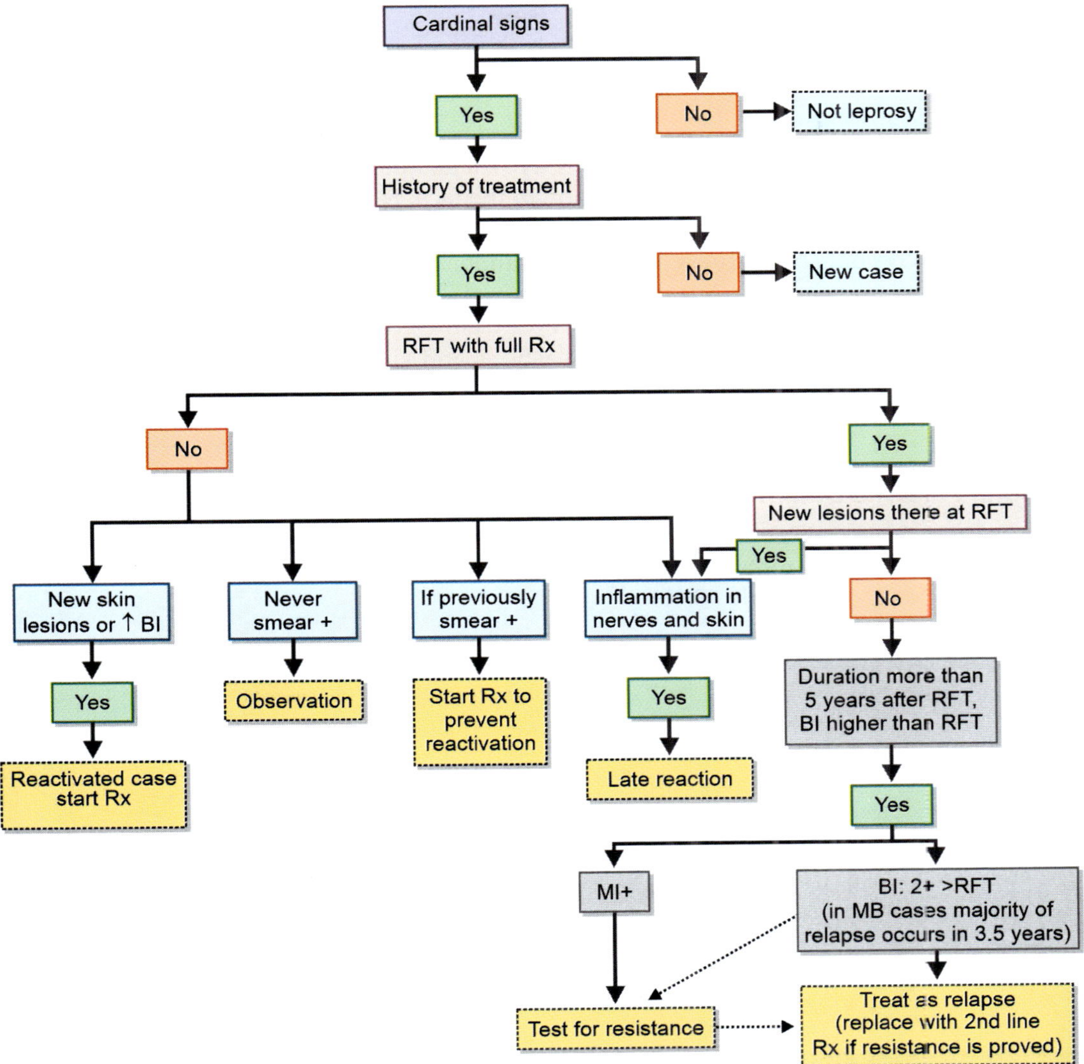

DISABILITY AND NERVE TESTING

- Deformity: A visible alteration in form, shape and appearance of a part of the body.
- Disability: Deterioration in one's ability or capacity. It is felt only by the patient.

Types of Deformities (Table 18.17)

I. *Specific Deformities*

Occur directly as a result of leprosy involving a particular part wherein it is *infiltrated*, *damaged* or *destroyed* by the **granuloma**. Most common in the face. For example:

- Loss of **eyebrows**—atrophy of hair follicles due to leprous granuloma.
- **Ear lobules** become huge due to heavy infiltration, and hang down during regression due to permanent stretching of skin (Buddha ear).
- **Nose deformity**—supporting structures of nose destroyed by granuloma and superinfection.
- Hand involvement following repeated reactions and subsequent dermal and subdermal fibrosis leading to stiffness and non-paralytic clawing of fingers (frozen hand).
- Banana fingers: Due to heavy infiltration followed by atrophy and deposition of fat under the skin.

II. *Motor Paralytic Deformities*

In these cases, leprosy is not a direct cause of deformity but only an indirect cause; the direct cause being unbalanced motor paralysis. For example, claw hand resulting from ulnar nerve damage due to leprosy **(Table 18.18)**.

TABLE 18.17: Overview of deformities in leprosy

	Specific	Motor paralytic	Anesthetic
Face	• Loss of eyebrows • Nasal deformity • Hanging ear lobes • Sagging face	• Lagophthalmos • Facial palsy	—
Hands	• Reaction hand or frozen hand • Twisted finger • Intrinsic plus fingers	• Claw hand • Drop wrist • Paralyzed thumb	• Shortening of digits • Mutilation • Contractures
Feet		• Claw toes • Drop foot	• Neuropathic disorganization of foot • Neuropathic plantar ulceration

TABLE 18.18: WHO grading of impairment (1998)

EHF score—total score of all 6 sites (2H, 2F, 2E)	**Hands and feet**	
	Grade 0	No anesthesia/no visible deformity
	Grade 1	Anesthesia present/no visible deformity
	Grade 2	Visible deformity present
	Eyes	
	Grade 0	No eye problem due to leprosy
	Grade 1	Eye problems due to leprosy present, vision ≥6/60
	Grade 2	Severe visual impairment <6/60, lagophthalmos, iridocyclitis, corneal opacity

BOX 18.6: Site of damage of nerves in leprosy

- Median nerve: Above the wrist joint
- Radial nerve: Above the elbow joint, in the radial groove
- Common peroneal nerve: At the neck of the fibula
- Posterior tibial nerve: Near the medial malleolus of the tibia
- Facial nerve: Above the zygomatic arch

The nerves affected in leprosy are approximately in the following order of frequency: Ulnar, posterior tibial, common peroneal, median, facial and radial **(Box 18.6)**.

III. *Anesthetic Deformities*

Damage to sensory nerves due to leprosy leads to anesthesia and analgesia. This increases chances of injuries leading to formation of ulcers, and negligence allowing them to get infected, further resulting in damage to the part and destruction of tissues. Combined tissue loss and scarring results in deformity.

For example, scar contracture of fingers and mutilation of hands and feet.

An overview of the consequences of nerve involvement is given in **Box 18.7**.

BOX 18.7: Consequence of nerve damage

Sensory fibers	→	Hypoesthesia or anesthesia	→	Ulcers on hand and foot
Motor fibers	→	Muscle weakness or paralysis	→	Claw hand, foot drop, etc.
Autonomic nerve fibers	→	Lack of sweat and sebum	→	Dry skin, cracked skin, ulcers, etc.

Preventable and Treatable Deformities

- Anesthetic deformities: Preventable and untreatable.
- Specific and motor paralytic deformities: Not preventable but treatable.
- Prevention depends on prevention of disease or at least prevention of advancement of disease to involve motor nerves.
- 'Not preventable' and 'untreatable' are not used in absolute meaning but relative sense.

Nerve and Muscle Testing

- **Muscles of the hand and their nerve supply:** It is essential to first understand the muscles and their nerve supply as shown in **Fig. 18.19**.

1. *Testing of Selected Intrinsic Muscles of Hand*

1. **Pen test for abductor pollicis brevis (median nerve)**
   - Lay hand flat on the table with palm upwards
   - Keep the pencil or pen above the palm
   - Ask the patient to first touch it without resistance and then with resistance **(Fig. 18.20)**.
2. **Test for opponens pollicis (median nerve)**
   Ask the patient to touch the proximal phalanx of 2–5 digits with the TIP of the thumb.
3. **Dorsal interossei (ulnar nerve)**
   Ask the patient to spread out (abduct) his fingers against resistance **(Fig. 18.21)**.
4. **Palmar interossei (ulnar nerve)**
   Card test: Place a paper between the fingers and see how firmly it can be held **(Fig. 18.22)**.

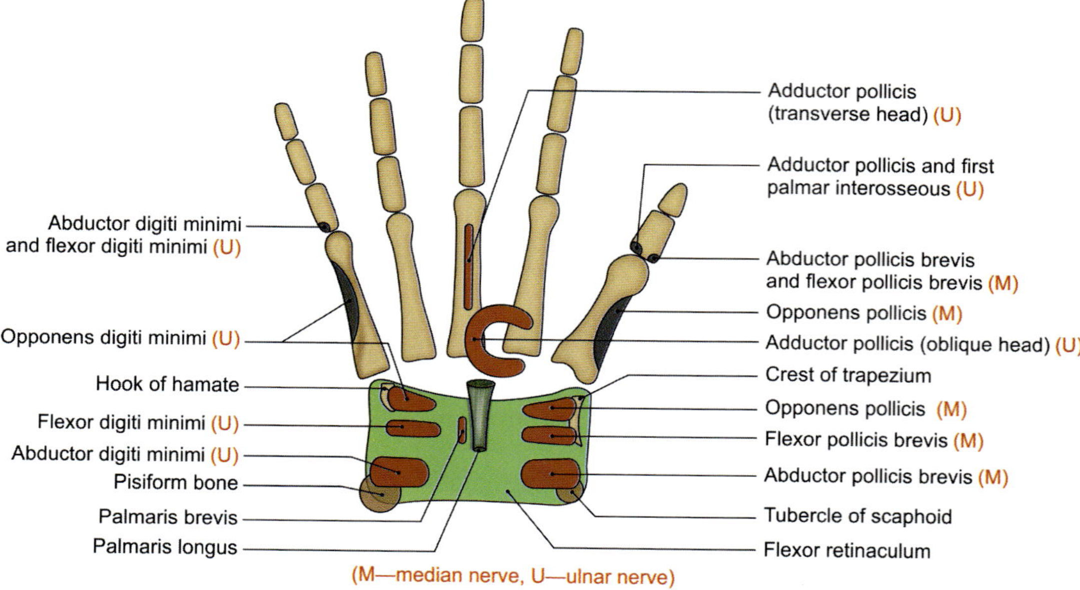

Fig. 18.19: Nerve supply of intrinsic muscles of the hand (*Courtesy*: BD Chaurasia's Human Anatomy, Volume 1, 9th edition)

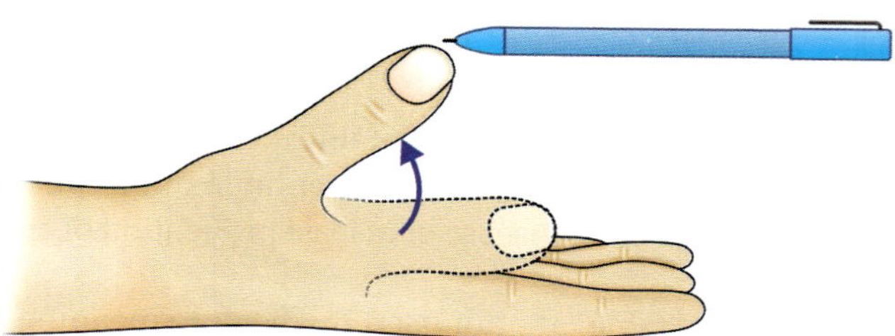

Fig. 18.20: Pen test (*Courtesy*: BD Chaurasia's Human Anatomy, Volume 1, 9th edition)

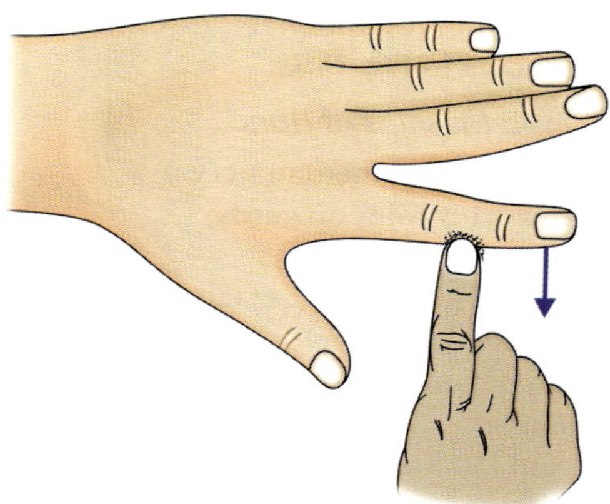

Fig. 18.21: Test for dorsal interossei (*Courtesy*: BD Chaurasia's Human Anatomy, Volume 1, 9th edition)

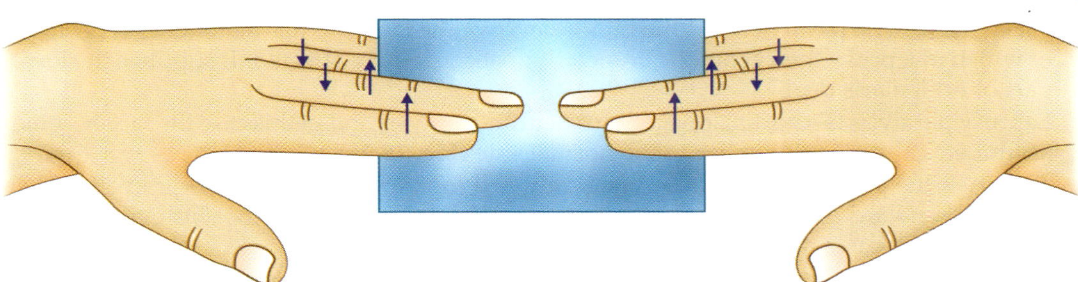

Fig. 18.22: Card test (*Courtesy*: BD Chaurasia's Human Anatomy, Volume 1, 9th edition)

5. **Froment's sign/book test (ulnar)**

   Tests the adductor pollicis **(Fig. 18.23)**
   - Ask the patient to hold a book firmly between the thumb and other fingers of the hand
   - In case of ulnar nerve palsy, the terminal phalanx of thumb will flex at the IP joint due to the action of the flexor pollicis longus supplied by the median nerve.

2. *Tests to Detect Nerve Damage in Other Nerves*

1. Radial nerve: Ask the patient to close his fist and extend the wrist against resistance and test for anesthesia of the dorsum of the hand.
2. Common peroneal nerve: Foot drop—ask the patient to dorsiflex and evert his foot against resistance.
3. Posterior tibial nerve: Ask the patient to plantar flex and invert his foot against resistance.

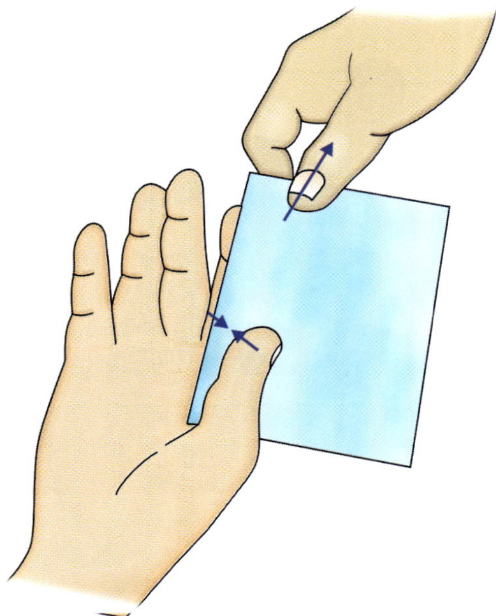

Fig. 18.23: Froment's sign test for adductor pollicis (*Courtesy*: BD Chaurasia's Human Anatomy, Volume 1, 9th edition)

4. Facial nerve: The facial nerve is the motor nerve of the face and has 5 branches **(Fig. 18.24)** of which in leprosy the zygomatic branch is most commonly affected. It supplies the lower part of orbicularis oculi.
   Leprosy paralysis is a partial lower motor neuron paralysis and in this case the face becomes asymmetrical and is drawn up to the normal side **(Fig. 18.25)**.
   Test: Ask the patient to close his eyes gently and look for a lag of the lower eyelid. Then apply downward pressure on the lower lid and ask the patient to close his eyes and then try to open them against resistance.
5. Trigeminal nerve: Test for corneal reflex. Touching the cornea (limbus) with cotton wool closes the eye as a protective mechanism. Tests both V (afferent) and VII (efferent) nerves.

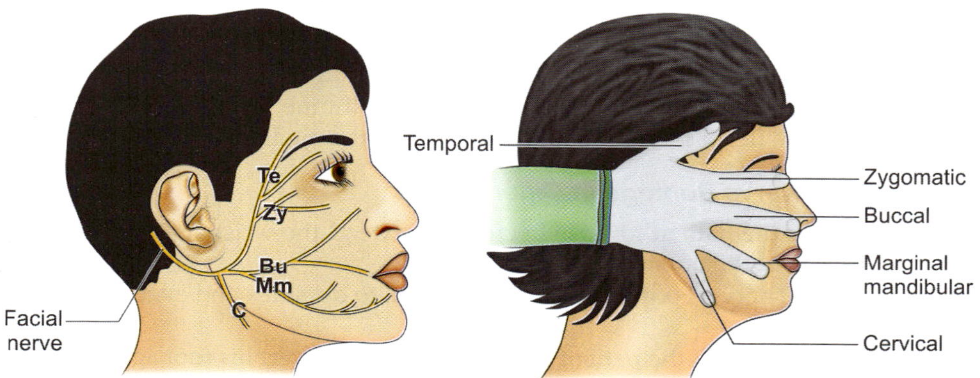

Fig. 18.24: Divisions of the facial nerve (*Courtesy*: BD Chaurasia's Human Anatomy, Volume 1, 9th edition)

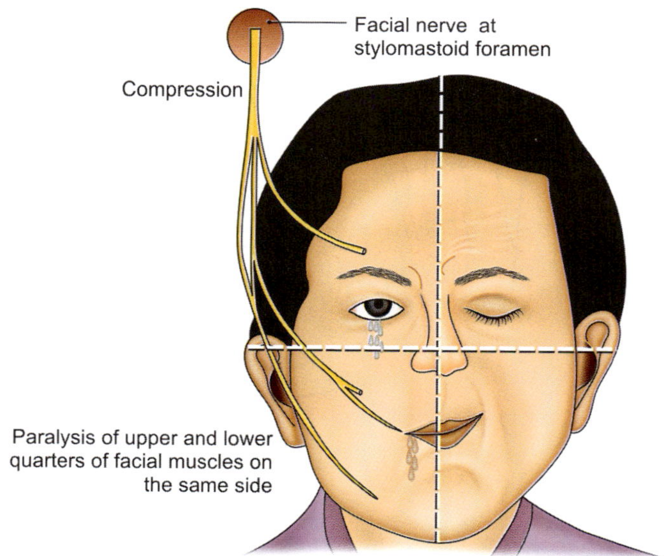

Fig. 18.25: Depiction of complete right facial nerve palsy (note that leprosy has a partial LMN) (*Courtesy*: BD Chaurasia's Human Anatomy, Volume 1, 9th edition)

SENSORY TESTING USING GRADED MONOFILAMENTS

The use of a standardized set of nylon filaments for sensory testing was first reported by Semmes, Weinstein, Ghent and Teuber in 1960. The filaments are made from polyhexamethylene dodecandiamide or nylon 612, which absorbs very little water (<3% in 100% humidity). These can be easily and safely cleaned by alcohol and have an indefinite shelf life and therefore can be stored for long periods without losing stiffness or bend recovery. The advantage of using graded monofilaments mainly lies in greater accuracy and much less inter-observer variability as compared to standard ballpoint pen testing and thus testing with the graded monofilaments is recommended for referral centers **(Table 18.19)** but should ideally be performed in field settings as well.

TABLE 18.19: Recommended nerve function assessment at primary care and referral centers (Ref: WHO)

	Primary care center	Referral center
Nerve	Palpation	• Palpation • Ultrasound
Sensory function	Temperature: Cotton swab with acetone (cold); hot/cold test-tubes Touch: 2 G monofilaments Touch pressure: 10 G monofilaments	Quantitative pain thresholds and temperature (QST) Semmes–Weinstein monofilament kit (0.05 G, 0.2 G, 2.0 G, 4.0 G, 10.0 G and 300 G) Pain scale gradation 0–10
Motor function	VMT: Strong/weak/paralyzed	MRC scale 0–5

Although sophisticated readymade testing sets are available **(Fig. 18.26)**, in field testing simpler and cheaper versions are made using aluminum rods or bicycle wheel spokes **(Fig. 18.27)**, wherein the length of the rod and filament needs to be as per standards described. The reproducibility of Semmes-Weinstein filaments (SWF) testing has been reported to be good when filament length and diameter are standardized. The complete set of SMF consists of 20 filaments which are colour coded as per the target force in grams **(Table 18.20)**. However, in daily practice, a set of 5–6 "pocket" monofilaments is commonly used **(Fig. 18.26)**.

SWFs should be applied perpendicularly to specified sites on the hands and feet to form a C-shaped curve. Most of the studies involving SW filament have assessed the sensory perception pertaining to hands and feet since sensory nerve function impairment affecting these sites amounts to Grade 1 disability; hence testing these sites requires a more sensitive test for early detection. The number of testing sites on hands and feet maybe between 4 and 10. Studies in different Asian countries determined that the 200 mg filament represents the normal threshold for the palm of the hand (median and ulnar nerves) while

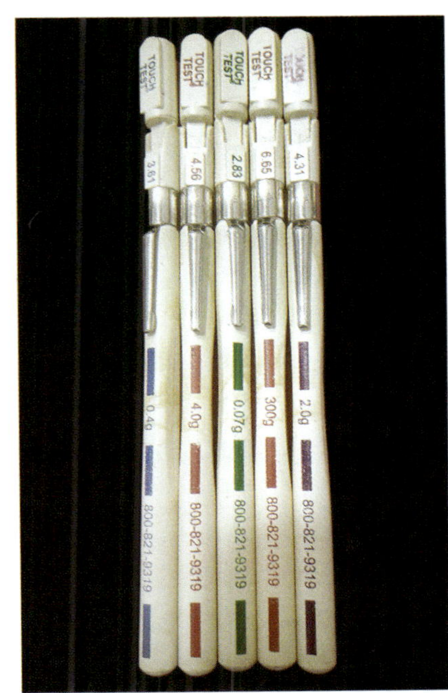

Fig. 18.26: A standard set of 5 pocket nylon monofilaments (*Courtesy*: Prashant Jakhmola)

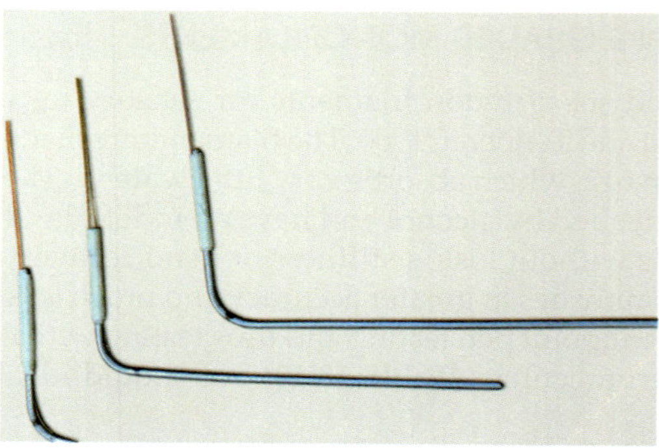

Fig. 18.27: Nylon monofilaments used in field settings, made using bicycle wheel spokes. The length of the rod used, including the bent portion and the length of monofilament used is as per standard recommendations

TABLE 18.20: Target force and color coding of the standard 20 set Semmes–Weinstein monofilments

Product number	Evaluator size	Target force* in grams	Representation	Palmar hand and dorsal foot thresholds	Plantar thresholds
NC12755-01	1.65	0.008	Green	Normal	Normal
NC12755-02	2.36	0.02			
NC12755-03	2.44	0.04			
NC12755-04	2.83	0.07			
NC12755-05	3.22	0.16	Blue	Diminished light touch	
NC12755-06	3.61	0.4			
NC12755-07	3.84	0.6	Purple	Diminished protective sensation	Diminished light touch
NC12755-08	4.08	1			
NC12755-09	4.17	1.4			
NC12755-10	4.31	2			
NC12755-11	4.56	4	Red	Loss of protective sensation	Diminished protective sensation
NC12755-12	4.74	6			
NC12755-13	4.93	8			
NC12755-14	5.07	10			Loss of protective sensation
NC12755-15	5.18	15			
NC12755-16	5.46	26			
NC12755-17	5.88	60			
NC12755-18	6.10	100			
NC12755-19	6.45	180			
NC12755-20	6.65	300		Deep pressure sensation only	Deep pressure sensation only

Invividually calibrated to within a 5% standard deviation.

the 2 g filament was normal for the plantar side of the forefoot (posterior tibial nerve). In those doing heavy laboring work the threshold on soles maybe taken as 10 g instead. Additionally, the 2 g filament should be taken as the normal threshold when testing the radial cutaneous nerve while the 4 g filament is the normal threshold for the sural nerve.

If the set of six is used, the usual practice is to start from the lightest (usually 0.07 gm) and go on to the heaviest (300 g), testing up to three times with each filament, at each site. The lightest filament that is felt is recorded as the sensory threshold for that site. The testing should be done in a quiet room with no disturbances and should be repeated over follow-up visits to detect early nerve function impairment (NFI). If ten sites are tested on each hand and foot, it requires a significant loss of sensation of at least two sites to diagnose NFI. IF only four sites are tested, loss of sensation at any one site confirms a diagnosis of NFI.

QUESTIONS AND ANSWERS IN LEPROSY (WHO)

The set of questions below have been culled from the popular but now difficult to source booklet of WHO. The last updated version was in 1997 and a recent updated one in 2018 is listed below and these serve as a compact summary of leprosy and are often asked in examinations **(Tables 18.21 and 18.22)**.

TABLE 18.21: Common questions on MDT

Is WHO-recommended multidrug therapy (MDT) the best combination available for treatment of multi-bacillary (MB) and paucibacillary (PB) leprosy in leprosy control today?	Yes • It cures leprosy • It is cost effective
What are the basic principles in using multidrug therapy for the treatment of leprosy?	• Rifampicin should be one of the components of MDT • Rifampicin 600 mg should be given at least once a month to all patients • At least two anti-leprosy drugs should be used in the MB regimen and one anti-leprosy drug should be used in the PB regimen, in addition to rifampicin, in order to prevent the occurrence of rifampicin resistant *M. leprae*
What is the evidence that MDT is effective in MB and PB leprosy?	The most important indicator for the effectiveness is the rate of occurrence of relapse following successful completion of MDT • RR for PB—0.1% per year • RR for MB—0.06% per year
Why is rifampicin given only once a month?	• Rifampicin is a potent bactericidal agent • A single dose of 600 mg is capable of killing 99.9% or more of viable organisms • Rate of killing is not proportionately enhanced by subsequent doses • It exerts a delayed antibiotic effect for several days
Why is clofazimine given once a month in addition to the daily dose?	• Clofazimine is a repository drug • Loading dose of 300 mg once a month ensures that the optimal amount of drug is maintained in the body tissue, even if daily dose is missed occasionally

Can MDT prevent the resistance of *M. leprae* to anti-leprosy drugs?	Yes, it can prevent the resistance
	• Maximum bacillary load in PB—6 logs MB—11 logs
	• Out of these, the proportion of naturally-occurring drug-resistant mutants
	  – Rifampicin—1 in 7 logs
	  – Dapsone—1 in 6 logs. Thus:
	  – Clofazimine—1 in 6 logs
	  – Any 2 drugs—1 in 13 logs
	  – Any 3 drugs—1 in 19 logs
	• So, chances of drug-resistant mutants are remote in combination

(Contd.)

TABLE 18.21: Common questions on MDT (*Contd.*)

Can MDT eliminate persisting *M. leprae*?	• No, MDT cannot kill persisting bacilli Persisting *M. leprae* are viable organisms in a dormant metabolic state • They probably have a role in relapse
Is there any evidence that the drugs included in MDT can antagonize each other's antibacterial activity?	No evidence
What is the reason for shortening the duration of MDT for MB patients to 12 months?	• Majority of rifampicin susceptible *M. leprae* are killed by *few monthly doses* of rifampicin • Daily combination of dapsone and clofazimine is highly bactericidal and is capable of eliminating any rifampicin-resistant mutants in an untreated MB leprosy patient *within 3–6 months*
Is there any problem foreseen in treating multibacillary patients with a **high bacteriological index (BI)** with 12-month MDT regimen?	• High BI patients have a higher risk of developing reactions and nerve damage during the 2nd year than those with low BI • *Clearance* of skin lesions is slow • Those who do not note improvement or have deterioration need additional 12 months of MDT
Will shortening the duration of MDT for multibacillary leprosy increase the risk of *M. leprae* developing resistance to rifampicin? How can we **minimize this risk to multibacillary patients** with high bacterial index?	No, there is no risk The combination of drugs cannot lead to resistance if taken properly • The proportion of MB patients with high BI is <15% among newly detected cases • 3–6 months kills all bacilli • Surveillance for 1–2 years for such patients Patient education about signs/symptoms of relapse at the time of stopping MDT • Additional 12 months MDT to any patient who shows signs of deterioration
How should we deal with multibacillary leprosy patients who are currently on treatment and have completed 12 or more monthly doses of MDT? What is the reason for giving MDT to PB patients for 6 months?	• Such patients regarded as cured and removed from registers • Patient education about signs/symptoms of relapse and reactions • Six months of rifampicin should be satisfactory to kill all the organisms • Dapsone has been added to *avoid rifampicin resistance* in patients wrongly classified as PB
Is it necessary to give MDT to PB patients until clinical inactivity is achieved?	No, it is not necessary • *Clinical activity is not directly correlated with bacterial multiplication* • It is not possible to achieve clinical inactivity in 6 months even though all the organisms are killed • Lesions become inactive gradually over a period of 1 to 2 years after the treatment has been discontinued

(*Contd.*)

TABLE 18.21: Common questions on MDT *(Contd.)*

What is meant by fixed duration treatment for MB and PB patients?	• After taking 12 monthly doses of MDT the person is cured and should be removed from the register • For PB patients, after taking 6 monthly doses of MDT the person is cured and should be discharged
Is it necessary to give MDT to MB and PB patients who were on dapsone monotherapy and are now bacteriologically and clinically inactive?	• Such patients can relapse and should be treated with WHO-MDT for 12 months • Should not be re-registered as new cases
Does MDT help to bring about skin smear negativity earlier than with dapsone monotherapy?	• The rate of clearance of dead bacilli is about 0.6 to 1.0 logs per year • Thus, clearance depends largely on the *individual's immune response* • Not enhanced by MDT
Is the threat of rifampicin-resistant leprosy a serious problem?	• No, it is not a serious problem • But selective non-compliance with dapsone and/ or clofazimine may facilitate it
Does MDT expose patients to a higher risk of serious side-effects?	• No serious side effects
Does MDT increase the frequency and severity of lepra reactions?	• Significant reduction in the frequency and severity of ENL (type II) reactions in MB leprosy • Higher reporting of reversal reactions (type I) in MB leprosy in the first year of MDT which then gradually declines
What should be done if a PB patient, 9 months after starting treatment, has not taken 6 monthly doses of MDT or if an MB patient has not completed 12 monthly doses of MDT 18 months after starting treatment?	• Regimen should be continued from where it was left off and the full course completed • Do not restart the regimen from the beginning
What kind of harm can be done if patients are irregular in taking MDT?	• Cure will be delayed or incomplete • Disease activity will progress and the patient may develop serious disabilities and deformities Source of infection to the community • There is a possibility of drug resistance to multiple drugs
What is a **defaulter**? What should be done if a defaulter comes back for treatment?	• Defaulter is a patient who has not collected treatment for *12 consecutive months* • Defaulter with signs/symptoms should be given a new course of MDT These signs are: 1. Reddish raised lesions 2. Appearance of new lesions 3. Appearance of new nerve involvement 4. Lepromatous nodules 5. Signs of reaction

(Contd.)

TABLE 18.21: Common questions on MDT *(Contd.)*

What treatment can be given to patients who do not tolerate MDT due to adverse reactions or contra-indications in MB leprosy?	• In place of **rifampicin**, ofloxacin 400 mg daily and minocycline 100 mg daily, along with daily clofazimine 50 mg for the first 6 months • It is followed by daily administration of clofazimine 50 mg, ofloxacin 400 mg or minocycline 100 mg for the next 18 months • Stop dapsone in case of its toxicity
What treatment can be given to patients who do not tolerate MDT due to adverse reactions or contra-indications in PB and MB leprosy?	• In case of *dapsone toxicity in PB leprosy, it is substituted by clofazimine* in the same dosage as that used for MB patients but for 6 months • In MB leprosy the two drugs rifampicin and clofazimine will suffice
How should patients who **refuse** to take **clofazimine** be managed?	• Patient education about advantages of the drug and reversible nature of the discoloration produced by it • In exceptional cases, **ofloxacin 400 mg or minocycline 100 mg daily** may be used under supervision in place of clofazimine
How serious are the **side-effects** of **clofazimine**, such as discoloration and ichthyosis and how can they be managed?	• No serious problem, except it may be cosmetically unacceptable • Ichthyosis may predispose to certain dermatitis • Can be reduced by moistening the skin, followed by regular application of Vaseline or vegetable oils and avoidance of unnecessary exposure to sunlight
How long does it take to reverse the discoloration caused by clofazimine?	• Discoloration caused by clofazimine is completely reversible – Starts to *appear by third month* of MDT – Reaches *maximum intensity by end of first year* – Starts to diminish noticeably in *6 months* after stopping MDT – Skin returns to its normal color at the end of *1 year* after stopping MDT
Will the widespread use of rifampicin for treating tuberculosis (TB) and sexually transmitted diseases (STDs) have any effect on the use of MDT in leprosy patients?	• If a leprosy patient with TB is treated for TB with a rifampicin-containing ATT, risk of developing rifampicin-resistant leprosy is there • Hence, treat both simultaneously • Use of rifampicin for STD for very short periods may have no significant effect on emergence of rifampicin resistance
Is MDT contraindicated in patients suffering from tuberculosis?	• No such contraindication • ATT given in addition to MDT • If daily rifampicin is part of ATT, no need to administer monthly rifampicin as a part of the MDT
Is MDT contraindicated in patients suffering from human immunodeficiency virus (HIV) infection?	• No such contraindication • Management and response to MDT is similar to that of any non-HIV infected leprosy patient

(Contd.)

TABLE 18.21: Common questions on MDT *(Contd.)*

Is MDT safe during pregnancy and lactation?	• Continue MDT because leprosy is exacerbated during pregnancy • Mild discoloration of infant due to clofazimine reported as small quantity of drugs are excreted through breast milk
Why a small number of patients do not show any clinical or bacteriological improvement with MDT?	• Very poor drug compliance • Concomitant, debilitating, intercurrent infection • HIV
Is it necessary to give MDT cover to patients who have to receive steroids (e.g. for late reversal reaction or other medical conditions) even after successful completion of the scheduled course of MDT?	• Very small risk of possible endogenous reactivation exists after completion of adequate chemotherapy • Start **50 mg clofazimine** daily as a prophylactic measure if duration of steroid therapy is expected to exceed 4 months, and continue until the course of steroids is complete • Do not re-entry of patient into case registry
After patients have stopped treatment, how does one recognize **relapse**? How can relapse be distinguished from the various types of **reactions**?	• Relapse, in MB leprosy, is defined as the multiplication of *M. leprae*, suspected by the marked increase (at least 2+ over the previous value) in the BI at any single site, usually with evidence of clinical deterioration (new skin patches or nodules and/or new nerve damage) • Non-response to therapeutic test with corticosteroids in 4 weeks favors the diagnosis of clinical relapse over reactions
In some control programmes, after completion of MDT, patients continue with a single drug, usually dapsone, for various lengths of time. Is it necessary?	• It is unnecessary and not recommended
Are skin smears a prerequisite for starting a patient on MDT?	• No, skin smears are not a prerequisite for starting a patient on MDT • The clinical system uses numbers of skin lesions and nerves involved as the basis for grouping the patients into MB and PB • Doubtful cases should be treated with MB regimen
How often should skin smears be taken during and after the completion of MDT?	• One examination at the start of treatment to prevent an MB case being treated as PB • With fixed-duration MDT, skin smears not needed either to stop treatment or as a routine follow-up measure after treatment completion • In suspected cases of relapse, skin smears taken from the most active sites • One should limit the number of skin smear sites and frequency of collection to minimum in view of rising HIV and hepatitis B infections
Is post-MDT surveillance of patients essential?	• Active post-MDT surveillance is not necessary Patient education about early signs of possible relapse/ reactions needed

(Contd.)

TABLE 18.21: Common questions on MDT (Contd.)	
Is there any way to accelerate the removal of the dead bacilli seen in skin smears after MDT?	• Immunotherapy using *M. leprae* or other mycobacteria-derived vaccines may be useful in accelerating the clearance of dead bacilli
Does the presence of dead bacilli in the skin and other tissues cause the patient any problems?	• <u>No problem</u> in most of the patients • In a very small proportion of patients, the antigens from dead bacilli can provoke immunological reactions, such as **(late) reversal reaction**, causing serious nerve damage and subsequent disabilities • Can be treated with prednisolone
What is the role of WHO in ensuring that MDT drugs are freely available for all leprosy patients in need?	• WHO supplies MDT to the endemic countries as blister packs for MB-adult, MB-child, PB-adult and PB-child • MDT in blister packs ensures free access, safe storage and prevents possible misuse of rifampicin
What is to be done if leprosy programmes run short of one or more drugs used in MDT?	• Avoid such a situation • Adhere to the principle of using three drugs in MB leprosy and two drugs in PB leprosy under all circumstances
What are the new anti-leprosy drugs available for treatment of leprosy?	• Ofloxacin • Minocycline • Clarithromycin
Why is dapsone continued even in patients known to be or suspected of being infected with dapsone resistant *M. leprae*?	• Known/suspected dapsone resistant case harbors several subcategories of dapsone-resistant organisms • Subcategories of low/moderate levels of resistance to dapsone can be killed by dapsone
Define **newly diagnosed leprosy** case.	A person who has been diagnosed as a leprosy case and who has not taken MDT in the past
Define **leprosy misdiagnosed** case.	A person who has been wrongly diagnosed as suffering from leprosy
Define **recycled leprosy** case.	A person usually with residual signs of leprosy who has completed a full or partial course of MDT but who has now been registered as a newly diagnosed case and has restarted MDT
Why does it not aim for **the eradication** of leprosy than elimination?	• Eradication would mean the complete absence of the disease and the organism that causes it throughout the world • There is a lack of tools to protect people from developing leprosy and to diagnose and treat the disease in its subclinical form • It would be impossible to justify the use of resources when set against the needs of the diseases having high mortality rates like TB and malaria

(Contd.)

TABLE 18.21: Common questions on MDT *(Contd.)*

What is the difference between **leprosy control and leprosy elimination**?	• Leprosy control is a more limited concept than elimination based on detecting and treating leprosy patients without necessarily attempting to achieve complete geographical coverage with MDT • Control services are usually provided by specialized staff rather than by general health workers • In contrast, the concept of leprosy elimination takes advantage of free availability of MDT and the willingness of the general health services to work
What are **good practices** in the context of leprosy management?	• Being friendly, reassuring and encouraging • Being well informed and give correct information about the disease • Answering questions and reliving doubts • Maintaining confidentiality • Keeping up-to-date records • Providing patients with choices about when and where to return for check up • Using accompanied MDT where appropriate • Providing leprosy services free of charge • Avoiding unnecessary investigations

TABLE 18.22: Guidelines for diagnosis, prevention and treatment of leprosy, 2018 (WHO)

Diagnosis of leprosy	Clinical examination, *with or without* slit-skin smears or pathological examination of biopsies
Drug-resistant leprosy	**Rifampicin resistance**—2 drugs (clarithromycin, minocycline or a quinolone (ofloxacin, levofloxacin or moxifloxacin) **+** clofazimine daily for 6 months ***followed by*** clofazimine + one of the second-line drugs daily for an additional 18 months **Rifampicin and ofloxacin resistance**—clarithromycin, minocycline and clofazimine for 6 months **followed by** clarithromycin or minocycline + clofazimine for an additional 18 months
Chemoprophylaxis for contacts of patients with leprosy	Single-dose rifampicin (SDR) *may* be used as leprosy preventive treatment for contacts of leprosy patients (adults and children aged 2 years and above), after excluding leprosy and tuberculosis (TB) disease, and in the absence of other contraindications. Only if one can ensure i. adequate management of contacts, and ii. consent of the index case to disclose his/her disease (conditional recommendation, moderate quality evidence)
Treatment of PB and MB leprosy	Recommend a 3-drug regime of rifampicin, dapsone and clofazimine for both PB (6 months) and MB (12 months). This change in PB has the advantage of using the same blister pack and reduces the impact of misclassification of MB as PB since all will receive 3 drugs

Acknowledgment

We would like to thank **Dr Krishna Garg** for her valuable inputs for the chapter in the 1st edition of the book.

BIBLIOGRAPHY

Books

1. A guide for surveillance of antimicrobial resistance in leprosy 2017 update. © World Health Organization, 2017.
2. Birke JA, Brandsma JW, Schreuders TA, Piefer A. Sensory testing with monofilaments in Hansen's disease and normal control subjects. Int J Lepr Other Mycobact Dis. 2000 Sep;68(3):291–8.
3. Guidelines for the diagnosis, treatment and prevention of leprosy. © World Health Organization, 2018.
4. Handbook of Leprosy, 5E (Pb-2015). WH Jopling AC McDougall CBS, 2015.
5. Hastings, Robert C 1994, Leprosy, 2nd ed, Churchill Livingstone, Edinburgh; New York.
6. Leprosy. In Diagnosis and Management of Skin Disorders an evidence based approach. LWW, 2016.
7. Santhanam A. Silent neuropathy: detection and monitoring using Semmes-Weinstein monofilaments. Indian J Dermatol Venereol Leprol. 2003 Sep-Oct;69(5):350–2.
8. Sardana K, Khurana A. Jopling's Handbook of Leprosy, 6th edition, CBS Publishers 2020, New Delhi.
9. Wagenaar I, Brandsma W, Post E, Richardus JH. Normal threshold values for a monofilament sensory test in sural and radial cutaneous nerves in Indian and Nepali volunteers. Lepr Rev. 2014 Dec;85(4):275–87.
10. WHO Report of informal consultation on treatment of reactions and prevention of disabilities, 11–13 December 2018, Chennai, India (available at https://apps.who.int/iris/handle/10665/325146)
11. World Health Organization. Action Programme for the Elimination of Leprosy, 1997. MDT: questions and answers, Rev. Geneva: World Health Organization.

Journals

1. A Darlong J, Nathan R, Maseey A. Molecular detection of multidrug-resistant.
2. Ali MK, Thorat DM, Subramanian M, Partha-sarathy G, Selvaraj U, Prabhakar V. A study on trend of relapse in leprosy and factors influencing relapse. Indian J Lepr. 2005 Apr-Jun; 77 (2): 105–15.
3. Alter A, A Alcais, L Abel, et al. Leprosy as a genetic model for susceptibility to common infectious diseases. HUM Genet.123: 227–35.
4. Anand V, Kunte R, Jathar S, Patrikar S. Evaluation of National Leprosy Eradication Programme in Pune city of Maharashtra from 2008 to 2019-A Record Based Study. Indian J Lepr. 2020; 92: 211–9.
5. Desikan KV, Sundaresh P, Tulasidas I, Rao PV. An 8-12 year follow-up of highly bacillated Indian leprosy patients treated with WHO multi-drug therapy. Lepr Rev. 2008 Sep; 79 (3): 303–10.
6. Desikan KV. Relapse, reactivation or reinfection. Indian J Lepr 1995; 67: 3–11.
7. Grosset JH. Progress in the chemotherapy of leprosy. Int J Lepr Other Mycobact Dis. 1994 Jun; 62 (2): 268–77. Review.
8. https: //www.who.int/neglected_diseases/news/Leprosy-new-data-show-steady-decline-in-new-cases/en/
9. Ji B, Perani EG, Petinom C, et al. Clinical trial of ofloxacinal one and incombination with dapsoneplus clofazimine for treatment of lepromatous leprosy. Antimicrob Agents Chemother. 38: 662–7 19948031029.
10. Ji B, Jamet P, Perani EG, et al. Powerful bactericidal activities of clarithromycin and minocycline against *Mycobacterium leprae* in lepromatous leprosy. J Infect Dis.168: 188–90 19938257487.
11. Lavania M, LalR, Joseph G, Darlong J, Abraham S, Nanda NK, Jadhav RS. Genotypic analysis of *Mycobacterium leprae* strains from different regions of India on the basis of rpoT. Indian J Lepr. 2009 Jul-Sep; 81 (3): 119–24.
12. Lavania M, Singh I, Turankar RP, Ahuja M, Pathak V, Sengupta U, Das L, Kumar. *Mycobacterium leprae* from Indian leprosy patients. J Glob Antimicrob Resist. 2018 Mar; 12: 214–219.
13. Naafs B. Bangkok Workshopon Leprosy Research. Treatment of reactions and nerve damage. Int J Lepr Other Mycobact Dis 1996; 64 (4, Suppl.): S21–8.
14. NH Van Veen, PG Nicholls, WC Smith, et al. Corticosteroids for treating nerve damage in leprosy. Cochrane Database Syst Rev. 2007 CD005491.
15. Pardillo FE, BurgosJ, Fajardo TT, et al. Powerful bactericidal activity of moxifloxacin in human leprosy. Antimicrob Agents Chemother. 52: 3113–7 200818573938.

16. PardilloFE, BurgosJ, Fajardo TT, et al. Rapid killing of M. leprae by moxifloxacin in two patients with lepromatous leprosy. Lepr Rev. 2009;80:205–209,19743625.
17. Phetsuksiri B, et al. *Mycobacterium leprae* isolates in Thailand and their combination with rpoT and TTC genotyping for analysis of leprosy distribution and transmission. JpnJ Infect Dis. 2012;65(1): 52–6.
18. Pocaterra L, Jain S, Reddy R, et al. Clinical course of erythema nodosum leprosum: an 11-year cohort study in Hyderabad, India. Am J Trop Med Hyg. 2006;74: 868–879.
19. Prabu R, Manickam P, Mahalingam VN, Jayasree P, Selvaraj V, Mehendale SM. Relapse and deformity among 2177 leprosy patients released from treatment with MDT between 2005 and 2010 in South India: Aretrospective cohort study. Lepr Rev. 2015 Dec; 86 (4):345–55.
20. Rambukkana A. Molecular basis for the peripheral nerve predilection of *Mycobacterium leprae*. Curr Opin Microbiol. 200;4:21–7.
21. RP Croft, PG Nicholls, EW Steyerberg, et al. A clinical prediction rule for nerve function impairment in leprosy patients. Lancet. 2000;355:1603–1606.
22. RP Croft, PG Nicholls, JH Richardus, et al. The treatment of acute nerve function impairment in leprosy: results from a prospective cohort study in Bangladesh. Lepr. Rev. 2000;71:154–168.
23. Sanghi S, Grewal RS, Vasudevan B, et al. Immune reconstitution inflammatory syndrome in leprosy. Indian J Lepr. 2011;83:61–70.
24. The Leprosy Unit, WHO. Risk of relapse in leprosy. Indian J Lepr. 1995;67:13–26.
25. van Brakel WH, Khawas IB. Nerve function impairment in leprosy: An epidemiological and clinical study, part 2. Results of steroid treatment. Lepr Rev. 1996;67:104–118.
26. Wagenaar I, et al. B; TENLEP study group, Nicholls P, Richardus JH. Effectiveness of 32 versus 20 weeks of prednisolone in leprosy patients with recent nerve function impairment: A randomized controlled trial. PLoS Negl Trop Dis. 2017 Oct 4;11 (10).
27. Zhang FR, Liu H, A Irwanto, et al. HLA-B*13: 01 and the dapsone hypersensitivity syndrome. N Engl J Med. 2013;369:1620–1628.

Chapter

19

Lichen Planus and Lichenoid Disorders

Surabhi Sinha, Kabir Sardana, Snigdha Saxena

LICHEN PLANUS (LP)

Epidemiology

- Cutaneous LP occurs in 0.2–1% adult population and mucosal LP in 1–4%
- Onset between fifth and sixth decades.
- Classically does not occur in infants and elderly.

Genetic Factors

Genetic susceptibility to idiopathic LP is known. HLA-A3 and HLA-A5, TNF-α gene polymorphism have been reported.

Environmental Factors

- **Postulated associated microorganisms**: Hepatitis C virus, hepatitis B virus, human herpes virus-6, human herpes virus-7, varicella zoster, hepatitis B vaccine (usually after second dose, associated with oral LP, and bullous LP in children). Hepatitis C: Strongly implicated in subset of oral (ulcerative/erosive) LP.
- **Drugs**—antimicrobials, antihypertensives, antimalarials, antidepressants, anticonvulsants, diuretics, metals, NSAIDs, imatinib, IVIg, etanercept and adalimumab.
- **Dental amalgam (mercury)**
  - Associated with oral LP
  - 95%/improve with removal of sensitizing metal
  - Even with <u>negative patch test</u>, 75% clear when metal is removed
- Betel nut
- Radiotherapy
- Anxiety, stress and depression (might be the cause or may result from LP).

Pathophysiology

T cell-mediated autoimmune disease targeting the basal keratinocytes, triggered by a variety of situations, including viruses, drugs and contact allergens.

The various steps of pathogenesis are elucidated in **Box 19.1** and are shown in **Fig. 19.1**. The varied theories encompass <u>three</u> major stages—antigen recognition, lymphocyte activation, and keratinocyte apoptosis and have firm data, but the most relevant to clinicians-resolution, is a new and emerging topic that awaits more data.

BOX 19.1: Overview of pathogenesis of LP

- Earliest change—increased numbers of LC.
- CD8 cells predominate in epidermis and CD4 in dermis.
  1. Initiation phase: Damage to keratinocytes results in stimulation of pDCs and release of IFN-α.
  2. Stimulated mDC present CD4-Th cells with the antigen (unknown as yet).
  3. LCs and other APCs in epithelium present Ag (currently unknown) via MHC-II to CD4 cells, while basal cells present Ag via MHC I to CD8 cells → activate CD8 cells.
- CD4 cells secrete IL-2 and IFN-γ → activate CD8 cells.
- Activated CD8+ T cells induce keratinocyte apoptosis through 1 of 3 mechanisms—[1]secretion of tumor necrosis factor (TNF)-α, secretion of granzyme[2] B, or Fas-Fas ligand interactions[3].
- Activated CD8+ T cells produce chemokines—IL-2, 4, 6, TNF-α, IFN-γ—that attract additional inflammatory cells, thereby promoting continued inflammation.
- Chemokines released by CD8 cells interact with keratinocytes and cause apoptosis.
- Mast cells sustain the inflammation and secrete MMP/Chymase/Tryptase → basement membrane damage.
- **Cytokines:** IFN-γ, IL-6, granulocyte-macrophage colony-stimulating factor (GM-CSF), and tumor necrosis factor alpha (TNF-α).
- **Major kill signals:** TNF-α, granzyme, and perforin. Fas and Fas ligand (Fas-L) are expressed on both keratinocytes and lymphocytes and causes apoptosis as well as disease resolution.

LC, langerhans cells; CTL, cytotoxic T lymphocyte; MDC, myeloid dentritic cells; pDC, plasmacytoid dendritic cells

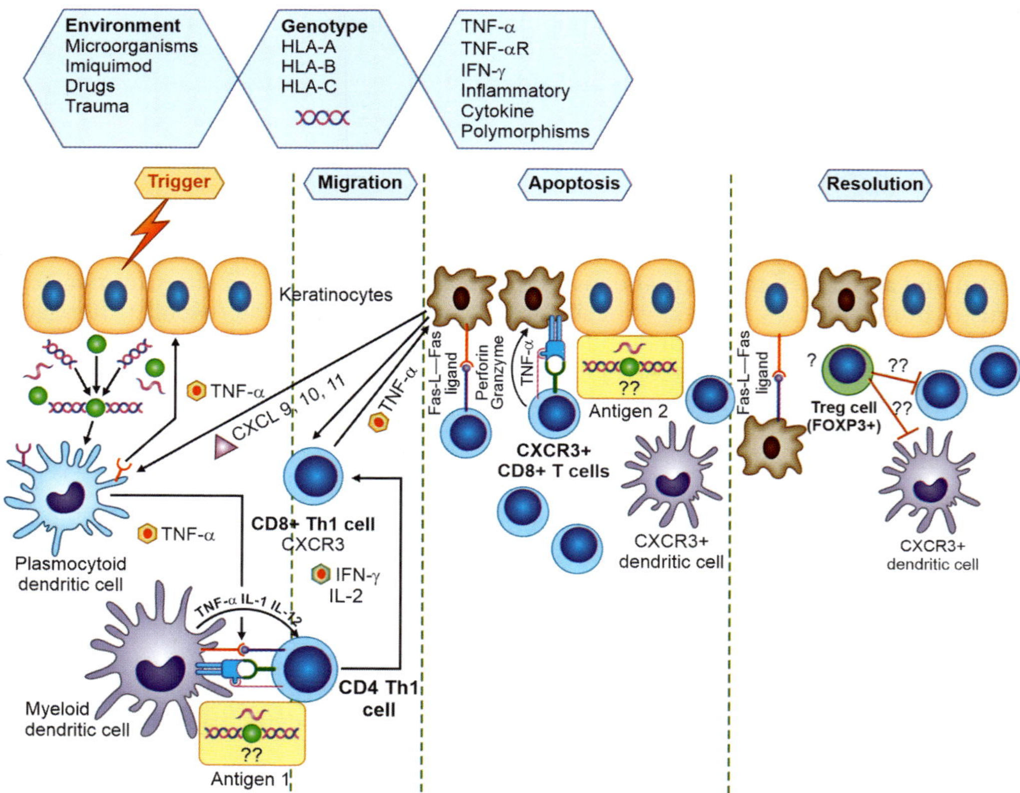

Fig. 19.1: Pathogenesis of LP: Numerous trigger factors have been implicated. The initiation phase leads to stimulation of plasmacytoid dendritic cells (pDC) with release of IFN-α. This leads to stimulation of CD4– T cells which in turn stimulate CD8– T cells which damage keratinocytes and can induce apoptosis

Clinical Features and Types of LP

Classical LP

- Shiny, polygonal, purplish (violaceous), pruritic, plane, 1–3 mm, papules which can be isolated or grouped, in a linear or annular distribution **(Fig. 19.2a)**.
- **Wickham striae** (thin white lines on the surface of the lesions) are seen on close observation **(Fig. 19.2b)**.
- Lesions heal leaving grayish-brown pigmentation due to melanin deposition in the superficial dermis.
- Sites: Mostly on volar aspects of the wrists, lumbar region and around the ankles.
- Hypertrophic lesions usually itch severely.
- Paradoxically patient tends to rub to gain relief (never scratch). Lesions usually not excoriated **(Fig. 19.2c)**.
- Some clinical variants are detailed in the sections that follow while others are listed in **Table 19.1**. LP—lupus erythematosus overlap syndrome and LP pemphigoides are rare variants.

The eruptive type has the *best* prognosis while the palmoplantar and ulcerative variants are the most *recalcitrant* types.

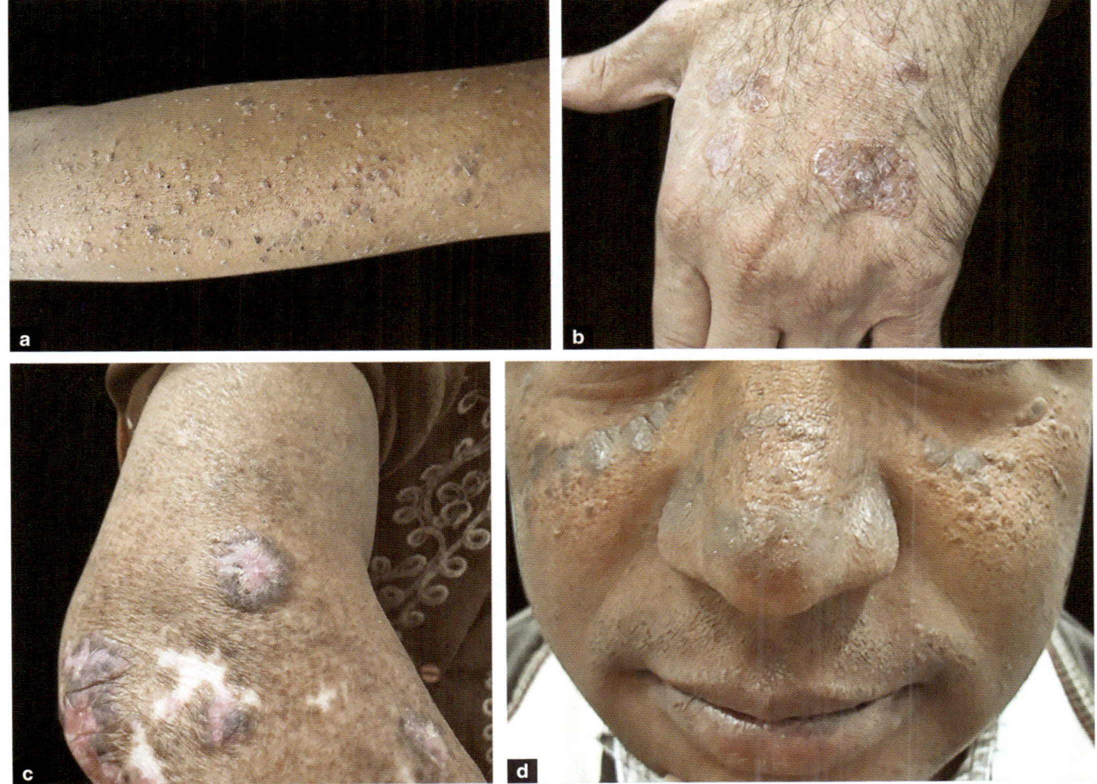

Fig. 19.2: (a) Multiple itchy violaceous papules in lichen planus; (b) Wickham striae seen on lichen planus lesion; (c) Hypertrophic LP; (d) Photosensitive LP (drug-induced)

TABLE 19.1: Clinical variants of LP	
Acute (exanthematous/ eruptive) LP	Rapid onset of disseminated lesions; heals with PIH; rapidly self-resolves (3–9 months)
Atrophic LP	May represent resolving phase of LP with centrally depressed/atrophic, hyperpigmented area
Drug-induced LP (Fig. 19.2d)	• Spares 'classic' LP sites; lesions more generalized and more eczematous or psoriasiform than classic morphology • Wickham striae absent • Frequently photodistributed (especially with thiazides) • Spares mucous membranes, usually scalp also spared • Average latency—12 months; delayed resolution in months • **Histology** like LP but frequently has parakeratosis, deeper infiltrate, eosinophils, apoptotic keratinocytes in higher levels of epidermis
Hypertrophic LP (also known as LP verrucosus)	Extremely pruritic, thick, scaly plaques; most commonly on dorsal feet and shins; symmetric; last longer (avg duration 6 years); may lead to multiple keratoacanthomas or follicular SCCs; biopsy may show many eosinophils
Inverse LP	Axilla > inguinal and inframammary folds > antecubital and popliteal fossae; hyperpigmentation usually present (thus may overlap with LP pigmentosus)
Linear LP	Lesions in a Blaschkoid distribution; favors younger patients (20–30 years), likely due to somatic mosaicism
Nail LP	Seen in 10% of LP patients; usually affects several nails; classic findings: Longitudinal ridging, nail plate thinning, fissuring, and dorsal pterygium; children lack these other nail findings but may present as twenty nail dystrophy (rare in adults)
Palmoplantar LP	Can be ulcerative (especially on soles); occurs in 30–40 years age group; extremely painful and recalcitrant to therapy; usually with typical LP elsewhere

Mucosal LP

Oral LP

- **30–70%** of cases.
- Buccal mucosa and tongue most common sites.
- Characteristic features are white streaks forming a lacework on the buccal mucosa on the inner surface of the cheeks, on the gum margins or on the lips.
- The tongue lesions are often slightly depressed, fixed, white plaques, especially on the upper surface and edges. Uncommonly ulcerative lesions are present which may be the site of malignant transformation.
- Diabetes, candidiasis—may coexist with LP.
- Clinical subtypes—**reticular (most common) (Fig. 19.3)**.
- Atrophic, hypertrophic, bullous, plaque, erosive and ulcerative. More than one type may be present. (Erosive and ulcerative forms have 0.5–1.0% risk of oral SCC, more in smokers and those with HCV infection.)
- **Esophageal LP:** Dysphagia and benign strictures.
- **Genital LP:** Usually characteristic, may be present on the penile shaft, glans penis, prepuce or scrotum. Ulceration—very unlikely. Circumcision may be required.
  - Lesions on the female genitalia are common which they may occur alone/along with lesions in the mouth/or may be part of widespread disease.

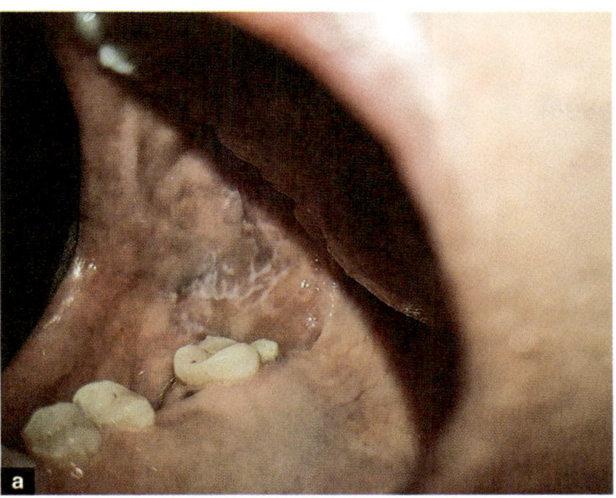

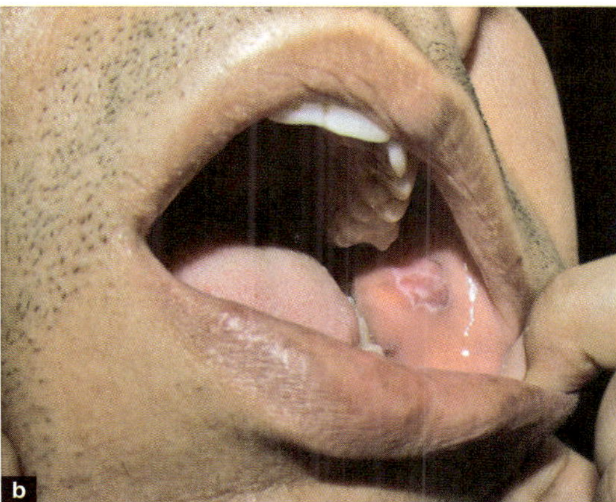

Fig. 19.3: Reticular pattern of oral LP

- Vulvar lesions vary from subtle, fine, reticulate papules to severe erosive disease resulting in dyspareunia, scarring and loss of the normal vulvar architecture.

Diagnostic criteria of vulvar LP

- Well-demarcated erosions/erythematous areas at the vaginal introitus.
- The presence of a hyperkeratotic border of lesions and/or Wickham striae in the surrounding skin.
- Pain/burning, scarring/loss of normal architecture.
- The presence of vaginal inflammation and the involvement of other mucosal surfaces.

Vulvovaginal–gingival syndrome: Association of erosive LP of the vulva and vagina with desquamative gingivitis.

Lichen Planopilaris (*see* also Chapter 11)

Characterized by follicular lesions **(Fig. 19.4)**.

Histopathology of lichen planopilaris

- Arrector pili muscles and sebaceous glands predominantly involved.
- A perivascular and perifollicular lymphocytic infiltrate in the reticular dermis and mucinous perifollicular fibroplasia within the upper dermis with an absence of interfollicular mucin.
- Superficial perifollicular wedge-shaped scarring.

Graham–Little–Piccardi–Lassueur syndrome

Triad of:

- Multifocal scalp cicatricial alopecia
- Non-scarring alopecia of the axillae and/or groin
- Keratotic lichenoid follicular papules.

Lichen Planus: Actinic

- Comprised of red-brown annular plaques or melasma-like patches (less common).
- Characterized by well-defined annular or discoid patches having a deeply hyperpigmented center surrounded by a hypopigmented zone.

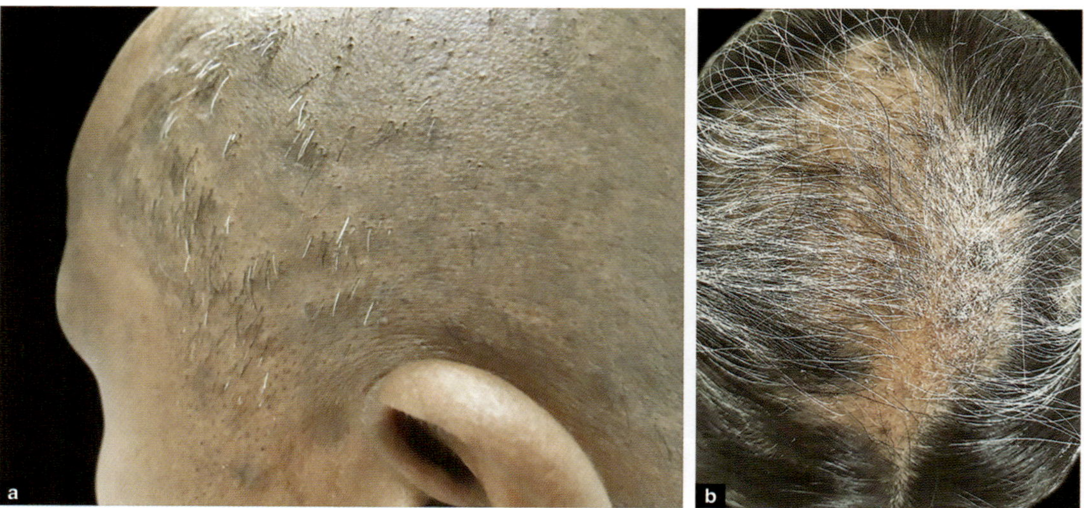

Fig. 19.4: Follicular LP: (a) Follicular lesion with scarring and areas with tufted hair; (b) Follicular papules on the scalp

- Most common in Middle Eastern and Indian patients (also Africans); young adults or children; onset in spring or summer.
- *Site*: On sun-exposed sites (face, forehead > dorsal extremities, neck, intertriginous sites).

Lichen Planus: Annular

Characteristically, a very narrow rim of activity and a depressed slightly atrophic center **(Fig. 19.5)**. Axilla is most common site, followed by penis.

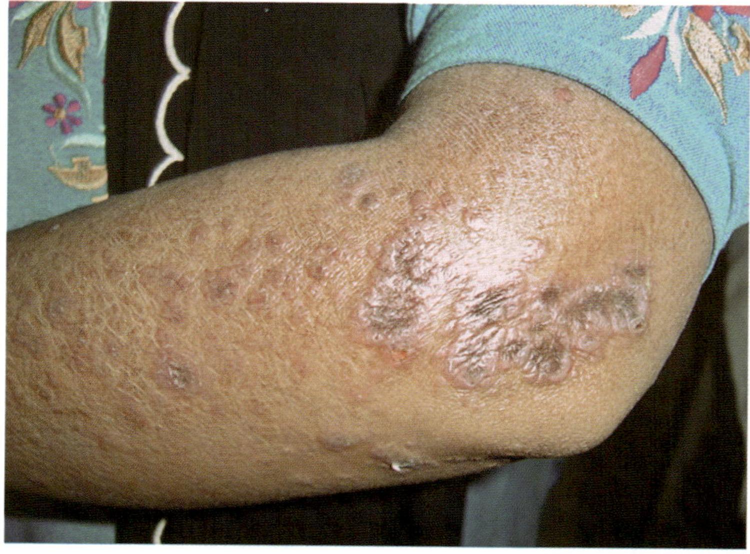

Fig. 19.5: Annular LP

Annular Lichenoid Dermatitis of Youth

Persistent, asymptomatic erythematous macules and round, annular patches with a red-brownish border and central hypopigmentation.

Site: Groin and flanks in children and adolescents.

Histology—lichenoid dermatitis with necrosis/apoptosis of the keratinocytes limited to the tips of rete ridges.

'Mixed' Lichen Planus/Discoid Lupus Erythematosus (Lupus Planus)

- Overlapping features of both disorders.
- Chronic atrophic DLE-like lesions on the head, neck and upper trunk may accompany reticular white lesions in the oral cavity.

Bullous LP and LP Pemphigoides

Bullous LP

- Blisters arise only on or near long standing lesions of LP as a result of severe liquefaction degeneration of the basal cell layer (expanded Max-Joseph spaces).
- Histology—there is sub-epidermal bulla formation with typical changes of LP.
- DIF and IIF—negative.

LP pemphigoides

- Sudden appearance of large bullae on both involved and uninvolved skin.
- Precipitated by psoralen and UVA (PUVA)
- Epidermal damage from liquefaction degeneration in LP exposes basement membrane antigens which results in stimulation of auto-antibody production.
- LP pemphigoides patients—*younger* than classic bullous pemphigoid, and the course of the disease is also less severe.
- Histology—a subepidermal bulla with no evidence of associated LP.
- DIF—linear basement membrane zone deposition of IgG and C3 in perilesional skin.
- Immunoelectron microscopic studies—deposition of IgG and C3 in the *base* of the bulla and not in the roof.
- Immunoblotting—circulating auto-antibodies in LP pemphigoides reacting with an epitope within the C-terminal NC16A domain of bullous pemphigoid *180 kDa* antigen, and also with a *200 kDa* antigen detected in bullous pemphigoid.

Nekam Disease

- Adults—20–40 years.
- Violaceous, papular and nodular lesions typically arranged in a *linear and reticulate* pattern, most marked on the extremities and buttocks often accompanied by a **rosacea-like or *seborrheic dermatitis-like* eruption** on the face in 75% **(Fig. 19.6)**.
- Individual lesions are erythematous verrucous papules covered by a hyperkeratotic plug that can only be removed with difficulty, revealing irregular indentations and prominent capillary loops.
- Symmetrical
- Sites—antecubital fossae, extensor forearms, lumbosacral area and buttocks, posterior thighs, popliteal fossae.

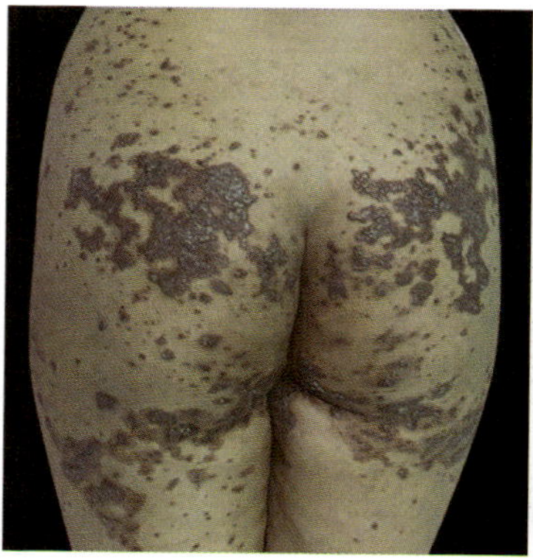
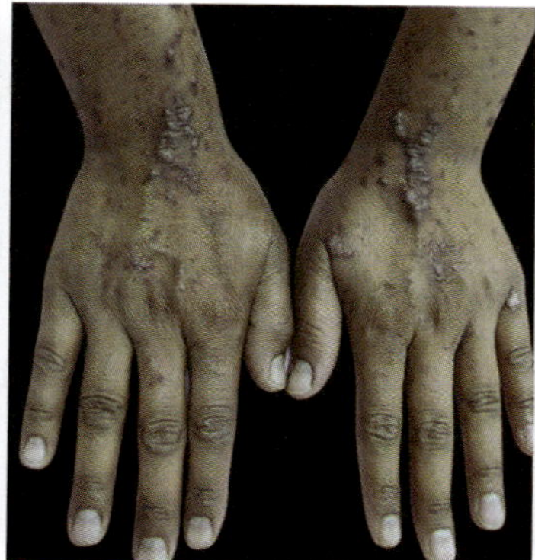
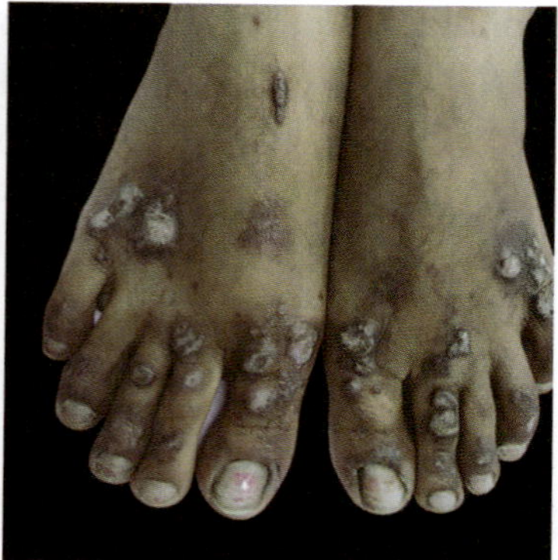

Fig. 19.6: A patient of Nekams diseases with reticulate lesions of LP recalcitrant to conventional agents

- Oral lesions: 50% of patients. Recurrent *aphthous ulcers* are the commonest oral features. Larger chronic ulcers or erythrokeratotic papules can also be found.
- Nails: Thickened, longitudinally ridged and 30% of patients—are prone to paronychia.
- Histopathology: Often nonspecific and consistent with chronic dermatitis, but lichenoid features can be seen.

Differential Diagnosis

Differential diagnosis of cutaneous and oral lichen planus are given in **Tables 19.2** and **19.3**, respectively. Lichenoid drug eruptions may closely mimic lichen planus and may cause diagnostic confusion. **Table 19.4** lists the important differentiating features between lichen planus and lichenoid drug eruptions.

Lupus erythematosus: More likely to have epidermal atrophy, follicular plugging, dermal mucin, and less likely to have hypergranulosis and colloid bodies. The dermal infiltrate is more perivascular and periadnexal than lichenoid (in LP it tends not to go down the adnexa except in LPP). Clinical, direct immunofluorescence, and serologic findings are different.

Complications

Hair

Scarring alopecia. More common in women.

TABLE 19.2: Differential diagnoses of cutaneous LP

Clinical variant of LP	Differential diagnoses
Classical	Verruca plana, guttate psoriasis, secondary syphilis, pityriasis rosea, lichenoid drug eruption, graft-versus-host disease, secondary syphilis, pityriasis rosea
Annular	Tinea corporis, pityriasis rosea, granuloma annulare, EAC
Linear	Blaschkoid dermatoses—lichen striatus, inflammatory linear verrucous epidermal nevus (ILVEN), linear psoriasis, linear Darier disease, Koebnerization of verruca plana, creeping eruption
Hypertrophic	CCLE, LSC, prurigo nodularis, papular amyloidosis, Kaposi sarcoma
Eruptive	Lichen nitidus, guttate psoriasis, lichenoid drug eruptions, papular viral exanthems

TABLE 19.3: Differential diagnoses of oral LP	
Oral candidiasis	• Discrete/confluent patches on buccal mucosa, tongue, palate and gingivae • Friable pseudomembrane resembles cottage cheese • Easily scraped off leaving beneath a brightly erythematous surface
Leukoplakia	• Whitish thickening of epithelium of mucous membranes on lips, gums, buccal mucosa, edges of tongue (common sites) • Lactescent superficial patches of various shapes and sizes coalescing to form diffuse sheets • Surface-glistening, opalescent, reticulated. White pellicle is adherent to underlying mucosa, attempts to remove it forcibly causes bleeding
White sponge nevus	• Thick white velvety lesions in oral mucosa • Buccal mucosa commonly affected • Mutation in keratin 4 and 13

TABLE 19.4: LP versus lichenoid drug eruption

	LP	Lichenoid drug eruption
Clinical features		
• Lesions	Smaller	Larger, scaly, more psoriasiform
• Extent	Less	More extensive
• Skin appendages—hair and nail	More frequent, scarring alopecia, nail shedding	Involvement +/–
• Mucosa involvement	Present	Absent usually
• Wickham striae	Present	Absent usually
• Sites	Flexures	Sun-exposed/generalized, spares 'classic LP' sites
HPE features		
• Parakeratosis	Absent	Present (focal)
• Colloid bodies	Lower down in epidermis	Higher up in stratum granulosum, more frequent
• Eosinophils and plasma cells	Less	Much more
• Infiltrate (perivascular)	Mostly around superficial vessels	Around deeper blood vessels too

Nails *(see also Chapter 22)*

- In up to 10% of cases. Majority during the fifth and sixth decades.
- Fingernails are more frequently affected.
- Exaggeration of the *longitudinal lines* and *linear depressions* due to slight thinning of the nail plate—most common.
- *Dorsal pterygium unguis*: Adhesion between the epidermis of the dorsal nail fold and the nail bed causing partial destruction of the nail.
- Trachyonychia/TND.
- Longitudinal melanonychia: LP of the nail bed.
- Hyperpigmentation, subungual hyperkeratosis or onycholysis or changes mimicking the yellow nail syndrome.

Mucous Membranes

- Squamous cell carcinoma on oral lesions is uncommon, occurs especially with ulcerated lesions. Site: Lips, buccal mucosa and the gum margin.
- Postulated that the high expression of cyclo-oxygenase 2 reported in oral LP may be of etiological significance in the development of squamous cell carcinoma.
- Rarely, squamous cell carcinoma arises on ulcerated cutaneous lesions of LP and anogenital lesions.
- Cicatricial conjunctivitis and lacrimal canalicular obstruction.

Investigations

See **Table 19.5** for the important investigations in LP. A summary of the salient aspects of pathology of LP is given in **Box 19.2**.

Management

Flowcharts 19.1 and 19.2 summarize the management of cutaneous and oral LP. The main drugs used with their level of evidence are listed in **Table 19.6**. As IFN-γ signals are one of the main mediators of LP and these signal via the JAK pathway JAK inhibitors are a useful drug, including upadacitinib, tofacitinib, baricitinib and Ruxolitinib [Motamed-Sanaye A].

TABLE 19.5: Investigations for diagnosis of LP

Dermoscopy	A reticular network of whitish striae with red vessels at the periphery
HPE (Fig. 19.7)	• A focal increase in thickness of the granular layer and infiltrate (corresponds to the presence of Wickham striae) • Colloid bodies—15–20 μm diameter, degenerating basal epidermal cells, appear singly or in clumps • The rete ridges may appear flattened or effaced giving a characteristic **'saw-tooth' appearance** and focal separation from the dermis may lead to **Max Joseph spaces** • A **band-like infiltrate** of lymphocytes and histiocytes, rarely admixed with plasma cells, obliterates the DEJ • **Pigmentary incontinence** with dermal melanophages is characteristic
DIF (Fig. 19.8)	Globular deposits of immunoglobulin M **(IgM)** and occasionally IgG and IgA, representing apoptotic keratinocytes, around the DEJ and lower epidermis, with **'shaggy' fibrinogen deposition** at the region of the DEJ (order of frequency from highest to lowest—fibrin, C3, IgG, IgM, and IgA within the dermoepidermal junction, as well as IgM, IgG, IgA, and C3 in cytoid bodies, have been described)

BOX 19.2: Important factoids about HPE of LP

1. **Lacks eosinophils**
   Exceptions: Drug-induced LP, hypertrophic LP
2. **Lacks parakeratosis**
   Exceptions: Drug-induced LP, oral LP
3. Dyskeratotic keratinocytes are **NOT** present in higher levels of epidermis (spinous and granular layers) → differentiates from EM, FDE, and SJS/TEN (all have suprabasilar keratinocyte apoptosis)
   Exceptions: Drug-induced LP

Flowchart 19.1: Treatment ladder for cutaneous LP (JEADV, 2020)

1st line
- **Limited**
  Clobetasol propionate ointment (0.05%) or I/L triamcinolone
- **Widespread**
  Prednisolone (0.5–1 mg/kg/day)

↓

2nd line*
- Topical calcineurin inhibitors
- Prednisolone (0.5–1 mg/kg/day) until improvement
- Acitretin (25 mg/day) for 8 weeks
- PUVA or UVB therapy (2–3 times/week) for 1–2 months, alone or in combination with systemic retinoids
- Excimer light

**Note:* Other systemic drugs: Griseofulvin, metronidazole, SSZ, MTX, cyclosporine, apremilast, thalidomide

Flowchart 19.2: Management of oral LP (JEADV, 2020)

1st line

Symptomatic oral LP
- Clobetasol propionate ointment (0.05% TDS) until remission, then maintenance
- Soluble prednisolone tablets (5 mg in 15 mL water for mouthwash TDS) or betamethasone soluble tablets (0.5 mg)

Severe erosive LP: Prednisolone (0.5–1 mg/kg/day) until improvement or I/L triamcinolone in erosive lesions

↓

2nd line

Papules and plaques in absence of erosive lesions:
Topical retinoids/topical calcineurin inhibitors

Resistant to topical corticosteroids:
Prednisolone (0.5–1 mg/kg/day) until improvement

↓

3rd line

Cortico-dependent/cortico-resistant erosive oral LP:
Azathioprine, mycophenolate mofetil, methotrexate, cyclosporine, topical cyclosporine

Note: USFDA states that topical pimecrolimus and tacrolimus should be used with caution in oral LP due to risk of malignant transformation

Management of Other Variants of LP

Anogenital LP

- Early superpotent corticosteroid (0.05% clobetasol propionate ointment) once daily/potent corticosteroid—to resolve symptoms and prevent synechiae and scarring.
- Hydrocortisone suppositories, foam or cream alternate day for vaginal LP.
- Foreskin retraction or removal surgery in uncircumcised men and vaginal dilators in women-prevent synechiae formation.
- Surgery—if adhesion occurs after complete resolution.

TABLE 19.6: Salient drugs used in LP

Agents	Comments
Topical steroids	• First-choice therapy • Different types of vehicles can obtain better outcomes with less amount of active drug
Tretinoin	• Useful for lichen planus pigmentosus
Topical calcineurin inhibitors	• Along with topical steroids, they are effective particularly in oral LP • Evidence is weak for cutaneous LP • Relapses are likely after cessation of treatment so that a long-term application is required to maintain the initial improvement
Oral retinoids	• **Acitretin**—useful for hypertrophic, palmoplantar and nail LP • **Alitretinoin**—female patients need optimal contraception
Oral steroids	• Reserved for severe and widespread lesions or unresponsive to topical steroids • The use of mini-pulse reduces the likelihood of side effects
Methotrexate	• Not indicated in patients with elevated serum IL-6 • May be combined with topical steroids and tacrolimus with lower weekly dose and enhanced effectiveness • Useful for actinic and annular atrophic LP not responding to or in combination with other therapies • Slow response
Dapsone	• Useful for bullous, erosive and generalized LP not responding to other therapies
Azathioprine	• Useful for severe, erosive and generalized LP not responding to other therapies

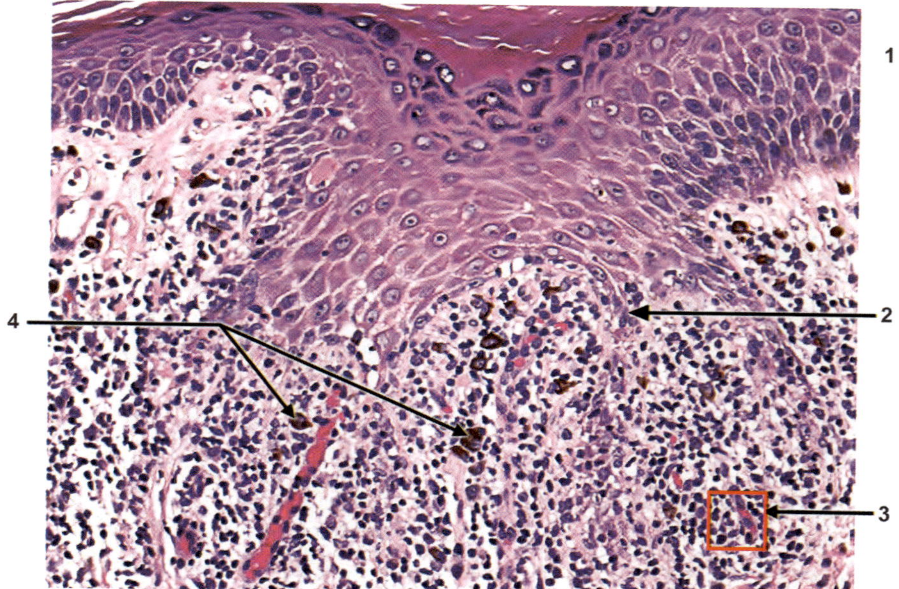

Fig. 19.7: Pathology of lichen planus. (1) Hyperkeratosis, hypergranulosis, irregular acanthosis; (2) Saw toothing of rete ridges with a lichenoid infiltrate; (3) Civatte bodies; (4) Pigment incontinence due to basal cell degeneration

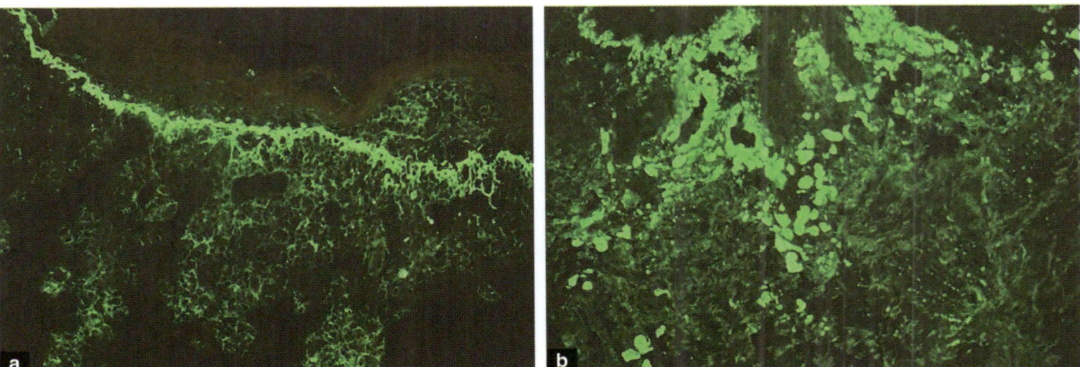

Fig. 19.8: DIF of LP showing (a) shaggy basement membrane zone which signifies fibrinogen; (b) scattered and clumped cytoid bodies with immunoglobulin M (IgM)

Lichen Planopilaris

- Potent corticosteroids (e.g. 0.05% clobetasol propionate ointment) twice daily.
- Monthly intralesional injection of triamcinolone acetonide (0.5–10 mg/mL) or systemic oral corticosteroids (prednisolone 1 mg/kg/day).
- HCQ 200 mg/day.

Nail Lichen Planus

- Less than four nails—twice daily application of superpotent corticosteroids (e.g. 0.05% clobetasol propionate ointment, or monthly intralesional injection of triamcinolone acetonide (0.5–10 mg/mL) in the periungual sites.
- More than four nails—systemic corticosteroids: Oral prednisolone (0.5–1 mg/kg/day) for 4–6 weeks. Etanercept reported in a case report.

Severe Erosive LP

- Systemic corticosteroids
- Systemic immunosuppressive agents (e.g. azathioprine, mycophenolate mofetil and methotrexate) and griseofulvin
- Extracorporeal photochemotherapy.

LP/DLE Overlap Syndrome

Cyclosporine, acitretin.

Actinic LP

Acitretin + topical corticosteroids + cyclosporine.

Bullous LP and Lichen Planus Pemphigoides

Systemic steroids, azathioprine, corticosteroids + acitretin.

Prognosis of LP

- The spontaneous remission rate is 65% one year after onset of the disease in the cutaneous variants.
- Nail and scalp forms usually lead to scarring.
- Oral form can become chronic (oral lichen planus is self-limiting in only 3% of cases).

LICHEN PLANUS PIGMENTOSUS (LPP) (*see also Chapter 28*)

LPP may overlap with Ashy dermatosis (AD), erythema dyschromicum perstans (EDP), Riehl melanosis (RM), idiopathic eruptive macular pigmentation (IEMP), and these entities have overlapping clinical and histopathological features. An overview is given in **Table 19.7** and differences with similar entities are given in **Table 19.8**.

LICHEN NITIDUS (LN)

- Discrete or closely grouped pinpoint to pinhead-sized papules, usually asymptomatic and flesh-colored or reddish-brown, with a flat or dome-shaped shiny surface **(Fig. 19.9)**.
- Children and young adults.
- Sites: Forearms, penis, abdomen, chest and buttocks.
- Nails: Affected nails may appear rough due to increased linear striations and longitudinal ridging, sometimes nail pitting.
- Mucous membrane lesions much rarer than in LP.

TABLE 19.7: A summary of clinical and histopathological features of lichen planus pigmentosus

Skin type	• Darker skin phototypes III to VI, with phototype IV being the commonest
Cause	• Similar immunopathogenesis to LP
Postulated triggers	• Mustard oil containing a photosensitizer (allyl-thiocyanate), amla oil, henna, hair dye, cold cream, and environmental causes, including sunlight
CF	• **Site:** Face and neck (most common). Face—temporal and preauricular areas, whereas on the neck it affects all areas. Arms > legs and trunk. Flexural areas are affected in 20% of cases, mainly the axillae, followed by the inframammary folds and the inguinal creases. Rarely affects the oral mucosa and scalp • **Morphology:** Symmetrical distribution of dark brown to gray or gray-blue, round or oval macules with irregular and poorly-defined borders, which eventually enlarge and coalesce. Rarely, incipient LPP manifests as entirely erythematous macules which represent an active phase that rapidly resolves • **Morphological variants:** Diffuse (most common), reticular, blotchy, perifollicular, and annular • **Symptoms:** The lesions are usually asymptomatic • **Note:** If the hyperpigmentation is limited to known areas of previous lichen planus lesions, or current visible and palpable lesions of lichen planus, such cases should be labelled as lichen planus with post-inflammatory hyperpigmentation and not LPP
HP	• Vacuolar degeneration of the epidermal basal cell layer, band-like lichenoid or perivascular lymphocytic infiltrates in the papillary dermis, as well as superficial pigmentary incontinence and melanophages are seen in LPP • Histology may be similar to EDP/AD with presence of dermal melanophages with or without interface dermatitis at some stage
Treatment	1. Avoid triggers: LPP: Avoid mustard oil, amla oil, henna, hair dyes, cold cream, products with nickel or nickel-containing food, cosmetics suspected as contactants, and sun exposure LPP-inversus: Avoid friction and tight clothing 2. Topical treatment: Medium to high potency CS, tacrolimus, and skin lightening creams containing hydroquinone and retinoids 3. Systemic: Corticosteroids in pulse doses or continuous administration with gradual tapering, dapsone, isotretinoin

TABLE 19.8: Common differentials of LPP	
Idiopathic eruptive macular pigmentation	• Occurs in **younger patients,** usually ages 10–30 • Brown to brown-gray macules, start in the middle area of the **trunk** and then spread to proximal areas of the limbs, spontaneous resolution common • Histopathology reveals pigmentation of the basal layer, few melanophages, and mild perivascular inflammatory infiltrate
Ashy dermatosis/erythema dyschromicum perstans	• Trunk and limbs. Macules are slate gray and may present with an *erythematous firm*, evanescent, *string-like halo* • AD and EDP can be considered to be synonymous except for the presence of raised erythematous border in the active stage of EDP • Interface dermatitis may be present but is not a feature necessary to diagnose these conditions
Riehl melanosis/pigmented contact dermatitis	• Face (forehead temples, neck), adults, common with facial cosmetics • Reticulate, acquired macules of pigmentation of uncertain etiology
Ochronosis	• History of hydroquinone use at high concentration for a prolonged period, most commonly on the face. Usually does not affect neck and flexural areas

- Associated with Crohn's disease, trisomy 21, congenital megacolon and Niemann–Pick disease type B.
- **Variants:** Morphology—actinic, perforating, spinous follicular, purpuric, vesicular, lichen nitidus and site—palmoplantar, linear, generalized.

HPE

- Well circumscribed intense infiltrate immediately below epidermis **(Fig. 19.10)**.
- Lymphohistiocytic, occasional Langhans giant cells.
- Overlying epidermis flattened and liquefactive degeneration of stratum basale.
- Rete ridges at the margin elongated and encircle the infiltrate—**'Ball in clutch' appearance.**

Differential Diagnosis (Table 19.9)

TABLE 19.9: Differential diagnosis of lichen nitidus

Lichen nitidus	Lichen scrofulosorum	Keratosis pilaris
Discrete or closely grouped pinpoint to pinhead-sized asymptomatic papules which are flesh-colored or reddish-brown, with a flat or dome-shaped shiny surface	Follicular papules grouped in small patches on the trunk, evidence of TB elsewhere	Horny follicular papules mainly on the extensor surface of the limbs

Treatment

- Self-limiting, fluorinated topical corticosteroid preparations—if treatment demanded by patient.
- Sun exposure, PUVA, narrow-band UVB phototherapy and astemizole, acitretin (palmoplantar), intramatricial steroid (nail).

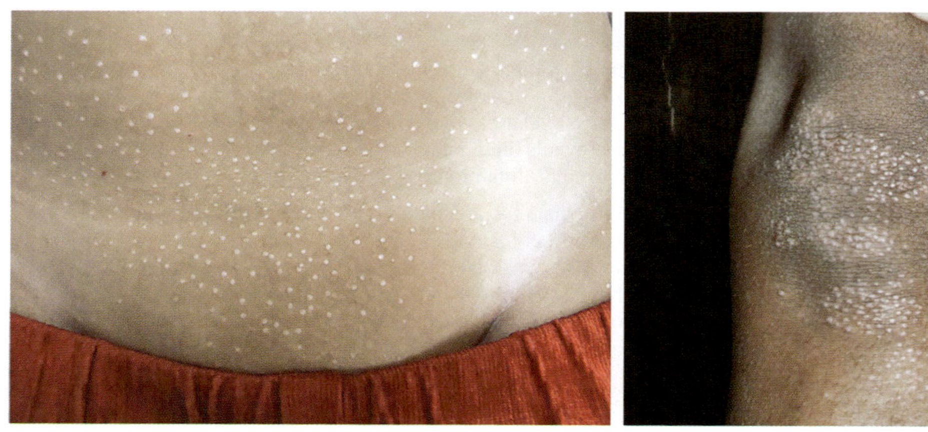

Fig. 19.9: Lichen nitidus showing grouped shiny flat topped papules

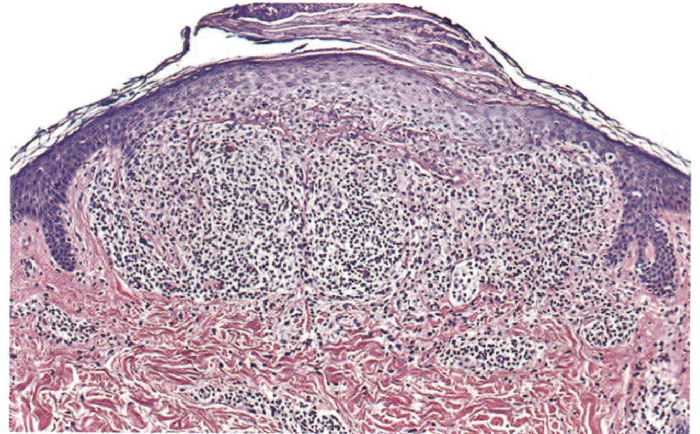

Fig. 19.10: Lichen nitidus: The lichenoid infiltrate constitutes the 'ball' that is engulfed by the epidermis (the 'claw') and this infiltrate is composed of lymphocytes and histiocytes and occasional giant cells

LICHEN STRIATUS

Epidemiology

- Age: 5–15 years
- Sex: Females > males
- History of atopy in **40%**

Clinical Features

- Sudden appearance of small discrete pink lichenoid flat-topped papules in linear distribution.
- Coalesce over 1–2 weeks—dull red to brown slightly scaly linear band.
- Unilateral over a limb.
- Papules may be hypopigmented in dark skins/post-inflammatory hypopigmentation may persist in dark skins.

- Nails—longitudinal ridging, splitting, onycholysis, nail shedding.
- Spontaneous resolution over 6–12 months, may be longer.

Differential Diagnosis

- Blaschkoid / linear lesions
  - ILVEN—always pruritic, persistent, no spontaneous resolution
  - Linear psoriasis
  - Liner LP
  - Linear porokeratosis
  - Linear Darier disease
  - Linear hypomelanosis (if hypopigmentation)

Treatment

See **Flowchart 19.3** for a treatment ladder for LS.

Flowchart 19.3: Treatment ladder of lichen striatus

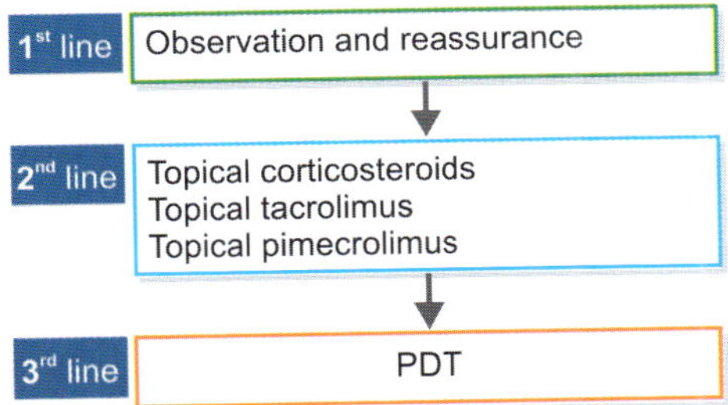

Acknowledgments

The authors thank **Dr Manu Sehrawat**, MD, for her work on this chapter in the previous edition of this book.

BIBLIOGRAPHY

Book

1. McKee's Pathology of skin (https://expert consult.inkling.com/read/mckees-pathology-of-the-skin-calonje-brenn-lazar-mckee-4th/Chapter-7).

Journals

1. Ioannides D, et al. European S1 guidelines on the management of LP: A cooperation of the EDF with the EADV. JEADV 2020;34:1403–14.
2. Kumarasinghe SPW. A global consensus statement on ashy dermatosis, erythema dyschromicum perstans, lichen planus pigmentosus, idiopathic eruptive macular pigmentation, and Riehl's melanosis. Int J Dermatol. 2018 Sep 3. doi:10.1111/ijd.14189.
3. Motamed-Sanaye A, Khazaee YF, Shokrgozar M, Alishahi M, Ahramiyanpour N, Amani M. JAK inhibitors in lichen planus: a review of pathogenesis and treatments. J Dermatolog Treat. 2022 Dec;33(8):3098–3103.
4. Robles-Méndez JC. Lichen planus pigmentosus and its variants: review and update. Int J Dermatol. 2018 May; 57(5):505–14.
5. Żychowska M, Woźniak Z, Baran W. Immunohistochemical analysis of the expression of selected cell lineage markers (CD4, CD8, CD68, c-Kit, Foxp3, CD56, CD20) in cutaneous variant of lichen planus. Int J Dermatol. 2021 Feb 20. doi: 10.1111/ijd.15437.

Chapter

20

Mastocytosis

Kabir Sardana, Surabhi Sinha, Bhavya Sangal

INTRODUCTION

- Mastocytosis is a group of rare conditions characterized by an abnormal accumulation of mast cells in one or more organs.
- It usually presents in the skin, but may affect other tissues, especially the bone marrow and gastrointestinal tract.
- Its clinical spectrum ranges from a solitary, self-healing, cutaneous nodule to a leukemic form that may have no associated skin lesions.
- The classification is given in **Table 20.1**.

EPIDEMIOLOGY

- Most cases are in children, with 60–80% presenting within the first year of life.
- Mastocytosis limited to the skin is primarily a disease of children, whereas systemic mastocytosis is more common in adults.
- This disorder has no gender preference, and it has been reported in all races.

PREDISPOSING FACTORS

- Temperature extremes, towelling, massage or alcohol are various physical stimuli that can exacerbate these symptoms.
- Potential triggers of mast cell degranulation include known allergens, non-steroidal anti-inflammatory drugs, insect and snake venoms, radiocontrast media, plasma expanders, opiates, and some muscle relaxants.

PATHOGENESIS

The symptoms of mastocytosis are primarily due to mast cell mediator release.

- **c-KIT mutations:** There is increasing evidence that mast cells accumulate in tissues as a direct consequence of acquiring a gain of function mutation of *KIT*, which encodes transmembrane receptor for stem cell factor (KIT). The KIT receptor is expressed on mast cells, melanocytes, primitive hematopoietic stem cells, primordial germ cells, and interstitial cells of Cajal.

TABLE 20.1: Updated World Health Organization classification of mastocytosis and basic demographics[a]			
Variant and subvariant	**Mostly found in (children/adults)**	**Estimated prevalence in mastocytosis[a]**	**Estimated median survival (years)**
Cutaneous mastocytosis (CM)			
Maculopapular CM (MPCM), also known as urticaria pigmentosa (UP)	Children	30–60%	>50[b]
Diffuse CM (DCM)	Children	10%	>50[b]
Mastocytoma of skin	Children	<5%	>50[b]
Systemic mastocytosis (SM)			
Nonadvanced forms SM			
Bone marrow mastocytosis (BMM)	Adults	<10%	>20[b]
Indolent SM (ISM)	Adults	30–50%	>20[b]
Smoldering SM (SSM)	Adults	5%	>10
Advanced forms of SM			
SM with an associated hematologic neoplasm (AHN)	Adults	5%	1–5
Aggressive SM (ASM)	Adults	<5%	2–5
Mast cell leukemia (MCL)	Adults	<1%	<2[c]
Localized aggressive mast cell tumor			
Mast cell sarcoma (MCS)	Adults	<0.1%	<2

[a]Mastocytosis is a rare disease with an estimated incidence of approximately 1/100,000 per year in industrialized countries.
[b]In these groups of patients, the life expectancy is normal or near normal.
[c]In chronic MCL, defined by the absence of SM-induced organ damage, the survival time is more than 2 years unless the patient progresses to acute MCL within a short time.

- c-KIT encodes KIT (CD117) on mast cells; stem cell factor is the ligand for KIT and essential for survival of mast cells.
- **Somatic** activating mutations in ***KIT* involving codon 816** represent the most common genetic abnormality in patients with sporadic mastocytosis. The result is a substitution of the amino acid aspartic acid (D) with valine (V), (i.e. D816V) or another amino acid. This leads to constitutive activation of KIT, resulting in continued mast cell growth and development.
- These mutations lead to accumulation of abnormal mast cells which are round to fusiform in shape, have long polar cytoplasmic processes with hypogranular cytoplasm, atypical nuclei and monocytoid appearance.

CLINICAL FEATURES OF CUTANEOUS MASTOCYTOSIS

Usually seen in children **(Fig. 20.1)**. Rare in adults.

Cutaneous mastocytosis is most common in children in the form of urticaria pigmentosa. Systemic mastocytosis occurs most commonly in adults, and ISM is the most common form.

Systemic symptoms such as pruritus, flushing, abdominal pain, diarrhea, palpitations, dizziness and syncope may be present. They occur due to release of mast cell mediators, such

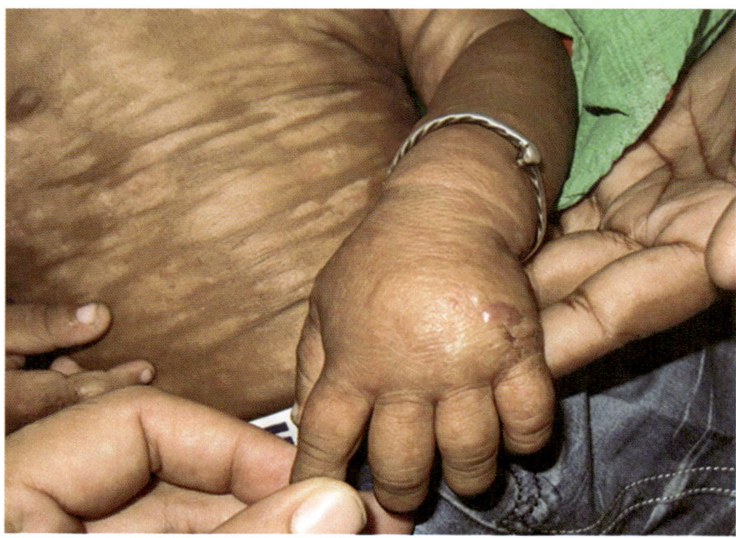

Fig. 20.1a: Multiple urticated papules and plaque with an occasional bulla in urticaria pigmentosa

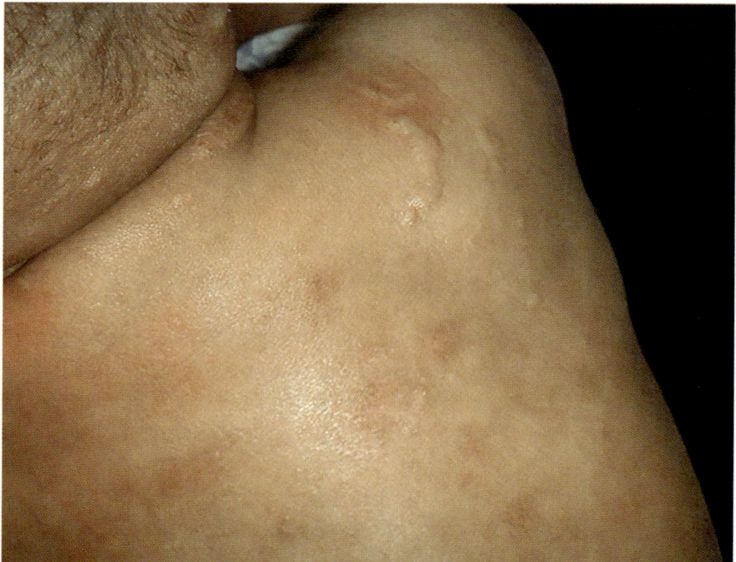

Fig. 20.1b: An urticated lesion overlying a plaque seen after rubbing the lesion—the Darier's sign

as histamine, eicosanoids and cytokines. An overview of the types is given in **Table 20.2** and the differences between adult and childhood disease in **Table 20.3**.

DIAGNOSIS

An approach to a patient of mastocytosis is given in **Flowchart 20.1** while **Table 20.4** lists the various investigations in a suspected case of cutaneous mastocytosis.

TABLE 20.2: Types of mastocytosis	
Urticaria pigmentosa	• **Most common pattern** of cutaneous mastocytosis in children and adults • It is characterized by numerous reddish brown or pale monomorphic maculopapules, plaques or nodules that appear in a symmetrical distribution anywhere on the body except the palms and soles **(Fig. 20.1a)** • These lesions may be present at birth or arise during infancy • In adults, lesions are relatively smaller in size (approx. 5 mm) and more numerous on trunk or proximal extremities • Blistering (bullous mastocytosis) in about one-fourth patients • Darier's sign is positive • No systemic involvement can be detected in most patients of UP, but systemic manifestations can still occur. If they do—diarrhea, abdominal pain, and wheezing/dyspnea are most common symptoms; anaphylaxis is rare, but possible. • Symptoms improve by early adolescence, but skin lesions may not completely resolve
TMEP	• Usually appears in adults • Patients develop crops of numerous, itchy, ill-defined, *telangiectatic*, brown macules, 3–8 mm in size, primarily on the trunk • Darier's sign and dermatographism are often present
Solitary mastocytomas	• Represent localized disease • Present with red, pink, tan brown or yellowish nodules or plaques in infancy or early childhood • MC site: Distal extremities • If multiple, the lesions can be difficult to distinguish from nodular urticaria pigmentosa • They tend to blister if rubbed • Mast cell concentration is 150 times of normal skin, therefore vigorous rubbing/ trauma is associated with flushing and hypotension • Generally self-resolve over 1–3 years
Diffuse cutaneous mastocytosis	• Characterized by a diffuse infiltration of virtually the entire skin by mast cells • It usually presents in the neonatal period, although may persist till adulthood • The skin tends to be thickened and doughy in consistency (peau d'orange look) and yellowish brown discoloration. • Blistering after minor trauma or scratching is common and pruritus + • Patients may have systemic disease and severe complications including anaphylaxis and diarrhea
Systemic mastocytosis	• Cutaneous and gastrointestinal manifestations are the most prominent chronic manifestations • UP is the most common cutaneous manifestation • The bone marrow, liver, spleen, lymph nodes, and gastrointestinal tract are the usual sites • Episodes of flushing lasting for about 15–30 minutes and are often accompanied by palpitations • Organ involvement: 70–80% of patients have gastrointestinal symptoms including abdominal pain, diarrhea (MC), nausea, and vomiting. Hepatomegaly—72%, peripheral lymphadenopathy—20–40%, bone involvement—70%

*Tumor like growths have been described in an adult mastocytosis patient, in whom mast cells expressed V560G c-KIT mutation.

TABLE 20.3: Difference between adult onset and childhood onset mastocytosis

Parameter	Adult onset mastocytosis	Childhood onset mastocytosis
Most common type of mastocytosis	ISM	Cutaneous mastocytosis
Typical course of disease	Chronic	Temporary
% Frequency of anaphylaxis	50	<10
Typical tryptase level (ng/mL)	>20	<20
Typical location of KIT mutation	KIT D816V	Exon 8, 9, 11 or 17
Typical morphology of maculopapular lesions	Monomorphic	Polymorphic
Typical size of maculopapular lesions	Small	Large
Typical distribution of maculopapular lesions	Thigh, trunk	Trunk, head, extremities

Flowchart 20.1: Approach to a patient of mastocytosis

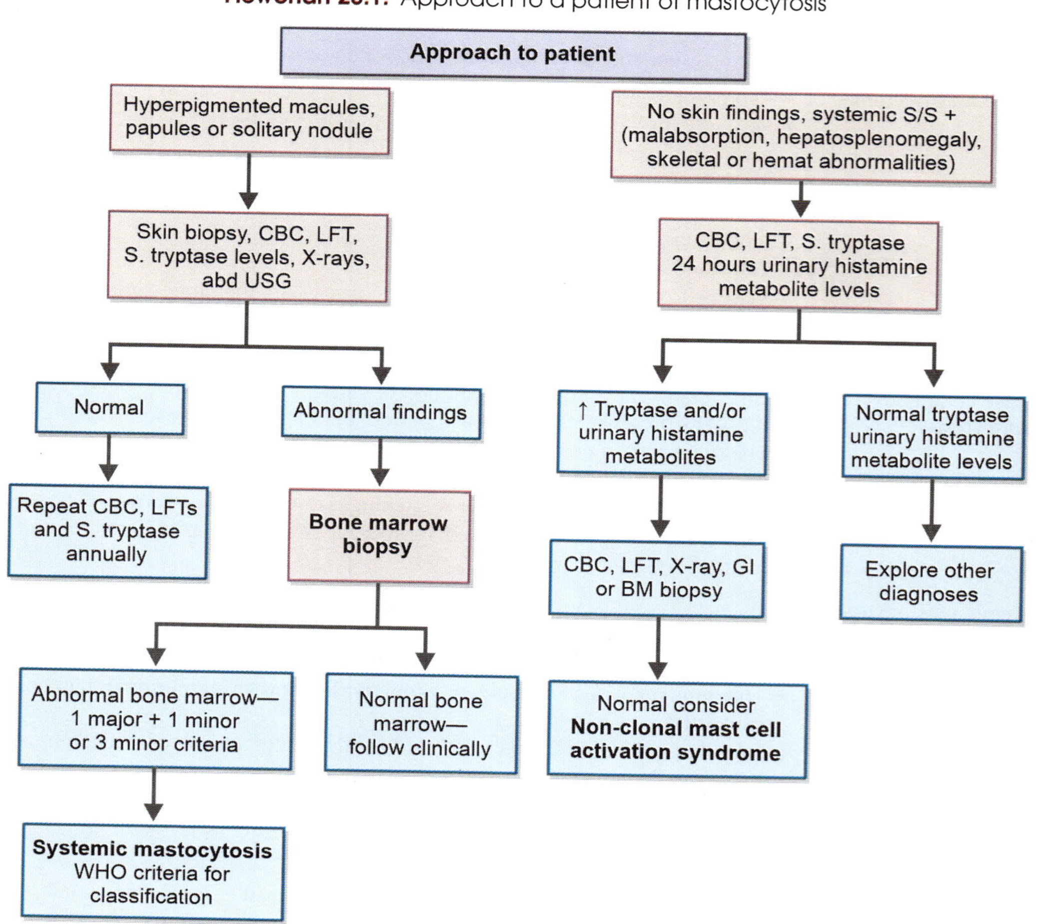

TABLE 20.4: Investigations in cutaneous mastocytosis

Dermoscopy	Vano-Galvan et al. (2011) identified four dermatoscopic patterns: Light brown blot, pigment network, reticular vascular pattern (consisting of thin reticular telangiectasias) and yellow-orange blot
HPE	• Histopathologically, all forms of mastocytosis are characterized by the dermal accumulation of mast cells particularly around blood vessels. Mast cells may appear elongated, like fibroblasts, or cuboidal. They are basophilic and granular • The epidermis shows increased melanization • In diffuse cutaneous mastocytosis, the infiltrate is dense and band-like near the epidermis • In TMEP, the infiltrate tends to be predominantly perivascular, and there is also vascular ectasia • The blister in bullous forms is subepidermal and the blister cavity often contains numerous eosinophils • In systemic mastocytosis, the liver, spleen, bone marrow, lymph nodes, and other organs may also be infiltrated
Special stains	• With toluidine blue or Giemsa stains, the granules stain metachromatically • **Others:** Giemsa, Leder, tryptase, and CD117 (KIT) antibodies
Other tests	• A full blood count, liver profile and tryptase • Bone marrow examination, abdominal ultrasound scan, X-rays (skull, spine and pelvis) and mutation analysis (*KIT*D816V) • Bone marrow biopsy should be performed when considering systemic disease • Serum tryptase may be elevated but is often normal (total serum tryptase >20 ng/ml is abnormal); urinary histamine and histamine metabolites (1,4-methylimidazole acetic acid and N-methylimidazole acetic acid) may be detectable. (Avoid intake of spinach, egg plant, cheese and red wine which are high in histamine)

Diagnosis of Systemic Mastocytosis

Table 20.5 gives the criteria for diagnosis of systemic mastocytosis.

TABLE 20.5: World Health Organization criteria for systemic mastocytosis (2016): 1 major + 1 minor, or 3 minor criteria on bone marrow biopsy

Major	Multifocal aggregates of at least **15 mast cells** in bone marrow or other organ (not skin)
Minor	• >25% of mast cells in infiltrates are spindle-shaped in bone marrow biopsy or other tissue or >25% of mast cells in bone marrow aspirate smears are immature or atypical • Activating mutations in *KIT* (at codon 816) in bone marrow, blood or other tissue (not skin) • Coexpression of CD117 with CD2 and/or CD25 in mast cells in bone marrow, blood or other tissue (not skin) • Serum tryptase >20 μg/L (unless associated with clonal myeloid disorder)

Differential Diagnosis

Table 20.6 lists the common differentials of the different types of CM.

TABLE 20.6: Differential diagnosis of cutaneous mastocytosis

Diffuse or localized hyperpigmented papules/macules
• Urticaria • Multiple nevi • Langerhans cell histiocytosis • Juvenile xanthogranulomas • Nodular scabies • Café au lait spots • Multiple cutaneous lentiginosis • Post-inflammatory hyperpigmentation
Bullous lesions
• Linear immunoglobulin A dermatosis • Bullous impetigo • Epidermolysis bullosa • Arthropod bite reaction • Toxic epidermal necrolysis • Incontinentia pigmenti
Solitary papule or nodule
• Congenital nevus • Juvenile xanthogranuloma • Pseudolymphoma

CLINICAL COURSE AND PROGNOSIS (Box 20.1)

BOX 20.1: Clinical course and prognosis

- Around 50% of children with urticaria pigmentosa clear by adolescence.
- Spontaneous resolution of cutaneous mastocytosis is observed in about 10% of adults.
- Serum tryptase, cardiovascular/constitutional symptoms, osteoporosis (independent predictors of progression to SM in CM) (Fuchs D, 2020)
- The main problems likely to be experienced by patients are related to the risks of anaphylaxis and osteoporosis.
- Anaphylaxis leading to death, osteonecrosis, malignancy are the major complications.
- Up to 50% of adults and 20% of children experience one or more episodes of anaphylaxis.
- Systemic mastocytosis may be associated with dysplastic and neoplastic disorders of myeloid cells.
- Mast cell leukemia is fatal, with a mean survival of less than 6 months.

TREATMENT

Avoid mast cell degranulators (e.g. alcohol, anticholinergics, NSAIDs, aspirin, narcotics, polymyxin, and systemic anesthetics).

The treatment of CM and noncutaneous manifestations of mastocytosis is listed in **Flowcharts 20.2** and **20.3**, respectively.

Cytoreductive therapy is restricted to patients with aggressive variants of mastocytosis (SM with AHN, ASM and MCL). The various cytoreductive drugs that are used in mastocytosis are cladribine, imatinib, midostaurin, masitinib, dasatinib, nilotinib. Oral midostaurin has response rates of ~60% in patients with aggressive SM and is the only FDA-approved drug (2018) for SM with AHN, ASM and MCL.

Flowchart 20.2: Treatment of cutaneous mastocytosis

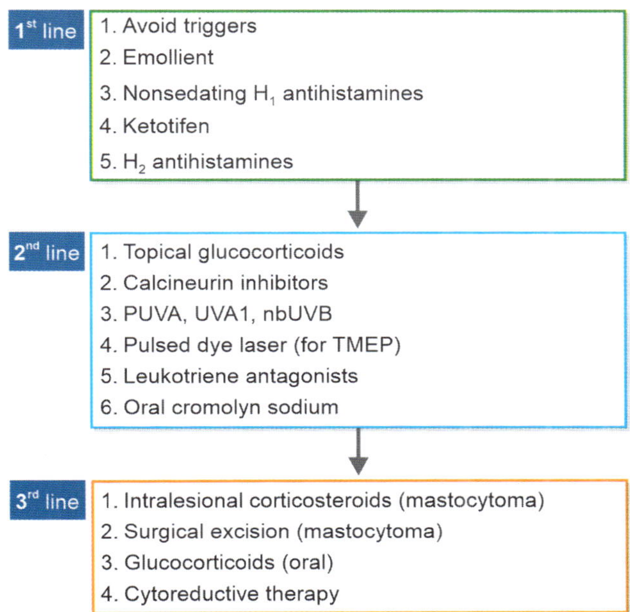

Flowchart 20.3: Treatment of noncutaneous mastocytosis

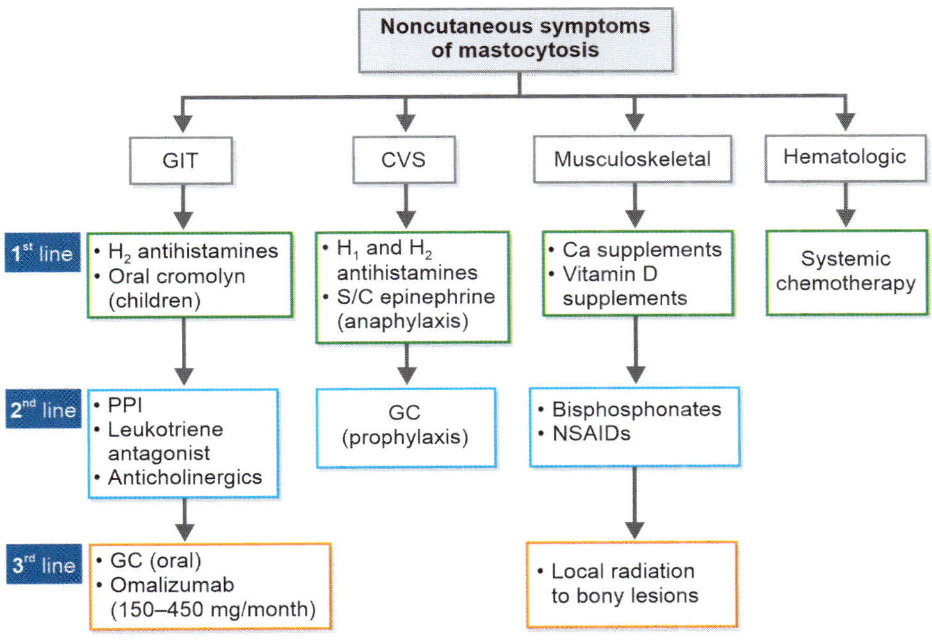

*GC, glucocorticoid

Acknowledgments

The authors thank **Konchok Dorjay**, MD, for his work on this chapter in the previous edition of this book.

BIBLIOGRAPHY

Books

1. Grattan CEH, Radia DH. Mastocytosis. Editors. In: Rook's Textbook of Dermatology (ninth edition) UK. Blackwell Publishers. Part 4, Chapter 46: p46.1–10.
2. Tharp MD, Sofen BD. Mastocytosis. Bolognia JL, Schaffer JV, Cerroni L, Editors. In: Dermatology (fourth edition). Elsevier, 2018. Section 18, Chapter 118:p2102–11.
3. Tharp MD. Mastocytosis. Kang S, Amagai M, Bruckner AL, Enk AH, Margolis DJ, McMichael AJ, Orringer JS, Editors. In: Fitzpatrick's Dermatology (ninth edition). McGraw Hill Education. Chapter 42:p-710–22.

Journals

1. Fuchs D, et al. Scoring the Risk of Having Systemic Mastocytosis in Adult Patients with Mastocytosis in the Skin. J Allergy Clin Immunol Pract. 2020 Dec 23:S2213-2198(20)31354-4. doi: 10.1016/j.jaip.2020.12.022. Epub ahead of print. PMID: 33346151.
2. Hartmann K, et al. Cutaneous manifestations in patients with mastocytosis: Consensus report of the European Competence Network on Mastocytosis; the American Academy of Allergy, Asthma and Immunology; and the European Academy of Allergology and Clinical Immunology. J Allergy Clin Immunol, 2016 Jan;137(1):35–45.
3. Horny HP, Metcalfe DD, Akin C, et al. Mastocytosis. In: SH Swerdlow, et al., eds. *WHO Classification of Tumors of Hematopoietic and Lymphoid Tissues*. Lyon, France: International Agency for Research and Cancer (IARC); 2017: 62–9.
4. Vano-Galvan S, Alvarez-Twose I, Heras ED, Morgade JM, Matito A, Sanchlz-Munoz L, et al., Dermoscopic features of skin lesions in patients with mastocytosis. Arch Dermatol 2011;147(8):932–40.

Chapter 21

Morphea and Lichen Sclerosus

Surabhi Sinha, Kabir Sardana, Sinu Rose Mathachan

MORPHEA

Epidemiology

- **Age**
  - **Childhood** onset: **2–14 years. Linear type** > plaque > generalized > deep
  - **Adult** onset: **40–50 years. Plaque type** > generalized > linear
- **Sex**
  - F:M = 2.6:1 to 7:1 (more marked in adults)
  - Children: F:M = 1.5:1
  - **Adult pansclerotic morphea:** Males > Females

Classification

- Peterson et al.—most widely used. But contains some controversial non-morphea entities and does not include "mixed" morphea (15–23%).
- Rook's Textbook of Dermatology—more inclusive classification.
- **Table 21.1** provides both the classification systems.

Predisposing and Triggering Factors

- **Genetics:** HLA-DRB1*04:04 and HLA-B*37—especially associated with generalized and linear morphea. HLA-DRB1*04:04—also associated with systemic sclerosis.
- **Infections:** *Borrelia burgdorferi sensu stricto* (USA) and *B. afzelii*/*B. garinii* (Eurasia). However, no conclusive evidence to prove causal association.
- **Trauma:** Accidental trauma/surgery/insect bite reactions/vaccinations/injections (more in linear and deep morphea, less in generalized)
  - **Vaccination**—hepatitis B, MMR, DPT, BCG, pneumococcal vaccine
  - **Injections**—vitamin B_{12}, vitamin K
  - **Mechanical trauma**
    - **Isotopic** (morphea developing in same area as previously healed skin disease/injury)—in 6%.
    - **Isomorphic** (morphea developing at sites of repeated trauma—Koebner's phenomenon)—in 9%.

TABLE 21.1: Classification of morphea

Peterson et al.	Rook's Textbook of Dermatology (9th Ed.)*
Plaque morphea • Morphea en plaque • Guttate morphea • Atrophoderma of Pasini–Pierini • Lichen sclerosus • Keloidal morphea	**Limited type** • Limited plaque morphea • Guttate morphea • Atrophoderma of Pasini-Pierini • Keloidal/nodular morphea • Limited deep morphea
Generalized morphea (lesions at 3 or more anatomical sites)	**Generalized type** • Disseminated plaque (isomorphic and non-isomorphic patterns) • Pansclerotic morphea • Eosinophilic fasciitis
Linear morphea • Linear morphea of limbs or trunk • En coup de sabre morphea • Progressive hemifacial atrophy-Parry–Romberg syndrome	**Linear type** • Head/neck variant – Morphea en coup de sabre – Progressive hemifacial atrophy • Trunk/limb variant – Linear morphea – Linear atrophoderma of Moulin – Linear deep atrophic morphea
Bullous morphea	**Mixed types** (most commonly linear + plaque, more common in childhood onset)
Deep morphea (inflammation and sclerosis in deep dermis, subcutaneous fat, fascia, muscle) • Subcutaneous morphea • Morphea profunda • Eosinophilic fasciitis • Disabling pansclerotic morphea	**Lichen sclerosus with morphea**

*Based on Padua Consensus classification

- **Radiation and radiotherapy**—especially radiotherapy for breast cancer—1/500 breast Ca patients may develop morphea within a year of completion of radiotherapy.
- **Drugs**—bleomycin, pentazocine, progestin, vitamin B_{12} vitamin K, cocaine, D-penicillamine, interferon-β1a, paclitaxel, methysergide, gemcitabine, bromocriptine, bisoprolol, L-hydroxytryptophan with carbidopa, ibuprofen, mitomycin C, balicatib. (**Balicatib** is used in treatment of osteoporosis and osteoarthritis. Inhibits collagenolytic activity of cathepsin K within lysosomes in skin fibroblasts → morphea.)

Pathogenesis

3 major components: Vascular damage, activated T cells, and altered connective tissue production by fibroblasts.

Role of microRNAs: MicroRNAs (miRNAs)—small non-coding RNAs that bind to mRNA and inhibit their translation to proteins. Downregulated miRNAs (especially miR-7 and miRNA-196a) → allow increased type I collagen expression in morphea fibroblasts → fibrosis of morphea. Thus, miRNA upregulation may be a potential therapeutic avenue.

Prevalent autoantibodies—anti-fibrillin-1, MMP-1, histone antibodies and ANA (18–68%, mostly speckled), and, less frequently, topoisomerase and centromere.

Immunological: There is also a role of **Th1/Th17 → Th2 shift** in the pathogenesis of morphea (**Figs 21.1** and **21.2**), which seems to be the prevalent hypothesis.

Clinical Features

Classic Lesion of Morphea

- Begins with erythematous edematous inflammatory 'bruise-like' change in texture of skin.
- Central sclerosis → skin becomes thickened waxy yellowish-white in center and surrounded by erythematous to violaceous 'lilac' ring. +/– Loss of hair, loss of sweating **(Fig. 21.3a** and **b)**.

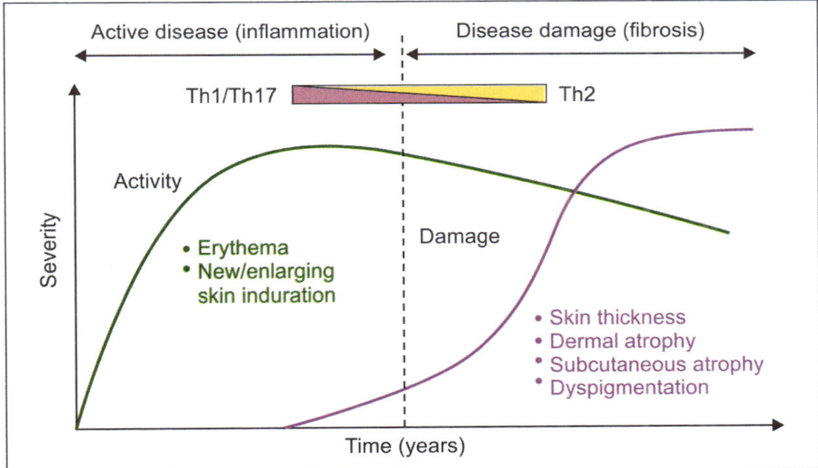

Fig. 21.1: Proposed conceptual model of morphea—transition from Th1/Th17 in the early stages to Th2 in the later stages

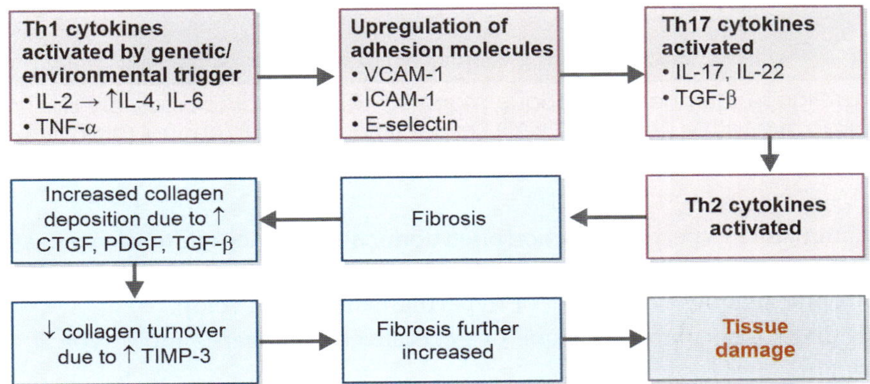

Fig. 21.2: Pathogenesis and role of Th cell subsets in morphea

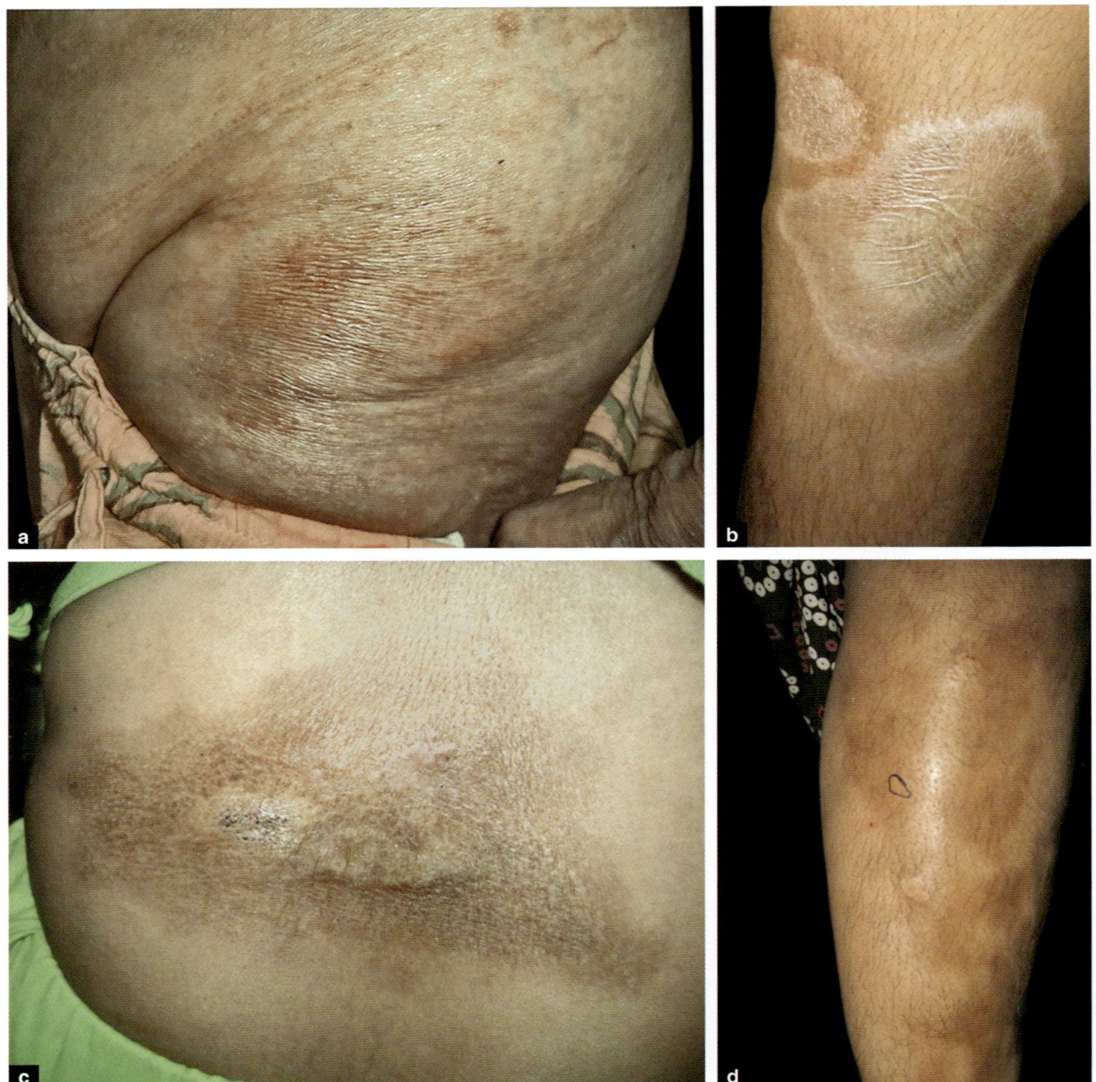

Fig. 21.3: (a) Plaque morphea; (b) Plaque morphea with central sclerosis, dry skin, loss of hair, peripheral lilac hue with a band of PIH; (c) Keloidal morphea with central raised firm lesion; (d) Limited deep morphea

- Post-inflammatory hyperpigmentation often dominates over the white sclerosis as the lesions mature.
- Later, atrophic plaques with hypo- or hyperpigmentation develop.
- Delay in diagnosis—more in plaque or generalized as linear is more typical and easily detected.

Table 21.2 describes the various clinical types of morphea.

TABLE 21.2: Clinical types of morphea

Type	Site	Typical lesions	Important differential diagnosis
Limited			
• Limited plaque	Up to 2 out of 7 anatomical regions*, usually trunk, breasts often (but always spare nipple-areolae complex)	• Round-oval >1 cm lesions • Induration +	• Granuloma annulare • Extragenital lichen sclerosus • Mycosis fungoides • Necrobiosis lipoidica • Pretibial myxedema • Post-inflammatory hyperpigmentation • Lipodystrophy • Steroid-induced atrophy
• Guttate	Trunk	• Multiple small <1 cm, erythematous-yellowish white, superficial, atrophic wrinkled appearance • Mild induration • Heal with hyperpigmentation	• Extragenital lichen sclerosus
• Atrophoderma of Pasini-Pierini	Trunk	• Symmetrical non-indurated blue-gray to brown hyperpigmented sharply demarcated depressed plaques with 'cliff-drop' border • May be hypopigmented or skin colored • May coexist with morphea	• Post-inflammatory hyperpigmentation • Actinic LP • Café au lait macule • Post-FDE hyperpigmentation
• Keloidal/nodular	Upper trunk, breasts common	• Keloid-like nodules in patients with morphea/SSc **(Fig. 21.3c)**	• Keloid
• Limited deep	—	• Diffuse taut bound-down skin (morphea profunda) **(Fig. 21.3d)**	• Lipoatrophy
Generalized (3 or more of 7 anatomical regions)			
• Disseminated plaque	Trunk, thighs, lumbosacral area (chronic friction)	• Multiple symmetrical discrete/coalescent plaques • Isomorphic phenomenon + • Start as limited plaque morphea	
• Pansclerotic	Trunk, centrifugal spread to near-total body surface area, typically sparing fingers, toes (distal to MCP and MTP joints) and nipples	• Rare • M > F • Severe, rapidly progressive • Circumferential involvement • Deep fibrosis common but not present in all	• Systemic sclerosis • Sclerodermoid GVHD • Scleredema • Scleromyxedema • PCT • Primary systemic amyloidosis

(Contd.)

***7 anatomical regions**—head and neck, each of 4 limbs, anterior trunk, posterior trunk.

TABLE 21.2: Clinical types of morphea *(Contd.)*

Type	Site	Typical lesions	Important differential diagnosis
		• Complications—joint contractures, chronic ulcers, SCC, dysphagia and dyspnea (due to skin tightening)	• Nephrogenic systemic fibrosis • Carcinoid syndrome • Drug-induced morphea • Chemical induced • Occupational skin sclerosis
• Eosinophilic fasciitis/Schulman syndrome	Lower limbs > upper limbs, typically spares fingers and face	• Other subtypes of morphea coexist in 29–40% • Extensive, deep, symmetrical • May follow unaccustomed severe exercise in 50% • Painful burning erythema and pitting edema of limbs → induration and fibrosis → peau d' orange, negative vein sign/groove sign (guttering) • Eosinophilic infiltrate in early stages • Complications—joint contractures	(Same as for pansclerotic morphea)
Linear (head and neck) (***see* Table 21.3** for differentiation between PHA and ECDS)	More in children (42–67%) • Limb/trunk twice as common as head/neck • Upper limb and lower limb of same side—common U/L mostly, B/L in 5–25%, Blaschkoid 25%—mixed (with plaque type)	—	—
• Morphea *en coup de sabre* (ECDS) **(Fig.21.4a)**	Frontoparietal area of scalp and face in paramedian distribution, Blaschkoid pattern	• More common than PHA (87% of head/neck morphea) in children • Sclerosis, hyperpigmentation, atrophy • Scarring alopecia of eyebrows, eyelashes, scalp • Linear depression in skull • Complications—neurological, ocular, auditory	• Post-traumatic atrophy

(Contd.)

TABLE 21.2: Clinical types of morphea *(Contd.)*

Type	Site	Typical lesions	Important differential diagnosis
• Progressive hemifacial atrophy (PHA)/Parry–Romberg syndrome	Area supplied by trigeminal nerve (now believed to be Blaschkoid pattern) **(Fig. 21.4a)**	• U/L progressive atrophy of skin, fat, muscle, cartilage and bone • With brownish/bruise-like pigmentation • Facial asymmetry due to loss of fat and bone—mouth and nose deviated towards affected side • Complications—ocular, dental, neurological	• Hemifacial microsomia (first and second branchial arch syndrome) and its variant *Goldenhar syndrome* (congenital and non-progressive) • Post-traumatic atrophy
	Blaschkoid	• Erythema, sclerosis, hyperpigmentation, atrophy • May coexist with plaque type on trunk, U/L • Complications—joint contractures, muscle atrophy, limb girth (adults)/length (children) asymmetry	• Post-traumatic atrophy
• Linear atrophoderma of Moulin	Limbs **(Fig. 21.4b)**	• A linear Blaschkoid form of atrophoderma of Pasini-Pierini	—
• Linear deep atrophic morphea	Limbs	• Linear limb form of PHA	—
Mixed	4% adults, 15–25% children	• Linear + Plaque most common	—
Lichen sclerosus with morphea overlap (**see Table 21.4** for differentiating features)	Extragenital and genital LS both may be present. Thus, always do genital examination in morphea—more commonly seen in limited plaque type and disseminated plaque type	• Increased prevalence of LS in morphea (odds ratio >18) • LS believed by some to be a superficial form of morphea Others say—a distinct disease	—

TABLE 21.3: PHA versus ECDS

PHA (progressive hemifacial atrophy)	ECDS (*en coup de sabre*)
Unilateral atrophy	Unilateral frontoparietal sclerotic band
Minimal/absent induration or previous inflammation	Usually preceded by skin induration
Cutaneous atrophy (normal hair)	Scarring alopecia possible
Half face involved	Usually does not go below eyebrow
Complications—enophthalmos, choroidal and retinal folding, hyperopia, uveitis, retinal vasculitis, glaucoma, third nerve palsy, headache, epilepsy, dental malocclusion and hemiatrophy of tongue	Neurological, ocular, auditory complications

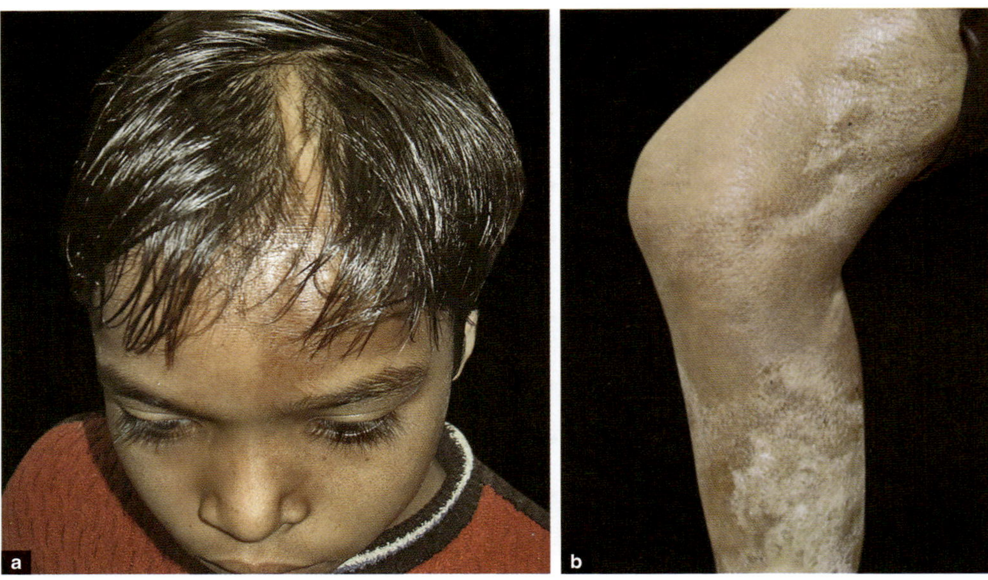

Fig. 21.4: (a) *En coup de sabre*; (b) Linear morphea

TABLE 21.4: Differentiation between morphea and LS

	Morphea	Lichen sclerosus
Clinical appearance	• Thicker larger plaques with inflammatory/lilac border • Sclerosis more apparent	• Porcelain white papules/plaques with follicular plugging/telangiectasia/purpura and atrophy • Sclerosis minimal
Histopathology	• Normal upper dermal elastic fibers more likely • Lichenoid infiltrate (–) • Basal layer vacuolization (–)	• Loss of elastic fibers • Lichenoid infiltrate (+) • Basal layer vacuolization (+)
Antibodies associated	• Antibodies to fibrillin-1 (also an extracellular matrix protein) likely	• Antibodies to extracellular matrix protein-1 (EMP-1)

Extracutaneous Manifestations

- In 20–25% of morphea patients:
  - **Linear**
    - Neurological (31%)—headache, migraine, seizures.
    - Ophthalmological (8%)—episcleritis, anterior uveitis, keratitis.
    - Dental/oral—malocclusion, tongue hemiatrophy, TMJ involvement.
  - **Generalized**
    - Arthritis and joint limitations
- Vascular—Raynaud's phenomenon
- Gastrointestinal—esophagitis, GERD. Rare. More likely due to skin immobility.
- Respiratory—dyspnea. Rare. More likely due to severe skin immobility.

Associated Diseases

- **Autoimmune diseases**
  - Mostly with generalized morphea
  - More common in adults—family history of AICTDs seen
  - Diseases:
    - AICTDs (autoimmune connective tissue diseases)—RA, SLE
    - AITD (autoimmune thyroid disorder)
    - Vitiligo
    - Diabetes mellitus
    - Psoriasis
    - Multiple sclerosis
    - IBDs (inflammatory bowel diseases)
- **Lichen sclerosus (Table 21.2)**
- **Melanoma and NMSC**–reported to occur at higher incidence in morphea and SSc.

Investigations

Table 21.5 lists the important investigations in morphea while **Tables 21.6** and **21.7** give a histopathological comparison of early/late morphea and morphea/SSc, respectively.

Scoring

LoSCAT (localized scleroderma cutaneous assessment tool) **(Fig. 21.5)**.

TABLE 21.5: Investigations in morphea

Types of investigation	Finding
Dermoscopy	• Morphea—fibrotic beams, pigmentary structures • Lichen sclerosus—patchy white structureless areas, comedo-like openings, purpuric globules, scale, ice slivers and sparse, thin vessels
ESR, CRP, IgG, eosinophil count	• High in eosinophilic fasciitis
Imaging	• Cranial MRI—MRI of the brain with contrast is recommended in all patients with morphea affecting the face, head and neck area, regardless of the presence of characteristic neurological symptoms (headaches/migraine, seizures, hemiparesis • CT scan—before surgery planned for unequal lengths of limbs • EEG • USG: USG in the 20-MHz range, can be used to accurately assess the activity and damage of skin lesions in morphea, with results comparable to the clinical validated score localized scleroderma cutaneous assessment tool (LoSCAT)
Measurement of skin thickness	• Photography • Cutometer • Thermography • Computerized skin score • USG (15–20 MHz) • Durometer • Scanning laser Doppler
HPE	• Deep incisional ellipse (to include muscle and fascia) • From erythematous border if present/otherwise from central sclerosis area • Depth of involvement—variable in morphea. Best measured by deep tissue biopsy and MRI

(Contd.)

TABLE 21.5: Investigations in morphea *(Contd.)*

Types of investigation	Finding
	• Detailed histopathological comparison of morphea (early versus late) and morphea versus SSc is given in **Tables 21.6** and **21.7**. • **Patterns of inflammation** (Walker et al., 2017) – **Top heavy**—hyalinized collagen bundles exclusively in the papillary to superficial reticular dermis with absence of these changes in the lower layers. – **Bottom heavy**—hyalinized collagen bundles in deep dermis and subcutaneous fat sparing the papillary through mid-dermis. Associated with higher functional impairment, pain and tightness. • **Full thickness**—throughout dermis. • **Severe inflammation**—associated with pain and functional impairment • **Types of lesions and patterns of inflammation** – Linear/limited plaque: Top = Bottom = Full – Deep: Bottom, full – LS with morphea: Top – Disseminated: Bottom, top
Serology	Positive ANA titers are a/w a higher risk for extracutaneous, deeper involvement and disease relapse ANA (18–68%), ENA, RA factor, *Borrelia serology* (in areas with high prevalence), anti-single strand DNA (ssDNA)—topoisomerase IIα, phospholipid, fibrillin-1, MMP-1, and histone antibodies (AHA)
Scoring of severity	**LoSCAT score (Fig. 21.5)**
Referrals	ENT, ophthalmology, dental, orthopedics, plastic surgery, physiotherapy

TABLE 21.6: Histopathological comparison of early and late morphea

	Active inflammatory phase	Late sclerotic phase
Epidermis	Normal/flattened with loss of rete ridges/acanthotic	Flattened usually
Papillary dermis	Occasionally edema and infiltrate may be present	Fibrosis may extend into papillary dermis too
Reticular dermis	• Edema, dense perivascular infiltrate—lymphocytes, plasma cells, macrophages, occasional eosinophils • Swollen collagen bundles parallel to the skin surface	• Inflammation minimal • Collagen bundles—closely packed, horizontal, highly eosinophilic
Eccrine glands and hair follicles	Infiltrate may encompass them	Entrapped by collagen → appear higher up in dermis, eventually lost
Subcutaneous fat	Infiltrate may spill into fat Thickened newly formed wavy collagen bundles (type III collagen and fibrillin 1)	Replaced by collagen
Blood vessels of dermis and fat	Mild changes. Edema of walls and endothelial swelling	Fewer blood vessels, walls thickened
Fascia, striated muscles	Inflammation +/–	Fibrosis +

Site		mLoSSI (localized scleroderma skin activity index) *New/enlarge (within 1 mo)* 0 = None 3 = N/E	*Erythema* 0 = None 1 = Pink 2 = Red 3 = Dark red/ Violaceous	*Skin thickness* 0 = None 1 = Mild 2 = Moderate 3 = Marked	LoSDI (localized scleroderma skin damage index) *Dermal atrophy* 0 = None 1 = Shiny 2 = Visible Vessel 3 = Obvious cliff drop	*Subcutaneous atrophy* 0 = None 1 = Flat 2 = Concave 3 = Marked atrophy	*Dyspigmentation (hypo/hyperpig.)* 0 = None 1 = Mild 2 = Moderate 3 = Marked
Scalp/face							
Neck							
Chest							
Abdomen							
Upper back							
Lower back							
RT	Arm						
	Forearm						
	Hand						
	Thigh						
	Leg						
	Foot						
LT	Arm						
	Forearm						
	Hand						
	Thigh						
	Leg						
	Foot						

Total score: mLoSSI (activity) ______________ LoSDI (damage) ______________

Please mark with a straight line:

Physician global assessment of disease activity

____

0 Inactive — 100 Markedly active

Physician global assessment of disease damage

____

0 No damage — 100 Markedly damage

Comment: ____

Fig. 21.5: Localized scleroderma cutaneous assessment tool

TABLE 21.7: Histopathological comparison of morphea and systemic sclerosis

	Morphea	Systemic sclerosis
Inflammatory infiltrate	More intense	Less
Perineural inflammation	More likely	Less
Extent of fibrosis	More diffuse, may involve papillary and reticular dermis both	Less

Differential Diagnosis

Table 21.8 lists the disorders associated with skin sclerosis which may need to be differentiated from morphea on a few occasions.

Treatment (Flowcharts 21.1 and 21.2)

The therapy is based on various aspects and include General Measures, Pharmacotherapy and Emerging therapies.

The **General measures** include psychosocial support, physiotherapy, massage, lymphatic drainage, interdisciplinary consultations (rheumatology, physical medicine and rehabilitation, orthopedics, plastic and oral maxillofacial surgery) and surgery.

The **Pharmacotherapy** is detailed below and is dependent on various aspects including

1. **Subtype of morphea**
   a. **Limited superficial**—topical agents, topical tacrolimus 0.1%, 5% imiquimod cream (3–7 times weekly for 9-month period), calcipotriol/calcipotriene 0.005%, low-dose

TABLE 21.8: Disorders associated with skin sclerosis/sclerodermoid disorders

Types of disorder	Examples
Autoimmune disorders	Systemic sclerosis, sclerodermoid GVHD
Metabolic disorders	PCT, PKU, muscle glycogenosis, hypothyroidism, carcinoid syndrome, diabetic cheiroarthropathy with skin thickening
Deposition disorders	Scleredema, scleromyxedema, primary systemic amyloidosis
Genetic disorders	GEMSS syndrome, Werner syndrome, progeria, acrogeria, poikilodermatous EB, melorheostosis, scleroatrophic Huriez syndrome
Associated with hematological diseases	POEMS syndrome, myeloma
Occupational causes	Vinyl chloride, perchloroethylene, trichloroethylene, organic solvents, pesticides, epoxy resins, silicone
Chemical induced	Eosinophilia myalgia syndrome (L-tryptophan), toxic oil syndrome (rapeseed oil), nephrogenic systemic fibrosis (gadolinium exposure in renal failure)
Drug induced	Bleomycin, pentazocine, progestin, vitamin B_{12} and vitamin K, cocaine, D-penicillamine, interferon-β1a, paclitaxel, methysergide, gemcitabine, bromocriptine, bisoprolol, L- hydroxytryptophan with carbidopa, ibuprofen, mitomycin C, balicatib

PCT, porphyria cutanea tarda; PKU, phenylketonuria; GEMSS syndrome, glaucoma, ectopia, microspherophakia, stiff joints, Short stature; POEMS syndrome = polyneuropathy, Organomegaly, Endocrinopathy, Myeloma protein, and Skin changes

Flowchart 21.1: Therapeutic algorithm for morphea* (active stages) (Knobler et al., 2017)

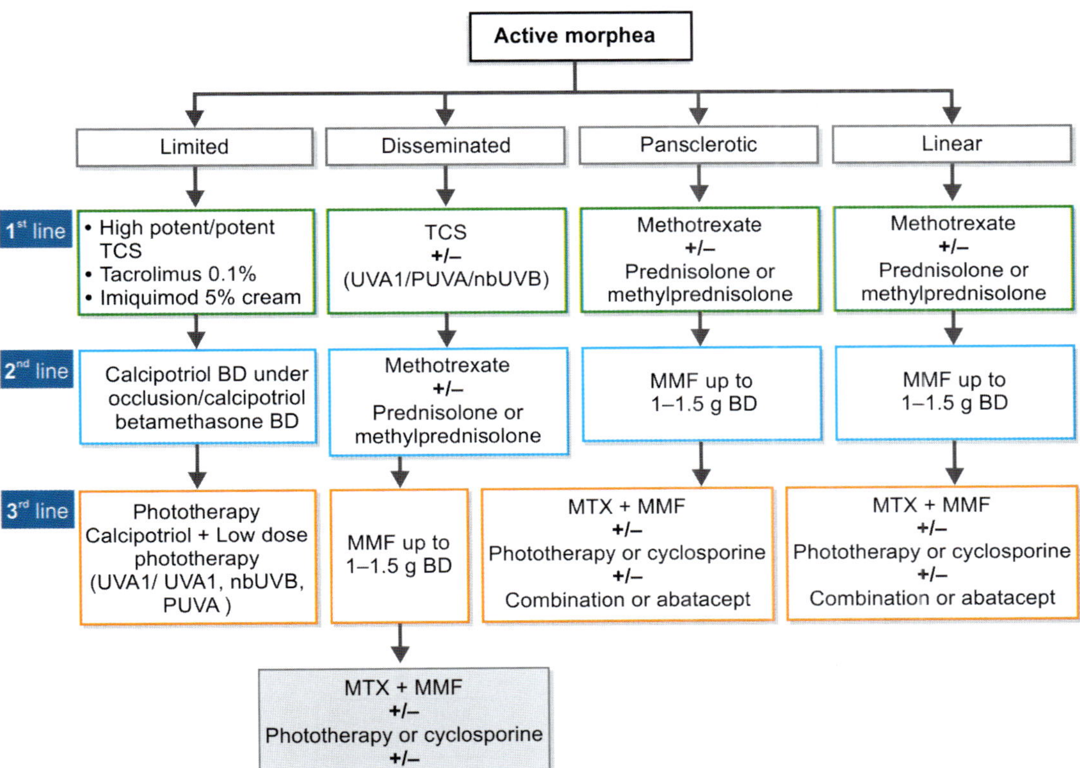

*Go to the next step if no response after 8–12 weeks.
For inactive morphea—autologous fat transfer, dermal fillers, surgical correction (epiphysiodesis of healthy extremity to adjust leg length inequality).
For all cases—psychological support, physiotherapy, manual lymphatic drainage.

UVA-1 phototherapy (children) and topical and intralesional corticosteroids. Steroids reserved for early inflammatory stages of disease or if there are pronounced epidermal changes.

b. **Disseminated forms**—phototherapy, preferably UVA-1, but when this is not available, broad-band UVA, narrow-band UVB or topical psoralen and UVA (PUVA).

Why phototherapy? UVA and UVB can induce MMPs such as collagenase, UVA-1 → upregulate antifibrotic haemoxygenase-1, cause T cell apoptosis, deplete dermal Langerhans and mast cells, induce interferon-γ (INF-γ), IL-1 and IL-6 production, ↓TGF-β production, ↑antifibrotic protein-decorin.

Ideal light—UVA wavelength (320–400 nm) as they penetrate deeper and **UVA-1** (340–400 nm) is less erythemogenic and penetrates deeper than UVA-2 (320–340 nm).

Dose: Low dose (10–20 J/cm^2), medium dose (>20–70 J/cm^2) and high dose (>70–130 J/cm^2), UVA-1 have all shown efficacy, significantly reducing skin thickness and stiffness

Flowchart 21.2: Treatment of newly diagnosed or refractory patients with **juvenile localized scleroderma** according to the clinical subtype (Zulian et al., 2019).

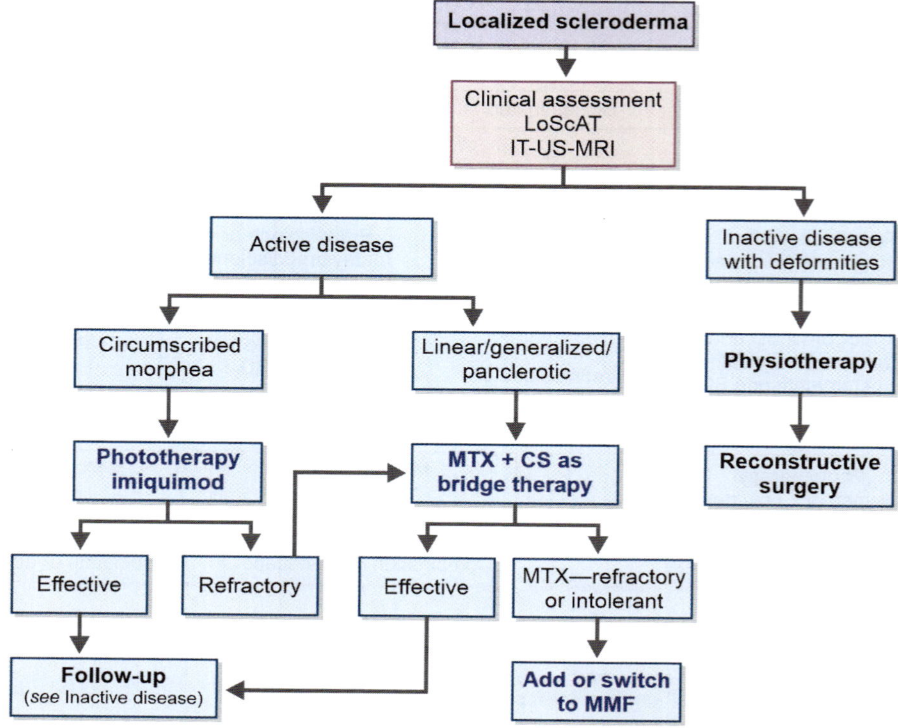

CS, corticosteroid; IT, infrared thermography; LoSCAT, localized scleroderma cutaneous assessment tool; MMF, mycophenolate mofetil; MTX, methotrexate; US, ultrasound.

in adults and children with all forms of morphea. Use **high doses** because of the lower cumulative UV exposure.

Others: Broad-band UVA, bath PUVA, cream PUVA and NBUVB.

c. **Progressive and severe types:** Combinations of pulsed intravenous and/or oral steroids with methotrexate should be used as first line.

(i) Steroids: (0.5–1 mg/kg/day for 6 weeks then taper over a mean of 18 months).

Dose = 0.3–0.6 mg/kg/week (15 mg/m^2/week) in children and 15–25 mg/week in adults. Methotrexate treatment should be for at least 1 year before tapering as this leads to longer remission periods. The drug should be stopped only when the patient is in remission and off steroids for at least 1 year.

(ii) Methotrexate—ideal drug.

Action: ↓IL-8, ↑IL-1 receptor antagonist and soluble TNF receptor p75, ↓in serum IL-2, -4 and -6, ↓mast cell numbers and levels of tenascin.

Combination: Pulse steroids + Methotrexate

(iii) Other drugs: Mycophenolate mofetil, abatacept, infliximab. High dose intravenous immunoglobulin in resistant cases.

2. **Disease activity**
3. **Age of the patient:** Zullian et al recently proposed an algorithm **(Flowchart 21.2)** for treatment of morphea in pediatric patients.
4. **Sequelae**

Emerging Therapies

i. *Antifibrotic Drugs*

Imatinib, a tyrosine kinase inhibitor that interferes with both signaling pathways by blocking the activity of c-Abl, c-Kit and PDGF receptors, respectively, showed beneficial results in numerous case reports of morphea patients.

Connective tissue growth factor (CTGF) is a profibrotic peptide that acts downstream of TGF-β and is highly expressed in morphea lesional skin and iloprost, a prostaglandin analogue, which is already used in SSc patients for the treatment of severe Raynaud's syndrome, can suppress the secretion of CTGF by fibroblast.

ii. *Anti-inflammtory Drugs*

IL-6 plays a crucial role in the pathogenesis of morphea. It exerts both inflammatory and profibrotic effects by binding to its membrane receptor (IL-6R) and activating the downstream Janus kinase (JAK)-STAT. The latter leads to the stimulation of collagen and MMP production by fibroblasts, and the differentiation of naïve CD4+ to pathogenic TH17 cells via the putative TGF-β axis. **Tocilizumab** is a potentially useful drug as it inhibits the IL-6 pathway.

A more useful pathway is the **JAK/STAT** signaling pathway, which acts downstream of the central TGF-β axis. Thus JAK inhibitors can be use to block the TGF-β-driven skin fibrosis. Tofacitinib, a JAK1 and JAK3 inhibitor, has been shown to show improvement in both clinical and histological skin thickness and also joint mobility in numerous cases of refractory, generalized morphea. Therapeutic response is seen in the first month, with a maximum response between 11 and 16 months [Papara C, et al., 2023].

Course and Prognosis

- In most patients, morphea progresses over 3–5 years, then stabilizes and eventually resolves spontaneously.
- Residual atrophy and dyspigmentation +
- Recurrences may occur months—years after quiescent disease
- Older age of initial onset and ANA positivity are potential markers for risk of relapse.
- 30–50% linear morphea have osteoarticular complications.
- Juvenile may behave more aggressively.
- Morphea → SSc rarely.
- Linear morphea → SSc in 0.9–1.3%.

Markers of disease activity are given in **Box 21.1**.

Some common questions that are useful in clinical practice and examinations are listed in **Box 21.2.**

BOX 21.1: Markers of disease activity

Clinical

1. New lesions in last 3 months (documented).
2. Expansion of pre-existing lesions in last 3 months (documented).
3. Moderate/severe erythema/skin lesions with erythematous borders.
4. Violaceous lesions/borders.
5. Increased induration of border.
6. Worsening of hair loss on scalp/eyebrow/eyelash.
7. Extracutaneous manifestations

Investigation*

8. Progression to deeper tissue by MRI/USG.
9. Elevation of laboratory markers (CPK, aldolase, ANA).
10. Skin biopsy suggestive of active disease.

*Of the investigative measures, only the computerized skin score, ultrasonography and MRI have been validated.

BOX 21.2: Factoids about morphea[Q]

Are skin biopsies useful for diagnosis?	Skin biopsies are recommended for the diagnosis of localized scleroderma
Are blood tests useful for the diagnosis and evaluation of disease activity?	No blood test findings are highly disease-specific and useful for diagnosis of this condition. Anti-ssDNA antibodies are positive in approximately 50% of cases, and there is often a correlation between disease activity and antibody titer
What imaging tests are useful for evaluating the spread of lesions?	Contrast magnetic resonance imaging (MRI) and Doppler ultrasound are useful for evaluating the extent of the spread of localized scleroderma in the skin and into the underlying tissue (adipose tissue, muscle, tendons and bone) Computed tomography (CT), MRI, electroencephalogram (EEG) for brain involvement in en coup de sabre
Does disease activity ever spontaneously resolve?	The disease activity in localized scleroderma generally disappears in approximately 50% of cases within 3–5 years, but relapses can occur
What findings are useful for differentiating localized scleroderma from systemic sclerosis?	The findings including sclerodactyly, Raynaud phenomenon, abnormalities in the nail-fold capillaries, visceral lesions and absence of autoantibodies that are specific to systemic sclerosis
Can localized scleroderma transform into systemic sclerosis?	Localized scleroderma does not transform into systemic sclerosis

[Q], commonly asked questions for postgraduages.

LICHEN SCLEROSUS (LS and BALANITIS XEROTICA OBLITERANS)

Epidemiology

- F >> M, whites >non-whites
- Any age, but has bimodal peaks:
  - Major peak = 40–50 years post-menopausal females
  - Second peak = Prepubertal girls (8–13 years)

- Associated with autoimmune diseases (especially in women)
  Most common: Autoimmune thyroid disease (15%)
  Others: Pernicious anemia, localized scleroderma/morphea (6%), psoriasis, and vitiligo
- **Autoantibodies:** Extracellular matrix protein-1 (ECM-1)
- **Site:** Most commonly affects male and female anogenital region (85%)
- Extragenital LS accounts for only 15%
- Extragenital sites—neck, shoulders, flexor surfaces of the wrists, and sites of physical trauma or continuous pressure.
- Male penile involvement = Balanitis xerotica obliterans (BXO).

Clinical Features (Extragenital LS)

- Classic lesions: Sclerotic, ivory-white, atrophic, and flat-topped papules coalescing into plaques (**Fig. 21.6**).
- Follicular plugging (follicular delling) more prominent in extragenital LS. The **Ink Test** is useful to highlight the follicular plugging, where marking ink is applied on the lesion then cleaned with isopropyl alcohol , the ink remains in FP and can be visualized by dermoscopy.
- Genital LS is usually symptomatic (itching, pain, and burning), whereas extragenital LS is typically asymptomatic.

Clinical Features (Genital LS)

Males

- Phimosis may be asymptomatic.
- Symptoms—itching, burning, bleeding, tearing, splitting, rash, hemorrhagic blisters, sexual dysfunction or dyspareunia, discomfort with urination and narrowing of the urinary stream.

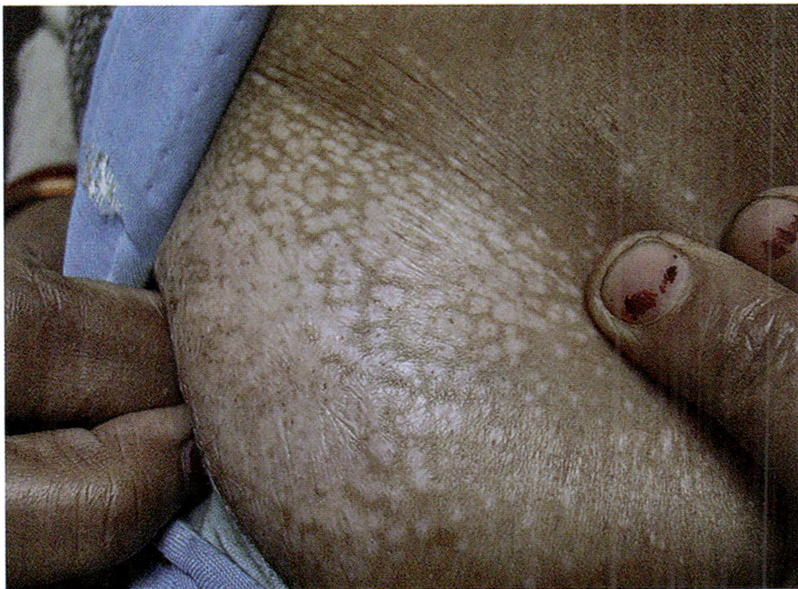

Fig. 21.6: Lichen sclerosus: Ivory-white lesions with follicular plugging

- Signs—atrophic leukodermic patches or plaques, telangiectasia and sparse purpura, incomplete paraphimosis or 'waisting' due to a constrictive posthitis, signs of dysplasia, carcinoma *in situ* or of a frank cancer.
- Posthitis xerotica obliterans—prepuce damage, balanitis xerotica obliterans—glans penis.

Females

- Flat, atrophic, whitened epithelium, may become confluent, extending around the vulval and perianal skin in a 'figure-of-eight' configuration. Vaginal lesions do not occur, as LS seems to spare mucosal epithelium **(Fig. 21.7)**.
- Symptoms—severe pruritus and soreness. Leading to dysuria, dyspareunia, or pain upon defecation (often manifesting as constipation in children). Scarring can lead to burying of the clitoris and fusion of the labia minora to the labia majora.

Differential Diagnosis

- Morphea (extragenital LS)
- Erosive lichen planus or erythroplasia of Queyrat (genital LS)
- Chronic GVHD
- SCC

Histopathology

- Epidermis is atrophic with basal cell hydropic degeneration.
- Superficial dermis is edematous and hyalinized. Deep to the hyalinized zone is a band-like lymphohistiocytic infiltrate. Lymphocytes are noted between sclerotic collagen bundles in

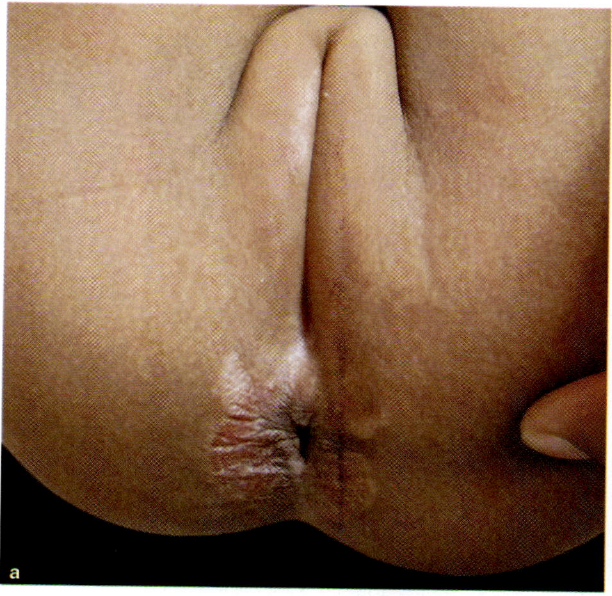

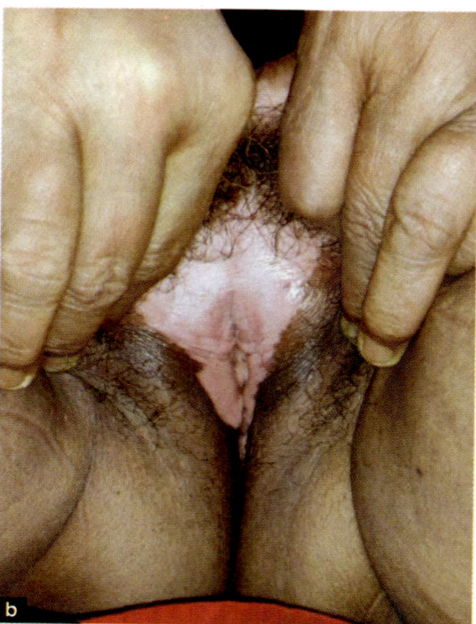

Fig. 21.7: Genital LS—atrophic wrinkled plaques with loss of appendages. Associated soreness and itching is pronounced

majority of the slides and is referred to as the "Lymphocyte-peppered sclerotic collagen" [Yadav D, et al., 2021].

- **'Red, white, and blue sign'**
  - Orthohyperkeratotic stratum corneum **(pink-red)**
  - Hyalinized/edematous papillary dermis **(pale-white)**
  - Band-like lymphocytic infiltrate **(blue)**

Treatment (Table 21.9)

- Contact with soap and urine should be avoided by use of a soap substitute and a barrier preparation.
- General measures like the avoidance of mechanical irritation (e.g. rough paper towels or hard bicycle saddles).
- Usually, clobetasol propionate is effective.

***Principle of use of potent steroids*:** The plasticity of the male genital epithelium seems to allow significant remodeling without long-term sequelae.

TABLE 21.9: Therapy of lichen sclerosus (Akel et al., 2018)
Extragenital lichen sclerosus
• UVA-1 (30–60 J/cm^2) phototherapy for 10 weeks
• Potent to ultrapotent topical steroids
• Tacrolimus ointment (0.1%) twice daily
• Systemic steroids/methotrexate
Genital LS
Female
• CP (0.05% ointment—OD × 30 days; alternate day × 30 days, 2/week × 30 days. Maintenance 2/week) Efficacy—70%
• Resolution of skin thickening and ecchymosis, but not pallor, as pallor does not always resolve completely
• More effective than tacrolimus 0.1%, testosterone 2% in petrolatum, ultraviolet A1 home-based phototherapy
• As efficacious as mometasone furoate 0.1%
• Treatment failure—poor compliance or coexistent vulvodynia, malignancy (SCC risk—5%)
Male
• Circumcision—first-line therapy
• CP (0.05% ointment OD) for 1–3 months with an emollient soap substitute and barrier
• 50% of male patients with LS respond to CP
• Surgery—boys, complete circumcision is the treatment of choice, adult males may require surgery
• Subdermal injection of poly deoxyribonucleotide (a mitogen for fibroblasts, endothelial cells and adipocytes) is an interesting new approach
• Treatment failure—tight phimosis, obesity and burying of the penis, SCC risk 0–12.5%

CP, clobetasol propionate

BIBLIOGRAPHY

Books

1. Martin Rocken and Kamran Ghoreschi. Morphea and Lichen sclerosus. Bolognia LJ. Schafler VJ. Cerroni L Editors. In: Dermatology (4th Edition). Elsevier publishers. Ch 44: p 707–72.

2. Morphea (localized scleroderma) Part 4, Chapter 57: Rook's Textbook of Dermatology, Ninth Edition. Wiley Blackwell Publishing, 2016, UK.

Journals

1. Akel R, Fuller C. Updates in lichen sclerosis: British Association of Dermatologists guidelines for the management of lichen sclerosus 2018. Br J Dermatol. 2018 Apr;178(4):823-824. doi: 10.1111/bjd.16445. PMID: 29668094.
2. Boozalis E, Shah AA, Wigley F, Kang S, Kwatra SG. Morphea and systemic sclerosis are associated with an increased risk for melanoma and nonmelanoma skin cancer. J Am Acad Dermatol. 2019 May;80(5):1449–51.
3. Giuggioli D, Colaci M, Cocchiara E, Spinella A, Lumetti F, Ferri C. From Localized Scleroderma to Systemic Sclerosis: Coexistence or Possible Evolution. Dermatol Res Pract. 2018 Jan 30;2018:1284687.
4. Kirtschig G. Lichen sclerosus-presentation, diagnosis and management. Deutsches Ärzteblatt International. 2016 May;113(19):337.
5. Knobler, et al. European Dermatological Forum S1—guidelines on the diagnosis and treatment of sclerosing disease of the skin. Part I—localized scleroderma, systemic sclerosis and overlap syndromes. JEADV 2017; 31:1401–24.
6. Kurzinski KL, Zigler CK, Torok KS. Prediction of disease relapse in a cohort of paediatric patients with localized scleroderma. Br J Dermatol. 2019 May;180(5):1183–9.
7. Papara C, De Luca DA, Bieber K, Vorobyev A, Ludwig RJ. Morphea: The 2023 update. Front Med (Lausanne). 2023 Feb 13;10:1108623.
8. Ramos-Rodríguez D, Arteaga-Henríquez M, Lukoviek V, Markthaler M. Ink test: A useful technique to enhance extragenital lichen sclerosus diagnosis. Pediatr Dermatol. 2022 Jul;39(4):648–649.
9. Walker, et al. Histopathological changes in morphea and their clinical correlation: Results for the Morphea in Adults and Children cohort (MAC) V. J Am Acad Dermatol 2017;76:1124–30.
10. Yadav D, Agarwal S, Thakur S, Ramam M. Lymphocyte-Peppered Sclerotic Collagen: An Additional Histological Clue in Lichen Sclerosus, Morphea, and Systemic Sclerosis. Am J Dermatopathol. 2021 Dec 1;43(12):935–938.
11. Zulian F, Culpo R, Sperotto F, et al. Consensus-based recommendations for the management of juvenile localised scleroderma. Ann Rheum Dis. 2019 Aug;78(8):1019–24.

Chapter 22

Nail Disorders

Surabhi Sinha, Kabir Sardana, Sweta Singh

Nail changes are an important cutaneous finding—both isolated and as a part of a disorder. Few important nail disorders are discussed in the sections that follow.

TRACHYONYCHIA

First described in 1950 by Alkeiwicz.

Trachyonychia, also called 'rough nails', 'twenty-nail dystrophy' or 'sandpaper nails', is used to describe brittle, thin nails with diffuse longitudinal ridging, usually accompanied by loss of nail lustre. However, the term 'twenty-nail dystrophy' is a misnomer as trachyonychia can affect any number of nails.

Etiology

- Idiopathic: Presents as an isolated nail abnormality. More common in children.
- Can be caused by an inflammatory disease which mildly affects the nail matrix keratinization.
  - Alopecia areata (most common association—trachyonychia seen in 3.6% cases (AU > AT)
  - Lichen planus (seen in 10% nail LP cases)
  - Psoriasis
  - Eczema including atopic dermatitis
- Uncommon associations
  - Dermatologic
    - Amyloidosis
    - Darier's disease
    - Ichthyosis vulgaris
    - Palmoplantar keratoderma
    - Pemphigus vulgaris
    - Vitiligo
  - Systemic
    - Amyloidosis
    - Autoimmune hemolytic anemia

- Chemotherapeutic agents
- Down syndrome
- Hematologic abnormalities (i.e. idiopathic thrombocytopenia)
- IgA deficiency
- Immune dysregulation polyendocrinopathy enteropathy X-linked syndrome (IPEX)
- Incontinentia pigmenti (Bloch–Sulzberger syndrome)
- Primary biliary cirrhosis
- Reflex sympathetic dystrophy
- Sarcoidosis

Clinical Features

- More commonly seen in childhood.
- Involves whole of the nail plate and when all the 20 nails are involved, it is known as 'twenty nail dystrophy (TND)'.
- Clinically asymptomatic
- Two types (Baran):
  - **Opaque (sand-blasted nails)**—more severe and more common type, grey roughened **'sandpaper'** surface of the nail plate, extensive longitudinal ridging, cuticles thickened and ragged, nail plate thickened/thinned. Due to waxing and waning nail matrix inflammation that never ceases.
  - **Shiny (Fig. 22.1)**—less severe and less common type, shiny opalescent nails with numerous pits that reflect light. Mostly in alopecia areata. Due to intermittent recurrent nail matrix inflammation with periods of normal function in-between.

The investigations and differential diagnoses (DDs) are listed in **Boxes 22.1** and **22.2**.

BOX 22.1: Investigations in trachyonychia

1. **Onychoscopy**
   - Opaque: The nail plate shows multiple fine and superficial longitudinal fissures covered by thin scales.
   - Shiny: The nail plate shows superficial ridging and a myriad of small geometrical pits.
2. **Histopathology**
   - Longitudinal nail matrix biopsy is needed rarely to ascertain the cause of inflammation in severe, recalcitrant cases. (After ruling out fungus by PAS stain.)
   - Isolated form shows lymphocytic infiltrate and exocytosis into the epidermis and spongiosis within the matrix. Findings of other specific causes may be seen.
   - The histopathologic changes observed in trachyonychia, regardless of underlying cause, appear to be more prominent in the proximal nail matrix and ventral proximal nail fold.

BOX 22.2: Differential diagnosis of trachyonychia

Brittle nails: Will not exhibit the typical excessive longitudinal ridging and roughness but will have some longitudinal and superficial splitting of the nail.

Senile nails: Have mild longitudinal ridging, but this abnormality will not involve the entire nail plate as in trachyonychia.

Alopecia areata: One-third have nail pitting, but only 12% can be classified as having trachyonychia.

Lichen planus: Longitudinal fissures and pterygium, which are not seen in trachyonychia.

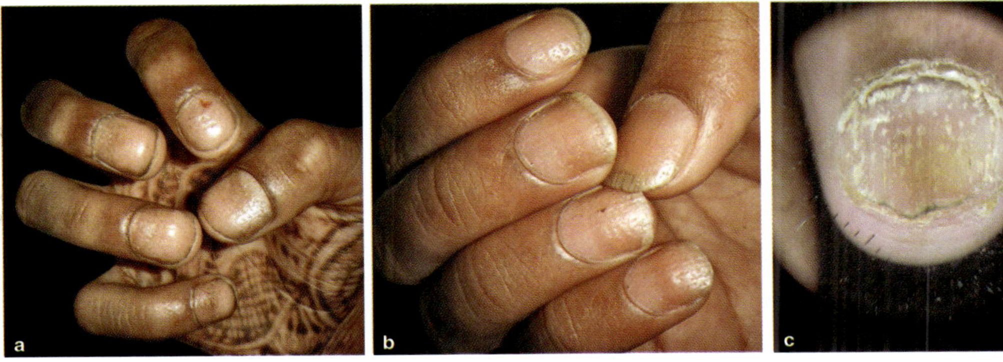

Fig. 22.1: (a and b) Trachyonychia (shiny type); (c) Trachyonychia (onychoscopic image of opaque type)

Treatment

Principle: A variety of treatment options exist, and the treatment should be conservative since this is a nonscarring condition. Counseling, active nonintervention and reassurance are effective. A lower threshold for treatment can be employed in adults. **Table 22.1** lists the treatment options that have been tried, though none has been very effective.

Mild emollients are helpful in severe trachyonychia and nail polish in less severe, shiny trachyonychia. A summary of the clinical course is given in **Box 22.3**.

TABLE 22.1: Treatment options for trachyonychia

Topical	• Calcipotriol/betamethasone dipropionate ointment—4–8 months • Topical tazarotene gel—3 months • 5% 5-fluorouracil cream—4 months • Alitretinoin: 30 mg of alitretinoin daily for at least 3 months
Systemic	• Biotin (20 mg/day)—6 months • Chloroquine phosphate (250 mg twice daily)—30 weeks • Cyclosporine (3 mg/kg)—3 months • PUVA therapy—6–7 months • Acitretin (0.3 mg/kg)—3 months • Tofacitinib citrate (5 mg twice daily)—3–6 months • Prednisolone (0.5 mg/kg)—4 weeks
Intralesional	Intralesional injection of triamcinolone into proximal nail fold

BOX 22.3: Clinical course of trachyonychia

- Nonscarring condition
- Children—shorter disease, 50% spontaneous resolution in 6 years.
- Mostly self-resolving, nails usually improve over time even in adults.

ONYCHOMYCOSIS

Onychomycosis (OM) refers to the fungal infection of the nail plate. It can be caused by dermatophytes (tinea unguium), nondermatophyte moulds and *Candida* species. The most common dermatophytes isolated are *Trichophyton rubrum*, *T. interdigitale* and, infrequently, *E. floccosum*.

Epidemiology

- Prevalence of dermatophytic onychomycosis: 6–25%
- Age—rare in children
- Sex—equal distribution
- **Toenails** are more frequently involved than finger nails (TN > FN)

Predisposing Factors

- Tinea pedis
- Nail trauma
- Geriatric age—due to slow linear growth of nail
- Immunocompromised state/diabetes.

Pathogenesis

Flowchart 22.1 is a schematic diagram outlining the pathogenesis of OM.

Neoscytalidium species produce keratinases which help in penetration of the stratum corneum.

Flowchart 22.1: Schematic diagram showing the pathogenesis of OM

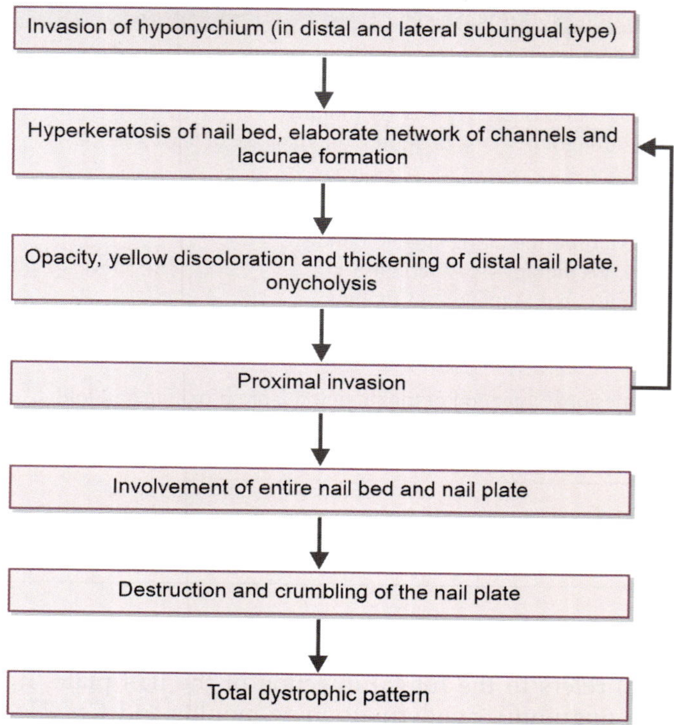

Clinical Types/Variants

Onychomycosis is divided into seven main patterns **(Table 22.2)** depending on the site of nails apparatus involvement and how the infection is initiated. **Figure 22.2** shows two clinical variants of onychomycosis. The diagnostic parameters are listed in **Box 22.4** and the differential diagnosis are listed in **Boxes 22.5** and **22.6**.

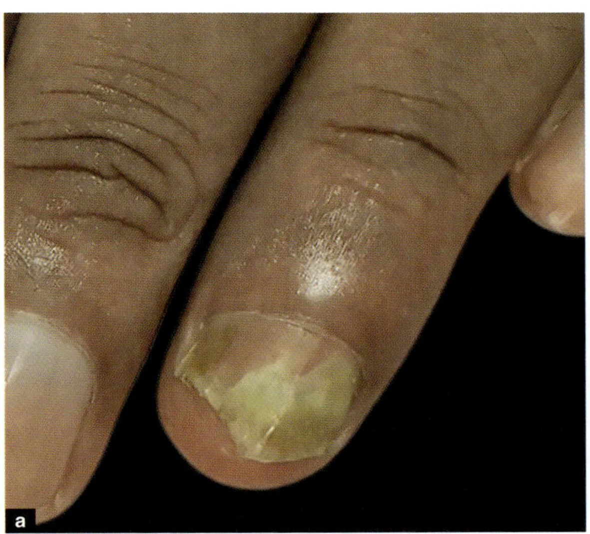

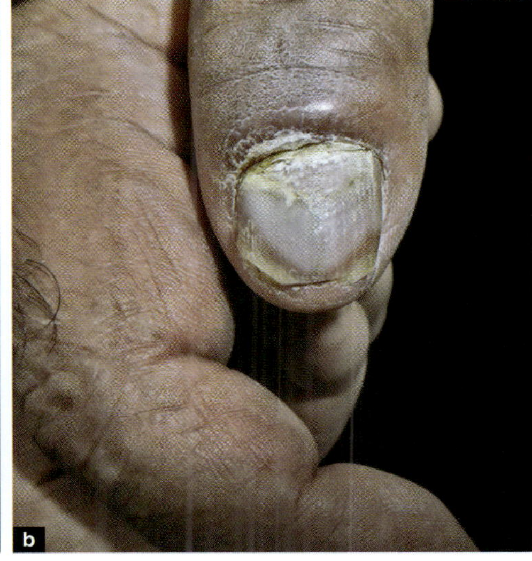

Fig. 22.2: (a) DLSO; (b) Mixed OM (DLSO + PSO)—paronychia can also be seen in the image

TABLE 22.2: Patterns of onychomycosis

S. No.	Patterns of onychomycosis	Subtypes	Causative fungi	Clinical features
1.	**Distal and lateral subungual onychomycosis (DLSO)**		• Dermatophytes—(*Trichophyton rubrum*, *T. mentagrophytes*) • *Candida albicans*, • *Fusarium spp.*, • *Neoscytalidium* spp., • *Scopulariopsis brevicaulis*	**Most common pattern** • Present as streak or a patch of white or yellow discoloration near the free edge of the nail plate and lateral nail fold • In nondermatophytic infection—extensive undermining of nail plate from lateral and distal edges, leading to transverse fracture of nail plate
2.	**Superficial onychomycosis (SO) (white or black)**	Patchy	• *T. mentagrophytes*, • *T. rubrum*, • *Fusarium* spp., • *Acremonium* spp., • *Neoscytalidium* spp.	• Classical—well circumscribed, powdery white patches due to erosion of dorsal surface of nail plate Easily scrapable. • Black discoloration (in nondermatophytic infections)

(*Contd.*)

TABLE 22.2: Patterns of onychomycosis *(Contd.)*

S. No.	Patterns of onychomycosis	Subtypes	Causative fungi	Clinical features
		Transverse	• *T. rubrum*, • *Fusarium* spp.	• Frequently in immunocompromised state, e.g. AIDS • Linear transverse streaks, away from free edge
3.	**Proximal subungual onychomycosis (PSO)**	Patchy, striate (transverse), longitudinal	• *T. rubrum*, • *Fusarium* spp.	• Very uncommon • Present as linear bands or patches near proximal nail fold • Due to rapid deeper invasion of the nail plate from proximal nail folds **Frequently in immunocompromised state, e.g. AIDS**
4.	**Endonyx onychomycosis**		• *T. soudanense*, • *T. violaceum*	• Pits and lamellar splits in the nail plate • Invasion occurs from superficial nail surface deep into nail plate
5.	**Totally dystrophic onychomycosis (TDO)**		• Dermatophytes, • *C. albicans*, • *Neoscytalidium* spp.	Total nail plate destruction and crumbling in severe infection
6.	**Mixed onychomycosis**	DLSO plus SO SO plus PSO DLSO plus PSO	• *T. rubrum*, • *Fusarium* spp. • *T. rubrum*, • *Fusarium* spp. • *T. rubrum*	Presence of ≥2 different patterns on same nail
7.	**Paronychia**	**With** onychomycosis	• *Candida* spp., • *Fusarium* spp., • *Neoscytalidium* spp.	• Loss of cuticle • Detachment of proximal and lateral nail fold from dorsal nail plate • Swelling and redness of nail folds and discharge • Nail dystrophy with buckling of nail plate, onycholysis • Common cause of onychomycosis in children <3 years
		Without onychomycosis	• *Candida* spp., • *Fusarium* spp., • *Neoscytalidium* spp.	• Loss of cuticle • Detachment of proximal and lateral nail fold from dorsal nail plate • Swelling and redness of nail folds and discharge

BOX 22.4: Diagnosis of onychomycosis

Careful examination of skin of palms and soles

- **Bedside tests:** Nail clipping (as proximal as possible) or scraping (subungual debris under the nail with no. 15 blade or 1–2 mm serrated curette) for direct microscopy.
  - **Direct microscopy:** KOH (10–30%), can be heated if required to soften the nail.
  - Sodium sulfide solution (10%)—no heat required.
  - Jagged edge of proximal margin of onycholysis, with sharp spikes directed proximally towards proximal nail fold (PNF).
  - White-yellow longitudinal striae in the onycholytic nail plate.
  - Affected nail plate with parallel bands of fading colors resembles the aurora borealis **(aurora borealis pattern)**.
- **HPE**
  - Special stains: Periodic acid-Schiff (PAS) stain.
- **Culture:** Sabouraud dextrose agar.
  - Duplicate cultures on media.
  - With cycloheximide—for dermatophytic infection.
  - Without cycloheximide—for nondermatophytic molds.

BOX 22.5: Differential diagnosis of dermatophytic OM

Disease	Dissimilarity
• Eczema	• Irregularly buckled nail • Pits may be present
• Lichen planus	• Onychorrhexis (longitudinal splitting), thinning and longitudinal ridging of the nail plate • Trachyonychia, pterygium, anonychia • Fingernails > Toenails
• Psoriasis	• Nail pits, splinter hemorrhages, oil staining

BOX 22.6: Differential diagnosis of nondermatophytic OM (*Neoscytalidium* spp.)

Disease	Similarity	Dissimilarity
1. Dry type *T. rubrum* infection	Onycholysis Distal and lateral involvement	• Extensive undermining of nail plate from lateral and distal edges, leading to transverse fracture of nail plate • Relatively less thickening of nail plate
2. Candida paronychia	Distal and lateral nail fold involvement, loss of cuticle	• Onychomycosis with paronychia, blackish discoloration of nail plate

Treatment

The various treatment options are listed in **Table 22.3** and **Flowchart 22.2** gives a treatment algorithm for the management of onychomycosis.

Treatment of Dermatophytic Onychomycosis

We will dwell on this as this is a common variant of onychomycosis. The therapy in clinical practice can be either generic as given in **Table 22.3** or can be based on the severity.

1. **Mild-to-moderate dermatophyte onychomycosis:** (For example, distal lateral subungual onychomycosis involving ≤50% involvement of the nail and sparing the matrix/lunula)
   - Oral terbinafine.

- Topical agents: Efinaconazole (10% solution is applied directly to the nails once daily for 48 weeks), amorolfine (amorolfine 5% nail lacquer once a week), tavaborole (5% solution once daily) and ciclopirox (8% nail lacquer daily).
- Topical preferred if:
  - Contraindications to systemic anti-fungal therapy
  - Patients at risk for drug-drug interactions with systemic anti-fungal drugs
  - Patients who prefer to avoid systemic treatment (especially with three or fewer nails involved).
  - Children

2. **Moderate-to-severe dermatophyte onychomycosis:** For example, dermatophyte onychomycosis involving >50% of the nail **or** involving the matrix or lunula, proximal subungual onychomycosis, or total dystrophic onychomycosis.

Systemic terbinafine or itraconazole as given in **Table 22.3**. In children (NOT adults), body weight adjusted doses are given in **Boxes 22.7** and **22.8**.

TABLE 22.3: Treatment options for OM according to causative agents

	First line (standard adult dose)	Second line (standard adult dose)
Dermatophytic onychomycosis (mild DLSO/patchy SO)	• Topical – Amorolfine – Ciclopirox	
Dermatophytic onychomycosis (moderate–severe)	• Terbinafine (250 mg/day) – FN—6 weeks – TN—12 weeks • Itraconazole (200 mg/day) – FN—6 weeks – TN—12 weeks • Pulse itraconazole (200 mg twice daily—1 week/month) – FN—2–3 pulses* – TN—3–4 pulses	Griseofulvin (500 mg twice daily—4–8 months)
White superficial onychomycosis	• Mechanical removal of the involved area (i.e. scraping the superficial nail plate) followed by a topical antifungal agent	
***Neoscytalidium* spp.**	• Same as above but seldom responds to drugs. Voriconazole has been shown to be more effective than itraconazole and terbinafine	The topical therapies (efinaconazole, amorolfine, tavaborole, and ciclopirox) have some activity against yeasts and nondermatophyte molds
Scopulariopsis brevicaulis	• 40% urea paste for chemical nail avulsion → an azole anti-fungal cream or lotion to be applied daily to the nail bed • Itraconazole 200 mg/twice a day for 1 week/month Duration: 2–3 months for fingernails 3–4 months for toenails	

(Contd.)

TABLE 22.3: Treatment options for OM according to causative agents *(Contd.)*

	First line (standard adult dose)	Second line (standard adult dose)
Fusarium onychomycosis	• Oral itraconazole and terbinafine are commonly used	• Newer triazoles, voriconazole and posaconazole, have greater *in vitro* activity against *Fusarium* spp. than itraconazole • Voriconazole (loading dose of 400 mg orally every 12 hours for two doses, followed by 200 mg orally twice daily) • Adjunctive nail avulsion with topical amphotericin B can be used in patients who do not respond to systemic antifungal therapy, but is usually avoided in severely immunocompromised patients
Candidal paronychia	• Azole solution to be used twice daily for 2–4 months depending on clinical response + A medium strength topical corticosteroid applied to the nail fold skin once daily • **Itraconazole** 100 mg/day for 1–2 months • **Fluconazole** 100 mg/day for 1–2 months	4% thymol solution

*Pulse itraconazole only approved for fingernail OM.
FN, fingernail; TN, toenail.

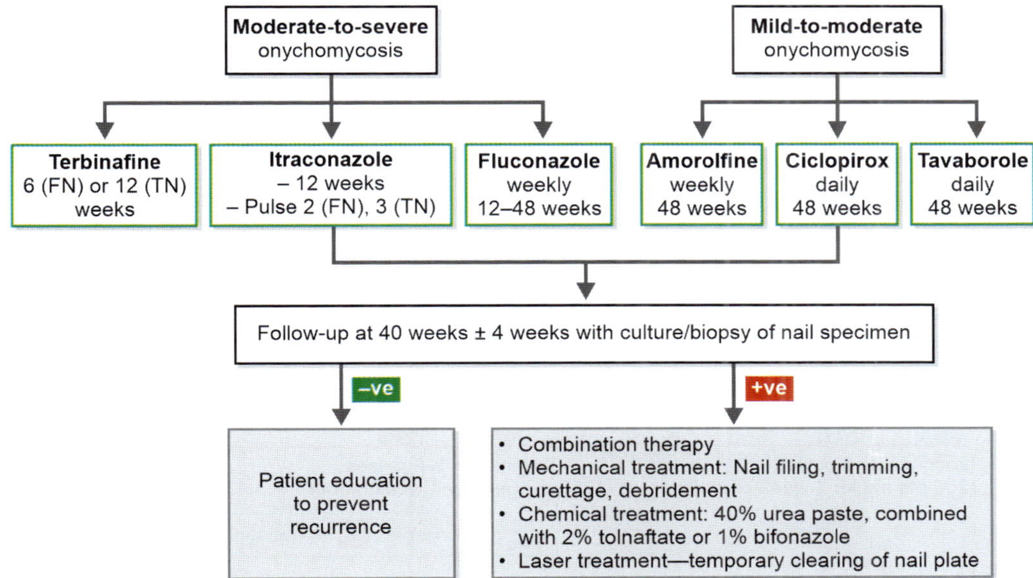

Flowchart 22.2: Treatment algorithm for onychomycosis (*modified from* Thomas et al. 2010)

BOX 22.7: Dosage of terbinafine according to body weight

Weight	Dose
<20 kg	62.5 mg/day
20–40 kg	125 mg/day
>40 kg	250 mg/day

Box 22.8: Dosage of pulse itraconazole according to body weight

Weight	Dose
<20 kg	5 mg/kg for 1 week/month
20–40 kg	100 mg/day for 1 week/month
40–50 kg	200 mg/day for 1 week/month
>50 kg	200 mg twice daily for 1 week/month

Regimens to Improving Efficacy

1. **Booster or supplemental therapy for onychomycosis:** In this a second anti-fungal is given at months 6–9 after the start of treatment **(Fig. 22.3)**.

   The objective of this supplemental dosage is to maintain a drug concentration greater than the minimal inhibitory concentration (MIC) for a longer period of time than with standard therapy duration, thus increasing the chances of eliminating infection.

   Booster therapy may be considered at 3–6 months after completing the initial 3-month course of oral terbinafine or itraconazole if any of the following conditions are met:

   - There is poor nail outgrowth (<50% reduction in the initial nail plate area that was diseased at baseline)

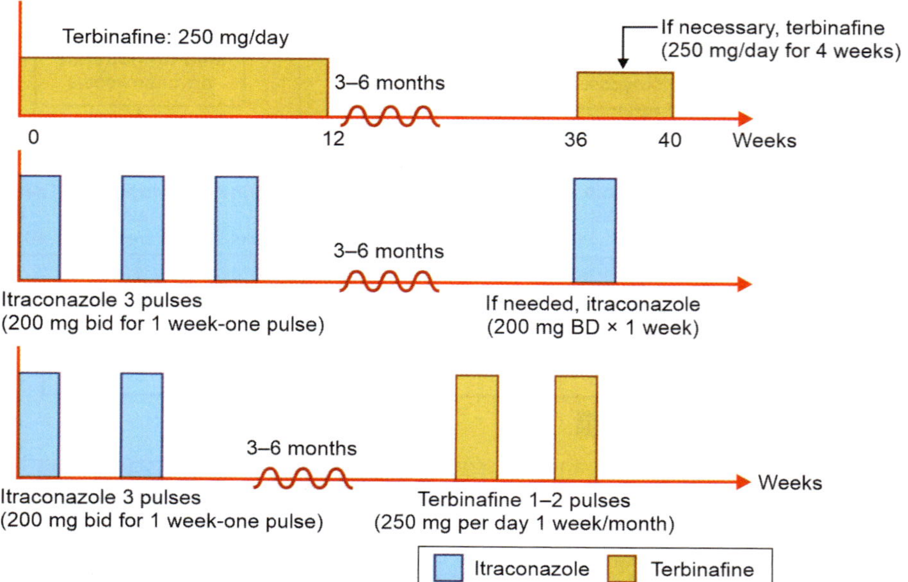

Fig. 22.3: Suggested booster therapy regimens, usually the same drug is given after a gap of 3–6 months but a switch to another drug may also be considered

- The nail plate is thickened (>2 mm thickness).
- There is a positive culture at month six post-initiation of oral antifungal therapy.
- Severe onychomycosis was present at baseline (proximal involvement or >75% of nail plate or bed is diseased).
- There is dermatophytoma, lateral onychomycosis, severe onycholysis, or immunosuppression; or there is a history of relapse.

2. **Boosted therapies (BATT and BOAT):** It has been hypothesized that complete cure is not achieved because of dormant chlamydospores and arthroconidia present inside the infected nail plate which are less susceptible to antifungal drugs compared with fungal filaments. Boosting their germination using agar may increase response to treatment and reduce recurrence. This is the basis of boosted antifungal topical treatment (BATT) and its counterpart, boosted oral antifungal treatment (BOAT).
3. **Combination therapies:** This entails combining oral and topical agents.

Prevention of Relapse

Long-term recurrence rates of onychomycosis range from approximately **20–50%**. An overview of the causes of treatment failure is listed in **Box 22.9**. Methods that are sometimes tried in an attempt to prevent recurrence include intermittent oral antifungal therapy and the application of topical antifungal creams, powders, or ciclopirox to affected nails after clinical cure is attained. There is little objective evidence to support these attempts at preventing relapses.

BOX 22.9: Causes of treatment failure in onychomycosis

- Total dystrophic onychomycosis
- Dermatophytoma (mass of hyphae below nail plate seen as linear opaque streaks)
- Involvement of proximal nail bed
- Subungual hyperkeratosis >2 mm thick
- Lateral involvement
- >50% involvement of nail
- Old age
- Immunosuppression
- Peripheral vascular disease
- Diabetes mellitus
- Mixed disease (e.g. psoriasis with OM)
- Inadequate antifungal choice or delivery modality
- Early termination of treatment, missed doses
- Presence of dormant conidia, sequestrated mycelium pockets or resistant species

NAIL PSORIASIS

Epidemiology

- Nail involvement can be seen in up to 50% of psoriasis patients.
- Nail involvement in children with psoriasis can be in 7–39% cases.

Pathogenesis

- The etiological factors are the same as cutaneous psoriasis with the nail plate being affected consequent to the localized skin changes.

- High degree of correlation of the nail matrix inflammation with the inflammation of the adjacent DIP and the enthesitis of the extensor tendon of the same joint.

Clinical Features

Nail psoriasis presents variably depending upon the predominant part of nail involved. **Table 22.4** enlists the various clinical manifestations of nail psoriasis which are depicted in **Figs 22.4** and **22.5**). The severity of involvement is assessed with the NAPSI score and more recently, the modified NAPSI **(Box 22.10** and **Fig. 22.6)**.

A summary of the differential diagnosis **(Box 22.11)**, histopathological changes **(Box 22.12)** and clinical course **(Box 22.13)** can be referred to for better understanding of the topic.

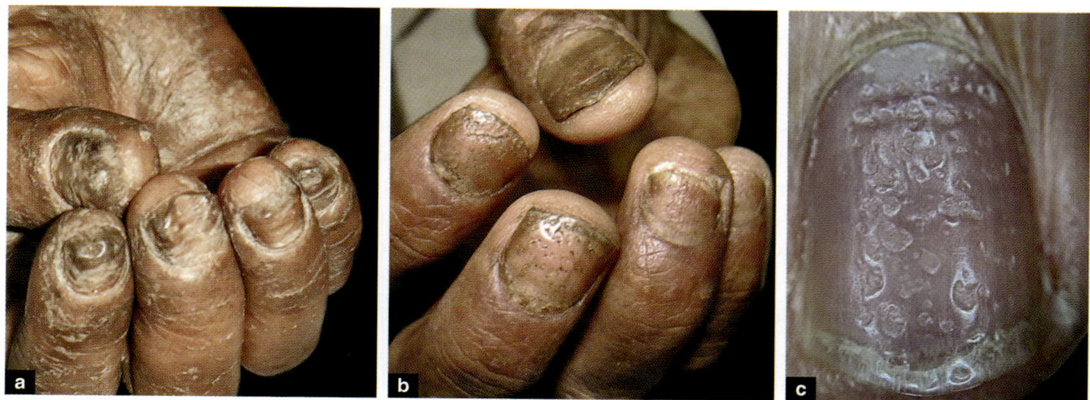

Fig. 22.4: Clinical photographs of nail psoriasis with: (a) nail plate thickening and discoloration with subungual hyperkeratosis; (b) extensive nail pitting with mild nail plate thickening; (c) magnified view of a thumb nail showing the deep, randomly placed, irregularly shaped and large pits seen in psoriasis (Mnemonic—DRIL)

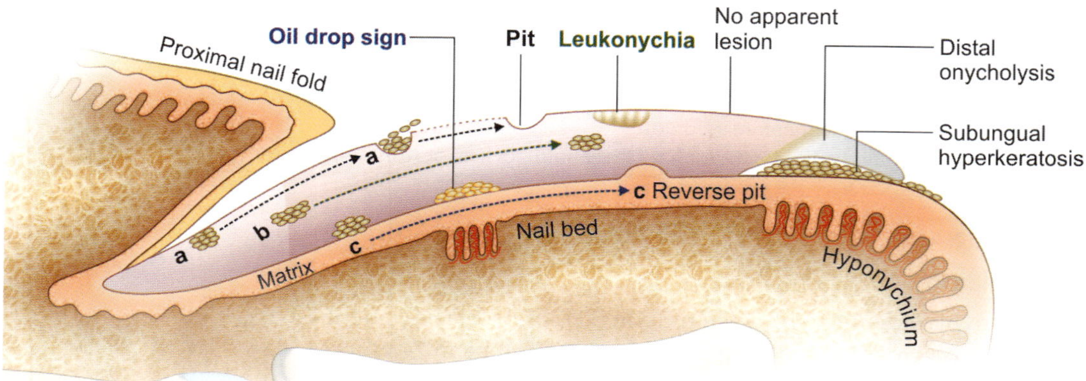

Fig. 22.5: Overview of nail findings in psoriasis depending on the defect on the (a) Proximal; (b) Intermediate; (c) Distal matrix and nail bed

TABLE 22.4: Nail psoriasis manifestations according to the predominant anatomical structure involved

Nail changes	Clinical presentation	Part of nail involved	Duration of disease
Matrix and nail plate abnormalities	**Pitting (most common)** **FN > TN** Random, shallow or large, a punched out defect +/– (elkonyxis)	Proximal matrix (inflammation of the proximal nail matrix causes parakeratosis and the parakeratotic cells fall, leaving the pits on the nail plate. >60 pits confirms psoriasis)	Short
	Splitting, crumbling, thickening	Entire matrix	Prolonged
	Transverse furrows **Leukonychia** with rough surface	Proximal matrix Middle or distal matrix (parakeratotic cells remain within the nail plate in leuconychia?)	1–2 weeks Variable
Nail bed changes	**O**il spot/salmon patch (specific nail finding)	Focal nail bed parakeratosis (lymphocytes, parakeratotic cells, and neutrophils and accrual of glycoprotein contribute to the oil spots)	Prolonged
	Onycholysis–extension of oil spot to free edge/ disruption of onychocorneal band	Nail bed parakeratosis (an erythematous border around the onycholytic area in fingernails is diagnostic for psoriasis)	Prolonged
	Subungual hyperkeratosis—most marked distally with proximal extension	Nail bed disease	
	Splinter hemorrhages red lunula	Fragility of nail bed dermis and increased capillary prominence vessel dilatation or changes	Short
Miscellaneous	Yellow/green discoloration of nail bed	Candidal/pseudomonal infection. Can also be secondary to nail plate thickening	Prolonged
	Acropustulosis-associated erythema with pain at the distal end of the digit	Sterile pustules involving either the nail bed or the nail matrix	Variable with long-term loss of nail

FN, fingernail; TN, toenail

Nail Psoriasis Severity Index (NAPSI)

The target nail is graded for nail matrix psoriasis and nail bed psoriasis. The sum of these two scores is the total score for that nail.

Nail matrix psoriasis consists of any of the following: Pitting, leukonychia, red spots in the lanula and nail plate crumbling.

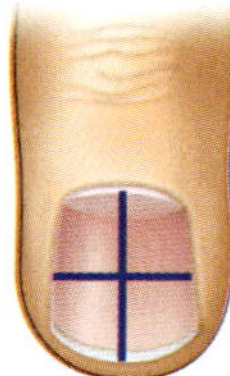

Score for matrix psoriasis ___
0 = None
1 = Present in 1/4th nail
2 = Present in 2/4th nail
3 = Present in 3/4th nail
4 = Present in 4/4th nail

Nail bed psoriasis is the presence or absence of any of the following: Onycholysis, splinter hemorrhages, oil drop (salmon patch) discoloration, and nail bed hyperkeratosis

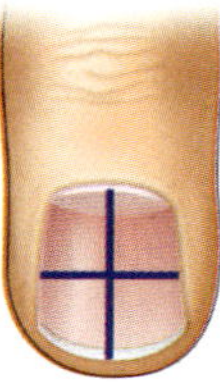

Score for nail bed psoriasis ___
0 = None
1 = Present in 1/4th nail
2 = Present in 2/4th nail
3 = Present in 3/4th nail
4 = Present in 4/4th nail

Total for nail ________ **(0–8)**

Fig. 22.6: NAPSI

BOX 22.10: What is modified NAPSI (mNAPSI)?

For calculating NAPSI, each nail is divided into four quadrants. Each quadrant is evaluated for the presence of any manifestation of psoriasis in the nail matrix or nail bed **(Fig. 22.6)**. The lesion(s) of nail matrix and nail bed are given a score of 1 in each quadrant, so that there is nail matrix score of 0–4 and nail bed score of 0–4 per nail with a maximum score of 8 and a minimum score of 0 per nail. Maximum NAPSI score of all fingers and/or toes are 80 and 160, respectively.

mNAPSI is modified NAPSI which would give a degree of gradation for each parameter of 0–3 (0, none; 1, mild; 2, moderate; 3; severe) in each quadrant, for better measurement of clinical improvement. This same grading system is used for all 8 parameters, giving the target nail score a range of 0–96.

BOX 22.11: Differential diagnosis of pits in nail psoriasis

Psoriatic pits—are deeper than the pits observed in other nail disorders, because the inflammation involves the intermediate and ventral nail plate. It has been suggested that one should consider psoriasis in the differential diagnosis if at least **20 pits** are present, while over **60 pits** confirm it.

- **Pits in AA:** Pits in alopecia areata are small, superficial and often arranged in geometric patterns, associated with punctate leukonychia, onychomadesis and trachyonychia.
- **Pits in eczema:** Coarse, very irregular and associated with cross ridging.
- **Onychomycosis:** Toenails > fingernails with a few digits involved.
- **Lichen planus:** Pitting is rarely seen, dorsal pterygium formation, pup tent sign.
- **Parakeratosis pustulosa:** Single digit involved, erythema and scaling of periungual area, self-resolving, pustules rarely seen.
- **Reactive arthritis:** Difficult to differentiate from psoriasis.

BOX 22.12: Histopathology of nail psoriasis

- Presence of granular layer in matrix and nail bed
- Loss of granular layer in hyponychium
- Mounds of parakeratosis in the nail bed with neutrophils
- Presence of Munro's microabscess
- Pits within the nail plate are lined by parakeratotic cells.

BOX 22.13: Clinical course and prognosis of nail psoriasis

Nail changes are present in up to 50% of psoriasis cases.
Nail psoriasis is associated with more extensive psoriasis, longer disease duration, family history of psoriasis and the presence of psoriatic arthritis.

Management

Usually most of the systemic agents work well for nail psoriasis. Apart from the list of treatment options given in **Table 22.5**, even biological drugs, lasers and PDT have been tried. **Flowchart 22.3** gives an algorithm for nail psoriasis based on number and part of nails involved. Common questions on the topic are given in **Box 22.14**.

TABLE 22.5: Treatment options for nail psoriasis

General	Topical	Intralesional	Systemic
Avoid local trauma to nails	Topical **nail lacquer** hardened by table top UV lamp	Intramatricial **Trimacinolone** Injection: 10 mg/mL—0.1 mL at each site	Photochemotherapy in the form of localized PUVA to nail unit
Treat the associated fungal infection if present	• High potency steroid application—**Clobetasol propionate** • **Vitamin D analogues** like calcipotriol (not effective for proximal nail fold inflammation but avoids risk of atrophy) (Effective maintenance therapy for pustular psoriasis) • **Tacrolimus** 0.1% ointment • **Tazarotene** 0.1% gel • **5-FU** in 20% urea base/propylene glycol		**Acitretin**—can cause nail plate thinning **Methotrexate** and cyclosporine—can be used but *not recommended* for the disease of nail unit alone, *effective* in acrodermatitis continua of Hallopeau

Differential Diagnosis of Nail Psoriasis

The commonest differential diagnosis is onychomycosis which may sometime coexist with nail psoriasis **(Table 22.6)**.

TABLE 22.6: Differentiation of nail psoriasis and onychomycosis

Feature	Nail psoriasis	Onychomycosis
Skin lesions	Psoriatic lesions	Tinea pedis/mannum
No. of nails	Several usually	Usually great toenails only
Fingernails/toenails	FN > TN	TN > FN
Nail plate surface	Pitting, many surface abnormalities	Normal surface texture
Nail plate color	Oil drop sign, erythematous halo at proximal edge of onycholysis	White to yellow to orange or brown (resemble aurora borealis on dermoscopy-aurora borealis pattern)
Dermoscopy	Proximal margin of detachment has a slightly dented edge	Typical ragged edge with sharp spikes directed proximally
Subungual hyperkeratosis	Silvery white color	White to yellow to green to brown color
Proximal nail fold	May show psoriatic plaques	Normal, may be inflamed if molds are the cause

FN, fingernail; TN, toenail

Flowchart 22.3: Treatment algorithm for nail psoriasis according to the number and part of nail involved (*modified from* Rigopoulos et al)

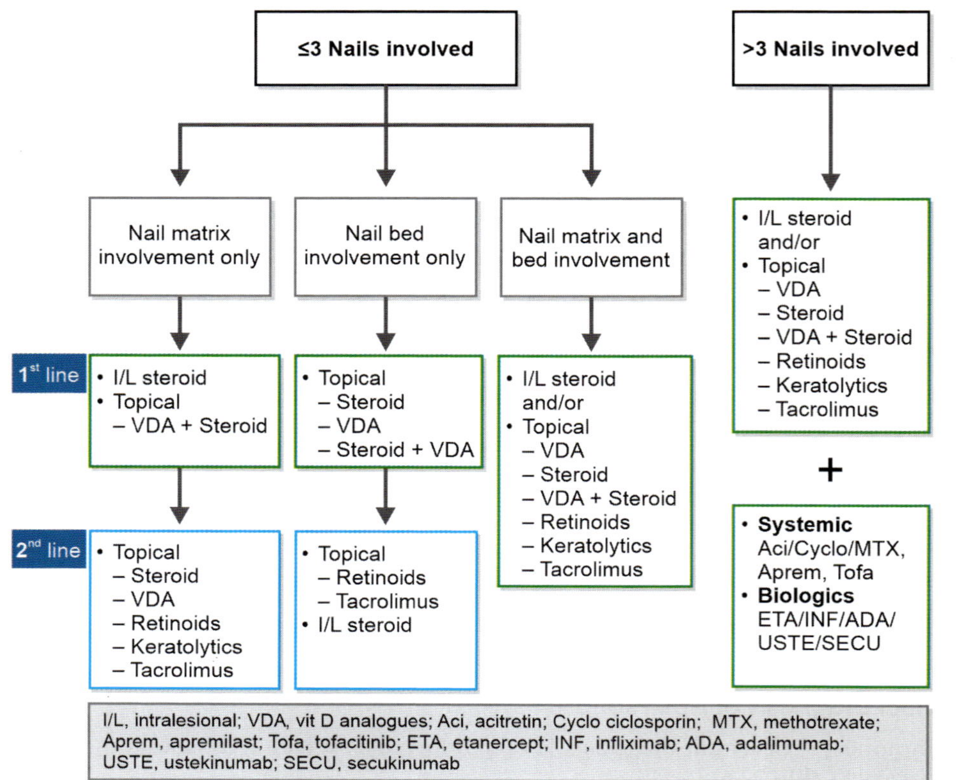

BOX 22.14: Factoids about nail psoriasis[Q]

- Does nail psoriasis predispose to onychomycosis?
  Yes. Compact orthokeratotic nail plate is replaced by loose parakeratotic plate + nail bed detached from nail plate leaving moist subungual space which is easily invaded by microbes
- Does psoriasis paradoxically protect against OM also?
  - Rapid turnover of affected nail prevents invasion of nail keratin by fungus.
  - Serum-like glycoprotein in oil spots—inhibits dermatophyte growth.
  - AMP (e.g. psoriasins)—upregulated in psoriasis → protect against infections.

  However, studies are still inconclusive. Some show increased OM in psoriasis, some show decreased incidence. OM due to non-dermatophyte molds and *Candida* spp.—more common than dermatophyte OM in psoriasis.
- Does treatment of nail psoriasis predispose to OM?
  Yes. Topical CS, systemic cyclosporin-A and methotrexate, anti-TNF-α, esp. infliximab—all predispose.
- Can OM increase severity of nail psoriasis?
  Yes, by koebnerization.

[Q], commonly asked questions in postgraduate examination.

NAIL LICHEN PLANUS

Disseminated LP has nail involvement in 10% of the cases.

Isolated nail LP is uncommon but equally distressing.

Clinical Features

Depending on severity of the inflammatory damage and its localization, nail LP may clinically present as different variants:

- **'Typical' nail lichen planus** (of matrix, of nail bed, or of matrix + nail bed), accounting for about 80% of the cases
- **Trachyonychia,** responsible for about 8% of the cases
- **Idiopathic atrophy** of the nails, accounting for less than 5% of patients
- **Yellow nail syndrome (YNS)—like LP,** rare
- **Bullous—erosive LP,** extremely rare.

The list of manifestations is shown in **Table 22.7** and is depicted in **Fig. 22.7**.

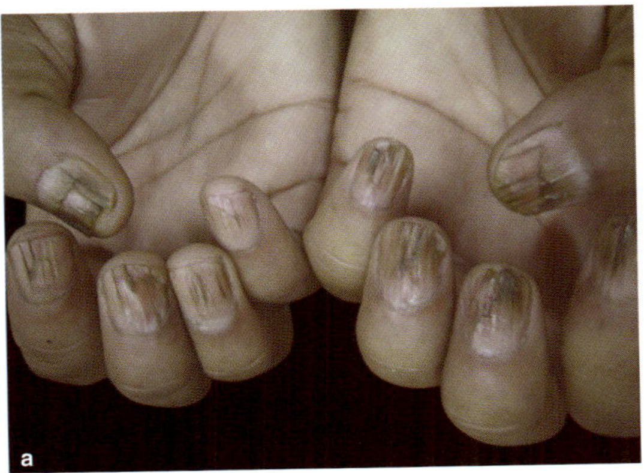

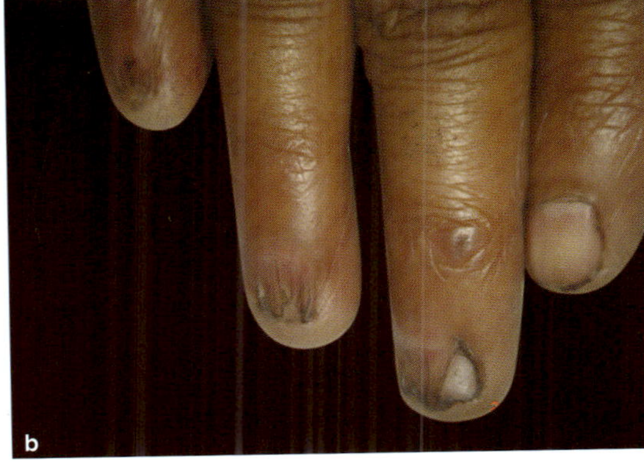

Fig. 22.7: Lichen planus of nails. Longitudinal ridging and fissuring with nail plate thinning. Matrix Slow but potentially scarring. Longitudinal ridging and fissuring

TABLE 22.7: Nail LP manifestations

	Type	Clinical features
Typical nail lichen planus	Matrix	Longitudinal ridging and fissuring with nail plate thinning
		Slow but potentially scarring. Longitudinal ridging and fissuring Dorsal pterygium, anonychia Mottled lunulae
	Bed	Onycholysis Diffuse nail bed hyperkeratosis (hypertrophic LP)
Atypical Nail Lichen Planus	Trachyonychia	Thin longitudinal striations of the nail plate covered by minute scales
	Idiopathic atrophy of the nail	Total or subtotal absence of the nail plate with dorsal pterygium
	YNS-like	Severe nail thickening and yellow discoloration of the toenails
	Bullous-erosive LP	Absence of the nail plates, nail bed erosions and marked inflammation of the periungual skin
	Nail degloving	Partial or total avulsion of the nail and surrounding tissue
	Nail LP with involvement of the periungual tissues	Erythematous hyperkeratotic plaques in the proximal nail fold and distal pulp

YNS, yellow nail syndrome.

A severity assesment of nail LP is detailed in **Box 22.15** and the basic investigations are detailed in **Box 22.16**.

BOX 22.15: Grading of severity of nail LP

Mild: Nail thinning, longitudinal ridging, distal splitting of <3 mm in length, onycholysis <25%, and no nail bed hyperkeratosis.

Moderate: Partial fissuring, longitudinal grooves, distal splitting of 3–5 mm in length, onycholysis between 25% and 50%, mottled erythema of the lunula, and subungual hyperkeratosis.

Severe: Complete fissuring, deep grooves, splitting of >5 mm in length, onycholysis >50%, and diffuse erythema of the lunula. Pterygium and anonychia belong to this last stage and do not respond to any treatment.

BOX 22.16: Investigations

- Nail matrix/nail bed biopsy: Biopsy is not necessary in all cases but it is essential to rule out destructive LP to prevent scarring and permanent loss of nails.
  Histopathology: Hypergranulosis of the nail bed gives rise to the nail plate changes and subungual hyperkeratosis, Saw toothing of rete ridges, colloid bodies rarely present.

Differential Diagnosis

A detailed list of differential diagnosis is given in **Table 22.8**.

Treatment

The various treatment options are detailed in **Box 22.17** while **Flowchart 22.4** gives an algorithm for treatment of nail LP according to the number and parts of nail involved.

TABLE 22.8: Differential diagnosis of nail LP

Longitudinal ridging and fissuring:		
• Nail ageing	• Psoriasis	• Systemic amyloidosis
• Graft-versus-host disease	• Dyskeratosis congenita	• Lichen striatus
Dorsal pterygium:		
• Bullous diseases	• Digital ischemia	• Trauma/burns
Nail thickening of hypertrophic nail LP and toenail LP:		
• Nail psoriasis	• Onychomycosis	• Yellow nail syndrome (YNS)
Trachyonychia:		
• Nail psoriasis	• Eczema	• Alopecia areata of the nails
Bullous LP:		
• Bullous diseases	• Pyogenic grauloma of the nail bed	• Squamous cell carcinoma
• Melanoma		

BOX 22.17: Treatment options for Nail LP

- Initial stage of erythema of the nail fold with mild nail plate changes—**potent topical steroids** like clobetasol propionate applied daily for 2–3 months.
- **Injection triamcinolone acetonide** into the nail fold.
- In cases of severe ulcerative and scarring LP systemic steroids like **prednisolone** (up to 60 mg/day) or I/M inj of triamcinolone acetonide (0.5–1 mg/kg/month) for 3–6 months.
- **Dapsone** can be added to acitretin and systemic steroids to arrest the ulcerative and scarring variant
- **Acitretin, alitretinoin**
- **Methotrexate and JAK inhibitors**
- **Cyclosporine**

Flowchart 22.4: Treatment of nail lichen planus according to the number and part of nails involved

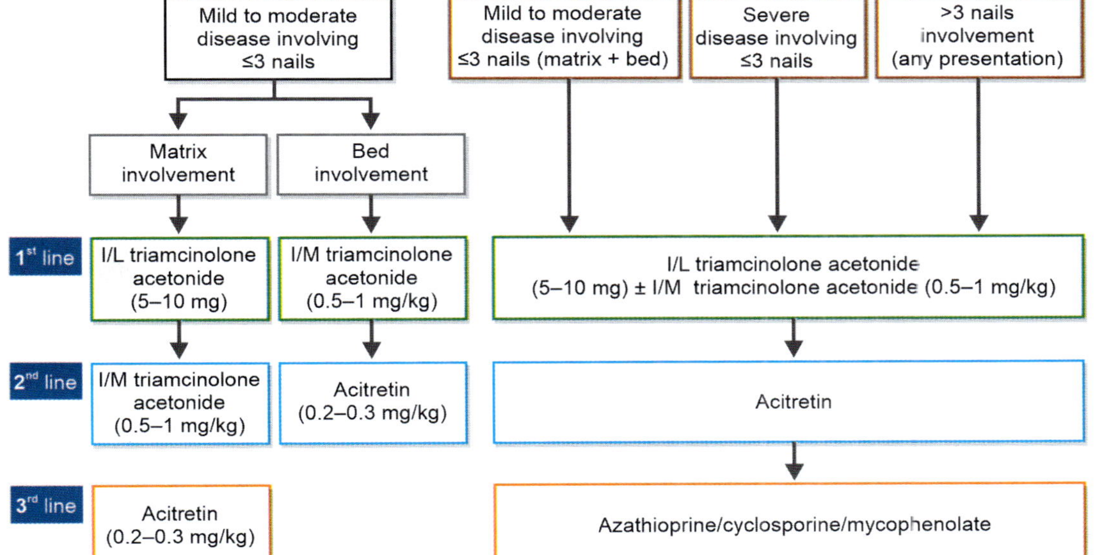

MELANONYCHIA STRIATA

Clinical presentation: Tan, brown, or black longitudinal streak within the nail plate that runs from the proximal nail fold to the distal part of the nail plate.
More common in adults with Fitzpatrick skin types IV, V, and VI.

Causes

Melanonychia striata is due to either increased activity of melanocytes or melanocytic hyperplasia in the nail matrix with subsequently increased melanin deposition in the nail plate. Most common cause—ethnic melanonychia which occurs in dark-skinned individuals. **Figure 22.8** shows for clinical appearance of racial/ethnic melanonychia and **Table 22.9** for common causes of melanonychia.

Nail apparatus/subungual melanoma should be suspected if there is an abrupt onset after middle age, personal or family history of melanoma, rapid growth, darkening of a melanonychia band, pigment variegation, blurry lateral borders, irregular elevation of the surface, a bandwidth >3 mm, proximal widening, associated nail plate dystrophy, single rather than multiple digit involvement, and periungual spread of pigmentation onto the adjacent cuticle and/or proximal and/or lateral nail folds **(Hutchinson sign)**. **Table 22.10** summarizes the difference between nail melanoma and melanonychia—two conditions that often need to be distinguished in clinical settings.

An overview of diagnosis and differential diagnosis of melanonychia is given in **Boxes 22.18** and **22.19**.

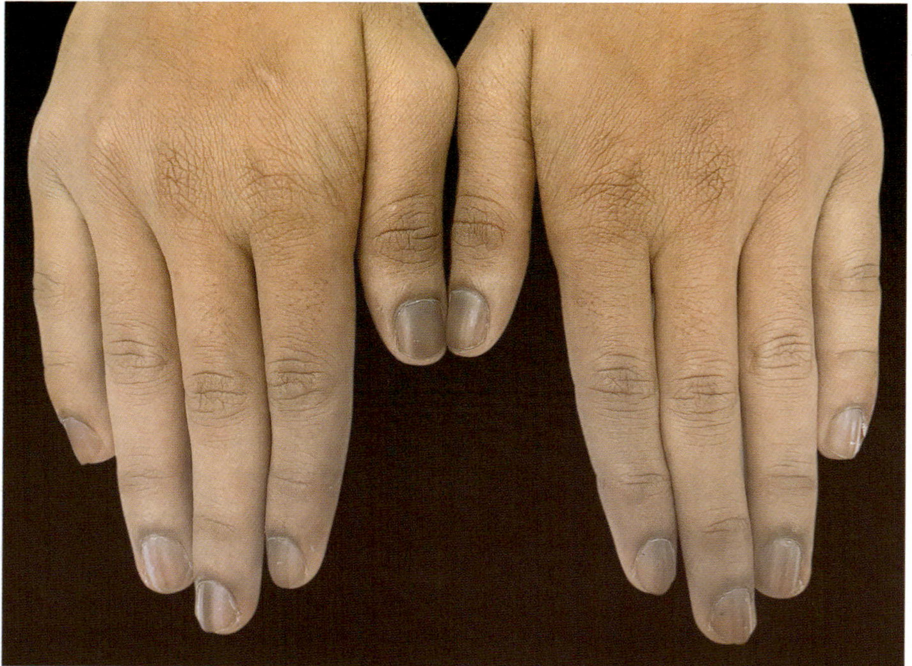

Fig. 22.8: Clinical image showing racial/ethnic melanonychia striata in fingernails of an Indian female with type V skin

TABLE 22.9: Causes of melanonychia		
Melanocytic activation in the nail matrix	Infection	Onychomycosis by *Trichophyton rubrum* var. *nigricans, Aspergillus niger, Fusarium oxysporum, Candida*, and *Neoscytalidium dimidiatum*
	Drugs	Minocycline, clofazimine, chloroquine
	Skin disorders	Lichen planus, nail psoriasis, SLE, localized scleroderma, chemotherapeutic agents
	Endocrine disorders	Addison disease, Nelson syndrome, Cushing syndrome, acromegaly, thyrotoxicosis
	Others	**Ethnic**, pregnancy, trauma, vitamin B_{12} deficiency, Alkaptonuria, Laugier-Hunziker syndrome
Melanocytic hyperplasia in the nail matrix		1. Nail matrix melanocytic nevus 2. Nail lentigo 3. Nail apparatus *in situ* and invasive melanoma 4. Subungual pigmented Bowen disease 5. Subungual pigmented squamous cell carcinoma

TABLE 22.10: Clinical characteristics differentiating melanonychia striata from subungual melanoma

Clinical characteristics	Melanonychia striata	Subungual melanoma
Onset	Gradual	Abrupt
Age of onset	Usually before middle age	Usually after middle age
Race	Dark-skinned individuals	Fair-skinned and dark-skinned individuals
Family history	Melanonychia striata +/–	Melanoma/subungual melanoma +/–
Growth rate	Stationary or very slow growing	Rapid growth
Digit(s) involved	Most common in the thumb; may have multiple digit involvement	Single rather than multiple digit involvement; may involve any digit
Darkening of melanonychia band	–	+
Pigment variegation	–	+
Blurry lateral borders	–	+
Irregular elevation of the surface	–	+
Bandwidth >3 mm	–	+
Proximal widening (triangular shape)	–	+
Associated with plate dystrophy	–	+
Hutchinson sign	Not common	Highly suggestive of subungual melanoma

BOX 22.18: Diagnosis of melanonychia

1. Mainly clinical
2. Bedside test: Onychoscopy
3. Nail matrix biopsy (confirmatory): Depending on the cause

BOX 22.19: Differential diagnosis of melanonychia

1. Subungual hematoma: Migrate distally as the nail grows, history of trauma +
2. Exogenous discoloration: Follows the shape of the proximal nail fold and can be scraped off the nail surface
3. Splinter hemorrhages: Longitudinal streaks corresponding to nail bed capillaries
4. Longitudinal erythronychia: Linear red band(s) seen in glomus tumor, warts, BCC, SCC, Bowen's disease, lichen planus, Darier disease, idiopathic.
5. Fungal melanonychia
6. Kawasaki disease—transverse orange brown chromonychia
7. Onychomatricoma: Yellow, thickened, longitudinal band with the rough ridging of the nail plate, often with proximal splinter hemorrhages.

Treatment

While no major intervention has been shown to be successful, an overview is given below.
1. Wait-and-see approach
2. Surgical excision—if malignant changes suggestive of subungual melanoma seen.

Prognosis

Good (benign condition) **(Box 22.20)**.

BOX 22.20: Prognostic factors

Factors for good prognosis: Early age of onset, stable character of the lesion, occurrence in dark-skinned individuals, and/or involvement of multiple digits.

Table 22.11 gives a list of some high-yield nail disorders.

TABLE 22.11: High-yield nail disorders

Nail sign/disorder	Cause/site of injury	Associations
Beau's lines	Matrix (proximal)—**temporary stoppage of growth**	Usually due to mechanical trauma or skin diseases of proximal fold; also **chemotherapy**, stress on body (e.g. childbirth), **systemic illness**, major injury
Onychomadesis	Matrix (proximal)—temporary stoppage of growth	Same as above: Also seen with **Coxsackievirus** infection (hand-foot-mouth disease)
Pitting	Matrix (proximal)	• **Psoriasis** • **Alopecia areata (geometric, regularly distributed** grid-like small superficial pits)
Onychorrhexis (brittle nails)	Matrix	• Lichen planus • Chronic wet work, frequent nailpolish use, eating disorders
Trachyonychia (sandpaper nails)	Matrix	• **Alopecia areata** (children > adults) • Lichen planus, psoriasis, and other autoimmune process
True leukonychia	Matrix	• Punctate: Usually from trauma in kids • Striate: Fingernails in women from manicures; great toenails from shoe trauma; • **Mee's lines** from arsenic and thallium • Diffuse: Rare, may be congenital

(Contd.)

TABLE 22.11: High-yield nail disorders *(Contd.)*

Nail sign/disorder	Cause/site of injury	Associations
Koilonychia	Matrix	Normal in kids; in adults may be associated with **iron deficiency** (e.g. **Plummer-Vinson syndrome**)
Onycholysis	Nail plate detachment (distal)	**Psoriasis**
Onychauxis	Subungual hyperkeratosis → thickened nail	• **Onychomycosis** • Trauma (e.g. great toenails with shoes), drugs (e.g. **photo-onycholysis with TCN/fluoroquinolones/chloramphenicol/psoralens + UV**) Systemic causes (e.g. thyroid issues)
Onychocryptosis (ingrown nail)	Excess lateral nail growth into nailfold → pseudo-foreign body reaction/inflammation	• Causes include psoriasis, onychomycosis, eczema • May be mimicked by periungal pyogenic granuloma (which may be due to isotretinoin, protease inhibitors, and EGFR inhibitors)
Apparent leukonychia	Nail bed edema (color that **fades with pressure**)	• Chemotherapy • Chronic hypoalbuminemia (**Muehrcke's nails** = transverse white bands parallel to lunula) • Liver cirrhosis (**Terry's nails**—leukonychia of most of nail plate) • Chronic renal disease with hemodialysis (**half and half nails**—leukonychia of half nail plate)
Longitudinal erythronychia	Erythema from matrix to distal onychodermal band	Seen in inflammatory conditions (e.g. lichen planus, **Darier disease**)
Splinter hemorrhages	Damage to nail bed capillaries	Distal (usually from trauma, psoriasis, onychomycosis) Proximal (**endocarditis**, vasculitis, trichinosis, APLS)—rarer
Hutchinson sign	Pigmentation in proximal nail fold with longitudinal melanonychia	May be **sign of nail melanoma**, particularly in adults
Green nail syndrome	Green staining of nail plate due to **pyocanin** from ***Pseudomonas***	Factors → infection are wet work (e.g. barbers, dishwashers), nail trauma, harsh exposures of note, **black nails may be caused by *Proteus*** or *Trichophtyon rubrum*
Red lunulae	Erythema of lunulae	**SLE, alopecia areata, rheumatoid arthritis, dermatomyositis, cardiac failure,** cirrhosis, lymphogranuloma venereum, psoriasis, vitiligo, chronic urticaria, LS&A, **carbon monoxide** poisoning, COPD
Brachyonchia	Shortening of distal phalynx → racquet thumb	Congenital finding—may be seen in **Rubinstein-Taybi** syndrome

(Contd.)

TABLE 22.11: High yield nail disorders *(Contd.)*

Nail sign/disorder	Cause/site of injury	Associations
Nail-patella syndrome	**Mutation of LMX1B** (autosomal dominant)	Manifestations include: Nail abnormalities (radial side of thumbs most commonly—triangle-shaped lunula may occur), bone findings (e.g. absent/underdeveloped patellae, iliac horns), nephropathy/renal insufficiency, Lester iris (pigmentation of pupillary margin of iris)
Clubbing	Soft tissue growth in distal digit → curved, enlarged nail plate	Various causes, but **pulmonary** most common in acquired type; HIV is another reported cause
Yellow nail syndrome	Arrest in nail growth → yellow color, absent cuticle, thickening/ curved (transversely and longitudinally)	Associated with **lymphedema, pleural effusions, bronchiectasis,** chronic pulmonary infection/ sinusitis
Acute paronychia	***S. aureus*** or *S. pyogenes* infection → inflamed tender digit	Usually due to trauma Treat with drainage of abscess and treatment of infection
Chronic paronychia	Inflammation of proximal nail fold → fingernail issues and cuticle loss	Usually due to continuous contact exposure/ wet work (e.g. food handlers) **Secondary infection with *Candida* common**
Habit-tic deformity	Due to manipulation of mid-cuticle of thumb → central longitudinal depression	**Median canaliform dystrophy** may be a subtype with inverted fir tree appearance
Pincer nails	Overcurvature of nail plate	Cause—pain due to pinching of distal nail bed Hereditary *vs* acquired (trauma from shoes) **Lateral matricectomy is treatment of choice:** r/o subungual exostosis
Onychomatricoma	Tumor → thickening of nail plate with multiple longitudinal hollow spaces	Middle-aged patients on fingernails typically Frontal view of nail—**holes in thick margin** Yellow-white thick longitudinal nail with spinter hemorrhages
Subungual exostosis	Subungual bony growth → nodule → nail plate elevation	Usually due to trauma in young patients, most commonly on hallux. **X-ray** confirms diagnosis
Myxoid cysts (digital mucous cyst)	Outpouching of DIP joint space via a tract	**Most common nail tumor** Classic appearance is small **translucent nodule close to proximal nail fold** with nail plate groove distally
Pterygium unguis	Scarring between eponychium and matrix	Classically seen in **lichen planus**
Pterygium inversum unguis	Attachment of distal nail bed to ventral nail plate	Associated with CTDs, esp. **scleroderma**

R/o, rule out

Acknowledgment

We would like to acknowledge **Dr Sidharth Tandon**, Consultant Dermatologist, for his valuable contribution in the preparation of this chapter in the first edition.

BIBLIOGRAPHY

Books

1. Fitzpatrick's Dermatology 9th ed. Mc Graw Hill Education. Chapter 32: Lichen Planus.
2. Nail Unit Lichen Planus Springer International Publishing AG, part of Springer Nature 2018 Al. Rubin *et al.* (eds.), Scher and Daniel's Nails, accessed on 2 January 2019.
3. Nail Unit Psoriasis Dimitris Rigopoulos and Stamatis Gregoriou. © Springer International Publishing AG, part of Springer Nature 2018A. I. Rubin *et al.* (eds.), Scher and Daniel's Nails, accessed 2 January 2019.
4. Nirmal B. Onychoscopy pp 89–93. In: Dermoscopy in darker skin. Chatterjee M, Neema S, Malakar S., Eds. Jaypee Bros. New Delhi, India.
5. Rook's Textbook of Dermatology 9th ed. Wiley Blackwell. Chapter 35: Psoriasis and Related Disorders.
6. Trachyonychia© Springer International Publishing AG, part of Springer Nature 2018. Al Rubin *et al.* (eds.), Scher and Daniel's Nails, accessed on 2 January 2019.

Journals

1. Alessandrini A, Starace M, Piraccini BM. Dermoscopy in the Evaluation of Nail Disorders. Skin Appendage Disord 2017; 3:70–82.
2. Christenson JK, Peterson GM, Naunton M, *et al.* Challenges and Opportunities in the Management of Onychomycosis. J Fungi (Basel). 2018 Jul 24;4(3):87. PMC6162761.
3. Gordon KA, Vega JM, Tosti A. Trachyonychia: A comprehensive review. Indian J Dermatol Venereol Leprol 2011; 77:640–5.
4. Haber JS, Chairatchaneeboon M, Rubin AI. Trachyonychia: review and update on clinical aspects, histology and therapy. Skin Appendage Disord 2017; 2:109–15.
5. Iorizzo M, Tosti A, Starace, M, Baran, R, Daniel, CR, Di Chiacchio, N, … Piraccini, BM (2020). Isolated Nail Lichen Planus—an expert consensus on treatment of the classical form. J Am Acad Dermatol doi:10.1016/j.jaad.2020.02.056.
6. Kolbach-Rengifo M, Navajas-Galimany L, Araneda-Castiglioni D, Reyes-Vivanco C. Efficacy of acitretin and topical clobetasol in trachyonychia involving alltwenty nails. Indian J Dermatol Venereol Leprol. 2016 Nov-Dec; 82(6):732–4.
7. Natarajan V, Nath AK, Thappa DM, Singh R, Verma SK. Coexistence of onychomycosis in psoriatic nails: A descriptive study. Indian J Dermatol Venereol Leprol 2010; 76:723.
8. Parrish *et al.* Modification of the nail psoriasis severity index. https://doi.org/10.1016/j.jaad.2004.11.044.
9. Rigopoulos D, Baran R, Chiheb S, *et al.* Recommendations for the definition, evaluation, and treatment of nail psoriasis in adult patients with no or mild skin psoriasis: A dermatologist and nail expert group consensus, J Am Acad Dermatol 2019; doi:https://doi.org/10.1016/ j.jaad.2019.01.072.
10. Salomon J, Szepietowski JC, Proniewicz A. Psoriatic nails: A prospective clinical study. J Cutan Med Surg 2003; 7:317–21.
11. Scher RK, Baran R. Onychomycosis in clinical practice: Factors contributing to recurrence. Br J Dermatol. 2003;149(suppl 65):5–9.
12. Thappa DM. Current treatment of onychomycosis. Indian J Dermatol Venereol Leprol 2007;73:373–6.
13. Thomas J, Jacobson GA, Narkowicz CK, *et al.* Toenail onychomycosis: An important global disease burden. J Clin. Pharm. Ther. 2010;35:497–519. doi: 10.1111/j.1365-2710.2009.01107.x.
14. Zaias N. Psoriasis of the nail: A clinical-pathological study. Arch Dermatol 1969; 99:567–79.

Chapter

23

Necrobiotic Disorders

Kabir Sardana, Seema Rani, Bhavya Sangal

Necrobiotic disorders are characterized by a necrobiotic or collagenolytic granuloma where granulomatous infiltrate develops around a central area of altered collagen and elastic fibers.

1. Granuloma Annulare (GA)

- Granulomatous disease of the skin and subcutaneous tissue characterized by annular plaques, nodules or papules on the extremities, which slowly enlarge and fade over months or years.
- It may occur at any age and is approximately twice as common in women as in men.
- Children and young adults most commonly affected.
- **Genetics:** Increased prevalence of **HLA-Bw35** amongst individuals with **generalized GA**.

Clinical Types

Localized, generalized, subcutaneous and perforating and patch (macular)

- **Localized GA** most common variant, children and adults both.
- **Generalized GA** adults with a mean around 50 years.
- **Subcutaneous GA** seen predominantly in children.
- **Perforating GA** both adults and children.
- **Patch GA** seen in adult women.

Associated Diseases

- Generalized GA is more commonly associated with hyperlipidemia (up to 45%), type 1 diabetes, HIV, thyroid disease, and malignancy.
- There are isolated reports of the coincidence of temporal arteritis, morphea, necrobiosis lipoidica and sarcoidosis.

Pathophysiology

- GA represents a reaction pattern (most likely Th1-type delayed hypersensitivity reaction) to a variety of triggers like scabies, hepatitis B, *Mycobacterium tuberculosis*, human papillomavirus, varicella/zoster, Epstein-Barr virus, parvovirus, hepatitis C, HIV and *Borrelia burgdorferi*.
- Traumatic triggers include a variety of immunizations, tuberculin testing, animal and insect bites, waxing, saphenectomy and tattoo (red pigment).

- A number of medications have been implicated in triggering GA including TNF-α inhibitors, allopurinol, topiramate and gold therapy. Localized GA has been reported after injection of collagen for soft tissue augmentation and mesotherapy.
- Sunlight exposure has been implicated in seasonal GA
  - Trigger → Th1 reaction → monocyte accumulation in dermis → release of lysosomal enzymes → degradation of elastic fibers.

Clinical Features

Localized GA (Fig. 23.1)

- Accounts for about three-quarters of cases.
- Typically presents as a ring of small, smooth, flesh-colored or erythematous or violaceous papules.
- With intact overlying skin of papules and without scaling. They may be solitary or multiple.
- Commonest sites are the **dorsa of the hands, knuckles, fingers and feet**.

Generalized or disseminated GA

- Accounts for **10–15%** of cases, seen predominantly in adults, is the **most common** form seen in **HIV patients (Fig. 23.2)**.
- Pruritus may be the presenting feature.
- Lesions are often ill-defined with skin-coloured or erythematous macules, papules and/or plaques in an annular pattern surrounding a faintly violaceous central area on the trunk and limbs.
- Lipid abnormalities in 45%; diabetes in 21% (*vs* only 10% in localized GA); ↑prevalence of HLA-Bw35.
- Self-resolves over 3–4 years.

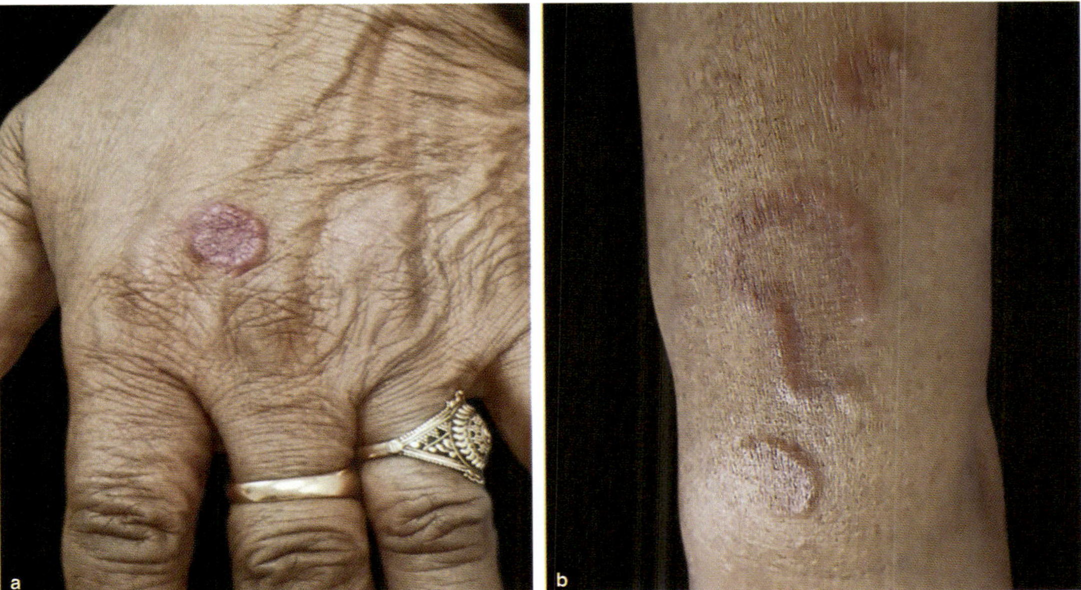

Fig. 23.1: (a) Localized solitary granuloma annulare over dorsum of hand; (b) Multiple lesions of granuloma annulare over dorsum of hand

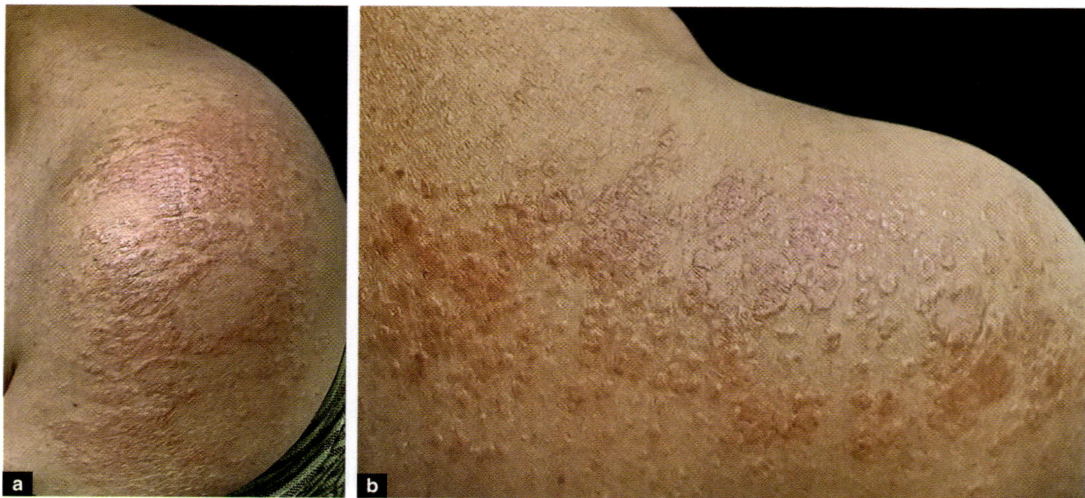

Fig. 23.2: (a) Generalized granuloma annulare, erythematous macules, papules and/or plaques in an annular pattern on shoulder and arm; (b) Generalized granuloma annulare over the back

Perforating GA

- Uncommon but has been described in all ages including infancy and in HIV.
  Site: Dorsal hands and fingers.
  It is characterized by transepidermal elimination of necrobiotic collagen.
- Localized or generalized papules develop yellowish centers and discharge clear, viscous fluid that dries to form a crust, eventually separating to leave a hypo- or hyperpigmented scar.

Subcutaneous GA

- Uncommon, occurs predominantly in children (<6 years).
- Also known as benign rheumatoid nodules, pseudorheumatoid nodules, deep granuloma annulare, subcutaneous palisading granuloma, isolated subcutaneous granuloma and subcutaneous necrobiotic granuloma.
- Nodular lesion occurring predominantly on the scalp and legs, particularly in the pretibial region, unusual locations include the periorbital area, palm and penis.
- About 50% patients of subcutaneous GA can have associated classic lesions of GA.
- Magnetic resonance imaging features are diagnostically helpful.

Patch GA

Symmetrical erythematous patches commonly on bilateral dorsal feet (or trunk and extremities).

- Often lacks annular configuration.
- Histology shows interstitial GA.

GA-like eruptions

May be seen in association with solid organ tumors, B- and T-cell lymphomas, HIV (generalized > localized), or at sites of prior herpes zoster scars.

Pathology

- The most characteristic histological lesion in GA is the **necrobiotic granuloma**.
- There are **three histological patterns** seen **(Table 23.1)**:
  (i) Necrobiotic palisading granulomas (25%), (ii) Interstitial form (70%), and (iii) Sarcoidal or tuberculoid type (5%)
  - Marked reduction in or absence of elastic fibers in approx 20% of generalized GA and 35% of localized GA.
  - Immunofluorescence shows vascular changes include fibrin, C3 and IgM deposition in vessel walls and occlusion of vascular lumina. If granulomatous vasculitis or thrombosis is present, there is ↑risk of systemic disease (probably represents PNGD variant-palisaded neutrophilic granulomatous dermatitis).
- **Table 23.1** summarises features of the three different histological variants of GA.

Differential Diagnosis

Differential diagnosis of variants of GA is summarized in **Table 23.2**.

Disease Course and Prognosis

- In about 50% of patients, the lesions resolved within 2 years.
- Recurrence rate is 40%, in the majority of cases at the same sites as the original lesions.

Treatment

While a overview is given in the **Flowchart 23.1**, it is useful to understand if the treatments and their success mirror the etiopathogenetic theories of GA.

TABLE 23.1: Histological variants of granuloma annulare

1. Necrobiotic palisading type (25%)	• Single or multiple foci of inflammation with a central necrobiotic core, surrounded by palisaded histiocytes • Mucin (colloidal iron or alcian blue) and lipid +
2. Interstitial type (nonpalisaded) (70%)	• Swollen collagen fibres tend to alternate with normal collagen fibers with increased mucin, lymphocytes and histiocytes in between
3. Tuberculoid type (5%)	• Presence of lymphocytes, epitheloid cells and Langhans giant cells with or without central necrosis • Increased mucin and eosinophils

TABLE 23.2: Differential diagnosis of different variants of GA

Localized GA (classical GA)	• Tinea or erythema multiforme, subacte cutaneous LE, annular lichen planus, NLD
Subcutaneous GA	• Trauma, infection, tumors, sarcoidosis, rheumatoid nodules, erythema nodosum and dermoid cyst
Perforating GA	• Molluscum contagiosum, insect bite, pityriasis lichenoides, other perforating disorders, sarcoidosis and papulonecrotic tuberculid
Patch type	• Morphea, erythema annulare centrifugum, parapsoriasis

Flowchart 23.1: Summarised overview of treatment

Granuloma annulare

	Localized	Generalized
1st line	• Await spontaneous resolution • Potent topical CS • I/L steroid (2.5 mg/mL) • Cryotherapy	• NB UVB, PUVA • Antimalarial, dapsone, ciclosporin, MTX • Triple antibiotics (rifampicin, ofloxacin, minocycline)
2nd line	• Tacrolimus • Pimecrolimus • Imiquimod 5% • Tofacitinib (JAK inhibitor)	
3rd line	• Photodynamic therapy • Laser (pulse dye, excimer, Nd:YAG, CO_2)	

The moderate success of corticosteroids, and other agents like dapsone, methotrexate, pentoxifylline and sulphasalazine, is consistent with the long-established inflammatory nature of GA. But many cases do not respond to these drugs and thus in severe cases these drugs often fail. Also the relative inefficacy of antimicrobials supports the putative non-infectious etiology of GA. The use of antibiotics like dapsone and doxycycline are probably working via their anti-inflammatory action. The excellent response of GA to anti-TNFα therapy seen seems to implicate the Th1 pathway in GA. Certain drugs have been shown to be useful including dupilumab, which suggest a Th2 pathway. Lately JAK ib drugs have been used, including tofacitinib and upadicitinib, which probably are effective as the JAK receptors are expressed on Th lymphocytes cells and thus may serve as a pan cytokine drug class in GA. Clearly, GA pathogenesis is not amenable to simple explanation and further studies are needed to better understand the immunology underpinning GA.

2. Annular Elastolytic Giant Cell Granuloma (AEGCG, Actinic Granuloma of O'Brien, and Atypical Facial NLD)

- GA variant affecting chronically sun-exposed-skin (face, neck, upper trunk, and arms).
- Possibly caused by inflammatory response to UV; most commonly middle-aged women **(Fig. 23.3)**.
- Start as flesh-colored to pink papules → coalesce into annular plaques 1–10 cm in diameter; with raised erythematous border and slightly atrophic, hypopigmented center; normally <10 total lesions.
- **Histopathology: Interstitial** (well-formed palisaded) granulomatous infiltrate with more multinucleated **foreign body giant** cells than typically seen in GA); phagocytosed elastic fibers within histiocytes and giant cells (**elastophagocytosis**); no collagen alteration or lipid deposition, lacks mucin; VVG stain shows absence of elastic fibers and loss of solar elastosis in affected areas. There is sparse perivascular lymphocytic infiltrate but no vascular changes.
- There are four histopathological variants described by O'Brien: The giant cell variant, the necrobiotic variant, the histiocytic variant and the sarcoid variant.

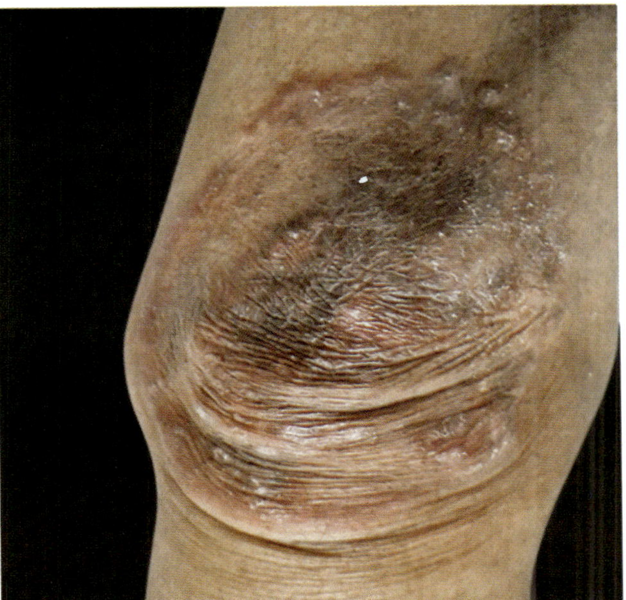

Fig. 23.3: Annular elastolytic giant cell granuloma over elbow

Disease Course and Prognosis

Lesions last for months to years after which they undergo spontaneous remission. They leave behind mottled dyspigmentation or normal appearing skin.

Differential Diagnosis

- Erythema annulare centrifugum, annular lichen planus, secondary syphilis, tinea corporis and granulomatous infections.
- **Rx:** Typically persistent; poor response to standard GA treatments.

3. Interstitial Granulomatous Dermatitis and Arthritis (IGDA) and Palisaded Neutrophilic Granulomatous Dermatitis (PNGD)

- Palisaded neutrophilic granulomatous dermatitis, interstitial granulomatous dermatitis, and interstitial granulomatous drug reaction represent cutaneous reaction patterns that occur in the setting of a systemic trigger.
- Systemic triggers include connective tissue diseases (lupus, vasculitis, other), arthritides (rheumatoid arthritis, other inflammatory and reactive arthritides), malignancy (hematologic more often than solid organ), and medications.

a. **Palisaded neutrophilic and granulomatous dermatitis:**
   - Symmetric erythematous papules on the *extremities*
   - Histology—includes neutrophilic inflammation with possible frank vasculitis, cellular debris, altered collagen, and variable palisaded histiocytes and granulomas.

   Associated with systemic diseases, such as connective tissue diseases, inflammatory arthritis, hematologic disorders, and rarely with infections or medications.

b. Interstitial granulomatous dermatitis

i. Classic IGD
- Palpable linear cords on the trunk.
- Histologic findings of interstitial epithelioid histiocytes surrounding small foci of altered collagen, often leading to the ***floating sign***, with absent mucin and no vasculitis.
- Systemic diseases: Arthritis, connective tissue diseases, hematologic disorders, malignancies, and rarely with infections or medications.

ii. Drug induced: Clues may be histologic findings of tissue eosinophilia, an interface reaction, and occasional lymphoid atypia, in addition to features of classic IGD.
- Most commonly caused by CCBs and ACE inhibitors (usually months to years after drug initiation).
- *Others*: TNF-α inhibitors in RA patients, statins, furosemide, β-blockers, anti-histamines, HCTZ, anakinra, and thalidomide.

A comparison of the three entities is given in **Table 23.3**.

4. Necrobiosis Lipoidica

- Necrobiosis lipoidica is relatively uncommon.
- Reported prevalence range from 0.3 to 1.2% in patients of diabetes.
- Most commonly seen in young adults and in early middle age. The female-to-male ratio is 3:1 **(Fig. 23.4)**.

Associated diseases
- Diabetes, although only about 1% of diabetics develop it.
- 22% of patients with NLD have or will develop diabetes/glucose intolerance.
- Diabetics with NLD have ↑risk of peripheral neuropathy, retinopathy, and joint immobility.
- May be associated with smoking, thyroid dysfunction.
- Ulcerative colitis, Crohn disease and after jejunal bypass surgery.

TABLE 23.3: Classic descriptions of PNGD, IGD, and IGDR

	PNGD	IGD	IGDR
Clinical morphology	Symmetric umbilicated papules on the elbows	Linear erythematous cords on the trunk	Erythematous macules and patches symmetrically on the trunk and proximal extremities
Histology	Intense neutrophilic inflammation, ± leukocytoclastic vasculitis, degenerated collagen, palisading granulomas, minimal mucin	Spares interstitial histiocytes, rosettes of degenerated collagen ± **floating sign**, absent vasculitis and no mucin	Similar to IGD with addition of a vacuolar interface reaction and prominent dermal eosinophilis, variable lymphoid atypia
Associations	Connective tissue diseases, inflammatory arthritis, hematologic disorders	Inflammatory arthritis, connective tissue diseases, hematologic disorders, medications	Medications (CCBs, β-blockers, ACE inhibitors, statins, other)

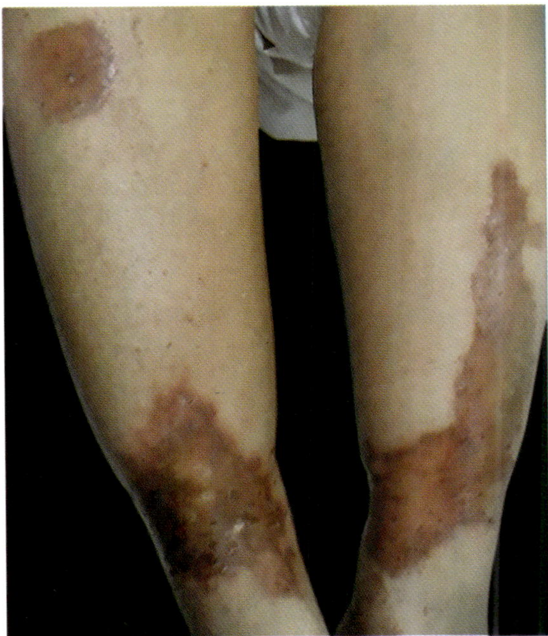

Fig. 23.4: Necrobiosis lipoidica, yellowish atrophic plaque with erythematous edge, glazed surface over lower extremity

- It has also been reported in association with granuloma annulare, sarcoidosis, possible random association with systemic sclerosis, rheumatoid arthritis.

Pathophysiology

- Vascular changes to be important: These might explain the association with diabetes.
- Other contributory factors are altered plasma protein profile, elevated factor VIII-related antigen and fibronectin.
- Vascular compromise from immune complex deposition in vessel walls or diabetes-related microangiopathic changes → subacute **dermal ischemia** → dermal collagen degeneration → secondary granulomatous inflammatory response.

Pathology

- The epidermis is normal or atrophic, and absent if there is ulceration.
- There are changes involving the full thickness of the dermis and these often extend into the subcutaneous fat. (Unlike GA, which tends to have patchy, predominantly superficial dermal inflammation.)
- Horizontally arranged **('layered') palisaded granulomatous** inflammation with horizontal tiers of degenerated collagen fibers (irregular size and shape) and **dermal sclerosis**.
- Early lesions show a perivascular and interstitial mixed inflammatory cell, plasma cells infiltrate.
- There is degeneration of collagen and elastin within the lesions. Histiocytes border the areas of necrobiosis.

- There are variable numbers of plasma cells and Langhans or foreign body giant cells (not seen in GA).
- Lipid can be demonstrated in the necrobiotic areas, and cholesterol clefts may be present.
- Mucin may be present in the dermis, but it is not as prominent as in granuloma annulare.
- Small superficial blood vessels are increased in number and are telangiectatic. Deeper dermal blood vessels often show thickening of their walls and proliferation of endothelial cells.
- The walls are often infiltrated with periodic acid-Schiff positive, diastase-negative material.
- Histologically, comedo-like plugs at the periphery of lesions represent the elimination of necrotic material through hair follicles.
- Decreased number of nerve and fibrosis in the dermis and subcutis leads to anesthesia in lesion and atrophic lesion, respectively.

Clinical Features

- Well-defined red-brown indurated plaques with an atrophic yellow center.
- Seen on the legs-pretibial skin (MC site), can occur on other parts of the body, including the trunk and penis, and rarely may diffuse.
- Begin as a firm, dull red papule or plaque that enlarges radially to become a yellowish atrophic plaque with an erythematous edge.
- The surface is often glazed in appearance and telangiectatic vessels may be prominent. Hypohidrosis and hypoaesthesia or anesthesia may develop.
- Comedo-like plugs may occur at the periphery of lesions.
- In most cases, lesions are bilateral, and they are similar in appearance whether occurring in diabetic or non-diabetic individuals.
- They tend to be persistent and may ulcerate causing pain. Ulceration occurs in one-third of lesions (13–35% of cases), usually following minor trauma.
- Squamous cell carcinoma may develop in long-standing lesions.
- Koebnerization at sites of trauma may also occur.
- Dermoscopic features:
  - Comma-shaped vessels—in early lesions
  - Irregular pattern of arborizing vessels—in advanced lesions
  - Whitish areas—correspond to degenerated collagen
  - Yellow to orange patches—correspond to granulomatous inflammation.

Disease Course and Prognosis

Slow extension over many years is usual, but long periods of quiescence or resolution with variable atrophy and scarring may occur.

Differential Diagnosis

Granuloma annulare, necrobiotic xanthogranuloma, sarcoidosis, diabetic dermopathy, lipodermatosclerosis, morphea, lichen sclerosus, and sclerosing lipogranuloma.

Management

The response of necrobiosis lipoidica to therapeutic intervention is generally disappointing **(Flowchart 23.2)**.

Flowchart 23.2: Summarized overview of treatment

Necrobiosis lipoidica

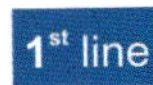
1st line

- Topical or I/L steroids
- Topical tacrolimus

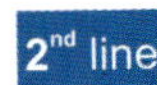
2nd line

- PUVA
- UVA1

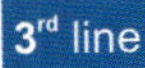
3rd line

- **Topical** : Tretinoin 0.5%, GM-CSF
- **Systemic** : Thalidomide, chloroquine, clofazimine, high dose nicotinamide, fibrinolytic, PGE1, aspirin, ciclosporin, MMF, infliximab, IVIG
- Hyperbaric oxygen
- Pulse dye laser
- Split thickness autografting
- Photodynamic therapy

BIBLIOGRAPHY

Books

1. Chapter 93: Non-infectious granulomas. Dermatology. Fourth Edition. Edited by Jean L. Bolognia, Julie V. Schaffer, Lorenzo Cerroni.
2. Fitzpatrick's Dermatology ninth edition. Part 5, Chapter 34: Granuloma annulare.
3. Rook's Textbook of Dermatology, 9th edition. Part 8, Chapter 97: Granulomatous Disorders of the Skin.

Journals

1. Coutinho I, Pereira N, Gouveia M, Cardoso JC, Tellechea O. Interstitial Granulomatous Dermatitis: A Clinicopathological Study. Am J Dermatopathol. 2015 Aug; 37(8):614–9.
2. Pietta EW, Rosebach M. Granuloma annulare: Pathogenesis, disease associations and triggers, and therapeutic options. J Am Acad Dermatol. 2016 Sep;75(3):467–79.
3. Rosenbach M, English JC 3rd. Reactive Granulomatous Dermatitis: A Review of Palisaded Neutrophilic and Granulomatous Dermatitis, Interstitial Granulomatous Dermatitis, Interstitial Granulomatous Drug Reaction, and a Proposed Reclassification. Dermatol Clin. 2015 Jul; 33(3): 373–87.

Chapter

24

Neutrophilic Dermatoses

Kabir Sardana, Seema Rani, Sweta Singh

This term is used to describe noninfective dermatoses that exhibit a predominantly neutrophilic inflammatory infiltrate and promptly respond to corticosteroid therapy. **Flowchart 24.1** gives a comprehensive overview of these disorders (clinically important entities will be discussed in the text below).

SWEET SYNDROME

- Sweet syndrome is an inflammatory dermatosis characterized by non-itchy, tender, erythematous plaques and nodules most commonly distributed on the arms, upper body, head and neck.
- Associated fever and peripheral leucocytosis are commonly seen.
- Age group most commonly between 30 and 60 years and females are more frequently affected (F:M = 4:1).

Associated Syndromes

- **Infections:** *Streptococcal* respiratory tract infections, gastrointestinal infections by *Salmonella* and *Yersinia* and mycobacterial infections, viral infections—CMV, hepatitis B and C, HIV and fungal—sporotrichosis, coccidiomycosis are all confirmed triggers.
- **Inflammatory bowel disease:** Ulcerative colitis and Crohn's disease.
- **Endocrine:** Pregnancy, thyroid disorders.
- **Immunological disorders:** Include collagen vascular disorders: Lupus erythematosus, Sjögren syndrome.
- **Malignancy:** 10–20% of cases, majority of them are hematological and others are solid organ.
- **Medications:** Antibiotics (minocycline), antiepileptics (carbamazepine), highly active antiretroviral therapy (HAART), antihypertensives (hydralazine), diuretics, nonsteroidal anti-inflammatory drugs (NSAIDs) and retinoids, G-CSF, GM-CSF, ATRA, TMP/SMX, other hematological treatments (imatinib mesylate, bortezomib), contraceptives, propylthiouracil. PAradoxical drug reaction in the form of Sweet syndrome may be caused by—azathioprine, adalimumab, abatacept and tocilizumab.
- **Others:** Sarcoidosis, rheumatoid arthritis, Behçet disease and erythema nodosum.

Flowchart 24.1: Approach to diagnosis of neutrophilic dermatosis

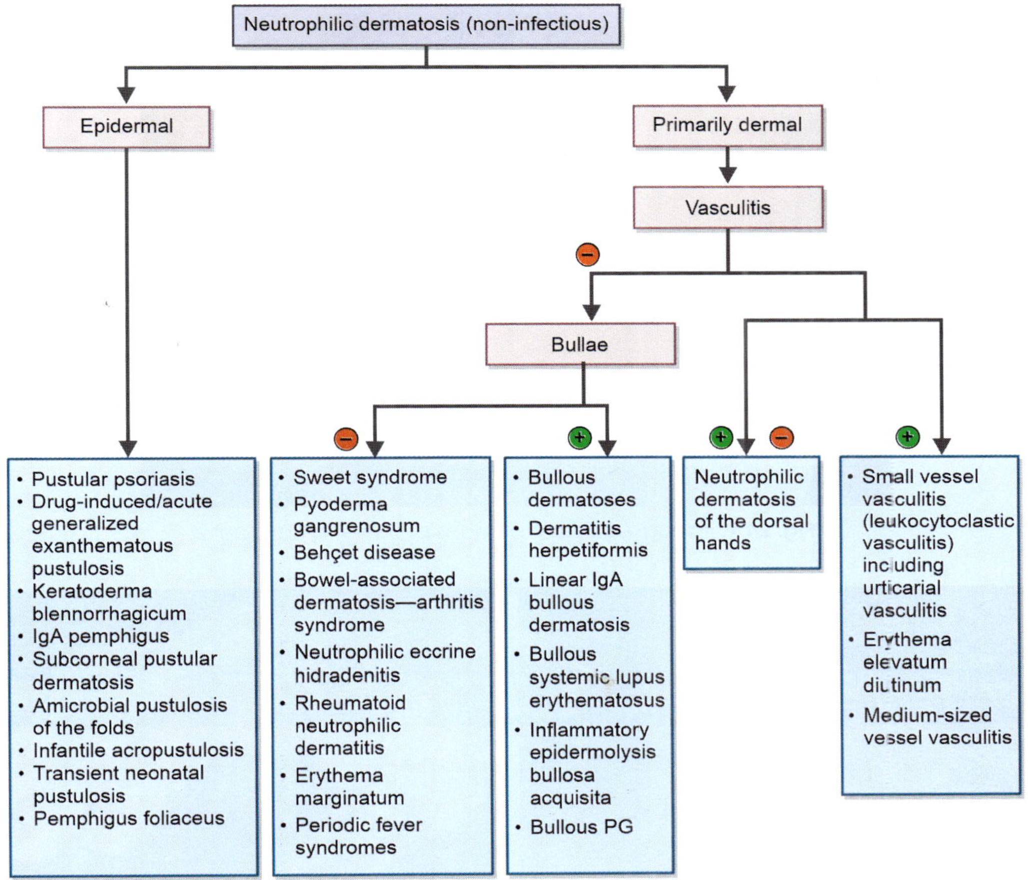

Clinical Features

Three main types of Sweet syndrome are now recognized:

- Classical-associated with infections, inflammatory bowel disease and pregnancy
- Malignancy associated
- Drug induced-granulocyte-colony stimulating factor (G-CSF) is the most frequently reported causative agent.

History of prior infection, malignancy or drug intake should be taken. The classical appearance is of tender red papules, nodules and eventually plaques distributed over the head, neck, upper trunk and upper arms **(Fig. 24.1)**. Cases of definite malignancy-associated Sweet syndrome may have a more widespread distribution.

- The plaques are often edematous and as the process develops, they may become studded with *pseudovesicles* or *pseudopustules* due to prominent papillary dermal edema. Associated arthralgia, myalgia, fever and arthritis have been described.
- Ocular involvement is also relatively common with conjunctivitis and episcleritis. Oral and genital involvement is uncommon.

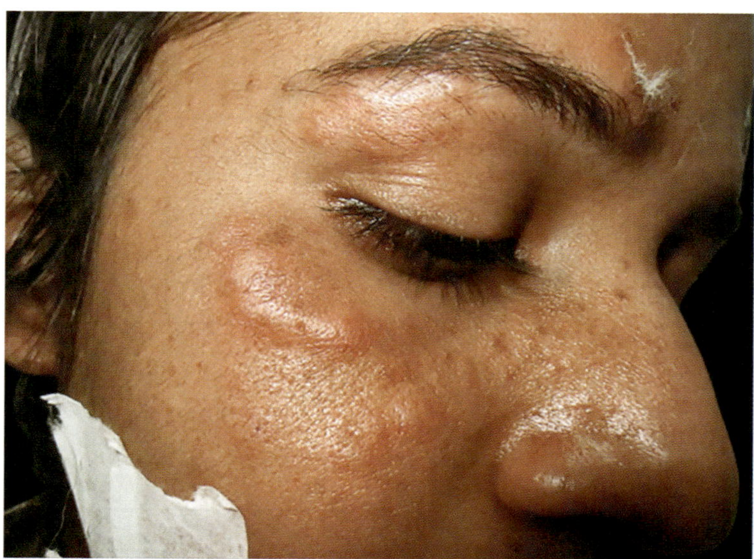

Fig. 24.1: Pseudovesicular plaques of Sweet syndrome

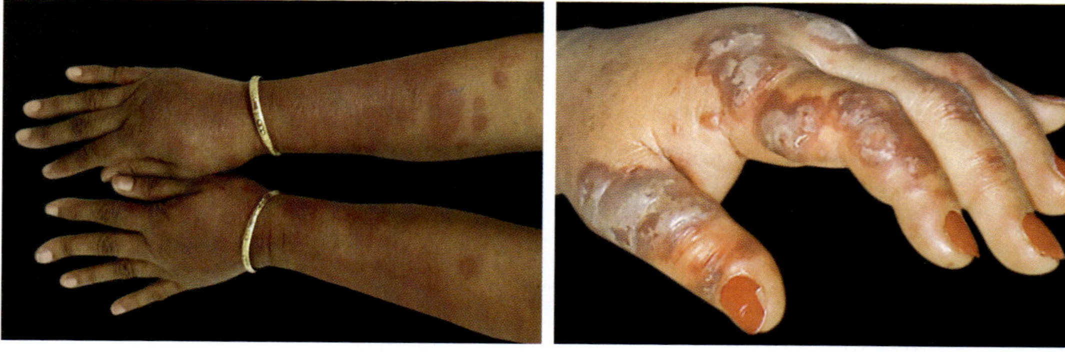

Fig. 24.2: (b) Pseudovesicular plaques of Sweet syndrome. Edema of the dorsa of hands can be seen; (c) Neutrophilic dermatoses of the hand

- Central nervous system involvement (neuro-Sweet syndrome) may involve benign encephalitis, aseptic meningitis, brainstem lesions and psychiatric symptoms amongst others.
- Respiratory involvement may include neutrophilic inflammation of the bronchi or aseptic pulmonary effusion.
- Neutrophilic dermatosis of the dorsal hands—ulcerative red-violaceous plaques on dorsal hands **(Fig. 24.2)**.
- The diagnostic criteria of Sweet syndrome are given in **Table 24.1**.

Clinical Variants

- Subcutaneous Sweet syndrome.
- Histiocytoid Sweet syndrome.

TABLE 24.1: Diagnostic criteria for Sweet syndrome (needs both major criteria and at least 2 minor criteria) [Walker & Cohen, 1996]

Major

1. Acute onset of typical lesions (painful erythematous plaques or nodules)
2. Histopathological evidence of a dense neutrophilic infiltrate without evidence of leukocytoclastic vasculitis

Minor

1. Fever >38°C.
2. Association with malignancy, inflammatory disorder or pregnancy, or antecedent respiratory or gastrointestinal infection or vaccination.
3. Excellent response to systemic corticosteroids or potassium iodide (KI).
4. Abnormal laboratory values at presentation (3 of 4 required: ESR >20 mm; leukocytes >8000; neutrophils >70%; positive C-reactive protein).

Investigations

- Histopathology
  - Diffuse dermal **neutrophilic infiltrate karyorrhexis**
  - Massive papillary dermal edema (responsible for **pseudovesicular** clinical morphology)
  - Generally, *lacks LCV* (although some bystander damage is done to vessels).
  - **Variants**
    1. **Subcutaneous Sweet:** Neutrophils infiltrate subcutis in a lobular pattern; (deep-seated red nodules on extremities)
    2. **Histiocytoid Sweet (variant):** Dermal and/or subcutaneous infiltrate of neutrophils and "histiocytoid" cells (immature myeloid cells that stain positively for myeloperoxidase); that this form may have a stronger association with hematologic malignancy.
- Routine blood tests, full blood count, liver and kidney function test, C-reactive protein
- Additional tests should be guided by the clinical findings and may include thyroid function test, rheumatoid factor and antistreptolysin O antibody titre.
- All suspected malignancies should be investigated according to local guidelines.

Differential Diagnosis

Common differential diagnosis of Sweet syndrome is given in **Table 24.2**.

TABLE 24.2: Differential diagnosis of Sweet syndrome

Inflammatory dermatoses	Infections	Neoplasms
• Pyoderma gangrenosum (bullous) • Neutrophilic dermatosis of the dorsal hands • Neutrophilic eccrine hidradenitis • Rheumatoid neutrophilic dermatitis • Schnitzler syndrome • Autoinflammatory diseases • Erythema multiforme • Urticarial vasculitis • Cutaneous small vessel vasculitis • Erythema elevatum diutinum • Granulomatosis with polyangiitis (Wegener's granulomatosis)	• Cellulitis, pyoderma, furunculosis • Septic vasculitis • Erythema migrans • Cryptococcosis and dimorphic fungal infections • Mycobacterial infections (atypical and leprosy) • Leishmaniasis	• Lymphoma cutis (T- and B-cell lymphomas including mycosis fungoides, cutaneous angiocentric lymphomas) • Leukemia cutis • Metastatic carcinoma

(Contd.)

TABLE 24.2: Differential diagnosis of Sweet syndrome *(Contd.)*

Inflammatory dermatoses	Infections	Neoplasms
• Behçet disease • Bowel-associated dermatosis—arthritis syndrome • Panniculitis, including erythema nodosum • Halogenoderma (iododerma or bromoderma) • Wells syndrome • Autoimmune connective tissue diseases—lupus erythematosus • Granulomatous diseases	As above	As above

Complications and Comorbidities

In the vast majority of cases, Sweet syndrome resolves with no sequelae. Severe skin lesions with ulceration or with delayed treatment can lead to scarring.

Disease Course and Prognosis

Without treatment, the disease will often resolve within 3 months. Approximately one-third of cases will recur.

Treatment

Topical/systemic corticosteroids and potassium iodide are the mainstay of treatment. **Flowchart 24.2** shows a treatment ladder which can be followed. Systemic corticosteroids are the treatment of choice for most patients with Sweet's syndrome. They provide prompt relief-skin lesions begin to resolve within 48 hours and clearing frequently occurs within a week to 10 days.

Flowchart 24.2: Treatment ladder for Sweet syndrome

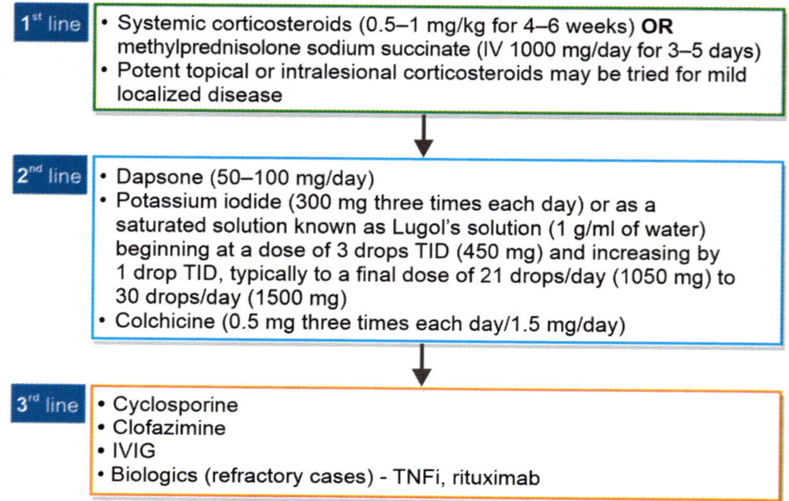

PYODERMA GANGRENOSUM (PG)

- Adults (20–60 years); F > M.
- Almost half the cases are associated with a systemic inflammatory disorder (IBD most common, up to 30%), hematologic disorder (e.g. IgA monoclonal gammopathy, AML, CML, hairy cell leukemia, and polycythemia vera), or inflammatory arthritis.
- PG is a diagnosis of exclusion and the histology is not specific; thus rule out infection, vasculitis, vasculopathy, and malignancy.

Pathogenesis

- Likely immunologic disorder
- Genetic: Some cases are caused by a mutation in CD2-binding protein 1 (PAPA syndrome)
- Pathergy (30%): May initiate and/or aggravate disease.

It is beleived to be a T helper 17/T helper 1-skewed inflammation with a exaggerated inflammasome activation that leads to a dysregulated neutrophil-dominant milieu with high levels of tumor necrosis factor-α, interleukin (IL)-1β, IL-1α, IL-8, IL-12, IL-15, IL-17, IL-23, and IL-36.

Clinical Features

Major types include *classic* (ulcerative), *bullous* (less destructive than ulcerative type; strongly associated with myeloproliferative disorders), *pustular*, and *superficial granulomatous* (vegetative; cribriform superficial ulcers on trunk).

Classic (Ulcerative) PG

- Starts as inflamed **papulopustule/bulla** → forms a painful undermining ulcer with overhanging, irregular, violaceous border and purulent/vegetative floor; satellite lesions arise at periphery of ulcer → break down and fuse with central ulcer **(Figs 24.3 and 24.4)**.
- Heals with atrophic *cribriform scar*.
- Most commonly on lower extremities (pretibial).

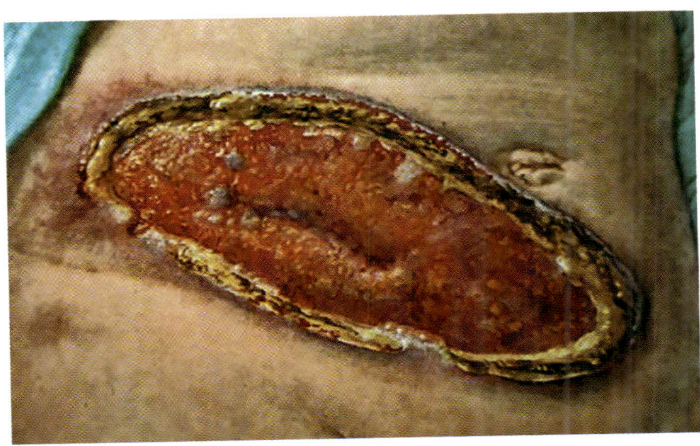

Fig. 24.3: Depiction of PG: The elevated border zone is described in three parts: Linear culminating ridge; peripheral red areola, with a gentle slope and gradual fading towards healthy skin; and inner border vertically cut (80–85°), compared to a steep cliff. The walls of this 'cliff' are riddled by small abscesses. Gentle pressure causes purulent oozing, compared to a sponge

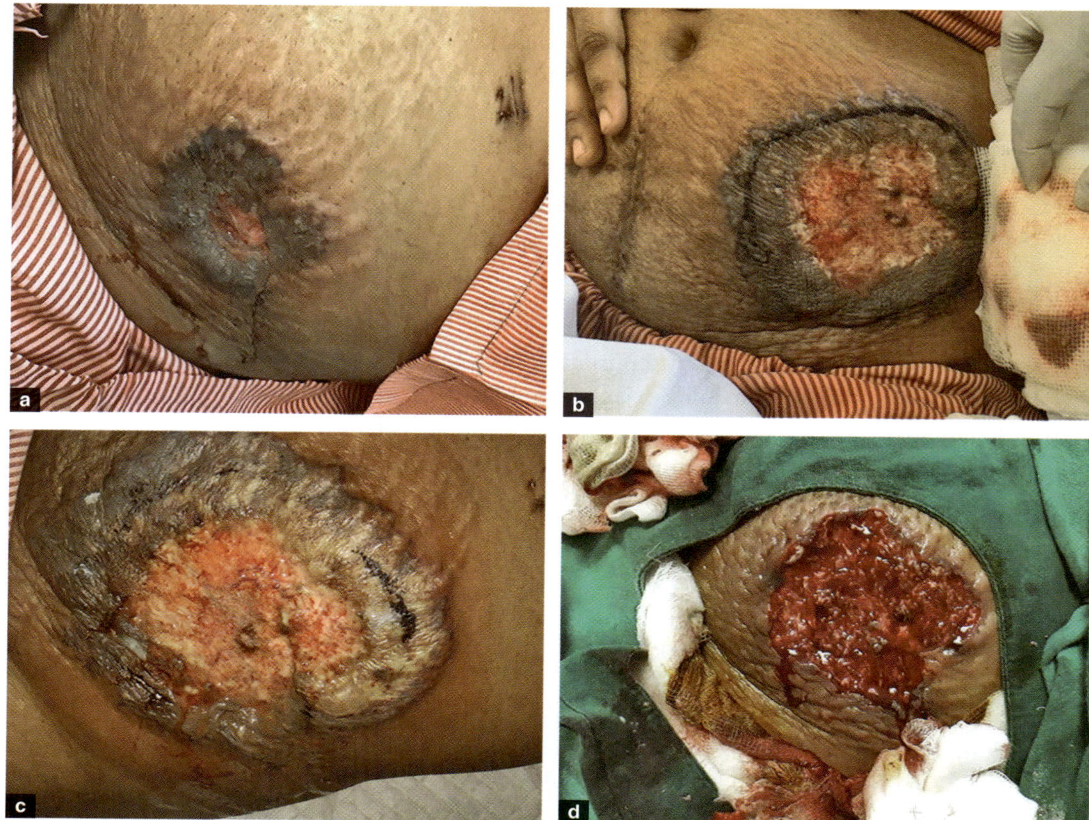

Fig. 24.4: Postoperative pyoderma gangrenosum: (a) Post-nephrectomy (8 days) ulcer at incision site; (b) progressive increase in size of ulcer; (c) Large ulcer with bluish well-defined undermined edges with central necrosis and peripheral erythema; (d) Wound dehiscence and rapidly progressive necrosis at site of abdominal surgery (*Courtesy*: Dr Aditi Gupta, IBS, Delhi)

Variants of classic PG

- Pyostomatitis vegetans: Chronic vegetative pyoderma of oral mucosa associated with IBD.
- Peristomal PG: Painful, undermined lesions around ostomy; associated with IBD.

Classic PG in children (rare): Most common on head and anogenital region; usually associated with IBD or leukemia.

Pustular PG

Multiple small pustules that do not progress to ulcers and occur with IBD in most cases.

Bullous PG

- More superficial, less destructive than classic PG.
- The more widespread distribution (face, dorsal hands, arms) → overlaps with bullous Sweet syndrome → but bullous PG ulcerates and heals with scarring.
- More strongly associated with hematologic malignancy (AML, CML, MDS, polycythemia vera).

Vegetative PG

- Least aggressive form
- Present with superficial, painless cribriform ulcers on trunk; responds well to conservative treatment.
- Usually arises as a result of trauma (e.g. surgery).
- Not associated with underlying systemic diseases.

Histopathology

- Epidermal ulceration with dense *underlying superficial and deep dermal neutrophilic infiltrate* (*inflammation deeper than Sweet syndrome*), leukocytoclasis, epidermal pustules, and dermal edema.
- Neutrophilic infiltrate extends laterally beyond overlying ulcer (undermining infiltrate).

Diagnosis

Diagnostic criteria are given in **Table 24.3**.
Approach to a patient of PG is outlined in **Flowchart 24.3**.

TABLE 24.3: Diagnostic criteria for classic ulcerative pyoderma gangrenosum*

	Criteria	Comments
Major criteria	Biopsy of ulcer edge demonstrating a neutrophilic infiltrate ↓ Yes	• Biopsy demonstrating leukocytoclastic vasculitis was not thought to exclude a diagnosis of PG because this finding can be seen in PG lesions • Atypical cases may be missed, in particular, cases in which a biopsy was obtained after initiation of immunosuppressive therapy or during spontaneous resolution
		Absence of infection was deemed helpful but not required in diagnosing PG
Minor criteria	**Histology:** Exclusion of infection **History** • Pathergy (ulcer occurring at sites of trauma) • Personal history of IBD/inflammatory arthritis • History of papule, pustule, or vesicle that rapidly ulcerated within 4 days of appearing	20–30% of PG show pathergy
	Clinical examination • Peripheral erythema, undermining border, and tenderness at site of ulceration • Multiple ulcerations (at least 1 occurring on an anterior lower leg) • Cribriform or wrinkled paper scar(s) at sites of healed ulcers	
	Treatment Decrease in ulcer size within 1 month of initiating immunosuppressive medication(s)	
In addition to a biopsy demonstrating a neutrophilic infiltrate, patients must have at least **4 minor** criteria to meet diagnostic criteria.		

*JAMA Dermatol. 2018 Apr 1; 154(4):461–466.

Flowchart 24.3: Approach to the patient with pyoderma gangrenosum

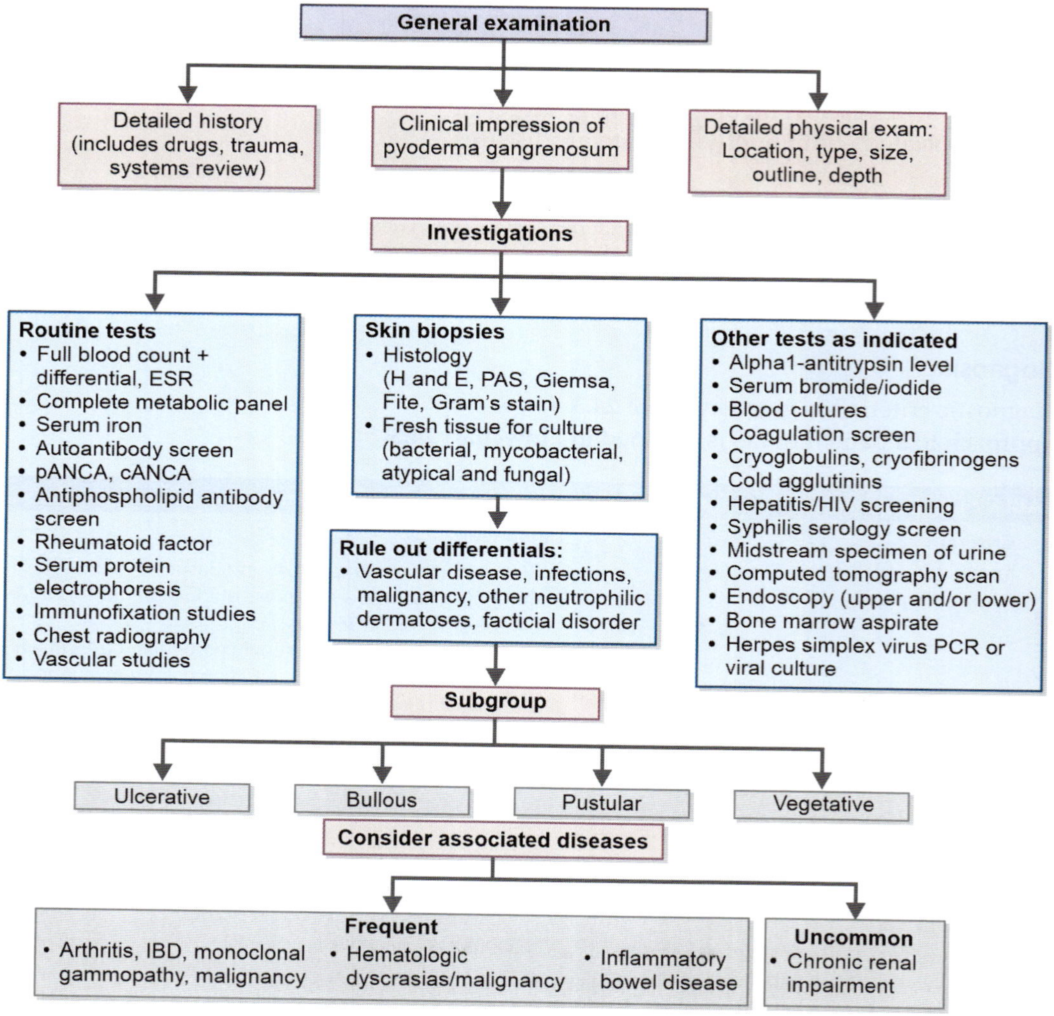

General examination

- Detailed history (includes drugs, trauma, systems review)
- Clinical impression of pyoderma gangrenosum
- Detailed physical exam: Location, type, size, outline, depth

Investigations

Routine tests
- Full blood count + differential, ESR
- Complete metabolic panel
- Serum iron
- Autoantibody screen
- pANCA, cANCA
- Antiphospholipid antibody screen
- Rheumatoid factor
- Serum protein electrophoresis
- Immunofixation studies
- Chest radiography
- Vascular studies

Skin biopsies
- Histology (H and E, PAS, Giemsa, Fite, Gram's stain)
- Fresh tissue for culture (bacterial, mycobacterial, atypical and fungal)

Rule out differentials:
- Vascular disease, infections, malignancy, other neutrophilic dermatoses, facticial disorder

Other tests as indicated
- Alpha1-antitrypsin level
- Serum bromide/iodide
- Blood cultures
- Coagulation screen
- Cryoglobulins, cryofibrinogens
- Cold agglutinins
- Hepatitis/HIV screening
- Syphilis serology screen
- Midstream specimen of urine
- Computed tomography scan
- Endoscopy (upper and/or lower)
- Bone marrow aspirate
- Herpes simplex virus PCR or viral culture

Subgroup

Ulcerative | Bullous | Pustular | Vegetative

Consider associated diseases

Frequent
- Arthritis, IBD, monoclonal gammopathy, malignancy
- Hematologic dyscrasias/malignancy
- Inflammatory bowel disease

Uncommon
- Chronic renal impairment

Treatment

Flowchart 24.4 depicts treatment of PG. The treatment of PG revolves around a emergent therapy aimed at controlling the inflammation which is achieved by CS and cyclosporine. Among biologics, TNFi, especially infliximab and adalimumab have demonstrated the maximum efficacy in classic PG. Adalimumab has been approved for PG in Japan. IL-17i and IL-23i have shown results in reports but paradoxically, have induced PG in some reports as well.

A useful sign that indicates healing and transition to a lower dose of ISA is the "Gulliver" sign where the ulcer which usually is depressed from the surrounding skin, starts healing, by approaching the peripheral margin, with strands of epithelial overgrowth over the ulcer.

Flowchart 24.4: Treatment ladder for pyoderma gangrenosum

1st line	• Wound care • Topical: Corticosteroid or tacrolimus • Intralesional: Corticosteroid
2nd line	• Oral: Corticosteroid, cyclosporine, corticosteroid and cyclosporine combination, methotrexate, mycophenolate, cyclophosphamide, azathioprine, dapsone, thalidomide • Pulse intravenous methylprednisolone
3rd line	• Biologics: Infliximab, adalimumab, etanercept, ustekinumab, anakinra • IVIG
	Alternative: Skin graft, granulocyte apheresis, topical sodium cromoglycate, topical nicotine, hyperbaric oxygen

BEHÇET DISEASE

Epidemiology

- Japanese, middle Eastern, and an Mediterranean (highest prevalence in Turkey)
- Usually 20–35 years
- M > F
- May be familial in a subset of cases.

Pathogenesis

- Multifactorial; circulating immune complexes and neutrophil dysregulation → vascular injury.
- Strongly associated with HLA-B51 allele.

Clinical Features

The ISG criteria for Behçet disease are given in **Table 24.4**. The clinical features include:

- **Recurrent oral ulcerations**
- **Recurrent genital ulceration:** Large, irregular aphthae on scrotum, penis, and vulva.

TABLE 24.4: International study group criteria for the diagnosis of Behçet disease

Major criterion	Required features
Recurrent oral ulceration	Aphthous (idiopathic) oral ulceration observed by physician or patient, recurring at least three times in a 12-month period
Plus any two of the following minor criteria:	
Recurrent genital ulceration	Aphthous genital ulceration or scarring, observed by physician or patient
Eye lesions	Anterior or posterior uveitis; cells in the vitreous by slit lamp examination; or retinal vasculitis observed by ophthalmologist
Cutaneous lesions	Erythema nodosum-like lesions papulopustular lesions or pseudofolliculitis; acneiform nodules in postadolescent patient not on corticosteroids
Pathergy test	Interpreted at 24–48 hours by physician

- **Ocular lesions (90%):** Uveitis (posterior > anterior), conjunctivitis, iridocyclitis, and retinal vasculitis (may → blindness).
- **Cutaneous lesions** (facial/acral papulopustules, purpura, EN-like lesions on legs/buttocks, and positive pathergy test).
- **Pathergy test:** Needle stick or intradermal injection of saline → papulopustule at site of trauma within 24–48 hours.
- **Vascular:** Superficial migratory thrombophlebitis (30%) and, less frequently, SVC thrombosis.
- **Other:** Joints (50% develop arthritis), neurologic (meningoencephalitis, MS-like symptoms), cardiopulmonary, renal (glomerulonephritis), and GI.

Histopathology

Dermal perivascular neutrophilic infiltrates and edema as well as a lobular neutrophilic or septal panniculitis thrombosis is also seen.

Treatment

Flowchart 24.5 shows a stepwise approach to treatment.

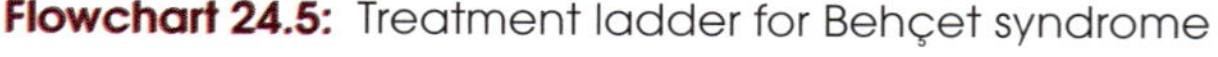
Flowchart 24.5: Treatment ladder for Behçet syndrome

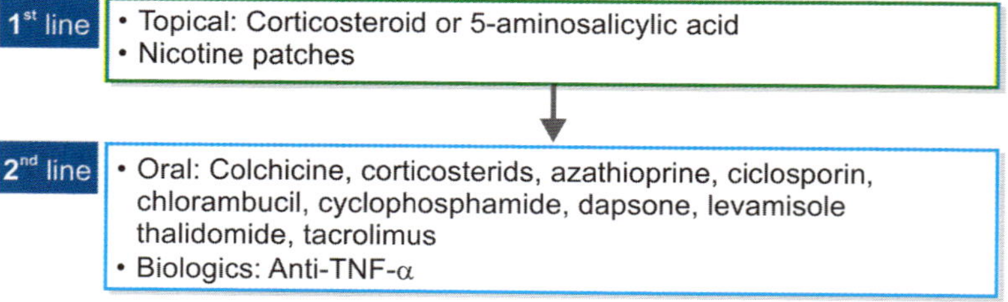

BIBLIOGRAPHY

1. Anatomy D. Ormesod and Philip J. Hampton. Neutrophilic Dermatoses. In: Rook's Textbook of Dermatology (9th edition). UK. Blackwell Publisher. Part 4; Ch 49: 1377–94.
2. Landis ET, Taheri A, Jorizzo JL. Gulliver's sign: A recognizable transition from inflammatory to healing stages of pyoderma gangrenosum. J Dermatolog Treat. 2015 Apr;26(2):171–2.
3. Samuel L Moschella and Mark DP Davis. Nuetrophilic Dermatoses. Bolognia LJ. Jorizzo L.J. Scheaffer VJ. Editors. In: Dermatology (4th edition); London. Elsevier Publishers Chap 26: p.423–37.
4. Natanel Jounabchi, Gerald S Lazarus. Pyoderma Gongrenosum. Fitzpatrick Dermatology (9th ed). New York McGraw Hill Education. Past 6; Chapter 37: 605–15.

Chapter 25

Nevi

Seema Rani, Kabir Sardana, Bhavya Sangal

Congenital nevi are hamartomas caused by a somatic mutation in a cell that resides in or will eventually reside in the skin. They are typified by the following:

- A part of the skin is affected.
- Most nevi are cutaneous mosaics.
- The phenotype will depend on the normal function of the **gene** during development. A working classification is given in **Flowchart 25.1** with the respective gene defect while a more comprehensive classification is given in **Table 25.1**.

Flowchart 25.1: An overview of nevi (Vercrica A Kinsler and Neil J Sebire, 2016)

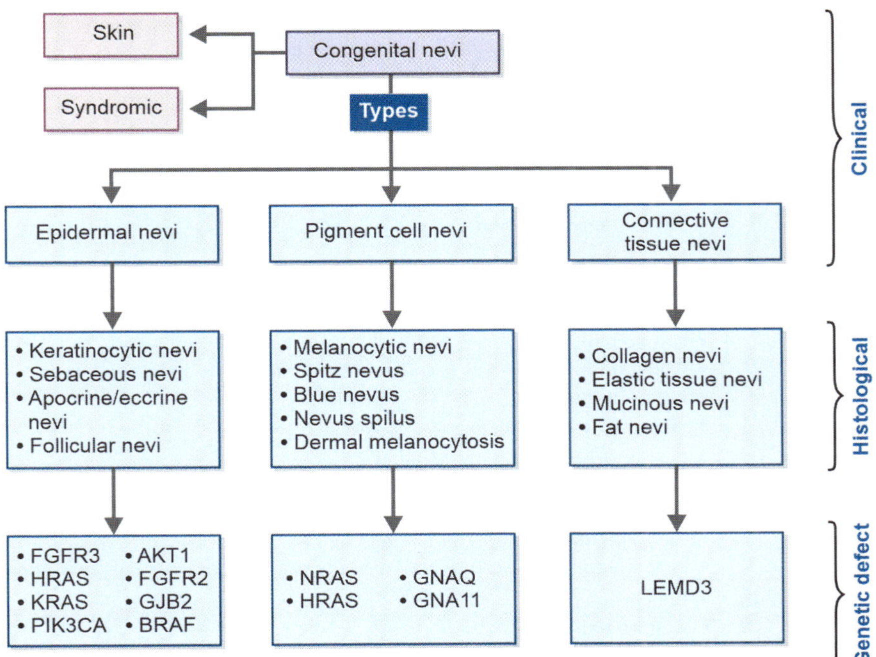

TABLE 25.1: List of nevi and 'nevoid' lesions (i.e. not histologically nevi but linear or segmental in distribution)

Epidermal nevi	• Keratinocytic hyperkeratotic verrucous epidermal nevus* • Epidermolytic hyperkeratotic verrucous epidermal nevus* • Inflammatory linear verrucous epidermal nevus (ILVEN)* • CHILD nevus (as part of CHILD syndrome) • Papular epidermal nevus with 'skyline' basal cell layer (PENS) • Sebaceous nevus* • Linear syringocystadenoma papilliferum • Comedo nevus* • Hair follicle nevus • Linear basaloid follicular hamartoma • Hairy malformation of the palms and soles • Nevus trichilemmocysticus • Apocrine nevus • Eccrine nevus • Porokeratotic eccrine ostial and dermal duct nevus (PEODDN)
Pigment cell nevi	• Congenital melanocytic nevus* • Congenital blue nevus • Congenital nevus spilus* • Congenital Spitz nevus • Mongolian blue spot (dermal melanocytosis)*
Connective tissue nevi	• Familial cutaneous collagenoma* • Eruptive collagenoma • Shagreen patch* • Isolated collagenomas* • Elastic nevus • Juvenile elastoma • Nevus anelasticus • Proteoglycan nevus • Mucinous nevus • Mixed connective tissue nevus
Muscle nevi	• Congenital smooth muscle hamartoma • Diffuse smooth muscle hamartoma (can lead to 'Michelin tyre baby') • Congenital leiomyoma • Striated muscle nevus
Fat nevi	• Nevus lipomatodes cutaneous superficialis* • Lipoblastoma • Encephalocraniocutaneous lipomatosis • Congenital lipoma • Congenital lipomatosis (can lead to 'Michelin tyre baby') • Neurolipomatosis • Nevus psiloliparus
Nevoid entities	• Linear atrophoderma of Moulin • Linear scleroderma/morphea* • Lichen striatus* • Incontinentia pigmenti and other X-linked conditions with expression mosaicism* • Linear Darier disease and other nevoid presentations of usually non-linear disorders
Currently **unclassifiable** nevi	• Becker nevus* • Angora hair nevus

*The **starred ones are important and commonly seen in clinical practice**.

CONGENITAL EPIDERMAL NEVI (CEN)

- Congenital epidermal nevi is a descriptive term for congenital hamartomas of epidermal structures.
- Single post-zygotic mutations in an epidermal precursor cell, leading to epidermal mosaicism, with or without mosaicism in other organs.
- Single CEN lesions can be either round or linear, but larger or multiple lesions are Blaschkoid (usually linear) in distribution. Exception—nevi of the **PENS** (papular epidermal nevus with 'skyline' basal cell layer) syndrome which are multiple but round/ovoid.

1. **Keratinocytic CEN** can be caused by mutations in
   - The fibroblast growth factor receptor 3 **(FGFR3)** gene (in isolated nevi and as part of the FGFR3 epidermal nevus syndrome).
   - **FGFR2 gene**
   - **PIK3CA** (in isolated nevi and as part of the CLOVES syndrome).
   - **HRAS** and **KRAS** (in isolated nevi and as part of unique epidermal nevus syndromes).
   - **AKT1** (as part of the *Proteus* syndrome)
   - **KRT1** and **KRT10** (epidermolytic nevus subtype).

   Importance of mutations: To diagnose epidermolytic subtype, as this is associated with gonadal mosaicism.

   Mosaic mutations can only be passed on if they affect the gametes of the individual, and are also compatible with life. They are passed on as a germline heterozygous trait in the affected offspring (i.e. the whole skin will be involved).

   Rarely, CEN are a feature of germline conditions, e.g. CHILD (congenital hemidysplasia with ichthyosiform erythroderma and limb defects) syndrome and Cowden syndrome.
2. **Sebaceous nevi**—mutations in HRAS or KRAS (both in individual nevi and as part of phakomatosis pigmentokeratotica (HRAS)/Schimmelpenning syndrome (HRAS or KRAS)).
3. **Follicular nevi** (nevus comedonicus or acne nevus) can result from mutations in FGFR2—explains acne sometimes seen in Apert syndrome (caused by germline FGFR2 mutations).
4. **Porokeratotic eccrine nevi** can be due to mutations in GJB2.

Syndromes

1. HRAS mosaicism: Schimmelpenning–Feuerstein–Mims syndrome/phakomatosis pigmentokeratotica-RASopathy.

CF: Linear sebaceous epidermal nevi with or without the following: Areas of keratinocytic epidermal nevus, nevus spilus or areas of café au lait macular pigmentation, neurological abnormalities, ocular abnormalities, developmental skeletal abnormalities and hypophosphataemia leading to rickets.

2. *Proteus* syndrome: Mosaic disorder of overgrowth, mutation in AKT1 lesions—keratinocytic epidermal nevi, connective tissue nevi, lipomas, vascular nevi and patchy lipohypoplasia or dermal hypoplasia.

3. PIK3CA-related overgrowth spectrum: *CLOVES* syndrome—**c**ongenital **l**ipomatous **o**vergrowth, **v**ascular **m**alformation, **e**pidermal nevi (keratinocytic type) and **s**keletal abnormalities.

- Associated with neurological, somatic mosaicism for PIK3CA mutations.

4. PENS syndrome: Round/ovoid, papular, white/yellowish, keratotic lesions of 0.1–1.5 cm diameter. They are present at birth or develop shortly after, and have a characteristic histological appearance of a 'skyline' basal cell layer.

5. CHILD syndrome: Unliteral, bilateral cutaneous involvement has rarely been described and limb defects are **not** always seen. May be mosaic ichthyosis, defect in NSDHL, X-linked dominant, seen in females.

6. Happle–Tinschert syndrome: Segmental basaloid follicular hamartomas with extracutaneous abnormalities, most notably in the dental, osseous and neurological systems.

7. Follicular nevus/nevus comedonicus syndrome: Nevus comedonicus has been described in association with cataracts, skeletal abnormalities and neurological abnormalities, FGFR2.

Approach to Diagnosis

- History, examination and relevant investigations for non-cutaneous associations.
- Biopsy of the epidermal nevus is required to make an exact diagnosis, particularly for keratinocytic CEN of any size, to look for epidermolysis. If epidermolytic CEN, look for gonosomal mosaicism.
- Extracutaneous abnormalities investigated depending on the type.
- Associated with hypophosphatemia: Baseline electrolyte and calcium/phosphate/alkaline phosphatase measurement.

Treatment (Box 25.1)

BOX 25.1: Treatment of epidermal nevi

- Small single nevi: *Full thickness* surgical excision or ablative laser therapy or cryotherapy. Others—*corticosteroids, retinoic acid, tars, anthralin, 5-fluorouracil and podophyllin.*
- ILVEN: Laser has a variable response, topical calcipotriol, etanercept and oral retinoids can be used.
- Extensive epidermolytic, hyperkeratotic, epidermal nevi: Systemic retinoids, and topical vitamin D analogues have been used.
- Topical sirolimus was found to reduce the thickness of the skin nevi in a patient with FGFR3 mutation.

BECKER NEVUS

Becker nevus (or Becker melanosis or Becker hamartoma) is a relatively common hyperpigmented, generally non-linear lesion.

Becker nevus is currently unclassifiable within the classification given in **Table 25.1**, as it shows features of lentiginous melanocytic hyperplasia, epidermal hyperplasia and smooth muscle hyperplasia.

- Incidence of around **0.25%**, and is commoner in **males** than females. Male-to-female ratio is 6:1.
- Rarely congenital, with the majority of lesions appearing in the first two decades (at puberty).

Clinical Features

- It presents as a hyperpigmented macular or speckled area, commonest configuration is block like and can be in linear pattern **(Fig. 25.1)**.
- Lesions are most often unilateral and commonly in the scapular region, upper arms and chest.
- They also have been described on the forehead, face, neck, lower trunk, extremities and buttocks.
- It is frequently hypertrichotic.

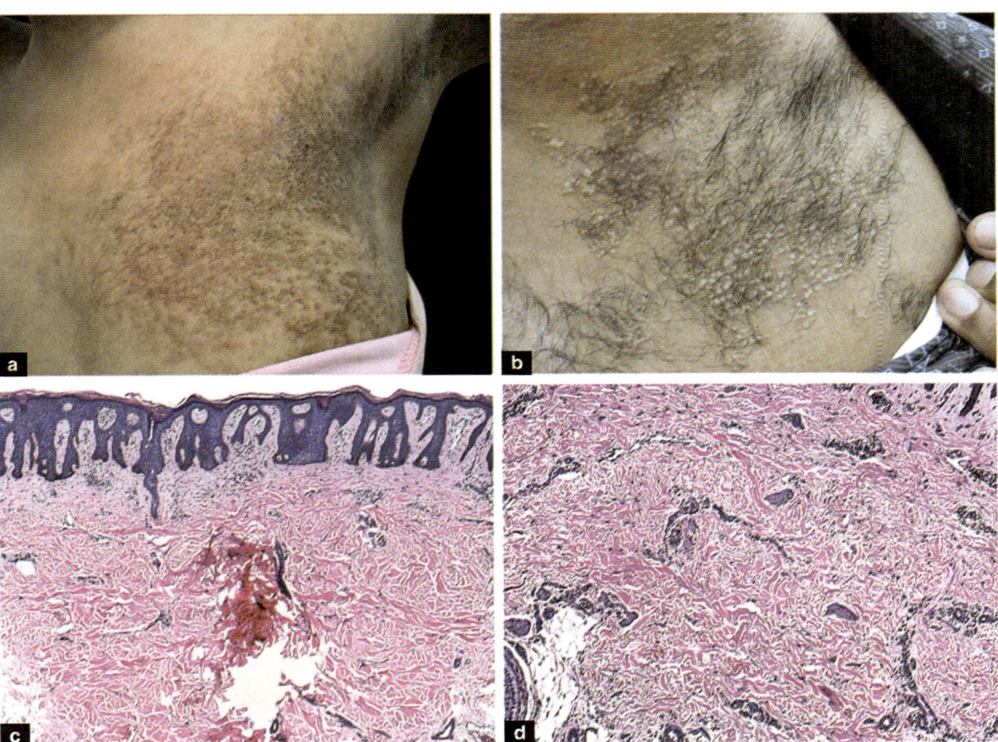

Fig. 25.1: (a) Becker nevus, hyperpigmented, hypertrichotic lesion over upper trunk; (b) Perifollicular papules seen over the Becker nevus; (c) Becker nevus showing the characteristic irregular elongation of rete, ridges increased basal layer pigmentation, mild acanthosis, and hyperkeratosis; (d) Becker nevus showing areas of hypermelanosis with smooth muscle hyperplasia in dermis that is not associated with follicular units

- Perifollicular papules, due to coexistent proliferation of the arrector pili muscle. Acneiform lesions strictly limited to the area of hyperpigmentation have also been reported **(Fig. 25.1)**.
- An increase in androgen receptors and sensitivity to androgens have been postulated.
- Becker nevus syndrome, here the **male-to-female ratio is reversed (2:5)**, associated with extracutaneous abnormalities, which can involve underlying structures:
  - Aplasia or hypoplasia of the underlying breast tissue or pectoralis major muscle
  - Lipoatrophy
  - Ipsilateral limb growth disturbance
  - Supernumerary nipples, **'SNUB syndrome'**—supernumerary **n**ipples, **u**ropathies and **B**ecker nevus
  - Scoliosis, lumbar spina bifida

Histopathology

- Epidermal acanthosis, hyperkeratosis and elongated rete ridges.
- Normal numbers of melanocytes, but increased levels of melanin in the basal epidermal layer are demonstrated.

- Slight increase in smooth muscle fibers exist in nearly all cases.
- When associated with smooth muscle hamartoma, irregularly arranged, thick bundles of smooth muscle are present in the dermis.

Dermoscopy

Findings differ between center and periphery of the lesion.
Center: Prominent pigmentary network, blotchy hyperpigmentation with terminal hairs, and parafollicular hyperpigmentation.
Periphery: Normal pigmentary network with no hyperpigmentation, but with terminal hairs and parafollicular hyperpigmentation.

Differential Diagnosis

Differential diagnosis is summarized in **Box 25.2.**

BOX 25.2: Differential diagnosis of Becker nevus

- CALM
- Plexiform neurofibroma
- Congenital hairy nevus
- Congenital melanocytic nevus
- Nevus of Ito
- Congenital smooth muscle hamartoma

*Congenital smooth muscle hamartoma—tends to be smaller in size, some authors consider Becker melanosis and congenital smooth muscle hamartoma to be two ends of a clinical spectrum.

Treatment (Box 25.3)

BOX 25.3: Treatment of Becker nevus

- Electrolysis, waxing, depilation
- Camouflage makeup
- *Lasers*:
  1. For hyperpigmentation: Long pulsed and picoseconds alexandrite laser, QS: Nd:YAG, QS ruby laser
  2. For hypertrichosis: Diode, Nd:YAG laser
  3. For The Nevi: Fractional Er:YAG

Lasers

- Results are inconsistent as the target is variable.
- Hypertrichotic BN have the worst results.
- Ablative lasers, specially Er:YAG is ideal as there is less chance for scarring.
- One option is to use both QS-1064 followed by QS 532 in the same session. This will ensure targeting both the dermal and the epidermal components at the same session.
- Despite some successes, failures and recurrences are frequent.

VERRUCOUS EPIDERMAL NEVUS (VEN)

- Verrucous epidermal nevi represent a heterogeneous group **(Table 25.2** and **Fig. 25.2)**.
- May possibly result from post-zygotic mutations in genes.

a. **Epidermolytic verrucous epidermal nevi**, often present since birth, 80% in first year of life, may occasionally become apparent during adulthood, are tan to brown warty lesions distributed along Blaschko lines, may have an abrupt midline demarcation, commonly present on trunk, extremities and neck.
   - A heterozygous mutation is present in keratinocytes **(KRT1, KRT10)** within the nevus but not in adjacent uninvolved skin. Heterozygous mutations in KRT2 have also been reported recently.

TABLE 25.2: Overview of VEN	
Epidermolytic VEN	**Nonepidermolytic VEN**
• Sporadic occurrence, mutations in **KRT1 and KRT10**	• Chromosomal abnormalities in 1q23 and mutations in **FGFR3, R248C, PIC3CA, PTEN, K16, ch6 trisomy**
• **HP** – Epidermolytic hyperkeratosis, acanthosis – Papillomatosis, hypergranulosis – *Perinuclear vacuolization* of keratinocytes – Premature, irregular keratohyaline granules	• **HP** – Sharply demarcated hyperkeratosis, acanthosis – Papillomatosis, parakeratosis – 10%—Church-spire pattern – 5%—seborrheic keratosis

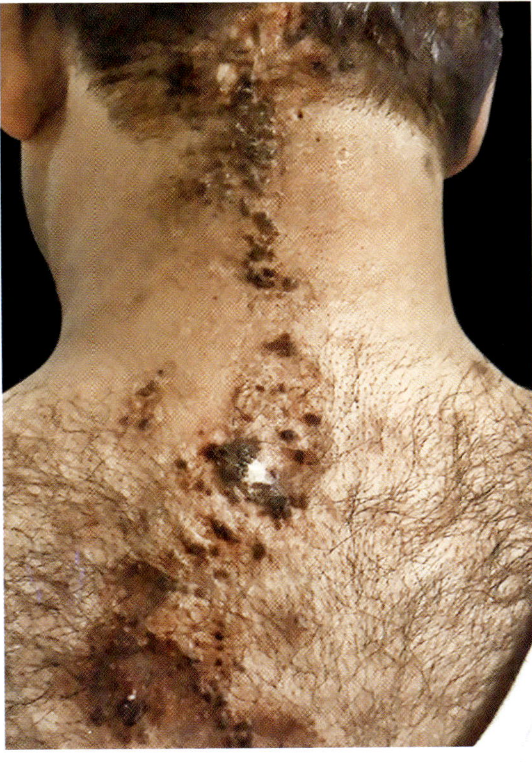
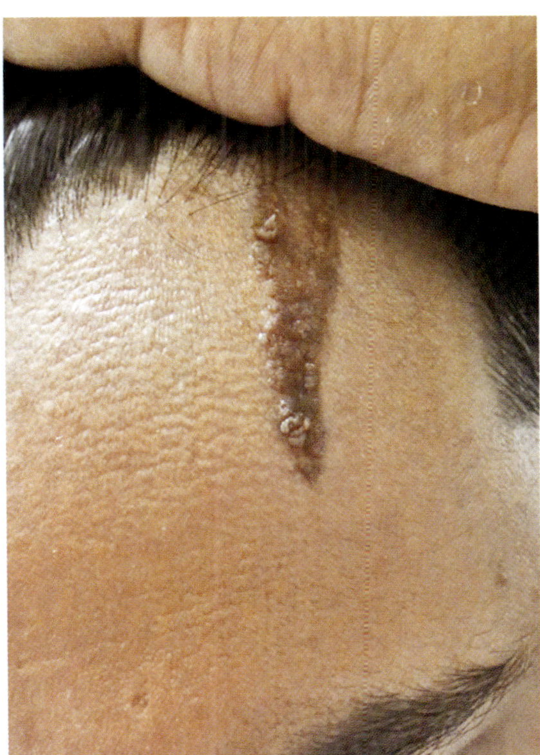

Fig. 25.2: Verrucous epidermal nevus, linear warty lesion (left-epidermolytic) (right nonepidermolytic) with papillomatous morphology

b. Nonepidermolytic verrucous epidermal nevi

– Mosaicism for a particular heterozygous activating mutation (R248C) in the fibroblast growth factor receptor 3 gene (FGFR3).

– Non-epidermolytic verrucous epidermal nevi, most often thick papillcmatous lesions, are associated with macrocephaly and additional segmental manifestations.

– A systematized epidermal nevus refers to a more extensively distributed variant of keratinocytic epidermal nevi. The unilateral subtype is termed nevus unius lateris but the bilateral subtype is known as icthyosis hystrix **(Box 25.4)**.

BOX 25.4: Differential diagnosis

- Nevus sebaceous
- Porokeratotic eccrine ostial and dermal duct nevus
- Linear lichen planus
- Lichen striatus
- Small lesions—seborrheic keratosis, verruca vulgaris
- X-linked dominant chondrodysplasia punctata

Epidermal Nevus Syndrome

The various components of this are listed below:

1. **Skin:**
   - Epidermal nevi (usually more than 2–3 cm in length, more than 0.5–2 cm in width)
   - ILVEN (most common): Long, linear, verrucous plaques on limbs; with/without scale, erythema
   - Ichthyosis hystrix: Extensive verrucous plaques in whorl-like pattern on trunk
   - Linear nevus sebaceous: Linear, orange-tan, waxy plaques on scalp extending onto the face
2. **Central nervous system (associated with head and neck or extensive nevi):** Mental retardation, seizures, spastic hemiparesis/paralysis, sensorineural deafness, cerebral hemangiomas, vascular malformations
3. **Skeletal (associated with location of nevi):** Hemihypertrophy, kyphoscoliosis, ankle/foot deformities, vitamin D-resistant rickets
4. **Eyes:** Extension of nevus to lid and bulbar conjunctiva, lipodermoids, colobomas, corneal opacity, nystagmus, cortical blindness
5. **Neoplasms (rare):** Variety of tumors reported; syringocystadenoma papilliferum, Wilms' tumor, astrocytoma, rhabdomyosarcoma, salivary gland adenocarcinoma

Complications

- Maceration: More common in intertriginous sites
- Infection
- Paronychia
- Megalopinna
- Malignancy—rarely (BCC, SCC and keratoacanthoma)

Management

The management is listed in **Box 25.5**. **Burosumab** (KRN23), is an IgG1 monoclonal antibody that binds to the FGF23 receptor and inhibits the activity of FGF23 has been recently used.

BOX 25.5: Management of VEN

- Topical: Salicylic acid, retinoic acid, lactic acid, 5FU, calcipotriol, calcitriol.
- Surgical excision can be suitable for small, single, epidermal nevi, but not for more extensive lesions.
- Lasers: Ablative laser therapy to reduce thickness and/or hyperkeratosis of the lesion.
- Cryotherapy and radiofrequency ablation for smaller verrucous lesions.
- Genetic counseling is recommended in epidermolytic VEN.

INFLAMMATORY VERRUCOUS EPIDERMAL NEVUS (ILVEN)

ILVEN is a clinical descriptor for a heterogenous group of mosaic inflammatory disorders.

- Commonly appears in the <u>first few years</u> of life and spreads gradually in a classic Blaschko-linear distribution.

- It is characterized clinically by inflamed, erythematous and hyperkeratotic skin that can be pruritic **(Fig. 25.3a** and **b)**.
- It is usually confined to a single limb, but can be more extensive.
- Clinically and histologically, there is a significant overlap between ILVEN and psoriasis.

Histopathology

- Hypergranulosis with orthokeratotic hyperkeratosis alternating with well-defined columns of agranulosis and parakeratotic hyperkeratosis **(Fig. 25.3c)**.
- Marked inflammatory component—superficial dermal inflammatory infiltrate.

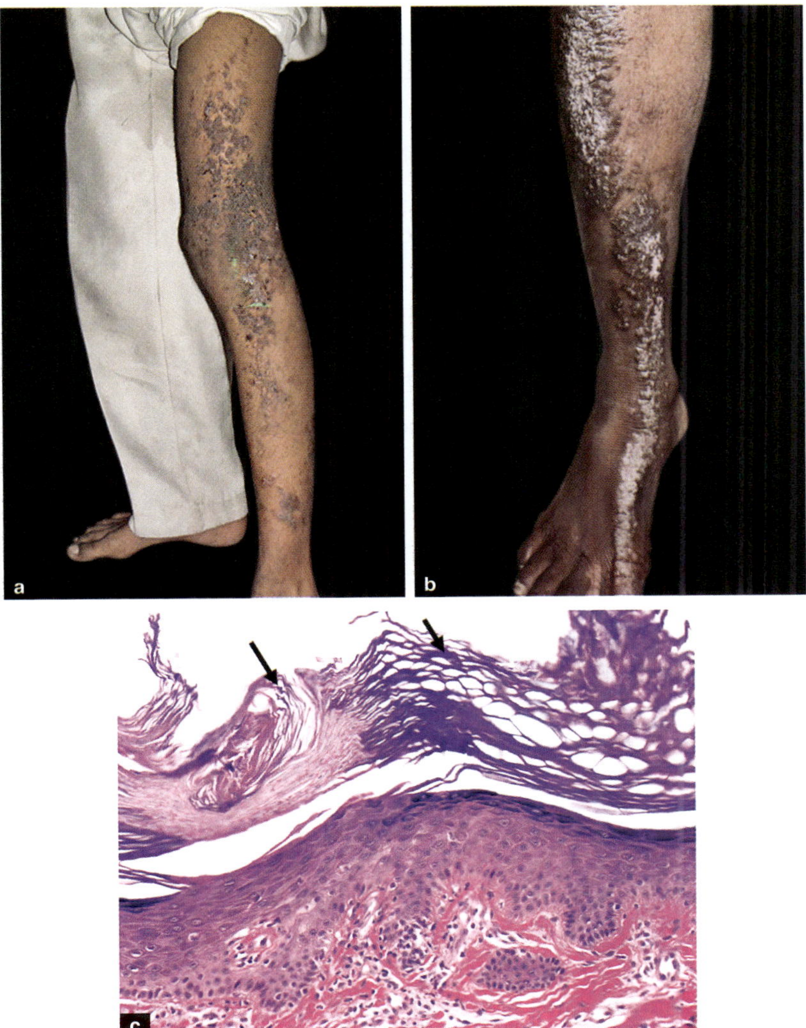

Fig. 25.3: (a and b) ILVEN is itchy and psoriasiform in appearance and there are often excoriation marks visible on the lesion; (c) Hyperkeratosis alternating with parakeratosis with acanthotic epidermis on histopathology of ILVEN

Differential Diagnosis (Box 25.6)

BOX 25.6: Differential diagnosis of ILVEN

- Inflammatory variants of epidermal nevus
- Lichenoid epidermal nevus/linear lichen planus
- Psoriasis superimposed on an epidermal nevus
- CHILD syndrome (congenital hemidysplasia with ichthyosiform nevus and limb defects)
- Lichen striatus
- Guttate psoriasis
- Blaschkitis
- Incontinentia pigmenti stage 2
- Linear porokeratosis
- Linear Darier disease

Treatment (Box 25.7)

While varied treatment have been tried, recently, an IL-17α receptor inhibitor was tried as studies have shown increased levels of IL-17 receptor expression in ILVEN keratinocytes. Thus **brodalumab** can be an effective treatment option for widespread ILVEN (Green R, et al., 2022).

BOX 25.7: Treatment options of ILVEN

- **Topical agents**
  - Potent topical corticosteroids under occlusion
  - Topical tretinoin, 5FU, calcipotriene, tacrolimus + fluocinonide, crisaborole[1]
- **Systemic agents:** Thalidomide[2], etanercept
- **Cryotherapy**
- **Surgical excision**
- **Lasers:** CO_2 laser, pulse dye laser, excimer laser[3]

Makins C, et al., 2020; Ossoria-Garcia L, et al., 2018; Wang RF et al., 2019.

NEVUS SEBACEOUS OF JADASSOHN

- Sebaceous nevi can be caused by mutations in HRAS or KRAS (both in individual nevi and as part of phakomatosis pigmentokeratotica (HRAS)/Schimmelpenning syndrome (HRAS or KRAS)) or NRAS. Thus it is beleived to be a neurocutaneous disorder caused by somatic gain-of-function mutations in KRAS or HRAS. LNSS brains have neurodevelopmental defects, including cerebral defects and epilepsy. Even mosaic FGFR2-activating mutation has been recently reported.
- Epidermal hamartomas of predominantly sebaceous glands on scalp and face.
- Seen in 0.3% of neonates.
- Equal male-female prevalence.
- Typically sporadic, but familial cases have been described.

Clinical Features

Sites—head and neck, scalp, around ears, temples, forehead, central face.

Prepubertal

- Solitary, circumscribed, smooth, pinkish yellow to orange velvety plaques on scalp and face **(Fig. 25.4)**.
- Nevus may present as bald patch on the scalp at birth
- Remains unchanged till puberty.

Post-pubertal

- Thickened, enlarged, waxy, greasy, nodular plaque.
- May present for the first time in this stage.

Prophylactic excision is recommended at this stage as most patients develop malignant degeneration after the age of 40 years. However, NS should be removed earlier if atypical morphological changes are seen and biopsy confirms malignant change.

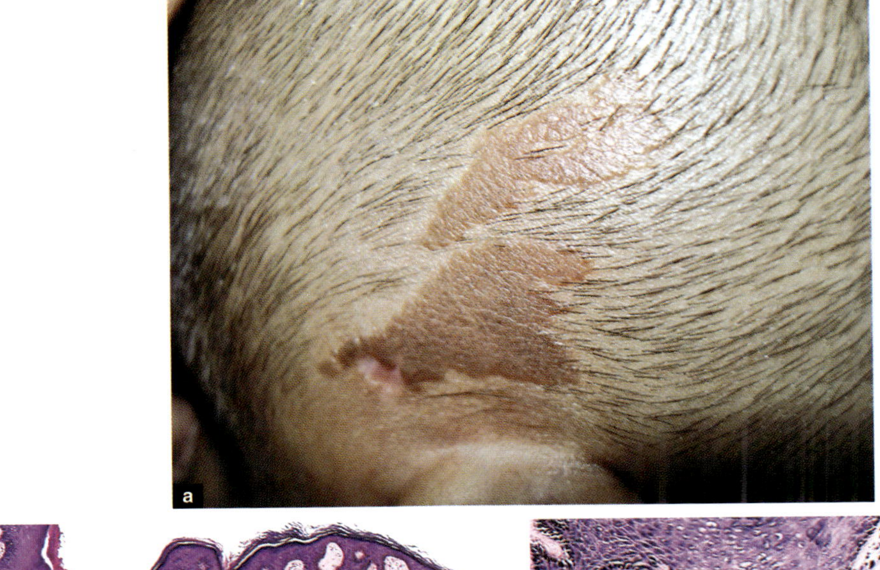

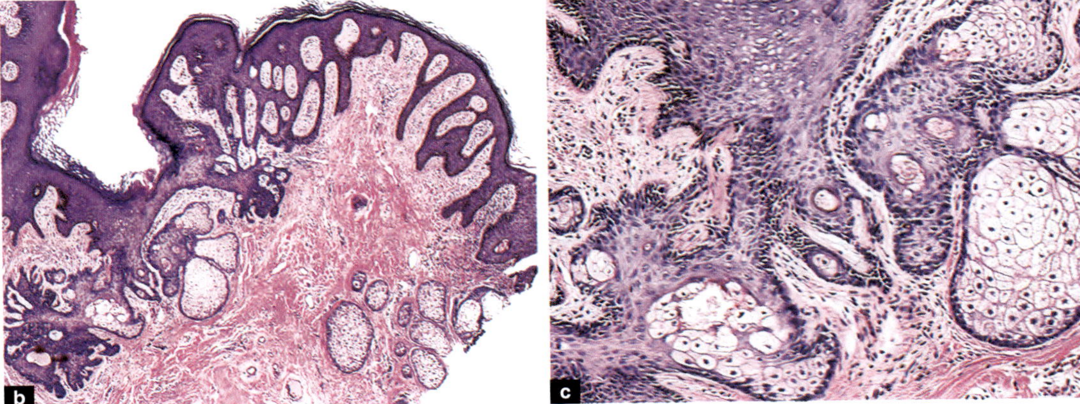

Fig. 25.4: (a) Nevus sebaceous—solitary, circumscribed, smooth alopecia, pinkish yellow to orange velvety plaques on scalp; (b and c) Hyperkeratosis, papilomatosis, pronounced sebaceous glands, with basaloid proliferations

Neoplastic changes

- Rapid, circumscribed enlargement and ulceration.
- Lesions occur singly (most common), but can be multiple or extensive.
- Risk of malignant transformation occurs at a rate of approximately **1%**.
- Basal cell carcinoma occurs in less than **1%** and squamous cell carcinoma is rarer.
- Risk factors suggested for malignant transformation include older age (usually >40 years), tumor on scalp, positive familial BCC history, HRAS mutation, and Fitzpatrick skin types I and II.
- Malignant degeneration is accompanied by morphological changes-rapid color change (black/brown/erythematous), protruding mass, ulceration, itching and discharge.
- Punch or incisional biopsies may miss malignant change in an NS and hence large specimen or 2–3 specimens must be taken from the area showing morphological changes.
- To differentiate BCC in an NS from benign trichoblastoma, IHC markers-cytokeratins-5, 19 and 20, and CD-10 should be used.

A list of tumors that can develop in it are listed in **Table 25.3**.

TABLE 25.3: Tumors seen in nevus sebaceous

Benign	Malignant
• **Syringocystadenoma papilliferum (M/C)**	• **Basal cell carcinoma (most common)**
• **Trichoblastoma**	• SCC
• Syringomas	• Sebaceous cell CA
• Trichoadenoma	• Apocrine CA
• Apocrine cystadenoma	• Eccrine CA
• Tricholemmoma	
• Nodular hideradenoma	
• Keratoacanthoma	

Pathology

Prepubertal

- Sebaceous and apocrine glands sparse and underdeveloped.
- Cords and buds of poorly differentiated epithelial cells representing primodial pilosebaceous follicles.

Post-pubertal

- Massive development and maturity of sebaceous glands.
- Papillomatous hyperplasia of epidermis, inconspicuous hair follicles **(Fig. 25.4b)**.

Differential Diagnosis (Box 25.8)

BOX 25.8: Differential diagnosis of nevus sebaceous

- Aplasia cutis (neonatal period)
- Viral warts
- Mastocytomas
- Epidermal nevi
- Juvenile xanthogranuloma

Management

- Surgical excision
- CO_2 laser
- Regular monitoring for hypophosphatemic rickets.

COMEDO NEVUS

- **Nevus comedonicus** (NC)
- Nevus acneiformis unilateralis

Definition: Rare type of epidermal nevus, presenting as a group of comedo-like lesions, due to abnormality of follicular infundibulm. May present at birth or in adult life, no sex predilection.

- FGFR2 mutations involved.
  (FGFR2 also involved in Alagille syndrome, Apert syndrome, cardiocranial syndrome, and Crouzon syndrome.)

Clinical Features

- Seen mainly on the head and neck area and appear as a cluster of comedones or as a single giant lesion **(Fig. 25.5)**.
- Unusual presentation over palm and wrist may also occur which represent variants of sweat duct nevus.
- **Two types** of NC have been identified; the first is non-inflammatory/nonpyogenic NC with acne-like characteristics and inflammatory characterized by formation of cysts, papules, pustules, and abscesses in various stages of development.
- There are various patterns of distribution: Unilateral, bilateral, linear, interrupted, segmental, or blaschkoid.
- In nevus comedonicus syndrome, nevus comedonicus is associated with non-cutaneous developmental abnormalities, including ipsilateral cataract, skeletal malformation, CNS abnormalities, and trichilemmal cysts.

Histology

The hallmark histologic findings are keratin-filled epidermal invaginations in association with atrophic pilosebaceous glands or follicles **(Fig. 25.6)**.

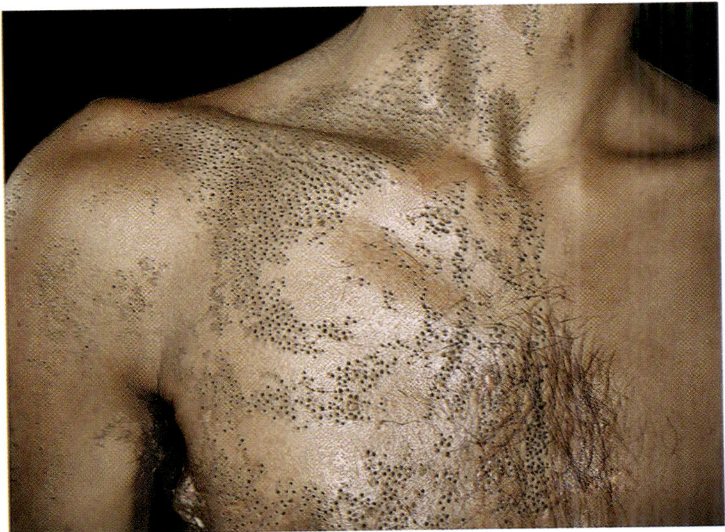

Fig. 25.5: Nevus comedonicus

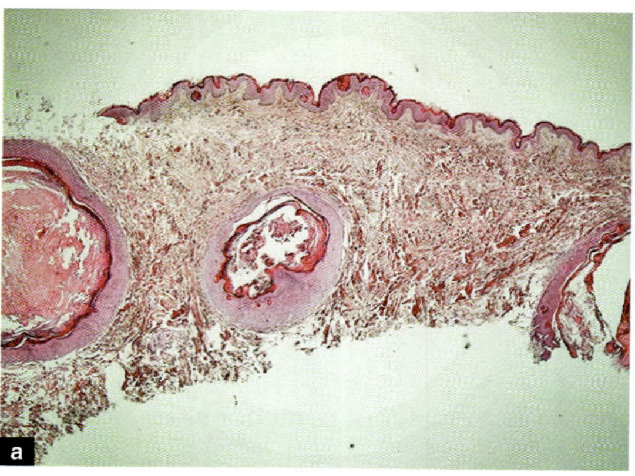

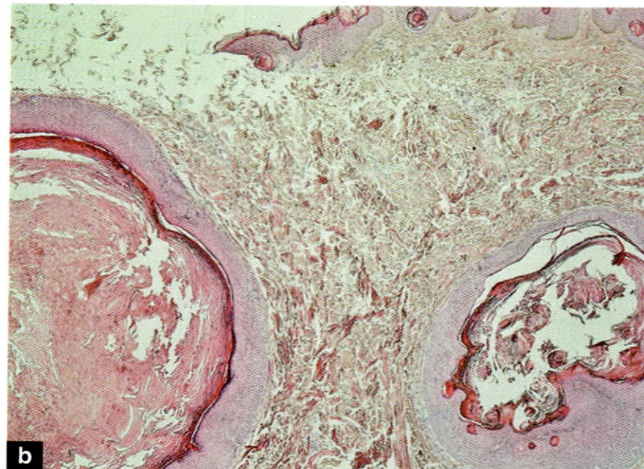

Fig. 25.6: Histopathology of nevus comedonicus. (a) Overview (hematoxylin and eosin stain (HE) × 2); (b) Details with large follicles containing lamellated keratin but absent hair shafts (HE × 4). Dermatol Ther (Heidelb). 2013 May 25;3(1):33–40.

Differential Diagnosis (Box 25.9)

BOX 25.9: Differential diagnoses

- Chloracne, acne vulgaris
- Dilated pore nevus
- Linear Darier disease
- Familial dyskeratotic comedones
- Porokeratotic eccrine ostial and dermal duct nevi

Treatment (Box 25.10)

BOX 25.10: Therapy options of nevus comedonicus

- Conservative: Topical emollients and moisturizes, topical corticosteroids (inflammatory lesion), salicylic acid, 12% ammonium lactate, topical retinoids (limited data).
- Surgical excision
- Lasers: 2,940 nm erbium YAG, 10,600 nm ultrapulsed CO_2, or 1,450 nm diode lasers.

What's New?

γ-secretase is another interesting drug target; absence of this enzyme results in complete conversion of hair follicles to epidermal cysts. Stimulators of this enzyme such as general control nonderepressible 2 (GCN2)—a subunit of eukaryotic translation factor 2 kinase—might be a future therapeutic option.

NEVUS SPILUS

- Congenital nevus spilus (or speckled lentiginous nevi).
- Pigmented lesions with a café au lait macule background and superimposed, more darkly pigmented areas (or speckles).
- In congenital nevus spilus, the superimposed pigmented areas are usually small, may increase in number over time and background may not be apparent at birth.

Epidemiology

- May present at birth or during childhood without any sex-predilection.
- Associated with multiple disorders.
  - **S**peckled **l**entiginous **n**evus syndrome **(SLN syndrome)**, with hyperhidrosis.
  - Ipsilateral dysaesthesia, underlying muscular defects and neurological abnormalities.
  - **Phakomatosis pigmentovascularis (PPV)**, coexistence of a macular SLN with a pale pink telangiectatic nevus.
  - **Phakomatosis pigmentokeratotica (PPK)** presence of a sebaceous nevus and a papular SLN, with or without skeletal and neurological disturbances.

Pathology

- Histologically, nevus spilus is lentigo simplex. The background macule shows a subtle increase of melanocytes.
- The darkly pigmented speckles present a 'lentigo' pattern, benign junctional or compound melanocytic nevi.
- Papular lesions correspond to superimposed dermal or compound melanocytic nevi, blue, Spitz, and/or atypical nevi.

Clinical Features

- Generally single lesion. Multiple lesions may be present and have segmental distribution.
- Flat macule on a tan background, often faintly appearing, and more darkly pigmented lentigo-like lesions or nevi **(Fig. 25.7)**.
- Other nevi, blue nevi, Spitz nevi or rarely congenital melanocytic nevi can occur within the lesion.
- Common sites are trunk, upper and lower extremities.
- May show zosteriform appearance or distribution.

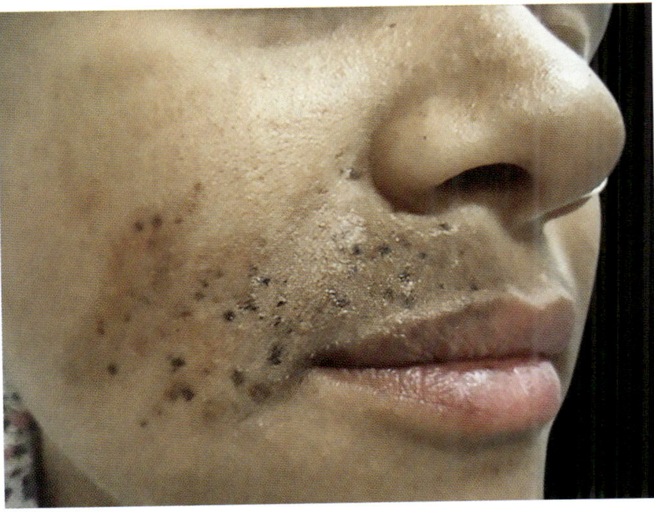

Fig. 25.7: Nevus spilus—multiple small darkly pigmented macules or papules on a light tan-pigmented background

Dermoscopy

- Dark speckled foci with a reticuloglobular pattern in a background light brown and reticular pattern.
- Mixed pattern may include combinations of homogeneous, reticular, globular, granular, and spitzoid patterns.

Differential Diagnosis (Box 25.11)

BOX 25.11: Differential diagnosis of nevus spilus

- CALM
- Agminated nevomelanocytic nevi
- Congenital melanocytic nevi
- Becker nevus
- Segmental lentiginosis

Disease Course and Prognosis

Melanoma arising from SLN have been reported. It is likely that the risk increases with size of nevus spilus, particularly with larger segmental lesions more than 40 cm.

Treatment

- Excision
- Ablative and nonablative lasers
- NS can be effectively treated with QS lasers but recurrences are not rare. Macular type appears to respond better than papular NS.
- Dermabrasion

LINEAR AND WHORLED NEVOID HYPERPIGMENTATION (LWNH)

- Benign skin condition, onset in infancy characterized by streaky hyperpigmented regions along the lines of Blaschko without preceding inflammation or atrophy, on the trunk and limbs **(Fig. 25.8)**.
- Soles, palms, face, eyes and mucous membranes are spared.
- Usually sporadic, epigenetic mosaicism, due to a clone of skin cells with increased pigment production.
- May be associated with extracutaneous findings, which can involve the CNS, musculoskeletal system, ocular, dental and (occasionally) heart.
- Skin histology shows increased pigmentation of the basal layer and prominence or vacuolization of melanocytes. Pigment incontinence is usually absent.
- Clinical course and prognosis: Onset of lesions in first few weeks of life with progression during the initial years. Pigmentation may fade gradually with advancing age.

Differential Diagnosis (Box 25.12)

BOX 25.12: Differential diagnosis of LWNH

- Hyperpigmented stage of incontinetia pigmenti (stage 3)
- Epidermal nevi (early stage)
- Disorders with linear hyperpigmentation

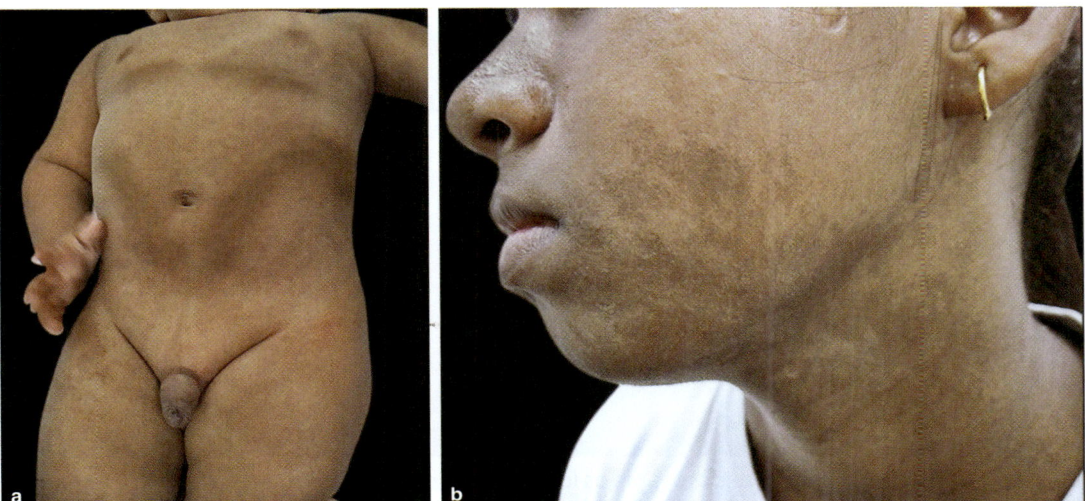

Fig. 25.8: Linear and whorled naevoid hypermelanosis

Treatment

- No effective treatment except camouflage.
- The 532 nm and the 755 nm QS laser were found to be both effective but long-term results and recurrences data is awaited.

NEVUS DEPIGMENTOSUS

Incidence: Seen in 1:50 of children.

Hypopigmented skin condition that may be a result of cutaneous mosaicism like hypomelanosis of Ito. It is believed to be due to functional defect of melanocytes with morphological abnormalities of melanosomes.

- Although classically present at birth, sometimes becomes apparent later in childhood, especially in lightly pigmented individuals.
- Associated conditions include seizures, mental retardation, unilateral limb hypertrophy, atopic dermatitis and abnormal systemic features.

Clinical Features

a. **Classical/solitary form:** It presents as a localized, hypopigmented patch that breaks apart into smaller macules at its periphery (resembling a splash of paint), that do not cross the midline **(Fig. 25.9)**.

b. **Segmental:** Unilateral, band-shaped lesions, sometimes Blaschkoid distribution.

Systematized: Extensive whorls and streaks of hypopigmentation, following the lines of Blaschko which mimic the cutaneous findings in HOI with midline demarcation and less distinct lateral borders.

Histopathology

Histological studies on lesional skin compared with perilesional normal skin shows a marked reduction in melanin, but variable results in the number of melanocytes (normal to reduced).

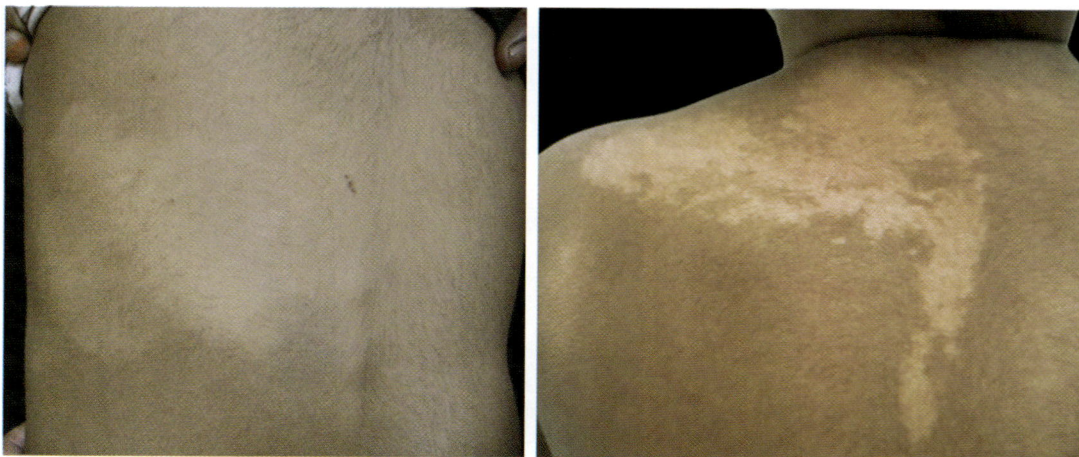

Fig. 25.9: Nevus depigmentosus, presents as localized, hypopigmented patch that breaks apart into smaller macules at its periphery ('splash of paint appearance') and does not cross the midline

Diagnostic Features (Box 25.13)

BOX 25.13: Diagnotic features of nevus depigmentosus

- Leukoderma present at birth or of early onset
- No alteration in the distribution of leukoderma throughout life
- No alteration in texture or change in sensation in the affected area
- Absence of hyperpigmented border

Differential Diagnosis (Box 25.14)

BOX 25.14: Differential diagnosis of nevus depigmentosus

- Nevus anemicus
- Hypomelanosis of Ito
- Incontinentia pigmenti
- Vitiligo
- Hansen disease
- Piebaldism

Treatment

In most cases no treatment is offered. Excimer laser (Zeng Q, 2018) and surgical techniques akin to that used for vitiligo have been tried (melanocyte-keratinocyte transplantation and suction blister) (Mulekar SV, 2011; Kar BR, 2013).

NEVUS ANEMICUS

Present since birth.

Clinical Features

- Nevus anemicus presents as a pale area of variable size (often 3–6 cm) with an irregular, 'broken up' outline, noticeable when there is surrounding vasodilation due to heat or emotional stress **(Fig. 25.10)**.

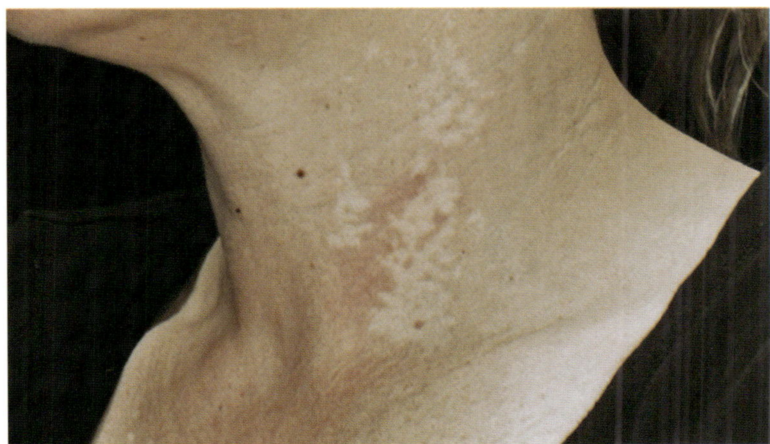

Fig. 25.10: Nevus anemicus, presents as a pale area with an irregular, 'broken up' outline. The contrast is more obvious when the surrounding skin is erythematous

- On diascopy, the lesion becomes indistinguishable from surrounding skin.
- Conversely, application of heat or an ice cube will often accentuate the lesion.
- More visible after emotional stress or after physical activities.
- It is usually unilateral and located on the trunk.

Pathology

- Local blood vessels within the lesional skin are permanently vasoconstricted because they are very sensitive to endogenous catecholamines. A decrease of E-selectin expression has also been reported.
- Histologically, there are no abnormalities in the melanocytes or melanin content.
- Islands of sparing may be present within the lesion, and skin transplanted within the nevus anemicus retains the characteristics of the donor site (donor-dominance).

Association

Sometimes associated with port-wine stains. Nevus anemicus and juvenile xantogranuloma have been found in higher frequency in patients with type 1 neurofibromatosis, and can be useful for early diagnosis of this genetic disorder.

Differential Diagnosis

- Nevus depigmentosus
- Vitiligo

Treatment

No treatment is required or effective.

CONGENITAL MELANOCYTIC NEVI (Fig. 25.11)

- Congenital melanocytic nevi (CMN) are benign, pigmented, melanocytic nevi present at birth.
- Definitely present since birth.

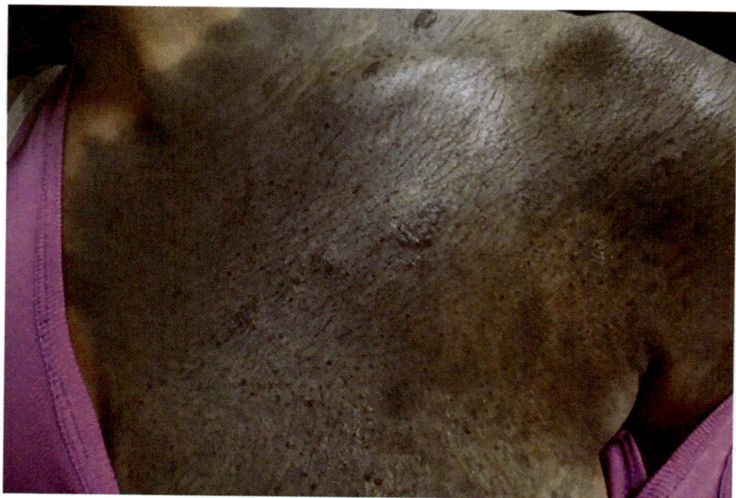

Fig. 25.11: Congenital melanocytic nevi, dark brown color, flat or elevated, with smooth to mammillated to verrucous surface, well-defined borders with coarse hair

- Slight preponderance of females to males of 1.2 :1.
- Mutation in NRAS or BRAS is known to occur.

Pathology

- CMN are almost always compound nevi with junctional and predominant dermal components.
- Composed of bland melanocytes that characteristically extend around adnexal structures and often into the underlying muscle and fat.

Types

- Small (<1.5 cm)
- Medium (1.5–20 cm)
- Giant (>20 cm)

Clinical Features

- Light to dark brown color, flat or elevated, with smooth to mammillated to verrucous surface and well-defined borders; may acquire coarse hair.
- After birth, benign proliferative nodules may form in the lesion which are of two types:
  1. Classic proliferative nodules: Present at birth. Well circumscribed, symmetrical, round or oval, soft to firm and of any uniform color. Can be resected easily if required.
  2. Diffuse neuroid proliferations: Not present at birth, develop during childhood and increase in size with time. They have ill defined edges, firm consistency and difficult to resect with tendency recur.

Dermoscopy

- Reticular, globular or mixed pattern
- Milia like cysts

- Perifollicular hypo- or hyperpigmentation black or brown dots/globules
- Hypertrichosis may be present.

Complications

- Risk of **neurological** and **malignant** complications, if more than one CMN.
- **Neurocutaneos melanosis (NCM):** May present with seizures, hydrocephalus or raised ICT. Prognosis is poor in symptomatic NCM.
- **Melanoma** (0.1–2%): High risk in giant CMN. The lifetime risk of melanoma development in lesions exceeding 40 cm (projected adult size) with satellite nevi has been estimated at 10 to 15%. Increased intensity of pigmentation, ulceration, or bleeding should raise suspicion of melanoma.

A **recent study found** that the risk ratio of melanoma incidence densities was 21.9 in large to giant CMN compared with small to medium CMN at 15 years of age. It was commoner with truncal location and in untreated or partially treated versus complete excision (Scard C, et al., 2023).

Disease Course and Prognosis

Lesions are darkest at birth, and lighten to some degree over first few years of life.

Differential Diagnosis (Box 25.15)

BOX 25.15: Differential diagonosis

- Becker nevus
- Aquired melanocytic nevus
- Nevus spilus
- Pigmented epidermal nevi
- Plexiform neurofibroma
- Melanoma
- Café au lait macules
- Congenital blue nevus
- Nevus of Ota/Ito
- Dermal melanocytosis (Mongolian spot)
- Congenital smooth muscle hamartoma

Investigations

- Skin biopsy
- If >1 CMN or neurological signs and symptoms—MRI brain with contrast.

Treatment

Depends upon risk of melanoma, cosmetic and functional considerations.

- Small CMN **<1.5 cm**: Observe
- Medium **(1.5–20 cm)**: Observation/surgical excision if on amenable area.
- Giant **(>20 cm)**: Management of patients with large and giant CMNs must be individualized. Serial excision or large scale excision using balloon skin expansion techniques.

Principles of Treatment

Today, the long-term aesthetic outcome is at the center of any therapeutic endeavor, whereas melanoma prevention plays only a minor role. The premise of 'removal at any cost' no longer holds (Ott H, 2019). Laser by itself does not lead to good results and surgical excision is at present the most reasonable option (ALMutairi HM, 2020).

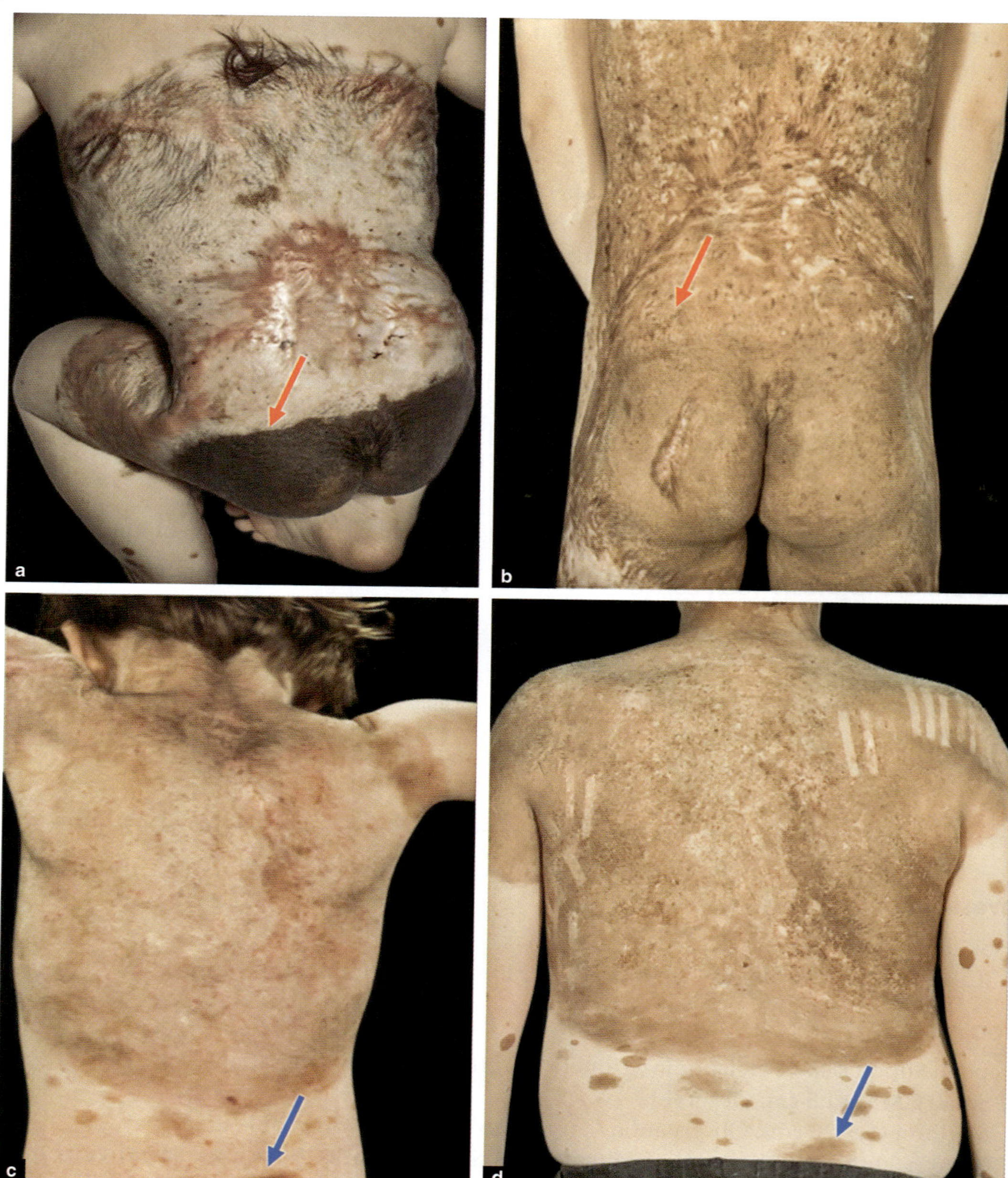

Fig. 25.12: Final congenital melanocytic naevus (CMN) color is entirely unaffected by superficial removal techniques. Patients immediately post-intervention compared with final CMN color, following intervention with curettage at (a) 9 months and (b) 7 years, and ablative laser at (c) 8 years and (d) 13 years. In (a) and (b) **red arrows** areas indicate the junction of treated and untreated CMN, and in (c) and (d) **blue arrows** indicate untreated areas, indicating that the final colour of treated and untreated naevi is the same. Note the scarring from the curettage in Figure "a" (*Modified from* Br J Dermatol. 2020 Mar;182(3):721–8.)

Final CMN color in childhood is significantly associated with the individual's normal skin color, and with *MC1R* genotype, and is therefore genetically determined. Final CMN color is not predictable from CMN color in the first 3 months of life. Superficial removal techniques do not alter the final color of CMN and a study has shown that gradual diminution in color gives comparable cosmetic results as surgical interventions (Polubothu S, 2020) **(Fig. 25.12)**.

HALO NEVUS (Fig. 25.13)

(*Leukoderma acquisitum centrifugum, Sutton nevus, leukopigmentary nevus, perinevoid vitiligo, and perinevoid leukoderma*)

Halo nevus is a melanocytic nevus (junctional, compound or dermal) surrounded by a depigmented halo.

- Dense lymphocytic infiltrate in the early phase and subsequent elimination of nevus cells.
- Central nevus exhibits the globular and/or homogeneous patterns, surrounded by a white rim.

Clinical Features

- Usually asymptomatic, often multiple, approximately 25–50% of affected individuals have two or more halo nevi.
- Most commonly affect the trunk of teenagers.
- The halo phenomenon signifies self-immunologic regression of a pre-existing melanocytic nevus.

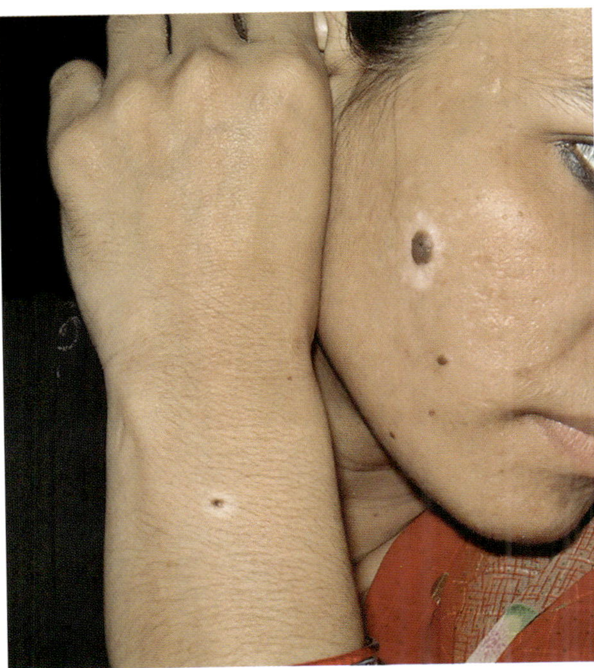

Fig. 25.13: Halo nevus, a melanocytic nevus surrounded by a depigmented halo

- Associations:
  - Concurrent or subsequent development of vitiligo (20%) or other autoimmune disease.
  - Turner syndrome
  - Atypical nevi, melanoma

Treatment

Individualized and depends upon clinical settings clinically atypical halo nevi should be examined histologically. Halo nevi with a benign clinical appearance need not be removed.

BIBLIOGRAPHY

Books

1. Celia Moss and Fiona Browne. Mosaicism anellinear lesions. Bolognia LJ, Schafler VJ, Lorenzo Cerroni (Editors). In: Dermatology, 4th ed. London. Elsevier Publisher; Ch 62:1011–12.
2. Cuda JD, Moore RF, Busam KJ. Melanocytic nevi. Kang S, Amagai M, Bruckner AL, Enk AH, Margolis DJ, McMichael AJ, Orringer JS (Editors). In: Fitzpatrick's Dermatology, 9th edition. McGraw Hill Education. Chapter 115:p1944–81.
3. Vercrica A Kinsler and Neil J Sebire. Congenital nevi and other developmental abnormalities affecting the skin. Griffiths EMC, Basker J, Bleiker T, Chalmers R, Creame D (Editors). In: Rook's Textbook of Dermatology 9th Edn, 2016. UK. Blackwell Publishers. Part 6.

Journals

1. ALMutairi HM, The outcome of using different surgical modalities and laser therapy in the treatment of small- and medium-sized congenital melanocytic nevi: A systematic review. Int J Dermatol. 2020 May;59(5): 535–42.
2. Green R, Hunter C, Chia JC. A case of inflammatory linear verrucous epidermal nevus successfully treated with Brodalumab. Pediatr Dermatol. 2022 Sep;39(5):757–760.
3. Kar BR. Nevus Depigmentosus Treated with Suction Blister Grafting: Follow-up After 10 Years. Indian J Dermatol. 2013 Mar;58(2):158.
4. Makins C, Sanghera R, Grewal PS. Off-Label therapeutic potential of crisa borole. J Cutan Med Surg. 2020 May/Jun;24(3):292–296.
5. Mulekar SV. Nevus depigmentosus treated by melanocyte-keratinocyte transplantation. J Cutan Aesthet Surg. 2011 Jan;4(1):29–32.
6. Ott H. Multidisciplinary long-term care and modern surgical treatment of congenital melanocytic nevi-recommendations by the CMN surgery network. J Dtsch Dermatol Ges. 2019 Oct;17(10):1005–16.
7. Ossorio-Garcia L, Jimenez–Gallo D, Collantes-Rodriguez C Balz-Perea JM, Lineares Barrios M. Treatment of inflammatory linear verrucous epidermal nevus pruritus with thalidomide. J Dtsch Dermatol Ges. 2018 Sep;16(9):1141–1142.2.
8. Polubothu S. Final congenital melanocytic naevi colour is determined by normal skin colour and unaltered by superficial removal techniques: A longitudinal study. Br J Dermatol. 2020 Mar;182(3):721–8.
9. Scard C, Aubert H, Wargny M, Martin L, Barbarot S. Risk of melanoma in congenital melanocytic nevi of all sizes: A systematic review. J Eur Acad Dermatol Venereol. 2023 Jan;37(1):32–39.
10. Tchernev G, Ananiev J, Semkova K, Dourmishev LA, Schönlebe J, Wollina U. Nevus comedonicus: An updated review. Dermatol Ther (Heidelb). 2013 May 25;3(1):33–40.
11. Wang RF, Milam PB, Chung C, Kaffen berges BH. Successful treatment of ILVEN with 308-nm excimer laser patient required. Photodermatol Photoimmunol Photomed. 2019 May; 35(3):193–196.
12. Zeng Q. Facial nevus depigmentosus getting remarkable repigmentation by treatment with a 308 nm excimer laser: A case report. Dermatol Ther. 2018 Sep;31(5):e12662.

Chapter 26

Panniculitis

Seema Rani, Sinu Rose Mathachan, Kabir Sardana

These are a group of inflammatory diseases involving the subcutaneous fat.

CLASSIFICATION

A detailed classification is given in **Table 26.1** and we will focus on the most common entity that is erythema nodosum.

TABLE 26.1: Classification of the panniculitides

Histopathological type	Clinical condition
A. Predominantly septal panniculitides	
1. With vasculitis	
• Veins	• Superficial migratory thrombophlebitis
• Arteries	• Cutaneous polyarteritis nodosa
2. No vasculitis	
a. *Lymphocytes and plasma cells predominantly*	
• With granulomatous infiltrate in septa	• Necrobiosis lipoidica
• No granulomatous infiltrate in septa	• Deep morphea
b. *Histiocytes predominantly* (*granulomatous*)	
• With mucin in center of palisaded granulomas	• Subcutaneous granuloma annulare
• With fibrin in center of palisaded granulomas	• Rheumatoid nodule
• With large areas of degenerate collagen, foamy histiocytes and cholesterol clefts	• Necrobiotic xanthogranuloma
• Without mucin, fibrin or degeneration of collagen, but with radial granulomas in septa	• Erythema nodosum
B. Predominantly lobular panniculitides	
1. With vasculitis	
• *Small vessels*	
– Venules	• Erythema nodosum leprosum • Erythema induratum of Bazin
• *Large vessels*	
– Arteries	• Erythema induratum of Bazin

(Contd.)

TABLE 26.1: Classification of the panniculitides *(Contd.)*

Type	Clinical condition
2. No vasculitis	
a. *Few or no inflammatory cells*	
• Necrosis at the center of the lobule	• Sclerosing panniculitis
• With vascular calcification	• Calcific uremic arteriolopathy (calciphylaxis)
b. *Lymphocytes predominant*	
• With superficial and deep perivascular dermal infiltrate	• Cold panniculitis
• With lymphoid follicles, plasma cells and nuclear dust of lymphocytes	• Lupus panniculitis • Panniculitis associated with dermatomyositis
c. *Neutrophils predominant*	
• Extensive fat necrosis with saponification of adipocytes	• Pancreatic panniculitis (high serum lipase, calcium soap formation)
• With neutrophils between collagen bundles of deep reticular dermis panniculitis	• Alpha1-antitrypsin deficiency (splaying of neutrophils)
• With bacteria, fungi or protozoa	• Infective panniculitis
• With foreign bodies	• Factitious panniculitis
• Neutrophilic lobular panniculitis	• Subcutaneous Sweet syndrome
d. *Histiocytes predominant* (granulomatous)	
• No crystals in adipocytes	• Subcutaneous sarcoidosis • Traumatic panniculitis
• With crystals in histiocytes or adipocytes	• Subcutaneous fat necrosis of the newborn (associated hypercalcemia, localized nodules, favorable prognosis) • Poststeroid panniculitis (due to rapid steroid withdrawal in children) • Sclerema neonatorum (premature infants, diffuse hardening, poor prognosis) • Gouty panniculitis • Fungal panniculitis (zygomycosis, mucormycosis and aspergillosis)
• With cytophagic histiocytes	• Cytophagic histiocytic panniculitis (bean bag cells) • Subcutaneous panniculitis-like T cell lymphoma
• With sclerosis of the septa	• Sclerosing postirradiation panniculitis

ERYTHEMA NODOSUM

Most common panniculitis.
2nd–4th decade, Female > Male

Pathogenesis

- *Delayed hypersensitivity response (Th1 cytokine pattern) to various antigens.*

Causes

- Idiopathic—most common cause, followed by streptococcal infections, other infections (bacterial GI infections—*Yersinia, Salmonella, Campylobacter*), viral URIs, coccidioidomycosis, tuberculosis, and histoplasmosis).

- *Drugs* (estrogens/OCPs, sulfonamides, and NSAIDs)
- Sarcoidosis, Behçet disease, pregnancy
- IBD (Crohn > UC)
  Positive prognostic factor in sarcoidosis and coccidioidomycosis.

Clinical Features

Acute, tender subcutaneous nodules **(Fig. 26.1)** on pretibial areas (most commonly) bilaterally with overlying erythema resolving within 1–6 weeks by turning to bruise-like patches (erythema contusiformis), ulceration/scarring or atrophy is not seen, systemic symptoms—arthralgia, fever, malaise.

Chronic forms (subacute nodular migratory panniculitis/erythema nodosum migrans) can occur. Seen in women, mainly unilateral, migrating centrifugally, nodules (are less tender than EN).

Investigations

Box 26.1 lists the investigations required in erythema nodosum.

Histology

- Septal panniculitis with thickening/fibrosis of septae. No vasculitis.
- Neutrophils seen particularly in early lesions.
- Miescher microgranulomas: Small histiocytic aggregates surrounding a central stellate cleft; located in fat septa +/– thrombophlebitis (more common in EN-like lesions seen in Behçet disease).
- In later stages, the septa become fibrotic, partially replacing the fat lobules

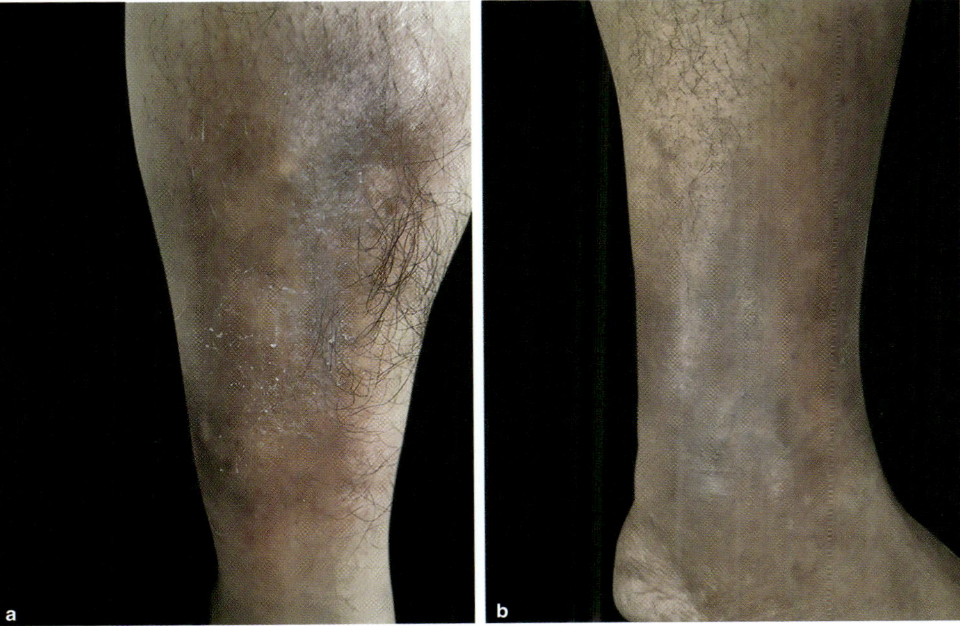

Fig. 26.1: Erythema nodosum

BOX 26.1: Investigations required in erythema nodosum

Complete blood count with ESR, CRP, throat swab culture, ASLO titers, Tuberculin skin test or IGRA, sputum for AFB, stool examination for cysts/ ova, chest X-ray, pregnancy testing in women of child-bearing age.

Treatment (Table 26.2)

TABLE 26.2: Depends upon etiology
• Rest and foot end elevation • Aspirin, NSAIDs • Supersaturated potassium iodide solution (SSKI)—2–10 drops (1 drop = 0.03 mL = 30 mg), three times per day in water or orange juice • Colchicine (especially for Behçet disease) • TNF-alpha inhibitors etanercept, infliximab (especially for IBD-associated) • Others—thalidomide, cyclosporine, HCQS, dapsone, systemic corticosteroids (rarely used, after ruling out underlying infections)

BIBLIOGRAPHY

1. Luis Requena. Ponniculitis Griffiths EMC. Basker J. Bleiker J. Chalmers R. Creamer D. Editors. In: Rook's Textbook of Dermatology (9th ed). UK Blackwell Publisher. 2016. Part 8; Chapter 99: P2629–89.

Chapter 27

Perforating Dermatoses

Surabhi Sinha, Kabir Sardana, Sinu Rose Mathachan

INTRODUCTION

A group of disorders with perforation or elimination of dermal connective tissue components through the epidermis (also known as transepidermal elimination).

Transepidermal Elimination (TEE)

- Proposed by Mehregan in 1970.
- **Definition**—this is a pathologic dermoepidermal reactive phenomenon incited by exogenous substances or altered dermal constituents characterized by pseudoepitheliomatous hyperplasia of epidermis and/or follicular epithelium and formation of multiple transepithelial perforating channels, facilitating the extrusion of the altered dermal material or foreign substances to the exterior.
- TEE can occur as a primary disorder or secondary to other pathologic processes **(Table 27.1)**.

TABLE 27.1: Classification of TEE disorders

Classical conditions with TEE* (Primary)	Unspecified conditions with TEE (Secondary)
Elastosis perforans serpiginosa	Collagenoma perforant verruciforme
Reactive perforating collagenosis (inherited)	Chondrodermatitis nodularis helicis chronica
Acquired perforating dermatosis (acquired reactive perforating collagenosis—Kyrle disease)	Non-infective granulomatous disorders—perforating granuloma annulare, necrobiosis lipoidica, rheumatoid nodule, sarcoidosis
Perforating folliculitis	Infections—cutaneous TB, botryomycosis, chromoblastomycosis, schistosomiasis, leishmaniasis, lobomycosis, histoid leprosy
	Calcifying dermatoses—PXE, calcified hair follicle tumors, calcinosis cutis, osteoma cutis
	Foreign materials—silica, wood splinter

*Confusion over most terminologies. Acquired perforating dermatosis is now used for most acquired conditions earlier labeled as RPC/ Kyrle disease. Perforating folliculitis—this term is also going out of favor.

Epidemiology

Acquired perforating dermatosis—most common associated with **diabetes mellitus/chronic kidney disease** with/without dialysis.

Predisposing Factors

- Basic pathology: Transepidermal elimination of degenerated collagen/elastin/other connective tissue elements.
- **Diabetes mellitus**—strongly associated.
- **Chronic kidney disease**—strongly associated.

Clinical Features

Even though it is now believed that most of the older 'named' disorders can essentially be clubbed under APD, these dermatoses should still be known and are listed in **Table 27.2** and depicted in **Fig. 27.1**.

TABLE 27.2: Differential diagnosis of common perforating dermatoses

	Inherited EPS	Inherited/familial RPC	Acquired perforating dermatosis	Perforating folliculitis
Morphology	Non-follicular papules—linear/arcuate/serpiginous patterns with keratotic papules along rim	Small eroded papules with central hyper-keratotic plug	Pruritic dermatosis with keratotic dome-shaped papules with central crusts	Pruritic keratotic follicular papules
Age of onset	2nd decade	1st decade	5th–6th decades	3rd decade
Sites	Nape and sides of neck, face, upper limbs, lower limbs	Dorsae of hands, fore-arms, elbows, knees, lower legs, face	Extensors of limbs, trunk, head and neck	Hair-bearing parts of limbs
Precipitating factors/course	Scratching, insect bites May spontaneously resolve but tend to persist longer	Scratching, cold spontaneous resolution over 6–10 weeks	—	—
Koebner phenomenon	Occasionally +ve	Often +ve	Occasionally +ve	–ve
Associated diseases	**MAD PORES** • **M**arfan • **A**crogeria • **D**own syndrome • **P**enicillamine • **P**XE • **O**steogenesis imperfecta • **R**othmund–Thomson • **E**hlers–Danlos • **S**cleroderma	—	• **Diabetes mellitus** • **Chronic kidney disease** • Natalizumab therapy • Dermatomyositis • Congestive heart failure • Liver disease	None
Differential diagnosis	• Granuloma annulare • Tinea • Actinic granuloma • Perforating PXE • Familial inherited RPC • Porokeratosis of Mibelli	—	• Prurigo nodularis • Arthropod bites • Dermatofibroma • Folliculitis	—

(Contd.)

TABLE 27.2: Differential diagnosis of common perforating dermatoses *(Contd.)*

	Inherited EPS	Inherited/familial RPC	Acquired perforating dermatosis	Perforating folliculitis
Histopathology	Keratotic crusted plug surrounding epithelial hyperplasia **('crab-claw')** grabbing pink elastic fibers in superficial dermis (*VVG stain*: Elastic fibers stain black *vs* pink collagen)	Shallow cup-shaped epidermal invagination with degenerated collagen bundles—extruded through vertically oriented fine slits (VVG stain, Masson trichrome stain)	• Cup-shaped epidermal invagination with degenerated collagen bundles—extruded through vertically oriented fine slits • Resembles RPC most commonly (may also resemble perforating folliculitis or less commonly EPS)	Suppurative folliculitis Collagen fibers and elastin fibers and degenerated fibers surrounding follicles
Important Factoids	• Associated with inherited disorders of connective tissue and Down syndrome	• Sites of minor trauma • Collagen perforates out • Upper extremities	• Almost always a/w **diabetes** or **renal failure** (10% of dialysis patients) • Lower extremities (extensor) • Possible role of fibronectin/advanced glycation end product (AGE) modified collagen I and III in causing perforation	—

a/w, associated with; EPS, elastosis perforans serpiginosa

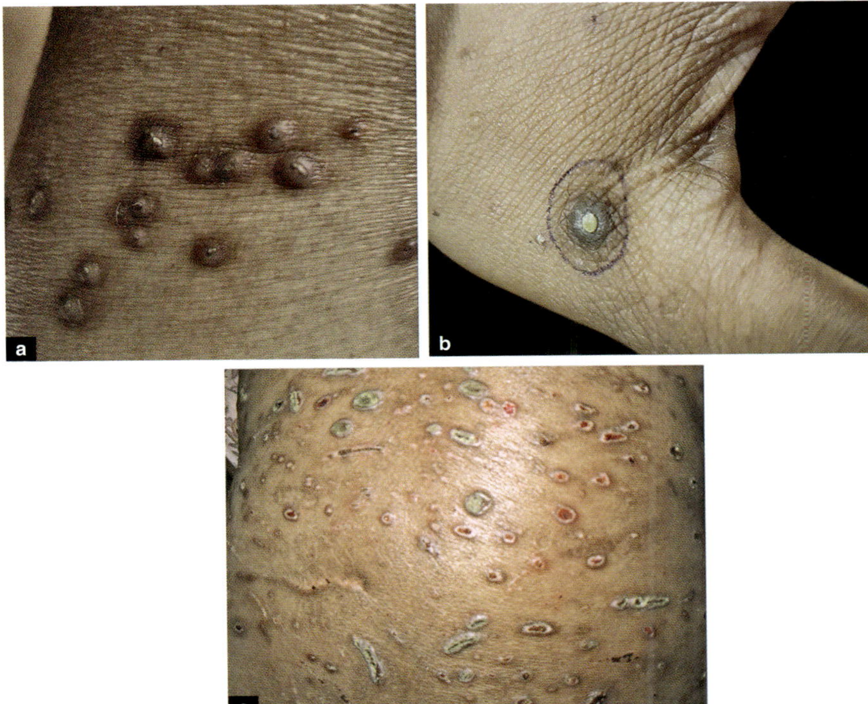

Figs 27.1: (a) Discrete papules and nodules with a central keratotic plug in APD; (b) Close up of lesions in acquired perforating dermatoses; (c) A case of APD with widespread lesions in a case with chronic renal failure

Treatment

Treatment of APD is listed in **Table 27.3** and a therapeutic algorithm for perforating dermatoses is shown in **Flowchart 27.1**.

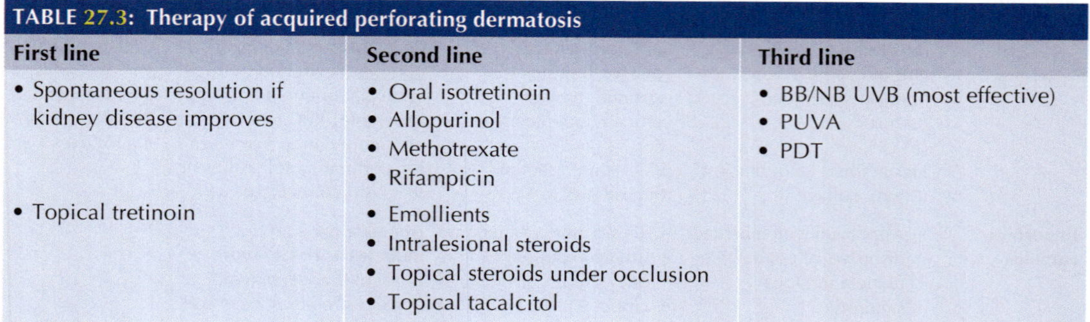

TABLE 27.3: Therapy of acquired perforating dermatosis

First line	Second line	Third line
• Spontaneous resolution if kidney disease improves	• Oral isotretinoin • Allopurinol • Methotrexate • Rifampicin	• BB/NB UVB (most effective) • PUVA • PDT
• Topical tretinoin	• Emollients • Intralesional steroids • Topical steroids under occlusion • Topical tacalcitol	

Flowchart 27.1: A summarized therapeutic algorithm for perforating dermatoses

RPC | EPS | PF | KD

1st line
Emollients +/– topical steroids +/– oral antihistamines +/– keratolytic agents [salicylic acid (5–7%) or urea (10–15%)]

2nd line

RPC — **Topical:**
- Tretinoin (0.1% cream or 0.025% gel)
- Intralesional triamcinolone

EPS — **Topical:**
- Tazarotene (0.1%)
- Imiquimod

PF — **Topical:**
- Tazarotene 0.1%

KD — **Topical:**
- Tretinoin 0.1%

3rd line

RPC — **Systemic treatment:**
- Colchicine (1mg/day)
- Steroids
- Acitretin (25 mg/day)

Phototherapy:
- PUVA
- NB-UVB

EPS — **Systemic treatment:**
- Acitretin (25 mg/day)
- Allopurinol (100 mg/day)

Phototherapy:
- PUVA
- NB-UVB
- PDT
- Pulsed dye laser

PF — **Systemic treatment:**
- Isotretinoin (30 mg/day)

Phototherapy:
- PUVA
- NB-UVB
- PDT

KD — **Systemic treatment:**
- Acitretin (25 mg/day)

Phototherapy:
- PUVA
- NB-UVB
- PDT

Others:
- Electrocautery
- Cryotherapy
- CO_2 laser

Treatment of coexisting systemic diseases (DM, HTN, CRF, etc.)
Drug-induced APD (biologic treatment) → Stop the drug

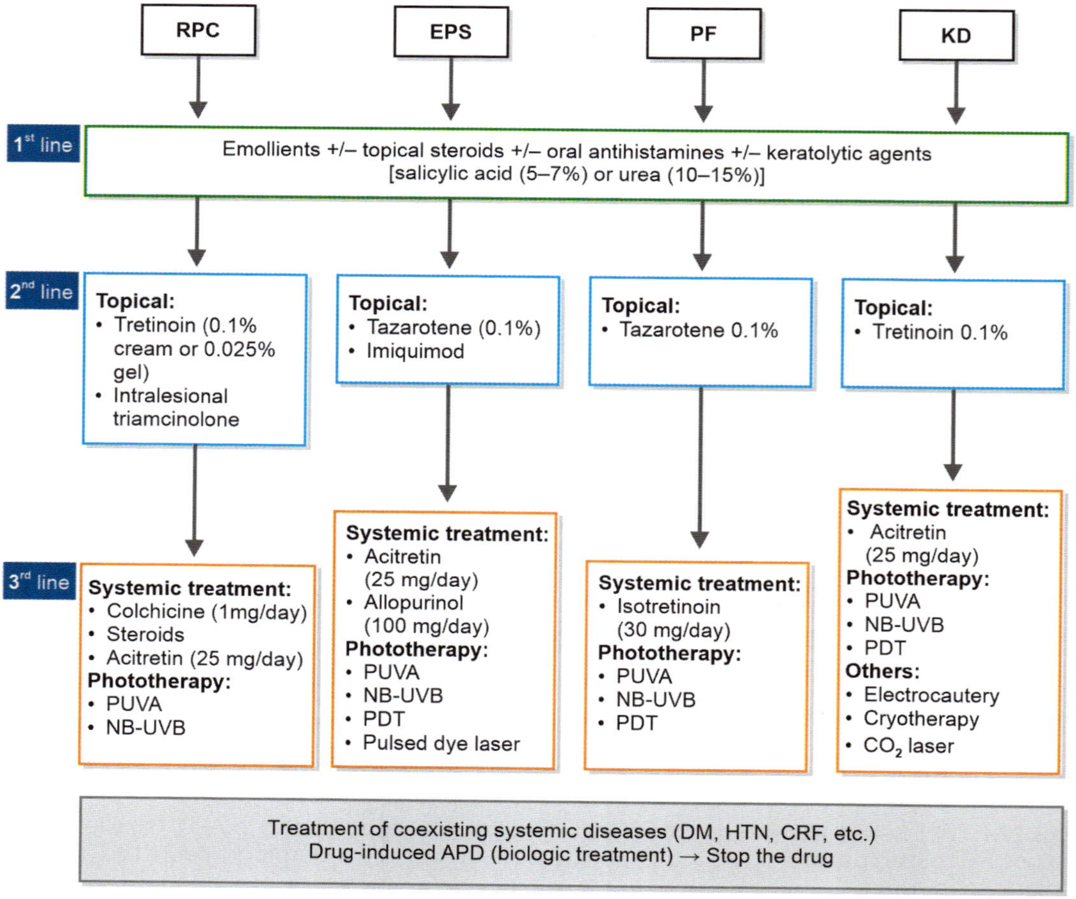

BIBLIOGRAPHY

Books

1. Dermatology (Bolognia). 4th Edn. Elsevier. Chapter 96.
2. Granulomatous, necrobiotic and perforating dermatoses. In. McKee's Pathology of the Skin. 4th Edition.
3. Rook's Textbook of Dermatology. 9th Edition. Wiley Blackwell. Chapter 96. Acquired disorders of dermal connective tissue.

Journals

1. García-Malinis AJ, Del Valle Sánchez E, Sánchez-Salas MP, Del Prado E, Coscojuela C, Gilaberte Y. Acquired perforating dermatosis: clinicopathological study of 31 cases, emphasizing pathogenesis and treatment. J Eur Acad Dermatol Venereol. 2017 Oct; 31(10):1757–63.
2. Shah H, Tiwary AK, Kumar P. Transepidermal elimination: Historical evolution, pathogenesis and nosology. Indian J Dermatol Venereol Leprol 2018; 84:753–7.

Chapter

28

Pigmentary Disorders

Surabhi Sinha, Kabir Sardana, Sweta Singh

Disorders of pigmentation can be divided into two types—hypermelanosis and hypomelanosis (including amelanosis). They can be acquired or inherited. We shall cover the following entities in this chapter:

- Disorders of **hyperpigmentation**
  - Acquired
    - Facial melanosis
    - EDP/Ashy dermatosis
  - Genetic
    - Nevus of Ota
    - Nevus of Ito
- Disorders of **hypopigmentation**
  - Acquired
    - Vitiligo
    - Idiopathic guttate hypopigmentation
    - Chemical leukoderma
    - Progressive macular hypomelanosis
  - Genetic
    - Nevus depigmentosus
    - Hypomelanosis of Ito
    - Incontinentia pigmenti
- Disorders with **reticulate pigmentation**

We shall first discuss disorders of hyperpigmentation in the section below.

DISORDERS OF HYPERPIGMENTATION

There are various methods to classify these disorders including a clinical approach based on the extent and pattern of pigmentation **(Flowchart 28.1)** and a histopathological classification based of predominant epidermal and dermal involvement **(Flowcharts 28.2** and **28.3)**, respectively.

Flowchart 28.1: Approach to diagnosis of common hyperpigmentation disorders based on extent and pattern

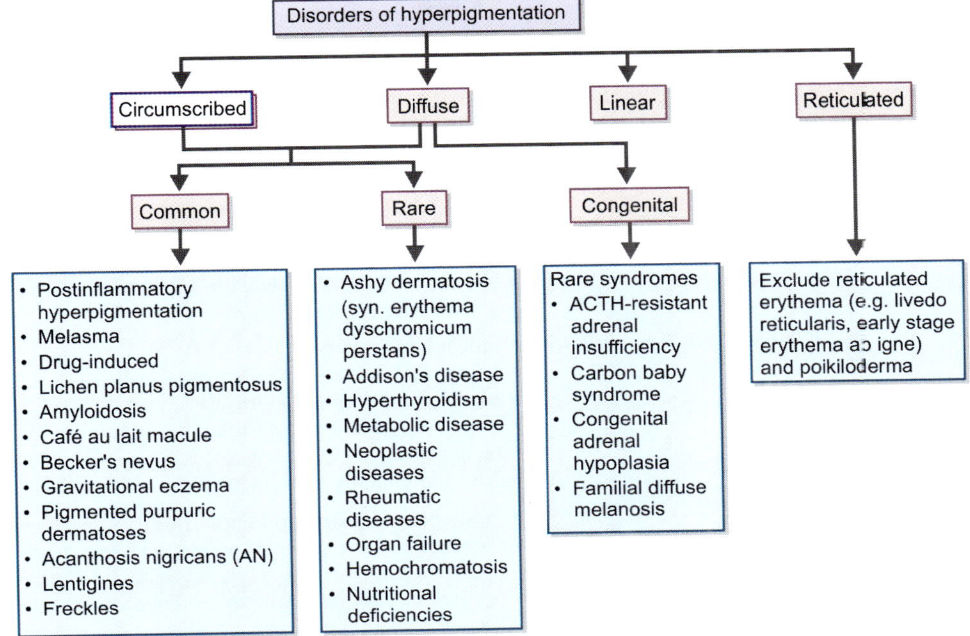

Flowchart 28.2: Classification of epidermal hyperpigmentation disorders

Hyperpigmentation (epidermal)

Melanocytotic

Lentigines

Melanotic

- Freckles
- CALMs
- Reticulate pigmentation disorders
- Becker's nevus
- Nevus spilus
- Melasma
- Drug-induced pigmentation*
- Pregnancy
- Nutritional#
- PIH
- Collagen vascular disorders

*Clofazimine, phenytoin, OCPs, hydroxy chloroquine, PUVA, arsenic, 5-FU, cyclophosphamide, bleomycin, AZT, vitamin B_{12} deficiency, kwashiorkor, pellagra
#Vitamin B_{12} deficiency, kwashiorkor, pellagra

Flowchart 28.3: Classification of dermal hyperpigmentation disorders

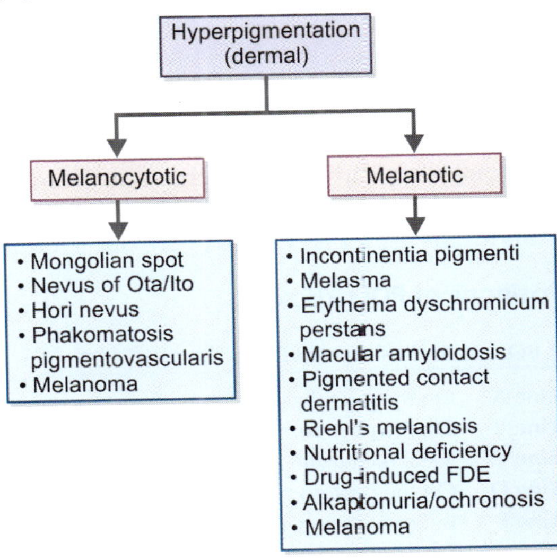

As linear hyperpigmentation disorders are commonly encountered, a list is given in **Table 28.1**. Before we discuss the common entities, we will discuss PDLs here as they are common and largely physiological.

TABLE 28.1: Causes of linear hyperpigmentation disorders

Lesions follow Blaschko's lines	Early onset, often during infancy or early childhood	• Linear and whorled nevoid hypermelanosis (LWNH) • Third stage of incontinentia pigmenti • Goltz syndrome (focal dermal hypoplasia) • X-linked hypohidrotic ectodermal dysplasias • CALMs in McCune–Albright syndrome • Linear morphea • Becker nevus • Conradi–Hünermann–Happle syndrome • Early subtle epidermal nevus
	Acquired and often later age at onset	• Linear lichen planus • Linear lichen planus pigmentosus • Linear fixed drug eruption • Linear atrophoderma of Moulin • Lichen striatus • Postinflammatory hyperpigmentation due to blaschkitis
Lesions that do not follow Blaschko's lines		• Pigmentary demarcation lines • Flagellate hyperpigmentation (e.g. bleomycin, shitake mushrooms) • Serpentine supravenous hyperpigmentation (hyperpigmentation overlying veins, e.g. after 5-FU chemotherapy) • Linear lichen planus (with koebnerization) • Linear postinflammatory hyperpigmentation after Berloque dermatitis/phytophotodermatitis • Linea nigra • Cryofibrinogenemia

PIGMENTARY DEMARCATION LINES

They are also known as Futcher's or Voigt's lines and are physiological, abrupt transitions from deeper pigmented skin to lighter pigmented skin. These are most notable in dark skinned individuals. Lines A–E (body) are depicted in **Fig. 28.1** and Lines F–H (face) in **Fig. 28.2**.

Positions of PDLs (Box 28.1)

BOX 28.1: Positions of PDLs

Line A	On the lateral aspect of the upper arm extending over the pectoral area.
Line B	On the posteromedial portion of the lower limb.
Line C	Mediosternal line, a vertical hypopigmented line in the pre-and/or para-sternal area (median/paramedian).
Line D	On the posteromedial area of the spine.
Line E	Bilateral hypopigmented streaks, bands or lanceolate areas over the chest in the zone between mid-third of the clavicles and the periareolar skin.
Line F	V-shaped hyperpigmented lines between the malar prominence and the temple.
Line G	W-shaped hyperpigmented lines between the malar prominence and the temple.
Line H	Linear bands of hyperpigmentation from the angle of the mouth to the lateral aspects of the chin.

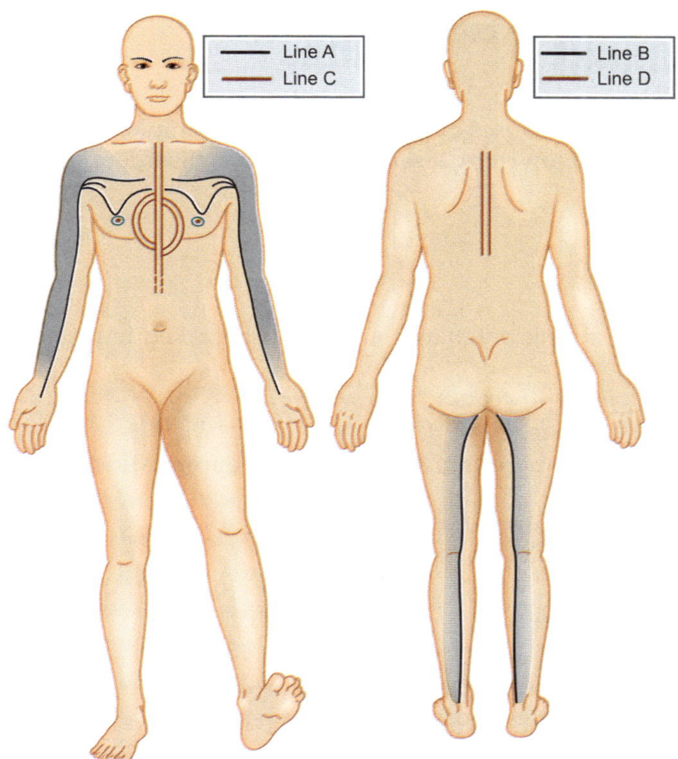

Fig. 28.1: A depiction of PDLs on the body (*see* Box 28.1 for details)

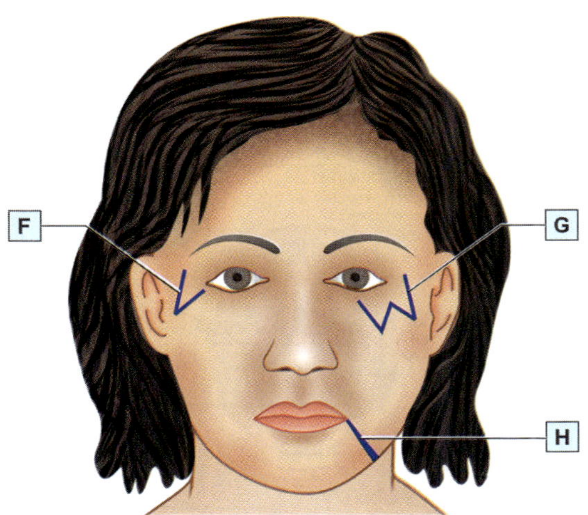

Fig. 28.2: A depiction of PDLs on the face (*see* Box 28.1 for details)

On the face, three lines **(Fig. 28.2)** have been described and are relevant as they are frequently misdiagnosed and treated as melasma. Some of the lines, specially type 'F' and 'G' often have an infraorbital extension.

ACQUIRED DISORDERS OF HYPERPIGMENTATION

FACIAL MELANOSIS

Though there are numerous causes of facial melanoses, a simple overview of the commonly seen disorders is given in **Flowchart 28.4** and a few select disorders will be discussed here.

MELASMA

Epidemiology

- Common condition.
- Commonly presents during pregnancy and is most marked in brunettes and women on oral contraceptives.
- Age of presentation is 20–40 years.
- F > M but up to 10% in men.
- More common in Latin Americans, Asians and those from Middle East with light brown skin types.
- About 30% have positive family history.

Predisposing Factors

- UV exposure (sun exposure)
- Hormonal factors
  - Believed to be due to the raised levels of estrogen and progesterone (which stimulate the activity of melanocytes), hormone replacement therapy, pregnancy and oral contraceptives.

Flowchart 28.4: Clinical approach to facial melanosis (EDP, erythema dyschromicum perstans; LPP, lichen planus pigmentosus)

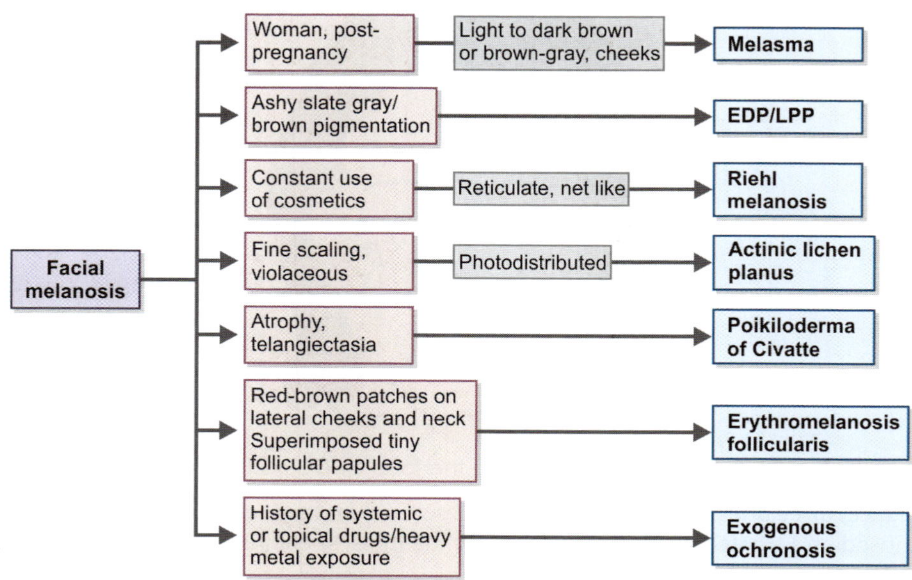

Pathogenesis

- Exact pathogenesis is unknown.
- It is hypothesized that exposure to UV radiation stimulates the hyperfunctional melanocytes to produce increased amounts of melanin.
- Role of increased expression of KIT and stem cell factor within the lesional epidermis and dermis, respectively, has also been mentioned.
- Medications like phenytoin, phototoxic drugs and disorders like autoimmune thyroid disease may aggravate the condition.

Clinical Features

- Characterized by light to dark brown or brown-gray patches with irregular borders, usually bilaterally symmetrical.
- *Site*: Mainly on the face involving the upper lip, the malar regions, forehead and chin and sometimes forearm.

Clinical Types/Variants

Based on site of involvement

1. Centrofacial (most common)—involving the forehead, cheeks, nose, upper lip (sparing the philtrum) and chin.
2. Malar—affecting the cheeks and nose.
3. Mandibular—along the jawline.

Based upon the primary location of the pigment

1. Epidermal
2. Dermal
3. Mixed
4. Indeterminate

This categorization is important as it may guide the treatment options and the extent of response that can be expected. Generally, dermal melasma is less responsive to therapies specially to the topical therapies.

Recent studies have shown that almost all cases of melasma are mixed.

Clinical Course

- Variable course
- After parturition the pigmentation usually lightens up but may persist for months or years.
- Similarly, the pigmentation takes a long time to become lighter after discontinuing oral contraception but sometimes it may never fade completely.
- The lesions become more prominent/more obvious just before menstruation in some women.

Complications

Cosmetically bothersome.

Diagnosis

No investigations are necessary as it is a clinical diagnosis. However, in doubtful cases, certain investigations can help in diagnosis **(Box 28.2)**.

BOX 28.2: Investigations in a case of melasma

Bedside tests	**Wood's lamp** (done to determine the type of melasma As majority are mixed, it has uncertain value in most cases)	• **Epidermal melasma:** Light brown in color and shows enhanced color contrast with Wood's lamp • **Dermal melasma:** Appears slightly gray or bluish on gross examination and shows less color contrast with Wood's lamp
	Dermoscopy	• Brown-black pseudoreticular network with dark brown colored globules, dots and blotches with perifollicular sparing. • Pseudoreticular pattern of pigmentation with diffuse dark brown to grayish pigmentation and involvement of follicular openings.
Histology	• Increased melanin deposition in all layers of the epidermis. • An increased number of melanophages may also be seen. • Epidermal melanocytes are enlarged with prominent dendrites.	
Ultrastructural study	• An increased number of melanosomes in the lesional melanocytes. Additionally, the mitochondria, Golgi apparatus and rough endoplasmic reticulum are increased in number or amount.	

Differential Diagnosis

Table 28.2 summarizes the common acquired causes of facial melanosis that form the differential diagnosis of melasma.

TABLE 28.2: Various causes of facial melanoses—differential diagnosis of melasma

Disease	Clinical features	Investigations
Poikiloderma of Civatte	• Middle aged fair-skinned females • Exposure to sunlight, cosmetics • Poikilodermatous (reticulate hyperpigmentation, atrophy and telangiectases) on face, neck, upper chest	• Patch testing • HPE: Melanin in lower epidermis and melanophages in dermis. Prominent solar elastosis of papillary dermis. Dilated blood vessels.
Erythromelanosis follicularis faciei et colli	• Predominantly young males • Triad of hyperpigmentation, follicular plugging and erythema on lateral cheeks and neck • Keratosis pilaris +/–	• Dermoscopy: Follicular plugs, some with a central hair, surrounded by blue-gray dots or peppering in a reddish-brown background. • HPE: Follicular hyperkeratosis, increased basal pigmentation, vaso-dilation, pigmentary incontinence.
Peribuccal pigmentation of Brocq	• Middle aged females • Exposure to cosmetics • Diffuse brownish-red pigmentation symmetrically around the mouth with a narrow zone of peri-oral sparing	—

(Contd.)

TABLE 28.2: Various causes of facial melanoses—differential diagnosis of melasma *(Contd.)*

Disease	Clinical features	Investigations
Lichen planus pigmentosus (LPP)	• Clinically, irregularly shaped or oval, brown to gray-brown macules and patches in sun-exposed areas • Often begins on the temples/in the preauricular area and involves the neck ± intertriginous sites • Might have lesions of classic LP (20% of cases)	• **Dermoscopy:** – Reticular network is accentuated uniformly – Pigment deposition is seen as grey to brown dots and globules which are evenly spaced – Typical case shows hem-like pattern • **Histopathology:** Vacuolar degeneration of basal layer; variable lichenoid infiltrate and epidermal atrophy
Pigmented contact dermatitis (Riehl's melanosis/ photocontact facial melanosis)	• Middle-aged females • Brown-gray pigmentation develops quite fast on the face affecting the forehead and temples more • Occurs at the sites of application, especially cosmetics (tar derivatives and fragrances) • May be reticulate in pattern • Brown-gray color due to dermal melanin deposits	• **Dermoscopy:** Regular array of brown and bluish-gray pigment globules giving a reticular network with finer and smaller globules than LPP. • **Histopathology:** Vacuolar degeneration of basal layer and lichenoid infiltrate in early lesions. But later epidermis appears normal with many melanophages in the upper dermis.
Exogenous ochronosis	• Pigmented macules on face in the same distribution as melasma • Positive history of application of hydroquinone to areas of hyperpigmentation followed by progressive darkening • Superimposed small pigmented papules may also be found	• **Dermoscopy:** Brown-black reticular pattern is seen, with pigment deposition as blue-gray dots and globules in a **"caviar like"** appearance. • Obliterated follicular openings and confetti-like depigmentation with elongated and curvilinear **"worm-like structures"** are seen conjoined together in a reticulate pattern **(mimics melasma and nevus of Ota)** • **Histopathology: Gold standard. Ochre-colored, banana-shaped,** fibers in the dermis.
Acquired bilateral nevus of Ota-like macules (Hori's nevus or ABNOM)	Hyperpigmented bilateral blue-gray or brown small macules on face	• Asian women are predisposed • Usually in fourth or fifth decade of life • Multiple brown-gray to brown-blue macules • Primarily in the malar region but other less common sites: Lateral forehead, temples, upper eyelids, nasal root or alae • Lack of ocular or mucosal involvement • **Histopathology:** Pigment-producing dermal melanocytes

Treatment

Difficult to treat condition due to the refractory and recurrent nature **(Flowchart 28.5)**. A plethora of varied therapies that include varied HQ free products , tyrosine inhibitors , lasers and varied oral drugs have been tried and this is a classic condition that fits the bill that "A Disease for Which There Is No Cure has multiple treatments!"

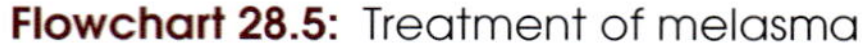

Flowchart 28.5: Treatment of melasma

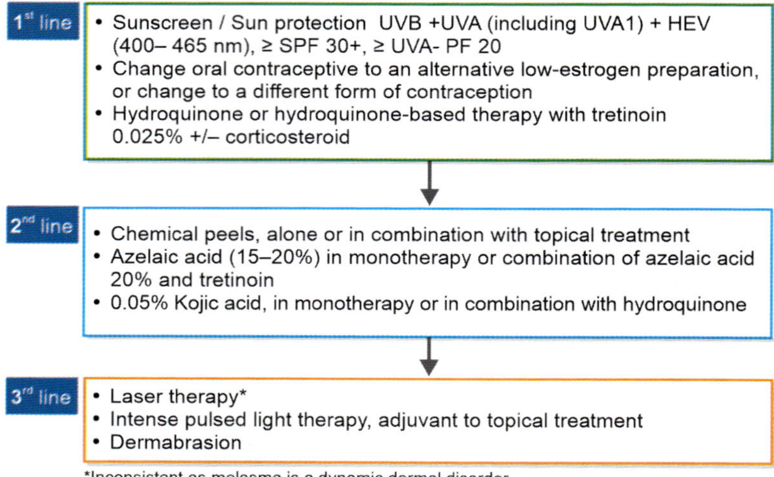

RIEHL'S MELANOSIS/PIGMENTED CONTACT DERMATITIS

- Both terms are used interchangeably in most studies.
- Also known as melanodermatitis toxica/pigmented cosmetic dermatitis.

While ashy dermatosis, erythema dyschromicum perstans, Riehl's melanosis, lichen planus pigmentosus and pigmented contact dermatitis are all now believed to be difficult to differentiate and are clubbed under the term "acquired dermal macular hyperpigmentation", there are cases where some of these entities can differ and we do not concur with the lumping as that does not add to the existent problem of treating these disorders.

History

- The term "pigmented contact dermatitis" (PCD) was first used by Osmundsen in 1970 to describe an epidemic of contact dermatitis in Copenhagen due to the optical whitener Tinopal (CH 3566) used in washing powders.
- Soon afterwards, in 1976, Nakayama described "pigmented *cosmetic* dermatitis" in women using certain cosmetics on the face and demonstrated positive patch tests with certain cosmetic allergens.
- In 1917, after World War I, Riehl had described "Riehl's melanosis" in Germany with follicular pigmentation on the forehead and zygomatic/temporal areas "of a toxic nature". He, however, could not link it to cosmetic use and attributed it to some "nutritional deficiency". Many years later, Pierini described Riehl's melanosis after repeated use of cosmetics containing mineral oils and concluded it too was a form of PCD.

Epidemiolopgy

Middle-aged females.

Pathogenesis

PCD is a variant of noneczematous contact dermatitis with a lichenoid reaction on histopathology. Lichenoid reaction has been described by Nakayama as a scaled down Type IV hypersensitivity reaction with positive patch tests possible as it is a form of contact dermatitis. Persistent contact with low levels of allergenic chemicals are believed to incite the type IV allergy, leading to basal layer cytolysis and thus pigment incontinence and dermal melanophages. Cutaneous inflammation increases the number and size of melanocytes and enhances their enzymatic activity, thus explaining the association of pigmentation with contact dermatitis.

Predisposing Factors

Numerous agents have been implicated and a list is provided in **Box 28.3**. In India, various allergens have been implicated including **PPD** (hair dyes) and **red Kumkum** from South India but a recent study implicated cetrimonium, gallate mix, and thimerosal in North India.

Clinical Features

- PCD presents as reddish brown/brown/slate gray macules in a fine/reticulate/patchy/blotchy/bizarre pattern. Macules that are smaller in size and perifollicular may extend beyond the defined margins **(Fig. 28.3)**.
- There is no preceding inflammation/no major scaling though mild itching and fine scaling may be seen in initial stages.
- Face followed by neck is the most common site. More commonly involved sites (Patch test more often positive) are hair margins (especially in hair dye associated), outer surface, helix and lobule of ears, preauricular area, temples, dorsum of neck, upper back.
- It is believed to occur around 2 months to 2 years after the contact sensitizer, though temporal correlation is often difficult to establish.

Diagnosis

Box 28.4 lists the important investigations in PCD.

BOX 28.3: List of agents implicated in the causation of PCD

Fragrances	Benzyl salicylate, benzyl alcohol, cinnamic alcohol, ylang-ylang oil, canaga oil, jasmine, synthetic sandalwood, lavender oil, geraniol, musk-ambrette, musk moskene, lemon oil and hydroxycitronellal
Textiles	Azo dyes, optical whiteners (Tinopal CH3566), naphthol AS, Biocheck60®, PPP-HB
Lipsticks	Diisostearyl malate, lanolin, alcohol
Cosmetics	Phenyl salicylate, propolis, 2-bromo-2-nitropropane-1,3-diol (bronopol), methyl-dibromo glutaronitrile (MDBGN)
Oils	Mustard and amla oil
Hair dyes	PPD
Miscellaneous agents	Potassium dichromate, colophony, balsam of Peru, paraben mix, sorbitans esquioleate 5%, quaternium 15 (Dowicil 200), Nickel sulfate, cobalt chloride hexahydrate, cetrimonium bromide, gallate mix, thimerosal and skin lightening creams.

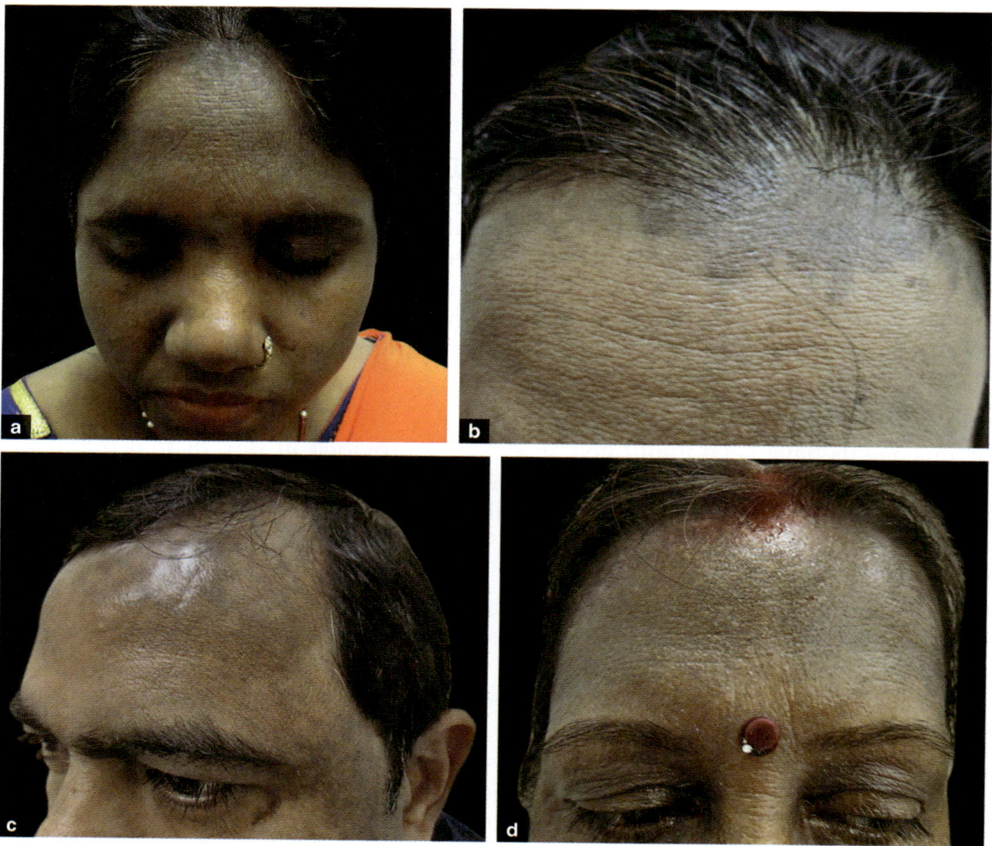

Figs 28.3: Various presentations of pigmented contact dermatitis

BOX 28.4: Important investigations in PCD

Bedside tests	Patch testing with standard, cosmetic and fragrance, textile, hairdressers and footwear series.
Dermoscopy	Pseudonetworks, grey dots/globules.
HPE	Early lesions show liquefaction degeneration in the basal layer of the epidermis and a mild perivascular dermal infiltrate with pigmentary incontinence while in later stages, the epidermis appears normal but many melanophages and some eosinophils are present in the upper dermis.
Ultrastructural studies	Intercellular and intracellular edema of keratinocytes with a multilayered basal lamina, along with many melanophages in the dermis are seen.

Differential Diagnosis

- The closest clinical, dermoscopic and histological differential diagnosis is LPP. Nakayama had suggested that patch test should be performed in Indian patients with "LPP" to diagnose them as "contact dermatitis" and if it is positive, they could be labelled as PCD. However, due to lack of any consensus on these terms, both have continued to be in use and so patients of LPP have also had positive patch tests and patients of PCD have been described as having interface dermatitis and lichenoid inflammation.

- Due to the considerable overlap, some authors consider them variations of the same disease process and others split them into different conditions. Clinical, dermoscopic, histopathological features have been studied but there is no single reproducible feature which can distinguish between these. Recently, there have been attempts to clump the conditions PCD, LPP, EDP and ashy dermatosis together into an "umbrella term"—to include dermatosis presenting as non-scaly macular lesions with interface dermatitis with pigment incontinence, known as "acquired dermal macular hyperpigmentation" (Kumarasinghe et al. 2018). The dermoscopic examinations also revealed similar findings in all three conditions—gray-brown dots/globules and pseudoreticular network.

Treatment of PCD (Flowchart 28.6)

It is a difficult-to-treat condition where allergen avoidance is the mainstay. However, identification of causative agent is difficult and pigmentation may take a long time to start reducing after cessation of allergen exposure.

LICHEN PLANUS PIGMENTOSUS

History

Lichen planus pigmentosus (LPP) was first described by Bhutani in 1974 in Indian patients.

Pathogenesis

It is a disease of unknown etiology with an insidious and prolonged course. Potential etiologic factors-mustard oil (photosensitizer allyl thiocyanate), amla oil (photosensitivity may be caused by fragrances), cosmetic agents such as kumkum, hair dyes, etc.

Clinical Features

It is characterized by dark brown macules—mostly in the sun-exposed areas and has a female preponderance **(Fig. 28.4)**.

- It has been reported to occur predominantly in persons with darker skin. Cases have been reported from India, Japan, Korea, the Middle East, and Latin America.
- Often begins on the temples/preauricular areas and involves the neck and intertriginous areas too.
- Up to 20% may have classic LP lesions.
- Mucosal hyperpigmentation may coexist.

Flowchart 28.6: Treatment of PCD

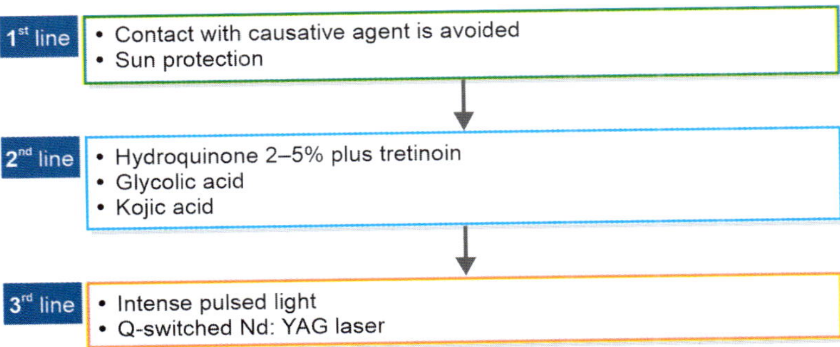

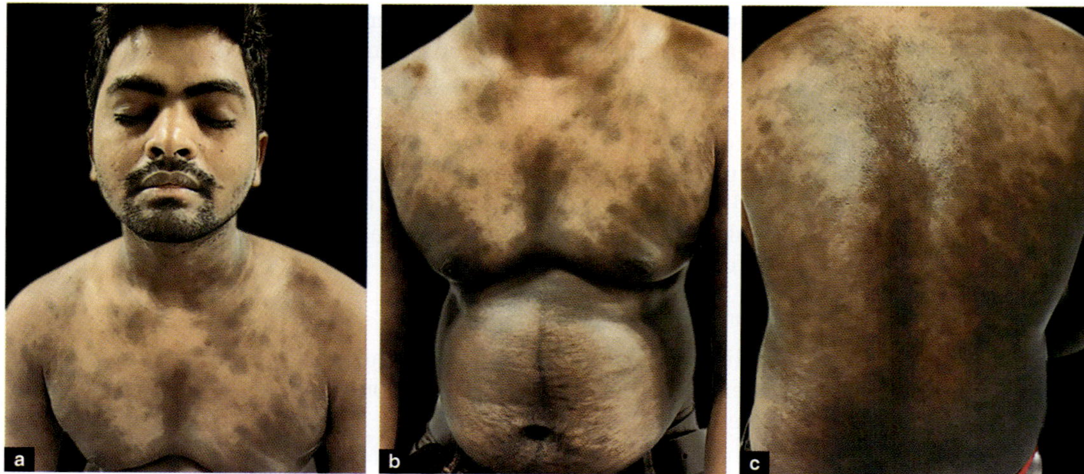

Fig. 28.4: Extensive lichen planus pigmentosus involving the face and trunk

Diagnosis

Dermoscopy: Large dots/globules showing brownish color because of the location of melanophages/melanin situated in the superficial dermis as a result of the dermoepidermal junction damage caused by the lichenoid infiltrate located just below the epidermis.

Histopathology: Vacuolar degeneration of basal layer; variable lichenoid infiltrate and epidermal atrophy.

Treatment

Difficult-to-treat condition. Topical tacrolimus, isotretinoin, cyclosporine, dapsone and systemic corticosteroids have been tried with variable results.

ERYTHEMA DYSCHROMICUM PERSTANS (EDP) AND ASHY DERMATOSIS

History

Ramirez first described ashy dermatosis (AD) in 1957. Convit et al later used the term erythema dyschromicum perstans in 1961 to highlight the erythematous halo around pigmented macules.

Epidemiology

- The majority of the cases are reported from central and South America or East Asia.
- Young adults (during the second to third decade) are mainly affected but it can occur at any age.
- F > M
- Skin types III–IV
- HLA-DR4 positive, Mexicans.

Predisposing Factors

No causal agent or triggering factor has been found. Different case reports of EDP following the ingestion of ammonium nitrate, oral X-ray contrast media and medications like penicillin and benzodiazepine, pesticide exposure, endocrinopathies including thyroid disease, whipworm infection and HIV have been published.

Pathogenesis

- Etiology of EDP is unknown.
- A cell-mediated immune reaction to an ingestant, contactant or microorganism has been postulated for the discrete areas of pigmentary incontinence.

Clinical Features

- In the early stage, lesions have erythematous thin, raised borders showing signs of inflammation initially which resolve afterwards.
- Circular, oval or irregular shaped, discrete or coalescent, slate-gray to blue-brown macules of various sizes distributed symmetrically over trunk, limbs and face.
- The lesions start developing initially from trunk and later spread to the neck, proximal upper limbs and sometimes face.
- Macules of hypomelanosis or hypermelanosis are found against a general greyish background.
- The condition is persistent and slowly extends.
- The condition is mostly asymptomatic, persistent and extends gradually. But sometimes mild pruritus develops.
- Mucous membranes are spared.

Differential Diagnosis (Box 28.5)

BOX 28.5: Differential diagnosis of EDP

- Lichen planus pigmentosus.
- Postinflammatory hypermelanosis secondary to identifiable cause.
- Late pinta, which should be excluded in endemic areas.

Clinical Course

The initial erythematous phase tends to settle after several months. The pigmentation is persistent with a tendency to extend gradually over years.

Diagnosis

Box 28.6 lists the important investigations.

BOX 28.6: Important investigations in EDP

Dermoscopy	Gray-bluish small dots over a bluish background corresponding to melanophages/melanin deposits in deeper dermis.
HPE	• Epidermis: Increased melanin and melanophages with pigmentary incontinence. • The dermal vessels are sleeved with an infiltrate of lymphocytes and histiocytes. • The active border in cases of erythema chronicum perstans shows vacuolar degeneration of the basal cells. • Colloid bodies and dermal hemosiderin may be present. • In later ("inactive") lesions, the dermal melanophages number is raised with no hydropic changes in the basal layers and minimal mononuclear cell infiltrate.
Ultrastructural studies	Vacuoles within the cytoplasm of basal and suprabasal keratinocytes that contain many melanosome complexes.

Treatment (Flowchart 28.7)

No effective and consistent treatment so far.

Flowchart 28.7: Treatment of EDP

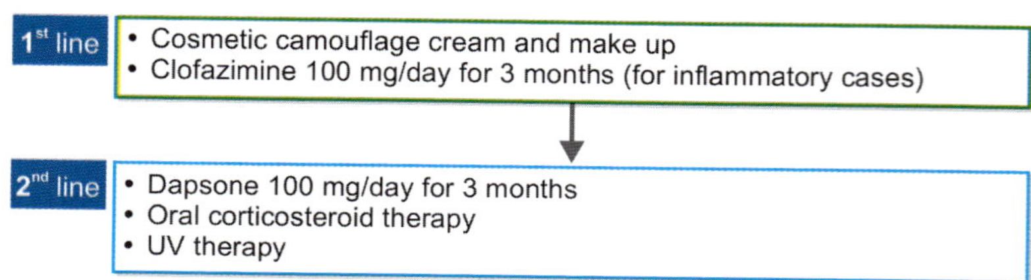

NEVUS OF OTA AND ITO

Nevus of Ota: An extensive, bluish, patchy, dermal melanocytosis that affects the region of the trigeminal nerve usually in a unilateral distribution (V1 and V2 most frequently). The sclera and the skin adjacent to the eye are often involved. Extracutaneous lesions may also present in the uveal tract, dura, nasopharynx, tympanum and palate.

Nevus of Ito is very similar to nevus of Ota except it differs in the territory of distribution-unilateral lateral cutaneous brachial nerves of the shoulder and posterior supraclavicular nerves.

Epidemiology

- Asians and Blacks mostly, but also in Caucasians (high in Japanese).
- Bimodal peaks of onset: At birth or during infancy and second peak at puberty.
- More common in females (F:M = 5:1).
- Rarely familial but the condition is not hereditary generally.

Associated Diseases

- Nevus of Ito.
- Extensive Mongolian spots with cases of bilateral nevus of Ota.
- Sturge–Weber and Klippel–Trénaunay syndromes (infrequently associated).

Pathogenesis

- During embryogenesis, the melanoblasts migrate to skin and uvea causing the typical bluish-gray pigmentation in these sites. Melanin-producing melanocytes in the dermis are responsible for the blue to blue-gray color.
- The female preponderance is thought to be due to hormonal influence.
- 6% have a GNAQ mutation which is a genetic link between nevus of Ota and uveal melanoma. Monosomy of chromosome 3 and gain of the long arm of chromosome 8q is a significant risk factor for uveal melanoma and poor outcome.
- The genes BRAF and NRAS of the MAP kinase pathway have been implicated. G-coupled protein, GNAQ is found to be mutated causing the G-coupled protein to be constitutively turned on.

Clinical Features

- Most commonly, they present at birth, but lesions can also appear in puberty or during pregnancy due to hormonal changes.
- Ueda et al classified nevus of Ota into various types based on the color as brown, brown-violet, violet-blue, and blue-green (Ueda S, et al., 2000) while Tanino classified it into Types I (mild), II (moderate), III (scalp, forehead, nose) and IV (bilateral) based on extent (Tanino H, 1939).
- Brown pigmentation is superficial and patchy with a reticular or geographical pattern while blue pigmentation is deeper and more diffuse, usually distributed along the ophthalmic and maxillary divisions of the trigeminal nerve, and thus present in the periorbital region involving the bulbar and palpebral conjunctiva and the sclera, and the temple, forehead, scalp, nose, ears, palate and malar area.
- Round, oval or serrated irregularly demarcated and often mottled macules composed of blue and brown components that may not coalesce and the size of individual macules may vary from few millimeters to extensive unilateral and sometimes bilateral involvement **(Fig. 28.5)**.
- About 2/3 have ipsilateral sclera involved, with the rare involvement of cornea, iris, fundus oculi, retrobulbar fat, periosteum, retina and optic nerve. About 10% of the patients have iris mammillations and glaucoma, but usually vision is not affected.
- Other sites are tympanum (55%), nasal mucosa (30%), pharynx (25%) and palate (20%), external auditory canal, mandibular area, lip, neck and thorax.
- 5–15% have bilateral lesions where the sclera appears blue and the conjunctiva appears brown.

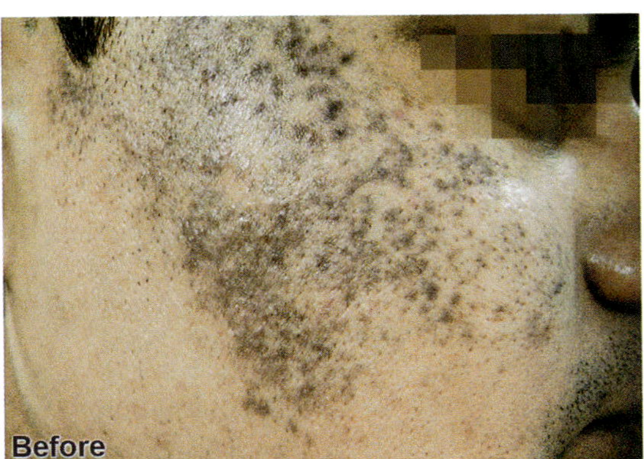

Fig. 28.5: Male patient with a blue-colored nevus of Ota (left) and after 12 sittings of Qs Nd:YAG (1064 nm) (Lasers and energy devices in aesthetic dermatology practice 2019)

Differential Diagnosis (Box 28.7)

BOX 28.7: Differential diagnosis of nevus of Ota

Disease	Differentiation from nevus of Ota
Hori nevus	• No mucosal involvement in Hori's nevus • Acquired later on in life • B/L
Café au lait macule	Brown colored, no mucosal involvement, any site on body
Nevus spilus	Any site on body, darker brown smaller macules superimposed on a background light brown macule

Clinical Course

- Overall good prognosis.
- The lesions of nevus of Ota may enlarge gradually and persist forever.
- The intensity of color fluctuates especially during menstruation, puberty or menopause.
- Rare cases of developing malignancy within nevus of Ota lesions is reported in 1 in 400 Caucasians and there is 10.3% risk of glaucoma. Hence annual ophthalmologic screening for intraocular pressure and dilated indirect ophthalmoscopy is recommended.

Complications

- Cutaneous melanoma.
- Uveal melanoma and glaucoma.
- Other tumours that may arise in nevus of Ota are atypical and borderline cellular blue nevi and primary melanoma of the choroid, orbit, iris, chiasma and meninges. Thus, regular ophthalmological monitoring should be done and a close eye on skin nodule development should be kept for melanoma.

Diagnosis

Box 28.8 lists the important investigations in nevus of Ota.

BOX 28.8: Investigations in nevus of Ota

Ocular investigations	• Visual acuity testing • Intraocular pressure measurement • Slit-lamp examination of the anterior segment—sub-conjunctival melanosis and episcleral pigmentation • Dilated fundus examination with an indirect ophthalmoscope—to rule out any choroidal mass/choroidal melanoma in peripheral retina. • Gonioscopy should be performed to note the hyperpigmentation of trabecular meshwork. • Stereoscopic examination of the optic nerve head should be done to document any optic nerve head cupping.
HPE (to rule out malignancy)	• Pigmented, elongated, dendritic melanocytes are found scattered among the collagen bundles in the non-infiltrated areas of nevus of Ota. • The melanocytic cells are more numerous and are located in the upper third of the reticular dermis and sometimes in the papillary dermis or even deep in the subcutaneous fat **(Fig. 28.6)**. • NOA has been classified histologically into five types based on the locations of the dermal melanocytes, which are superficial, superficial dominant, diffuse, deep dominant, and deep. This correlates clinically with the finding that the more superficial lesions tend to be located on cheeks, while deeper lesions occur on periorbital, temple, and forehead. • Hypermelanosis of the lower epidermis and an increase in basilar melanocytes may occur. • The melanocytes can also be found-clustering around blood vessels and sweat and sebaceous glands and occasionally seen within vessel walls or in sweat ducts.
Special stains	The DOPA reactivity of the melanocytes varies: Strong reaction is seen with less pigmented cells while heavily pigmented cells do not show much reactivity indicating minimal residual enzymatic activity.

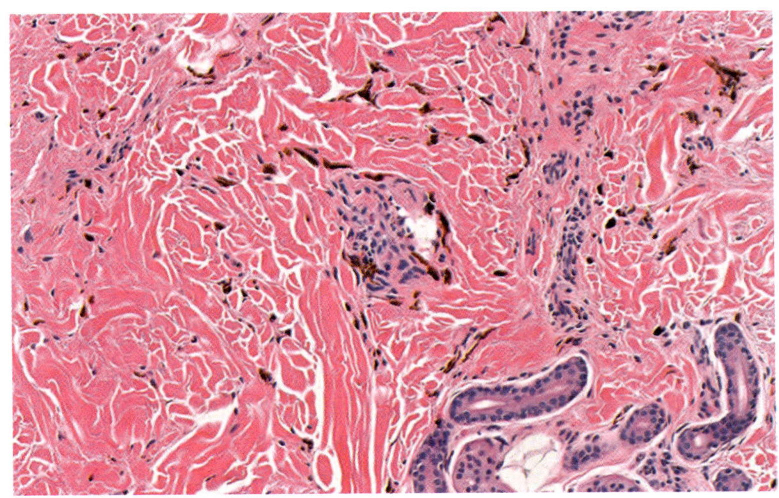

Fig. 28.6: Elongated and pigmented dendritic melanocytes seen on high power in nevus of Ota

Treatment (Flowchart 28.8)

While the treatment has been listed as largely lasers there are multiple variables that determine the response to therapy and it is uncommon to achieve complete improvement.

Some of the variables are listed in **Box 28.9**.

Flowchart 28.8: Treatment of nevus of Ota

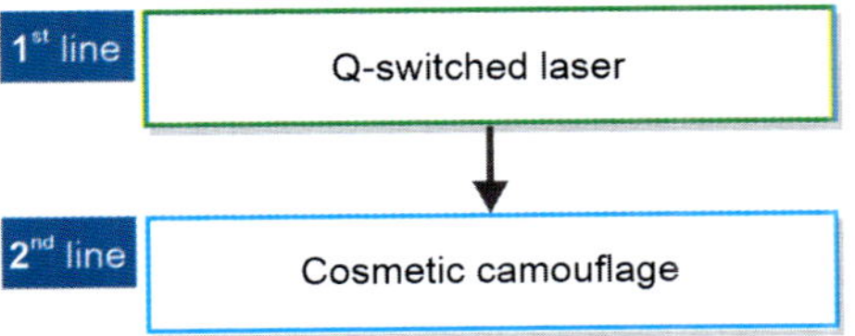

BOX 28.9: Variables that determine response with QS lasers

Laser wavelength	Q-switched Nd:YAG 1064 nm is ideal for pigmented skin but as the depth of the pathology varies QS-532 nm, Alexandrite-755 nm have also been tried.
Dose	6–10 J/cm^2, one to seven treatments, interval of 12 weeks.
Spot size	Larger spot size to achieve maximum depth (with lowest fluences).
Pulse duration	Pico are as good as QS lasers in pigmented skin.
Interval of sessions	3 months
Site	**Periorbital** involvement has been found to be associated with **more treatment** sessions. Nevi of Ota with the depth of 1 mm or less were associated with excellent or good results.
Color	**Brown-colored** lesions have more superficial dermal melanocytes, **blue** have deeper dermal melanocytes, and **gray** have both deep and diffuse dermal melanocytes. This affects the treatment responses, thus brown rather than blue lesions are a good predictive factor of response to treatment.

Rani S, Sardana K, et al., 2019.

Ir is important to appreciate that a "cook book" approach is rarely of use in NOA and the pulse duration and wavelength both determine the ideal settings. The optimal pulse duration is between **15** and **150 ns** to limit heat transfer inside the hyperplastic melanin, and 50 ns is recommended to decrease the energy absorption by normal melanin in epidermis. For the same NOA, the therapy window of the 755-nm laser is larger than that of 1064-nm. For NOA with shallow depth the 755-nm laser is recommended to make the treatment more stable owing to its lager therapy window. For deeper depth or higher volume fraction, the 1064-nm laser is recommended to avoid thermal damage of epidermis (Xiao C, 2022).

LENTIGINES

Common melanocytic lesions developing at birth or childhood or adulthood. Occur on the skin, conjunctivae or mucocutaneous surfaces. Little or no relationship to sun exposure.

- Juvenile lentigo–develop in the first decade of life
- Partial/segmental lentigines–unilateral, agminated (clustered) distribution
- Lentigines profuse–generalized distribution
- Syndromic–LEOPARD syndrome, Carney syndrome, Peutz–Jeghers syndrome, Laugier–Hunziker syndrome, centrofacial lentiginosis.

Clinical Features

Lentigo simplex are sharply circumscribed macules with uniform light brown to black pigmentation **(Table 28.3)**.

Pathogenesis

Not well understood. Increased density of melanocytes with melanin macroglobules in melanocytes. It lacks FGFR3, PIK3CA or BRAF mutations frequently seen in solar lentigo, PUVA lentigines or nevi respectively.

Histology

Moderate elongation of rete ridges, melanocytic hyperplasia, increased epidermal pigmentation and dermal melanophages. Rarely, melanin macroglobules (giant pigment granules) may be seen. A lymphohistiocytic infiltrate may be seen. Solar elastosis is not prominent or is absent.

Differential Diagnosis

- Solar lentigo
- Frecnkes
- Junctional nevomelanocytic nevus
- Atypical melanocytic nevus
- Café-au-lait macule
- Lentigo maligna.

Prognosis

Relatively stable. May increase in number during pregnancy. Do not undergo malignant transformation.

TABLE 28.3: Lists the clinical features of disorders associated with multiple lentigines present in a localized or generalized distribution

Name	Inheritance	Clinical features
Localized distribution		
Peutz–Jeghers syndrome	AD, STK11 mutation	Perioral, oral mucosal, hands lentigines, longitudinal melanonychia + multiple hamartomatous GI polyps + pancreatic/ovarian/testicular cancer
Laugier–Hunziker syndrome	—	Similar distribution as PJ syndrome Not associated with malignancy
Centrofacial lentiginosis	AD	Lentigines in a butterfly distribution, onset in infancy, increase in childhood. Possible association with neuropsychiatric illness and bony abnormalities.
Cowden disease	AD, PTEN mutation	Periorificial and acral lentigines, hamartomas
Cronkhite–Canada syndrome	—	Older males, lentigines of buccal mucosa, face, hands and feet, diffuse non-scarring alopecia, nail dystrophy, intestinal polyposis, diarrhea, malabsorption
Bannayan-Riley-Ruvalcaba syndrome	AD, mutation in PTEN	Penile > vulvar lentigines
Xeroderma pigmentosum	AR, mutations in DNA repair pathway genes	Lentigines on body, more on sun-exposed sites, multiple skin cancers
Partial/segmental unilateral lentiginosis **(Fig. 28.7)**	—	Multiple lentigines in segmental distribution, CALMs too in same distribution
Generalized distribution		
LEOPARD syndrome/ Noonan syndrome with multiple lentiginosis	AD, mutation in PTPN11 > RAF1 > BRAF	Lentigines in infancy/early childhood, Café-noir macules + ECG changes (conduction defects, hypertrophic cardiomyopathy) + ocular hypertelorism +pulmonary stenosis + abnormal genitalia + growth retardation + deafness
Carney complex (NAME/LAMB syndrome)	AD, mutation in PRKAR1A	Lentigines, mucocutaneous myxomas, blue nevi + aatrail myxoma + myxoid mammary fibroadenoma + testicular/thyroid/pituitary tumors

Management

- Do not require therapy
- Cryotherapy, QSNYL–if treatment desired
- Sunscreens and sun avoidance.

A recent reveiw compared the various treatments and found that **combination-based treatments** showed the best efficacy (65%) followed by laser-based treatments (43%), topical retinoids (21%), cryotherapy (15%) and peels (6%). Thus it is obvious that by iitself the use of peels and cryotherapy is markedly inferior to the use of combination therapy and lasers (Mukovozov I, 2023).

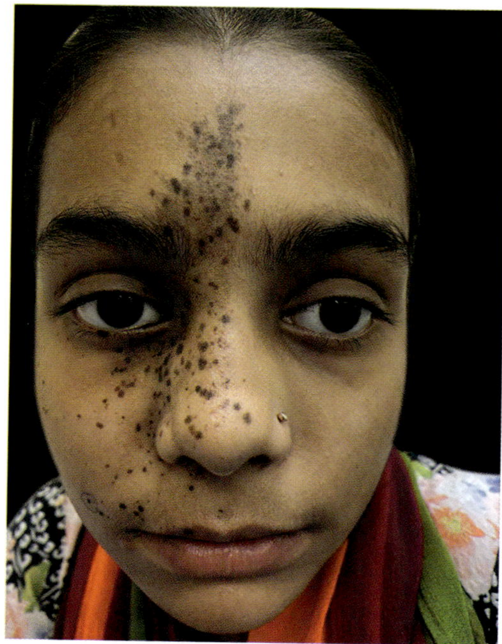

Fig. 28.7: Unilateral segmental lentiginosis

SOLAR LENTIGO

Solar lentigines are strongly associated with old age and photodamage. Also with facial freckles, tanning capacity, concurrent OCP use. They are known to occur with actinic keratoses, SCC, BCC and melanoma. Type 2 diabetes mellitus has an independent association.

PUVA may induce PUVA lentigines especially with a higher number of treatments, in male fair-skinned older individuals.

Clinical Features

Solar lentigo-Light to dark brown macules with well-defined irregular borders. Mostly occur on sun-exposed skins of face and dorsal forearms of light -skinned persons. Multiple lentigines occur on the face in type III-IV skins. May tend to coalesce when multiple.

PUVA lentigines- on sun-exposed sites but also on sun-protected sites like buttocks and genitalia exposed to phototherapy or artificial sunbeds.

Lentigines need to be differentiated from Freckles which are small uniformly pigmented macules on the central face in children and may disappear on cessation of continued sun exposure.

Pathogenesis

They occur due to proliferation of melanocytes and increased melanin production. Keratinocytes are in fact more sensitive to UVR than melanocytes and lead to activation of melanocytes through ROS release, MC1R and MITF activation (a key transcription factor for melanin production in melanocytes).

Histology

Elongated rete ridges extending in to the papillary dermis with club-like endings. Melanocytes may be normal or slightly increased in number with markedly increased melanin production. Dermis shows solar elastosis. Occasionally small horn cysts may form. A scant to moderate perivascular inflammatory infiltrate is present in the dermis with melanophages.

Differential Diagnosis

- Freckle
- Lentigo simplex
- Junctional nevomelanocytic nevus
- Lentigo maligna
- Reticulated seborrheic keratosis
- Pigmented actinic keratosis
- Large cell acanthoma.

Prognosis

Solar lentigines may enlarge or darken, persist or regress over time. They may evolve into lichenoid keratosis. May rarely evolve into BCC, SCC, melanoma.

PUVA lentigines may persist years after treatment cessation. May evolve into melanoma.

Management

- Do not require therapy
- Cryotherapy, QSNYL–if treatment desired
- Prevention with sunscreens and sun avoidance.

DISORDERS OF HYPOPIGMENTATION

INTRODUCTION

There are two ways of classifying the hypopigmentation disorders.

The first is a clinical classification based on the regional involvement and arrangement **(Flowchart 28.9)** while the second is based on the pathology based on the defect, either at the level of the melanocyte-melanocytopenic (defective melanocyte or function) and melanopenic (defect in melanin formation) and miscellaneous hypopigmentation disorders **(Fig. 28.8)**.

Some of the disorders that are mentioned here are covered in other chapters. The differentials of punctate leukoderma are given in **Box 28.10** and those that follow a linear arrangement are detailed in **Box 28.11**.

GENETIC DISORDERS OF HYPOPIGMENTATION

While we will discuss the common disorders, a few uncommon disorders are listed in **Figs 28.9** to **28.12**. They are uncommon and a working knowledge would suffice for diagnosis while the other disorders are described in the next page.

HYPOMELANOSIS OF ITO

A rare neuroectodermal disorder +/– mental retardation +/– epilepsy.

Flowchart 28.9: Approach to diagnosis of hypopigmented disorders based on the regional involvement

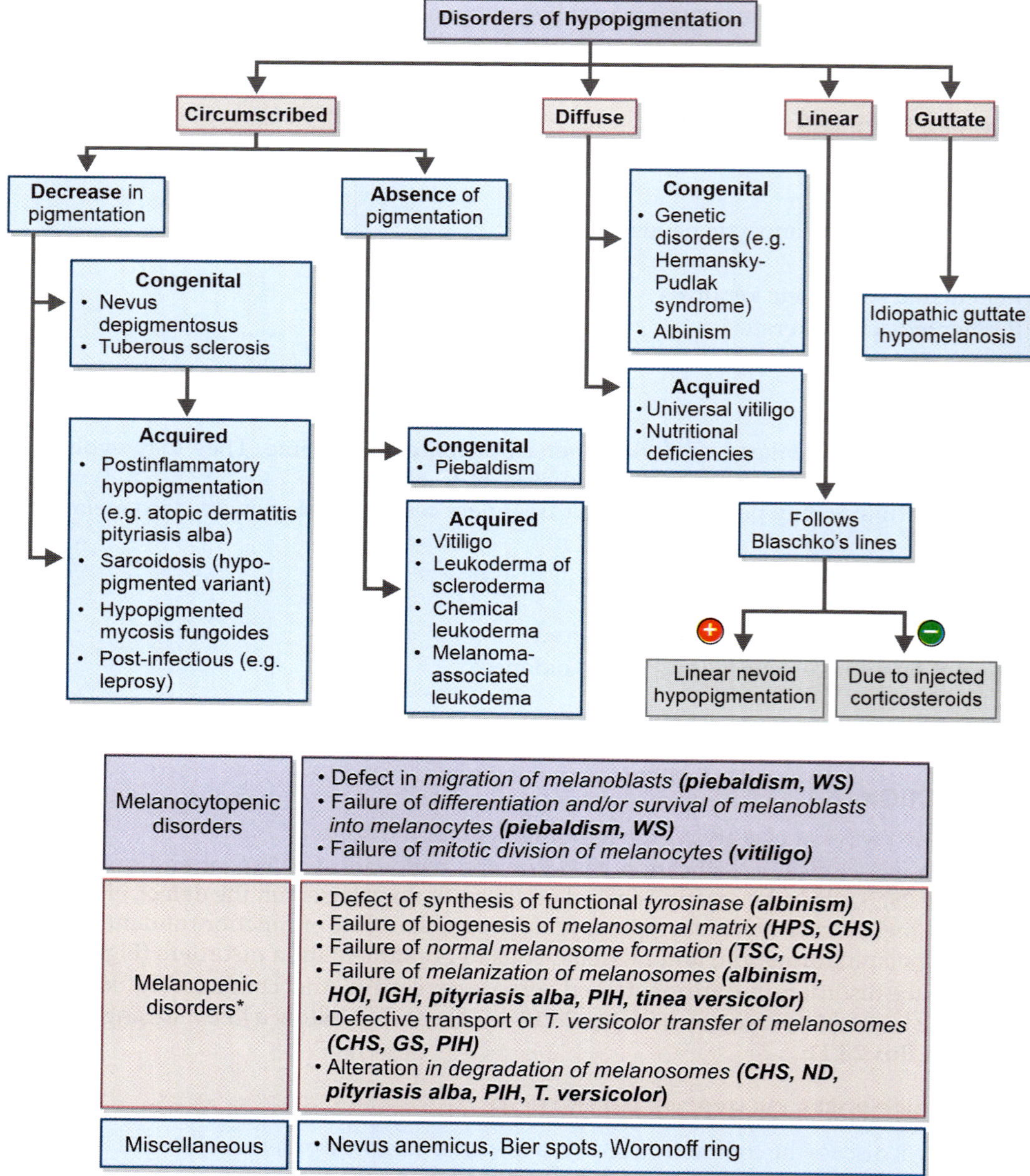

CHS, chédiak-Higashi syndrome; GS, griscelli syndrome; HOI, hypomelanosis of Ito; HPS, Hermansky–Pudlak syndrome; IGH, idiopathic guttate hypomelanosis; ND, nevus depigmentosus; PIH, postinflammatory hypopigmentation; TSC, tuberous sclerosis complex; WS, Waardenburg syndrome.

*Other causes are leprosy, PKDL, nutritional deficiency, drugs (HQ, arsenic, steroids) and endocrine causes.

Fig. 28.8: Classification of hypopigmentation disorders based on the pathogenic defect

BOX 28.10: Guttate hypomelanosis/leucoderma

Common	• Idiopathic guttate hypomelanosis • Pityriasis lichenoides chronica • Lichen sclerosus • Confetti-like lesions of tuberous sclerosis • Early tinea versicolor (especially face) • Achromic verruca plana • Frictional lichenoid dermatosis • Clear cell papulosis • Vitiligo ponctué • Darier disease • Xeroderma pigmentosum • In association with chromosomal abnormalities • Following PUVA therapy

BOX 28.11: Linear hypopigmentation disorders

Lesions that follow Blaschko lines	• Linear nevoid hypopigmentation (macular, early onset) • Lichen striatus (mildly elevated, seen in children) • Linear lichen sclerosus (shiny wrinkled surface, follicular plugging) • Goltz syndrome (dermal atrophy, fat 'herniation,' early onset) • Linear Darier disease (guttate hypopigmented macules, crusted papules) • Incontinentia pigmenti stage 4 (hairless and atrophic, favors calves)
Lesions that do not follow Blaschko lines	• Injected corticosteroids (irregular outline, along lymphatics) • Pigmentary demarcation lines, type C (vertical or curved on mid-chest and abdomen)

Epidemiology

- Incidence is found to be between 1/8500 and 1/10000 but prevalence is unknown.
- Almost all cases are sporadic.
- Appears at birth or during infancy or early childhood.

Predisposing Factors

- Chromosomal anomalies (sometimes)
- Postzygotic mutation (hence not inherited).

Pathogenesis

Cutaneous mosaicism is considered as the cause for the condition as the lesion follows Blaschko lines.

Clinical Features

- Unilateral or bilateral cutaneous hypopigmented whorls, streaks and patches along the Blaschko lines **(Figs 28.13** and **28.14)**.
- Along with neurological, ophthalmological and skeletal defects.

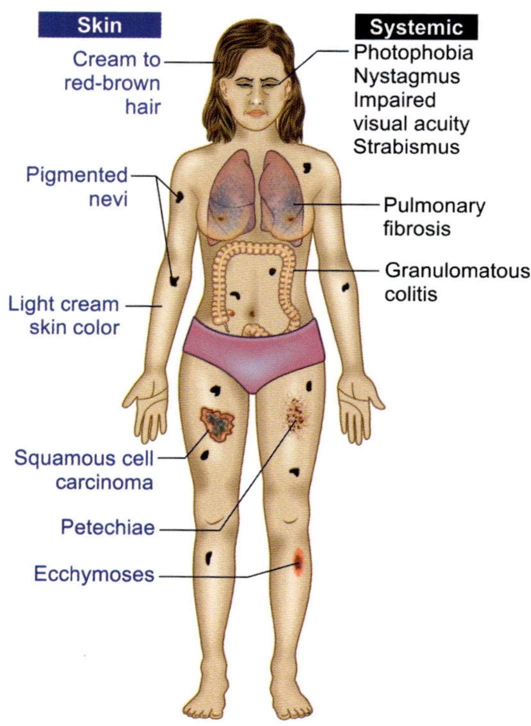

Fig. 28.9: Hermansky–Pudlak syndrome

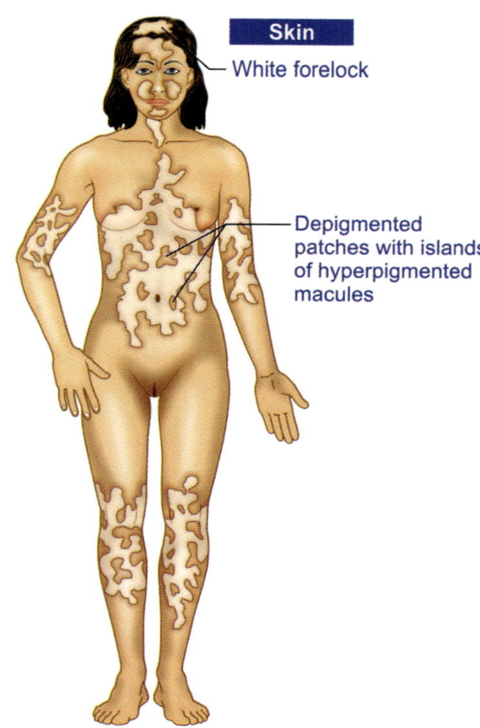

Fig. 28.10: Piebaldism (*see* also Table 28.4)

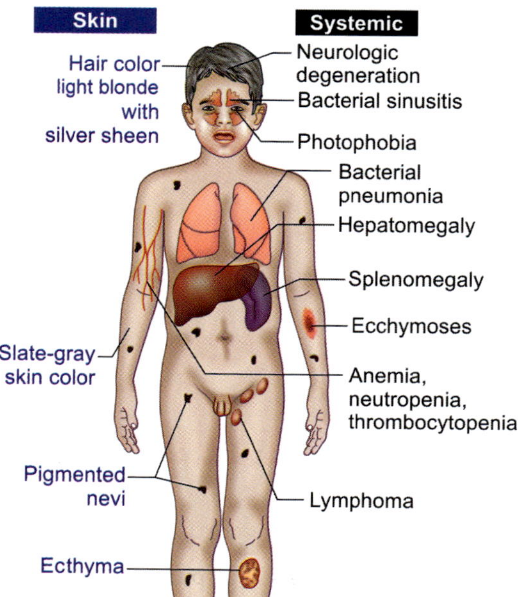

Fig. 28.11: Chédiak–Higashi syndrome

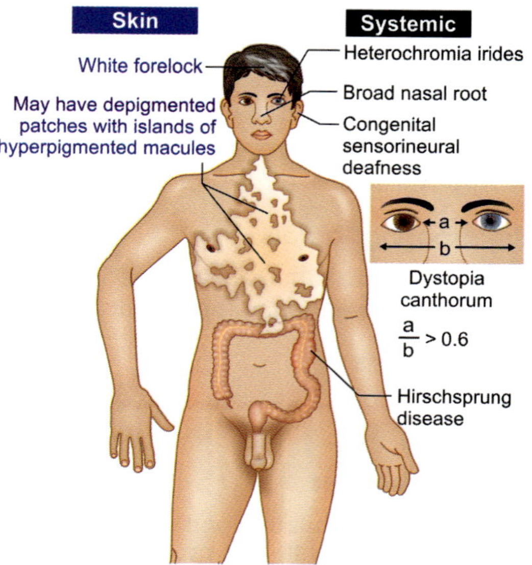

Fig. 28.12: Waardenburg syndrome

Skin
Alopecia
Marble-cake hypopigmentation

Systemic
Epilepsy
Mental retardation
Motor retardation
Strabismus hypertelorism
Anodontia
Scoliosis
Limb length discrepancy

Fig. 28.13: Hypomelanosis of Ito

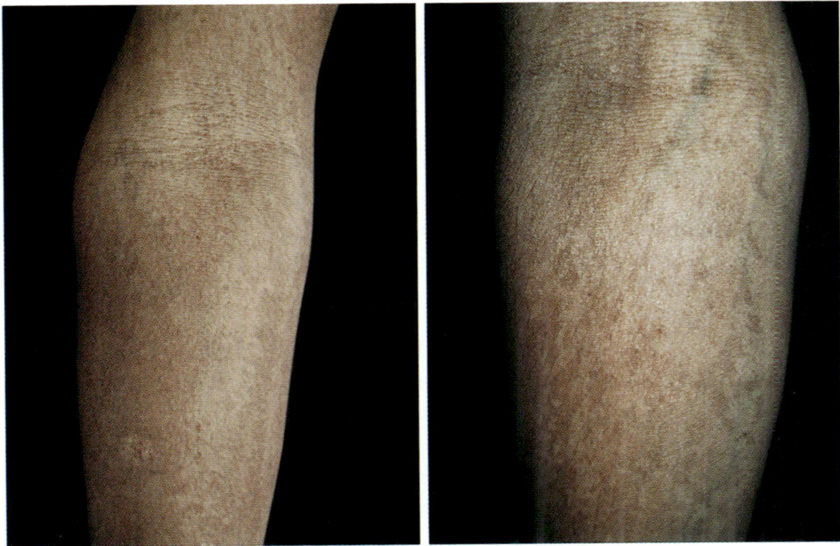

Fig. 28.14: Whorled hypopigmentation on the limbs: A mosaic pattern of pigmentation seen in HOI

TABLE 28.4: Factoids on piebaldism	
Cause	• Rare autosomal dominant disorder. • Due to mutations in *KIT gene* (encodes c-KIT–a tyrosine kinase receptor responsible for cell proliferation and migration) → impaired migration of melanocytes to skin → hypopigmented patches. • Other gene mutations seen-zinc finger transcription factor SNAI2.
Clinical features	• A white forelock of hair with a V-shaped area of leukoderma on mid-forehead. • Hypopigmented patches usually on anterior trunk and mid-portions of limbs, bilateral but not always symmetrical. • Small hyperpigmented macules within the hypopigmented patches or on normal skin. • Usually no extracutaneous features, rarely deafness or mental retardation.
Differential diagnosis	• Vitiligo • Waardenburg syndrome • Nevus depigmentosus (if focal involvement)
Histopathology	• Absent melanocytes/reduced number of large abnormal melanocytes in hypopigmented lesions. • Normal as well as abnormal spherical and granular melanosomes in melanocytes in hyperpigmented islands.
Management	• Sunprotection • Surgical–epidermal cell suspension or skin grafting • Topical steroids, phototherapy–inefficacious.

Differential Diagnosis

Table 28.5 depicts differential diagnosis of HOI.

TABLE 28.5: Differential diagnosis of HOI

Disease	Differentiation from HOI
Focal dermal hypoplasia	Skin shows atrophic changes
Nevus depigmentosus	Extent is limited and usually no extracutaneous associations

Diagnosis

HPE shows

- ↓ number of melanocytes and melanosomes on both light and electron microscopy.
- Various cytogenetic abnormalities in lymphocytes and/or lesional fibroblasts.

Treatment

No treatment is required for cutaneous lesions. Pigmentation appears in many cases eventually with time but if not, then cosmetic camouflage may be used.

INCONTINENTIA PIGMENTI (IP)

- A rare X-linked dominant multisystem disorder presenting predominantly in females with skin lesions, dental abnormalities, alopecia, nail dystrophy, and ocular and neurological manifestations.
- Lethal in males.

Epidemiology

- Birth prevalence is 0.6–0.7/1000000.
- The female to male ratio is 20:1.

Pathogenesis

The disorder is consequent to a defect in the Nuclear Factor Kappa B Kinase Regulatory Subunit Gamma **(IKBKG)** gene located at the Xq28 chromosomal region, which encodes for NEMO/IKKgamma, a regulatory protein involved in the nuclear factor kappa B (NF-κB) signaling pathway. NF-κB plays a prominent role in the modulation of cellular proliferation, apoptosis, and inflammation. IKBKG mutation that results in a loss-of-function or dysregulated NF-κB pathway contributes to the pathophysiology of IP. Thus, IP is considered as a proapoptotic state with epidermal cells destruction and progressive replacement of normal cells with the cells with mutant X-chromosome **(Fig. 28.15)**.

Clinical Features (Figs 28.16 and 28.17)

Stage 1

Onset: Within the first few weeks of life up to 18 months.
Bullous stage: It presents perinatally with an erythematous vesicular rash following Blaschko lines commonly present on limbs, scalp and trunk and rarely on face.

↓

Evolves over months

Stage 2

Onset: Within the first few months of life and lasts for a few months.
Verrucous stage: Mainly on limbs.

↓

Within months

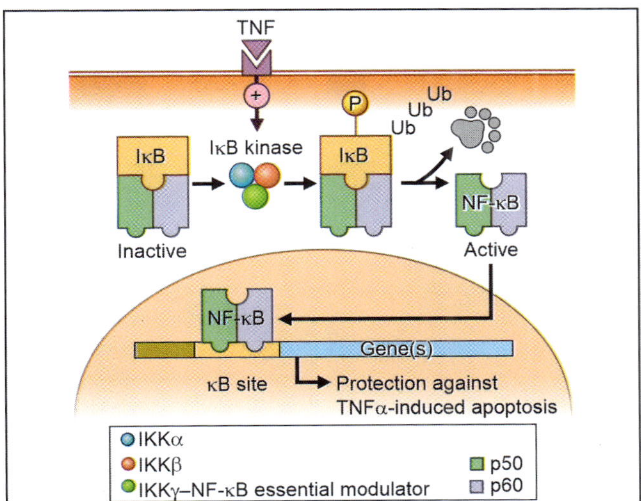

Fig. 28.15: Functions of NEMO. In incontinentia pigmenti, lack of NF-κB essential modulator (NEMO) results in failure to activate NF-κB, which normally protects against tumor necrosis factor alpha (TNF-α) induced apoptosis

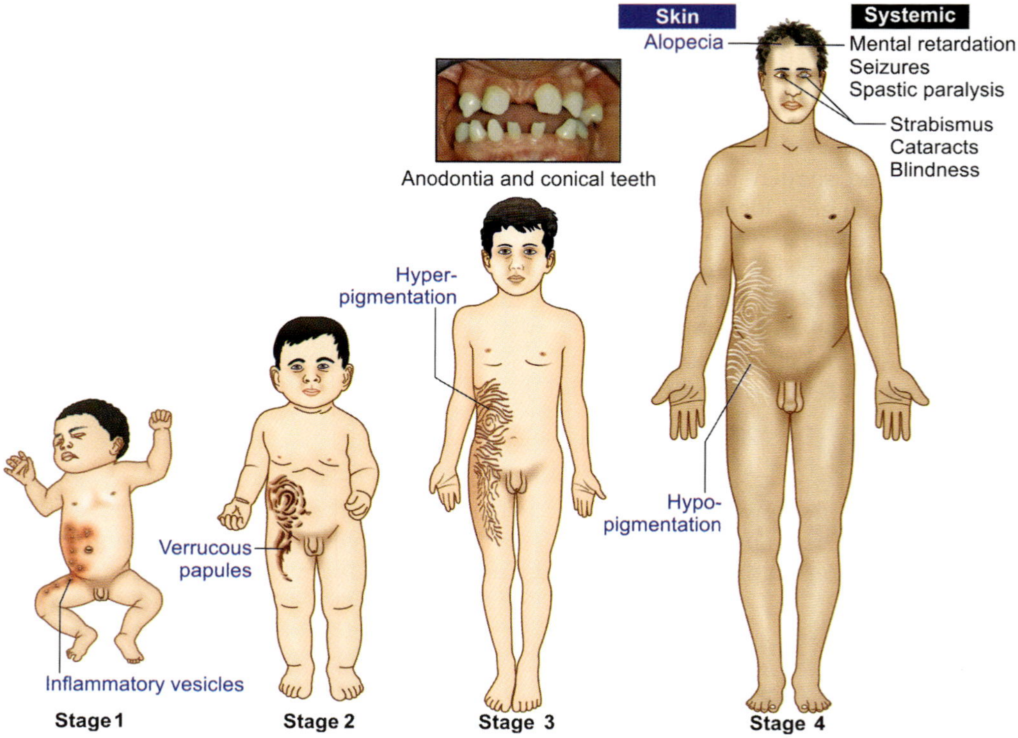

Skin
Alopecia

Systemic
Mental retardation
Seizures
Spastic paralysis
Strabismus
Cataracts
Blindness

Anodontia and conical teeth

Hyper-
pigmentation

Hypo-
pigmentation

Verrucous
papules

Inflammatory vesicles

Stage 1
Stage 2
Stage 3
Stage 4

Fig. 28.16: Incontinentia pigmenti

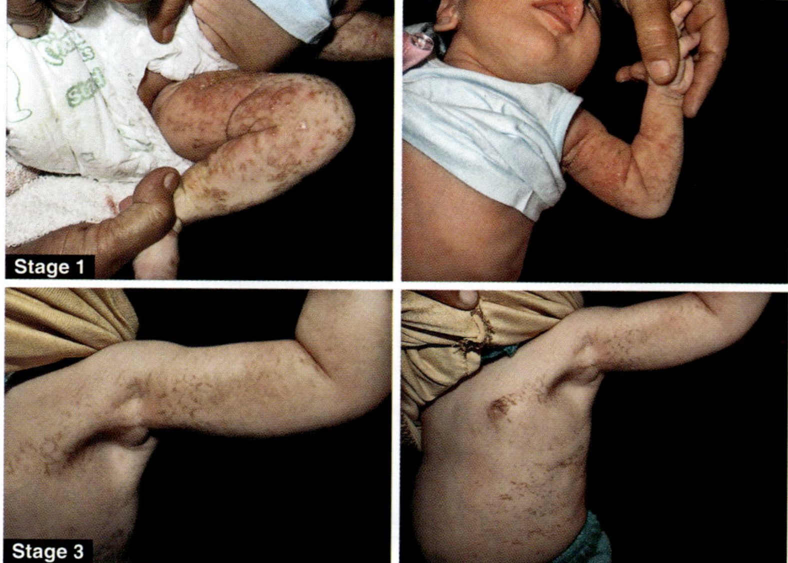

Fig. 28.17: A child who presented with stage 1: Vesicles/bullae (first 2 weeks of life) and on the follow-up came with stage 3: Hyperpigmentation along the lines of Blaschko

Stage 3

- *Hyperpigmented streaks and whorls*: Along Blaschko lines but fade in adolescence.
- Lesions have scalloped edges which are considered to be there because of the growth of normal keratinocytes into the affected skin.
- Predilection for the trunk and intertriginous sites.

Stage 4

- *Hypopigmented stage*: It presents at adolescence as pale, hairless, atrophic linear streaks or patches usually on the lower extremities (on the posterior aspects like calves).
- The lesions resembling stage 1 may also recur on the pigmented areas during febrile illness in infancy and later in childhood.
- The diagnostic criteria are given in **Box 28.12**.

BOX 28.12: Updated diagnostic criteria for IP from the criteria of Landy and Donnai (J Med Genet 1993,30:53–59)*

Major criteria	• Typical neonatal rash with erythema and vesicles (stage 1) • Verrucous papules or plaques along Blaschko's lines (stage 2) • Typical hyperpigmentation along Blaschko's lines fading in adolescence (stage 3) • Linear, atrophic, hairless lesions on limbs (stage 4) or scarring alopecia of the vertex (stages 3 or 4) • Teeth: Dental agenesis (hypodontia or oligodontia), shape anomalies (peg-shaped incisors, conical teeth, molar cusp pattern alteration) and delayed eruption • Common recurrent rearrangement (deletion rearrangement of exons 4–10 of IKBKG gene)
Minor criterion	• Eosinophilia (stage 1) • Hair: Alopecia or woolly hair (dull and dry) • Nails: Punctuate depressions, onychogryphosis (or ram's horn nails) • Mammary gland involvement (hypoplasia, asymmetry, hypogalactia) and/or nipple involvement (inverted nipples, supernumerary, difficulty in feeding) • Characteristic skin histology • Retina: Peripheral neovascularization

*In the absence of a family history, the presence of at least one major criterion is sufficient for the diagnosis of IP. If a first-degree female parent is affected, one minor criterion is sufficient for IP diagnosis. The complete absence of minor criteria should induce some doubt about the diagnosis.

Extracutaneous Findings

- Delayed dentition, missing or malformed cone-shaped teeth
- Onychodystrophy
- Alopecia
- Ophthalmological abnormalities with retinal neovascularization including strabismus, cataracts, microphthalmia, optic atrophy.
- Central nervous system abnormalities: Microcephaly, seizures and neurocognitive and motor impairments. Almost 60% are neurologically normal.
- Asymmetric breast development or super-numerary nipples.
- Skull anomalies, scoliosis.
- Pulmonary hypertension

Differential Diagnosis

Differentials of different stages of IP are given in **Table 28.6**.

TABLE 28.6: Differential diagnosis of IP

Disease	Similarity IP	Dissimilarity with IP
Stage 1* Bullous impetigo	Vesiculobullous lesions	Lesions distributed randomly and not along Blaschko lines H/E • Split in the epidermis just below the stratum granulosum • Migration of the neutrophils through a spongiotic epidermis into the blister cavity, which may also contain cocci • Inflammatory infiltrate composed of neutrophils and lymphocytes found the upper dermis
Herpes/varicella	Vesicular lesions	• Etiology is viral infection • No distribution along the Blaschko lines • Tzanck smear is done for the diagnosis which shows multinucleated giant cells
Stage 2 Warts	Smooth, flat or slightly elevated, usually skin-colored or grayish yellow round or polygonal plaques varying in size from 1 to 5 mm or more in diameter	HPE • Hyperplasia of all layers of the epidermis • Hyperkeratosis with areas of parakeratosis, especially above the papillomatous projections • Both spinous and granular layers are thickened • Rete ridges are elongated and flattened and are bent inwards towards the center of the wart • Foci of koilocytes in the disordered granular layer
Verrucous epidermal nevus	Verrucous lesions distributed along Blaschko lines	Hyperkeratosis, thickened epidermis and papillomatosis
Stage 3 Linear and whorled nevoid hypermelanosis	• Onset is in infancy • The hyperpigmented lesions follow the lines of Blaschko on the trunk and limbs • Soles, palms, face and mucous membranes are spared	• No preceeding inflammatory phase • Histopathology: Predominantly epidermal hyperpigmentation
Stage 4 Hypomelanosis of Ito	• Almost all cases have postzygotic mutation • Clinically, lesions are unilateral or bilateral macular hypopigmented whorls, streaks and patches, following the Blaschko lines • Neurological, ophthalmological involvement and skeletal defects are found and thus mental retardation and epilepsy are associated	• No preceeding inflammatory phase • Decreased number of melanocytes and melanosomes on both light and electron microscopy • Various cytogenetic abnormalities in lymphocytes and/or lesional fibroblasts

*Stage 1 also Goltz syndrome, Stage 2 also chondrodysplasia, Stage 3 also pigmentary mosaicism.

Clinical Course

- Normal life expectancy
- Normal physical and cognitive development in patients with no central nervous system involvement.

Diagnosis

HPE

Stage 1: Early inflammatory phase showing eosinophilic spongiosis and scattered dyskeratotic keratinocytes.
Stage 2: The epidermis is acanthotic with hyperkeratosis and foci of dyskeratosis.
Stage 3: Pigmentary incontinence and variable vacuolization of basal keratinocytes.
Stage 4: Dermis and epidermis are thinned out with no adnexa.

Hemogram

Peripheral eosinophilia and leukocytosis in neonates.

Treatment

- No specific treatment
- Symptomatic treatment
  a. Dermatological management
    - Careful monitoring in the first months of life
    - Every three months in the first year
    - Every year until the age of 5 years
    - Then according to disease progression
    - 1 annual visit in a referral centre, with a multidisciplinary assessment if needed, until adulthood.
    - Increased frequency of visits in cases of prolonged and profuse inflammatory lesions and disabling verrucous lesions.

  b. Ophthalmological follow-up for monitoring and treatment of retinal neovascularization through laser photocoagulation or cryotherapy; retinal detachment.
  c. Dental problems: Follow-up with pediatric orthodontist along with speech therapy and a pediatric nutrition program.
  d. Neurological
    - If no neurological manifestation is observed at birth:
      - Neurocognitive examination: At 9 months and at 24 months
      - Brain MRI: At 2½ years (30 months)
    - If neurological manifestation is observed at birth:
      - EEG: During neonatal period, at 4 months and at 24 months
      - Brain MRI: During neonatal period and at 30 months.

ACQUIRED DISORDERS OF HYPOPIGMENTATION

IDIOPATHIC GUTTATE HYPOMELANOSIS

Epidemiology

- Up to 80% are affected after 70 years of age.
- F = M, more reported in females because of cosmetic reasons.
- More in light skinned people.

Predisposing Factors

- Normal aging.
- Photoaging process.

Clinical Features

- Asymptomatic single or multiple porcelain-white macules with smooth non-atrophic surface and sharply defined borders, may be angular or irregular, 2–6 mm in size but may be larger, with skin furrows delineating them. Macules never increase in size or coalesce.
- Distributed over pretibial area and forearms usually. Other sites: Face, neck and shoulders may be affected.
- Hair present over macules is unaffected.

Differential Diagnosis

Table 28.7 provides differential diagnosis of macular hypopigmentation.

TABLE 28.7: Differential diagnosis of macular hypopigmentation

Disease	Characteristic findings	Clinical features
Atrophie blanche	Site of predilection: Shin and ankle	Lesions present as porcelain white depressed scars encircled by papular telangiectasias
Guttate vitiligo	Milky white sharply demarcated macules	• Site of involvement can be anywhere • Any age of presentation • Repigmenation can occur with treatment or spontaneously • Macules may increase in size and coalesce • Hair overlying the affected areas may be affected • Wood's lamp: Bright bluish-white patches • Dermoscopy: Dense/glowing white shade • HPE: Lack of DOPA-positive melanocytes in the basal layer of the epidermis
Extragenital lichen sclerosus	• All races • Ivory colored sclerotic papules and plaques with shiny and or wrinkled surface, sometimes with pink or light-violet hue	• Involves all ages • Can occur anywhere • Mucosa can also be involved • Sclerotic ivory white lesions are preceded by polygonal, bluish-white, shiny, slightly elevated, interfollicular papules in early stages • Itching may be present • Telangiectases and interfollicular plugging are seen in advanced stages • HPE: Epidermis—atrophy DEJ: Lichenoid infiltrate Dermis: Fibrosis and homogenization of acid mucopolysaccharides infiltrate at the dermal-epidermal junction in late stages while papillary edema in early lesions

(Contd.)

TABLE 28.7: Differential diagnosis of macular hypopigmentation *(Contd.)*

Disease	Characteristic findings	Clinical features
Leukoderma punctata (after PUVA therapy)	• Multiple small punctate macules of size 0.5–1.5 mm distributed symmetrically over shins, extensors of the arms • No relation to hair follicles	• Develops in young adults • Phototoxicity from sun exposure or UV therapy is the etiological factors • Clinically, the macules are smaller than IGH and may have repigmentation • Variable amount of damage to keratinocytes and melanocytes ultrastructurally
Pityriasis versicolor	Hypopigmented macules in seborrheic distribution	• Caused by *Malassezia* spp a commensal fungus • Hyperpigmented areas can also be seen • Macules have fine scales and there might be slight itching • Woods's lamp: Yellow-green fluorescence • Dermoscopy: A well-demarcated white area with fine scaling
Hypochromic vitiligo	• Dark skinned people • Earlier lesions may present as hypopigmented macules which may be discrete or coalescent distributed anywhere on the body	• Presents at any age • Coexistence with typical depigmented vitiligo, macules • Wood's lamp: Bright bluish-white patches • Dermoscopy: Dense/glowing white shade • HPE: Lack of DOPA-positive melanocytes in the basal layer of the epidermis
Postinflammatory hypopigmentation of pityriasis alba	• Asymptomatic ill-defined round or oval irregular hypopigmented patches ranging in size from 0.5 to 2 cm or larger • Larger lesions are present on trunk • Dermoscopy: Dense/glowing white shade	• Predominantly in children (3–16 yr) • Often a manifestation of atopic dermatitis • Distribution: Face (cheeks, around mouth and chin), trunk, neck, arms and shoulders • Earlier lesions have erythema followed by hypopigmentation and fine scaling • Persist for a few months to a few years

Clinical Course

Numbers increase with age and no spontaneous repigmentation.

Complications

UV-damaged skin.

Diagnosis

Essentially a clinical diagnosis. **Box 28.13** lists the relevant investigations.

BOX 28.13: Investigations in IGH

Dermoscopy	"Cloudy sky-like" pattern: Multiple small irregular coalescing macules with different shades of white having both well-defined and ill-defined edges, surrounded by patchy hyperpigmented network.
HPE	• Slight basket-weave hyperkeratosis with epidermal atrophy and flattening of rete ridges. • Significant reduction in the number of melanin granules in the basal and the suprabasal layers. • The superficial dermis shows fibrosis in 90% of cases
Special stains	Marked reduction in DOPA-positive melanocytes and melanin content and irregularly distributed pigment granules.

Treatment

- Usually no treatment required
- Sunscreens and physical barrier are recommended
- Systemic and topical retinoids
- Topical steroids
- Cryotherapy
- Topical tacrolimus
- Superficial dermabrasion (carbon dioxide laser)

PROGRESSIVE MACULAR HYPOMELANOSIS

Epidemiology

Commonly misdiagnosed, under reported, seen mostly in adolescents and young adults of all races.

Predisposing Factors

Propionibacterium spp might play a role in its development.

Clinical Features (Fig. 28.18)

Multiple asymptomatic ill-defined nummular nonscaly macules distributed mostly in the truncal areas more or less in a seborrheic distribution converging towards the midline. Rarely proximal extremities and head and neck are involved.

Clinical Types/Variants

Presenting as large circular lesions.

Clinical Course

Stabilize or progress slowly with time, rarely undergo spontaneous regression.

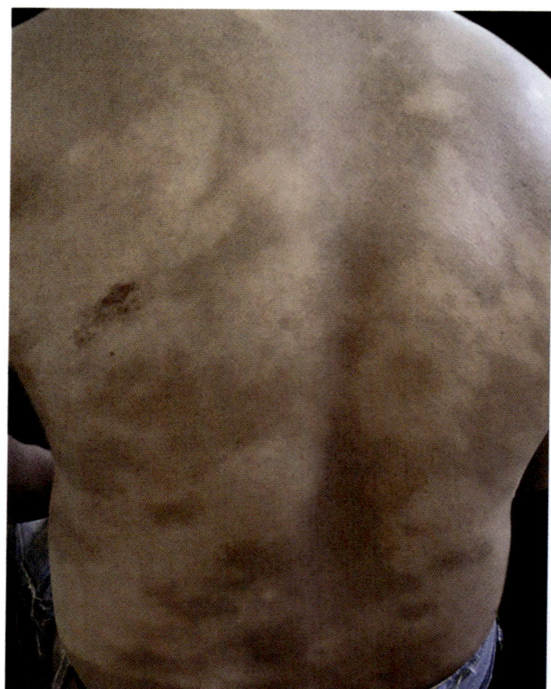

Fig. 28.18: Progressive macular hypomelanosis is usually mistaken for leprosy and PKDL

Diagnosis (Box 28.14)

BOX 28.14: Investigations in PMH

Bedside tests	Wood's lamp: Orange-red fluorescence
Dermoscopy	Ill-defined smooth whitish area
HPE	• Epidermis: Decreased pigment • Dermis: Normal
Electron microscopy	Transition from large melanosomes in normal skin to multiple aggregates of small membrane-bound melanosomes is demonstrated.

Treatment (Flowchart 28.10)

Flowchart 28.10: Treatment of progressive macular hypomelanosis

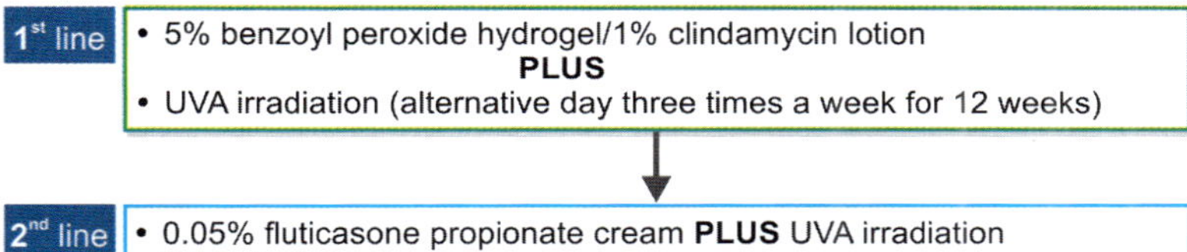

VITILIGO

Epidemiology

- Incidence: 0.5–2% worldwide
- Age: 20–30 years
- Sex: Same, some studies show female preponderance.

Pathogenesis

Many theories put forward—they may be working together to cause vitiligo ("Convergence/ Integrated" theory). Prominent ones are as follows:

1. **Genetic theory**
2. **Autoimmune/autoinflammatory theory (Fig. 28.19):** This is the most prevalent theory and the success and failure of most therapies depend on the main mediators of this pathways, notably the T cell variants involved. Certain cytokines like **TNF-α**, **IL-23**, and **IL-17** have now been shown **not** to drive vitiligo.
   i. **T cells**
      a. **CD8 + T cells:** Early histology of human vitiligo lesions reveal lymphocytic infiltrates at the border of depigmented lesions, where disease is most active. These infiltrates are comprised predominantly of CD8+T cells **(Fig 28.19)**. Melanoma studies first identified several melanocyte-specific antigens that are recognized by self-reactive CD8+ T cells, including tyrosinase, Melan-A/MART-1, gp100, TRP-1, and TRP-2; and vitiligo patients have elevated numbers of these cells in their peripheral blood relative to healthy controls.
      b. T cells secrete IFN-γ, which induces CXCL9 and CXCL10 production by keratinocytes to recruit additional T cells and promote vitiligo progression. In addition to initiation

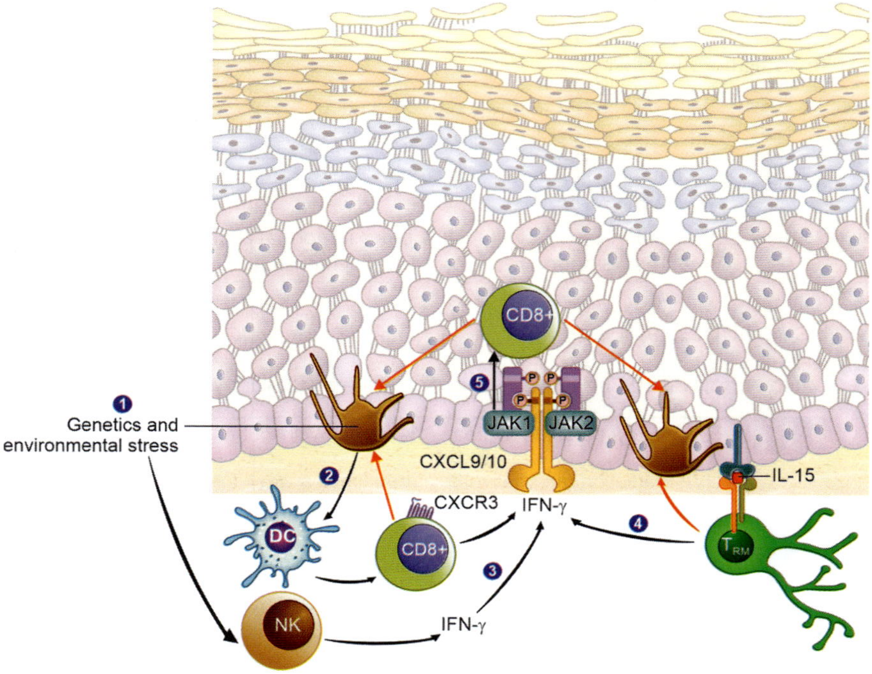

Fig. 28.19: Pathologies of vitiligo. In vitiligo, melanocytes are more susceptible to oxidative stress, which in turn targets antigens to nearby dendritic cells and induces their maturation into efficient antigen-presenting cells. Upon endogenous or exogenous stress, NK cells produce IFN-γ that induces the production of chemokines. Binding of IFN-γ to its receptor activates the JAK/STAT pathway and leads to T-cell recruitment and function, which induces melanocyte apoptosis. Established vitiligo is maintained by T RM cells, which remain long-lived in the skin through IL-15 -dependent signaling.

and progression of vitiligo, the IFN-γ-chemokine pathway is also required for maintenance of established lesions, as both depletion of CXCR3-expressing cells and neutralization of CXCL10 chemokine induced repigmentation of vitiligo, positioning the **IFN-γ-chemokine axis** as a potential therapeutic target that forms the basis of the rationale of using JAK inihibitors.

c. **Resident memory T cells in vitiligo:** Relapse of vitiligo is common, approximately 40% within the first year after stopping treatments and this has been linked to Trm (resident memory T cells). Multiple groups identified CD8+T cells possessing a Trm cell phenotype within vitiligo lesions, in both mouse models of disease and human patients **(Fig. 28.19)**. Therefore, Trm cells likely mediate longterm maintenance and potential relapse of vitiligo in human patients through cytokine-mediated recruitment of T cells from the circulation. Treatments that inhibit this pathway without affecting Trm cell number, which includes most conventional treatments including JAK inhibitors, effectively reverse disease, but relapse occurs after they are discontinued.

The most important cytokine that stimulates the formation of CD8+Trm cell is **IL-15**. This binds to three receptor chains, CD215, CD122, and CD132 (the common gamma chain), which can all be expressed by lymphocytes to bind IL-15 as a soluble cytokine. Lymphocyte recognition of IL-15 most often occurs by binding to CD122 and CD132, and these receptors are targets of novel therapies in vitiligo **(Fig. 28.19)**.

d. **T reg cells:** While it is unclear exactly how Treg cells are disrupted in human vitiligo, yet it seems that there is in vitiligo a Treg cell deficiency.

ii. Dysregulated innate and adaptive immune response-increasing evidence

iii. Increased **oxidative stress**—melanocyte stress [Mathachan SR]: The pro-oxidant state of vitiligo skin subjects melanocytes to oxidative stress, making them vulnerable to apoptosis, and disrupts their microenvironment, with the release of paracrine factors by epidermal keratinocytes and dermal fibroblasts. An important factor that mediates stress leading to vitiligo is the release of DAMPs and the possible formation of neoantigens. Intrinsic abnormalities and environmental phenols both induce melanocyte stress, leading to elevated ROS, UPR activation, autophagy, and exosome release. HSP70i stimulates PRRs to activate innate immune cells. Macrophages also infiltrate active vitiligo lesions and release IL-1β through inflammasome activation.

iv. Antibodies to human melanocytes

v. Innate immunity

3. **Self-destruction of melanocytes (autocyto-destructive) theory**
4. **Neurogenic theory**
5. **Immune-checkpoint inhibitor induced vitiligo:** Melanoma patients on immune checkpoint inhibitors who develop vitiligo are seen to have higher survival rates. Expansion and larger area of vitiligo may be predictive factors of prolonged survival during anti-PD-1 antibody treatment in melanoma patients.

Clinical Features

a. **Nonsegmental vitiligo (NSV)**—this is what is implied by the term "vitiligo" usually. Bilateral macules often distributed acrofacially/generalized. Includes the following variants:
   - **Localized**
     - Focal
     - Mucosal
   - **Generalized**
     - Acrofacial
     - Vulgaris
     - Universal

b. **Segmental vitiligo (SV):** Unilateral macules in a segmental/band-like distribution. Classified separately by Vitiligo Global Issue Consensus conference recently. More common in children (15–30% of childhood vitiligo)
   - Unisegmental
   - Bisegmental
   - Plurisegmental

c. **Mixed (SV + NSV)**

d. **Unclassified**

Sites: Areas of repeated friction/pressure/trauma. Hips, dorsa of hands/fingers, feet, elbows, knees, ankles

Margins: Convex, irregular

Hair: Normal/leukotrichia.

Clinical Variants

- **Trichrome**—presence of a narrow to broad intermediate color zone between a vitiligo macule and normal pigmented surrounding skin. Marker of unstable disease.

- **Quadrichrome**—fourth color in vitiligo lesions, usually seen in darker skin phenotypes. A macular perifollicular or marginal hyperpigmentation is its salient feature and denotes repigmenting disease.
- **Pentachrome**—infrequently encountered variant in which there is a sequential display of white, tan, brown, blue-gray hyperpigmentation and the normal skin. Black-skinned individuals are predisposed.
- **Inflammatory** vitiligo.
- **Hypochromic vitiligo/vitiligo minor**—described in skin types V/VI. Persistent hypopigmented macules in a seborrheic distribution on face, neck, trunk and scalp, with some additional achromic macules with decreased melanocytes on histology.
- **Follicular vitiligo**—leukotrichia in absence of depigmented epidermis.
- **Vitiligo punctata/confetti amelanotic macules** sometimes superimposed on a hyperpigmented macule.
- **Figurate papulosquamous type**.
- **Blue vitiligo**—vitiligo in areas of postinflammatory dermal pigmentation.

Clinical Course

- Unpredictable
- Peripheral hypopigmentation and poorly defined borders, spotty depigmentation—**predictors of active vitiligo**.

A study that evaluated clinical markers of vitiligo found a few markers to have high chance to correlate with activity of disease **(Box 28.15)**.

BOX 28.15: Clinical markers of activity of vitiligo (van Geel N, et al., 2019)

- Koebner's phenomenon ✓
- Tri- and hypochromic lesions ✓
- Itch
- Confetti-like depigmentation ✓
- Inflammatory borders/areas
- Leukotrichia

✓ Have the highest evidence

- Halo nevi and leukotrichia in segmental vitiligo (SV) → **increased chances of development of NSV (mixed vitiligo)**.

Scoring Systems

- **VASI** (vitiligo area and severity index)
- **VETF** (Vitiligo European Task Force) **score**

Comorbidities

- **Autoimmune thyroid disease (AITD)—5–15%**
- **Halo nevi**
- **Alopecia areata**
- **Diabetes mellitus**
- **Pernicious anemia**
- AICTDs—SLE, RA, Sjögren syndrome, dermatomyositis, systemic sclerosis
- Addison's disease
- IBDs

- Psoriasis—more in pediatric patients
- Atopic dermatitis—more in pediatric patients

Differential Diagnosis (Box 28.16)

BOX 28.16: List of differential diagnosis of vitiligo

- Halo nevi
  - Nevus depigmentosus
  - Nevus anemicus
  - Inherited hypomelanotic disorders
- Progressive macular hypomelanosis
- Secondary hypomelanosis (postinflammatory/post-traumatic)
- Post-infectious hypomelanosis
- Cutaneous lymphoma

Diagnosis

Relevant investigations needed to differentiate vitiligo from common differentials are listed in **Table 28.8.**

Treatment

Predictably for an autoimmune disease, immunosuppression is an important component of the treatment of the disorder. Topical corticosteroids and calcineurin inhibitors promote repigmentation, and systemic corticosteroid treatment helps to stabilize very active disease. However, successful repigmentation of vitiligo requires the accomplishment of two treatment goals:

1. The suppression of autoimmunity
2. Regeneration of melanocytes from their stem cell niche in the hair follicle.

Tables 28.9 and **28.10** give an overview of the treatment options.

TABLE 28.8: Investigations in vitiligo

Bedside	**Wood's lamp**	• Especially in lighter skins due to lack of contrast • Mostly on palmoplantar lesions and lip lesions	
	Dermoscopy	**Feature**	**Characteristics of stage of disease**
		Absence of satellite lesions, absence of micro-Koebner phenomenon	Most sensitive markers of stability (Nirmal B, 2019)
		Perifollicular pigmentation (PFP)	Stable disease
		Perilesional/marginal hyperpigmentation	Stable repigmenting disease
		Marginal reticular pigmentation	Stable repigmenting disease
		Polka dot	Progressive disease
		Starbust appearance	Progressive disease
		Comet tail appearance	Progressive disease
		Micro-Koebner's phenomenon	Progressive disease
		Tapioca sago appearance	Progressive disease
Histopathology	• Melanocytes absent/scanty in lesional skin • Immunohistochemistry for melanocyte markers: **Melan-A (MART-1), MITF, HMB-45, DOPA stains.**		

TABLE 28.9: Medical therapy for vitiligo vulgaris

Topical	Systemic	Implants	Phototherapy
Corticosteroids	Corticosteroids	Afamelanotide (synthetic analogue of α-MSH → binds to the melanocortin-1 receptor → stimulating melanocyte proliferation)—16 mg sub-cutaneous implant monthly	nbUVB
Topical calcineurin inhibitors	Anti-inflammatory antibiotics—minocycline		PUVA/PUVAsol
Topical vit D analogs	Statins–simvastatin		UVA1
Latanoprost (PGF2α analog)	Immunosuppressives		308 nm monochromatic excimer light (MEL)
Topical PUVA	Antioxidants		• Khellin UVA (KUVA)
	Biologics		• He–Ne laser
Topical JAKi - ruxolitinib (FDA approved)	JAK inhibitor • Tofacitinib		(632 nm) → increases melanocyte proliferation and melanogenesis

TABLE 28.10: Autologous grafting techniques

Tissue grafts	• Split skin thickness graft (SSTG)—thin manual dermatome	Mostly for small areas
	• Ultra-thin skin grafting (UTSG)—ultra-thin motorized dermatome	Works well for even larger areas
	• Full thickness punch grafting	
	• Mini-punch grafting (1–2 mm)	Good for sites with irregular contours (nipple-areolae complex) and sites with doubtful recipient bed (palms and soles)
	• Suction blister grafting	For smaller lesions
	• Flip-top grafting	
	• Smash grafting	Poor efficiency
	• Hair follicle grafts	
Cellular grafts	• **Noncultured** epidermal cell suspension **Same day transplant: Hot trypsinization** **Next day transplant: Cold trypsinization**	For larger areas **Donor : recipient = 1:10**
	• **Cultured** autografts Cultured melanocytes Cultured epithelial cell grafts	**Donor : recipient = 1:60**
	Hair follicle melanocyte and melanocyte precursors/stem cell transplantation	Superior efficiency not proven
	Combined epidermal and hair follicle cell suspensions—keratinocyte derived growth factors for melanocytes	
	NCES + FCS (noncultured epidermal cell suspension + follicular cell suspension)	Preferred modality nowadays, for acral areas, when repigmentation required quickly

Flowchart 28.11 gives an overview of the treatment options for non-segmental vitiligo.

Flowchart 28.11: Treatment of vitiligo vulgaris

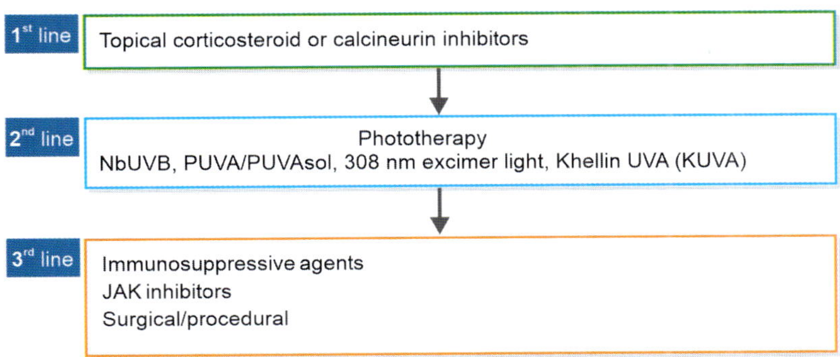

JAK Inhibitors: Role in Vitiligo

- **MOA** of JAK inhibitors
  1. INF-γ-induced expression of CXCL-10 is crucial for autoreactive T cell recruitment to the skin and destruction of melanocytes. Since IFN-γ-signal transduction occurs through JAK1/2, the JAK inhibitors can block the IFN signaling and downstream expression of CXCL-10.
  2. JAK: Promote sonic Hedgehog and Wnt signaling in epidermal pigmentation. The sonic Hedgehog pathway induces migration, proliferation and differentiation of melanocytes.
- **Tofacitinib (JAK 1/3 inhibitor)**—tried by Craiglow and King recently. 5–10 mg twice daily dose.
- **Ruxolitinib**—(JAK1/2 inhibitor). 20 mg twice daily for 5 months (unfortunately, most of the repigmented areas depigmented within 12 weeks of drug cessation).

Various other drugs in this class that have been used include ifidancitinib (JAK1/3), brepocitinib (TYK2/JAK1) barictinib (JAK1/2), ritlecitinib (JAK3) and cerdulatinib (SYK/JAK).

Phototherapy

PUVA utilizes UVA light to convert psoralen compounds into DNA-reactive, oxidative chemical products that both suppress immune function and stimulate melanocyte proliferation and repigmentation. The combined immunosuppressive and pigment-stimulating properties may explain the strong efficacy of PUVA as a vitiligo treatment but it has been replaced by narrow-band UVB (nbUVB) phototherapy which is believe to achieve better repigmentation of vitiligo lesions with fewer adverse side effects, such as an increased risk of skin cancer noted only with PUVA therapy. Most therapies combine nbUVB phototherapy with topical corticosteroids and/or topical calcineurin inhibitors.

- Rate of repigmentation, extent of repigmentation, color match—nbUVB > PUVA
- Longer duration (6 months instead of 3)—to determine responsiveness to nbUVB
- Longer duration needed for better response
- **Greatest results—face and neck > trunk > extremities > hands and feet**
- May be preceded by laser-assisted dermabrasion (erbium/CO_2)
- May be combined with pseudocatalase—doubtful efficacy
- **TCS alone and phototherapy in association with TCS/TCI have been found to have maximum short-term results (Cochrane review, 2016).**

Autologous Grafting Techniques

- Done only after lesional stability for 1 year or more.
- Effective in segmental, focal, non-acral lesions and at non-Koebner's sites.
- **Repigmentation starts by 4 weeks**
- **Maximal repigmentation—by 6 months**
- Color match—by 6 months
- Slower repigmentation continues-till 1–2 years (perigraft halo and leukotrichia may repigment during this time).
- **Therefore, try 2nd surgical endeavor only after 1 year has passed**.

Depigmentation Therapies

- Used in >40 years patients with more than 50% depigmentation of the areas to be treated and a desire for permanent depigmentation.
- MBEH (monobenzyl ether of hydroquinone) 20% cream applied twice daily for 9–12 months or longer.
- MMEH 20% cream.
- Q-switched ruby laser—faster depigmentation.
- Other measures
  - Photoprotection
  - Camouflaging
  - Psychological support.

Future Therapies

Varied novel therapeutic targets inlcude , drugs targeting microRNAs (miRNAs), (Tregs) and monoclonal antibodies that target the major cytokines implicated like IFN-gamma, CXCL10, CXCR3, HSP70i, IL-15, IL-17/23, and TNF.

CHEMICAL VITILIGO/CONTACT LEUKODERMA

Clinically, histologically and pathogenically indistinguishable from non-chemically induced vitiligo contact leukoderma following contact with chemicals may occur due to selective destruction of melanocytes, pigment transfer blockade or decreased melanogenesis. Some chemicals directly cause melanocyte destruction while some may, rarely, incite an irritant or allergic contact dermatitis which subsequently results in contact leukoderma. Phenolic/ catecholic derivatives are the most frequent triggers, inducing reactive oxygen species (ROS) during reactions catalyzed by tyrosinase-related protein-1 (Tyrp1). In genetically predisposed individuals, these ROS are not scavenged and lead to oxidative stress and melanocyte destruction. Most cases follow topical exposures, presumable due to the higher concentration of the offending chemical delivered to cutaneous melanocytes. Depigmentation limited to the site of contact with chemicals, often with confetti macules, is suggestive of contact leukoderma.

Causative Agents

A list of the common offending chemicals is given in **Box 28.17**.

Clinical Features

- Initial reaction may or may not look like irritant or allergic contact dermatitis
- Depigmented macules localized to the site of application and may rarely spread to remote, unexposed locations **(Fig. 28.20)**.

BOX 28.17: List of common offending agents in contact leukoderma

- Monobenzyl ether of hydroquinone (MBEH)—FDA approved for depigmentation therapy in vitiligo,
- 4-tert-butylcatechol (4-TBC)—present in lubricating oil
- 4-tert-butylphenol (4-TBP)—present in adhesive resin.
- 4-tert-amylphenol (4-TAP)—present in detergents
- para-phenylenediamine (PPD)—present in hair dyes
- Crocein Scarlet MOO or brilliant crocein—present in alta/red dye solution
- Rhodamine B, or tetraethyl rhodamine—present in alta/red dye solution
- Rhododendrol—present in cosmetics

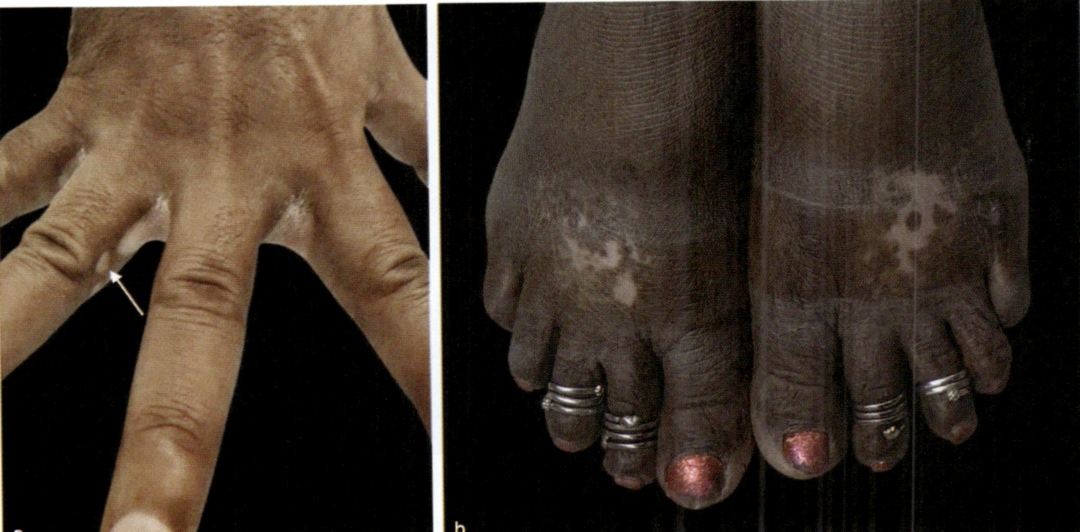

Fig. 28.20: (a) Chemical vitiligo following isopropyl alcohol based sanitizer. The arrows point towards confetti macules; (b) Chemical leukoderma due to footwear containing rubber

- Confetti macules may be present but are no longer considered specific to chemical vitiligo (considered markers for active disease now).

Clinical Course

May resolve partially or completely after withdrawing the depigmenting agent.

Treatment

- Avoid the depigmenting agent.
- Topical tacrolimus and topical steroids may help in repigmentation.

RETICULATE PIGMENTARY DISORDERS

Reticulate pigmentary disorder is a term, i.e. loosely defined to include a spectrum of acquired and congenital conditions with different morphologies that vary from the reticular or net-like pattern to the "freckle-like" hyper- and hypopigmented macules that are usually restricted to the true genetic reticulate pigmentary disorders. In this text we will harmonise the entities mentioned below as "mottled pigmentation" (Sardana K, et al., 2013).

a. Reticulate pigmentary disorders (acquired and congenital) **(Fig. 28.21)**
b. Dyschromatosis **(Fig 28.22)**.

Dyschromatoses are characterized by the presence of both hypo- and hyperpigmentation. Often, at least one component of the dyspigmentation is guttate.

Flowchart 28.12 covers the important classic true reticulate disorders and dyschromatoses. The other rare causes are detailed in **Box 28.18**. Salient features of the commonly encountered variants are listed in **Table 28.11**.

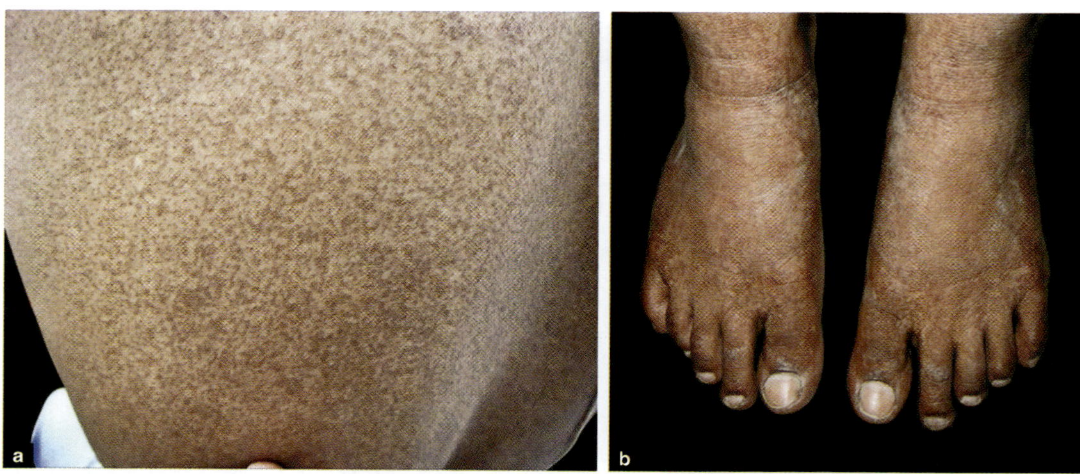

Fig. 28.21: Reticulate—hyperpigmentation wherein a "net like" hyperpigmentation is seen

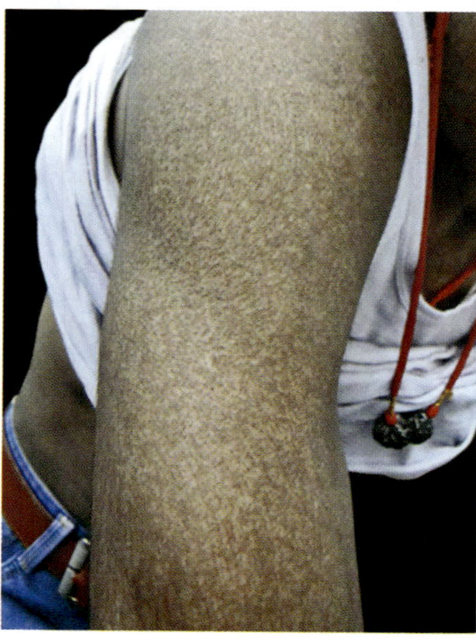

Fig. 28.22: Dyschromatosis—Hyper- and hypopigmented macules

Flowchart 28.12: Overview of reticulate disorders

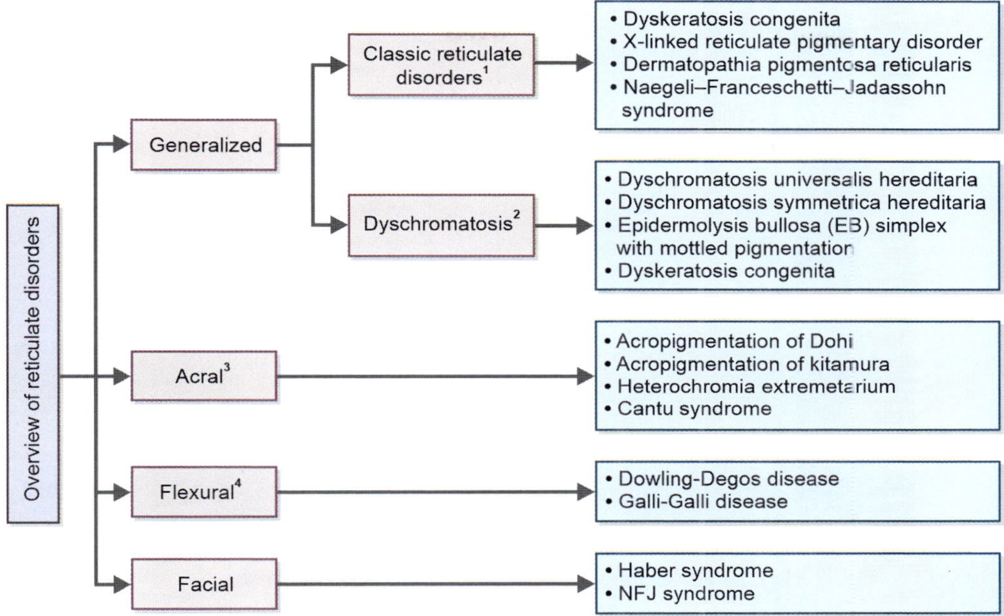

((NFJ syndrome: Naegeli-Franceschetti-Jadassohn syndrome) (1, 2, 3, 4—more disorders of the type)) (other disorders—[1] Fanconi anemia, Mendes de Costa syndrome, Berlin's syndrome, Cantu syndrome.[2] Arsenic, MBEH, DPCP, syphilis, amyloidosis.[3] Acromelanosis progressiva is another rare disorder.[4] Confluent and reticulate papillomatosis pigmentation reticularis faciei *et colli*)

BOX 28.18: Rarer causes of reticulate pigmentation

Confluent and reticulated papillomatosis (CARP) of Gougerot and Carteaud	• Elevated, favors neck and upper trunk; treated with minocycline • Often appears during adolescence **(Fig. 28.23)**
Erythema ab igne (later stage)	• Widely spaced net that corresponds to vascular pattern • Due to heat injury, including from heating pads (back) or laptop • Computer batteries (anterior thighs) **(Fig. 28.24)**
Atopic dirty neck	• Anterolateral neck, favors children
Prurigo pigmentosa	• Typically, young Asian women • Favors the back, neck, and chest • Recurrent crops of pruritic papulovesicles that resolve with a reticulated pattern of hyperpigmentation
X-linked reticulate pigmentary disorder	• XLR • Males present with generalized reticulated pigmentation, neonatal colitis, recurrent pneumonia, hypohidrosis, photophobia, ± amyloid deposits in adults • Female carriers present with hyperpigmented streaks along Blaschko lines
Fanconi anemia	• AR • More diffuse hyperpigmentation, radial ray bony defects, pancytopenia, leukemia
Galli-Galli disease	• Acantholytic variant of DDD
Haber syndrome	• Rosacea-like facial eruption plus the clinical features of DDD
Pigmento reticularis faciei *et colli*	• Possible variant of DDD • Hyperpigmentation of the face and neck plus multiple epidermoid cysts

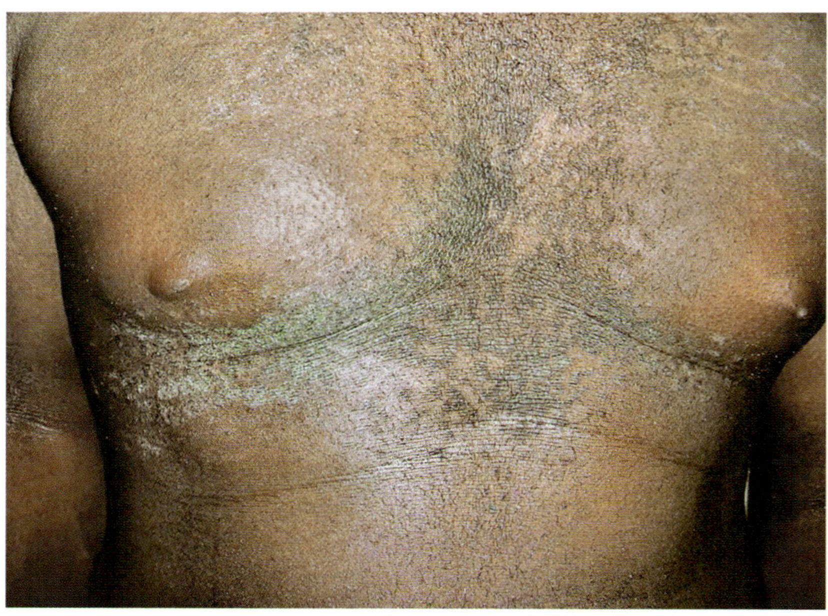

Fig. 28.23: Confluent and reticulated papillomatosis

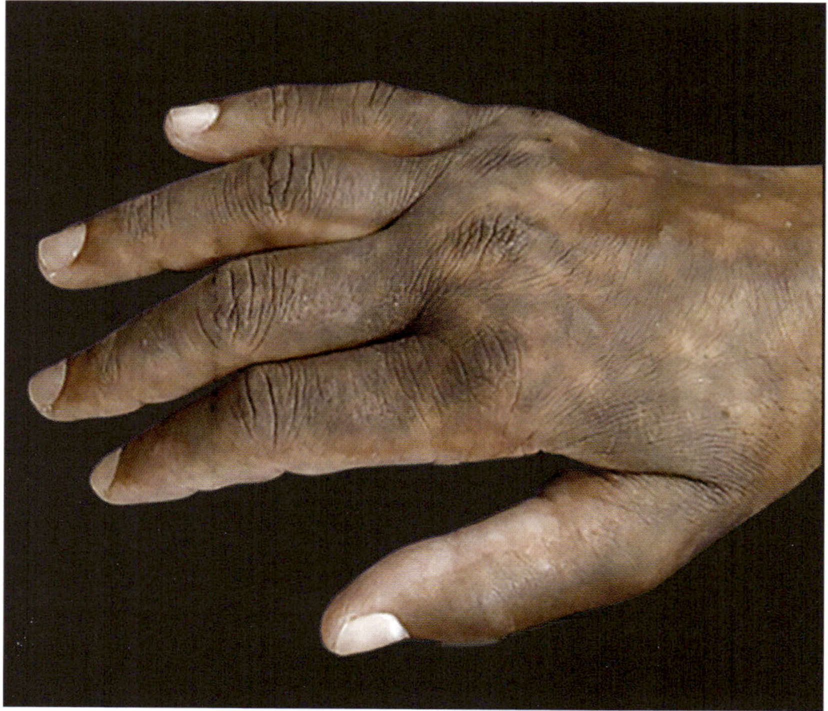

Fig. 28.24: Erythema ab igne

TABLE 28.11: Reticulate pigmentary disorders

Disease	Epidemiology and predisposing factors	Clinical features	Clinical course and complication	Investigations	Treatment
Dyschromatosis universalis hereditaria (DUH) (Fig. 28.25) **SASH 1 gene** **ABCB6, gene** **ABCB6 might play a role in the transport of melanosomes, thus explaining the pigmentary defects**	• AD, AR +/– at birth • Mostly in Japan • No seasonal change • No spontaneous regression with age	• Hypo- and hyperpigmented lesions • Mainly truncal, (+/–) whole body Palms and soles (+/–) Spares mucosae • Hair and nail abnormalities (+/–)	CNS, eye and hematological complications	**HPE:** Hyperpigmented macules: Focal increase in basal layer melanin content Hypopigmented: Focal decrease in melanin content of basal layer	No satisfactory treatment
Dyschromatosis symmetrica hereditaria (DSH) Also known as • Symmetrical dyschromatosis of the extremities • Symmetrical or reticulate acropigmentation of **Dohi** • Mutations in **DSRAD gene**	• AD • Begins in infancy/early childhood • Asians, (inc. Japanese, Chinese, Koreans and Indians)—more common	• Multiple freckle-like macules on face • Small hyper- and hypopigmented macules on back of the hands, feet, sparing the palms, soles and mucosae	No spontaneous clearing Darkening after sun exposure	**HPE:** Increased melanin in the basal keratinocytes is seen in the hyperpigmented macules, while decreased DOPA-positive melanocyes in hypopigmented ones	• No satisfactory treatment • Strict sun protection • Lasers including: Q-switched ruby, Q-switched Nd:YAG, Q-switched alexandrite, and the 510 mm pulsed dye lasers have been tried. Split-thickness skin autografts
Reticulate acropigmentation of Kitamura (Fig. 28.26) • Mutations in **ADAM10** (ADAM10 encodes for a zinc metalloprotease, a disintegrin and a metalloprotease domain-containing protein 10. It is known to be involved in the ectodomain shedding of various substrates in the skin) • Sunlight may aggravate the condition	• Autosomal dominant • Appear during childhood usually • Asians • Few familial cases	• Reticulate hyperpigmented **atrophic** macules on the hands → darken and spread proximally on extensor of limbs, neck, face and upper trunk • Pits break the epidermal ridge pattern on the palms and soles	The progression of lesions in number and in the intensity of color stops in the middle age	**HPE** • Epidermal thining • Elongation of the rete ridges with increased pigmentation (melanin) at their tips • Slight hyperkeratosis without parakeratosis is also seen **DIF/special stains** DOPA-positive melanocytes increased in the basal layer **Dermoscopy** Brownish reticular pigment networks	Not much has been seen to be effective. The following treatments are tried: • 20% azelaic acid • Hydroquinone, tretinoin, adapalene and corticosteroid topically • Er:YAG laser

(Contd.)

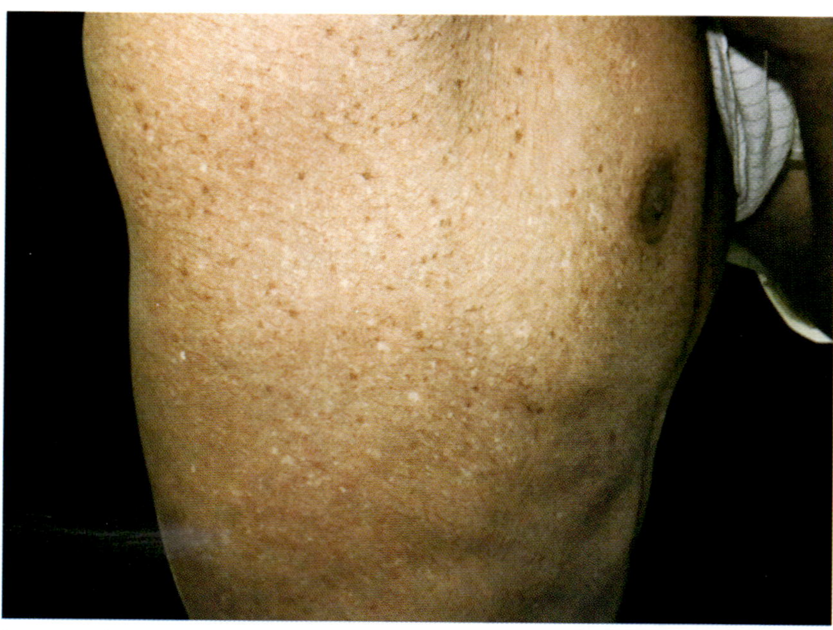

Fig. 28.25: Hypo- and hyperpigmented macules in a case of dyschromatosis universalis hereditarian

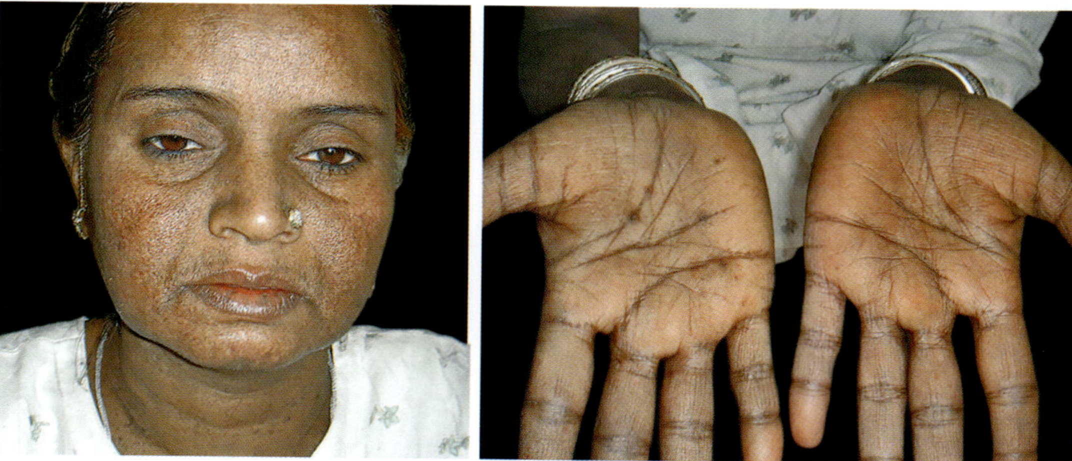

Fig. 28.26: Reticulate acropigmentation of Kitamura: Angular pigmented macules involve initially the extremities (dorsum of the hands and feet) then spreading to the limbs, neck, upper trunk, lower face with pits that interrupt the dermatoglyphics of the palm creases

TABLE 28.11: Reticulate pigmentary disorders *(Contd.)*

Disease	Epidemiology and predisposing factors	Clinical features	Clinical course and complication	Investigations	Treatment
Dyskeratosis congenita (DKC) (Fig. 28.27)	• X-linked (most common), AR and AD • 90% are males • AD cases show anticipation • Age of onset is 2nd decade	**Triad of** • *Reticular skin pigmentation* distributed over neck, upper chest and proximal parts of the limbs (starts developing in the 1st decade) • *Nail dystrophy*: In early childhood with longitudinal splitting and ridging leading to pterygium • *Leukoplakia* in oral mucosa in early adolescence. Sometimes involve urethra, vagina and anus Also, hypopigmented macules mixed with hyperpigmentation; poikiloderma; palmoplantar hyperhidrosis and hyperkeratosis; acrocyanosis; testicular atrophy; pulmonary fibrosis; liver cirrhosis, developmental delay; and immunologic dysfunction leading to opportunistic infections	• Bone marrow dysplasia: In 2nd or 3rd decade • Hematological and epithelial malignancies (SCC most common): In 3rd or 4th decade • Lacrimal duct atresia leading to continuous lacrimation	**HPE:** • Early stage: Hydropic degeneration of basilar keratinocytes and a band-like inflammatory infiltrate in the upper dermis • Late stage: Markedly thinned epidermis and flattened, and melanophages are present in the upper dermis • **Flow fluorescence**—Short telomere length in leukocytes	• Multidisciplinary approach and symptomatic treatment • Regular monitoring for development of malignancy • Sun protection • Blood transfusions, androgens, erythropoietin, G-CSF in bone marrow failure and hematopoietic stem cell transplantation in leukemias

(Contd.)

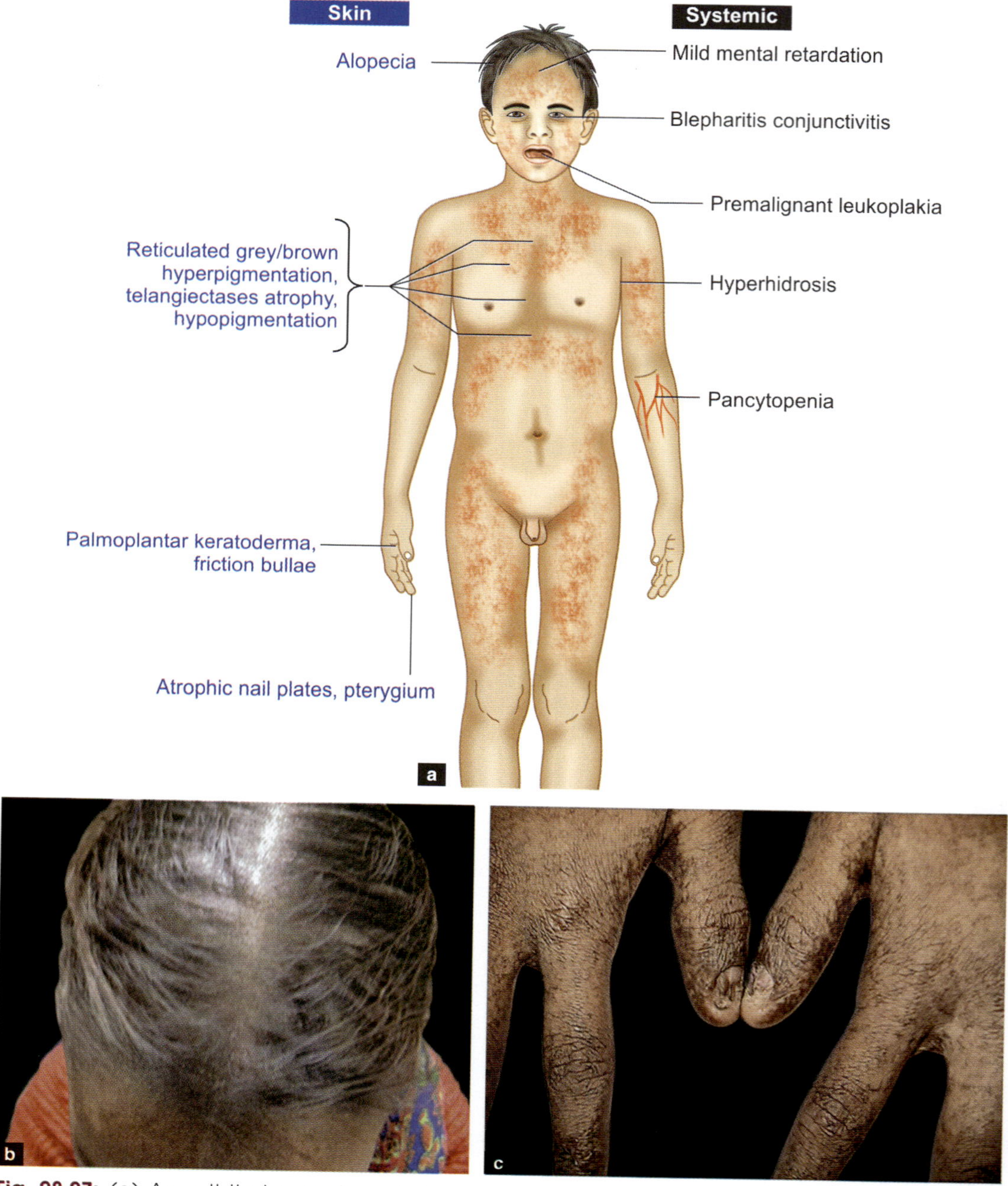

Fig. 28.27: (a) An artistic impression of clinical features of DKC; (b) A depiction of dyskeratosis congenita with reticulate hyperpigmentation visible; (c) Dystrophy of nails in DKC

TABLE 28.11: Reticulate pigmentary disorders *(Contd.)*

Disease	Epidemiology and predisposing factors	Clinical features	Clinical course and complication	Investigations	Treatment
Naegeli-Franceschetti-Jadassohn syndrome (NFJS) and dermatopathia pigmentosa reticularis (DPR)	**NFJS** • Mostly the Swiss and British families • Males = females **DPR** • AD ectodermal dysplasia syndromes • KRT14 gene sequence mutation: Makes keratinocytes more susceptible to pro-apoptotic stimuli	**NFJS** • Reticular cutaneous pigmentation starting in early life (by 2 years of age) and lightening during adolescence • Intolerance to heat with hypohidrosis, poor dentition and moderate palmoplantar hyperkeratosis **Dermatopathia pigmentosa reticularis** **Triad:** Persistent reticulate hyperpigmentation, non-cicatricial alopecia and onychodystrophy Common features: • Complete absence of dermatoglyphics • Reticulate skin pigmentation with trunk and face as primary sites of involvement • Palmoplantar keratoderma, sweating abnormality		**HPE** in both: Pigmentary incontinence of melanophages in hyperpigmented lesions	No satisfactory treatment Moisturizers for xerosis, maintenance of hydration, appropriate clothes, wet dressings, dental follow-up
Dowling-Degos disease (DDD) (Fig. 28.28) Loss of functional mutation of KRT5 gene	• AD • Incidence is worldwide. No racial or sex predilection • Age of onset is 30–40 years	• Progressive reticular pigmentation distributed in the *flexures* and in the genital and perianal areas, lentigo-like macules and brown papules with variable hyperkeratosis (+/–) • *Comedo-like* lesions of the neck and back • *Perioral* pitted scars		**HPE** • Increased basal layer pigmentation with finger rete ridges and thus thinning of suprapapillary epithelium giving *antler-like pattern* to the epidermal down-growths • A mild perivascular lymphohystiocytic infiltrate with dermal melanophages are seen	Varying results with: • Topical hydroquinone, tretinoin, adapalene and corticosteroids • Er:YAG laser

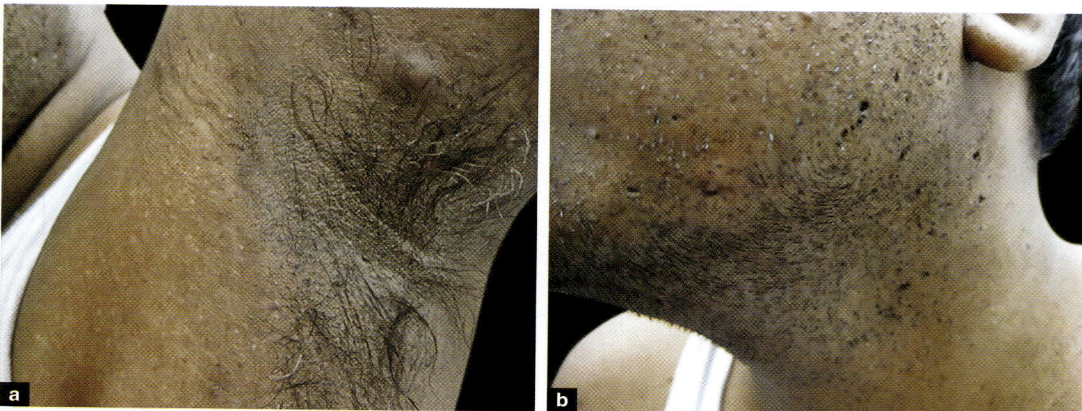

Fig. 28.28: (a) Dowling degos disease—reticulated pattern of pigmentation on axillae; (b) Comedolike, hyperkeratotic follicular papules on the neck and axillae

Acknowledgment

The authors wish to thank **Dr Manu Sehrawat**, MD, for her work on this chapter in the previous edition of this book.

BIBLIOGRAPHY

Books

1. Hideo Nakayama. Pigmented Contact Dermatitis and Chemical Depigmentation. JD Johansen, et al. (eds.): Contact Dermatitis, DOI: 10.1007/978-3-642-03827-3_19,© Springer-Verlag Berlin Heidelberg 2011.
2. Jean Bolognia Julie Schaffer Lorenzo Cerroni Dermatology: 2-Volume Set, 4th Edition. Elsevier, 2107. Chapters 66 and 67.
3. Kabir Sardana, Pooja Arora Mrig. Handbook of Pigmentary Disorders for Practitioners. CBS, 2018.
4. Rook's Textbook of Dermatology, 9th Edn. Wiley Blackwell. Chapters.

Journals

1. Bae, et al. Phototherapy for vitiligo: A systematic review and meta-analysis. JAMA Dermatol 2017; 153:666–74.
2. Craiglow and King. Tofacitinib citrate for the treatment of vitiligo. JAMA Dermatol 2015; 151:1110–2.
3. Dahir, et al. Comorbidities in vitiligo: comprehensive review. Int J Dermatol 2018; 57:1157–64.
4. Diagnosis and management of Skin Disorders. An Evidence based approach. LWW. 2012.
5. Gomes, et al. The role of interleukins in vitiligo: A systematic review. JEADV 2018; 32:2097–111.
6. Handbook of Pigmentary Disorders for Practitioners. CBS, 2018.
7. Harris, et al. Rapid skin repigmentation on oral ruxolitinib in a patient with coexistent vitiligo and alopecia areata. J Am Acad Dermatol 2016; 74:370–1.
8. Jha, et al. Dermoscopy in vitiligo: diagnosis and beyond. Int J Dermatol 2018; 57:50–4.
9. Kinsler VA, Boccara O, Fraitag S, Torrelo A, Vabres P, Diociaiuti A. Mosaic abnormalities of the skin: review and guidelines from the European Reference Network for rare skin diseases. Br J Dermatol. 2020;182 (3):552–63.
10. Mathachan SR, Khurana A, Gautam RK, Kulhari A, Sharma L, Sardana K. Does oxidative stress correlate with disease activity and severity in vitiligo? An analytical study. J Cosmet Dermatol. 2021 Jan;20(1): 352–9.

11. Molho-Pessach V, Schaffer JV. Blaschko lines and other patterns of cutaneous mosaicism. Clin Dermatol. 2011;29 (2):205–25.
12. Mukovozov I,. Treatment of Lentigines: A Systematic Review. Dermatol Surg. 2023 Jan 1;49(1):17–24.
13. Nirmal B, et al. Cross-Sectional Study of Dermatoscopic Findings in Relation to Activity in Vitiligo: BPLeFoSK Criteria for Stability. JCAS 2019;12:36–41.
14. Rani S, Sardana K. Variables that predict response of nevus of Ota to lasers. J Cosmet Dermatol. 2019 Apr;18(2):464–468.
15. Ruiz?Maldonado R, Toussaint S, Tamayo L, Laterza A, del Castillo V. Hypomelanosis of Ito: diagnostic criteria and report of 41 cases. Pediatr Dermatol. 1992;9 (1):1–10.
16. Sardana K, Goel K, Chugh S. Reticulate pigmentary disorders. Indian J Dermatol Venereol Leprol. 2013 Jan-Feb; 79 (1):17–29.
17. Sharma VK, Bhatia R, Yadav CP. Clinical Profile and Allergens in Pigmented Cosmetic Dermatitis and Allergic Contact Dermatitis to Cosmetics in India. Dermatitis. 2018 Sep/Oct; 29 (5):264–9.
18. T Razmi M, et al. Vitiligo surgery: a journey from tissue via cells to the stems! Exp Dermatol 2018;1–5.
19. Taibjee SM, Bennett DC, Moss C. Abnormal pigmentation in hypomelanosis of Ito and pigmentary mosaicism: the role of pigmentary genes. Br J Dermatol. 2004;151 (2):269–282.
20. Ueda S, Isoda M, Imayama S. Response of naevus of Ota to Q?switched ruby laser treatment according to lesion colour. Br J Dermatol. 2000;142(1):77–83.
21. van Geel N, Grine L, De Wispelaere P, Mertens D, Prinsen CAC, Speeckaert R. Clinical visible signs of disease activity in vitiligo: a systematic review and meta-analysis. J Eur Acad Dermatol Venereol. 2019 Sep;33(9):1667–1675.
22. Whitton, et al. Evidence-based management of vitiligo: summary of a Cochrane systematic review. Br J Dermatol. 2016 May; 174 (5):962–9.
23. Xiao C,. Aiming to personalized laser therapy for nevus of Ota: melanin distribution dependent parameter optimization. Lasers Med Sci. 2022 Dec 21;38(1):10.

Chapter

29

Pityriasis Rubra Pilaris

Seema Rani, Kabir Sardana, Snigdha Saxena

EPIDEMIOLOGY

- Papulosquamous dermatosis of unknown cause.
- In 1889, Besnier recommended the name pityriasis rubra pilaris.
- Five clinical types and recently a sixth type with HIV have been described.
- Bimodal age distribution with peaks in the first and fifth decades.
- Equal sex distribution.
- Mostly acquired, occasionally familial cases (up to 6.5%) with autosomal dominant inheritance.
- Associated diseases
  - Malignancy—solid tumors including carcinoma of the larynx, colon, kidney and lung
  - Autoimmune disorders-systemic sclerosis, autoimmune thyroiditis, myasthenia gravis, celiac disease, inflammatory arthritis.

ETIOPATHOGENESIS

- Unknown pathogenesis, earlier proposed due to vitamin A deficiency
- There have been reports of cases with preceding infections, UV exposure and various minor traumas to the skin implicating a physical trigger or superantigen.

CLINICAL FEATURES (Figs 29.1 and 29.2)

- Classically begins on head/neck → **progresses caudally**, scalp erythema with fine, diffuse scaling
- Multiple, well-defined, coalescing salmon red or orange red, dry scaly plaques which may be widespread and sometimes become erythrodermic.
- Typically islands of normal skin are present, the so-called 'islands of sparing'.
- Follicular hyperkeratosis on an erythematous base is a key finding.
- Especially seen over backs of the fingers, elbows and wrists—characteristic—'nutmeg grater' papules.
- Palm and sole become thickened and fissured with orange discoloration (sandal-like PPK)
- Pruritus and burning may be present in early stage.

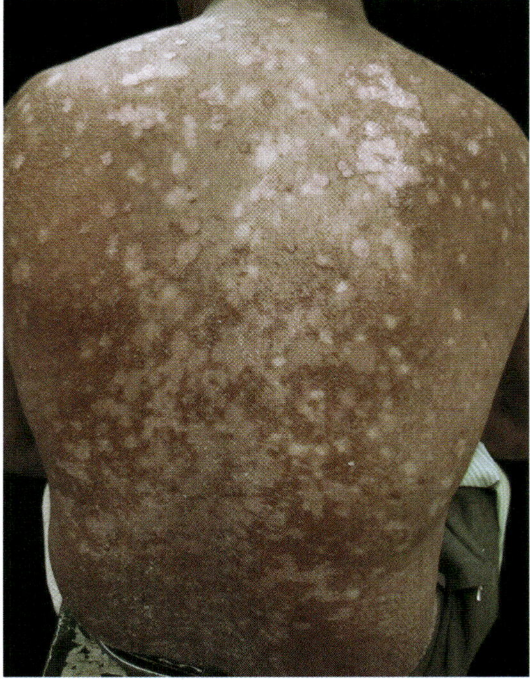

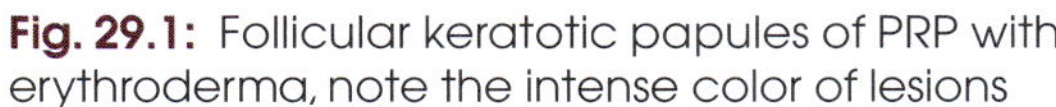

Fig. 29.1: Follicular keratotic papules of PRP with erythroderma, note the intense color of lesions

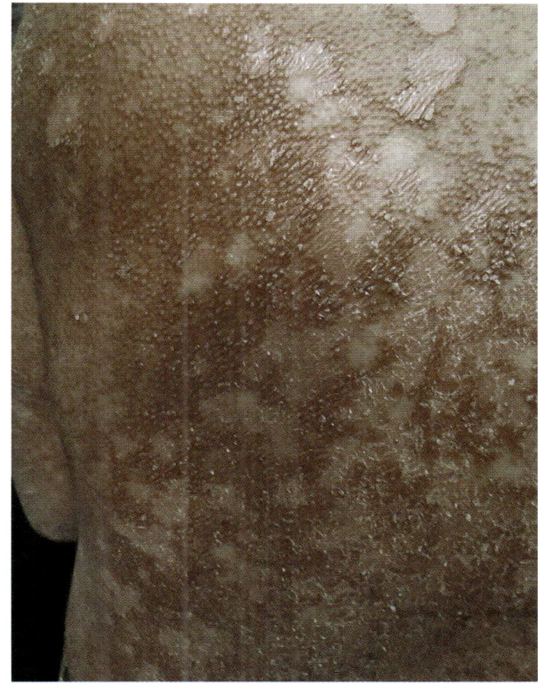

Fig. 29.2: A close-up view showing prominent follicular papules with islands of sparing

Clinical Variants (Flowchart 29.1)

All except type IV are generalized.

Six types

- **Classical adult onset PRP (type I)**
  - Most common form representing 50% of cases, seen in 40–60 years of age
  - Classical clinical presentation often progressing into erythroderma
  - Majority of affected patients eventually resolve within an average of 3 years (80%)
- **Atypical adult onset PRP (type II)**
  - Accounts for 5% of cases
  - Chronic form which may last longer.
  - Clinical picture does not evolve rapidly as compared to type I.
  - Erythroderma is less commonly seen.
  - Ichthyosiform leg lesions + Eczematoid lesions + Keratoderma with coarse and lamellated scale +/– alopecia
- **Classical juvenile onset PRP (type III)**
  - Most common childhood form of PRP with an onset between the ages of 5 and 10 years
  - Considered to be the juvenile counterpart of type I PRP
  - May evolve into type IV PRP
  - Undergoes spontaneous resolution in 1–2 years, recurrence can occur in adult life.

Flowchart 29.1: Classification and description of clinical types of pityriasis rubra pilaris

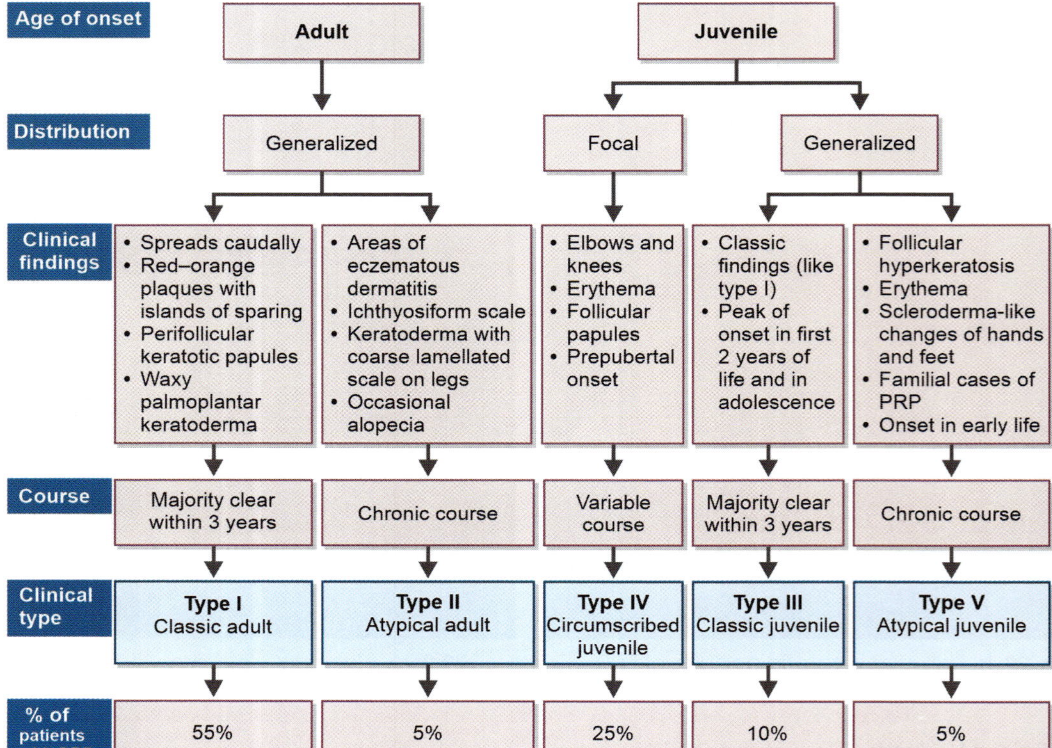

- **Circumscribed juvenile PRP (type IV)**
  - Represents 25% of cases of PRP
  - Seen in prepubertal age group, usually under 12 years of age
  - Commonly presents as well circumscribed plaques of erythema and follicular hyperkeratosis occurring on the elbows and knees with a few scattered plaques over trunk and scalp
  - Palmoplantar keratoderma may be present.
  - Prognosis is uncertain, may remit in teenage.
- **Atypical juvenile PRP (type V)**
  - Accounts for 5% of cases, mostly familial type
  - Type V PRP may be present at birth or start in early childhood with erythema and hyperkeratosis.
  - Prominent follicular hyperkeratosis and keratoderma + sclerodermoid changes of hands/feet
  - May be difficult to distinguish from ichthyoses and erythrokeratodermia.
- **HIV-related PRP (type VI)**
  - Apparent with onset of HIV
  - Tends to resemble type I
  - Generalized PRP in HIV patients with hidradenitis suppurativa, acne conglobata and elongated follicular spines
  - Treatment resistant, however, may respond to antiretroviral therapy.

Pathology

- Non-specific, changes with evolution of disease.
- Irregular hyperkeratosis and **alternating vertical and horizontal ortho- and parakeratosis (checkerboard pattern)** is distinctive.
- Hair follicles are dilated and filled with a keratinous plug, foci of parakeratosis in the perifollicular shoulder. **(Shoulder parakeratosis)**
- Patchy or confluent hypergranulosis. Dermal capillaries are dilated but are not tortuous as seen in psoriasis.
- Acantholysis and focal acantholytic dyskeratosis within the epidermis and irregular acanthosis with thickened suprapapillary plates which may help when distinguishing PRP from psoriasis.

Differential Diagnosis

The important differential diagnoses are given in **Table 29.1**.

TABLE 29.1: Differential diagnosis of PRP
• Seborrheic dermatitis—early PRP over scalp
• Psoriasis
• Erythrokeratodermia variabilis
• Sézary syndrome and other T-cell lymphomas
• Other forms of erythroderma
• Type IV PRP shares many clinical features with **keratosis circumscripta**

Complications and Comorbidities

Dependent edema and risk of high output cardiac failure especially in erythrodermic PRP.

Disease Course and Prognosis

Disease course and prognosis depends on the type of PRP

- Classical adult PRP (type I) may progress from limited disease to erythroderma.
- Classical juvenile PRP (type III) typically runs a shorter course with remission in an average of 1 year.
- Atypical PRP (types II and V) are chronic diseases but are usually more limited in extent than types I and III.
- Circumscribed juvenile PRP (type IV) is uncertain but may last indefinitely.

Investigations

Depend upon clinical features. Histopathology may be useful.

Management

Erythrodermic PRP may need intense supportive care to prevent hypothermia, electrolyte imbalance, protein loss and sepsis.

Treatment Ladder

The line of management is detailed in **Flowchart 29.2**, phototherapy has been tried but can also lead to a flare in the condition, hence we are not detailing it here.

Flowchart 29.2: Approach to therapy of pityriasis rubra pilaris (PRP)

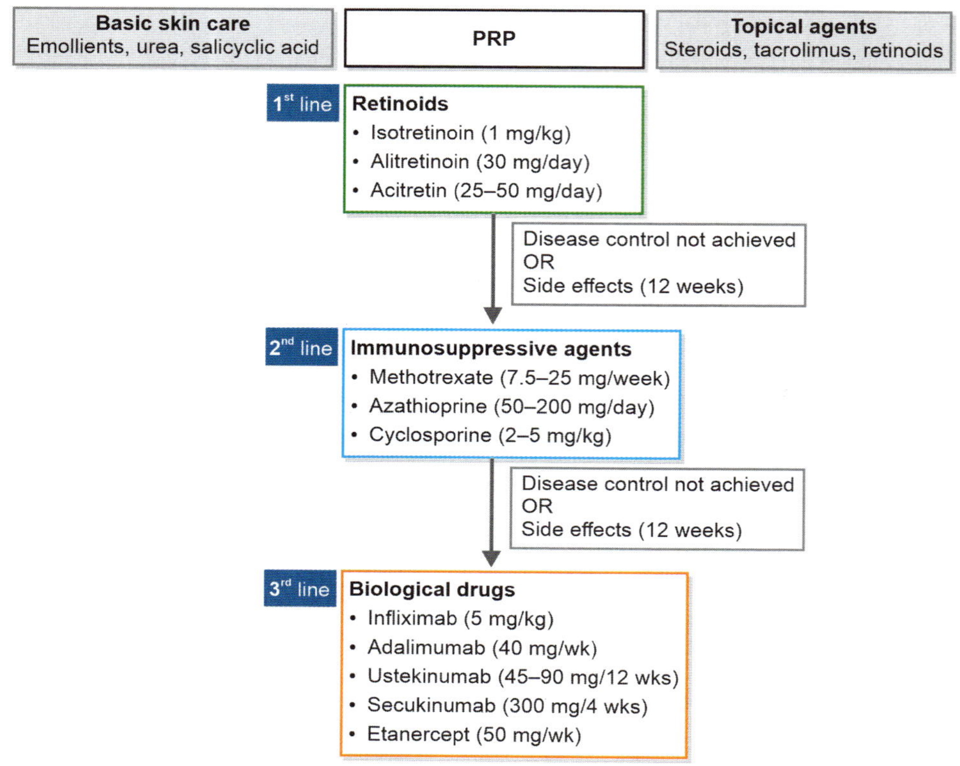

Note: *In case of underlying malignancy, apremilast can be an alternative therapy option.

What's New

Recent reports have shown the use of novel agents like **brodalumab, guselkumab, Ixekizumab imiquimod 5%** and risankizumab, a IL-23/p19 antagonist.

BIBLIOGRAPHY

1. Anthony C Chu. Pityriasis Rubra Piloris. In: Rook's Textbook of Dermatology (9th ed.). UK. Blackwell Publishers 2016. Part 4; Ch 36:1181–2.
2. Gary S Wood and George T Reizner. Papulo-squamous and Eczematous dermatoses. In: Dermatology (3rd ed.). London. Elsevier Publisher. 2012; sec 3: P162–5.

Chapter

30

Psoriasis

Surabhi Sinha, Snigdha Saxena

Psoriasis is a chronic inflammatory hyperproliferative skin disorder. **Table 30.1** gives a classification of psoriasis.

TABLE 30.1: Classification of psoriasis

Based on morphology (*see also* Table 30.2)	Based on specific sites (*see also* Table 30.3)	Based on age/precipitant
• Plaque • Acute guttate • Unstable • Erythrodermic • Pustular • Atypical	• Scalp • Follicular • Seborrheic/sebopsoriasis • Flexural/inverse • Genital • Nonpustular palmoplantar • Nail • Mucosal • Ocular	• Childhood/old age • Linear and segmental • Photo-aggravated • Drug induced/drug exacerbated • HIV induced/HIV exacerbated

TYPES OF PSORIASIS

PLAQUE PSORIASIS

Epidemiology

- **Prevalence:** 2–3% worldwide.
- **Age:** 2 peaks—16–22 years **(type I)** and 57–62 years **(type II)**. Onset before 20 years of age in one-third patients.
  - **Type I**—hereditary, strongly HLA-associated (especially HLA-C:06:02), early onset, more severe, thought to be linked to guttate psoriasis (which is invariably HLA-C:06:02 associated).
  - **Type II**—sporadic, HLA-unrelated, late onset, milder.
- **Sex**—M = F. Men may have more severe disease.

Predisposing and Triggering Factors

- **Genetics:**
  - Lifetime risk **4%**, **28%** or **65%** if neither, one or both parents affected, respectively.
  - 9 chromosomal loci PSORS1-PSORS9 (polygenic inheritance)
  - **PSORS1—major genetic determinant.** Located within MHC on chromosome 6p—most likely HLA-C: 06:02. Linked to guttate and type I psoriasis.
  - **PSORS2—chromosome 17q–gene CARD14.** Mutation of CARD14 → NF-κB activation → chemokines production by keratinocytes → PMNL recruitment.
- **Environmental**
  1. Infection
     a. Streptococcal infections esp. tonsillitis
        → Guttate > plaque psoriasis
  2. Drugs
     a. **Lithium, interferon-α, TNF-α inhibitors, antimalarials**—maximum evidence
     b. ACE inhibitors, beta-blockers, NSAIDs—seen in a few case series, not supported by larger studies, may be unlikely causes.
  3. Alcohol abuse
     a. Psoriasis—more prevalent and more severe in patients of alcoholic liver disease
     b. Psoriasis patients—more likely to misuse/abuse alcohol (in 30% psoriasis patients)
     c. Screen for alcohol misuse in severe psoriasis
  4. Smoking
     a. Plaque psoriasis patients, esp. women—more incidence of cigarette smoking
     b. Smokers—at higher risk of developing psoriasis, having more severe disease, developing psoriatic arthritis
     c. Strong association between smoking and palmoplantar pustulosis
  5. Psychological stress
     a. 80% patients—stress causes flares
  6. Sunshine
     a. Generally (80–95%)—sunshine beneficial to psoriasis plaques
     b. **5–20%**—sunshine provokes psoriasis and causes summer flares
  7. Physical trauma
     a. 25% patients—development of lesions on sites of trauma, esp. in type I psoriasis.

Pathogenesis

The involvement of T cells in psoriasis was already demonstrated in **1986**, when a study published by Fry and colleagues demonstrated clearance of psoriasis following administration of low-dose ciclosporin.

Now its is known that **IL-17** and **IL-22** represent key disease mediators, linking the adaptive immune response and epithelial dysregulation in psoriasis by inducing keratinocyte hyperproliferation via **Th17** and **LL-37** upregulation from activated keratinocytes.

Whereas Th1 cell development is driven by IL-12, development and maintenance of Th17 cells is linked to IL-23. IL-12 is composed of a p35 and a p40 subunit, while **IL-23** is composed of a p19 and a p40 subunit. Both cytokines therefore share the p40 subunit, and a therapeutic agent targeting the p40 subunit (ustekinumab) has shown clinical efficacy in patients with psoriasis.

In 2009, McGeachy et al. demonstrated that **IL-23** was required for *in vivo* Th17 cell differentiation in autoimmunity, inflammation and infection, thus indicating a more central role for IL-23 in Th17 function than previously thought. IL-23 appears to be critical in promoting the differentiation of pathogenic tissue-resident memory **(TRM)** T cells; this pathogenic subset of TRM cells has an important role in autoimmune inflammation in human skin.

In summary, the **IL-23/Th17** axis has a central role in the pathogenesis of psoriasis **(Fig. 30.1)**, as well as in psoriatic arthritis and other spondyloarthritides.

Dendritic Cells and Mononuclear Phagocytes in Psoriasis Immunopathology

Dendritic cells (DCs) are antigen-presenting cells that can be recruited from the circulation to modulate local immune responses at sites of skin inflammation or infection; Langerhans cells (LCs) are specialized DCs residing in the epidermal layer of the skin. A subset of these cells are known as epidermal DCs (eDCs) and epidermal-resident LCs in psoriasis where eDCs, which occurred only in psoriasis, were phenotypically different from normal DCs and were completely absent in resolved psoriasis.

The **eDCs** highly expressed genes involved in neutrophil recruitment and keratinocyte and T-cell activation. Additionally, while epidermal-resident LCs responded to Toll-like receptor (TLR) activation with increased IL-23 production, eDCs produced IL-23 together with IL-1β and TNF-α.

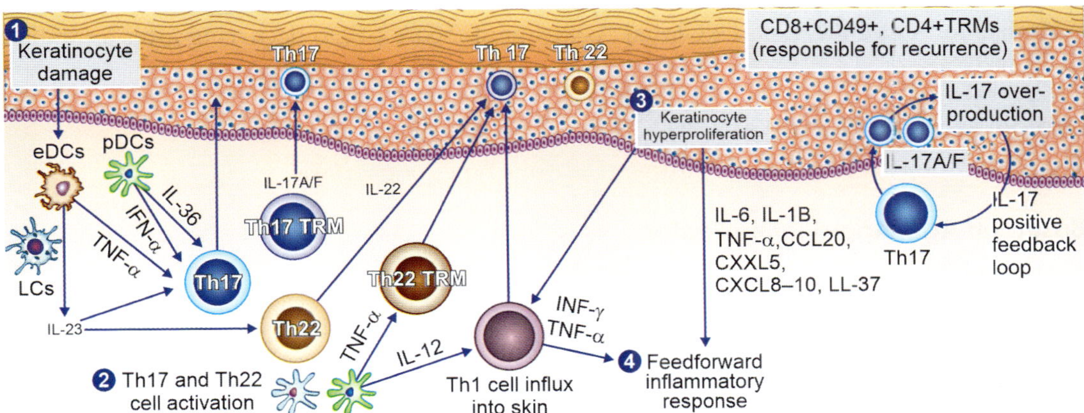

Fig. 30.1: Current model of psoriasis immunopathology (1) Activation of plasmacytoid dendritic cells (pDCs) and interleukin (IL)-23-producing epidermal DCs due to keratinocyte damage. (2) T helper (Th)17 cell polarization and clonal expansion is triggered. T-cell activation leads to production of proinflammatory cytokines. IL-23 promotes Th17 cell clonal expansion and differentiation. (3) IL-17 +/–tumour necrosis factor alpha (TNF-α) induces further inflammation with terminal keratinocyte differentiation and proliferation–forming a psoriatic plaque. (4) A feedforward inflammatory response is induced, with IL-17 inducing psoriasis-related gene expression in keratinocytes, driving further inflammation. eDCs, epidermal DCs; IFN, interferon; LC, Langerhans cell; LL-37, cathelicidin antimicrobial peptide; TRM, tissue-resident memory cell.
(Puig L, et al., 2022)

Tissue-resident Memory T Cells and Psoriasis

Resident memory T cells are of two types CD8 + and CD4 + subsets. **CD8+ TRM cells** are localized in the epidermis where they play a critical role in immune responses; **CD4+TRM** cells are less well characterized and potentially play a critical role in protective immunity against bacterial and fungal infections in the skin. Thus in resolved lesions, CD4+tissue-resident memory cells (TRMs) remain in the dermis, and CD8+TRMs and epidermal Langerhans cells (eLCs) remain in the epidermis **(Fig. 30.1)**. The majority of CD8+TRM cells express the cell marker CD103 (also known as integrin alpha-E), which is implicated in lodging TRM cells in the epidermis.

While varied drugs of IL-17 and IL-23 inhibitor classes have been used in psoriasis, it has also been shown that the clinical response is maintained slightly longer with IL-23 antagonists following treatment discontinuation. Thus the median time to loss of PASI 90 response after withdrawal of the IL-23 inhibitor guselkumab was 23 weeks while it was 20 weeks after withdrawal from IL-17A inhibitor ixekizumab. The maintenance of response with these agents was greater than might be anticipated based on their elimination half-lives of approximately 18 days and 13 days for guselkumab and ixekizumab. Also for the IL-23A inhibitor risankizumab, a median time of 30 weeks from withdrawal of treatment until loss of PASI 90 response was reported. For the IL-23 inhibitor tildrakizumab, the median time until loss of PASI 90 response was 16 and 20 weeks for patients withdrawing from a 100 mg and 200 mg dose, respectively.

For the IL-17A/F inhibitor bimekizumab, the median time to loss of PASI 90 response was approximately 20 weeks after the final dose. A somewhat shorter time to loss of response was reported for the anti-IL-17A receptor antibody brodalumab, with loss of response for static Physician's Global Assessment (score of ≥3) occurring after a median of 11 weeks.

Clinical Features (Tables 30.2 and 30.3)

Figure 30.2 depicts the clinical features of various types of psoriasis.

Based on Age/Aggravating Factor

Psoriasis in old age

- Less extensive disease
- Most common—**plaque psoriasis with scalp** involvement
- Inverse, erythrodermic, generalized pustular > Guttate

Psoriasis in childhood

- 0.7% prevalence
- Significant association with comorbidities—obesity, metabolic syndrome, diabetes
- No evidence that childhood onset predicts severe adult disease
- Infants—napkin psoriasis
- Older children—plaque psoriasis (**face and anogenital area)**
- Flexural > parakeratosis pustulosa
- Severe forms—rare

TABLE 30.2: Psoriasis of specific morphology

	Clinical features	Sites	Differential diagnosis	Preferred treatment
Plaque (Fig. 30.2a)	Well defined erythematous plaque with micaceous scales	Scalp, extensors of limbs, buttocks	LSC, discoid eczema, tinea corporis, PRP, Bowen disease	—
Acute guttate (12%) (Fig. 30.2b)	Sudden shower of small lesions, follows weeks after streptococcal pharyngitis (ASO +ve in 60%), <1 cm diameter, mild scaling, resolves over 3 months	Trunk and proximal limbs, face and scalp too +/–	Small plaque parapsoriasis, pityriasis rosea, secondary syphilis, lichen planus	—
'Unstable'	Plaques become larger and more erythematous, new smaller plaques develop, pain and pruritus >>, Koebner +, unpredictable course, serum IL-17 and IL-1 receptor antagonist >>	—	—	—
Erythrodermic (1–2%)	Psoriasis causes erythroderma in 25%, chronic (better prognosis) or acute (poorer prognosis)	≥90% body surface area	Other causes of erythroderma (*see* erythroderma chapter)	CsA, IFX (most rapid) Aci, MTX
Pustular	*See* later	—	—	Aci, MTX, ADA, Secu (GPP)
Atypical	Digital, interdigital, verrucous (legs), rupioid, elephantine, ostraceous	Limbs usually	—	—
Linear/ segmental	Isolated/superimposed on plaque psoriasis, more treatment refractory	Usually limbs	ILVEN, Koebner phenomenon in psoriasis or other disorders	—

IFX, infliximab; ADA, adalimumab; Secu, secukinumab; CsA, ciclosporin; Aci, acitretin; MTX, methotrexate

TABLE 30.3: Psoriasis of specific sites

	Clinical features	Sites	Differential diagnosis	Treatment
Scalp	Erythematous plaques with fine nongreasy scales	Limited to hairline with slight spillover beyond hairline	Seborrheic dermatitis, tinea capitis	TCS, VDA
Follicular	Smaller than guttate lesions, grouped/diffuse	Trunk and limbs	PRP	
Seborrheic/ sebopsoriasis (Fig. 30.2c)	Thin plaques, with plaque psoriasis or isolated	Seborrheic distribution	Seborrheic dermatitis	TCS
Flexural/ inverse	Thin, nonscaly plaques, characteristic glazed hue and color retained, sharp margins	Inguinal crease, axillae, submammary folds, gluteal cleft, umbilicus	Seborrheic dermatitis, candidal intertrigo, dermatophytosis, erythrasma, allergic contact dermatitis, Hailey-Hailey disease	TCI, TCS (low potency)
Genital	With inverse > plaque > isolated. Vulval—itchy	Glans and labia majora most common	Erythroplasia, plasma cell balanitis	TCI, TCS (low potency)
Non-pustular palmoplantar (Fig. 30.2d)	Typical psoriatic plaque/ eczematous plaque Sharply defined margins No vesicles	Strictly limited at wrist margin	Hyperkeratotic eczema	TCS (high potency), SA, TAZ
Nail	Grow more quickly, up to 73% plaque psoriasis have nail involvement. (*see* details under Nail disorders, Chapter 16)	—	—	TCS, TAZ, ADA, ETA, IFX, Aprem, CsA, MTX, Secu
Mucosal	Geographic tongue (benign migratory glossitis) and fissured tongue. Associated with HLA-C: 06:02. True mucosal involvement uncommon	—	—	

VDA, vitamin D analogue; TAZ, tazarotene; ADA, adalimumab; ETA, etanercept; IFX, infliximab; SA, salicylic acid; TCS, topical corticosteroid; CsA, ciclosporin; Secu, secukinumab; Aprem, apremilast

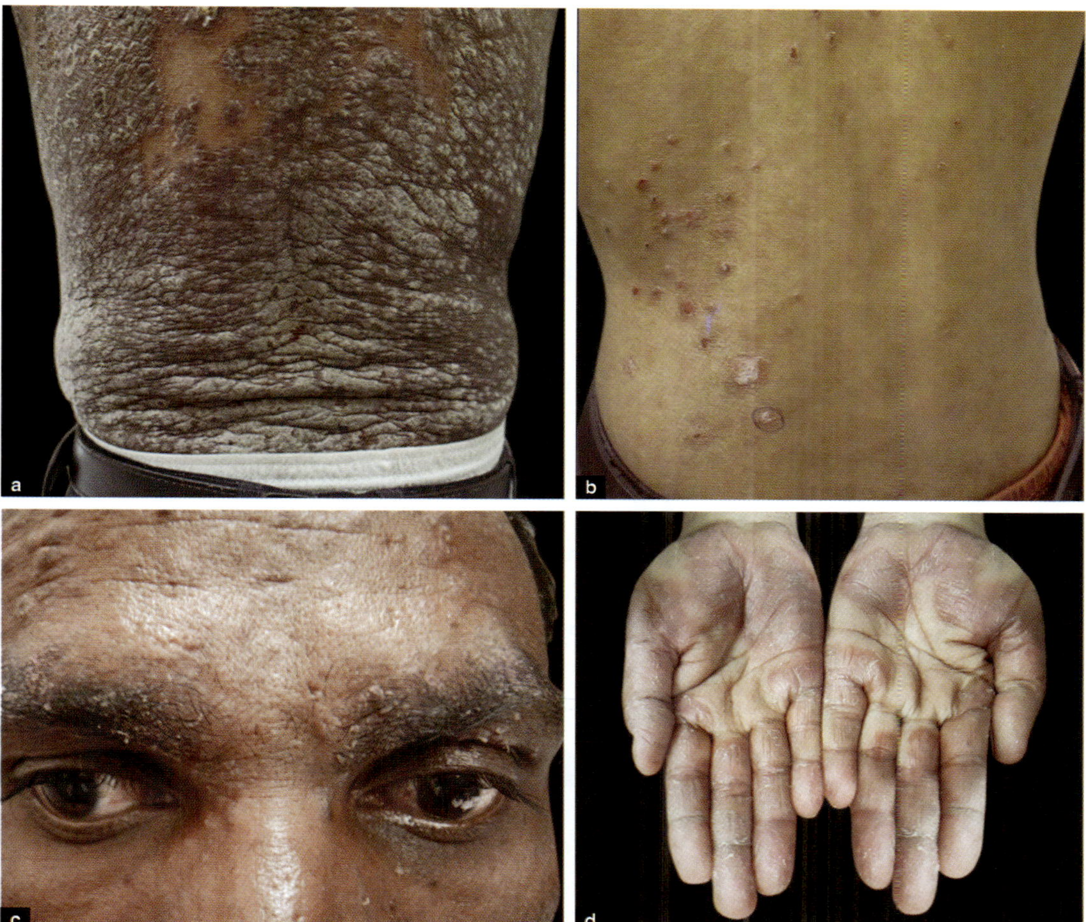

Fig. 30.2: (a) Chronic plaque psoriasis; (b) Guttate psoriasis; (c) Sebopsoriasis; (d) Palmar psoriasis

HIV-induced or exacerbated psoriasis

- Psoriasis—may be the presenting feature/may deteriorate in HIV.
- **Plaque—most common variant**
- Scalp and palmoplantar—most common sites

Comorbidities with Psoriasis

1. **Immune-mediated inflammatory diseases**
   a. Psoriatic arthritis (PsA)
   b. Inflammatory bowel disease
   c. Autoimmune thyroid disease
   d. Type 1 diabetes
   e. Celiac disease
   f. Alopecia areata, vitiligo, urticaria—esp. in PsA

2. Infections

a. Staphylococcal carriage on psoriatic plaques may occur. However, superinfection of psoriasis plaques is uncommon due to overexpression of AMPs.

3. Psychological distress

a. Higher risk of depression/anxiety/suicidality/alcohol dependence

4. Malignancy

a. **Nonmelanoma skin cancer (NMSC)**—strongest association

b. PUVA and immunosuppressive treatments—also increase risk of NMSC

5. Metabolic syndrome (MetS)

a. 34% psoriasis patients have MetS.

b. Strongest association—obesity, esp. **childhood psoriasis.**

6. Cardiovascular disease

a. Cardiovascular disease—accounts for majority of mortality in psoriasis

b. Higher risk of stroke, myocardial infarction, peripheral vascular disease, atrial fibrillation, venous thromboembolism

c. Higher risk in younger patients, severe psoriasis, psoriatic arthritis

7. Hepatobiliary disease

a. **Nonalcoholic fatty liver disease**—most common (50%)

b. Neutrophilic cholangitis—in pustular psoriasis

Diagnosis (Table 30.4)

TABLE 30.4: Diagnosis of psoriasis

Test	Findings
Bedside tests	Auspitz sign +ve (tiny bleeding points due to dilated dermal capillaries and suprapapillary thinning)
Dermoscopy	Dotted vessels in a regular arrangement over a light red background and white scales—highly predictive for diag. of plaque psoriasis (specificity 88%, sensitivity 84%)
HPE	• Parakeratosis with focal orthokeratosis with Munro microabscesses in S. corneum • Hypogranulosis/agranulosis • Regular acanthosis with spongiform pustules of Kogoj in S. spinosum • Suprapapillary thinning, dermis invaded by leukocytes, clubbed/fused rete ridges. Dilated, tortuous, papillary dermal vessels

Severity Scales of Psoriasis

- **Psoriasis area severity index (PASI)—0–72:** Absolute PASI is often used as an endpoint for evaluating therapy now as PASI 75 *or* PASI 90 have several limitations including dependency on a baseline severity assessment. Defining an absolute target disease activity endpoint in psoriasis has the potential to improve patient outcomes and reduce costs.
  - Absolute PASI ≤2 corresponds with PASI 90 response (Mahil SK, 2020)
  - Absolute PASI ≤2 and PGA clear/almost clear represent relevant disease endpoints to inform treat-to-target management strategies in psoriasis.

- SAPASI (self-assessed PASI)
- Static Physician Global Assessment (sPGA)
- DLQI
- Skindex-17
- 36-item Short Form Health Survey (SF-36)

'Severe psoriasis'—defined as PASI ≥10 *or* BSA >10% with DLQI >10.

Goal of treatment: PASI 75 (now PASI 90 or PASI 100 in some studies), low absolute PASI (≤3 *or* ≤2).

Disease Course (Table 30.5)

TABLE 30.5: Prognosis of psoriasis
Spontaneous remission – one-third to half cases
Untreated → Relapse is the rule
Guttate → better prognosis, longer remission
Severe plaque psoriasis – shortens lifespan by 4–6 years
PsA—morbidity ↑, Erythrodermic and pustular—mortality ↑↑

Treatment

As the treatment of psoriasis is complicated and cumbersome, we have detailed the various treatment options in **Tables 30.6** to **30.8**.

Systemic therapy, including phototherapy, should be offered to patients with any form of psoriasis meeting one of the following criteria:

- The disease is considered to be moderate-to-severe, defined as psoriasis covering over 10% of the body surface area (BSA), or resulting in a psoriasis area severity index (PASI) score >10 and/or a dermatology life quality index (DLQI) score >10;
- The disease has a significant impact on physical and social well-being, or on psychological well-being resulting in disease-related clinically relevant depression or anxiety;
- The disease is localized but cannot be controlled with topical therapy and is associated with significant functional impairment and/or high levels of distress, e.g. severe nail disease or involvement at high-impact sites (such as the palms and soles, genitals, scalp, face and flexures).

Biologics in Psoriasis

The sites of action of biological drugs are important, though there are region-specific recommendations of use, specially pertaining to the TNF-α biologicals due to their propensity for TB reactivation.

An updated pathogenesis of psoriasis is depicted in **Fig. 30.3** while the broad classes of drugs are depicted in **Fig. 30.4**. **Table 30.9** details the use of biologics in the treatment of psoriasis. Some salient aspects about biologicals are detailed in **Table 30.10**.

A recent study examined why some patients respond better than others to biological drugs. It is believed that the increased **Treg/CD8+TRM ratio** may be related to the superior long-term control of skin inflammation with guselkimab. Thus the effect of biological drugs depend on their action TRM cells.

TABLE 30.6: Topical treatments in psoriasis

Name of topical drug	Indications	Adverse effects	Remarks
Steroids	• First line topical treatment • DOC on face and neck, flexures and genitalia, in unstable, generalized pustular, erythrodermic	Atrophy, telangiectasia, striae, superinfections (fungal)	—
Vitamin D analogues	• Calcipotriol (50 μg/g) • Calcitriol (3 μg/g)—better tolerated on face and flexures than calcipotriol • Tacalcitol (4 μg/g)—less effective but only once daily application needed	Irritation, hypercalcemia (keep <50 g/week in children or <100 g/week in adult)	• Enhances efficacy of PUVA and UVB. UVA partially inactivates calcipotriol UVB absorbed by calcipotriol. So do *not* apply immediately <u>*before*</u> phototherapy
Dithranol (derivative of chrysarobin from Araroba tree bark) (Unna)	Short contact therapy can be used	Irritation esp. face and flexures, brown staining (resolves 2 weeks after stopping)	• Stability higher if combined with salicylic acid, part of *Ingram regimen* (tar + UVB + dithranol)
Coal tar (Goeckerman)	Higher efficacy for in-patient use	Folliculitis, contact allergic dermatitis	Modified *Goeckerman* regimen (coal tar 5 hours/day + UVB)
Retinoids (tazarotene → tazarotenoic acid)	For thick recalcitrant plaques	Irritation	—
Topical calcineurin inhibitors	Face and neck, flexures, genitalia	—	Safe, especially in children
Roflumilast (PDE4i) <u>(FDA approved 2022)</u>	Mild-to-severe psoriasis	—	Once daily application, ≥12 years
Tapinarof (arylhydrocarbon receptor modulator) <u>(FDA approved 2022)</u>	Mild-to-severe psoriasis	—	

DOC = Drug of choice

TABLE 30.7: Phototherapy for psoriasis

	NBUVB	PUVA
Wavelength	TL-01 lamps—311–313 nm	320–400 nm
Indication	Recommended first line for most moderate to severe psoriasis	Cost effective. However, it is falling out of favor nowadays
Contraindication	Photosensitive disorders, history of melanoma/NMSC	Pregnancy, lactation, children <12 years, photosensitive disorders, h/o melanoma/NMSC
Adverse effects	Erythema, pruritus, blisters rarely, less carcinogenic than PUVA	Erythema, blisters, PUVA itch (neurogenic pruritus), PUVA lentigenes, NMSC<with cumulative number of treatments, esp. after 250 total UVA doses, fairer skin type, immunosuppression with ciclosporin), teratogenic, ?malignant melanoma, ?cataract

(Contd.)

? = Questionable evidence

TABLE 30.7: Phototherapy for psoriasis *(Contd.)*

	NBUVB	PUVA
Dosage	According to MED, thrice weekly	8-MOP 0.6 mg/kg 2 hours before UVA, twice-thrice weekly. UVA 70% MPD with 20% increments till erythema develops
Efficacy	Clearance rates >90%, equal to PUVA but safer	Sessions to clearance 18 (avg.), remission lasts 6 months
Remarks	Can combine with methotrexate, acitretin, FAE, biologics **Avoid with ciclosporin due to accelerated carcinogenesis risk**	No more than 200 treatments recommended

MPD = Minimal phototoxic dose; MED = Minimal erythema dose; 8MOP = 8 Methoxypsoralen; FAE = Fumaric acid esters.

TABLE 30.8: List of systemic oral small molecules (OSMs) for treatment of psoriasis

Name of systemic drug	Dose	Adverse effects
Methotrexate (FDA approval 1972)	7.5–30 mg/week	Nausea, bone marrow suppression, mucositis, elevated transaminases, hepatotoxicity, pneumonitis, pulmonary fibrosis (rare), gastrointestinal ulcers
Ciclosporin (FDA approval 1997) 'the crisis drug'	2.5–5 mg/kg/day	Renal failure (dose-dependent), danger of irreversible renal damage (long-term therapy), hypertension, gingival hyperplasia, reversible hepatogastric complaints (dose-dependent), tremor, headache, burning sensation in hands and feet, reversibly elevated blood lipids, hypertrichosis, carcinogenesis
Acitretin (FDA approval 1997)	25–50 mg/day	Mucocutaneous xerosis, hyperlipidemia, hepatitis, teratogenic (women of childbearing age to avoid conception for 3 years), conjunctival inflammation (check contact lenses), hair loss, photosensitivity, hyperlipidemia
Fumaric acid esters (FAE)	Up to 240 mg three times/day	Diarrhea, flushing, proteinuria, transient eosinophilia, mild leukopenia, lymphopenia
Hydroxyurea/ hydroxycarbamide	0.5–1.5 g/day	Bone marrow toxicity, > actinic keratoses, > SCC
Apremilast (PDE4 inhibitor) (FDA approval 2014)	Up to 30 mg twice daily	Nausea, diarrhea, headache, bronchitis, upper respiratory tract infections, nasopharyngitis, decreased appetite, insomnia, migraine, depressive and suicidal ideation (rare)
Tofacitinib (JAK1/3 inhibitor) (FDA approval 2017 for PsA)	5–10 mg twice daily	Serious infections, viral reactivation, lymphocytosis, lymphopenia, neutropenia, anemia, elevated transaminases, gastro-intestinal perforations
Deucravacitinib (tyk 2 inhibitor) (FDA approval 2022 for psoriasis)	6 mg OD	Infections, rash, headache
Ponesimod (sphingosine-1-phosphate receptor S1PR inhibitor)	20–40 mg daily	Heart block, liver dysfunction

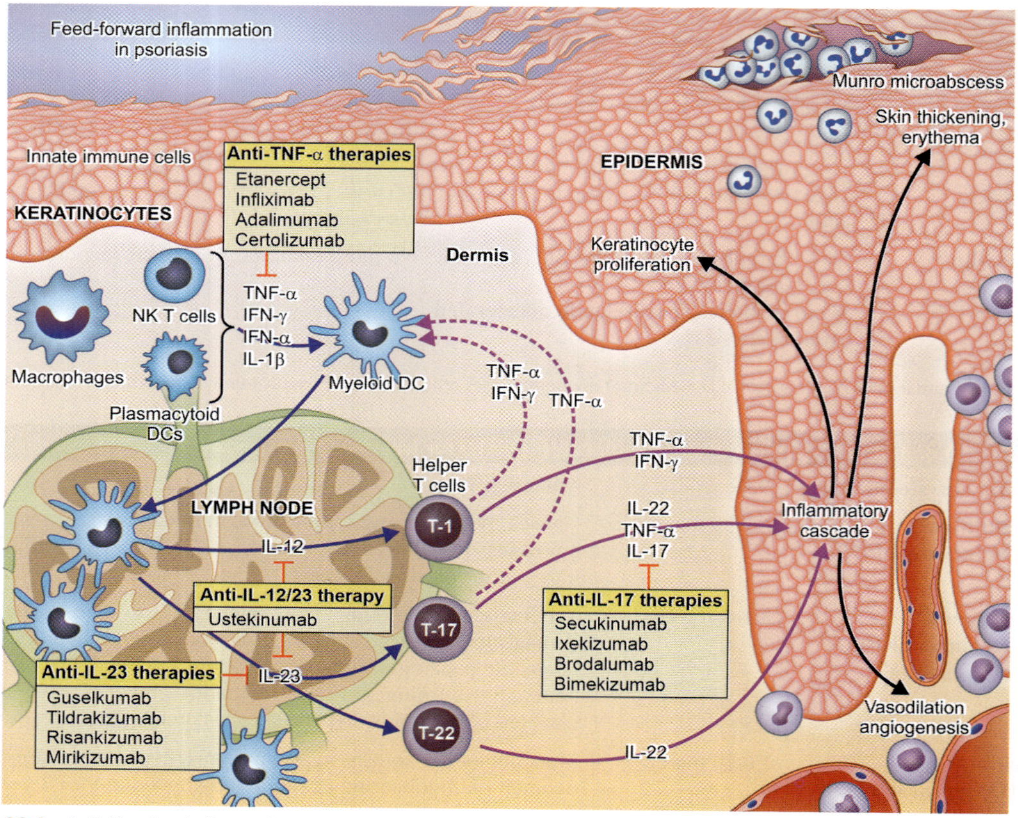

Fig. 30.3: Artistic depiction of immunopathogenesis of psoriasis and the sites of action of major classes of biological drugs

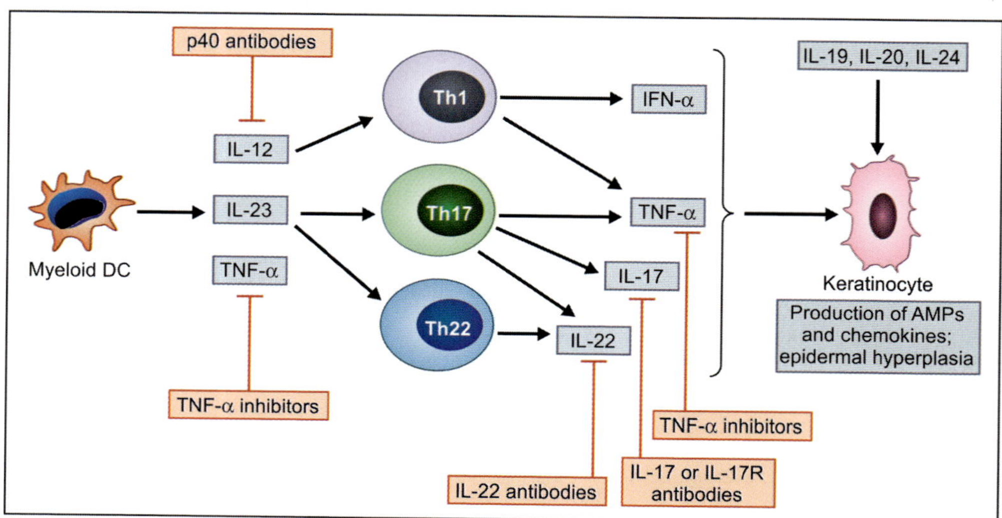

Fig. 30.4: Broad classes of biological drugs in psoriasis and their site of action

TABLE 30.9: List of biologics in treatment of psoriasis

Name of biologic	Mechanism of action	Route	Dose	Other approved indications	Remarks
Etanercept (2004)	• Recombinant human TNF-receptor fusion protein • Binds both soluble and membrane-bound TNF	SC	50 mg 2/weekly for 12 weeks → f/b 50 mg weekly	PsA, RA, JRA, AS	• **Approved for ≥4 years in 2016 by USFDA** • PASI 75 in 49% at week 12 • Safe for geriatric psoriasis
Infliximab (2006)	• Chimeric IgG1 Mab binds to and neutralizes TNF-α by binding both soluble and membrane-bound TNF-α	IV	5 mg/kg at weeks 0, 2, 6 then 8 weekly	PsA, RA, UC, CD, AS	• Chimeric composition renders it **more immunogenic** compared to other TNFi → Increased production of neutralizing **antidrug-antibodies (ADA)** and risk of infusion reactions.
Adalimumab (2008)	• Fully human Mab of the IgG1 isotype • Binds both soluble and membrane-bound TNF-α	SC	80 mg week 0 f/b 40 mg at week 1 f/b 40 mg every other week (EOW)	PsA, RA, AS	• **Approved by EMA for ≥4 years old** • PASI 75 in 71–80% at week 16
Certolizumab pegol (2008)		SC	400 mg at weeks 0, 2, 4 then 200 mg 2 weekly	RA, PsA, CD, AS	• Safe for use in pregnant and nursing patients
Ustekinumab (2009)	• Human IgG1 Mab targets shared protein **subunit p40 of IL-12 and IL-23** → inhibits the action of IL-12 and IL-23 • Specifically targets the **IL-12/Th1** and **IL-23/Th17** pathways for differentiation of naive T-cells into Th1-and Th17-cells.	SC	45 mg (≤100 kg) or 90 mg (>100 kg) at week 0, 4, then 12 weekly	PsA, UC, CD	• **First biologic to be first approved for psoriasis** (unlike TNFi that were first approved for rheumatologic conditions) • PASI 75 in 67% at week 12
Secukinumab (2015)	Fully human anti-IL-17A IgG1 Mab	SC	300 mg once weekly for 4 weeks starting at week 0, then every 4 weeks	PsA, AS	• **Label update** to include **scalp, nail,** palmoplantar **psoriasis and axial PSA**.

(Contd.)

F/b, followed by

TABLE 30.9: List of biologics in treatment of psoriasis *(Contd.)*

Name of biologic	Mechanism of action	Route	Dose	Other approved indications	Remarks
Ixekizumab	Humanized IgG4 anti-IL-17A Mab	SC	160 mg on day 0 f/b 80 mg every 2 weeks till 12 weeks then 4 weekly	PsA, AS	• FDA approved for ≥6 years with plaque psoriasis • The only biologic with FDA labeling specifically for genital plaque psoriasis • Very fast acting
Brodalumab (2017)	Fully human **anti-IL-17RA** IgG2 Mab → blocks IL-17 family	SC	210 mg at week 0,1, 2 then every other week (EOW)	—	• **BOXED WARNING**—risk of **suicidal ideation and suicidal events** (mostly with history of depression) • Frequently works where other biologics (including 1L–17i) have failed
Itolizumab (Biocon)	• A first in class humanized IgG1 Mab • Selectively targets **CD6,** a pan T cell marker	IV	1.6 mg/kg once every 2 weeks for 12 weeks, f/b 1.6 mg/kg every 4 weeks up to 24 weeks	—	
Guselkumab (2017)	IL-23i	SC	100 mg at week, 4 then weekly	PsA	The only IL-23i approved for PsA
Tildrakizumab (2018)	IL-23i	SC	100 mg at week, 0, 4 then 12 weekly	—	Provider–administered injections (so completely covered in medical insurance in the USA)
Risankizumab (2019)	IL-23i	SC	150 mg at week 0, 4 then 150 mg 12 weekly	—	• Very high efficacy • Very rapid onset of action

*Golilumab and certolizumab pegol—approved for psoriatic arthritis but not for psoriasis.

*PsA, psoriatic arthritis; RA, rheumatoid arthritis; JRA, juvenile rheumatoid arthritis; AS, ankylosing spondylitis; UC, ulcerative colitis; CD, Crohn's disease; TNFi, TNF inhibitors; MTX, methotrexate; Mab, monoclonal antibody.

Drugs in **Blue** are available in India.

Figures in parentheses refer to year of FDA approval for psoriasis.

TABLE 30.10: Salient aspects about biologicals in psoriasis

Parameters of response	Drugs
PASI 90 response	• Infliximab, all the IL-17 inhibitors (ixekizumab, secukinumab, bimekizumab and brodalumab) and IL-23 inhibitors (risankizumab and guselkumab) have equal efficacy
Fastest acting biologicals	• Ixekizumab and brodalumab, two agents that inhibit interleukin (IL)-17A, are the fastest-acting treatments
Short-term and long-term efficacy (10–16 weeks or 44–60 weeks)	• Brodalumab, guselkumab, ixekizumab, and risankizumab ideal drugs
Best drug survival	• Ustekinumab followed by secukinumab

Patients were categorized as being treatment refractory, treatment failure to ≥3 biologics targeting ≥2 different pathways.

Super-responders were patients treated with their first biologic for minimum 5 years without an absolute psoriasis area and severity index (PASI) > 3 between 6 months and 5 years of treatment.

The patients who were treatment refractory had a higher body weight (100.6 kg *vs* 90.6 kg) and higher mean BMI (32.2 *vs* 29.4,) while the fast responders had a higher socioeconomic status and fewer comorbidities.

Biosimilars in Psoriasis

Biosimilars are modelled after an already FDA-approved biologic medicine or biologic (also called the 'reference product'). **Biosimilars are highly similar to their biologic reference product in many ways. All biologics, including biosimilars** target specific parts of the immune system rather than impacting the entire immune system and are given as an injection or IV infusion.

Biosimilars of adalimumab, etanercept and infliximab are FDA approved for psoriasis and PsA.

Treatment of Psoriasis Subtypes and Scenarios

We are detailing the therapy of various types of psoriasis and the special scenarios in **Figs 30.5 to 30.7** and **Table 30.11**.

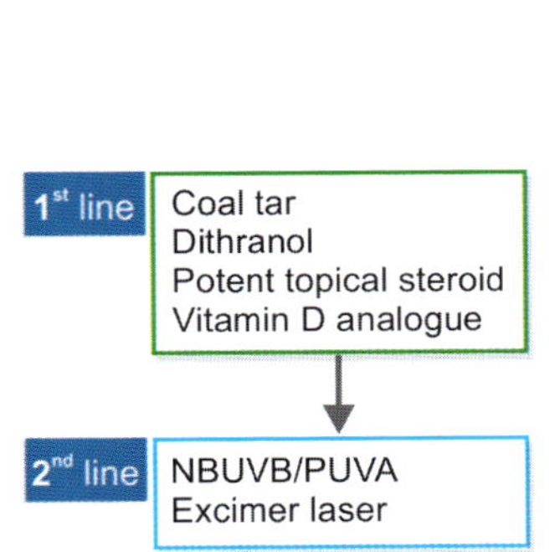

Fig. 30.5: Treatment of **mild plaque psoriasis** without PsA (BAD 2020)

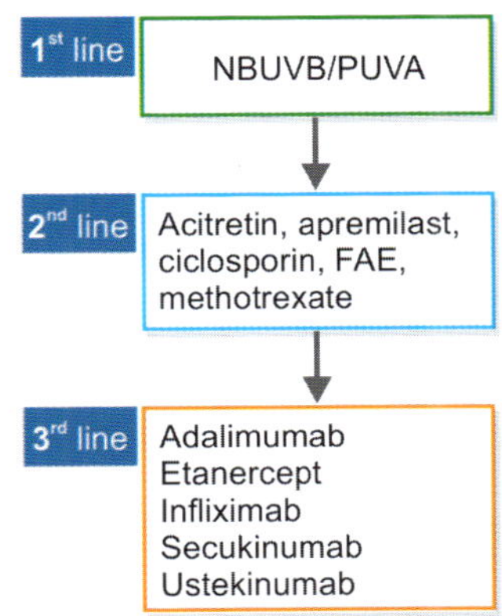

Fig. 30.6: Treatment of **moderate-to-severe psoriasis** without PsA (BAD 2020)

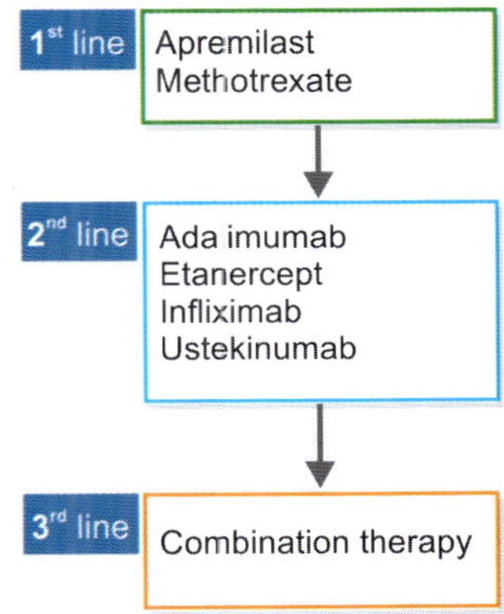

Fig. 30.7: Treatment of **moderate-to-severe psoriasis** with PsA (BAD 2020)

TABLE 30.11: Preferred treatment options in psoriasis according to age/precipitant/special situations (Menter A et al., 2019)

Category	Treatment
Children	MTX ADA, ETA (>4 years) ACIT
Elderly	ACIT, MTX, CYCLO, FUM ADA, ETA, IFX, APREM, SECU
Pregnancy	ADA, ETA, IFX, SECU (not in 3rd trim.)
Lactation	ADA, ETA, IFX, SECU
Males wishing to conceive	ACIT, CYCLO, APREM
HIV with undetectable viral load	ACIT, APREM (preferred) ADA, ETA, IFX, SECU
HIV with detectable viral load	ACIT, APREM
Hepatitis C	APREM, ADA, ETA, IFX
Hepatitis B	ACIT, CYCLO, APREM
LTBI	ACIT, APREM, FUM, SECU
NMSC	ACIT
Metabolic syndrome	FUM, APREM, ADA, ETA, IFX, SECU
Diabetes	ACIT, FUM, APREM, ADA, ETA, IFX, SECU
Obesity	FUM, APREM, IFX
Cardiovascular risk factors	MTX, FUM, APREM, ADA, ETA, IFX (C/I in heart failure)
Non-alcoholic fatty liver disease	CYCLO, APREM, ADA, ETA, IFX, SECU

MTX, methotrexate; CYCLO, cyclosporin; FUM, fumarates; ACIT, acitretin; APREM, apremilast; ADA, adalimumab; ETA, etanercept; IFX, infliximab; SECU, secukinumab; LTBI, latent tuberculosis infection; NMSC, non-melanoma skin cancer.

PUSTULAR PSORIASIS

- Microscopic pustules—feature of all psoriasis variants.
- Macroscopic pustules—features of pustular psoriasis only.

Types

1. **Generalized pustular psoriasis (GPP)**
   a. Acute GPP of von Zumbusch
   b. Subacute annular and circinate GPP
   c. Acute GPP of pregnancy (impetigo herpetiformis)
   d. Infantile and juvenile GPP
2. **Localized pustular psoriasis**
   a. Palmoplantar pustulosis
   b. Acrodermatitis continua of Hallopeau.

GENERALIZED PUSTULAR PSORIASIS

Epidemiology

- Rare
- Age: 40–60 years, earlier onset in patients who already have plaque psoriasis
- Sex: F:M = 2:1

Predisposing Factors

- **Genetic**
  - Deleterious germline mutations in ***IL36RN*** gene—in localized and generalized both
    - Encodes the IL-36 receptor antagonist (IL36Ra)—antagonist of proinflammatory cytokines IL-36 α, β, γ
- **Environmental triggers**
  - Infection
  - Irritating topical treatments—tar, dithranol
  - Withdrawal of systemic treatments—steroids, ciclosporin
  - Other implicated drugs—terbinafine, propanolol, bupropion, lithium, phenylbutazone, salicylates, potassium iodide
  - Psychological stress
  - Pregnancy
  - Hypocalcemia due to hyperparathyroidism

Clinical Features

Acute GPP (von Zumbusch)

- Most acute and severe form
- **Diagnostic criteria:**
  - Recurrent episodes of fever and malaise
  - Multiple isolated sterile pustules
  - Lab abnormalities—leukocytosis, ↑ESR, ↑CRP
  - HPE—Kogoj spongiform pustules

- Skin—burning sensation, dry, tender → fiery red skin with pinpoint pustules → sheets of erythema and postulation **(Fig. 30.8)**.
- **Flexures and genitalia**—particularly involved
- 'Lakes of pus' → dried pustules exfoliate → more waves of pustules may continue
- Nails—subungual pus, onychomadesis, onycholysis
- Oral mucosa—geographic tongue

Subacute Annular and Circinate GPP

- Common in infancy and childhood
- D/D—erythema annulare centrifugum

Acute GPP of Pregnancy

- Onset—**last trimester** usually
- Flexural onset **(inguinogenital region)** → GPP
- Constitutional symptoms—severe
- Cardiac/renal failure → death
- **More severe and more long-lasting disease** → placental insufficiency → stillbirth, neonatal death, fetal abnormalities
- Course—**recurs in subsequent pregnancies** and on OCP use too.

Infantile and Juvenile GPP

- Infantile—pustules confined to flexures, systemic symptoms usually absent, very rare
- Juvenile—2–10 years, annular and circinate > GPP von Zumbusch

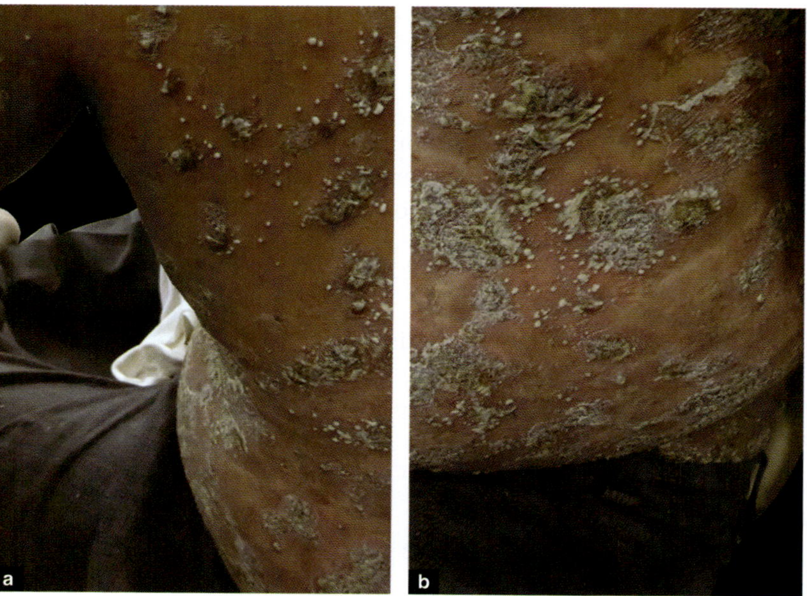

Fig. 30.8: Generalized pustular psoriasis involving the entire body with pustules coalescing with the classic "lake of pus" appearance

Differential Diagnosis

Most important differentials are AGEP, SPD variant of IgA pemphigus, Sneddon-Wilkinson disease, Reiter disease, candidosis **(Tables 30.12** and **30.13)**.

Complications

- Hypovolemia and oligemia—acute kidney injury
- Hypoalbuminemia—due to loss of plasma proteins into third space and malabsorption
- Hypocalcemia—due to hypoalbuminemia and malabsorption (hypocalcemia can be both a cause of and a complication of generalized pustular psoriasis)
- Cholestatic jaundice due to neutrophilic cholangitis
- Acute respiratory distress syndrome (psoriasis-associated aseptic pneumonitis)
- Telogen effluvium
- Amyloidosis

TABLE 30.12: Differentiation between pustular psoriasis and AGEP

	Pustular psoriasis	**AGEP**
History	History of psoriasis often present, absence of history of drug exposure	Abrupt onset of pustular rash hours or a few days after use of medication
Clinical features	Prolonged course—fever, pustular rash of longer duration than in AGEP, arthralgias in 1/3rd patients, starts in flexures usually	Hundreds of millimeter-sized non-follicular pustules, permeated by erythema and edema, more acute and more in flexures
Course	Prolonged, relapses, erythroderma/plaque psoriasis may ensue	Rapid resolution after drug suspension
Histopathology	Parakeratosis, neutrophilic macroabscesses in stratum corneum, spongiform pustules of Kogoj, epidermal spongiosis and papillary edema	Spongiform subcorneal or intraepidermal pustules, **eosinophils** in the pustules or in the dermis, **necrotic** keratinocytes, neutrophilic infiltrate, absence of tortuous or dilated vessels
Triggers	Infection, irritating topical treatments—tar, dithranol, withdrawal of systemic treatments—steroids, ciclosporin, other implicated drugs—terbinafine, propanolol, bupropion, lithium, phenylbutazone, salicylates, potassium iodide, psychological stress, pregnancy, hypocalcemia due to hyperparathyroidism	**Macrolides and beta-lactam based agents** (others—quinolones, sulfonamides, terbinafine, anti-malarials, calcium channel blockers, spider bites, infections by parvovirus B19, cytomegalovirus, coxsackie B4 and mycoplasma pneumonia)

TABLE 30.13: Differential diagnosis of generalized pustular psoriasis
AGEP
SCPD variant of IgA pemphigus
Sneddon-Wilkinson disease
Reiter disease
Candidosis

Diagnosis (Table 30.14)

TABLE 30.14: Investigations in pustular psoriasis

CBC with ESR	• ↓TLC • Absolute lymphopenia • Neutrophilia • ↑ESR
Blood biochemistry	• ↓S. calcium • ↓Albumin • ↓Zinc • ↑Liver enzymes
CRP	↑
Dermoscopy	May help especially in early cases when pustules cannot be made out on dermoscopy
HPE	• Earliest infiltrate—lymphocytic • Intense epidermal spongiosis and papillary edema • Neutrophils arrive → macroscopic abscesses in S. spinosum and S. corneum • S. corneum—parakeratotic scale shed off as turnover is accelerated

Disease Course and Prognosis (Table 30.15)

TABLE 30.15: Disease course and prognosis of pustular psoriasis

- Annular and circinate—good prognosis (children)
- Prognosis better when trigger identified
- GPP developing from acrodermatitis continua of Hallopeau—**worst prognosis** (?due to age)

Treatment (Fig. 30.9)

While a protocol of treatment is given below two new drugs that have potential use in GPP include, **Risankizumab**, a humanized immunoglobin G1 monoclonal antibody that specifically inhibits interleukin 23 by binding to its p19 subunit and **spesolimab**, a new interleukin-36 receptor antibody.

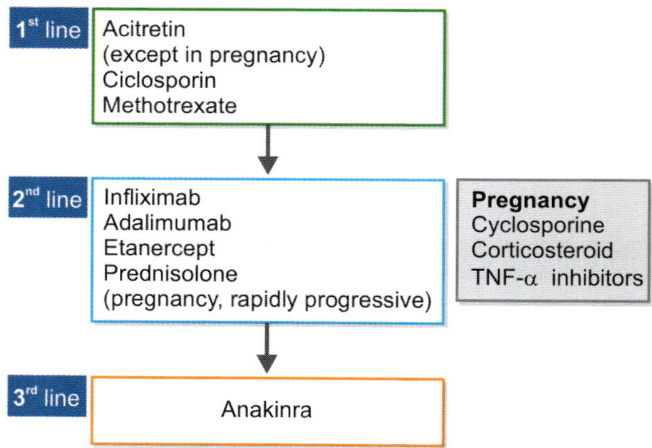

Fig. 30.9: Treatment of generalized pustular psoriasis (BAD, 2020)

LOCALIZED PUSTULAR PSORIASIS

Palmoplantar Pustulosis (PPP)

Epidemiology

- Very chronic, treatment resistant
- Palms and soles
- 18–24% palmoplantar pustulosis develop plaque psoriasis, usually PPP occurs in isolation
- Age—30–50 years
- Sex—F:M = 5:1

Predisposing Factors

- **Genetic:** Germline mutations in IL36RN gene
- **Environmental:**
  - Cigarette smoking—strong association (in >90%)
  - TNF-α inhibitors

Clinical Features

- Palms—thenar eminence most common site **(Fig. 30.10)**
- Soles—instep, medial/lateral border of foot at level of the instep, sides/back of heel
- Symmetrical lesions
- Pustules in all stages of evolution

Differential Diagnosis

- Tinea mannum/pedis
- Hand/foot eczema

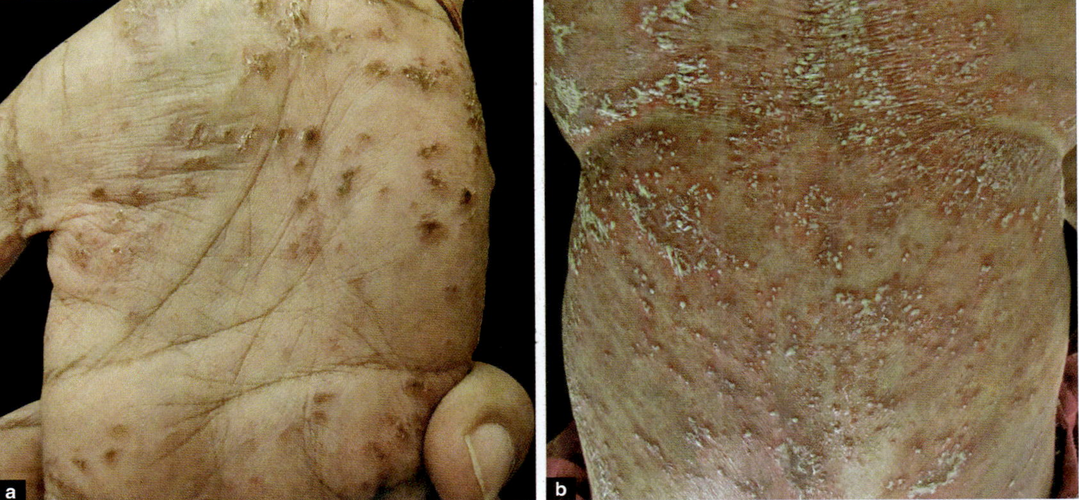

Fig. 30.10: Palmar pustular psoriasis in a case of GPP

Course and Prognosis

- Prolonged, chronic, treatment resistant
- Slow spread/extension

Treatment

Treatment of palmoplantar pustulosis and ACH is shown in **Fig. 30.11**.

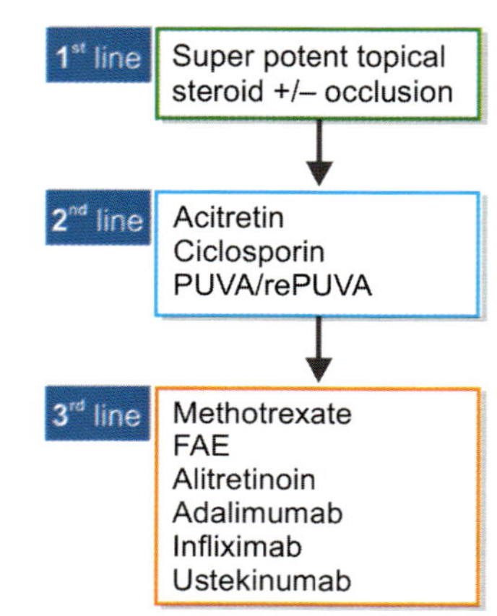

Fig. 30.11: Treatment of palmoplantar pustulosis and ACH

Acrodermatitis Continua of Hallopeau

Epidemiology

- Children, old age
- F > M

Associated Diseases

- Palmoplantar pustulosis
- May evolve into GPP

Predisposing Factors

- Trauma
- Infection
- Oral corticosteroids

Clinical Features

- Starts on finger/thumb more commonly than toe, extends proximally **(Fig. 30.12)**
- Red scaly pustules
- Nail fold and nail bed inflamed → nail dystrophy (nail almost always involved)

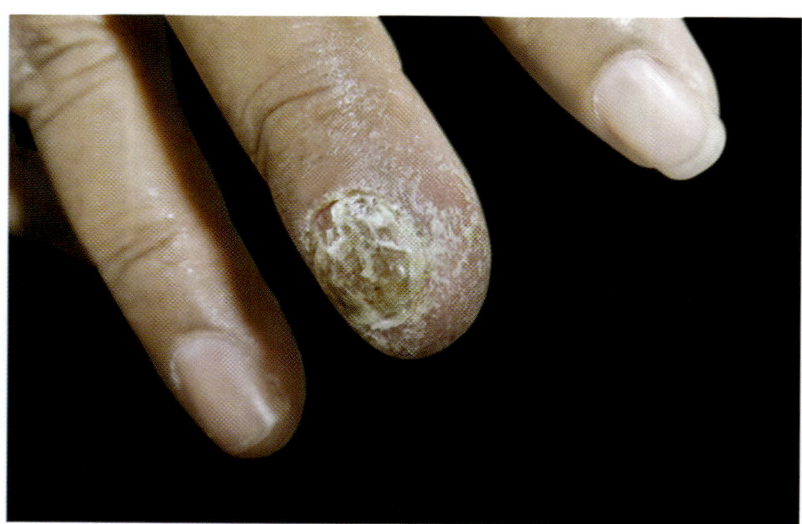

Fig. 30.12: Acrodermatitis continua of Hallopeau

- Proximal edge bordered by fringe of vesiculopustules
- Removal of scale → glazed surface
- Bone osteolysis of tuft of the distal phalanx–digit tip tapered like scleroderma

Differential Diagnosis

- Staphylococcal infection
- Herpetic whitlow
- Contact dermatitis
- Pulp infection
- Tinea
- Parakeratosis pustulosa

Course and Prognosis

- Prolonged
- Slow course and extension
- Treatment refractory

Treatment

Please *see* **Fig. 30.11**.

PSORIATIC ARTHRITIS (PsA)

Epidemiology

- In up to 40% patients with moderate–severe psoriasis
- 70%—skin before arthritis, 20%—skin after arthritis, 10% skin and arthritis concurrently.

Table 30.16 lists the **CASPAR criteria** for diagnosis of PsA and **Fig. 30.13** shows the clinical features of psoriatic arthritis with dactylitis.

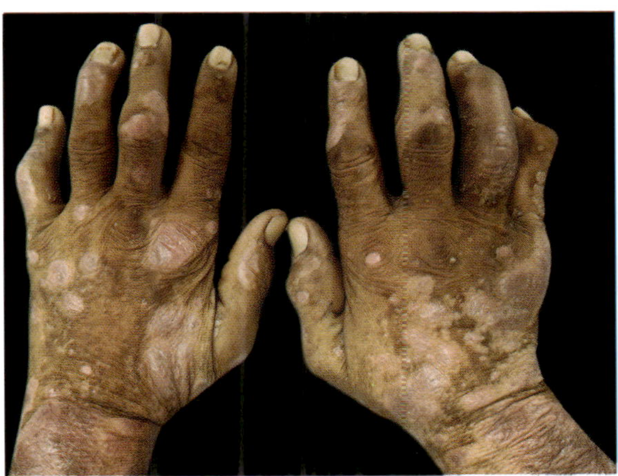

Fig. 30.13: Psoriatic arthritis with dactylitis

Moll and Wright classification for type of joint involvement

1. **Peripheral mono/oligoarthritis—commonest**
2. Symmetrical with predominant DIP joint involvement—second most common
3. Symmetrical RA-like pattern
4. Ankylosing spondylitis like and/or sacroiliac disease
5. Arthritis mutilans

Predisposing Factors and Triggers

- Trauma to joint/tendon (deep Koebner)
- Cigarette smoking
- Alcohol abuse
- HIV infection
- Metabolic syndrome

TABLE 30.16: Classification of psoriatic arthritis (CASPAR) criteria for diagnosis of PsA (Taylor et al. Ann Rheum 2006)			
S. No.	**Feature**		**Points**
1	Psoriasis	Current psoriasis Personal history of psoriasis Psoriasis in 1st/2nd degree relative	2 1 1
2	Typical psoriatic nail involvement		1
3	RA factor negative		1
4	Dactylitis	Current dactylitis	1
		History of dactylitis	1
5	X-ray evidence of juxta-articular new bone formation		1
			Inflammatory articular disease + 3/5 needed to diagnose as PsA

(91% sensitivity and 98% specificity)

Associated Diseases

- Severe cutaneous psoriasis, esp. nail and scalp involvement
- Ocular diseases—in 30% of PsA patients. Conjunctivitis with uveitis
- Metabolic syndrome

Differential Diagnosis (Table 30.17)

TABLE 30.17: Differential diagnosis of arthritis in patients of psoriasis	
Psoriatic arthritis	• Proximal and distal interphalangeal joints, small and large • Many patterns of involvement (m/c asymmetric oligoarthritis) • Dactylitis and enthesitis + • Nail involvement +
Rheumatoid arthritis	• Proximal interphalangeal and metacarpophalangeal joints, small and large • Symmetrical involvement • Dactylitis and enthesitis absent
Gout	• Toes, knees and ankles • Usually asymmetric involvement • Dactylitis and enthesitis absent
Osteoarthritis	• Weight bearing, distal hands • Could be symmetric • Dactylitis and enthesitis absent

Diagnosis

MRI—investigation of choice.

Treatment

Flowchart 30.1 shows the stepwise treatment of PsA.

(Biologics—indicated in active PSA affecting >3 joints that have failed at least 2 systemic medications or for axial arthritis that has failed NSAIDs and/or local steroids).

Flowchart 30.1: The EULAR 2019 algorithm for treatment of PsA (Gossec L, et al., 2020)

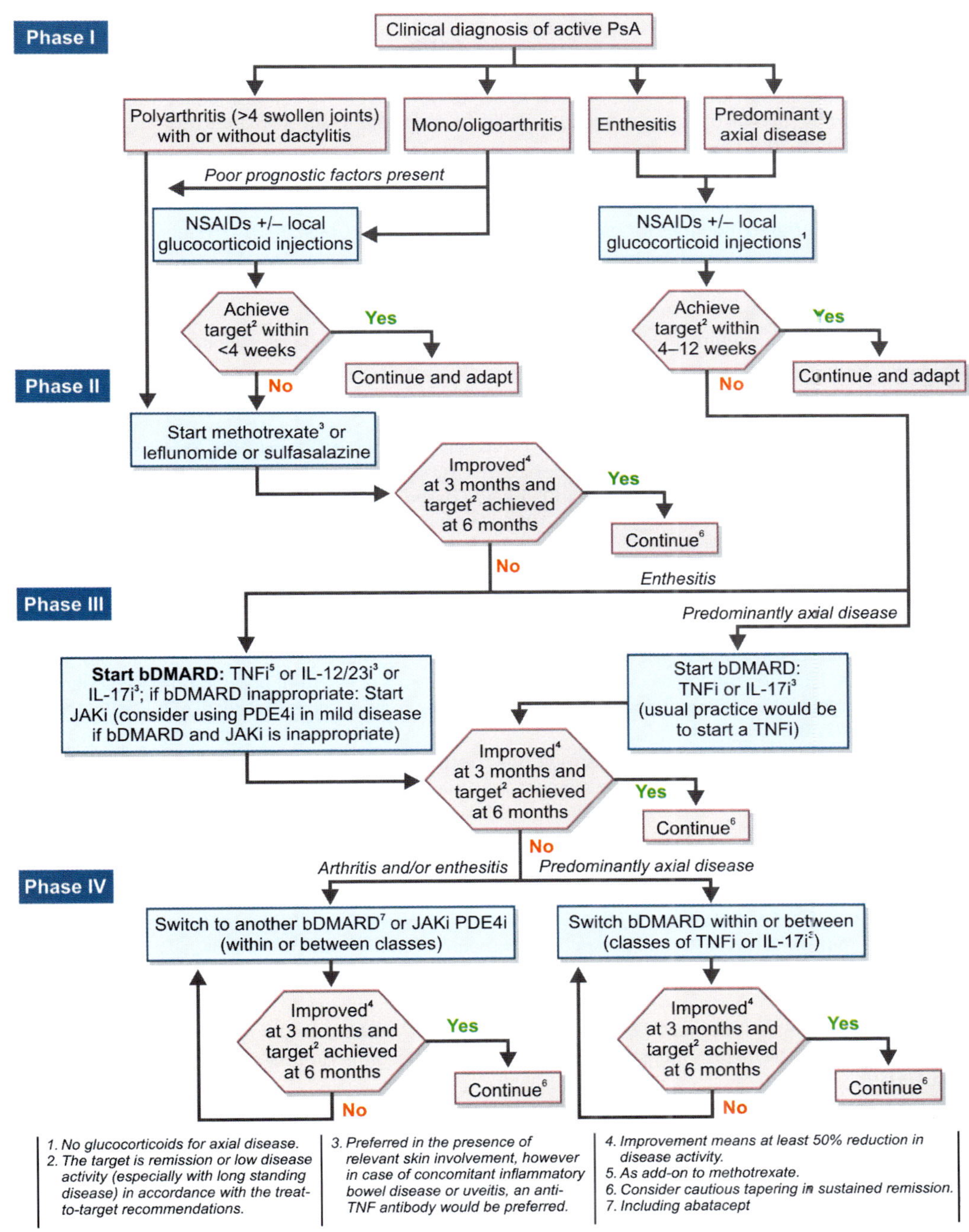

1. No glucocorticoids for axial disease.
2. The target is remission or low disease activity (especially with long standing disease) in accordance with the treat-to-target recommendations.
3. Preferred in the presence of relevant skin involvement, however in case of concomitant inflammatory bowel disease or uveitis, an anti-TNF antibody would be preferred.
4. Improvement means at least 50% reduction in disease activity.
5. As add-on to methotrexate.
6. Consider cautious tapering in sustained remission.
7. Including abatacept

bDMARDs, biological disease-modifying antirheumatic drugs; EULAR, European League Against Rheumatism; IL-12/23i, interleukin-12/23 inhibitor; IL-17i, interleukin-17 inhibitor; JAKi, Janus kinase inhibitor; NSAIDs, non-steroidal anti-inflammatory drugs; PDE4i, phosphodiesterase-4 inhibitor; PsA, psoriatic arthritis; tNFi, tumor necrosis factor inhibitor.

BIBLIOGRAPHY

Journals

1. Belge et al. Advances in treating psoriasis. F1000 Prime Reports 2014; 6:4.
2. Egeberg A, Ottosen MB, Gniadecki R, Broesby-Olsen S, Dam TN, Bryld LE, Rasmussen MK, Skov L. Safety, efficacy and drug survival of biologics and biosimilars for moderate-to-severe plaque psoriasis. Br J Dermatol. 2018 Feb; 178(2):509–19.
3. Geng W, Zhao J, Fu J, Zhang H, Qiao S. Efficacy of several biological therapies for treating moderate to severe psoriasis: A network meta-analysis. ExpTher Med. 2018 Dec; 16(6):5085–95.
4. Golbari et al. Current guidelines for psoriasis: a work in progress. Cutis. 2018;101(suppl 3):10–12.
5. Gossec L, Baraliakos X, Kerschbaumer A, et al. EULAR recommendations for the management of psoriatic arthritis with pharmacological therapies: 2019 update. Annals of the Rheumatic Diseases 2020;79:700–712.
6. Kolios et al. Swiss S1 Guidelines on the Systemic Treatment of Psoriasis Vulgaris. Dermatology 2016; 232:385–406.
7. Lallas et al. Accuracy of dermoscopic criteria for the diagnosis of psoriasis, dermatitis, lichen planus and pityriasis rosea. Br J Dermatol 2012 Jun; 166(6):1198–205.
8. Lambert JLW, Segaert S, Ghislain PD, Hillary T, Nikkels A, Willaert F, Lambert J, Speeckaert R. Practical recommendations for systemic treatment in psoriasis in case of coexisting inflammatory, neurologic, infectious or malignant disorders (BETA-PSO: Belgian Evidence-based Treatment Advice in Psoriasis; part 2). J Eur Acad Dermatol Venereol. 2020 Aug 13;34(9):1914–23. doi: 10.1111/jdv.16683. Epub ahead of print. PMID: 32791572; PMCID: PMC7496856.
9. Loft N. Prevalence and characterization of treatment-refractory psoriasis and super-responders to biologic treatment: a nationwide study. J Eur Acad Dermatol Venereol. 2022 Aug;36(8):1284–1291.
10. Mahil SK, Wilson N, Dand N, Reynolds NJ, Griffiths CEM, Emsley R, Marsden A, Evans I, Warren RB, Stocken D, Barker JN, Burden AD, Smith CH; BADBIR study group and the PSORT consortium. Psoriasis treat to target: Defining outcomes in psoriasis using data from a real-world, population-based cohort study (the British Association of Dermatologists Biologics and Immunomodulators Register, BADBIR). Br J Dermatol. 2020 May;182(5):1158–1166.
11. Menter A, Gelfand, JM, Connor C, Armstrong AW, Cordoro KM, Davis DMR, ... Elmets CA (2020). Joint AAD-NPF Guidelines of care for the management of psoriasis with systemic non-biological therapies. Journal of the American Academy of Dermatology. doi:10.1016/j.jaad.2020.02.044.
12. Puig L, López A, Vilarrasa E, García I. Efficacy of biologics in the treatment of moderate-to-severe plaque psoriasis: A systematic review and meta-analysis of randomized controlled trials with different time points. J Eur Acad Dermatol Venereol. 2014 Dec; 28(12):1633–1653.
13. Puig L, Costanzo A, Munoz-Elias EJ, Jazra M, Wegner S, Paul CF, et al. The biological basis of disease recurrence in psoriasis: A historical perspective and current models. Br J Dermatol 2022;186(5):773–781.
14. Rønholt K, Iversen L. Old and New Biological Therapies for Psoriasis. Int J Mol Sci. 2017 Nov 1; 18(11). pii: E2297.
15. Smith CH, Yiu ZZ, Bale T, Burden AD, Coates LC, ... Edwards, W. (2020). British Association of Dermatologists guidelines for biologic therapy for psoriasis 2020-a rapid update. British Journal of Dermatology. doi:10.1111/bjd.19039.
16. Gossec L, et al. The EULAR 2019 algorithm for treatment of PsA with pharmacological non-topical treatments. Ann Rheum Dis 2020;79:700–712. doi:10.1136/annrheumdis-2020–217159.

Chapter 31

Reactive Arthritis (Reiter's Disease)

Surabhi Sinha, Bhawuk Dhir

INTRODUCTION

Reactive arthritis (ReA), previously known as Reiter's disease, is a part of the spectrum of the spondyloarthropathies (usually RA factor seronegative).

It refers to an infection-induced systemic illness, characterized by a triad of urethritis, conjunctivitis/iritis, and arthritis (sterile synovitis) ("*can't see, can't pee, can't climb a tree*") occurring in a genetically predisposed individual, secondary to a bacterial infection localized in a distant organ/system, usually in the genitourinary (GU) or/and gastrointestinal (GI) tract.

Definitions

Reactive arthritis: Aseptic inflammatory arthritis, triggered by infection at a distant site, in genetically susceptible people.

Reiter's syndrome (classic definition): A triad of urethritis, conjunctivitis, and arthritis secondary to an infectious dysentery.

Reiter's syndrome (ACR definition): Episode of peripheral arthritis of more than one month's duration occurring in association with urethritis or cervicitis.

Uroarthritis: Reactive arthritis secondary to a urinary tract infection.

Sexually acquired reactive arthritis (SARA): Reactive arthritis associated with a recent sexually transmitted infection.

EPIDEMIOLOGY

ReA usually manifests itself as arthritis 2–4 weeks following GU or GI infections, sometimes up to 6 months, often with HLA-B27 positivity.

ReA is more frequent in males under 40-years-old.

ETIOPATHOGENESIS

The relationship between bacteria and genetics is well-illustrated in ReA.

The exact role of action of **HLA-B27** in spondyloarthropathies is not known; 30–40% of patients with ReA are positive for this antigen; one theory postulates that HLA-B27 presents arthritogenic bacterial peptides to T cells, stimulating an autoimmune response (molecular mimicry). Another theory is that HLA-B27 cells may act as an autoantigen that is targeted by the immune system. There also appears to be molecular mimicry between the infective organisms and a region of the HLA-B27α-I helix. The risk of developing ReA is 50 times higher in a HLA-B27 positive individual.

Toll-like receptors: TLR-4 can recognize lipopolysaccharides and could have a role in ReA. TLR-2 has also been associated with ReA.

Pathogens

A long list of bacteria has been described as triggers of ReA that can reach the joints through intestinal or genitourinary infections; these bacteria may reach the joints as a complete form or as fragments **(Table 31.1)**. Most are intracellular organisms. *Chlamydia trachomatis* is proposed to be the most common cause of ReA (genitourinary transmission); *Ureaplasma urealyticum* and occasionally *Neisseria gonorrohoeae* have been described.

CLINICAL FEATURES

Classified as acute (<6 months) and chronic (>6 months). Further subdivided into articular and extra-articular **(Table 31.2)**.

Diagnosis

The consensus diagnostic criteria as per Third International Workshop on Reactive Arthritis, 1995 are given in **Box 31.1**.

Differential Diagnosis

The commonest differential diagnosis is psoriatic arthritis (PsA). Though there are many similarities between the various types of SpA and even RA, **Table 31.3** lists some differentiating features and **Flowchart 31.1** shows a diagnostic algorithm of reactive arthritis and spondyloarthropathy.

TABLE 31.1: Arthritogenic agents associated with the development of reactive arthritis

Enteric infections	Urogenital infections	Respiratory infections	Others
Probable • *Shigella flexneri, S. dysenteriae, S. sonnei* • *Yersinia enterocolitica, Y. pseudotuberculosis* • *Campylobacter jejuni, C. coli* • *Salmonella enteritidis, S. typhimurium* ***Possible*** • *Clostridium difficile* • *Escherichia coli* • *Bacillus cereus* • *Cryptosporidium, Giardia lamblia* • *Helicobacter pylori, H. cinaeli* • *Strongyloides* spp. • *Tropheryma whipplei*	***Probable*** • ***Chlamydia trachomatis**** ***Possible*** • *Ureaplasma urealyticum* • *Mycoplasma genitalium* • *Neisseria gonorrhoeae*	***Possible*** • *Chlamydia pneumoniae* • Group A beta-hemolytic *Streptococcus*	• HIV • B-19 parvovirus • *Borrelia burgdorferi* • *Brucella abortus* • Bacillus Calmette-Guerin • Chikungunya virus

*Most commonly implicated urogenital pathogen causing ReA

TABLE 31.2: An overview of acute and chronic symptoms of reactive arthritis

Acute symptoms	Chronic symptoms
Articular Most commonly presents with **oligoarthritis**, but can also present with polyarthritis or monoarthritis i. **Axial** *Frequently involved* • Sacroiliac joints • Lumbar spine *Occasionally involved* • Thoracic spine (usually seen in chronic ReA) • Cervical spine (usually seen in chronic ReA) • Cartilaginous joints (symphysis pubis; sternoclavicular and costosternal joints) ii. **Peripheral** *Frequently involved* • Large joints of the lower extremities (especially knees) • <u>Dactylitis (sausage digit)</u>: <u>Very specific for a spondyloarthropathy</u>	**Articular** i. **Axial** • Sacroiliac joints • Lumbar spine • Thoracic spine • Cervical spine • Cartilaginous joints (symphysis pubis; sternoclavicular joints) ii. **Peripheral** • Large joints of the lower extremities (especially knees) • Dactylitis (sausage digit)—very specific for a spondyloarthropathy
Enthesitis Hallmark feature: Inflammation at the transitional zone where collagenous structures such as tendons and ligaments insert into bone Common sites: Plantar fasciitis, Achilles tendonitis ("Lover's heel"); but any enthesis can be involved	**Enthesitis** • Chronic inflammation can cause collagen fibers to undergo metaplasia forming fibrous bone Chronic enthesitis leads to radiographic findings: – Plantar/Achilles' spurs – Periostitis – Non-marginal syndesmophytes – Syndesmoses of the sacroiliac joints
Mucosal Oral ulcers (generally painless) Sterile dysuria (occurs with both post-venereal and post-dysentery forms) Predominant symptom in patients with enteric infection is diarrhea, which can be bloody	**Mucosal** • Sterile dysuria
Cutaneous (Fig. 31.1) **Keratoderma blennorrhagicum** (blennorrhagia = Excessive discharge of mucus): Pustular or plaque-like rash on the soles and/or palms. Grossly and histologically indistinguishable from pustular psoriasis. Can also involve nails (onycholysis, subungual keratosis, nail pits), scalp, extremities Develops in around 15% of patients **<u>Circinate balanitis</u>:** Erythema or plaque-like lesions on the shaft and/or glans of penis. These are erythematous, pustular, or plaque-like lesions that most often involve the glans of the penis, but they can include the shaft and rarely the scrotum	**Cutaneous** • Keratoderma blennorrhagicum • Circinate balanitis • Skin and mucosa: Aphthous ulcers (up to 60%) • Erythema nodosum (rare)
Ocular Conjunctivitis: Typically during acute stages only. Anterior uveitis (iritis): Often recurrent Rarely described: Scleritis, pars planitis, iridocyclitis, keratitis, retrobulbar neuritis, etc.	**Ocular** • Anterior uveitis (iritis): Often recurrent • Rarely described: Scleritis, pars planitis, iridocyclitis, and others
Cardiac Pericarditis (uncommon)	**Cardiac** • Aortic regurgitation • Valvular pathologies

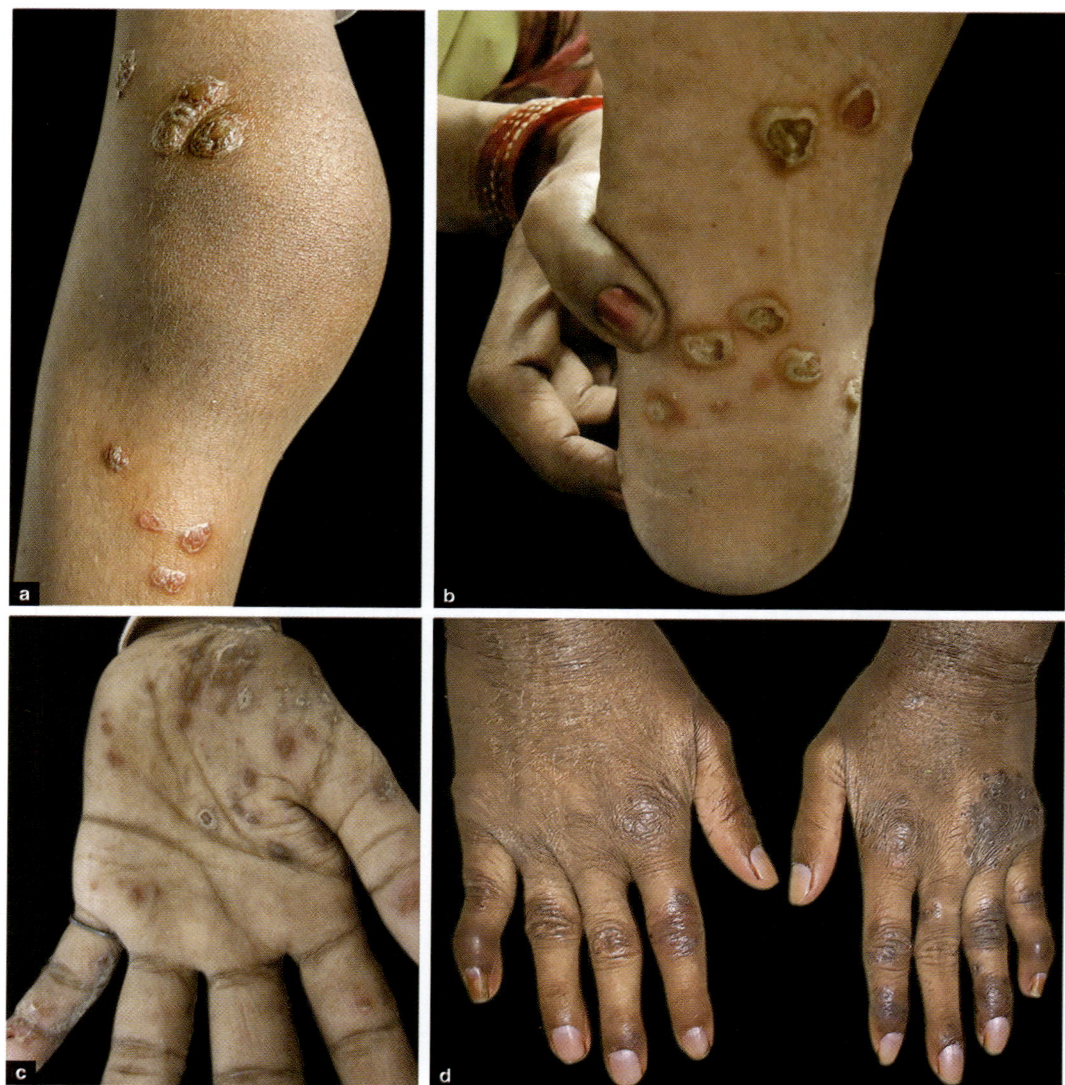

Fig. 31.1: (a) Heaped up crusted lesions typically seen in ReA; (b) Keratoderma blennorrhagicum; (c) Pustular lesions on the palms; (d) Swan-neck deformity with skin lesions

BOX 31.1: Diagnostic criteria for reactive arthritis (Kingsley and Sieper, 1995)

Typical peripheral arthritis

Predominantly lower limb, asymmetric oligoarthritis.

PLUS

Evidence of preceding infection

a. Where clear clinical diarrhea or urethritis within preceding 4 weeks, laboratory confirmation is desirable but not essential.
b. Where no clear clinical infection, laboratory confirmation of infection is essential.

(Contd.)

(*Contd.*)

Exclusion criteria

- Patients with other known causes of mono/oligoarthritis, such as other defined spondyloarthropathies, septic arthritis, crystal arthritis, Lyme disease, and streptococcal ReA, should be excluded.
- The diagnosis of ReA does not require the presence of HLA-B27 or extra-articular features of Reiter syndrome (conjunctivitis, iritis, skin lesions, non-infectious urethritis, cardiac and neurological features) or typical spondyloarthropathic features (inflammatory back pain, alternating buttock pain, enthesitis, iritis) but these, if present, should be recorded.

TABLE 31.3: Differential diagnosis of ReA

Feature	Psoriatic arthritis	ReA	RA	Ankylosing spondylitis
Distribution				
Sex	M = F	M = F (gastro-intestinal), M > F (genitourinary)	F > M	M > F
Predominant involvement	Hand ++ (cf all other SpA)	Mostly lower limb—foot > knee > ankle	Hand and foot ++	Mostly axial
• Nail involvement	+++	+/–	–	–
• Hand involvement	+++ (DIP/PIP)	–/+	+++ MCP/wrist	+
• Lower limb involvement	+++	+++ (MTP >> calcaneus > ankle > knee)	+++	+
Sacroiliac	++	++	+	+++
• Bilateral	+ (asymmetric)	++ (asymmetric)	+	+++ (symmetric)
• Unilateral	++	+++	+++	+
Spine	++ (cervical > lumbar)	+ (lumbar > cervical)	++ (cervical)	++– (lumbar)
Key signs				
Osteoporosis	–	+	+++	+++
Joint space	++ (widening)	+ (narrowing)	+++ (narrowing)	++ (narrowing)
Ankylosis	++ (coexistence of osteolysis with ankylosis within one region)	–	+	+++
Periostitis	+++ (fluffy)	+++ (fluffy)	+ (linear)	++
Tuft resorption	+++	–	–	–
Soft tissue swelling	++	++	+++	+
Laboratory				
ESR	+	++	+++	+++
RA factor	–	–	+++	–
HLA-B27	50% overall (10–20% peripheral disease, 60–70% spinal disease)	70–85%	6–8%	90–95%

Investigations

Unfortunately, there are no specific laboratory tests or biomarkers, except elevated CRP and ESR in acute febrile cases. **Table 31.4** lists some tests that would aid in arriving at the diagnosis of ReA.

Flowchart 31.1: Diagnostic algorithm of reactive arthritis and spondyloarthropathy

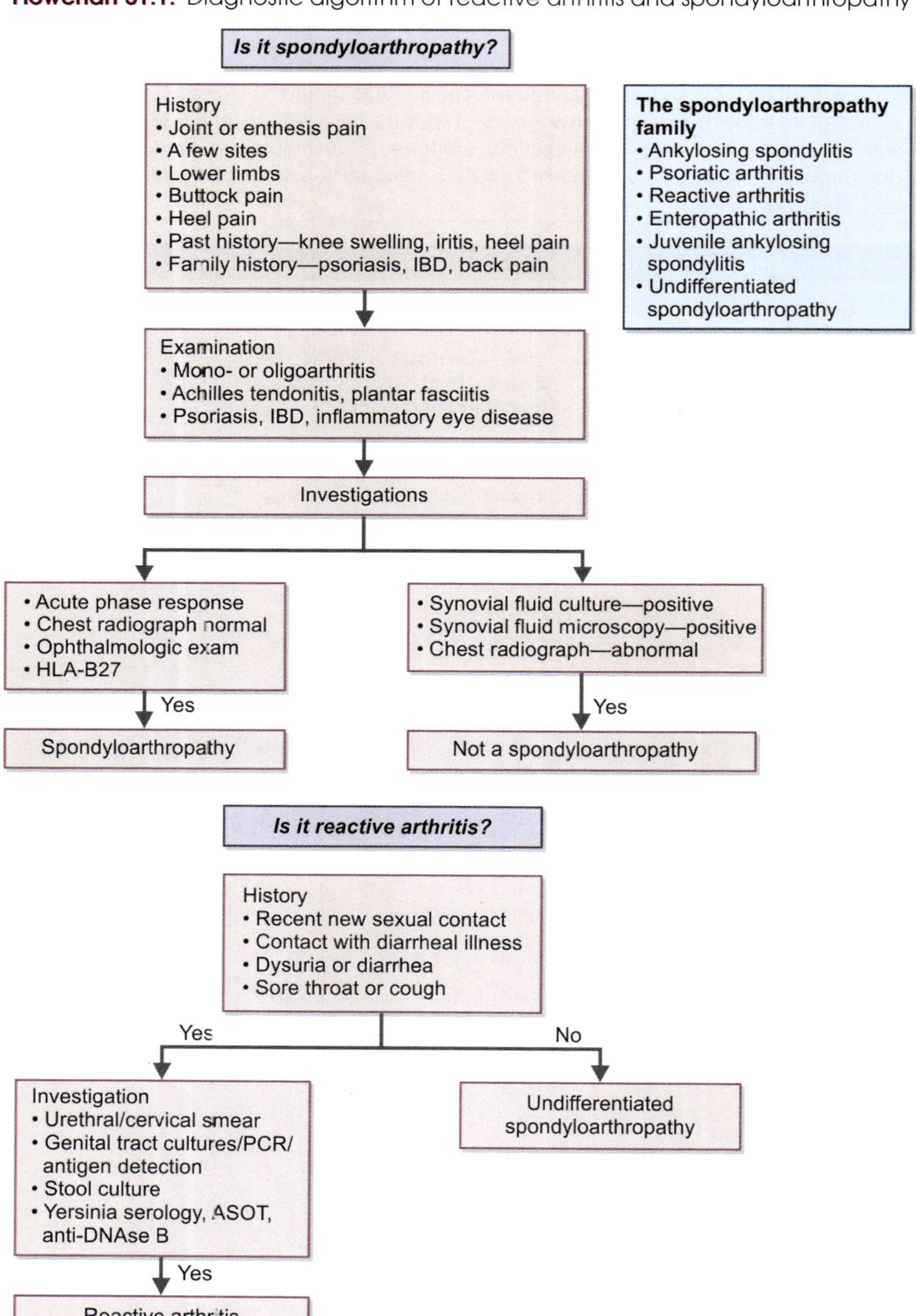

Anti-DNAse B, anti-deoxyribonuclease B; ASOT, antistreptolysin O titer; IBD, inflammatory bowel disease; MRI, magnetic resonance imaging; PCR, polymerase chain reaction

TABLE 31.4: Investigations in reactive arthritis

Investigations	Interpretation
Complete blood count	Neutrophilic leukocytosis, thrombocytosis, anemia of chronic disease
Acute phase response	ESR >60, raised C-reactive protein (may normalize with prolonged disease)
Autoantibodies	Negative
HLA-B27	+ve in 50–80%, associated with severe and protracted disease
Enteric	Stool culture/enzyme immunoassay: *Campylobacter*, *Salmonella*, *Shigella*, or *Yersinia*, PCR for *C. difficile*
Genitourinary	Nucleic acid amplification of urine or urethral swab—*Chlamydia trachomatis*
Urine analysis	Positive for leukocytes
Synovial fluid analysis	Polymorphs in acute disease followed by lymphocytes. No micro-organisms
Synovial biopsy	Polymorph infiltrate indistinguishable from other chronic rheumatic disease
Electrocardiogram	Often normal but may show variable degrees of heart block
Imaging	Non-specific. Include sacroiliitis, periostitis, syndesmophytes, joint erosions, joint space narrowing, and bone marrow edema

Treatment

Although there is an established link between pathogens and development of ReA, there is strong evidence against the efficacy of broad-spectrum antibiotic therapy. In the setting of acute or mild ReA, treatment is most often symptomatic and conservative. Acute ReA is usually self-limiting.

Principles of Treatment

- The initial treatment of choice for the arthritis is non-steroidal anti-inflammatory drugs (NSAIDs) not only for the analgesic anti-inflammatory effects but also because they retard the development of syndesmophytes.
- DMARDs such as sulfasalazine are effective for the peripheral manifestations, but not with the axial involvement. Most experts consider glucocorticoids for ReA contraindicated, except for an occasional intra-articular injection.
- Initial treatment of many extra-articular features of ReA includes topical corticosteroids. These have been utilized to treat iritis/uveitis, keratoderma blennorrhagicum, and circinate balanitis.
- Topical calcipotriene is a useful treatment modality for keratoderma. Emollients, keratolytics, coal tar, and phototherapy have also been advocated for keratoderma blennorrhagicum. In severe cases with cutaneous involvement, methotrexate (low-dose regimen as for psoriasis) and acitretin (0.5 mg/kg body weight) have been found to be beneficial but no formal clinical trials have been performed.
- Chlamydial replication is inversely proportional to TNF-α levels. There are no randomized trials in ReA to accurately assess the efficacy of anti-TNF therapy, but several case reports and a small open label study suggest clinical benefit with these drugs in the treatment of ReA.

  Flowchart 31.2 gives an overview of the treatment of ReA.

Prognosis

Although the majority of patients with ReA have a self-limited course within a few months of onset of the condition, relapses can develop in 30–50% leading to a chronic course (>6 months)

Flowchart 31.2: Treatment algorithm for ReA

Treatment of ReA

1st line	**Systemic** **Nonsteroidal anti-inflammatory drugs** (ibuprofen, indomethacin, naproxen, diclofenac, enteric coated salicylate) **Antibiotics** (If the inciting infectious agent is identified)	**Topical** Topical corticosteroids, emollients, keratolytics, coal tar
2nd line	**Intra-articular/systemic** Intra-articular corticosteroids	**Topical** Topical calcipotriene
3rd line	**Systemic agents** • **Acitretin (0.5 mg/kg)** • **DMARDs** – Sulfasalazine – Methotrexate – Azathioprine • **Anti-TNF-α agent**	**Phototherapy**

manifested by recurrent uveitis, urethritis or erosive arthritis. **Box 31.2** gives a list of predictors of severe disease.

BOX 31.2: Predictors of severe disease at presentation

- Onset <16 years of age
- Lumbar spine stiffness
- Oligoarthritis
- Poor response to NSAIDs
- ESR >30 mm in first hour
- Arthritis of hip
- Dactylitis
- Recurrent arthritis
- HLA-B27 positivity

Acknowledgment

The authors thank **Dr Akhilesh Thole**, for his work in this chapter in the previous edition of this book.

BIBLIOGRAPHY

Books

1. Dermatology (Bolognia). 4th Edn. Chapter 8. Reactive Arthritis (formerly Reiter Disease).
2. Fitzpatrick's Dermatology, 9th Edition, Chapter 65.
3. García-Kutzbach A, Chacón-Súchite J, García-Ferrer H, Iraheta I. Reactive arthritis: update 2018. *Clin Rheumatol*. 2018;37(4):859–74.
4. Hamdulay SS, Glynne SJ, Keat A. When is arthritis reactive? *Postgrad Med J*. 2006;82(969):446–53.
5. Kingsley G, Sieper J. Third International Workshop on Reactive Arthritis. 23–26 September 1995, Berlin, Germany. Report and abstracts. In: *Annals of the Rheumatic Diseases*. Vol 55. BMJ Publishing Group; 1996:564–84.
6. Rook's Textbook of Dermatology. 4th Ed. Wiley Blackwell.

Chapter 32

Sarcoidosis

Seema Rani, Kabir Sardana, Snigdha Saxena

Sarcoidosis is known as the great mimicker due to its myriad manifestations. It is characterized by noncaseating epithelioid cell granulomas in multiple organs. Increased incidence of sarcoidosis in spring and winter have been observed that may point towards an environmental/ infectious trigger.

PATHOGENESIS

- Sarcoidosis may represent a group of diseases, with a variety of environmental or infectious agents initiating the inflammatory process, which may vary.
- Upregulation of **CD4+ Th1** cells: Genetic predisposition (+), unknown antigen presented by monocytes with MHC class II molecules → activation of CD4+ Th1 cells → IL-2, **IFN-γ, TNF-α,** and monocyte chemotactic factor (MCF) → monocytes leave circulation and enter peripheral tissues, including skin, where they form granulomas → granulomas have potential to result in end-organ dysfunction.

  The function of programmed cell death receptor and ligand is to downregulate the immune system and promote self-tolerance. There is evidence to suggest that idiopathic sarcoidosis may be due to a hypoactive immune response with decreased T-cell proliferation and upregulation of programmed cell-death receptor 1 (PD-1) and ligand (PD-L).
- Drug-induced sarcoid:
  - Hepatitis C patients on treatment **(IFN-α, ribavirin)**
  - HIV patients on HAART
  - Other: TNF-α inhibitors, vemurafenib, ipilimumab, and alemtuzumab.

CLINICAL FEATURES

Skin lesions occur in 25% of patients with sarcoidosis.

Skin findings can be specific or nonspecific. The former has the classic histopathological sarcoid granulomas.

- **Specific:** Maculopapular, plaques, lupus pernio, scar sarcoidosis, subcutaneous sarcoid **(Table 32.1)**.
- **Non-specific:** Erythema nodosum—predicts a benign course

  Seen in 9–37% of cases, seen at the onset of disease. No prognostic significance.

  Predilection for face (especially lips and nose), neck, and upper half of the body.
- Variants **(Box 32.1)**

TABLE 32.1: Clinical features of common specific manifestations of sarcoidosis

Maculopapular form	• Acute form, good prognosis
Papules and papulonodules (Fig. 32.1)	• Most common morphology of the specific cutaneous manifestations of sarcoidosis • Color: Flesh-colored, yellow-brown, red-brown, purple-brown or hypo-pigmented • Location: Typically present on the face, but also on the trunk and extremities, can arise within scars
Plaques	• Description: Oval or annular in shape, often well demarcated, typically firm to the touch, scaly at times • Color: Red-brown to flesh-colored to purple-brown and sometimes yellow-brown • Location: Trunk, buttocks, shoulders, and arms; can arise within scars
Lupus pernio (Fig. 32.2)	• Upper respiratory tract may be involved • Can be disfiguring; tends to affect black Americans and women dispropor tionately; associated with a chronic and refractory course, often requiring aggressive systemic therapy • Description: Smooth shiny plaques, which may develop scale • Color: Brown to violaceous or erythematous • Location: Central face, specifically the nose, cheeks, lips, forehead, ears also
Subcutaneous nodules	• Description: Firm, mobile, round to oval nodules • Color: Erythematous, flesh-colored, violaceous, or hyperpigmented • Location: Extremities, mainly upper extremities; trunk

BOX 32.1: Variants of sarcoidosis

Lofgren syndrome	Acute form of sarcoidosis; erythema nodosum + hilar adenopathy + fever + migratory polyarthritis + acute iritis; most common in Scandinavian whites, rare in blacks; has a good prognosis
Heerfordt syndrome	**Uveitis + parotid gland enlargement + fever + cranial nerve palsy** (facial nerve most common)
Milkulicz syndrome	Outdated, non-specific term (may be seen in TB, sarcoid, Sjögren syndrome, lymphoma) refers to enlargement of salivary, lacrimal and parotid glands
Blau syndrome	Early onset (age <5 years) sarcoid-like disease; caused by **NOD2 mutation**; triad of skin, eye and joint disease
Drug-induced cutaneous sarcoid	**IFN-α (hepatitis C patients)**, HIV patients on HAART, TNF-α inhibitors

Other Areas of Involvement

- Lung disease (90%): Alveolitis, bronchiolitis, and pleuritis; **honeycombing** of lung, with fibrosis and bronchiectasis.
- Lymphadenopathy (90%): Hilar and/or paratracheal; typically asymptomatic.
- Ocular involvement (20–50%): **Anterior uveitis (most common)**, retinitis, lacrimal inflammation, and conjunctivitis → may result in blindness.
- Hypercalcemia (10%): Due to calcitriol synthesis by sarcoidal granulomas (convert 25-hydroxyvitamin D to more active 1,25-dihydroxyvitamin D) → hypercalcemia, hypercalciuria, and nephrocalcinosis → renal failure.

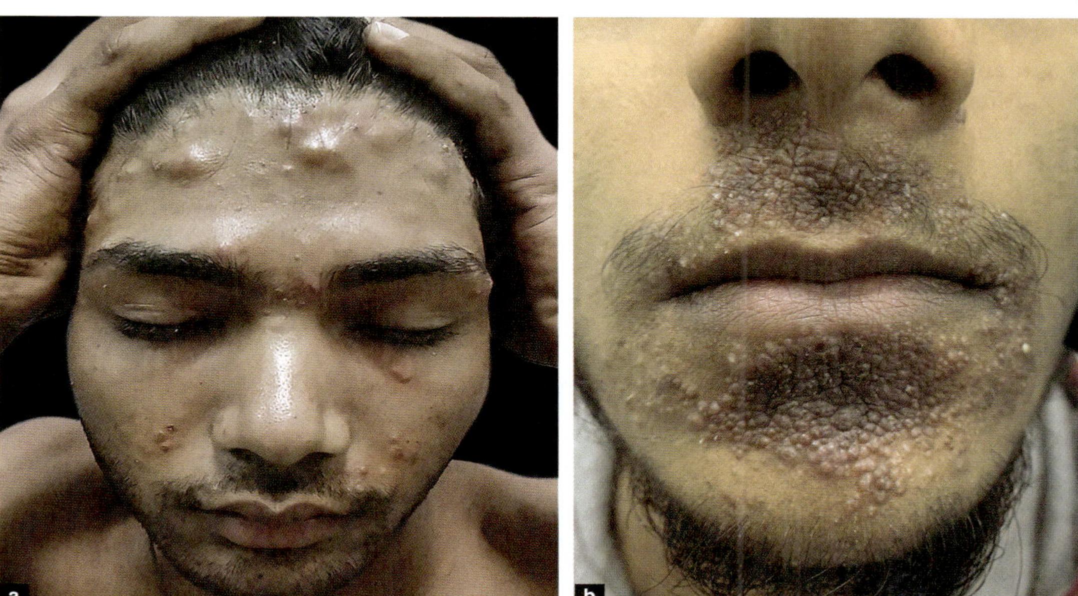

Fig. 32.1: (a) Specific lesions of cutaneous sarcoidosis with multiple papulonodular lesions on face; (b) Multiple papular lesions on perioral area

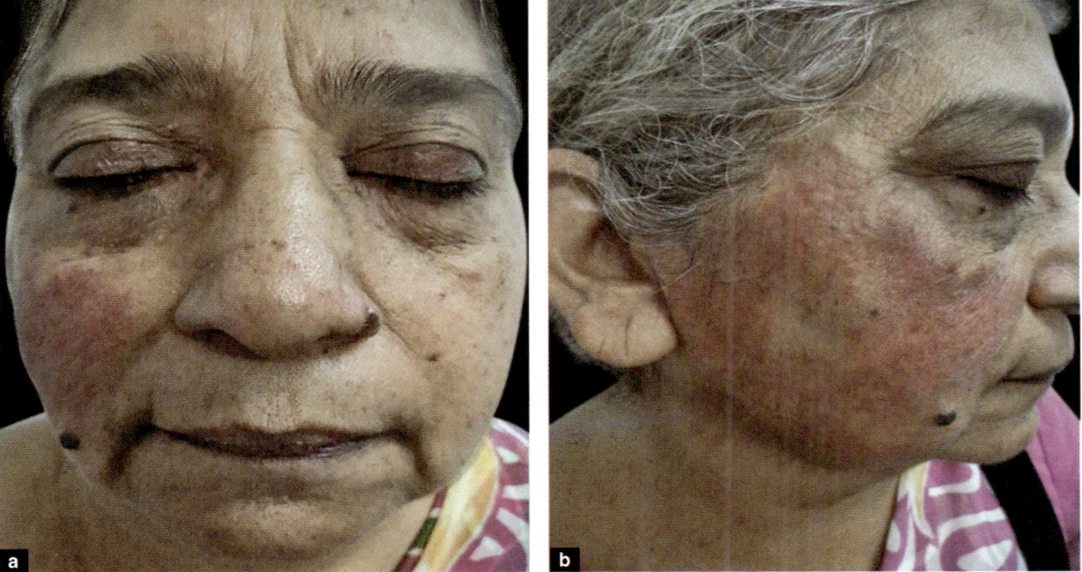

Fig. 32.2: Cutaneous sarcoidosis with lupus pernio type of lesions

- Others: Nail changes (clubbing, onycholysis, and subungual hyperkeratosis), oral involvement (salivary gland, gingiva, hard/soft palate, and tongue), liver, and heart involvement.

HISTOPATHOLOGY

- Granuloma in the dermis, occasionally follows nerves, well-formed, noncaseating, **'naked epithelioid granulomas'** (epithelioid granulomas lacking a significant inflammatory rim of lymphocytes or plasma cells).
- Langhans giant cells → seen in older lesions.
- Sometimes tuberculoid granuloma, rare caseation.
- Giant cells can contain inclusion bodies like **Schaumann bodies and asteroid bodies.** None of these is specific for sarcoidosis and are also seen in TB, leprosy, Crohn disease, berylliosis.
- Subcutaneous sarcoidosis—granulomas in subcutaneous tissue; appearance of lobular panniculitis.
- Polarizable foreign bodies are observed in 22–50% of cutaneous sarcoidosis.

DIFFERENTIAL DIAGNOSIS (Table 32.2)

Sarcoidosis must be approached as a diagnosis of exclusion and has to be distinguished from the numerous conditions that may be associated with a non-caseating granulomatous histology, including some forms of tuberculosis, tuberculoid leprosy, berylliosis, fungal infections, Crohn disease, and foreign body granulomatous reactions.

- Use special stains, including the Ziehl–Neelsen preparation for mycobacteria and the periodic acid-Schiff (PAS) and methenamine silver reactions for fungi.
- Depending on the clinical context, culture may also be required to exclude an infective etiology.
- Tuberculoid leprosy is characterized by nerve involvement, a feature that is usually absent in sarcoidosis. Granulomas follow nerves and therefore appear elongated and show small areas of central necrosis more often than sarcoidosis.
- **Lupus vulgaris**—lymphocytic infiltrate around granulomas and significant central necrosis.
- **Rosacea** granulomas are usually perifollicular.
- **Syphilis**—plasma cells, endarteritis and coagulative necrosis are features of syphilis.

INVESTIGATIONS (Table 32.3)

The diagnosis of sarcoidosis is based on a compatible clinical and radiological picture, demonstration of noncaseating granulomas with negative cultures for mycobacteria and fungus, and exclusion of other granulomatous diseases.

TABLE 32.2: Differential diagnosis of sarcoidosis

Maculopapular sarcoidosis	Rosacea, xanthelasmata, secondary syphilis, lupus erythematosus, sebaceous adenoma, granuloma annulare, trichoepitheliomata, syringoma
Nodular and plaque sarcoidosis	Lupus vulgaris, necrobiosis lipoidica, leprosy, leishmaniasis, DLE, granuloma annulare
Lupus pernio	Rosacea, DLE, lupus vulgaris
Subcutaneous sarcoidosis	Epidermal cysts, multiple lipomata, calcinosis, rheumatoid nodules, morphea, cutaneous metastases

Ref: Rook's 9th Ed.

TABLE 32.3: Investigations in a case of sarcoidosis

Investigations	Remarks
1. Routine investigations	CBC (↑ ESR, lymphopenia), S. Ca^{2+} (hypercalcemia) LFT, KFT, BUN, urine analysis
2. CXR or CT scan	Abnormal CXR >90%,CT scan—most sensitive Hilar/paratracheal lymphadenopathy +/– pulmonary infiltrates
3. Gallium-67 scanning	Useful in monitoring treatment response rather than diagnosis. Specific signs—*Panda* sign (bilateral lacrimal and parotid gland uptake) and *Lambda* sign (bilateral hilar and right paratracheal uptake)
4. PET with ^{18}F–fluorodeoxyglucose (^{18}F–FDG PET)	More sensitive than ^{67}Gallium scan for assessing the activity and extension of sarcoidosis
5. PFT, spirometry, DLco and KLco	Restrictive lung pattern → ↓ total lung capacity, ↓ diffusion capacity and ↓ vital capacity
6. ACE levels	↑ in 60% cases; more useful for monitoring response than for diagnosis
7. Biopsy	Transbronchial , skin, peripheral lymph nodes In cases of atypical clinical and radiological findings, especially with stage 0 chest radiographs, at least two positive biopsies should be obtained
8. Tuberculin skin test	Negative in >80% patients
9. Ophthalmological examination	Uveitis (most common)
10. Electrocardiogram	Cardiac arrhythmia or left venticular dysfunction

TREATMENT

The data on treatment of cutaneous sarcoidosis is derived from rheumatological literature.

The principle is—treatment directed at abolishing, or at least limiting, the inflammatory response, especially the effect of TNF-α, which is integral in the formation and organization of granulomas.

Flowchart 32.1: Treatment algorithm for sarcoidosis

1st line

1. Systemic involvement—**Oral prednisolone**; degree of lung, eye and other internal involvement determines how quickly steroids can be tapered
2. Cutaneous involvement—**Topical or I/L steroids**

↓

2nd line

1. **Anti-malarials, Methotrexate** (80% response—6 months)
2. **Minocycline**—Can be used in mild-to-moderate disease and as steroid sparing agent in patients with severe disfigurement or lupus pernio
(Initiate Rx with minocycline for 3 months → add HCQ → methotrexate may then be added to regimen.)

↓

3rd line

Infliximab and adalimumab—refractory cutaneous sarcoidosis

HCQS, 200–400 mg; MTX 7.5–25 mg/wk; Minocycline, 200 mg/day; Adalimumab 40 mg every 1–2 wk

The ISA agents like methotrexate and leflunomide, and others like thalidomide, indirectly inhibit TNF-α release and biologic agents can be used if these fail.

Patients who do not respond adequately to one TNF-α inhibitor can be changed to the other. All patients should be monitored for worsening disease while on TNF-α inhibitor therapy, as sarcoid can develop as a response to these medications. Etanercept is generally not used for sarcoidosis.

While an overview of treatment options is listed in **Flowchart 32.1;** a more elaborate algorithm is depicted in **Flowchart 32.2**.

Flowchart 32.2: Treatment algorithm for cutaneous sarcoidosis

Cutaneous sarcoidosis without significant systemic dysfunction

Erythema nodosum

T/t based on symptoms NSAIDs or prednisolone

Specific lesions

Asymptomatic, not disfiguring

No t/t or monitor

Symptomatic or disfiguring

Assess extent/severity of disease

Localized or mild disease

Inadequate response

Topical potent steroid/ intralesional steroids

Inadequate response

Add topical tacrolimus

Inadequate response

Short course of prednisolone (<1 month) if no CI

Inadequate response

Antimalarials or methotrexate or cyclines or pentoxyfylline or melatonin (alone or in combination)

Good response

Taper very slowly over months

Inadequate response

Symptomatic or disfiguring

Add low-dose prednisolone

Good response

Lupus pernio, severe/extensive

Corticosteroids (prednisolone 40–60 mg/day) + Steroid-sparing agent (MTX, MMF, Aza) + I/L steroid to prominent areas

Inadequate response

Add TNF-α inhibitor (adalimumab or infliximab) with low dose MTX to prevent antibody formation

Good response

Taper steroids slowly over several months. Then taper steroid-sparing agent slowly over several months

Consider experimental, surgical, or more toxic therapies

Ref: Fitzpatrick, 9th ed, Nat Clin Pract Rheumatol 2007;3(8):458

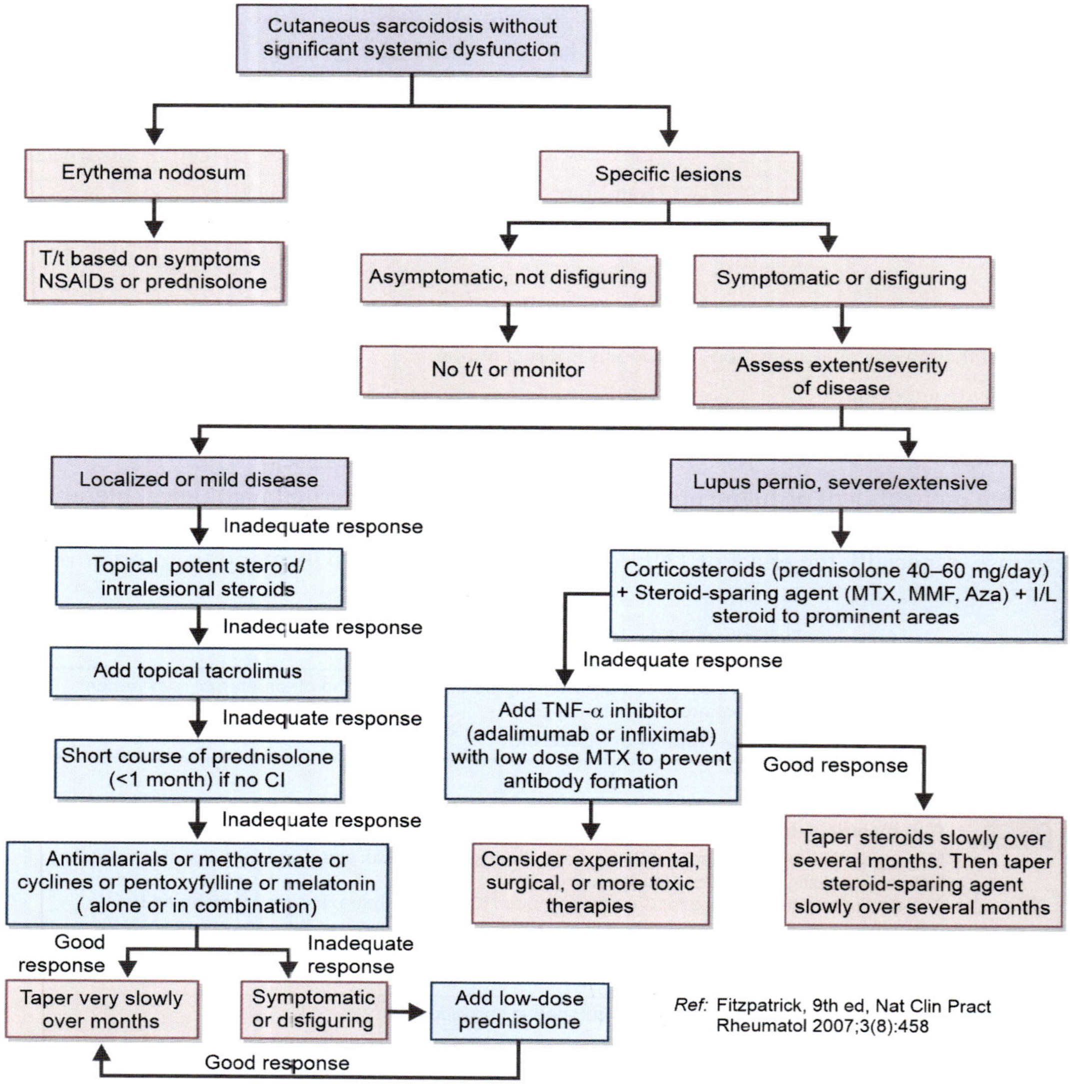

MTX, methotrexate; MMF, mycofenolate mofetil; Aza, azathioprine; CI, contraindication

Novel therapies being trialled include:

- CLEAR protocol (concomitant levofloxacin, ethambutol, azithromycin, rifampin)
- Nicotine
- JAK inhibitors

BIBLIOGRAPHY

Books

1. Fitzpatrick's Dermatology in General Medicine, 9th edition.
2. Joaquim Marcoval, Juan Mana. Sarcoidosis. Griffiths EMC, Barker J, Bleiker T, Chalmens R, Creamev D, Editors. In: Rook's Textbook of Dermatology. UK Black Well Publishers. 2016. Part 8; Chapter 98; P2611–2627.

Journals

1. Bargagli E, Olivieri C, Rottoli P. Cytokine modulators in the treatment of sarcoidosis. Rheumatol Int 2011; 31(12):1539–1544.
2. Caplan A, Rosenbach M, Imadojemu S. Cutaneous Sarcoidosis. Semin Respir Crit Care Med. 2020 Oct;41(5): 689–699.
3. Mallbris L, Ljungberg A, Hedblad MA, et al. Progressive cutaneous sarcoidosis responding to anti-tumor necrosis factor-alpha therapy. J Am Acad Dermatol 2003;48(2):290–293.

Chapter

33

Sexually Transmitted Diseases

Surabhi Sinha, Kabir Sardana, Sinu Rose Mathachan

INTRODUCTION

While STDs constitute a group of important and common disorders, the attempt here would be to delineate the common STDs that can be encountered by a dermatology student. We will initially discuss the approach to the common clinical presentations of STDs and after that discuss the important disorders: Notably, while syphilis is detailed exhaustively, it is not commonly seen and herpes genitalis, even though touted to be the most common cause of genital ulcer, is usually a transient condition. Hence, most of the cases that the student may encounter in an examination setting revolve around urethral discharge and genital warts. The chapter ends with a summary of syndromic approach which is often the most commonly practised treatment approach in clinical settings.

APPROACH TO A PATIENT WITH STD

History Taking and Examination in a Patient with STD

History taking in a patient with an STD should be conducted as for any dermatology patient, with special attention paid to the evolution of the lesions and sexual history. Likewise, examination should be conducted in entirety with greater emphasis on the genitalia, regional lymph nodes and perianal and perineal areas.

Presenting Complaints

1. **Genital ulcer**
   - Single/multiple, painful/painless, what is the primary lesion?
2. **Discharge**—urethral/vaginal (and/or cervical)
3. **Scrotal swelling and pain**
4. **Inguinal swelling**
   - Painful/painless
   - Unilateral/bilateral
   - Single/multiple
5. **Rash over body** +/– mucosal patches/ulcers
6. **Warty growths** (anogenital warts)
7. Flesh colored papules with central depressions (molluscum contagiosum)

HOPI (Including Sexual History) (*see* also Fig. 33.1 and Table 33.2)

- Promiscuous—Y/N, heterosexual/MSM/bisexual, unprotected/protected contact, type of contact, under influence of alcohol/illegal drugs.
- Last contact—how many days ago? (mainly relevant in single partners... still always take history)
  1. 1–7 days—GU, HPG (not recurrent HPG)
  2. 1 day–2 weeks—chancroid, NGU (7–14 days)
  3. 2–3 weeks—syphilis (primary)
  4. 3–30 days—LGV
  5. 8–80 days—donovanosis
- Evolution of the lesions. Other relevant history (rule out HIV, assess knowledge about STD).
- Past history—similar/different STD, stillbirth/abortion/HPV vaccination.
- Personal and occupational history—addictions, migrant, education and socioeconomic status.
- Family history—mainly relevant partner history, change in partners, frequency of change of partners.

Examination

Examine all these areas **(Table 33.1)**

TABLE 33.1: Examination of male and female STD patients

Male	Female
• Pubis • Penile shaft • Prepuce, glans, coronal sulcus • Urethral meatus • Scrotum-skin and contents • Perianal skin	• Pubis • Labia majora and minora • Urethral meatus • Vaginal opening • Vaginal walls • Cervical os • Perianal skin

PLUS Do not forget 'LPP OTP':

- **L**ymph nodes
- **P**er-rectal examination (except primary HPG)
- **P**erianal area
- **O**ral mucosa and lips
- **T**runk
- **P**alms and soles

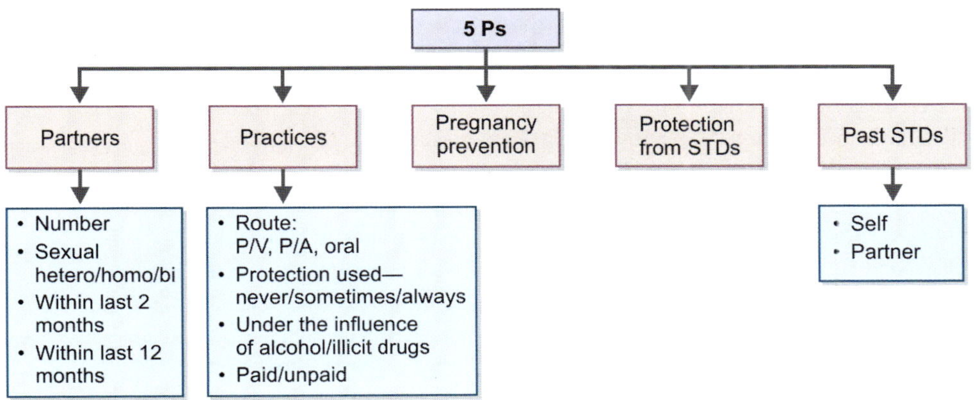

Fig. 33.1: 5 Ps of sexual history in a patient of STD

TABLE 33.2: Salient points in sexual history taking and its rationale (Int J STD AIDS 2020)

Sexual history	Rationale
Time interval since the last sexual contact (LSC) and previous sexual contact (PSC)	Need for repeat testing if still inside 'window' periods and assess need for emergency contraception or PEP for HIV infection
Gender of partner(s)	STI risk, eligibility for hepatitis/HPV screening and vaccination, other prevention options (HIV, PEP and PrEP), partner notification
Partnership type /whether partner can be contacted	To facilitate partner notification
Type of sexual contact/sites of exposure	To identify which sites need to be sampled
Condom use/barrier use (and whether properly used)	Condom promotion, risk assessment and HIV prevention options
Any symptoms or any risk factors for blood-borne viruses in the partner/risk of sexual infection	To identify STI or BBV diagnosis, or symptoms suggestive of an STI, in partners
The diagnosis of previous STIs and the approximate date of diagnosis and treatment	To allow the interpretation of positive syphilis serology in patients with a previous history of syphilis
Past medical and surgical history (specifically obstetrics and gynecology)	To identify conditions that may be associated with or influence the management of STIs and reproductive health
HPV vaccination history in women/men and MSM	Vaccination of those eligible if not started or not completed
Family history	Eligibility and contraindication for contraception
Drug history and history of allergies	To identify medication that may interfere with sexual function, potential drug interactions and drugs safety
Alcohol and recreational drug history/Chemsex*	Major factors in sexual risk taking
Smoking history	Modifiable risk factor (including cervical cancer) and alters eligibility status for some contraceptives
Identification of unmet need about difficulties with sexual performance and satisfaction	Provides opportunities for information giving, support and provision of referral pathways
Gender-based violence (GBV) or intimate partner violence (IPV)	Provision of support and access to referral pathways (risk for—STIs and unintended pregnancy)
Pregnancy risk	To avoid drugs contraindicated, provide post-coital contraception if indicated, advice about contraception, to support decision making
Contraception history	Information giving, motivational interviewing and to offer a more effective method of contraception
History of unusual or altered vaginal bleeding	Should prompt a cervical examination and a potential urgent colposcopy clinic referral
Obstetric history, including outcomes and complications	May have impact on the current presentation, assessment, examination and screening or to screen children or close contacts
Assessment of cyclical mood disorders, pelvic pain, dysmenorrhea or menorrhagia	Referral into secondary care or for further investigations (s/o premenstrual dysphoric disorder, endometriosis, PCOS or fibroids)
Cervical smears	To include in the risk assessment, smoking cessation advice and HPV vaccine recommendation
Current or past history of injecting drug misuse	Need for hepatitis B/C and HIV testing and hepatitis A and B vaccine
Sex with a partner from high HIV prevalence	To identify sexual partners at higher risk of HIV
HIV testing history	To determine whether HIV testing is appropriately timed
Previous use of HIV PEP and PrEP	Indicates past risk and risk reduction
Sex with cisgender MSM and transgender women#	To identify the need for hepatitis B, C and HIV testing and hepatitis A and B vaccination and offer risk reduction advice

*Chemsex—sex under the influence of psychoactive drugs.
#Cisgender—gender identity same as biological sex, transgender—gender identity opposite to biological sex.

1. GENITAL ULCER DISEASE

Sexually transmitted GUDs include the following pathogens:

a. HSV-1 and HSV-2
b. *Treponema pallidum*
c. *Haemophilus ducreyi*
d. *Chlamydia trachomatis* (L1, L2, L3 serovars)
e. *Klebsiella granulomatis*

(For a more detailed list, *see* later section on GUD). The history and examination of a GUD patient should be directed towards finding the most likely cause for the symptoms and examination findings **(Table 33.3** and **Fig. 33.2)**.

Bedside Tests

The following bedside tests **(Table 33.4)** are performed for a patient presenting with a genital ulcer:

- Gram stain
- Crush smear (with Giemsa stain)
- Tzanck smear
- Dark ground microscopy

Specimens for bedside tests are collected using sterile cotton, calcium alginate, Dacron rayon swabs or platinum loops.

TABLE 33.3: Comparison of clinical features of different genital ulcers

Characteristics	Syphilis	Herpes simplex	Chancroid	LGV	Donovanosis
Primary lesion	Papule	Vesicle	Pustule	Papule, vesicle pustule	Papule
Number of lesions	Single	Multiple	Multiple	Single	Variable
Diameter	5–15 mm	1–2 mm	Variable	2–10 mm	Variable
Edges	Sharply demarcated, elevated	Erythematous Polycyclic	Undermined Ragged	Elevated Round or oval	Elevated Irregular
Depth	Superficial or deep	Superficial	Excavated	Superficial or deep	Elevated
Floor	Smooth Non-purulent, serous exudate	Erythematous	Purulent, Dirty gray slough	Variable	Red, beefy, velvety, bleeds easily
Induration	Button-like	Non-indurated	Non-indurated	Non-indurated	Non-indurated
Pain	Absent	Present	Present	+/–	Absent
Lymph nodes	Bilateral Non-tender Firm, shotty Non-suppurative	Bilateral Tender Firm Non-suppurative	Unilateral Tender Suppurative Uni-locular	Unilateral Tender Suppurative Multi-locular Sign of groove	None Pseudobubo
Recurrences	No	50% (HSV-1) to 90% (HSV-2) (Corey L-JAAD 1988)	No	No	No

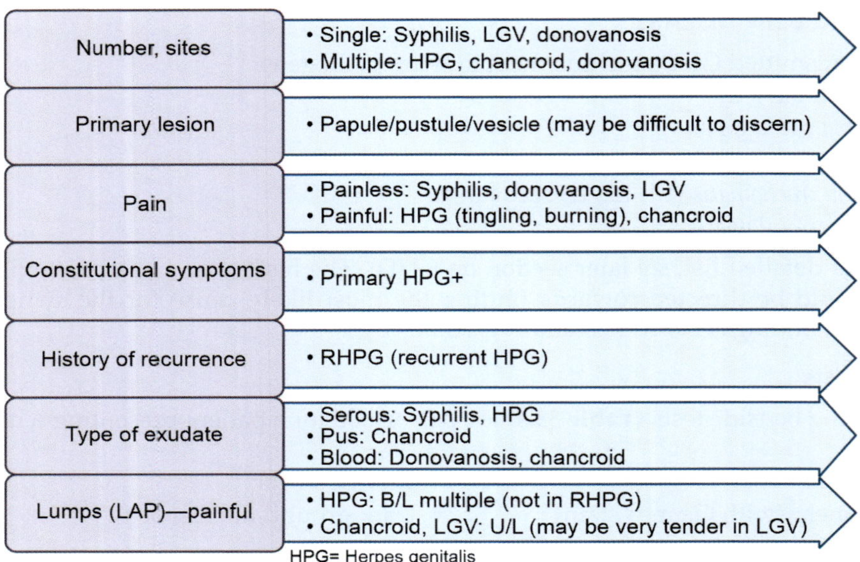

Fig. 33.2: History taking in genital ulcer disease (GUD)

TABLE 33.4: Summary of bedside tests in genital ulcers

Test	Chancroid	Donovanosis	Herpes genitalis	Syphilis
1. Gram stain	Gram-negative coccobacilli *Railroad or school of fish appearance*	—	—	—
2. Tzanck smear	—	—	*Ballooning degeneration, multinucleated giant cells*	—
3. Giemsa stain (on crush smear)	—	Large mononuclear cells with *intra-cellular Donovan bodies—safety pin appearance*	—	
4. DGI	—	—	—	Luminous self-motile slender organisms exhibiting corkscrew and angulation movements

Syphilis

Collection of specimen

1. Clean surface of the lesion with a sterile saline-soaked gauze.
2. Squeeze the base of the lesion to induce a serous exudate.
3. The first few drops of exudate, which may contain blood, are wiped away.

4. Serous exudate is obtained on the coverslip.
5. Invert onto slide.
6. Add drop of NS if fluid is less to make material homogenous.
7. Immediately examine slide under dark field microscope.

Lymph node aspirate

1. Overlying skin infiltrated with 1% lignocaine.
2. Skin stretched and LN held firmly between thumb and index finger.
3. 0.1 mL of sterile NS injected into LN.
4. LN massaged gently, fluid aspirated and expressed onto glass slide.

Chancroid

Specimens are collected from the undermined edge or the floor of the ulcer. Organisms are also usually demonstrable in the aspirate from an intact bubo. Wipe the lesion with saline-soaked gauze followed by dry gauze (thorough cleaning not essential) to remove the superficial debris and crusts. Roll a sterile swab in one direction beneath the undermined edge of the ulcer. Re-roll the swab in the reverse direction at 180° only once on a clean glass slide to maintain the arrangement of the bacteria and stain with Gram stain.

Herpes Genitalis

A fresh vesicle (<72-hour-old) is opened with a hypodermic needle or blade, the roof is folded back and the undersurface of the roof or the floor is scraped with a curette or scalpel (blunt side). An erosion is scraped with a cotton-tipped swab.

Donovanosis

Wipe the lesion with saline-soaked gauze, followed by dry gauze. Remove a small piece of tissue from the border of a well-defined ulcer using a curette/forceps/edge of a safety razor blade. Place this specimen on a clean grease-free microscopic glass slide and crush the specimen between two clean slides (Rajam and Rangiah method). Alternatively, a crush biopsy specimen may be used (Greenblatt and Barfield method). Impression smears from the lower surface of the biopsy specimen may also be used. The specimen is air-dried and stained with Giemsa or Leishman stain.

Lab Tests for Diagnosis of Genital Ulcers

Following bedside tests, laboratory tests can be utilized to confirm the diagnosis. Various lab tests and their respective findings in each of the causes of genital ulcers have been summarized in **Table 33.5** and **Figs. 33.3** and **33.4**.

Rapid Point-of-Care Test (POCT)—for GUD

- <30 min-results
- Require minimal training
- At peripheral clinic
- Whole blood based (no centrifuge/rotator)
- Ingredients at room temperature (no incubator/fridge)
- Battery dependent (no electricity)
- Not batched (less wait)

TABLE 33.5: Summary of lab tests for genital ulcers

Criteria	Syphilis	Herpes	Chancroid	LGV	Donovanosis
Specimen collection	Ulcer exudate or lymph node aspirate	Disruption of new vesicles—vesicle fluid, swabs from ulcer floor	Swabs from ulcer floor, lymph node aspirate	Swabs from ulcer floor, LN aspirate	Swabs from ulcer floor
Microscopy/ immuno-fluorescence	Dark ground microscopy or DIF	Tzanck smear	Gram stain	Micro-IF, IF-demonstrating inclusion bodies in WBC (LN aspirate)	Crush smear Giemsa stain
Culture	—	Human diploid fibroblast cell/ HeLa or McCoy cell culture	• Gonococcal agar base with 2% bovine hemoglobin, and 5% fetal calf serum • Mueller–Hinton agar base with 5% chocolate horse blood	Cell line inoculation • HeLa • McCoy • Yolk sac • Human diploid fibroblast cells	Difficult to culture, heat-inactivated fetal calf serum and pooled blood donor PBMC
Serology	VDRL TPHA FTA-Abs ELISA	ELISA Western blot	EIA, CFT, Immunoblot	CFT IF Micro-IF	—
Molecular techniques (NAATs)*	PCR	PCR	PCR	PCR	PCR
Skin biopsy (ulcer edge)	Do in HIV +ve patient	Do in HIV +ve patient	—	—	Do

*Additionally, HIV, HBsAg and VDRL testing must be done in all patients presenting to the STD clinic, NAAT: Nucleic acid amplification tests.

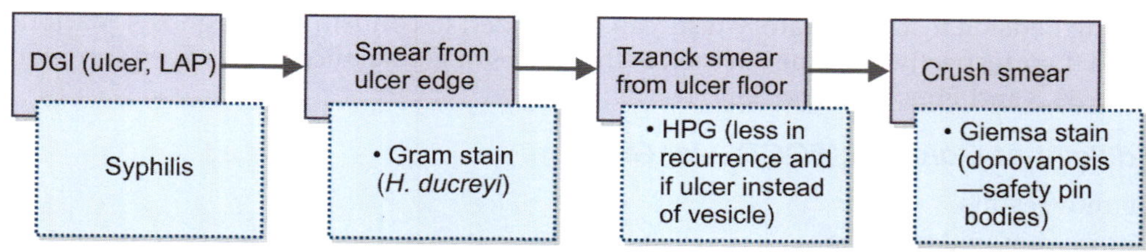

Fig. 33.3: Diagnostic algorithm for genital ulcers

Common POCTs

- Agglutination—flocculation and agglutination
- Immunochromatography (ICT)—lateral flow tests.

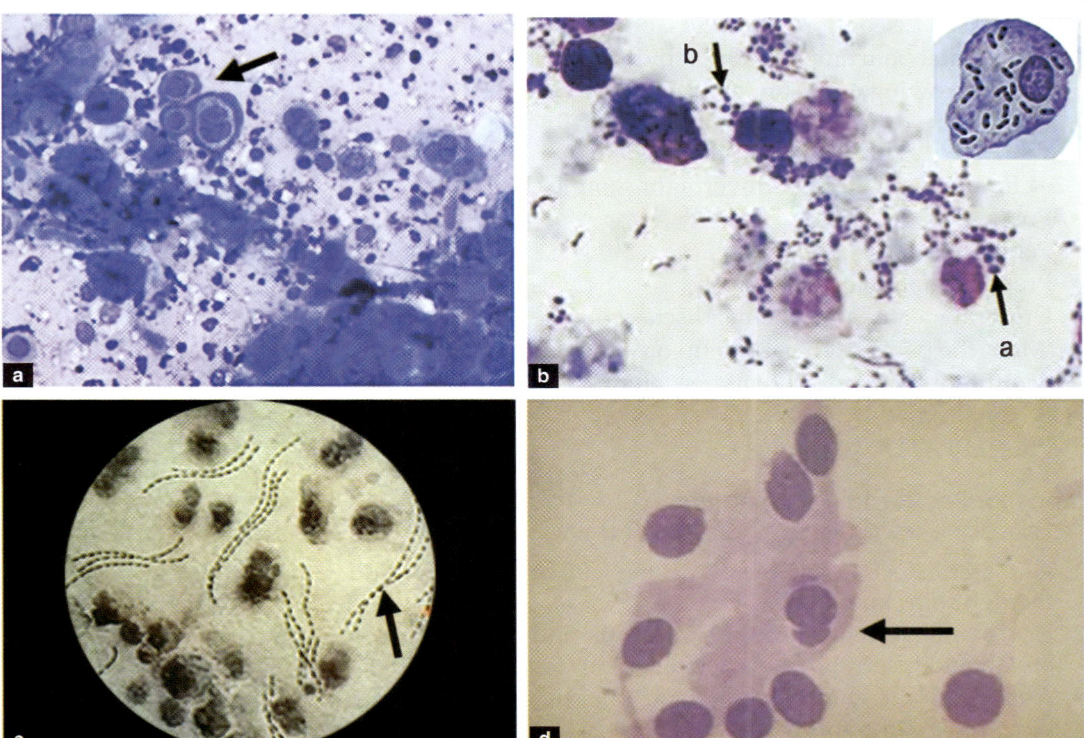

Fig. 33.4: (a) Multinucleated giant cells in a Tzanck smear in a case of genital herpes; (b) Donovan bodies in Giemsa stained smear in a case of donovanosis; (c) Depiction of school of fish appearance of *Hemophilus ducreyi* in Gram stained smear in a case of chancroid; (d) Intracytoplasmic elementary bodies in a Tzanck smear in a case of LGV

2. URETHRAL DISCHARGE

History Taking in Urethral Discharge

i. Type of discharge
   - Mucopurulent/purulent/greenish foul odor
   - Usually dysuria+
   - Onset, color, amount, smell of discharge
   - Rule out other causes for discharge (foreign body/trauma)

ii. Discharge at other sites
   - Rectal (MSM): Discharge+/–, pruritus+/–, pharyngitis+/–

iii. History suggestive of complications
   - Fever, constitutional symptoms
   - U/L tender abscess on 1 side of frenulum (Tyson's gland abscess)
   - Tender abscess in midline with deep pain (periurethral abscess)
   - U/L throbbing pain in perineum and painful defecation (Cowper's gland abscess)
   - Frequency, dysuria, terminal hematuria, suprapubic pain (prostatitis, seminal vesiculitis)

- Rectal discomfort, tenesmus, perineal pain (prostatic abscess)
- Scrotal pain and swelling (epididymitis)
- Narrowing of stream of urine (urethral fibrosis).

Examination of Urethral Discharge

>**2–4 hours** post-voiding or overnight sample

- Pubis
- Penile shaft
- Prepuce, glans, coronal sulcus
- Urethral meatus—erythema, discharge
- 'Milk' the penis from base to tip on ventral aspect 3–4 times
- Scrotum—skin and contents—swelling/tenderness
- Perianal skin

  Plus **'LPP OTP'** (*see* earlier)

Steps for Per Rectal Examination
(to be done in all cases of urethral/vaginal discharge)

1. Left lateral decubitus (Sims position): Patient lies on left side with left hip/leg straight and the right hip/knee bent
2. Use a small amount of lubricant on the index finger and ask the patient to take a deep breath and insert the finger facing down (6 o'clock position)
3. Appreciate the external sphincter tone, then ask the patient to bear down and feel for tightening of the sphincter
4. Palpate the prostate gland. Note the following:
   - Approximate size of the prostate gland (normally about the size of a walnut, 2–3 cm, but wider at the top)
   - Feel for tenderness (prostatitis)
5. Palpate the rectal wall starting from the 6 o'clock position clockwise to the 12 o'clock position. Then return to the 6 o'clock position and palpate the other half of the rectal wall feeling for masses, nodules and tenderness.
6. Examine the gloved finger to look for discharge/blood stains.

Lab Tests in Urethral Discharge (Fig. 33.5)

- **Serology (antibody detection)**—not usually employed
- **Antigen detection**
  - Enzyme immunoassay (EIA): NGU

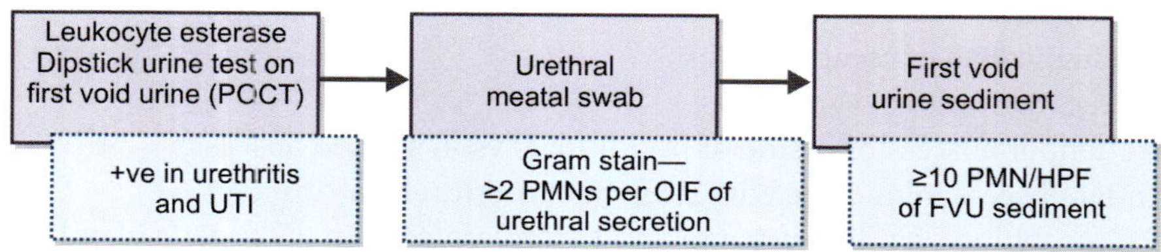

Fig. 33.5: STD clinic tests for urethral discharge (OIF, oil immersion field)

- **Culture**
  - Modified Thayer Martin medium: NG (gonorrhea)
  - Cell culture—CT (*Chlamydia*)
- **NAATs**
  - PCR—*C. trachomatis*, *N. gonorrhoeae*—LCR (ligase chain reaction)
  - TMA (transcription-mediated amplification)

Investigate for Alternative Pathogens

- **Persistent urethritis**—no improvement within 1 week of treatment for NGU.
- **Recurrent urethritis**—urethritis recurring within 6 weeks of previous episodes of NGU.

3. VAGINAL/CERVICAL DISCHARGE

History Taking in Vaginal (and/or) Cervical Discharge (Fig. 33.6)

Etiology—**vaginal discharge:** VVC, BV, TV; **cervical discharge:** NG, CT

- Vaginal discharge
- Itching/burning
- Spotting
- Dyspareunia
- Post-coital bleeding

Amount	Scanty/profuse
Consistency	**Homogeneous** (BV), **frothy** (TV), **curdy** (VVC)
Color	**White** (VVC), **greenish** (TV), **grayish** (BV)
Odor	BV: Characteristic fishy odor after unprotected intercourse
Vulval itching	VVC+
Complications of TV/BV	Preterm/LBW/post-operative infections
Lower abdominal pain (S/o PID)	Fever, menstrual irregularity, dyspareunia, dysuria, tenesmus
Risk assessment (for cervicitis)	Symptomatic partner, new partner, multiple partners, partner returned after long stay away
Symptoms of cervicitis	Dysuria, intermenstrual bleeding, bleeding after intercourse
Complications of cervicitis	Pharyngitis, tenesmus (proctitis), periurethral abscess, Bartholin's gland abscess

Fig. 33.6: History taking in vaginal discharge

(BV, bacterial vaginosis; VVC, vulvovaginal candidiasis; TV, *Trichomonas vaginalis*)

Examination of Vaginal Discharge (Fig. 33.7)

- Look for external **vulvitis**—*Candida albicans* most common cause (others—*Staphylococcus aureus, Streptococcus pyogenes*).
- Look for regional **LAP**
- Introduce **speculum** (except in unmarried or non-consenting females) → do all tests in a predetermined order so as not to leave out anything (Fig. 33.8)

Plus LPP OTP (*see* page 875)

Bedside Tests (Fig. 33.8)

1. *Litmus Testing for pH of Vaginal Fluid*

The pH of the vaginal fluid can be determined by placing a pH litmus paper (range at least 4–6.5) on the wall of the vagina or directly in pooled vaginal secretions. The normal pH of the vagina is typically between 3.8 and 4.5. A pH greater than 4.5 is consistent with a diagnosis of bacterial vaginosis.

2. *Saline Wet Mount*

Procedure: A drop of warm 0.9% saline and a drop of the vaginal discharge specimen are placed on a glass slide, a cover slip is placed over the solution on the slide, followed by immediate examination under a microscope at both low (10×) and high (40×) power within 10 minutes.

- Unstained—especially for *Trichomonas vaginalis*.
- Stained—1.8 mL normal saline plus 0.2 mL methylene blue—in syringe—add 1 drop to vaginal vault sample on slide—aids visualization.

Amount	Scanty/profuse
Consistency	Homogeneous (BV), frothy (TV), curdy (VVC)
Color	White (VVC), greenish (TV), grayish (BV)
Odor	BV-characteristic fishy odor/no odor
Vaginal ulcers/erythema	+/– (may occur in TV)
Cervical os	• IUD thread +/– • Erythema, pus, friable, bleeding—GC/CT • Strawberry cervix—TV
Urethral meatus	Inflamed—GC
Signs of PID	Lower abdomen guarding, tenderness

Fig. 33.7: Examination of vaginal discharge
(BV, bacterial vaginosis; VVC, vulvovaginal candidiasis; TV, *Trichomonas vaginalis*; GC/CT, gonococcal/*Chlamydia trachomatis*)

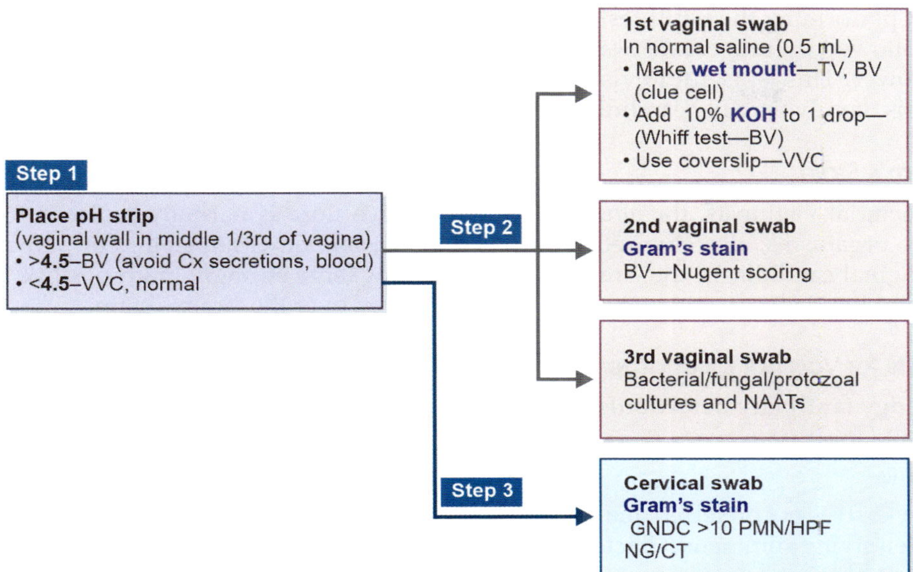

Fig. 33.8: Sequence of clinic tests for vaginal discharge (also *see* text below)
(BV, bacterial vaginosis; NG, *Neisseria gonorrhoeae*; CT, *Chlamydia trachomatis*; VVC, vulvovaginal candidiasis; Cx, cervical)

Interpretation of wet mount

- **Unremarkable**—polymorphous rods, only isolated WBCs, normal looking epithelial cells.
- **BV**—>20% clue cells of the total epithelial cells seen, absent lactobacilli, mixed bacterial rods and cocci, no increase in WBCs (*refer* to **Fig. 33.36**).
- **Inflammation**—more WBCs than epithelial cells or >25 WBCs at 400× (candidiasis or *Trichomonas* vaginitis)

Size comparison of important structures on wet mount

- *Trichomonas vaginalis*—≤25 microns
- Nucleus of epithelial cell—15 microns
- PMNL—10–15 microns
- RBC—6–8 microns
- Blastospore (*Candida* spp.)—5–7 microns

Description of structures on wet mount

- **Blastospores**—round/oval, half size of epithelial cell nucleus, present in groups, budding+/–
- **Pseudohyphae**—refractile delicate parallel walls, develop from blastospores.
- **PMNL**—same size as nuclei of epithelial cells but segmented nuclei.

3. *Potassium Hydroxide (KOH) Preparation and Whiff Test*

A second sample of vaginal fluid is placed on a slide and a 10% KOH solution is added. Soon after applying the KOH, bring the slide near the nose to perform the whiff test; the presence of a strong amine 'fishy' odor is considered a positive whiff test. A positive whiff test is consistent with a diagnosis of bacterial vaginosis.

After performing the whiff test, a coverslip should be placed over the preparation on the slide, followed by immediate examination under a microscope at both low (10×) and high (40×) power. This is useful to visualize yeasts or pseudohyphae and is consistent with the diagnosis of vulvovaginal candidiasis.

4. *Gram's Stain*

With bacterial vaginosis, the abundant gram-positive flora is partially replaced by gram-negative organisms; also clue cells are sometimes visible on Gram stain. For patients with vulvovaginal candidiasis, the Gram's stain may show large strongly gram-positive staining yeasts and hyphae, but a wet mount, KOH is preferred over the Gram's stain.

Lab Tests for Vaginal Discharge

- **Serology (antibody detection)**—EIA-TV
- **Antigen detection**
- **Culture**
  - VVC, BV—not preferred due to low sensitivity (less than 50%) and potential for mistakenly identifying commensal bacteria as pathogens, resulting in inappropriate treatment
  - TV—gold standard is culture
    - Inoculate InPouch® TV (bedside)/Amies transport medium
    - Kupferberg medium
    - Diamond's TV medium
  - NG culture
- NAATs
  - PCR—for *Candida*, *Gardnerella*, *Trichomonas*

POCTs for vaginal discharge (based on microbial byproducts)

1. **BV**
   - Proline aminopeptidase: QuickVue Advance GV® test
   - Trimethylamine and high pH: QuickVue Advance pH® and Amine test card
   - **OSOM BV Blue®**
     - Chromogenic, based on sialidase levels in vaginal fluid (produced by *Bacteroides*, *Prevotella*, *Gardnerella*).
2. **TV**
   - **OSOM *Trichomonas* Rapid test®**
     - FDA approved for vaginal swabs
3. **VVC**
   - Savvy Check® vaginal yeast assay

4. INGUINAL SWELLING (Chancroid, LGV)

History Taking in Inguinal Bubo

- Number, size, site, pain, history of breakdown.
- Elephantiasis—genital, anorectal syndrome.

Examination of bubo (Table 33.6)

- Number, site (U/L), size, scars, fistulae/sinuses, overlying skin, tethered to surrounding skin
- Horizontal/vertical/both groups ('sign of groove')
- Tenderness, warmth, discrete/matted, mobile/fixed, firm/soft/fluctuant
- Plus LPP OTP (*see* page 875)

Lab tests for bubo

LAP aspirate

- Serology
  - CFT >1:64
  - micro-IF >1:256
- Culture
- NAAT

5. SCROTAL SWELLING

History Taking in Scrotal Swelling and Pain

- Acute severe pain U/L
- Sudden swelling
- Dysuria/urethritis—preceding/concurrent
- D/D—testicular torsion

Examination

- Erythema/swelling/tenderness
- Rule out testicular torsion

STD clinic and lab tests

- Along the lines of urethritis

TABLE 33.6: Differences between the inguinal bubo in LGV and chancroid

LGV bubo	Chancroid bubo
Transient genital ulcer/not noticed	Genital ulcer present
Bubo less painful	Extremely painful
More common (66.7% cases)	In 50% cases
Unilateral in 2/3rds	Mostly U/L
Multilocular suppurative swelling	Unilocular suppurative swelling
Rupture to form multiple sinuses	Rupture to form single sinus
Does not tend to ulcerate	Tends to ulcerate to form chancroidal ulcer
Heals slowly with scarring	Less scarring

GENITOULCERATIVE DISEASE (GUD)

Predisposing Factors

- Low socioeconomic status
- Lack of circumcision
- High risk groups—MSM, IDU (injecting drug users)
- High risk sexual practices—multiple partners, unprotected contact
- Concurrent STDs
- Concurrent HIV infection

Etiology

Causes of sexually transmitted genitoulcerative disease include the following:

- *Herpes simplex virus* (both HSV-1 and HSV-2)
- *Treponema pallidum*
- *Haemophilus ducreyi*
- L-biovar of *Chlamydia trachomatis*
- *Klebsiella* (previously *Calymmatobacterium*) *granulomatis*

Other infective causes include

- *Pthirus pubis*
- *Trichomonas vaginalis*
- Mixed non-syphilitic spirochetes
- *Sarcoptes scabiei*
- *Entamoeba histolytica*
- Pyoderma

Non-infectious causes

- Trauma
- Malignancy
- Reiter disease
- FDE
- Behçet disease

GENITAL HERPES

Herpes (Gr.)—'to creep'

Genital herpes is caused by the herpes simplex virus 1 and 2.

Epidemiology

- HSV is the most common cause of genital ulcerations both in the developed and in the developing world, especially with the decline of *T. pallidum* and *H. ducreyi* infections.
- There is a wide disparity between antibody prevalence and clinical infections, indicating that many persons acquire subclinical infection.
- Rate of transmission of HSV is from 2–3% to 12% per year in a serodiscordant couple. Most transmission occurs during episodes of subclinical shedding from asymptomatic partners. Frequency of transmission of HSV-2 depends on:
  1. Gender: Females >males (due to greater surface area exposed)
  2. Past HSV-1 infection—more in HSV-1 seronegative
  3. Frequency of sexual activity:
     i. Median length of relationship before transmission—3 months
     ii. Median number of sexual encounters before transmission—24

- Only 40% of newly acquired cases of genital HSV-2 develop genitourinary complaints around the time of acquisition; prior HSV-1 infection protects against symptomatic acquisition of HSV-2.
- The incidence of HSV-1 induced genital herpes has also significantly increased amongst young people, women and MSM—due to decrease in oral acquisition of HSV-1 during childhood and frequent oral–genital contact.

Pathogenesis

- The structure of HSV is depicted in **Fig. 33.9**.

1. *Viral Latency*

- HSV penetrates susceptible mucosal surfaces or abraded cracks in the skin.
- It ascends the nerve endings and then the nerve axons through retrograde transport where HSV establishes persistent infection in the sacral ganglia and paraspinal ganglia.
- Because HSV is not cleared from neurons, the ganglia become lifelong reservoirs of virus.

2. *Viral Reactivation*

- Transcripton of viral genes
- Causes DNA replication, transcription/translation of viral proteins, and subsequent viral transport down the axon to epithelial cells.
- The viral replication leads to either asymptomatic viral shedding or clinically symptomatic genital ulcer disease.
- This occurs throughout the distribution innervated by the sacral ganglia, including the buttocks and thighs; thus viral shedding is more diffuse and can be detected throughout the genital region.

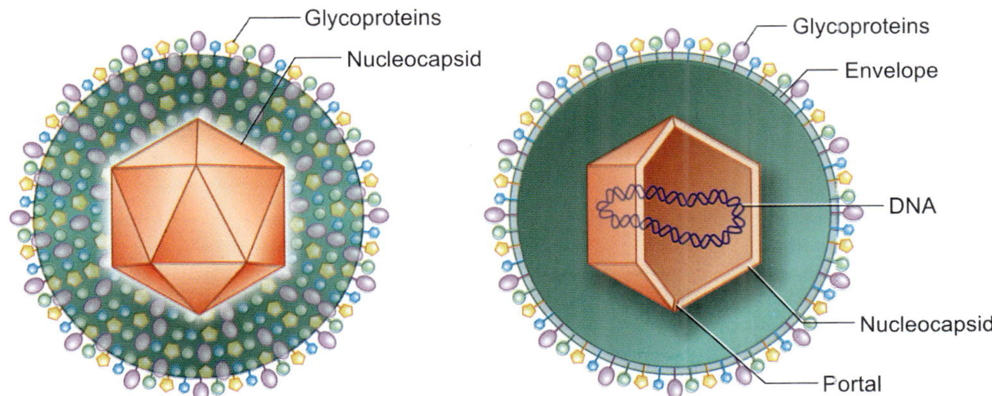

Fig. 33.9: Structure of herpes simplex virus: The envelope consists of a lipid bilayer membrane with 12 distinct types of glycoproteins which determine viral entry and elicit neutralizing antibodies. Differences in glycoprotein G (gG) between HSV-1 and HSV-2 are used for development of type-specific serologic testing.

3. ***Viral Shedding***

- Shedding is frequent but approximately 60% of the episodes are less than 24 hours in duration (median 13 hours).
- Tissue resident memory CD8+ T cells help to contain viral shedding.
- HSV-2—has increased genital tract inflammation, plus it selectively recruits CD4 cells (HIV target cells) to the genital skin and mucosa and likely accounts for the increased risk for HIV acquisition in HSV-2 seropositive persons.

4. ***Asymptomatic Viral Shedding***

- Most HSV-2 seropositive persons have asymptomatic viral shedding.
- In women, from the vulva and perianal area, whereas in men, it occurs from the penile skin and perianal area.
- The viral shedding is shorter than clinical recurrences, but the quantity of virus shed is similar in symptomatic and subclinical episodes. Days with asymptomatic HSV-2 genital shedding are highest in the first year after infection and gradually decreases over time.
- Majority of HSV-2 transmission is thought to occur with viral shedding in asymptomatic persons.
- Antiviral suppressive therapy dramatically reduces HSV-2 shedding by 70–80%, but it does not eradicate it.
- Genital HSV-1 shedding is less frequent than HSV-2 shedding, with shedding detected by culture on 2% of days.

5. ***Transmission***

- The transmission of HSV-2 **most often** involves asymptomatic shedding of HSV-2, often in persons unaware that they have HSV infection.
- It's more from men-to-women than from women-to-men.
- Fomite transmission of HSV is unlikely, although autotransmission of viral particles can occur from genital sites to other mucocutaneous sites, fingers, or eyes.

Clinical Features

- **Incubation period—2–7 days**
- *Types*: Primary, recurrent, asymptomatic shedders **(Fig. 33.10)**. Clinically, the three types of infections have variable healing times as seen in **Fig. 33.11**.

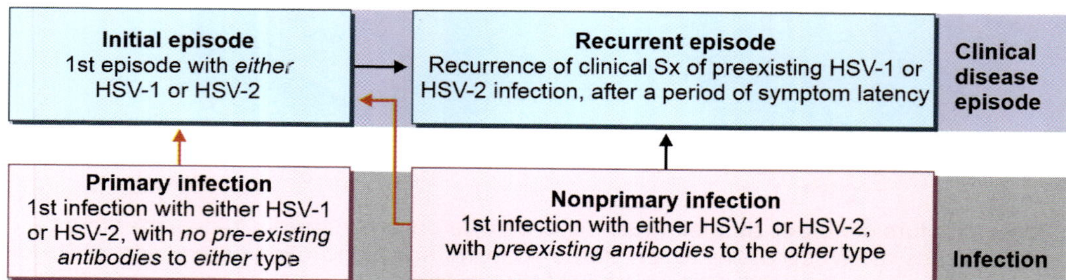

Fig. 33.10: A depiction of the definition of primary, recurrent, and initial episode of genital herpes

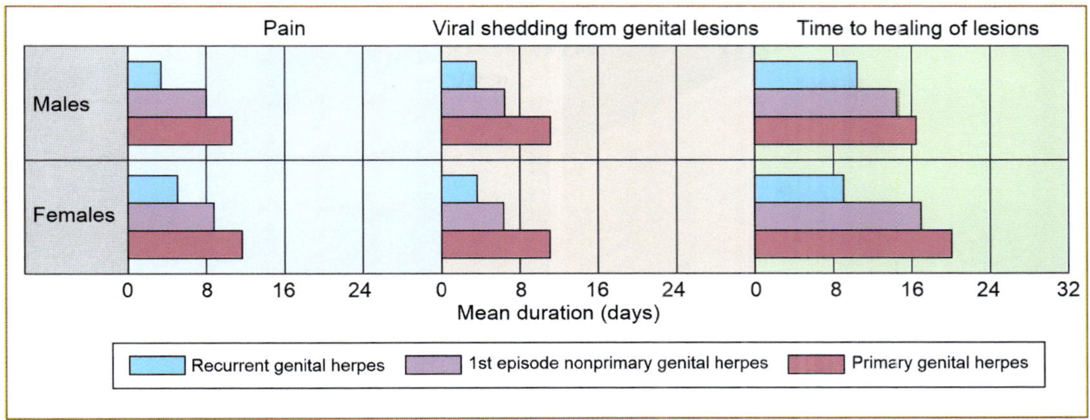

Fig. 33.11: Comparison of duration of pain, viral shedding and healing time in different types of genital herpes

i. *First (Initial) Episode of Genital Herpes*

Definition: The **first clinical episode** refers to the initial symptomatic occurrence of genital herpes.

Primary infection is defined as the first infection with either HSV-1 or HSV-2 with absence of antibody to either HSV type.

- First episodes of genital herpes often are associated with **systemic symptoms, a prolonged duration of lesions, and viral shedding**, and involve **multiple genital and extragenital sites (versus recurrent HPG).**
- True **primary infection** refers to infection occurring for the first time with either HSV-1 or HSV-2 (patient being seronegative for both).
- First episode may or may not be primary infection. Only **50% of persons** who present with their first episode of symptomatic genital herpes have **primary infection with either HSV-1 or HSV-2.**
- Most persons with **non-primary first episodes** have serological evidence of **past HSV-1 infection (75%).**
- **25%** of individuals with their **first clinical episode** already have antibody to **HSV-2,** indicative of a past **asymptomatic acquisition of HSV-2.**
- **Most genital HSV-1 infections are primary infections**, as genital HSV-1 acquisition is rare after HSV-2 infection.

  (In some settings, such as university campuses, HSV-1 has now replaced HSV-2 as the leading cause of first-episode genital herpes. One proposed reason for this shift is decreasing HSV-1 orolabial infection in childhood and early adolescence, with first exposure to HSV-1 occurring later in life with sexual activity. Changing sex practices in young adults, namely an increase in oral–genital sex, may also contribute to the changing epidemiology of genital herpes).
- Prior oral-labial HSV-1 infection appears to protect against the acquisition of genital HSV-1 disease.
- However, genital HSV-1 disease does not protect completely against acquisition of genital HSV-2.

C/F: Vesicular lesions or vesicular papules → breakdown to form multiple, bilateral, superficial, painful ulcers → polycyclic ulcer **(Fig. 33.12)**. Constitutional Sx+.

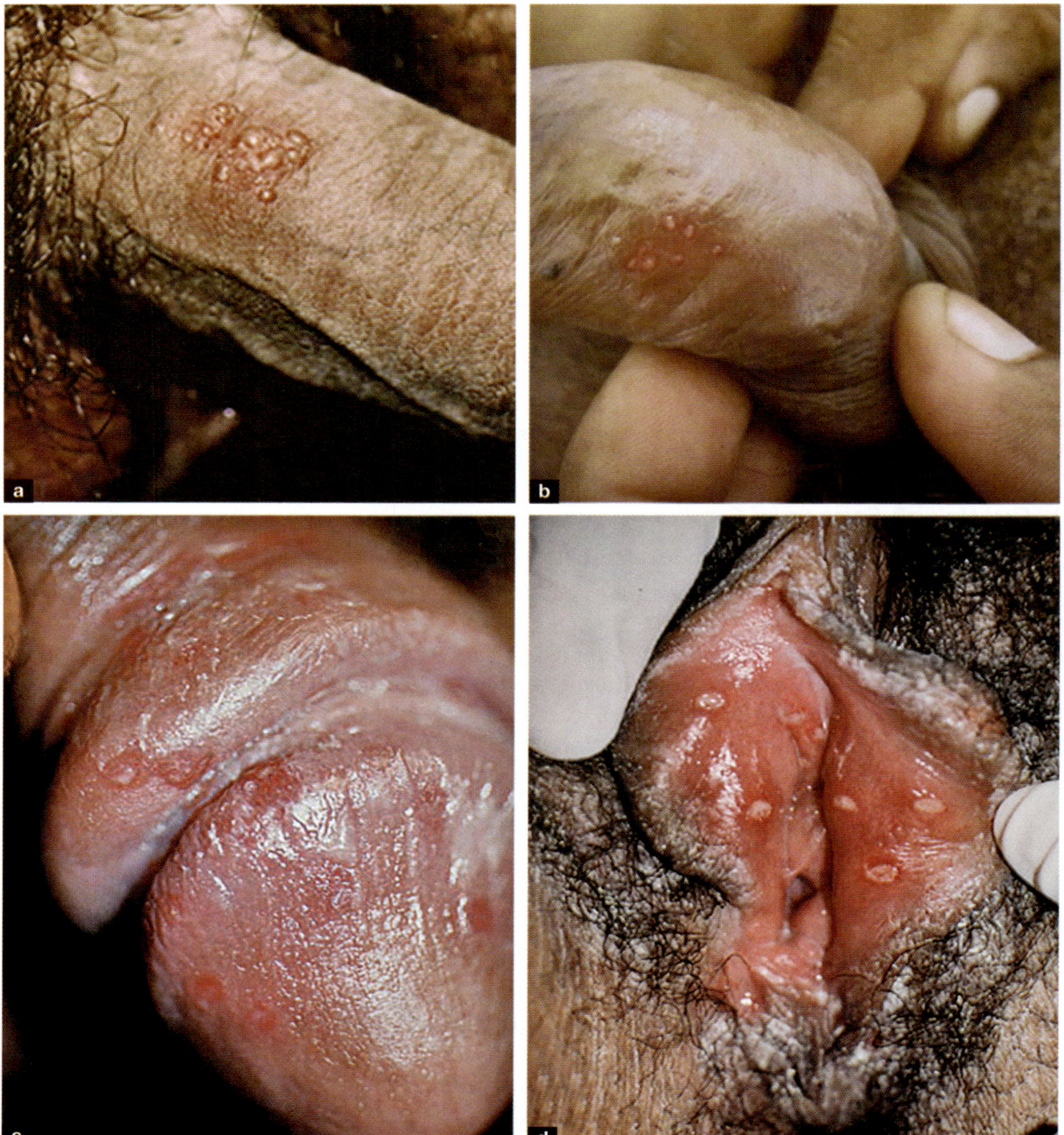

Fig. 33.12: Vesicles and erosions of herpes. The superficial level of erosions is diagnostic of herpes genitalis

- Herpetic urethritis (men)—clear mucoid discharge with dysuria out of proportion to amount of discharge.
- Herpetic cervicitis—primary HPG—70–90% develop cervicitis *vs* 15–20% in RHPG. May be symptomatic or asymptomatic—ulceration and necrotic cervicitis is highly correlated with HPG.

- Dysuria—more common in women than men.
- Inguinal lymphadenopathy—tender, second-third week.
- Median duration of viral shedding—12 days.

ii. *Recurrent Episodes and Subclinical Shedding*

- Causes of recurrences:
  - UV light
  - Immunosuppression
  - Fever
  - Pneumococcal pneumonia
  - Trauma to latently infected neurons
  - Menstruation
- Almost all HSV-2 seropositive persons reactivate HSV-2 in the genital region, over a large anatomic area.
- Around 90% of patients with genital HSV-2 develop recurrences in the first 12 months of infection.
- Reactivation is less common with genital HSV-1 (57% in the first year) versus genital HSV-2 (90% in the first year).
- HSV-2 reactivates 16 times more frequently than HSV-1 (Fitzpatrick)
- Median recurrence rate is 0.33 recurrences/month.
- Long-term studies indicate that the frequency of symptomatic recurrences gradually decreases over time.
- In the initial years of infection, reported recurrence rate decreases by a median of 1 recurrence per year.

C/F: A prodrome (local skin tingling, sciatic nerve pain) occurs in 50% of cases up to 48 hours before lesions appear. Lesions are similar to initial episode, and range from vesicles to erosions, unilateral, and lesions heal more quickly. Area of involvement one-third of primary herpes genitalis.

iii. *Asymptomatic Shedding*

- Approximately 80% of persons seropositive for HSV-2 have never received a diagnosis of genital infection
- Highest in the first year after acquisition.
- About 50% shedding occurs around the episode, while 50% occurs within 7 days of the episode.
- Shedding site: Men—penile skin, women—cervical secretions, MSM—perianal skin
- Risk of transmission is independent of lesions.
- If patients are counseled about the mild signs and symptoms of recurrent outbreaks, they can avoid sexual contact during these periods and prevent transmission to their partners.

Complications of Genital Herpes (Table 33.7)

1. Local extension of the disease
2. Super infection
3. Extragenital lesions
4. Disseminated infection
5. Central nervous system involvement

TABLE 33.7: Complications of genital herpes		
Complication	**Cause**	**Manifestations**
Local extension of disease	Spread of the virus to the uterine cavity and cervix—can cause pelvic inflammatory disease	Lower abdominal pain and adnexal uterine tenderness Laparoscopic evidence of vesicular lesions— fallopian tube
Superinfection	Bacterial superinfection (uncommon) Fungal infection (common)	Pelvic cellulitis of the perineal area Fungal vaginitis—change in character of the vaginal discharge, vulvar itching and irritation Potassium hydroxide examination of vaginal secretions—budding yeast cells
Extragenital lesions	Common complication of first-episode primary genital herpes and is seen more commonly in women than in men	Most frequently located in the buttock, groin, or thigh area, although finger and eye can also be involved. Extragenital lesions develop after the onset of genital lesions, often during the second week of disease
Disseminated infection	Blood-borne dissemination Pregnancy, atopic dermatitis predispose to severe visceral dissemination In immunosuppressed patients, especially those with impaired cellular immune responses, reactivation of genital HSV infection can be associated with viremic spread to multiple organs	Multiple vesicles over widespread areas of the thorax and extremities, aseptic meningitis, hepatitis, pneumonitis, or arthritis
Central nervous system involvement	Aseptic meningitis	Both HSV-1 and HSV-2 have been isolated from CSF. Aseptic meningitis—frequently associated with genital HSV-2 infection. HSV encephalitis in older children or adults—associated with oral HSV-1 infection Fever, headache, vomiting, photophobia, and nuchal rigidity are the predominant symptoms of HSV aseptic meningitis Lymphocytic CSF pleocytosis, increased glucose, increased protein
	Transverse myelitis • Occurs in association with primary genital HSV infection	Decreased deep-tendon reflexes and muscle strength in the lower extremities, as well as the above-described autonomic nervous system signs and symptoms, are present
	Sacral radiculopathy (Elsberg syndrome) • Viral invasion of CNS or immunological response	Hyperesthesia or anesthesia of the perineal, lower back, and sacral regions and urinary retention and constipation Electromyography usually reveals slowed nerve conduction velocities and fibrillation potentials in the affected area, and urinary cystometric examination shows a large atonic bladder. Most cases gradually resolve over 4–8 weeks

Diagnosis

In a patient presenting with multiple grouped vesicles or a history of lesions of similar size, duration, and character, HSV infection is the most likely cause. Moreover, lesions of genital herpes are typically tender and this sign may be useful in differentiating it from other etiologies of genital ulceration **(Tables 33.8** and **33.9; Fig. 33.13)**.

Serological Tests

Since the natural history and subsequent clinical course depends on whether HSV-1 or HSV-2 is the causative agent, the clinical diagnosis of genital herpes should be confirmed by laboratory

TABLE 33.8: List of investigations in herpes genitalis

Investigations	Comments
Tzanck smear	Multinucleate giant cells
HSV DNA PCR	*Four times more sensitive* than viral culture
Viral isolation or culture	Most specific, gold standard test, subtyping of the isolate → specificity 100%, sensitivity 75% (primary) to 50% (recurrent)
Serodiagnosis (see Table 33.9)	• Strong antigenic cross-reactivity between the two HSV subtypes—due to similar genetic make-up • The only exception is the gene that encodes **glycoprotein G of HSV-1 (gG-1)**, which is nearly 1500 base pairs shorter than the gene encoding HSV-2 gG (gG-2). Human antibody responses to these proteins are functionally type-specific, enabling differentiation between HSV-1 and HSV-2 infection • **Type-specific serologic assays (TSS)** have specificities of more than 98% for the detection of HSV-2 antibody and sensitivities of more than 90%-ELISA or Immunoblot • Western blot assay is the most accurate test for serologic diagnosis of HSV-1 and HSV-2 infection, with a sensitivity and a specificity of >98%
Complement fixation, indirect immunofluorescence or neutralization technologies	*Cannot* reliably distinguish antibodies to HSV-1 from those to HSV-2

TABLE 33.9: Clinical designation of genital herpes simplex virus (HSV) infection on the basis of serology

Direct viral test result*	Type-specific serologic status¶		Classification of genital HSV infection
	HSV-1 antibodies	**HSV-2 antibodies**	
HSV-1 detected	–	–	Primary HSV-1 infection
	–	+	Non-primary first episode HSV-1 infection$^{\Delta}$
	+	– or +	Recurrent HSV-1 infection
HSV-2 detected	–	–	Primary HSV-2 infection
	+	–	Non-primary first episode HSV-2 infection
	– or +	+	Recurrent HSV-2 infection

*Testing of the ulcerative lesion with culture, polymerase chain reaction, or direct fluorescent antibody.

¶Performed at the time of initial presentation with the ulcerative lesion.

$^{\Delta}$Non-primary first episode genital HSV-1 infection is rare.

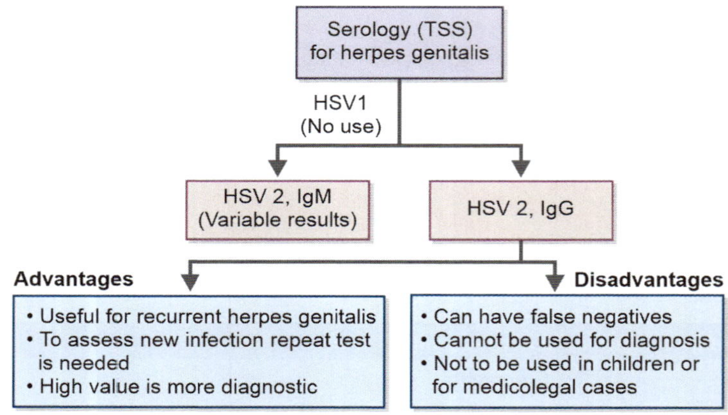

Fig. 33.13: Relative merits of type-specific serology (TSS) for genital herpes

testing, including HSV typing. As these tests are most commonly employed, we will detail these below. Here it is crucial to realise that the interpretation of these tests is contingent on using the type-specific serology as non-specific serological tests are not useful to confirm herpes genitalis.

The importance lies in using them to support the diagnosis of the different clinical presentations of herpes genitalis **(Table 33.9)**.

The drawbacks and salient features of the serological tests are listed in **Box 33.1** and an overview of the relative merits of serology in relation to the IgM and IgG is given in **Fig. 33.13**.

BOX 33.1: Factoids on serological tests of herpes genitalis

- Positive serologic testing for HSV-2 indicates anogenital infection, but positive serologic testing for HSV-1 can be consistent with either anogenital or orolabial infection.
- For **new infection**: Seroconversion from a negative result to a positive result with a subsequent specimen is needed and takes up to 6–12 weeks.
- Type-specific IgM testing is neither currently available nor reliable.
- IgM antibody testing is not useful for discriminating primary versus recurrent episodes of HSV infection.
- TSS in children under 14 years of age is not recommended.
- TSS-gG-based type-specific serology in medicolegal cases has several pitfalls and is not advisable.
- In India there is a high seroprevalence in controls, hence the diagnostic value of TSS is poor.

TSS, type-specific serology.

Treatment (Table 33.10)

Randomized trials have suggested that three antiviral medications provide clinical benefit for genital herpes: Aciclovir, Valaciclovir (valacyclovir), and Famciclovir. Valacyclovir, the valine ester of acyclovir, has a better absorption after oral administration. Famciclovir also has high oral bioavailability. Topical therapy with antiviral drugs offers minimal clinical benefit and is currently not recommended.

- Antiviral therapy reduces the severity and frequency of symptomatic genital herpes, however, **subclinical shedding remains unaffected**.

TABLE 33.10: Therapy of herpes genitalis (CDC 2021)		
First episode	Acyclovir Valacyclovir Famciclovir	– 400 mg orally TDS for 7–10 days – 1 g BD × 7–10 days – 250 mg TDS × 7–10 days
Episodic therapy for recurrent episode	Acyclovir Famciclovir Valacyclovir	– 800 mg orally BD for 5 days/800 mg TDS × 2 days – 125 mg BD for 5 days/1000 mg BD × 1 day – 1 g orally OD for 5 days/500 mg BD × 3 days
Suppressive therapy for recurrent episodes (≥6/year)	Acyclovir Famciclovir Valacyclovir	– 400 mg BD – 250 mg BD – 500 mg OD/1 g OD (for **≥10 episodes/year**—500 mg OD might be less effective)

- Suppressive or episodic therapy with oral antiviral agents is effective in decreasing the clinical manifestations of HSV among persons with HIV infection, **but it may or may not reduce the risk for HIV transmission or HSV-2 transmission to susceptible sex partners (Valaciclovir seen to reduce transmission in serodiscordant partners.)**.

  Suppressive Rx should be discontinued after a maximum of **12 months** to reassess symptom episode frequency. Suppressive acyclovir has been given to patients for up to **8 years** without adverse effects (Patel et al., 2017). Data for valacyclovir and famciclovir are available for up to **1 year**, and these drugs are also well tolerated.
- **Investigational therapy:** Tenofovir, when administered for HIV preexposure prophylaxis (PrEP) to an HSV-2 negative patient, may also reduce the risk of acquiring HSV-2. But additional studies are needed before these agents can be recommended for the purpose of HSV-2 prevention in routine care.

Prevention of Transmission

Multiple strategies, including suppressive antiviral therapy, consistent use of condoms, and disclosure of HSV status to partners and circumcision have been shown to reduce HSV transmission.

SPECIAL SITUATIONS

1. Antiviral-resistant HSV

All acyclovir-resistant strains are also resistant to valacyclovir, and most are resistant to famciclovir.

- Only drug FDA approved for acyclovir-resistant HPG is **Foscarnet** (40–80 mg/kg IV every 8 hours until clinical resolution is attained).
- Intravenous Cidofovir 5 mg/kg once weekly.
- Imiquimod and 1% Cidofovir gels are topical alternatives—once daily × 5 days.

2. Genital Herpes in Pregnancy

Course of HPG in Pregnancy

Most of the clinical manifestations of genital herpes, are similar in pregnant and non-pregnant women; however, a few key manifestations as outlined below are distinct:

- Inguinal adenopathy may be severe.
- Viral dissemination may occur leading to hepatitis, pneumonitis or encephalitis, especially if infection is acquired in third trimester.

- Asymptomatic viral shedding is common.
- Rate and severity of recurrence in pregnancy is—high around 80%.

Effect of HPG on Pregnancy

- Only primary infection leads to pregnancy morbidity (neonatal HSV, premature labor).
- Recurrent HPG usually does not affect pregnancy outcome.
- Mother—disseminated infection possible, spontaneous abortion (uncommon), risk of preterm delivery, vertical transmission.
- Fetus—uncommon—microphthalmia, microcephaly, chorioretinitis, intracranial calcification.

Transmission of Herpes to Fetus/Neonate

- High (30–50%) among women who acquire genital herpes near the time of delivery and low (<1%) among women with recurrent herpes or who acquire genital HSV during the first half of pregnancy.
- 70% neonatal herpes born to mothers without symptoms at delivery.
- Neonate—ranges from mild skin involvement (0% mortality) to eye and CNS to disseminated infection (>50% mortality).

How to avoid transmission of HSV in pregnancy?

- Female partners of men with HPG should avoid intercourse in presence of lesions.
- Avoid orogenital contact if oral herpes present in male partner.
- Suppressive therapy should be considered if the couple is discordant for antibodies to HSV-2.

If you have a pregnant woman with herpes, ask yourself:

- Is this a first episode or a recurrence? (Though this may be difficult to establish.)
- Which trimester?

The principles that govern the management are listed in **Box 33.2**.

BOX 33.2: Basic principles of management of genital herpes in pregnancy

- Maximum transmission occurs during *labor* and *delivery*.
- Highest risk—primary genital HSV infection acquired near the time of delivery.
- Type-specific *antibodies* to HSV generally develop within the first *12 weeks* after infection and last indefinitely.

Management of genital herpes in pregnancy (ACOG, 2020 and CDC, 2021):

- Prophylactic therapy with acyclovir (400 mg TDS) or valacyclovir (500 mg BD) beginning at 36 weeks gestation should be offered to all women with a history of genital herpes since it has been shown to reduce the risk of HSV recurrence at delivery by 75%, the risk of cesarean delivery for recurrent genital herpes by 40%, and the risk of HSV shedding at delivery.
- Primary episode in third trimester—continue antiviral till delivery.
- Suppressive dose-higher than in non-pregnant due to enhanced renal clearance. (400 mg TDS—36 weeks till delivery).

i. Indications of cesarean section (C/S)

- Active genital lesions/prodromal symptoms (e.g. pain, burning) of first episode/recurrent HPG (neonatal herpes occurs in 1.2% C/S and 7.7% vaginal deliveries; though may occur even after C/S, if membranes rupture before the C/S).

- Active genital lesions/prodromal symptoms (e.g. pain, burning) with ruptured membranes.
- Primary/non-primary first episode of HPG in third trimester esp. within 6 weeks prior to EDD—C/S may be offered (due to high rates of viral shedding and insufficient time for adequate antibody response).

ii. C/S can be avoided if:

- Primary/non-primary first-episode genital infection but have no active lesions at the time of labor.
- Nongenital lesions (rule out genital lesions → cover nongenital lesions with occlusive dressing before vaginal delivery).

iii. Preterm premature rupture of membrane (PROM before 37 weeks) and recurrent HSV infection

- Expectant management
- Glucocorticoids for fetal lung maturation
- Intravenous acyclovir (5 mg/kg every 8 hours) to shorten the duration of active lesions in the mother and to decrease viral burden.

iv. Women with active genital lesions at delivery: Cesarean section (ideally, before rupture of membranes) for any pregnant woman with active genital lesions or prodromal symptoms at the time of delivery. In addition, use of invasive monitors during delivery should be limited. Delivery by cesarean section does not completely eliminate the risk for HSV transmission to the infant.

3. Neonatal Herpes

- Newborn infants exposed to HSV during birth are at a risk of developing neonatal herpes.
- Viral cultures or PCR of mucosal surfaces of the neonate to detect HSV infection might be considered before the development of clinical signs, to guide the initiation of treatment.
- Additionally, treatment with acyclovir might be considered for neonates born to women who acquired HSV near term because of the high risk for neonatal herpes.
- All infants with neonatal herpes should be promptly treated with systemic acyclovir.
- Acyclovir 20 mg/kg IV every 8 hours for 14 days if disease is limited to the skin and mucous membranes, or for 21 days for disseminated disease and central nervous system involvement.

4. HIV Infection and Herpes Genitalis

Multiple epidemiologic studies have shown that there is synergy between the HIV and HSV-2 epidemics **(Fig. 33.14)**

Effect of HSV on HIV

- An ulcerative STD in the source partner may lead to a 5-fold increase in HIV transmission (Holmes).
- Genital HSV also facilitates HIV infection by recruitment of activated CD4+ cells, and HSV proteins ICP0 and ICP14 can induce HIV-1 replication.
- Seropositivity with HSV-2 increases risk of HIV infection 3-fold in females, 2-fold in men and 1.7-fold in MSM (Holmes).

Effect of HIV on HSV

- The most marked effect is an increase in the rate of viral reactivation, mostly subclinical, which persists even with HAART.
- HIV also increases risk of acquiring HSV-2.

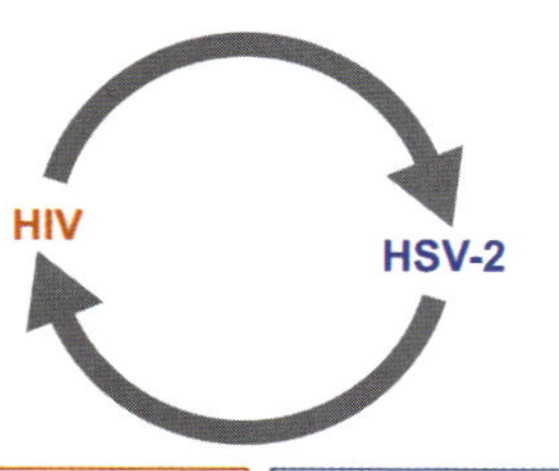

Effect of HSV-2 on HIV	Effect of HIV on HSV-2
↑ HIV transmission	↑ HSV-2 transmission
↑ HIV accuisition	↑ HSV-2 acquisition
↑ HIV level in	↑ Frequency of HSV-2 shedding
– plasma and genital tract	↑ Frequency of prolonged, atypical lesions
– affects disease progression	↑ Acyclovir resistance

Fig. 33.14: Epidemiologic and biologic synergy between HSV-2 and HIV infections

Table 33.11 lists the effects of HIV on clinical manifestations of HPG while the treatment is listed in **Box 33.3**.

[Notably unlike in HSV-2 sero-discordant couples without HIV, in whom antiviral treatment significantly reduces HSV-2 transmission to the susceptible partner, treatment of HIV-1 and HSV-2 coinfected individuals with daily suppressive antiviral therapy, does not reduce the transmission of HSV-2 to susceptible partners. Given the increased risk of HSV shedding and genital ulcers in those who start anti-retroviral therapy with a CD4 count less than 250 cells/mm^3, suppressive therapy may be considered to prevent immune reconstitution inflammatory syndrome (IRIS).]

TABLE 33.11: Effect of HIV infection on clinical manifestations of genital herpes

Number of lesions and symptoms	Lesions increased in number and size; more painful
Atypical **morphology**	Hyperkeratotic lesions, large ulcers, hemorrhagic and echthymatous lesions
Atypical **sites**	Buttock and lower back
Atypical **presentation**	Necrotizing lymphadenitis, urinary retention, intestinal obstruction, transverse myelitis, esophagitis, hepatitis, pneumonitis, pseudotumor of tongue and dissemination
Course	Increased chronicity and severity, increased number and severity of recurrent outbreaks, healing slow, subclinical HSV shedding increased
Investigations	Tzanck smear, culture, antigen detection, serology, PCR, biopsy
Treatment	Longer courses of antiviral therapy for resolution of genital ulcers and higher doses of antiviral therapy for suppression of recurrences

BOX 33.3: Therapy of herpes genitalis in HIV-infected individual (CDC 2021)

HIV+ (episodic therapy)

Acyclovir: 400 mg orally TID for 5–10 days

Famciclovir: 500 mg BID orally for 5–10 days

Valacyclovir: 1 g orally BID for 5–10 days

HIV+ (daily suppressive therapy)

Acyclovir: 400–800 mg orally BID to TID

Famciclovir: 500 mg BID

Valacyclovir: 500 mg orally BID

SYPHILIS

Epidemiology

Globally, there are an estimated 6 million new cases of syphilis annually, in persons aged 15 to 49 years, and over 300,000 fetal and neonatal deaths are attributed to syphilis. HIV has increased the incidence of syphilis.

Pathogenesis

- In 1905, Schaudinn and Hoffmann identified the causative agent of syphilis, *Treponema ('coiled thread') pallidum ('pale staining')*—a motile, corkscrew-shaped, microaerophilic prokaryotic bacterium with a flexible, helically coiled cell wall.
- An obligate human pathogen. Not reliably cultured on artificial media.
- Too slender to be observed using direct light microscopy, so dark field microscopy is used.

Clinical Features

Early Syphilis

- Primary stage (chancre)
- Secondary stage
- Relapses

Latent disease—early (<1 year) and late (≥1 year) stages. (CDC 2015 and European classification) or early (<2 years) and late (≥2 years) (as per WHO 2016 and UK classification) (French P, 2007).

Late Syphilis

Tertiary—cutaneous, cardiovascular, or neurologic involvement.

The course of syphilis is depicted in **Fig. 33.15**.

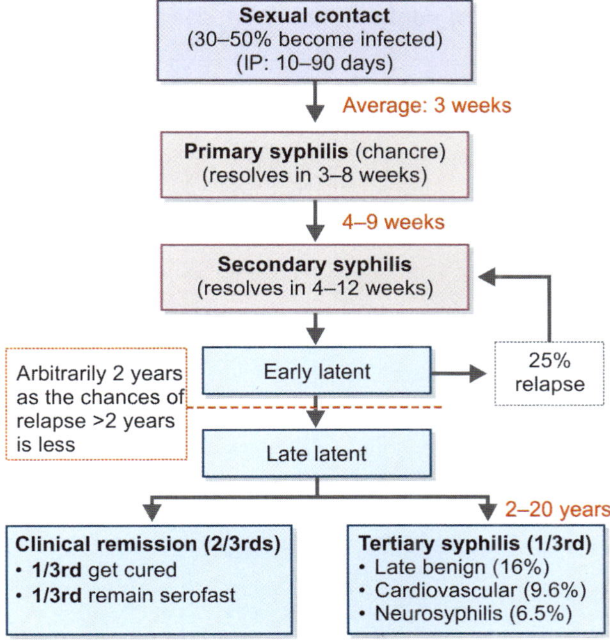

Fig. 33.15: Natural course of untreated syphilis

A. Primary Syphilis

- The initial lesion of syphilis is a papule that appears at the site of sexual contact, 10–90 days (average 3 weeks) after exposure.
- 0.5–1.5 cm in diameter → ulcerates after 1 week → classical/Hunterian chancre.
- Round/oval/slightly elongated, painless ulcer, 1–2 cm across, with an indurated base, rubbery to feel ('penny in a flannel'), clean 'ham colored' dull red floor or a wash-leather slough covering the floor **(Fig. 33.16)**.
- **Dory flop sign**—retraction of prepuce with chancre in its mucosal surface → causes prepuce to 'flop' briskly.
- Painless, firm, shotty bilateral lymphadenopathy 1–2 weeks later.
- Solitary lesion—typical, but multiple lesions frequently occur.
- Untreated—heals in 3–6 weeks, treated—heals within 1–2 weeks.
- 15–30%—chancre goes unnoticed
- 23–47%—multiple chancres
- **Sites:**
  - Males—**coronal sulcus (MC)**, glans, shaft, prepuce, frenulum, external urinary meatus.
  - Females—**labia majora/minora (MC)**, fourchette, clitoris, urethra, perineum, cervix, vaginal wall.
- **Types of chancres**
  - Classical Hunterian (43%)
  - Kissing chancre
  - Multiple chancres (23–47%)
  - Extragenital (12–14%)—lips (MC), anorectal (in MSM), fingers, breasts, trunk, etc.
  - Condom chancre—at root of penis
  - Intrameatal chancre

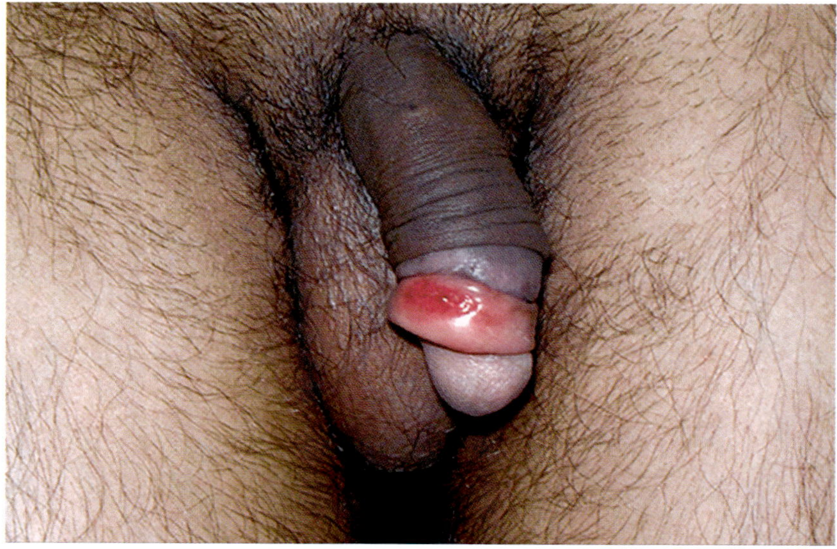

Fig. 33.16: Single firm painless ulcer (also called hard chancre) seen in a case of primary syphilis

- Edema indurativum—females, unilateral labial swelling
- Chancre redux (chancre at the site of healed chancre, *T. pallidum* present)
- **Pseudochancre redux**—gumma at the site of healed chancre (*T. pallidum* absent)
- Mixed chancre—chancre + chancroid.

Diagnosis
- A specific diagnosis can be made using a smear from the chancre seen under dark ground microscopy.
- It is important to note that most serological tests will take **3–4 weeks** to become positive.
- Order of positivity:
- **EIA (IgM)/19S IgM-FTA-ABS** followed by
  - **Rapid plasma reagin/venereal disease research laboratory (RPR/VDRL)**
  - **TPHA.**

Differential Diagnosis of Primary Syphilis

- **Other STDs**—chancroid, herpes simplex, granuloma inguinale
- **Non-STDs**—traumatic.

Complications of Primary Chancre

1. Edema
2. **Phagedenic chancre** (due to coinfection with fusospirochaetes) → penile gangrene, phimosis
3. Erosive balanitis
4. Lymphangitis
5. Thrombophlebitis of dorsal vein of penis
6. Intrameatal chancre → urethral obstruction/persistent urethritis/penile gangrene
7. **Syphilitic balanitis of Follman**—an inflammatory reaction of glans penis developing instead of/concurrently with/after primary chancre. Numerous *T. pallidum* in the lesion.

B. Secondary Syphilis

- 3–12 weeks after primary syphilis
- **Syphilis d'emblee**—secondary syphilis without primary syphilis (for example, after unsafe blood transfusion)
- **Cutaneous lesions**
  - Generalized symmetric polymorphic rash usually without pruritus (**except in African-Americans and immunocompromised** cases **follicular syphilid**)
  - Heals with/without treatment in 2–10 weeks
  - Morphological types:
    1. Macular (roseola/syphilitica/roseolar syphilid)
    2. Maculopapular—**most common**
       - Macules become thick and develop coppery hue
       - Lesions around hairline—**'Corona veneris'**
    3. Papular **(Fig. 33.17)**
       - Papulosquamous—coppery/erythematous, with thin white ring of scales on the surface **(Biette's collarette)**, on palms and soles, trunk, limbs, **'Clavi syphilitica'**—callus-like lesions on soles.

         [**Buschke–Ollendorff sign**—press palm/sole lesion with head of pin → on 'release' patient winces in pain due to obliterative endarteritis]

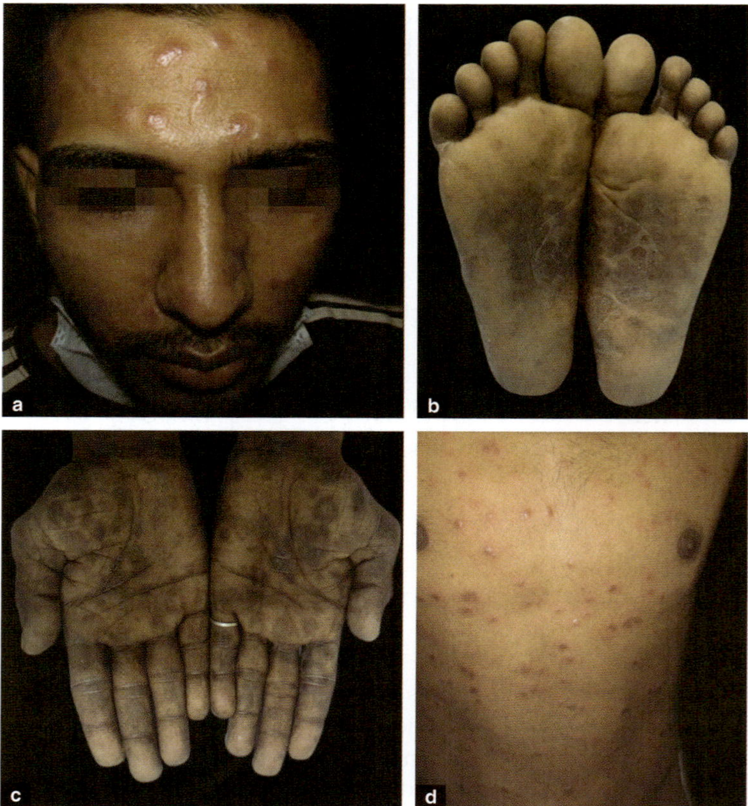

Fig. 33.17: Papular syphilis affecting the face and lips, soles and palms, and trunk

- Follicular/lichen syphilitica—in debilitated, may be itchy
- Lenticular—face, genitalia
- Corymbose/bombshell—rare, large central papule surrounded by multiple small satellite papules
- Annular—face, anogenital, flexures. **'Nickel and Dime syphilid'** (as lesions on face are like coins)
- Nodular

4. Pustular
   - Miliary
   - Acneiform/varioliform
   - Impetiginiform/ecthymiform
   - Malignant pustular/**'Lues maligna'**/rupial syphilis/pustuloulcerative syphilis
     - Prodrome—fever, headache, malaise
     - Widespread pustules 'necrotic' ulcers with thick oyster shell-like crusts
     - Face and scalp
     - In debilitated/immunocompromised/HIV patients

5. Pigmentary changes:
   - **'Necklace of Venus/leukoderma colli syphiliticum'**—post-inflammatory hypopigmentation on sides of neck in dark patients.
   - Post-inflammatory hyperpigmentation—especially on palms and soles.
6. Mucosal changes:
   - **Condyloma lata:** *Most infectious lesion of syphilis* **(Fig. 33.18)**
     - Flesh colored/erythematous/hypopigmented moist oozing flat macerated papules
     - Broad base and flat top (versus condyloma acuminata), highly infectious, teeming with treponemes.
     - Genitalia, perianal area, oral commissures, inframammary folds, interdigital web spaces.
   - Mucous patches:
     - Painless shallow rounded erosions covered with gray slough
     - Mouth-lips and tongue

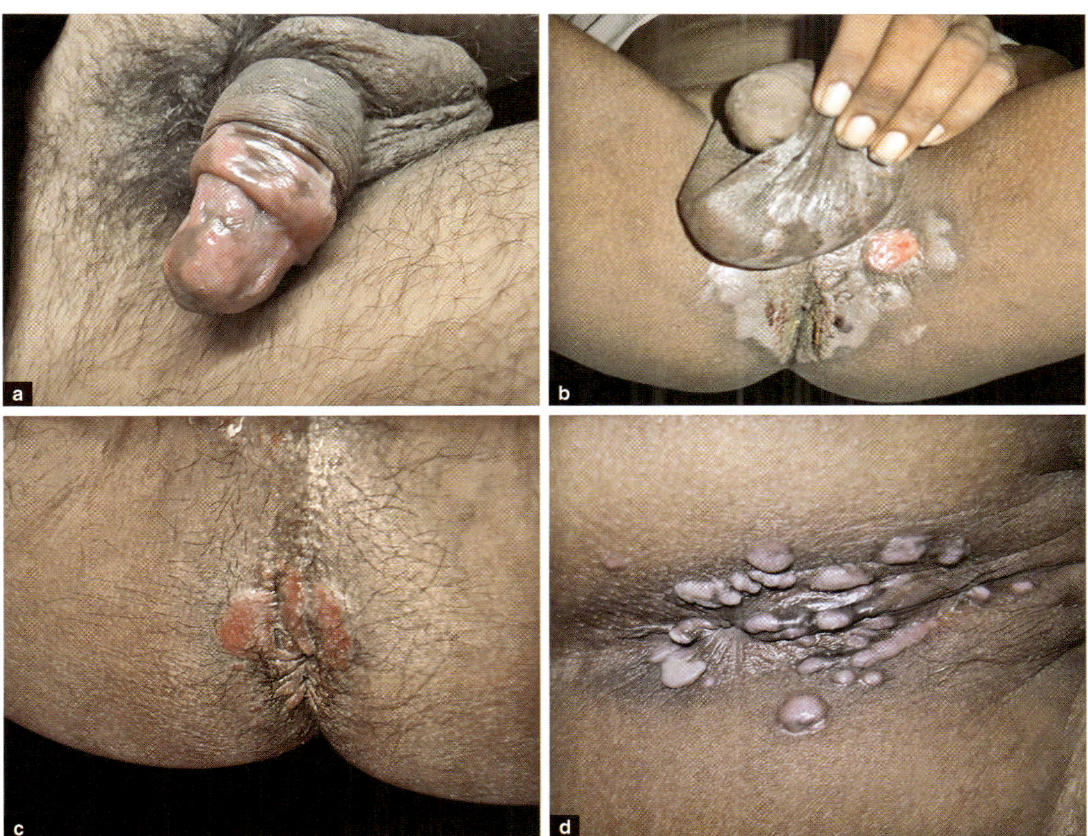

Figs 33.18: Lesions of condylomata lata on the genitalia, perianal area and inguir al folds, the lesions have a eroded, flat-topped, oozing surface

- Confluent denuded lesions on tongue—'*Plaques fauchees en prairie*'
- Split papules—elevated mucous patches with central fissure in oral commissures
- Pharyngitis
  - Diffuse redness and edema

Nail changes

- Nail plate—brittle, splitting, onycholysis, shedding, dystrophy, (amber-colored nail plate similar to artificial nails—characteristic of late secondary syphilis)
- Nail folds—paronychia, break down to form 'horseshoe ulcer'
- Cyanotic painful toes 'Blue toe syndrome'

Hair changes

- Alopecia—patchy noncicatricial 'moth-eaten alopecia'/trichotillomania like/alopecia areata-like/diffuse.

Reticuloendothelial system

- Lymphadenopathy—in 50–80%. Inguinal > axillary > cervical > epitrochlear > femoral > supraclavicular. Firm, mobile, non-tender, discrete, symmetrical.
- Mild splenomegaly

Eye

- Iritis, the most common eye complication, <3%
- Late in the course

Bones

- Periostitis, osteomyelitis, bone destruction, sclerosis on X-rays.

CNS

- Patients with secondary syphilis can develop neurosyphilis.
- Characterized by either asymptomatic infection of the central nervous system, or acute syphilitic meningitis, a basilar meningitis that typically causes headache and stiff neck and may involve cranial nerves, which may result in hearing loss, facial weakness, or visual disturbances. Strokes may also occur. Patients may also develop ocular or otic syphilis without basilar meningitis.

Hematological

- Anemia, leukocytosis, relative lymphopenia, and elevated ESR.

Diagnosis of Secondary Syphilis

- All serological tests are usually positive in high titers in secondary syphilis.
- Additionally, one can detect treponemes from smears made from lesions like condylomata lata.

Differential Diagnosis of Secondary Syphilis

Most likely

- Pityriasis rosea
- Condyloma acuminata (condyloma lata)
- Drug eruptions
- Viral exanthems
- Psoriasis

- Reiter's disease/reactive arthritis
- Leukoplakia (mucous patch)
- Glossitis (mucous patch)

C. Latent Syphilis

- An asymptomatic stage where the only evidence of the disease is reactive serologic testing.
- Early latent (<1 year): 75% go to late latent and 25% relapse to secondary. Infective to others.
- Late latent (>1 year): One-third get cured, one-third go to tertiary and one-third remain serofast indefinitely. Non-infectious to others.
- However, this determination of early and late may not always be possible, and the clinician must settle for a diagnosis of syphilis of unknown duration, which is treated in the same manner as late latent syphilis.

Diagnosis

EIA is the most sensitive test followed by FTA-ABS and then by TPHA/TPPA.

D. Relapsing Syphilis

Approximately 25% of untreated patients relapse, with more than two-thirds of the relapses occurring within 6 months and 90% within the first year. Relapses may present with the reappearance of chancres, or more frequently, an eruption of secondary syphilis. Even though the presentation is localized and less severe, the disease remains highly contagious even at this stage.

E. Tertiary Syphilis

Around one-third of patients with untreated latent syphilis develop tertiary syphilis, while the other two-thirds remain in latency. The three principal presentations during this stage are late benign syphilis, cardiovascular disease, and neurosyphilis.

Nowadays, tertiary syphilis is rare because of widespread availability and use of antibiotics. Without treatment, however, approximately 30% of patients eventually progress to the tertiary stage of syphilis within 1–20 years of the original infection.

Late benign syphilis includes any symptomatic syphilitic manifestation after the secondary and relapsing stages that does not involve the cardiovascular or nervous systems. The lesions are caused by a cell-mediated inflammatory response to a small number of treponemes present in the affected tissues. The more commonly involved organs are the skin (70%), mucous membranes (10.3%), and bones (9.6%), but gummas may appear in any organ.

a. *Late Benign Syphilis of the Skin*

Three types of lesions—granulomatous nodules, psoriasiform granulomatous plaques, and gummas.

'Precocious' lesions develop within the first 2 years after resolution of the secondary stage, and 'late' lesions at any time after that. Most lesions develop within 3–7 years, but gummas have appeared as long as 60 years after infection. The longer the interval before the appearance of the skin lesions, the more solitary and destructive the process.

- **Nodular and noduloulcerative tertiary lesions**—firm, painless, dull-red, shiny, flat cutaneous nodules that appear in a grouped configuration and coalesce into plaques, which break down forming irregular ulcers. Central healing and advancing borders produce plaques with annular or polycyclic configurations and are most commonly seen on the arms, back, and face and heal after several years, leaving atrophic scars.

- **Gummas**—non-tender, rarely contagious, dusky-red nodules or plaques that favor sites of trauma and more common on the scalp, forehead, buttocks, and presternal, supraclavicular, or pretibial areas. The nodule is initially firm but subsequently develops necrotic tissue. As the central gumma heals, new lesions may develop on the periphery, forming scalloped border and, in contrast to noduloulcerative lesions, gummas are deeper punched out ulcers, with wash-leather slough and more destructive.
- **Mucous membrane lesions of late benign syphilis:** Discrete gummas or diffuse gummatous infiltration may involve mucous membranes, especially the palate, nasal mucosa, tongue, tonsils, and pharynx. The lesions ulcerate and cause disfigurement. Destruction of the nasal cartilage and bone leads to a saddle nose and *perforation* of the nose and palate is considered pathognomonic of the disease.

b. *Cardiovascular Syphilis*

Very infrequent (probably due to widespread penicillin use) with 15–30 years latency. M:F = 3:1. Most cases are asymptomatic and diagnosed inadvertently at postmortem examination.

- Most common changes include aortitis, aortic aneurysm, aortic valve incompetence, coronary ostial stenosis, and myocardial gummatous disease. The changes occur predominantly in the *ascending aorta*.
- Atherosclerotic changes occur almost throughout the aortic intima ('Tree barking') and the diagnosis is suspected when **linear eggshell calcifications of the anterolateral aortic wall** are present in chest radiographs.

c. *Neurosyphilis*

It is the only tertiary syphilis encountered nowadays in the antibiotic era. Hematogenous invasion of the meninges by *T. pallidum* occurs early in syphilis. About 25% of patients with untreated primary or secondary syphilis do not clear the spirochetes from the CNS, and the organisms presumably remain dormant (as has been revealed by PCR). Experts have postulated that several decades of widespread use of antibiotics active against *T. pallidum* underlies the notable shift in clinical presentation from paresis and tabes dorsalis to meningeal and meningovascular syndromes and is marked in cases with HIV infection.

- Early neurologic manifestations include cranial nerve dysfunction (III, VI, VII and VIII), meningitis, stroke and auditory or ophthalmic abnormalities and usually present within the first few months or years of infection.
- Late neurologic manifestations (i.e. tabes dorsalis and general paresis) usually develop between 5 and 35 years after the initial infection.

Neurosyphilis has also been divided into (Merritt et al.):

- Asymptomatic—31%
- Meningeal—20%
  - Meningovascular
- Parenchymatous—48%
- Gummatous disease—1%

Among persons with HIV and syphilis, CSF abnormalities (mononuclear pleocytosis and elevated protein) are associated with a CD4 count of 350 cells/mm^3 or less and/or a non-treponemal serologic test titer of greater than or equal to 1:32. In general, persons with HIV infection tend to have more frequent CSF abnormalities in the absence of neurologic symptoms, and the presence of 20 or more white blood cells (WBC)/mm^3 might improve the specificity of probable neurosyphilis in this patient population.

Diagnosis of tertiary stage: For tertiary syphilis: Most sensitive is FTA-ABS, followed by TPHA/TPPA.
Neurosyphilis
- **Neurosyphilis: CSF-VDRL** is the investigation of choice and a positive test is considered highly specific for neurosyphilis.
- **CSF FTA-ABS** is the most sensitive test for neurosyphilis. If the CSF-VDRL is nonreactive, and neurosyphilis is suspected, a CSF FTA-ABS can be ordered and neurosyphilis is highly unlikely with a negative CSF FTA-ABS test.
- **CSF analysis following treatment:** Suspected treatment failure and suspected treatment failure with 4× or greater increase in non-treponemal test titer that persists longer than 2 weeks. An initially high titer (1:32 or higher) that fails to decline at least 4-fold within 12–24 months following treatment.

F. Congenital Syphilis

Transmission to the fetus in pregnancy can occur during any stage of syphilis, but the risk is much higher when a pregnant woman is in the primary or secondary stage of syphilis. Fetal infection can occur during any trimester of pregnancy and may range from mild to severe, with only severe cases manifesting clinically at birth.

If primary infection accompanies conception, many spirochetes cross the placenta, the fetus is damaged, and it usually aborts at 7–8 months. Additional testing at 28 weeks gestation and again at delivery is warranted for women who are at increased risk or live in communities with increased prevalence of syphilis.

It is divided into two stages and there are certain stigmata of syphilis that have been described:

- **Early congenital syphilis**—within the first 2 years of life. It is equivalent to adult secondary syphilis, is infectious **(Box 33.4)**, and is more common. Bone involvement is the most common specific manifestation and is seen in 60 to 80% of infected infants.
- **Late congenital syphilis**—this takes place after 2 years of life and resembles adult tertiary syphilis but CVS involvement is rare. It is non-infectious.
  - Interstitial keratitis: (10%) Usually bilateral; appears at age 10–30.
  - Sensory deafness: Develops at 10–20 years of age in 10–30%; usually bilateral.
  - Neurosyphilis: Late onset but affects 30–50%.
- **Stigmata (Box 33.5)**:

Bone lesions including frontal bossing, shortened maxilla, high palatal arch are the most common stigmata.

BOX 33.4: Features of early congenital syphilis

Present at birth	Low birth weight, abnormally large placenta, hepatosplenomegaly, blisters and erosions mainly on palms and soles (*Pemphigus syphiliticus*)
First month in untreated infants	• *Snuffles* (chronic runny nose, often bloody), periorificial rhagades • *Hepatosplenomegaly* with fibrosis and jaundice (*flintstone liver*) • Periosteitis and osteochondritis involving mainly long bones with so much pain that infants do not move limbs (*Parrot pseudoparalysis*—epiphyseal dislocation of the ulna, leaving a useless forearm). • Wimberger sign—loss of density of medial side of upper part of tibia.

BOX 33.5: Stigmata of congenital syphilis

1. **Saddle nose** (75%)
2. **Frontal bossing** (hot cross bun skull). Maxillary hypoplasia (85%)
3. **Higouménaki sign:** Thickening of medial end of clavicle
4. **Saber shins**
5. **Clutton joints:** Effusions into large joints
6. **Gothic palate** (high-arched palate): 75%
7. Periorificial furrowed scars **(parrot lines)**
8. **Dental changes:**
   - **Mulberry molars:** First molars with multiple rounded rudimentary enamel cusps on their surface; 65%.
   - **Hutchinson incisors:** Incisors-shaped like tip of a screwdriver, often notched; 65%.

Note: The Hutchinson **triad** consists of Hutchinson incisors, sensory deafness, and interstitial keratitis.

Diagnosis

Proven or highly probable congenital syphilis: Any neonate with:

1. An abnormal physical examination that is consistent with congenital syphilis.

OR

2. A serum quantitative non-treponemal serologic titer that is 4-fold higher than the mother's titer.

OR

3. A positive dark field test or PCR of lesions or body fluid(s).

Recommended Evaluation

- CSF analysis for VDRL, cell count, and protein.
- Complete blood count (CBC) and differential and platelet count.
- Other tests as clinically indicated (e.g. long-bone radiographs, chest radiograph, liver function tests, neuroimaging, ophthalmologic examination, and auditory brainstem response).

Laws of Congenital Syphilis

1. **Colles' law**—syphilitic infants can transmit the disease to previously healthy nurses but not to their own mothers.
2. **Profeta's law**—healthy infant born to a syphilitic mother is immune to the disease.
3. **Kassowitz' law**—the toll of the mother's syphilis decreases with successive pregnancies.

G. HIV and Syphilis

Both HIV and syphilis increase rate of transmission of the other infection and HIV may alter the course and morphology of syphilis **(Table 33.12)**. After appropriate therapy, persons with HIV infection more frequently demonstrate 'high serofast' values of nontreponemal serologic tests (often defined as RPR ≥1:8).

DIAGNOSIS OF SYPHILIS

Diagnosis of early syphilis can be done by the demonstration of spirochetes in lesional exudate or tissue either by dark field microscopy or by direct immunofluorescence. Other modalities include serological diagnosis and skin biopsy for suspected primary, secondary, and certainly, tertiary syphilis lesions. A presumptive diagnosis of syphilis requires use of two tests: a non-treponemal test and a treponemal test (CDC 2015). Diagnostic modalities are listed in **Table 33.13**.

The diagnostic value of these commonly used tests is given in **Box 33.6**.

TABLE 33.12: Effect of HIV on syphilis

• **Clinical features**	*Primary syphilis:* Multiple chancres, extensive chancre, painful lesions, persistence, gummatous lesions, extragenital chancre, chancre merging with secondary syphilis *Secondary syphilis:* Lues maligna *Late syphilis (tertiary)*: Neurosyphilis, ocular syphilis, syphilitic aortitis and encephalitis Relapse/recurrence
• **Course**	Rapid progression to tertiary stage and neurosyphilis
• **Serological response**	Atypical response: Biological false positive, seronegativity and delayed titer response, accelerated loss of antibody reactivity after treatment, antibody production to decrease antigens and return of titres to normal on advancing immunosuppression

TABLE 33.13: Investigations in syphilis

Investigations	Comments
Direct detection of *T. pallidum*	• Dark field microscopy • Direct fluorescent antibody test for *T. pallidum* (DFA-TP) (body fluids) • Direct fluorescent antibody tissue test for *T. pallidum* (DFAT-TP) (tissues) • Molecular methods/NAATs
Serological tests	• Non-treponemal tests • Treponemal tests
Histopathology	Endothelial swelling, perivascular plasma cells
Animal infectivity testing	Inoculation in rabbits (Nichol's strain)

BOX 33.6: Overview of the diagnostic tests in syphilis

Most **specific test:** DG microscopy

Most **specific blood test:** TPHA/TPPA

Most **sensitive blood test:** IgM-FTA-ABS/EIA

Test for **monitoring Rx:** VDRL

Seropositivity of common tests:

- EIA (IgM)/IgM-FTA-ABS—3 weeks
- VDRL/RPR—4 weeks
- TPHA/TPPA—4–6 weeks

A. Direct Detection of *T. pallidum*

1. *Dark Field Microscopy*

Must be done immediately after the specimen is obtained as movement of *T. pallidum* is imperative to visualize. Dark field examination is the diagnostic test of choice in chancres and also in condylomata lata.

Invalid for oral lesions because saprophytic treponemes of mouth cannot easily be differentiated from *T. pallidum*. (*T. microdentium*, *T. macrodentium*, *T. denticola*, *T. orale*, *T. vincentii*). (Do specific immunoperoxidase stains.)

Principle of dark ground microscopy

A contrast exists between object and field as the background is dark and the object appears bright against it. The objective and ocular lens are same as in light microscope and a **dark field patch** stop prevents the transmitted light from directly illuminating the specimen and only scattered light reaches the specimen and passes onto the lens **(Fig. 33.19)**.

T. pallidum appears as white, delicate organisms (6–15 μ length, 0.10–0.18 μ wide with 8–24 regular coils, at a regular interval of 1 μ) and demonstrates characteristic movements:

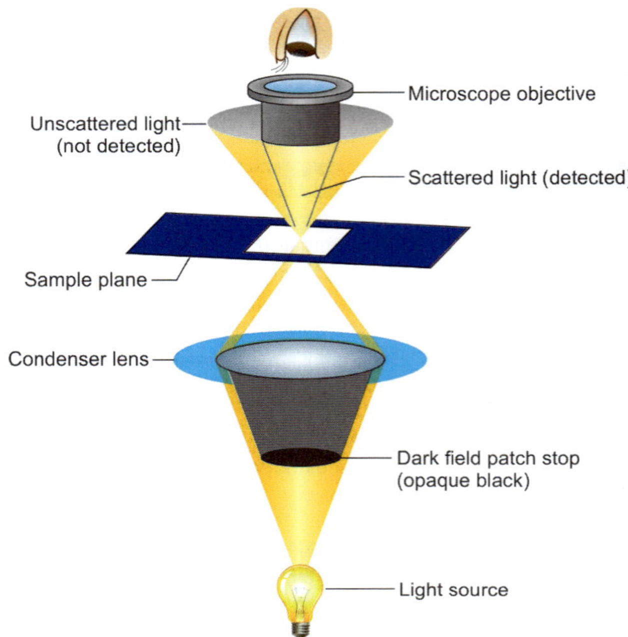

Fig. 33.19: Principle of dark ground microscopy

1. **Locomotion**—*rotation* and *propulsion*
2. **Change of shape**—*Angulation (most typical)*, *buckling*, *coil compression* and *expansion*, *looping* and *undulation*, *cork screw like movement*.

How to distinguish nonpathogenic treponemes from *T. pallidum*?

- Surface organisms, absent from the depth of lesion
- Thick, coarse and loosely coiled
- Writhing movement with marked flexion and frequent relaxation of coils
- Pathogenic treponemes lack locomotion in liquid media unlike saprophytic treponemes.

Table 33.14 depicts merits and demerits of DGI.

TABLE 33.14: Merits and demerits of DGI

Merits	Demerits
Specific	Not very sensitive (80%) Single examination <50%
Immediate diagnosis	Not recommended in: Oral and rectal lesions—commensal treponemes
Distinguishes from other spiral organisms	Difficult to differentiate from other pathogenic treponemes
Diagnosis before serological tests become reactive (early primary)	False negative if: Resolving lesion, previous topical/systemic applications, inadequate specimen collection
Useful if clinical symptoms s/o syphilis but serology negative	Special equipment (dark field microscope), has to be seen immediately (within 20 minutes)

2a. *Direct Fluorescence Antibody Test for Body Fluids*

It is easier to perform than dark ground microscopy. It detects antigen and, thus, does not require the presence of motile treponemes and can be used in rectal and oral specimens too. The lesional exudate is smeared on a glass slide and stained with fluorescein labelled anti-*T. pallidum* antibody as shown in **Fig. 33.20**.

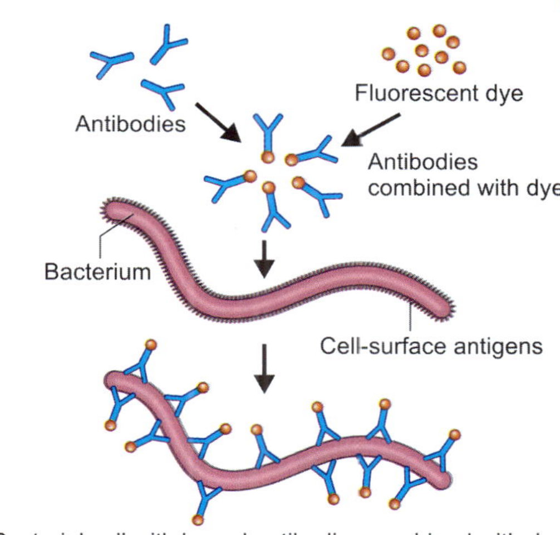

Fig. 33.20: DFA test for *T palladium*

2b. *Direct Fluorescent Antibody Test for Tissues*

A combination of the DFA-TP test and histologic stains may be used to examine biopsy and autopsy material for the presence of pathogenic *Treponema* spp. Tissue for paraffin-embedded sections are collected frequently from:

- Brain
- Placenta
- Skin
- Gastrointestinal tract
- Umbilical cord

3. *Molecular Tests (NAATs)*

- Have a high sensitivity (as low as 1–5 organisms) and high specificity.
- Body fluids and fresh and paraffin-embedded tissues are used for diagnosis.
- However, they are not standardized and not commercially available.
- Include PCR, RT-PCR

Sensitivity of these tests is compared in **Table 33.15**.

B. Serological Tests

These are primarily of two types:

- Non-treponemal tests (NTTs)
- Treponemal tests (TTs)

A comparison of NTT and TT is given in **Table 33.16**.

TABLE 33.15: Sensitivity of the methods for direct detection of *T. pallidum*

Method	Material examined	Minimum number of organisms present	Sensitivity (%)
Dark field microscopy	5 μL exudate	50	73–78
Direct fluorescent antibody test for *T. pallidum* (body fluids)	5 μL exudate	50	73–100
Direct fluorescent antibody tissue test for *T. pallidum* (tissues)	Tissue	50	86–88
PCR-DNA	5 μL exudate	1–10	100
RT-PCR	1 μL	1	100

TABLE 33.16: Comparison of non-treponemal and treponemal tests

Non-treponemal tests	Treponemal tests
Lipoidal antigens	*T. pallidum*-specific antigen
May be non-reactive (early infection and late stages of disease)	Reactive earlier than non-treponemal tests
Non-reactive after treatment of early infection	Remain positive for life (even after treatment)
Non-specific	Specific
Easy to perform	Difficult
Cheap	Expensive
Useful in screening and monitoring	Useful in confirmation of diagnosis

a. *Nontreponemal Serologic Tests*

Nontreponemal tests (NTTs) are rapid, simple and inexpensive. They can be used to monitor disease after treatment and to detect reinfection as they are quantitative tests. Their limitations include reduced sensitivity in primary syphilis and late latent syphilis, biological false-positive results and prozone phenomenon causing false-negative results.

1. VDRL—microflocculation, read under microscope, the only NTT that can be used on CSF
2. RPR—macroscopic flocculation
   a. TRUST—macroscopic flocculation
   b. USR—microflocculation, read under microscope
3. Indirect ELISA

1. **Venereal disease research laboratory (VDRL) test:**
   - Special slide with depressions of 14 mm diameter each
   - **0.05 mL of inactivated serum** (at 56°C for 30 min) is taken on a slide to which one drop of **freshly prepared cardiolipin antigen is added.**
   - The slide is then **rotated at 180 revolutions per minute** for 4 minutes and **examined under low power objective of microscope.**

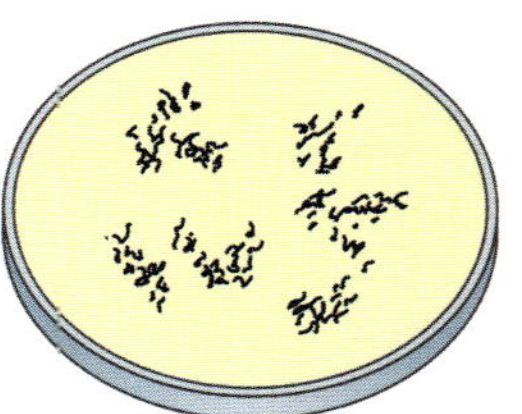

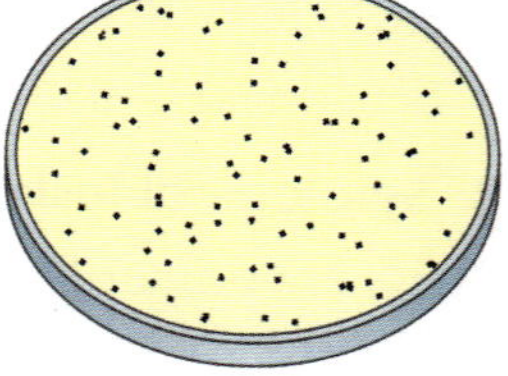

Fig. 33.21: Interpretation of VDRL in syphilis

   - **Presence of clumps signifies positive reaction (flocculation)** while uniformly distributed crystals indicate a negative reaction **(Fig. 33.21).**
   - If the test is **positive, it is quantitated** by performing the test with serial dilutions.

CSF VDRL

Quantitative VDRL is the test of choice on CSF specimens.

- The antigen is diluted in equal volumes with 10% saline.
- **CSF must not be heated (or inactivated)**
- Volume of antigen solution taken is 0.01 mL
- Rotation time is 8 minutes
- Results of VDRL are both qualitative and quantitative:
  - Medium or large clumps: Reactive

  - Small clumps: Weakly reactive
  - No clumping or slight roughness: Nonreactive
- Samples exhibiting any degree of reactivity should be quantitated.
- **Serial 2-fold dilutions** of the samples are prepared in 0.9% saline.
- Reported as: **Highest dilution giving a reactive result**.

2. **Rapid plasma reagin (RPR) test:** Performed on plastic coated cards onto which 18 mm circles have been imprinted. Undiluted serum + stabilized antigen preparation + charcoal particles, mixed within the card. Rotated at 100 rpm × 8 minutes. Flocculation of charcoal particles: Positive result
   Variations of RPR and VDRL:
   - **TRUST (toluidine red unheated serum test):** Better visualization
   - **USR (unheated serum reagin test):** Stabilized VDRL antigen
3. **Indirect ELISA:** Non-treponemal antibody test
   - VDRL antigen coats the wells of microtitre plates
   - Patient serum added (NT Ab attaches to the antigen)
   - Anti-human Ig conjugate labelled with enzyme is added:
     - At a specified time, stop solution added
     - Results read spectrophotometrically

Interpretation of Non-treponemal Tests

- Become reactive: **4–5 weeks after infection**
- **100% sensitivity** by approx. **12 weeks**
- A presumptive diagnosis is based on the presence of typical rash and reactive non-treponemal tests in a titer ≥1:8 in a patient with no previous history of syphilis.
- If history of syphilis is present, then the criteria should be a **4-fold** rise in titer. (A 4-fold change in titer, equivalent to a change of two dilutions (e.g. from 1:16 to 1:4 or from 1:8 to 1:32) is considered necessary to demonstrate a clinically significant difference.)
- High titres **(>1:16)** usually indicates **active infection**.
- Effect of **treatment:**
  a. For **primary syphilis:**
     - **Non-reactive in 60% by 4 months**
     - **Non-reactive in all patients by 12 months**
  b. For **secondary syphilis**: Non-reactive **12–24 months** after treatment.
  c. Latent syphilis (after treatment in **early latent stage):** May remain **reactive in low titers for up to 5 years** or longer. Late latent syphilis may have non-reactive test results, even without a history of treatment.
- **Serofast:** When a non-treponemal serological test shows persistent reactivity with no signs of decline in titer at 6 months after adequate therapy or fails to show a 4-fold decrease of an initial high titer within a year, it is considered a **seroresistance (serofast)**.
- **Treatment failure:** Patients with prior treatment and higher (but unchanged) non-treponemal titer are considered treatment failures unless there is clinical suspicion for reinfection.
- **Prozone phenomenon:** In a small percent of secondary syphilis cases, **very high antibody titers inhibit test reactivity**, producing a false-negative result, called the prozone phenomenon. To exclude the prozone phenomenon, the test must be repeated with diluted serum.

- **Biological false positivity:** Constitute 1–2% of all reactive non-treponemal tests. Titers are mostly <1:8.
  - Acute (<6 months)
  - Chronic (>6 months)

b. *Treponemal Serologic Tests*

These tests measure antibody directed against *T. pallidum* antigens by particle agglutination, immunofluorescence, or enzyme immunoassay and variably detect IgG only or both IgM and IgG. These qualitative tests most often remain reactive for life, even after adequate treatment, but 15–25% of patients treated during the primary stage revert to being serologically non-reactive after 2–3 years. Treponemal antibody titers correlate poorly with disease activity, and they should not be used to assess treatment response. Treponemal tests (TTs) are used mainly as confirmatory tests after nontreponemal tests. They cannot differentiate venereal syphilis from endemic syphilis (yaws and pinta). More technically demanding and expensive.

Treponemal tests

1. *Treponema pallidum* immobilization test **(TPI)**
2. Fluorescent treponemal antibody absorption assay **(FTA-Abs)**
3. *Treponema pallidum* passive particle agglutination **(TP-PA)** test
4. *T. pallidum* haemagglutination test **(TPHA)** and **MHA-TP**
5. EIA
   - Captia™ syphilis G—IgG
   - Captia syphilis M—IgM
   - SpiroTek—highest sensitivity of all TTs, esp. in untreated primary syphilis, recommended by CDC as confirmatory test.
6. IgM antibody tests
7. Western blot
8. Rapid tests (POCTs)

1. ***Treponema pallidum* immobilization (TPI) test**
   - Antibody present in the serum of a syphilitic patient.
   - Immobilization of actively motile *T. pallidum* obtained from testes of a rabbit infected with syphilis.
   - Highly specific but expensive and technically demanding
   - Not done now
2. **Fluorescent treponemal antibody absorption test (FTA-Abs):** It utilizes the indirect fluorescent antibody technique, and the *T. pallidum* subspecies *pallidum* (Nichol's strain) serves as the antigen. Serum diluted 1:5 in sorbent (extract from cultures of non-pathogenic Reiter treponeme) to remove non-specific treponemal antibodies.

   Method
   - Antigen (glass slides) + sera with Ab + FITC labelled anti-human Ig
   - Look for fluorescence under fluorescent microscope

   Advantages
   - Maximum sensitivity in primary syphilis (IgM)
   - Sensitivity approaches 100%

Disadvantages

- Technically difficult
- No indication of activity of disease.

3. **Treponema pallidum hemagglutination test (TPHA)**
   - Antigen: Ultrasonicated material from Nichol's strain of *T. pallidum* adsorbed onto surface of formalinized tanned sheep RBCs.
   - SERA: Patient's sera diluted 1:5 in sorbent.

   Method
   1. Serum placed in microtiter plates
   2. Antigen coated sheep RBCs added
   3. Specific antitreponemal antibodies if present, agglutinate RBCs

   Advantages
   1. Easier to perform than FTA-Abs
   2. Suitable for large number of samples

   Disadvantages
   1. Specificity same as VDRL, FTA-Abs
   2. Becomes positive a few days later than FTA-Abs.

   Modifications
   1. MHA-TP (micro-hemagglutination assay)—more cost effective
   2. Automated micro-hemagglutinization assay with *T. pallidum*
   3. Finger prick MHA-TP: Done in children
4. **Treponema pallidum passive particle agglutination (Tp-PA) test**
   - The test is a passive agglutination procedure based on the agglutination of gel particles sensitized with *T. pallidum* antigen by antibodies found in the patient's serum.
   - Smooth mat of agglutinated particles: +ve.
   - Compact button of agglutinated particles: –ve.
5. **ELISA:** It is recommended for screening.

   Antigen: Recombinant proteins:
   1. TmpA protein (membrane localized lipoprotein)
   2. Tmp B and Tmp C protein
   3. 47 kDa, 15.5 kDa, 17 kDa, 44.5 kDa protein

   Sensitivity shown to be similar/higher than TPHA in primary stage.

   Specificity and sensitivity in later stages need evaluation.

   Advantages
   - Capacity to process a large number of samples.
   - Automated reading—decreases manual error.
   - More useful in HIV-syphilis coinjection.

   Disadvantage: Time and cost—high if small number of samples.
6. **Western Blot**
   - Characteristic banding patterns
   - Uses recombinant antigens—47 kDa, 15.5 kDa, 17 kDa, 44.5 kDa protein
   - Reactive—antibodies to at least three of the four immunodeterminants
   - Highly specific and sensitive for syphilis.

7. **IgM antibody tests:** Detected within 2–3 weeks of infection. Indicator of active syphilis. May be useful in monitoring response to therapy.
   Does not cross placenta or blood–brain barrier, hence valuable in:
   - **Congenital syphilis**
   - **Reinfection**
   - **Early primary syphilis**
   - **Neurosyphilis**

   Sensitivity: S1—93%; S2—85%; Early latent—64%.
   i. **IgM FTA-Abs:**
      - Performed on serum
      - Poor sensitivity as:
        – ↑false-negative: Competitive binding of high titers of IgG
        – ↑false-positive: Autoantibodies in test sera.
   ii. **19S IgM FTA-Abs:**
      - 19S fragment of IgM
      - More sensitive and specific
      - But complicated and cumbersome
   iii. **IgM solid phase hemabsorption:**
      - Modification of TPHA
      - Simpler than IgM FTA-Abs and gives comparable results
   iv. **Captia™ Syphilis M:**
      - Detects 19S (IgM) against 37 kDa major axial filament
      - First serological test to become positive after infection
      - Highly specific
      - *Sensitivity*:
        – Congenital syphilis: 100%
        – Primary syphilis: 82%
        – Neurosyphilis: 34%
        – Treated syphilis: 11%

Sensitivity and Specificity of Serologic Tests

- Sensitivity of the non-treponemal tests is approximately 90%, up to 28% of patients with early primary syphilis will have non-reactive non-treponemal test results on the initial visit.
- Non-reactive non-treponemal tests seen in about 30% of cases of late untreated syphilis.
- Specificity for the non-treponemal tests is 98%.
- The overall sensitivity (about 98%) of the FTA-Abs test is greater than that of the other major treponemal tests.
- Approximately 20 to 30% of patients presenting with a chancre have been reported to have a non-reactive NTT for syphilis. Although TTs may or may not show a positive result in this setting, they are generally considered more sensitive than NTTs.
- The fluorescent treponemal antibody absorption (FTA-Abs) is thought to be most sensitive in primary syphilis (sensitivity of 98.2% versus 92.7% for RPR and 72.5% for VDRL test). The sensitivity of the enzyme immunoassay (EIA) is comparable to the FTA-Abs.

- If there is a high clinical suspicion for early syphilis, repeat serologic testing at a later time point (e.g. 2–4 weeks later) may be diagnostic. Presumptive therapy, rather than waiting for the results of additional testing, is appropriate in patients at high risk for syphilis.

The different tests have varying rates of positivity that are depicted in **Fig. 33.22**.

An overview of the interpretation of serological tests is given in **Tables 33.17** and **33.18**.

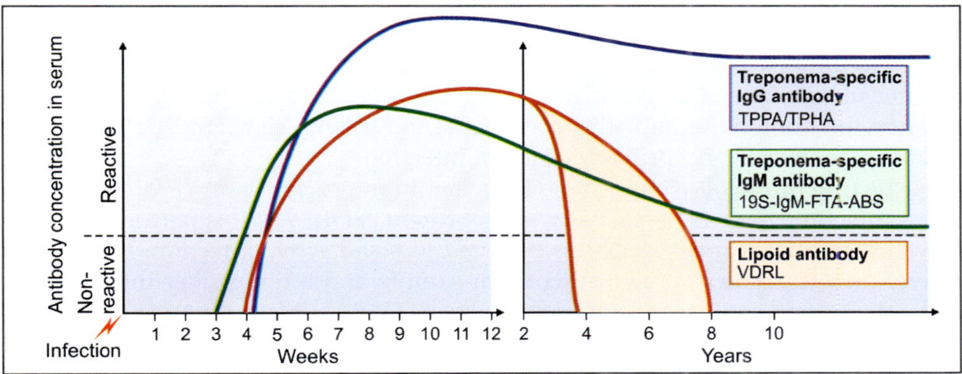

Fig. 33.22: A depiction of the positivity of serological tests depending on the time from the infective dose

TABLE 33.17: Sensitivity and specificity of tests in untreated case of syphilis (Seña AC, 2010)

Test	Primary	Secondary	Latent	Late	Specificity %
VDRL	78	100	95	71	98
RPR	86	100	98	73	98
FTA-Abs*	84	100	100	96	97
TP-PA	88 (86–100)	100	100	NA	96
ELISA (IgG)	100	100	100	NA	100

*FTA-Abs and TP-PA are generally considered equally sensitive in the primary stage of disease.

TABLE 33.18: Interpretation of serological tests

Treponemal	Nontreponemal	
Positive	Positive	Definitive diagnosis of syphilis
Negative	Positive	False positive NTT
Positive	Negative	• History of successfully treated syphilis • Very early untreated syphilis • Late syphilis • False positive TT (endemic treponematoses) Use a second treponemal test
Negative	Negative	• No syphilis • Very early syphilis (before seroconversion)

A reactive nontreponemal test with a reactive treponemal test gives a positive predictive value of approximately 97%, or only a 3% error factor. In contrast, if any one test is used, the positive predictive value, regardless of the method, is less than 50% in a low-prevalence setting.

Serology Testing Protocol

a. **Traditional method**—VDRL/RPR and if positive in significant titre ≥1:16, then perform EIA/TPPA for confirmation. If both are negative it rules out syphilis, except if there is a high clinical suspicion for syphilis where repeat serologic testing should be performed in 2–4 weeks **(Fig. 33.23)**.

   Major limitations with using a non-treponemal test for initial screening include the personnel time required to perform a labor-intensive test, biologic false positives (i.e. pregnancy, medication use, and other conditions) and, as with all diagnostic tests for syphilis, the inability to detect early primary or latent infection.

b. **<u>Reverse testing protocol</u>**—first EIA or CIA (chemiluminescent assay) is done. Positive EIA signifies infection, but can be past as well as present. VDRL/RPR is performed, and if it is positive in significant titre (titer), it is believed to be an active infection. If VDRL/RPR is negative, then it is taken to be a discordant sample and a tie-breaker third test is taken (CDC)—the second confirmatory treponemal test (TP-PA). If found positive and there is no history of prior, treated syphilis, the patient is diagnosed with syphilis **(Fig. 33.24)**.
   - If the patient has received prior treatment for syphilis and has no evidence (by history or examination) of recent infection with *T. pallidum*, then the patient does not require further evaluation or management (Workowski KA, 2015).
   - Patients without prior treatment and no evidence of recent infection are considered to have latent syphilis and require further evaluation and treatment.
   - If recent infection possibly occurred, then repeat nontreponemal testing should take place 2–3 weeks later; if this repeat testing is positive the patient likely has early syphilis and if the test is negative then further evaluation is usually not needed.

   Summary: This protocol is ideal for very early syphilis, those with prior treated syphilis, and those with late or late latent syphilis whose nontreponemal test has become non-reactive over time. Most false negative non-treponemal results occur when the test is performed prior to the development of humoral antibodies.

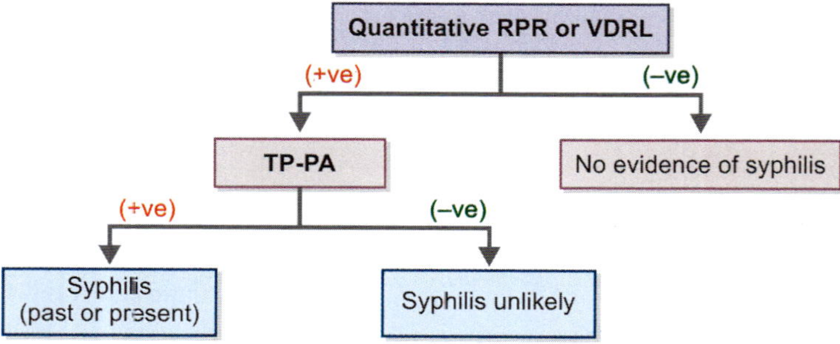

Fig. 33.23: Syphilis serologic screening—traditional sequence algorithm. The traditional (standard) serologic screening sequence algorithm uses a quantitative non-treponemal test (RPR or VDRL) for screening followed by a treponemal test for confirmation of positive screening tests.
(RPR, rapid plasma reagin; VDRL, venereal disease research laboratory; TP-PA, *Treponema pallidum* particle agglutination).

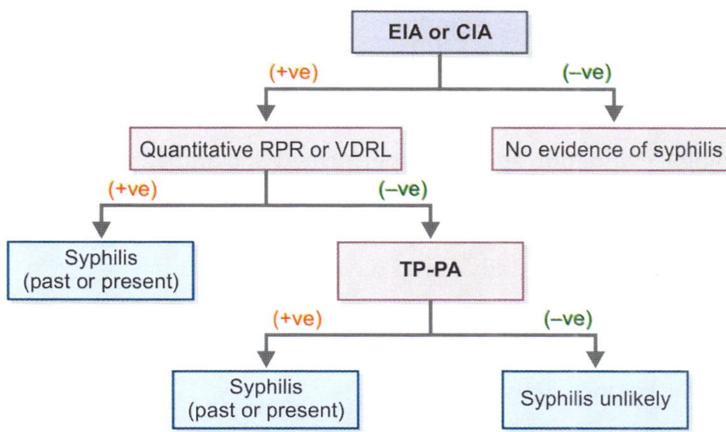

Fig. 33.24: Syphilis serologic screening—reverse sequence algorithm. The reverse serologic screening algorithm uses an initial treponemal test for screening, followed by a nontreponemal test confirmation. A specimen with reactive EIA/CIA results should be tested reflexively with a quantitative non-treponemal test (RPR or VDRL). (EIA, enzyme immunassay; CIA, chemiluminescent immunoassay)

C. Histopathology

The fundamental pathologic changes in syphilis are:
a. Swelling and proliferation of endothelial cells.
b. Perivascular infiltrate of lymphoid cells and often of **plasma** cells.
c. Granulomatous infiltrates: In secondary and tertiary syphilis.

D. Animal Infectivity Testing

This is rarely done nowadays, and is utilized mainly for experimental purposes.

Rabbit is the most practical option because of the following reasons:

- Local lesion at site of inoculation
- Tissues remain infective for life of animal
- Infection can be transferred from one animal to another
- Serological tests of syphilis become reactive.

Disadvantages:

- Technically demanding
- Expensive
- Up to 90 days to obtain a result
- Suitable only for research

Other options include chimpanzee and hamsters.

TREATMENT (CDC 2021)

1. Primary and Secondary Syphilis

Benzathine penicillin G, 2.4 million units IM in a single dose.

All persons who have primary and secondary syphilis should be tested for HIV infection and in areas with a high prevalence of HIV, persons who have primary or secondary syphilis should be retested in 3 months if the first HIV test result was negative.

Persons who have syphilis and symptoms or signs suggesting neurologic disease or ophthalmic disease should have an evaluation that includes CSF analysis, ocular slit-lamp and ophthalmologic examination, and auditory examination.

Follow-up

Clinical and serologic evaluation should be performed at 6 and 12 months after treatment.

Penicillin Allergy

In non-pregnant, penicillin-allergic persons who have primary or secondary syphilis:

Doxycycline 100 mg orally twice daily for 14 days

OR

Tetracycline (500 mg four times daily for 14 days)

OR

Ceftriaxone 1 g IM or IV once daily for 10 days.

2. Early Latent Syphilis and Late Latent Syphilis

Recommended regimens for adults

Early latent syphilis
Benzathine penicillin G 2.4 million units IM in a single dose.
Late latent syphilis or latent syphilis of unknown duration
Benzathine penicillin G, 7.2 million units total, administered as 3 doses of 2.4 million units IM each at 1-week intervals.

Follow-up

Quantitative non-treponemal serologic tests should be repeated at 6, 12, and 24 months. A CSF examination should be performed if:

1. A sustained (>2 weeks) 4-fold increase or greater in titer is observed,
2. An initially high titer (≥1:32) fails to decline at least 4-fold within 12–24 months of therapy, or
3. Signs or symptoms attributable to syphilis developed. In such circumstances, patients with CSF abnormalities should be treated for neurosyphilis. If the CSF examination is negative, retreatment for latent syphilis should be administered.

3. Tertiary Syphilis

a. *Normal CSF examination*:

Recommended regimen

Benzathine penicillin G, 7.2 million units total, administered as 3 doses of 2.4 million units IM each at 1-week intervals.

b. *Neurosyphilis/ocular syphilis/otosyphilis:*

Aqueous crystalline penicillin 3–4 MU IV—every 4 hours × 10–14 days (total of 18–24 MU/day)
Alternative: Procaine penicillin PLUS probenecid
Penicillin allergic: IV/IM ceftriaxone 2 g daily × 14 days

It is important to note that some experts believe the duration of neurosyphilis therapy is not sufficient for treatment of late latent syphilis. Therefore, intramuscular benzathine penicillin G, 2.4 million units once per week for up to 3 weeks can be considered after completion of a neurosyphilis regimen in order to provide a comparable total duration of therapy.

4. HIV Infection and Syphilis

Primary, secondary and early latent syphilis among persons with HIV infection.

Benzathine penicillin G, 2.4 million units IM in a single dose.

Late latent syphilis with HIV infection

Benzathine penicillin G at weekly doses of 2.4 million units for 3 weeks.

Follow-up

Persons with HIV infection and primary or secondary syphilis should be evaluated clinically and serologically for treatment failure at 3, 6, 9, 12, and 24 months after therapy; those who meet the criteria for treatment failure (i.e. signs or symptoms that persist or recur or persons who have a sustained (>2 weeks) 4-fold increase or greater in titer) should be managed in the same manner as HIV-negative patients (i.e. a CSF examination and retreatment guided by CSF findings).

In addition, **CSF examination** and **retreatment** can be considered for persons whose non-treponemal test titers do not decrease 4-fold within 12–24 months of therapy. Also if CD4 count <350/µL and (RPR >1:32).

5. Pregnancy and Syphilis

Some evidence suggests that additional therapy is beneficial for pregnant women. For women who have primary, secondary, or early latent syphilis, a **second dose** of benzathine penicillin 2.4 million units IM can be administered 1 week after the initial dose.

- When syphilis is diagnosed during the second half of pregnancy, management should include a sonographic fetal evaluation for congenital syphilis.
- At a minimum, serologic titers should be repeated at 28–32 weeks gestation and at delivery.
- Pregnant women who have a history of penicillin allergy should be desensitized and treated with penicillin.

6. Congenital Syphilis

a. Scenario 1: Congenital syphilis proven or highly probable

Any neonate with

- abnormal clinical examination consistent with congenital syphilis;
- serum NTT titer ≥4-fold greater than the mother's titer at delivery; or
- a positive DGI/PCR of placenta, cord, lesions or body fluids or a positive silver stain of placenta cord.

Recommended regimens:

Aqueous crystalline penicillin G, 100,000–150,000 units/kg/day, administered as 50,000 units/kg/dose IV every 12 hours during the first 7 days of life and every 8 hours thereafter for a total of 10 days.

OR

Procaine penicillin G, 50,000 units/kg/dose IM in a single daily dose for 10 days.

b. Scenario 2: Possible congenital syphilis

Any neonate with normal clinical examination and serum NTT titer ≤4-fold of the maternal titer at delivery PLUS one of the following:

- Mother was not treated/inadequately treated/no documentation available.
- Mother was treated with erythromycin or non-penicillin G regimen.
- Mother was treated <30 days before delivery.

Aqueous crystalline penicillin G, 100,000–150,000 units/kg/day, administered as 50,000 units/kg/dose IV every 12 hours during the first 7 days of life and every 8 hours thereafter for a total of 10 days.

OR

Procaine penicillin G, 50,000 units/kg/dose IM in a single daily dose for 10 days.
Benzathine penicillin G 50,000 units/kg body weight/dose IM single dose.

c. Scenario 3: Congenital syphilis less likely

Any neonate who has a normal physical examination and a serum quantitative non-treponemal serologic titer equal to or less than 4-fold the maternal titer and both of the following are true:

1. Mother was treated during pregnancy, treatment was appropriate for the stage of infection, and treatment was administered >4 weeks before delivery and
2. Mother has no evidence of reinfection or relapse.

***Recommended regimen*:**

Benzathine penicillin G, 50,000 units/kg/dose IM in a single dose.

d. Scenario 4: Congenital syphilis unlikely

Any neonate who has a normal physical examination and a serum quantitative non-treponemal serologic titer equal to or less than 4-fold the maternal titer and both of the following are true:

1. Mother's treatment was adequate before pregnancy and
2. Mother's non-treponemal serologic titer remained low and stable (i.e. serofast) before and during pregnancy and at delivery (VDRL <1:2; RPR <1:4).

***Recommended regimen*:**

No treatment is required, but infants with reactive non-treponemal tests should be followed serologically to ensure the non-treponemal test returns to negative. Benzathine penicillin G 50,000 U/kg as a single 1 M dose might be considered if follow-up is uncertain and the neonate has a reactive NTT.

Follow-up

All neonates with *reactive non-treponemal tests* should receive follow-up examinations and serologic testing (i.e. a non-treponemal test) every 2–3 months until the test becomes non-reactive.

In the neonate who was not treated because congenital syphilis was considered less likely or unlikely, nontreponemal antibody titers should decline by *age 3 months* and be non-reactive by age *6 months*, indicating that the reactive test result was caused by passive transfer of maternal IgG antibody.

7. Special Considerations

Penicillin Allergy

Infants and children who require treatment for congenital syphilis but who have a history of penicillin allergy or develop an allergic reaction presumed secondary to penicillin should be desensitized and then treated with penicillin.

Jarisch–Herxheimer Reaction

An acute febrile reaction to endotoxin like products released by *T. pallidum* on treatment.

- Clinical features—headache, myalgia, fever and a transiently increased prominence of lesions within the first 24 hours after the initiation of any therapy.
- The onset is within 4–6 hours after treatment, and it subsides within 24 hours.
- Jarisch-Herxheimer reactions are not an indication for discontinution of treatment.
- It occurs most frequently among persons who have early syphilis, presumably because bacterial burdens are higher during these stages.
- Also seen in other spirochete infections—Lyme disease, relapsing fever, leptospirosis, etc.
- Treat with oral NSAIDs and oral/IV prednisiolone.

Hoigne's reaction

Pseudoanaphylactic/pseudoallergic reaction after accidental IV injection of procaine penicillin G.

- Occurs due to vascular occlusion and embolization of the vessels by the large crystals.
- Clinical features—severe agitation, mental confusion, visual and auditory hallucinations and fear of impending death.
- Differentiate from penicillin anaphylactic reaction by a negative oral challenge test with penicillin.

Missed dose

Clinical experience suggests that an interval of 10–14 days between doses for late latent syphilis (or latent syphilis with unknown duration) might be acceptable, the pharmacokinetic profile of benzathine penicillin G suggests an interval of 7–9 days between doses would be optimal. Clinicians have differing practices within these limitations, but treatments with intervals greater than 14 days should always be restarted and pregnant women should repeat the full course if any doses are missed.

8. Management of Sex Partners

- Persons who have had sexual contact with a person who receives a diagnosis of primary, secondary, or early latent syphilis within **90 days** preceding the diagnosis should be treated presumptively for early syphilis, even if serologic test results are negative.
- Persons who have had sexual contact with a person who receives a diagnosis of primary, secondary, or early latent syphilis >90 days before the diagnosis should be treated presumptively for early syphilis if serologic test results are not immediately available and the opportunity for follow-up is uncertain. If serologic tests are negative, no treatment is needed. If serologic tests are positive, treatment should be based on clinical and serologic evaluation and stage of syphilis.

Treatment Failure

A key reason for close follow-up of patients treated for syphilis is to monitor signs, symptoms, or serologic changes that indicate possible treatment failure. Treatment failure cannot usually be differentiated from reinfection and thus persons suspected to have treatment failure or reinfection should be retested for HIV and should have a CSF evaluation for neurosyphilis (regardless of symptoms or prior CSF findings). Clues to probable treatment failure or reinfection include the following:

- A patient has **persistent or recurring** signs or symptoms.
- Repeat testing shows **sustained 4-fold increase in non-treponemal titer**. These patients should be retreated and re-evaluated for HIV infection. Because treatment failure may be a result of unrecognized central nervous system (CNS) infection, CSF examination should be considered.
- Failure of non-treponemal titers to **decline 4-fold** within 12 months after therapy for primary or secondary syphilis may be indicative of treatment failure. However, **15–20%** of persons with primary and secondary syphilis treated with the recommended regimen will not achieve the 4-fold decline in nontreponemal titer used to define response at **1 year** after treatment. Additional clinical and serological follow-up is necessary since the optimal management is unclear. Examination of CSF can be considered in these instances. If follow-up cannot be ensured, retreatment is recommended.

Management

When patients are retreated for primary, secondary, or latent syphilis (assuming no evidence of neurosyphilis), the recommended regimen is weekly intramuscular injections of benzathine penicillin G, 2.4 million units for **3 weeks**. If neurosyphilis is diagnosed, aqueous crystalline penicillin G, 18–24 million units per day is given as 3–4 million units IV every 4 hours (or as continuous infusion), for a total of 10–14 days.

CHANCROID

- Chancroid (soft chancre/ulcus molle)—causes by *Haemophilus ducreyi*—a gram-negative coccobacillus (virulence factors—cytolethal distending toxin (CDT) and haemolysin).
- Largely confined to resource-poor and developing countries, and contributes significantly to HIV acquisition.

Risk Factors

- Developing nations and resource poor regions.
- High risk groups such as MSM or CSWs and their contacts.
- Low socioeconomic status.
- Lack of circumcision.
- Exchange of drugs for sex and illicit drug use.

Clinical Features

- Incubation period: 1–14 days.
- Erythematous papule (24 hours) may resolve or → pustule within 3–5 days → ulcerate in 1–2 weeks → painful ulcers. **The estimated bacterial dose required to initiate infection is as few as 1–2 colony-forming units**.
- Single or multiple, **painful, well-circumscribed**, deep ulcers, **non-indurated with ragged** undermined margins and may **bleed to touch. The floor is covered with** foul smelling, yellowish-gray **purulent necrotic slough (Fig. 33.25)**.
- **Inguinal lymphadenopathy (bubo)—unilateral or bilateral, unilocular**, suppurative, painful swellings in 10–40%. They may rupture leading to single sinus formation, or may ulcerate to form a chancroidal ulcer.

Types of Chancroid (Fig. 33.26)

1. **Giant chancroid:** It extends rapidly and covers a large area; spread to the suprapubic region or the thigh via autoinoculation and may lead to the formation of a serpiginous ulcer.
2. **Dwarf:** Small irregular ulcer that may mimic herpetic ulcers.
3. **Papular:** An ulcer with elevated edges; may mimic chancre of primary syphilis.

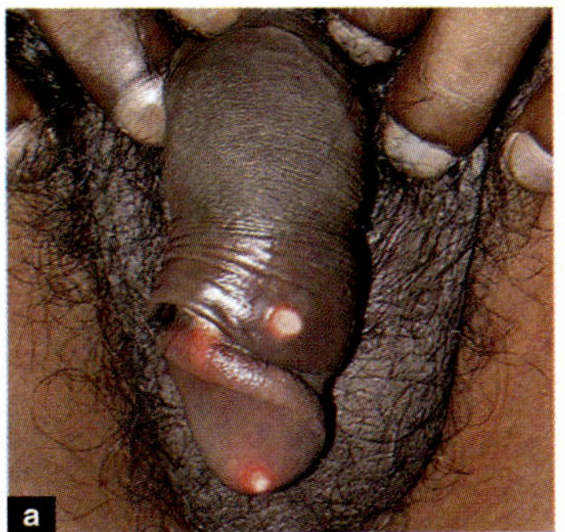

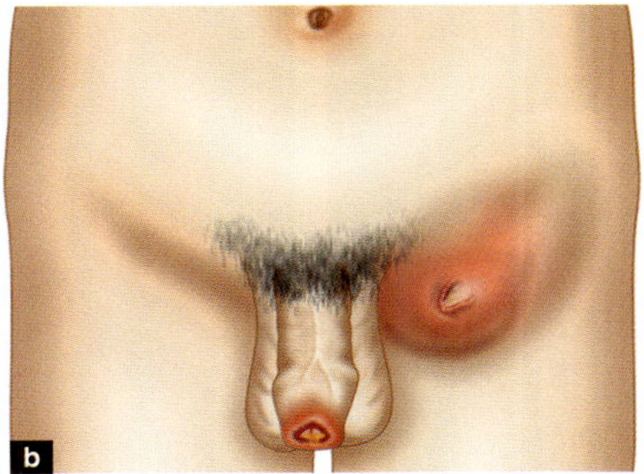

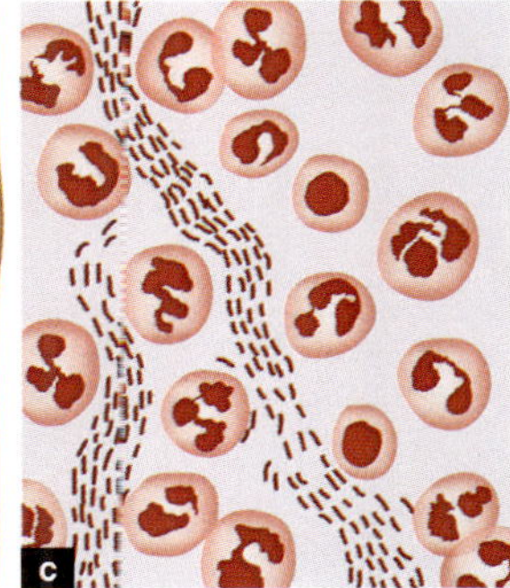

Fig. 33.25: Chancroid: (a) Painful multiple ulcers, necrotic base, with a red halo, bleeding on touch; (b) A depiction of the bubo that is classically unilateral, painful and unilocular; (c) A depiction of the gram-negative coccobacilli arranged in a linear 'school of fish' pattern

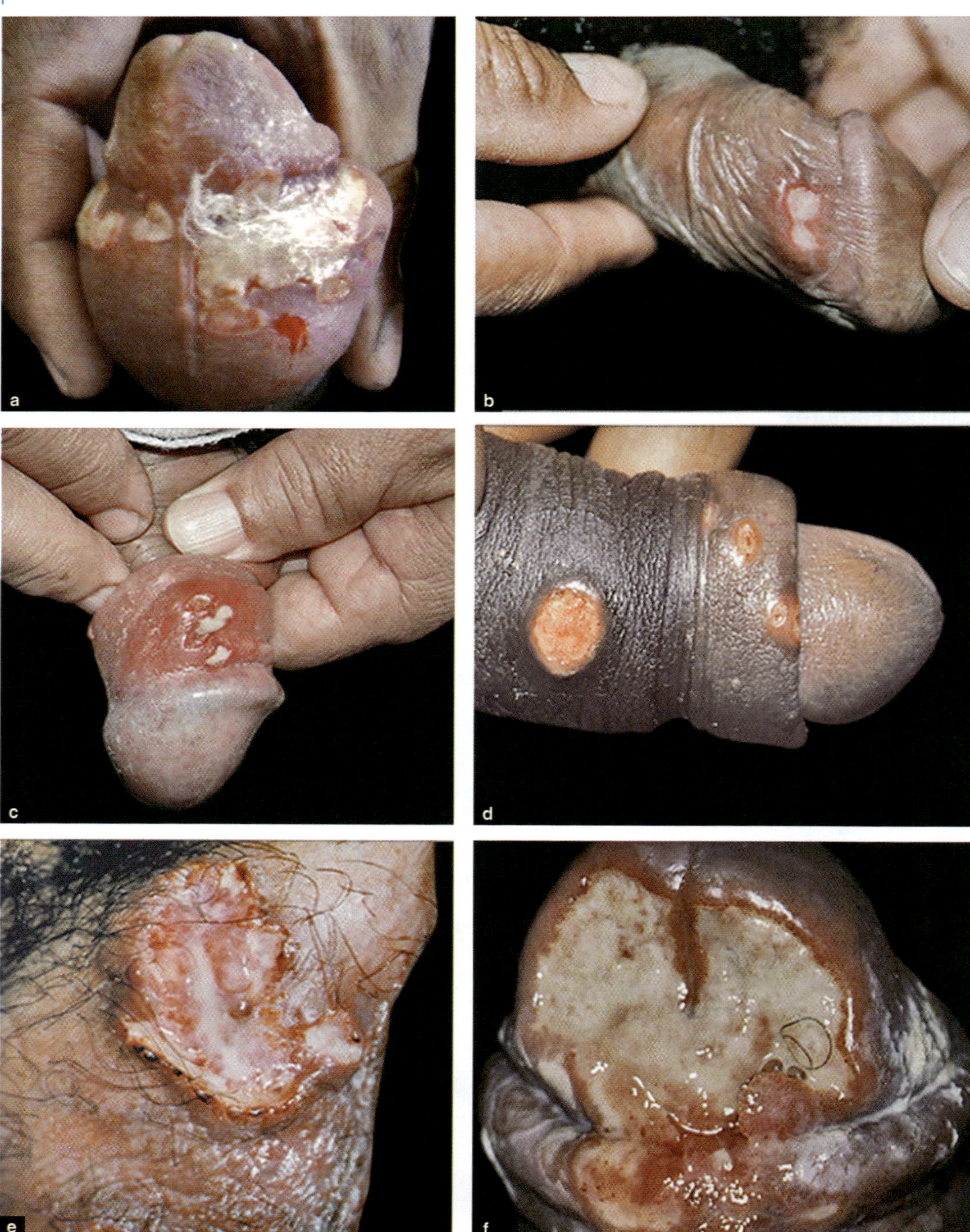

Fig. 33.26: (a) Large, deep, necrotic ulcers in chancroid; (b to f) A series of ulcers with characteristic deep necrotic floor seen in chancroid

4. **Transient:** It rapidly resolves and is transient; closely resembles LGV.
5. **Phagedenic:** It may start as a small lesion, but eventually becomes large and destructive (due to superinfection with fusospirochetes).
6. **Follicular:** These are superficial pustular lesions, which originate in the hair follicles and may resemble folliculity initially, but later tend to ulcerate.

According to CDC 2015 guidelines, a **probable diagnosis** of chancroid can be made if all of the following criteria are met:

1. The patient has one or more painful genital ulcers.
2. The clinical presentation, appearance of genital ulcers and, if present, regional lymphadenopathy are typical for chancroid.
3. The patient has no evidence of *T. pallidum* infection by dark field examination of ulcer exudate or by a serologic test for syphilis performed at least 7 days after onset of ulcers.
4. An HSV PCR test or HSV culture performed on the ulcer exudate is negative.

Most common sites

- Males—prepuce, frenulum, coronal sulcus, penile shaft.
- Females—vaginal entrance.
- Kissing ulcers can form on the lips of the labia majora.

Differential Diagnosis

- Chancroid must be differentiated from syphilis and genital herpes, which coexist with *H. ducreyi* in about 17.6% of chancroid cases. In contrast to syphilis, the ulcers of chancroid are more **tender** and, in contrast to genital herpes, they tend to be **deeper** and **not grouped (Fig. 33.27)**. However, only about **one-third** of genital ulcers are **classical** in appearance.

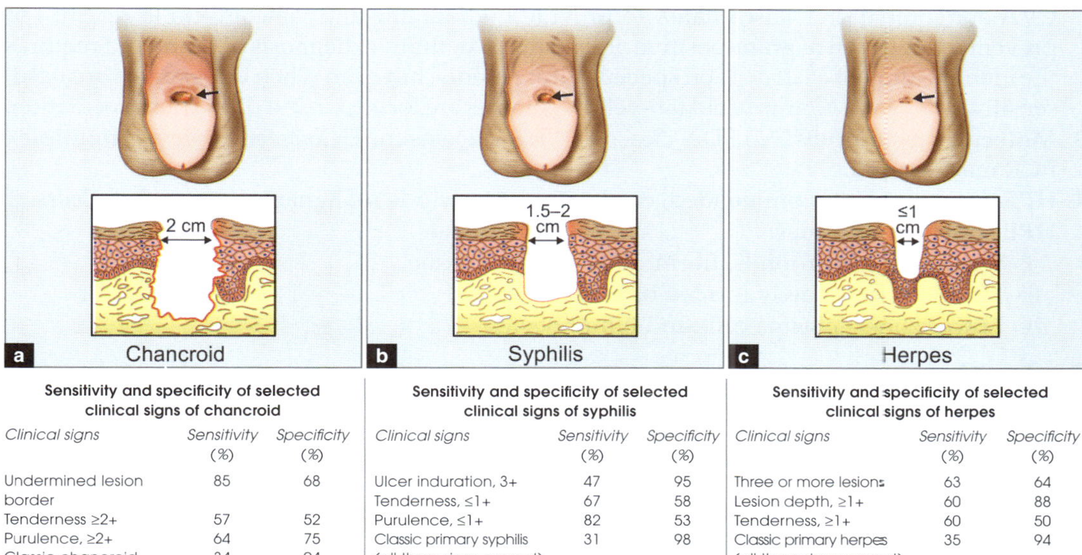

Sensitivity and specificity of selected clinical signs of chancroid

Clinical signs	Sensitivity (%)	Specificity (%)
Undermined lesion border	85	68
Tenderness ≥2+	57	52
Purulence, ≥2+	64	75
Classic chancroid (all three signs present)	34	94

Sensitivity and specificity of selected clinical signs of syphilis

Clinical signs	Sensitivity (%)	Specificity (%)
Ulcer induration, 3+	47	95
Tenderness, ≤1+	67	58
Purulence, ≤1+	82	53
Classic primary syphilis (all three signs present)	31	98

Sensitivity and specificity of selected clinical signs of herpes

Clinical signs	Sensitivity (%)	Specificity (%)
Three or more lesions	63	64
Lesion depth, ≥1+	60	88
Tenderness, ≥1+	60	50
Classic primary herpes (all three signs present)	35	94

Fig. 33.27: Sensitivity and specificity of a clinical diagnosis of genital ulcer disease based on selected clinical signs. (a) Chancroid; (b) Syphilis; (c) Genital herpes (DiCario RP, 1997)

- LGV may need to be differentiated from chancroid, particularly when lymphadenopathy is the prominent feature of the clinical presentation. The ulcer associated with LGV is transitory and precedes the appearance of lymphadenopathy.
- Donovanosis (granuloma inguinale), though causing destructive lesions in the genital area, is usually not associated with acute, painful ulcerations or lymphadenopathy.
- Traumatic lesion with secondary infection.

A dark field examination of the lesion, a serologic test for syphilis and a follow-up serologic test for syphilis should be performed, as therapy for chancroid does not treat syphilis.

Complications

Phimosis, paraphimosis, scar, fibrosis, contracture, fistula, phagedenic ulceration.

Diagnosis

Microscopy of exudates and antigen detection are neither sensitive nor specific enough to be clinically useful. Serology is only useful for prevalence studies. Culture and PCR-based tests are the cornerstones of diagnostic testing.

1. **Microscopy:** Swab from the ulcer base or an aspirate from the lymph node taken using a wide bore needle through healthy tissue. Gram stain from the exudate or an aspirate obtained from the bubo shows gram-negative coccobacilli in a typical **Railroad or School of fish appearance (Fig. 33.25c)**. This pattern occurs due to a tight intercellular adherence. Sensitivity 40–60%.
2. **Culture:** Cultures are obtained by swabbing the floor of the ulcer vigorously with a dry or moist cotton swab that becomes saturated with pus, which is immediately inoculated on the plates. Culture media—2 plates, one containing gonococcal agar base, 2% bovine hemoglobin, and 5% fetal calf serum (GC-HgS), the other containing Müller-Hinton agar base with 5% chocolated horse blood (MH-HB). These media are supplemented with 1% CVA enrichment or 1% IsoVitaleX to provide L-glutamine and vancomycin (3 µg/mL) to prevent overgrowth of gram-positive organisms. A definitive diagnosis of chancroid requires the identification of *H. ducreyi* on special culture media; but even when these media are used, sensitivity is <80%. Non-mucoid tan-yellow colonies are formed in 2–4 days after in oculation.
3. **Molecular techniques:** No FDA-cleared PCR test exists for *H. ducreyi*, however, multiplex PCR may be used.
4. **HPE**—not usually recommended, can be done to exclude malignancy in atypical ulcers.
   HPE shows three zones:
   i. Top zone—neutrophils, fibrin, RBC, necrotic tissue
   ii. Middle zone—newly formed blood vessels
   iii. Lower zone—plasma cells and lymphocytes

Treatment

Recommended Regimen (CDC 2021)

Azithromycin 1 g orally in a single dose
OR
Ceftriaxone 250 mg IM in a single dose
OR
Ciprofloxacin 500 mg orally twice a day for 3 days
OR
Erythromycin base 500 mg orally three times a day for 7 days

33

Follow-up

- Patient should be re-evaluated 3–7 days after initiation of therapy.
- Ulcers tend to improve symptomatically within **3 days** and objectively within **7 days** after successful therapy.
- Slower healing (>2 weeks) generally occurs in case of large ulcers and in case of uncircumcised men who have ulcers under the foreskin.
- If no clinical improvement is evident, the clinician must consider whether: 1. the diagnosis is correct, 2. the patient is coinfected with another STD, 3. the patient is infected with HIV, 4. the treatment was not used as instructed, or 5. the *H. ducreyi* strain causing the infection is resistant to the prescribed antimicrobial.
- Clinical resolution of fluctuant lymphadenopathy is even slower and may necessitate needle aspiration or incision and drainage from a non-dependent site. Although needle aspiration of buboes is a simpler procedure, incision and drainage might be preferred because of reduced need for subsequent drainage procedures.

HIV and Chancroid

HIV may alter the clinical presentation as given in **Table 33.19**.

TABLE 33.19: Effect of HIV on chancroid

Feature	Effect
Morphology	Longer ulcer duration, greater number of ulcers, necrotizing form, multilocular buboes, size unaffected
Atypical sites	Legs and digits
Course	Increased severity, slow healing and treatment failure
Investigations	Gram-stained smear, culture, biopsy and negative laboratory evaluation for *Treponema pallidum* and HSV

Pregnancy and Chancroid

There is no adverse effect on pregnancy outcome and pregnant females with chancroid can be treated with azithromycin 1 g single dose or a single dose injection ceftriazone 250 mg given intramuscularly or erythromycin 500 mg thrice a day for 7 days.

Doxycycline and sulphonamides are to be avoided during breastfeeding.

DONOVANOSIS (GRANULOMA INGUINALE/GRANULOMA VENEREUM/ULCERATING GRANULOMA OF PUDENDA)

Cause: ***Klebsiella granulomatis*** (formerly known as ***Calymmatobacterium granulomatis***)

Characterized by single or multiple, rounded, elevated, velvety, painless, friable beefy red ulcers, which typically bleed to touch.

Pathogenesis

- The characteristic inclusion bodies known as **Donovan bodies**, first identified by Goldzieher and Peckin in tissue sections—inside large mononuclear cells—**pathognomonic**. Rupture of these cysts releases the infective organisms.
- Incubation period—variable (1–360 days, average IP-17 days).

Epidemiology

- Male-to-female ratio—>6:1.
- An association between donovanosis and HLA-B57.
- A preponderance among uncircumscised men has also been noted.
- In India, it is endemic along the east coast, i.e. Odisha, Andhra Pradesh and Tamil Nadu.

Clinical Features

Begins with a firm papule or subcutaneous nodule that undergoes ulceration **(Fig. 33.28)**.

Most common sites: Genitals (90%), inguinal region (10%)

- men—prepuce, coronal sulcus, frenulum, and glans penis
- women—the labia minora and fourchette.

Extragenital lesions such as those involving the lip, gums, cheek, palate, pharynx, neck, nose, larynx, and chest occur in up to 6% of cases, and are often unnoticeable.

Types of Donovanosis

1. **Ulcerogranulomatous**—most common—painless, fleshy, exuberant, single or multiple, beefy-red ulcers that bleed easily when touched.
2. **Hypertrophic or verrucous type**, an ulcer or growth with a raised, irregular edge, sometimes completely dry with a walnut-like appearance.
3. **Necrotic**—a deeply excavated, foul-smelling ulcer associated with tissue destruction (D/D—carcinoma penis).
4. **Sclerotic or cicatricial type**—associated with extensive fibrosis and scar tissue formation.

Lymphadenitis is an uncommon finding, although subcutaneous granulomatous lesions may be seen in the inguinoscrotal region as pseudobuboes.

Haematogenous spread—liver/bone (rare)

Table 33.20 lists the effect of HIV infection on donovanosis.

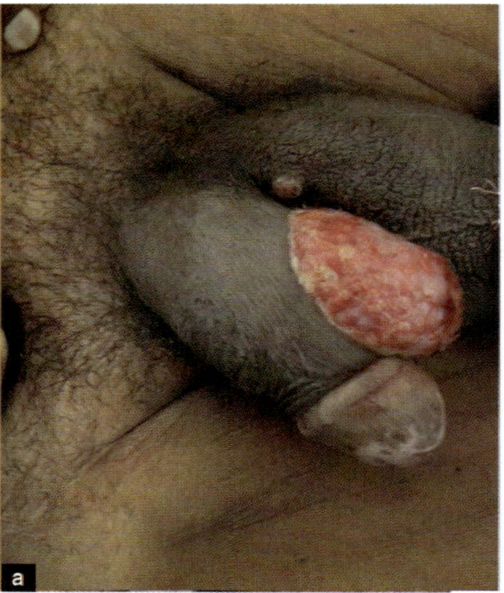

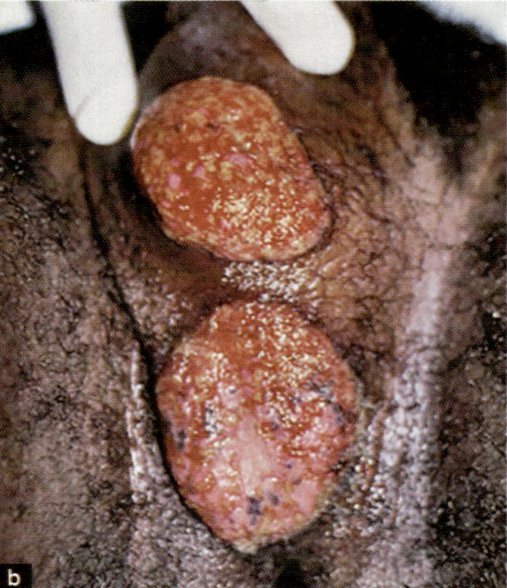

Fig. 33.28: Beefy red granulomatous ulcer of donovanosis

TABLE 33.20: Effect of HIV on donovanosis

Clinical features	Longer ulcer duration, greater tissue destruction
Atypical sites	Extragenital sites (chin)
Course	Increased severity, slow healing and treatment failure, may progress to SCC (case reports)

Differential Diagnosis

Syphilis, chronic HSV (pseudogranuloma herpeticum), amoebiasis, SCC.

Diagnosis

Klebsiella granulomatis—difficult to culture, and diagnosis requires visualization of dark-staining Donovan bodies on tissue crush preparation or biopsy.

- **Tissue smears:** Are considered to be the mainstay of diagnosis—usually by obtaining crush biopsy samples from the edges of lesions. The specimen is crushed between two slides and stained by the Leishman or Giemsa stains. Stains such as hematoxylin and eosin, Wright's and Papanicolaou may also be used. Donovan bodies are seen in 90% cases.
- **Histopathology:** Giemsa or silver stains are the most effective methods for visualizing the organisms in tissue sections. The characteristic histology shows chronic inflammatory infiltrate—**plasma cells** and neutrophils in the dermis. The epidermis may show surface ulceration and focal collections of polymorphonuclear leukocytes.
- **Serology:** Complement-fixation tests and indirect immunofluorescent technique have been utilized for the diagnosis of established lesions; but are not widely used.
- **Molecular methods:** Molecular techniques such as PCR are highly sensitive and specific. Multiplex-PCR is now available and can help detect mixed infections.

Treatment

Effective treatment halts the progression and leads to healing of the lesions, proceeding from the ulcer margins to the center, ultimately leading to re-epithelialization of the ulcers. If the treatment duration is inadequate, relapse can occur 6–18 months after apparently effective therapy.

Recommended Regimen (CDC 2021)

- **Azithromycin** 1 g orally once per week or 500 mg daily for at least 3 weeks and until all lesions have completely healed.

Alternative Regimens

- **Doxycycline** 100 mg orally twice a day for at least 3 weeks and until all lesions have completely healed.
- **Erythromycin** base 500 mg orally four times a day for at least 3 weeks and until all lesions have completely healed.
- **Trimethoprim-sulfamethoxazole** one double-strength (160 mg/800 mg) tablet orally twice a day for at least 3 weeks and until all lesions have completely healed.

Special Situations

Pregnant and lactating women—macrolide regimen (erythromycin or azithromycin).

Children with donovanosis should receive a short course of azithromycin 20 mg/kg.

Persons with both donovanosis and HIV infection should receive the same regimens as those who do not have HIV infection.

Complications

- Pseudoelephantiasis, particularly seen in women, is one of the most common complications.
- The sclerotic variant may lead to stenosis of the urethra, vagina, or anus.
- Secondary infection or mixed infection is also a common phenomenon.
- Squamous cell carcinoma of the penis is a rare occurrence, described in around 0.25% of 2000 cases. A higher incidence is seen in donovanosis–HIV coinfection.

LYMPHOGRANULOMA VENEREUM (Tropical/Climatic Bubo, Durand-Nicolas-Favre Disease)

Lymphogranuloma venereum (LGV) is one of the sexually transmitted diseases caused by *Chlamydia trachomatis*—serovars L1, L2 and L3.

It has both acute and chronic manifestations and passes through three stages. Left untreated, it may incite a chronic inflammatory response culminating in long-term complications such as fistulas, rectal strictures, and genital elephantiasis.

Pathogenesis

- *Chlamydia* cannot penetrate intact skin but gains entry through minute lacerations and abrasions.
- LGV is predominantly a disease of lymphatic tissue. The essential pathologic process is **thrombolymphangitis and perilymphangitis** with spread of the inflammatory process from infected lymph nodes into the surrounding tissue. Lymph nodes draining the site of primary infection rapidly enlarge and form small, discrete areas of necrosis. Inflammation mats the adjacent lymph nodes together by **periadenitis**, and as the inflammation progresses, abscesses coalesce and rupture, forming loculated abscesses, fistulae, or sinus tracts.
- Healing takes place by fibrosis, which destroys the normal structure of lymph nodes and obstructs lymph vessels. The resulting chronic edema and sclerosing fibrosis cause induration and enlargement of the affected parts. Fibrosis also compromises the blood supply to the overlying skin or mucous membrane, and ulceration occurs.

Clinical Features

Incubation period: 3–12 days.

Primary Stage: Ulcerative

- LGV may start as a papule, a transient painless or painful small ulcer, a small herpetiform lesion or a less commonly reported non-specific urethritis.
- The asymptomatic and transient herpetiform ulcer—most common manifestation and heals quickly with no scarring.
- Most common sites in men—coronal sulcus, frenulum, prepuce, penis, urethral glans, and scrotum. Women—posterior vaginal wall, fourchette, posterior lip of the cervix, vulva.
- Primary LGV lesions in men may be associated with a lymphangitis of the dorsal penis and formation of a large, tender lymphangial nodule—'Bubonulus'.

- Following rectal intercourse, acute colitis or proctocolitis is often seen as the main manifestation of primary infection and constitutes a common presentation in developed nonendemic nations. Urethritis and cervicitis are uncommon presentations at this stage.

Secondary Stage: *Inguinal Syndrome* (Fig. 33.29)

- Inflammation of the inguinal lymph nodes—most common manifestations of this stage and can present 10 days to 6 months following infection.
- The inguinal bubo is **unilateral in up to two-thirds** of the cases. In up to one-third of the cases, the bubo enlarges, and ultimately ruptures through the skin leading to sinus formation and discharge of thick, yellowish pus for days to weeks. Slow healing occurs with scar formation. In rest of the cases, slow involution of the bubo is seen, with no apparent sequelae. In about 20% of cases, the femoral lymph nodes may also be affected and may be separated from the enlarged inguinal lymph nodes by the inguinal ligament; this phenomenon is known as the **'sign of the groove', pathognomonic for LGV**. Women present less commonly with the inguinal syndrome. However, deep pelvic and lumbar lymph nodes may be involved and lead to lower abdominal and back pain.
- Constitutional symptoms such as fever, tachycardia, decreased appetite, etc. are associated with this stage and can be attributed to the systemic spread of the organism. Hepatitis, pneumonitis, arthritis and erythema nodosum.

Tertiary Stage: *Anogenitorectal Syndrome*

- The mechanism of spread to the rectal mucosa include the following—anal intercourse, lymphatic spread from posterior urethra, direct spread from vaginal secretions or lymphatic dissemination from the cervix or posterior vagina.
- Subacute manifestations—proctocolitis and hyperplasia of intestinal and perirectal lymphatic tissue **(lymphorrhoids)**.

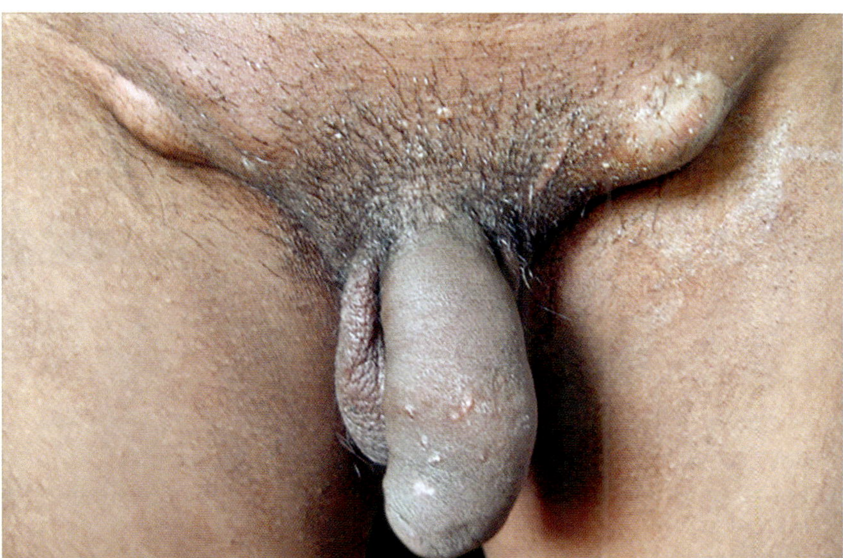

Fig. 33.29: A case of LGV with bilateral enlarged buboes (lymph node)

- Chronic or late manifestations—perirectal abscesses, ischiorectal and rectovaginal fistulas, anal fistulas, and rectal stricture or stenosis.
- Most commonly seen amongst women or homosexual men. Presents with ulcerative or granulomatous inflammation of the rectum and colon.
- Symptoms—anal pruritus, mucous rectal discharge, rectal bleeding, mucosal ulceration which may result in strictures and partial stenosis.
- Proctocolitis presents with fever, pain and tenesmus.
- Obstruction of the lymphatic and venous drainage of the lower rectum produces perianal outgrowths of lymphatic tissue that grossly resemble hemorrhoids but are called **lymphorrhoids**.
- Rectal cancer in LGV rectal stricture: **2–5%**.

Extragenital manifestations—ocular manifestations (follicular conjunctivitis, episcleritis, keratitis and iritis). Cutaneous manifestations include 'Id eruptions' and iliopsoas abscess.

Complications

- Epididymo-orchitis, prostatitis, seminal vesiculitis.
- Genital elephantiasis (**'Esthiomene' or vulval elephantiasis** in females and **'Ram-rod/Ram-horn/saxophone penis'**—elephantiasic enlargement of the scrotum and distortion of the penis in males).
- Rectal carcinoma (2–5%).

Differential Diagnosis

Primary stage	Secondary stage	Tertiary stage
Genital herpes	Chancroid	Trauma
Primary syphilis	Syphilis	Actinomycosis
Chancroid	Genital herpes	Tuberculosis
Traumatic ulcer	Bubonic plague	Schistosomiasis
Non-gonococcal urethritis	Tuberculosis	Inflammatory bowel disease
	Septic lymphadenopathy	Rectal cancer

HIV and LGV (Table 33.21)

TABLE 33.21: Effect of HIV on LGV

Morphology	No effect
Atypical features	Parinuad's syndrome, reactivation with multiple abscesses
Course	Disease duration prolonged

Diagnosis

The diagnosis of LGV is usually based on:

1. A positive **Frei skin test:** Skin hypersensitivity test which becomes positive 2–8 weeks after infection; this test is now not available commercially.
2. A positive **complement–fixation (CF)** or other serologic test for LGV (in general, active LGV infections have CF titers of 1:64 or greater).

3. **Micro-IF** test more sensitive and specific than the CF test; however, not available commercially.
4. **Isolation of** *Chlamydia* on tissue culture using **HeLa-229 and McCoy** cell lines. Pus obtained from a bubo is most commonly used for isolation of *Chlamydia*.
5. **Histologic or cytological identification of *Chlamydia*** in infected tissue—the elementary and inclusion bodies of *Chlamydia* can be visualized by using Giemsa, iodine, and fluorescent antibody staining methods.
6. Demonstration of *Chlamydia* by polymerase chain reaction (PCR) or other nucleic acid amplification test (NAAT) in infected secretions or tissues—one of the most sensitive and specific techniques.

Treatment (CDC 2021)

Recommended Regimen

Doxycycline 100 mg orally twice a day for 21 days.

Alternative Regimen

- Erythromycin base 500 mg orally four times a day for 21 days.
- Azithromycin 1 g orally once a week × 3 weeks (a test of cure with Chlamydia trachomatis NAAT 4 weeks after treatment completion can be considered)

Special Considerations

Pregnancy

Pregnant and lactating women should be treated with erythromycin.

HIV Infection

Persons with both LGV and HIV infection should receive the same regimens as those who are HIV negative. Prolonged therapy might be required, and delay in resolution of symptoms might occur.

URETHRITIS

Definition: Urethritis is diagnosed on the basis of any of the following signs or laboratory tests:

- Mucoid, mucopurulent or purulent discharge on examination.
- Gram stain of **urethral secretions** demonstrating ≥2 WBC per oil immersion field (according to CDC 2021); or
- ≥10 WBC per HPF of sediment from a spun **first void urine** sample or a positive leukocyte esterase on first void urine sample.

Classification of Urethritis (Table 33.22)

1. **Gonococcal urethritis (GU) (approx. 30%):** Gram stain showing GN diplococci with PMN.
2. **Nongonococcal urethritis (NGU) (approx. 70%):** *Chlamydia trachomatis* accounts for 15–40% of NGU. It has been suggested that mucopurulent non-gonococcal cervicitis is the female equivalent with approximately 20–40% of cases being due to infection with *Chlamydia trachomatis* and 5–20% *Mycoplasma genitalium*.
3. **Nonchlamydial, nongonococcal urethritis** (this is now commonly merged with NGU—**Box 33.7**): Commonly caused by *Mycoplasma genitalium* and *Trichomonas vaginalis*. Other organisms include Epstein–Barr virus, *N. meningitidis*, *Haemophilus* spp., *Candida* spp. In males >40 years UTI is a common cause.
4. **Nonspecific urethritis (NSU):** Contact dermatitis and immunologic disorders, trauma and catheterization.
5. **Persistent and recurrent urethritis:**
   - Persistent urethritis that fails to resolve or substantially improve within 1 week of initiating therapy.

TABLE 33.22: Causes of urethritis

Common causes	
1. *Neisseria gonorrhoeae*	
2. *Chlamydia trachomatis*	
3. *Mycoplasma genitalium*	
4. *Trichomonas vaginalis*	
Other causes	
Infectious	*Non-infectious*
1. *Ureaplasma urealyticum*	1. Reactive arthritis
2. *Neisseria meningitidis*	2. Urethral stricture
3. *Candida albicans*	3. Catheterization
4. Herpes simplex viruses	4. Stevens-Johnson syndrome
5. Adenovirus	5. Chemicals
6. *Hemophilus* species	6. Tumors
7. *Bacteroides ureolyticus*	7. Condom allergy
8. Exposure to bacterial vaginosis	

BOX 33.7: Prevalence of the most common pathogens isolated from patients with nongonococcal urethritis (NGU) (CDC 2015)

Organism	Comments
C. trachomatis	15–40%
M. genitalium	15–25%
Ureaplasma spp.	11–26%
T. vaginalis	1–20%: *T. vaginalis* isolation is greater in men aged over 30 years and may not always be associated with symptoms
Adenoviruses	2–4%: Associated with conjunctivitis and intense dysuria
Herpes simplex virus	2–3%: Dysuria
No pathogen identified	around 50%

- Recurrent urethritis is return of urethritis within 6 weeks following an initial response to therapy → r/o reinfection

6. **Chronic urethritis:** Persistent or relapsing NGU ≥30 days post-treatment.

Some general principles that govern treatment are given below.

Principles of select drug treatment of urethritis (CDC 2021)

- Ideally, treatment should be effective (microbiological cure >95%), easy to take (not more than twice daily), with a low side-effect profile, and cause minimal interference with lifestyle.
- In gonorrhea—dual therapy is **no longer** recommended as there is a low incidence of ceftriaxone resistance and increased incidence of azithromycin resistance (elevated MICs) in *N. gonorrhoeae, Mycoplasma genitalium* and other sexually transmissible enteric pathogens (e.g. *Shigella*).
- *M. genitalium*: Ideal drug is azithromycin 500 mg or 1 g stat, then 250 mg daily for a further 4 days or moxifloxacin 400 mg OD for 14 days.
- *Ureaplasma*: Both macrolides and tetracyclines are more than 80% effective, so is moxifloxacin.
- Give empirical antibiotics for a presumed UTI according to local prescribing policies and local knowledge of antibiotics ensitivities.

GONOCOCCAL URETHRITIS

- ***Neisseria gonorrhoeae*** is one of the most common causes of urethritis, second only to *Chlamydia trachomatis*.
- Prevalence in India—3–20%.
- *Neisseria gonorrhoeae* are gram-negative, non-motile and nonspore forming intracellular diplococci (GNID) measuring 0.8 µm × 0.6 µm in size. The organism divides every 20–30 minutes by binary fission **(Fig. 33.30a)** and infects mucous-secreting epithelial cells.
- The organism adhere to different types of epithelial cells via a number of structures located on the surface **(Fig. 33.30b)**. Ultrastructurally, *Gonococcus* has:
    i. Pili
    ii. Polyphosphate capsule (not a true capsule like *N. meningitidis*)
    iii. Trilaminar membrane—composed of 1. outer membrane, 2. peptidoglycan layer, 3. cytoplasmic membrane.

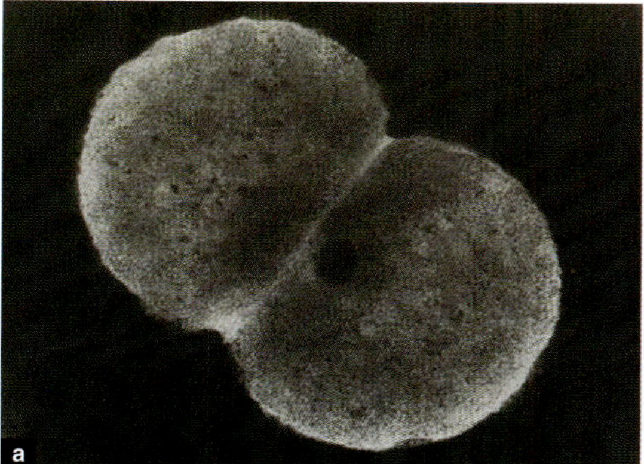

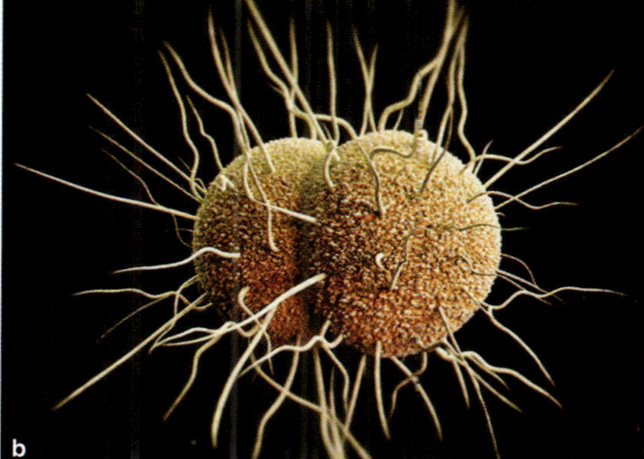

Fig. 33.30: (a) Division of *N. gonorrhoeae* by binary fission; (b) An artistic depiction of *N. gonorrhoeae* division

- Gonococci are immobile, aerobic, and nutritionally fastidious and grow best at a temperature range of 35–37°C, in an atmosphere of 3–5% CO_2 and a pH of 7.2–7.6.
- *N. gonorrhoeae* ferment glucose but not maltose, sucrose, lactose, fructose, and mannose. They are catalase and oxidase positive.

Pathogenesis

- Transmission
  - Male-to-female transmission via semen occurs—50–70% per episode of vaginal intercourse with ejaculation (Hooper RR, et al., 1978)
  - An infected woman can transmit *N. gonorrhoeae* to the urethra of a male sex partner; the rate of transmission is approximately 20% per episode from vaginal intercourse, and it increases to approximately 60 to 80% after four or more intercourse exposures (Lin JS, et al., 1998).
- The various **surface proteins** which facilitate infection:
  - Pili (adhesion to host cell)
  - pilus-related outer membrane protein pil C (adhesion)/Pil Q/pil T
  - Opa (adhesion)
  - Rmp proteins (blocking antibodies that prevent serum bactericidal activity directed against this antigen)
  - Por proteins (invasion)
  - LOS (endotoxin)—role in DGI
  - IgA protease (evasion of mucosal IgA1 immunity).
  - Integrins (inhibit mucosal cell shedding)
- *N. gonorrhoeae* has a predilection for columnar and cuboidal epithelium. Following adherence, the organism is enfolded by pseudopods and pinocytosed by the epithelial cells. The Por protein is translocated from the bacterial cell membrane to the epithelial cell membrane. Epithelial cell damage is mediated by release of certain enzymes like phospholipase and peptidase or due to LOS and peptidoglycan. The LOS antigen elicits the C5a-dependent chemotactic response.
- When the attack is prolonged, there is formation of stratified layers and eventually, keratinization and fibrosis occur, leading to stricture formation.

Antimicrobial Resistance

Gonococci is rapidly developed anti-microbial resistance as evidenced by the following data:

- 1980s—penicillin and tetracycline—no longer recommended for gonorrhea
- 2007—ciprofloxacin—no longer recommended
- 2012—cefixime—no longer recommended
- 2016—first global treatment failure with CDC-recommended dual therapy reported
- 2018—first isolates with combined ceftriaxone resistance and high-level azithromycin resistance reported.

Chromosomal mutations are the most frequent mutations observed, and may alter the affinity of the drug for its target and increase efflux of drug from the bacterial cell, or decrease permeability of gonococci **(Box 33.8)**. 30% of new cases of gonorrhea each year are resistant to at least one drug (CDC).

BOX 33.8: Resistance in gonorrhea

Type of resistance	Anti-microbial agent
Chromosomal (genes located on the chromosome)	Sulphonamides Penicillin Tetracycline Spectinomycin Macrolides Fluoroquinolones Cephalosporins
Plasmid-mediated (genes located on plasmids)	Penicillin (PPNG) Tetracycline (TRNG)

Clinical Features

- Sites
  - In males: The urethra, Littre's and Cowper's glands, the prostate, seminal vesicles and epididymis.
  - In females: The glands of Skene and Bartholin, part of the urethra and the urethral glands, the cervix and fallopian tubes.
  - The rectum is susceptible in both sexes, but bladder, upper urinary tract, preputial sac, vulva, vagina and uterus are less often involved.
- Incubation period 1–14 days, with an average of 2–5 days.
- Men: Characterized by a profuse, cloudy, thick, yellow, foul smelling urethral discharge (80%) associated with dysuria **(50%)**, meatal itching, burning, and frequency of micturition.
  - Meatal erythema/edema—may be so much as to cause entire distal penis to be swollen 'bull head clap'.
  - In 3–12% (average 10%) of men, asymptomatic urethral infection is present *without symptoms*, representing an important group in the transmission of the infection.
  - Rectal infection is usually asymptomatic but may cause anal discharge (12%) or perianal/anal pain or discomfort (7%).
  - Testicular pain (orchitis/epididymitis)—less than in chlamydial NGU.
- Women: In women endocervical infections are mostly asymptomatic. **Increased or altered vaginal discharge** is the **most common** symptom (up to 50%) and dysuria (12%).
  - Asymptomatic in 50%
  - Endocervicitis—mucopurulent vaginal discharge
  - Proctitis—through autoinoculation from cervical discharge/anoreceptive intercourse
  - 70–90% of women with genital gonococcal infection have laboratory evidence of urethral infection (urethritis).
- MSM:
  - Proctitis—in unprotected anoreceptive intercourse.

Complications

Depending on the site and the duration of disease, various complications can be seen that **(Table 33.23)** and have peculiar and characteristic features, though not all are seen nowadays. **Figures 33.31** and **33.32** show diagrammatic depictions of the male and female genital tract for better understanding of the various complications.

- Transluminal spread of *N. gonorrhoeae* from the urethra or endocervix may occur to cause epididymo-orchitis or prostatitis in men and pelvic inflammatory disease (PID) in 10–40% women.
- Hematogenous dissemination may also occur from infected mucous membranes to cause only asymmetric arthralgia/oligoarticular septic arthritis or petechial/pustular skin lesions, polyarthritis and tenosynovitis (arthritis–dermatitis syndrome), and occasionally perihepatitis, endocarditis and meningitis as part of disseminated gonococcal infection.
- Increased risk of HIV acquisition, esp. in MSM with GU (damaged anorectal mucosal integrity and recruitment of HIV-target cell types such as CCR5/CD4+ T cells).

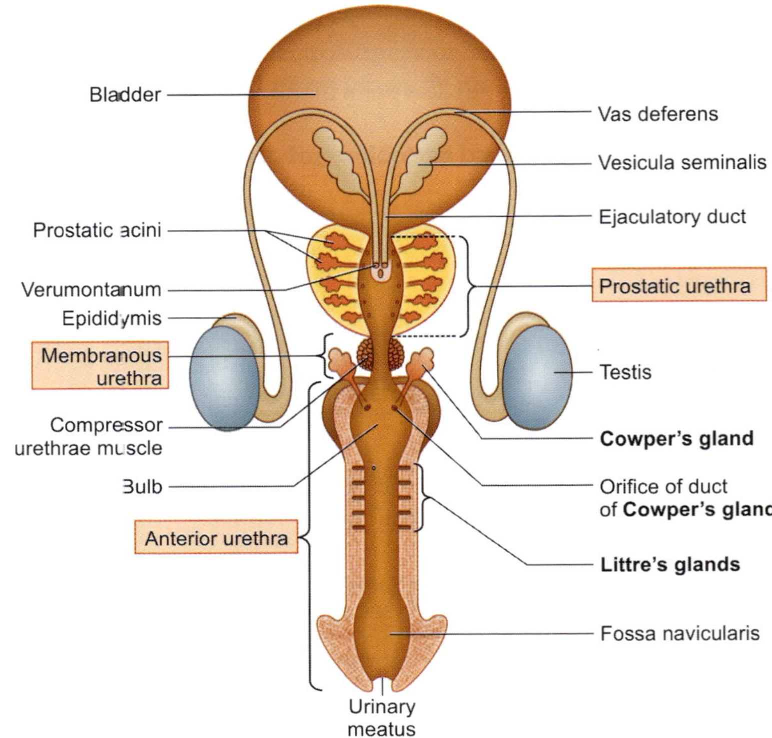

Fig. 33.31: A diagrammatic depiction of the male genital tract

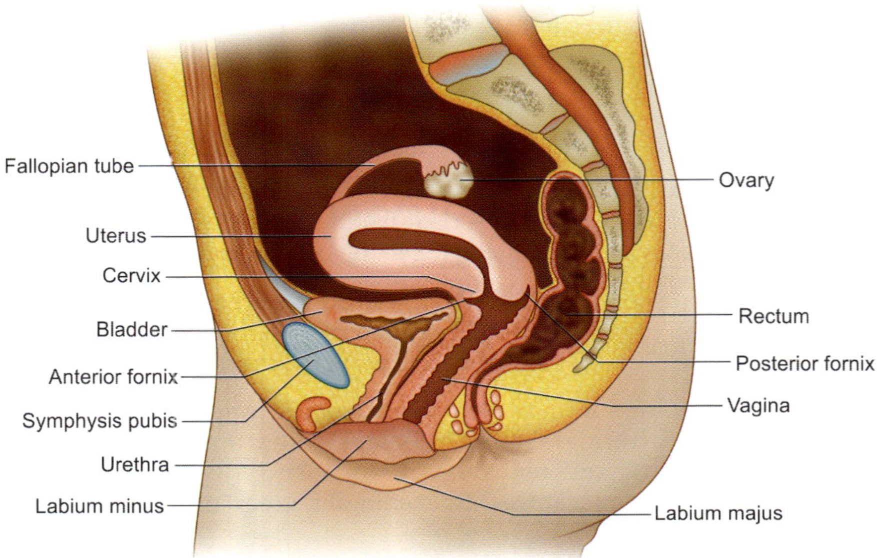

Fig. 33.32: A diagrammatic depiction of the female genital tract

TABLE 33.23: Overview of complications seen in gonorrhea

Males	**Anterior urethra**	• **Tysonitis:** Red swelling on one side of frenulum • **Paraurethral duct:** Inflamed opening inside the meatus expressing a bead of pus • **Periurethral abscess:** Pain, difficult micturition, chordee, tender swelling opening in midline on frenulum or root of penis • **Littritis:** Threads in urine (in first glass) • **Urethral stricture** (chronic): Water can perineum • **Cowperitis:** Aching pain in perineum, pain on defecation, frequency of micturition, acute retention of urine
	Posterior urethra (infection ascends in 10–14 days if untreated)	• **Prostatitis:** – Acute: Pain—suprapubic, perineal – Abscess: Severe, pain on defecation, tenesmus, *urethral discharge will decrease*! • **Epididymitis:** Retrograde passage of urine, the acute urethritis is relieved! • **Seminal vesiculitis:** Terminal hematuria, frequent erections (if chronic—presents as morning gleet) • **Trigonitis**
Females	Urethra Cervix, uterus and fallopian tubes Bartholin gland	• Skenitis • Periurethral abscess • Salpingitis • PID → ectopic pregnancy, infertility • Parametritis • Pelvic abscess • **Perihepatitis** • Abscess
Males and females	Anorectum Conjunctivae Oropharynx	• Pain, discharge, bleeding—P/R • Conjunctivitis • Pharyngitis • Disseminated gonococcal infection (arthritis–dermatitis syndrome or localized septic arthritis)

Disseminated Gonococcal Infection (DGI)

- Women > Men (0.5–3% of infected women).
- Due to asymptomatic infections that remain untreated.
- Most strains—porin 1A (promotes host cell invasion and diminishes host inflammatory response).
- Either as—acute arthritis—dermatitis syndrome (polyarthritis + dermatitis + tenosynovitis) or as acute septic oligoarthritis alone.
- Most common systemic complication of acute gonorrhea.
- In half of affected women, symptoms begin 7 days after menstruation.
- Risk factors for DGI—pregnancy, pharyngeal gonorrhea, menstruation, complement deficiency, IUD, prior pelvic surgery.
- Clinical features
  - Skin—tender necrotic pustules on erythematous base on distal extremitites <30 in number, mostly palms and soles, hemorrhage and necrosis give the 'gun metal gray' appearance to DGI lesions.

– Joints—wrist, MCP, ankle, knee. Arthralgias may occur before arthritis. With/without tenosynovitis.

Diagnosis of DGI

- **Proven DGI**—positive culture from blood/joint fluid/skin lesions/otherwise sterile sources.
- **Probable DGI**—appropriate signs and symptoms with positive culture from primary mucosal site of infection/from sexual partner in absence of blood or sterile site culture.
- **Possible DGI**—appropriate signs and symptoms with expected response to treatment but negative cultures for *N. gonorrhoeae*.
  Responds to treatment rapidly—within 48 hours.
  Recommended treatment (CDC 2021):
  – Ceftriaxone 1 g IV or IM 24 hourly
    Plus
  – Doxycycline 100 mg BD × 7 days (if chlamydial infection not ruled out).

Fitz-Hugh-Curtis Syndrome (FHCS)

- Perihepatic capsulitis—in one-fourth women with pelvic inflammatory diseases (PID).
- Probably due to hematolymphatic and peritoneal spread of pelvic infections to the liver and hyperimmune response to gonococcal/*Chlamydia* infection; with both processes leading to perihepatic and liver capsular inflammation.
- D/D—acute viral hepatitis
- FHCS is caused more frequently by *Chlamydia* than by gonococci.
- NAATs are preferred diagnostic tests (multiplex PCR for GC and CT).

Investigation of Urethritis

Urinary tract infection symptoms may overlap with those of urethritis, thus if there are symptoms of severe dysuria, visible hematuria, nocturia, urinary frequency, urgency, an STI is unlikely. The various sites of sampling are given in **Table 33.24**.

1. **Bedside tests**

Two-glass test (Fig. 33.33a)

This is a time-honored test, that was performed in UK-GU medicine clinics, considered by some to be of debatable value. It certainly can help to differentiate a pure urethritis (usually sexually acquired) from a urethritis in association with a cystitis (i.e. a UTI, and not sexually acquired).

TABLE 33.24: Clinical samples for the diagnosis of gonorrhea

Patient	Sample of choice	Secondary sample
• Women • Heterosexual men • Homosexual men	• Endocervix • Urethra • Urethra, rectum[c], pharynx[a]	• Rectum[c], urethra, pharynx[a]
• **For disseminated gonococcal infection** Women Men	 • Blood, endocervix, joint blood • Blood, urethra, joint liquid, rectum[c]	 • Pharynx[a], skin lesions[b], rectum[c] • Pharynx[a], skin lesions[b]

a, If there has been orogenital contact; b, If present; c, If there has been anogenital contact.

Principle

- Ant. urethra—requires about 60 mL to be washed off
- Ant. urethra drains outside, post. urethra into the bladder
- Patient is asked to hold urine overnight and come in the morning (without any active Rx).
- He is asked to pass urine in two glasses (approximately 50 mL each)
- Any remaining urine is passed into the urinal.

The following are the interpretation of urine results:

1. First: clear; second: clear = **normal**.
2. First: Pus (seen as threads, flakes, general haze); second: Clear = **Anterior urethritis** [e.g. non-gonococcal urethritis (NGU), gonorrhea] **(Fig. 33.33a)**.
3. First: Pus; second: Pus = **Posterior urethritis or cystitis** (e.g. *E. coli*, etc.). Send the first glass urine or mid-stream urine (MSU) for culture. The addition of acetic acid will clear the urine when excess phosphates are causing haziness, whereas the **haze remains in cases of pyuria** (phosphaturia is a common cause of cloudy urine) **(Fig. 33.33b)**.

Three-glass test

- Ant. urethra irrigated with a colorless antiseptic solution till clear—this is taken as the **1st glass**
- Patient asked to pass urine in three glasses:
  a. **2nd**—pus-posterior urethra infection
  b. **3rd**—bladder infection
  c. **4th**—prostate infection

There is another variation of this test four glass test done for diagnosing prostatic involvement which is better done by urologists.

2. **Direct microscopy of Gram's stained smear**

- As per the definition, urethritis is diagnosed when ≥2 polymorphonuclear leukocytes (PMNL) per oil immersion field (×1000 magnification) are present in >5 fields of a Gram stained smear of urethral secretions. It reveals gram-negative diplococci, typically kidney or bean shaped, found both intra as well as extracellularly **(Fig. 33.33c)**.
  - Positive—gram-negative diplococci with typical morphology within or closely associated with PMN.
  - Equivocal—if extracellular organism or morphologically atypical intracellular gram-negative diplococci.
  - Negative—no gram-negative diplococci.

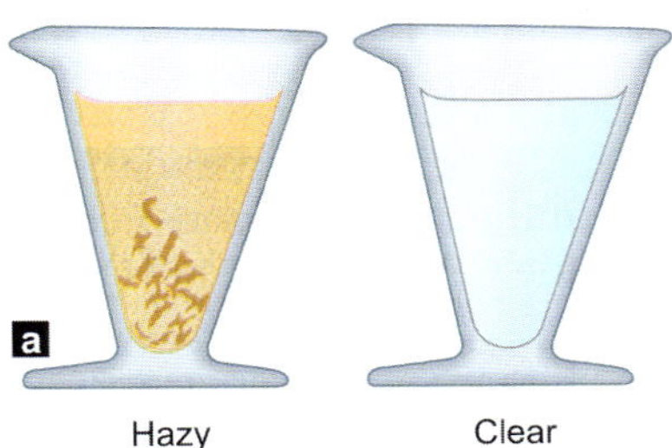

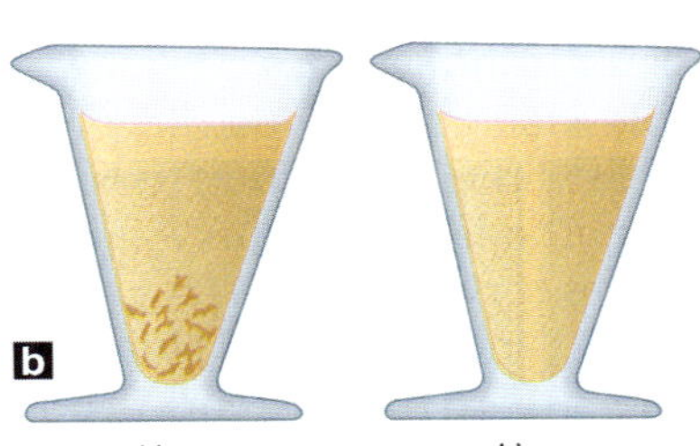

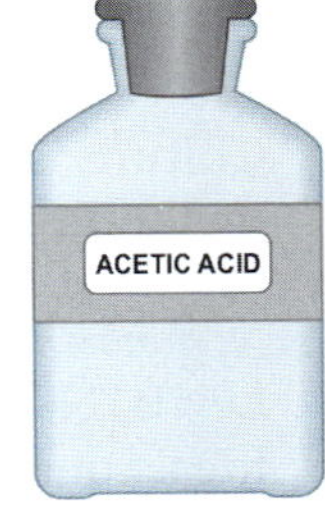

Fig. 33.33a and b: A depiction of the 2-glass test. (a) Suggestive of anterior urethritis; (b) Posterior urethritis, add acetic acid to remove haziness due to phosphates in the urine

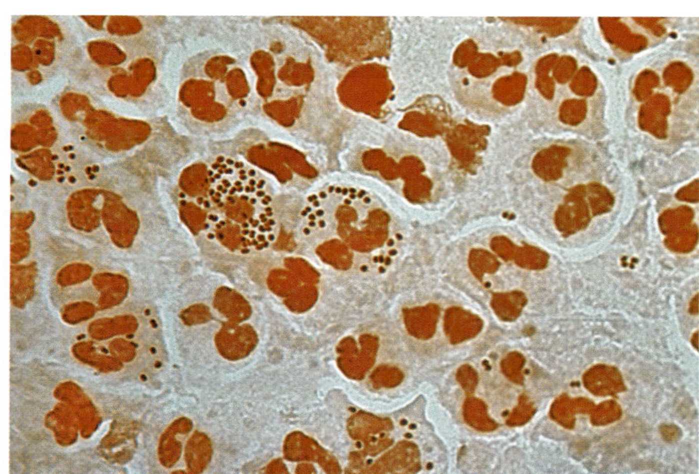

Fig. 33.33c: Gram-negative diplococci within the PMNs

- In men with urethral discharge: The sensitivity varies from 80 to 95% and specificity from 95 to 99%.
- In women, the sensitivity and specificity of endocervical smears vary from 25 to 65% and 90 to 100%, respectively. Performing a Gram's stain is not recommended on endocervical, pharyngeal, or rectal specimens due to poor sensitivity.
- Procedure for taking smear: A 1–5 mm plastic loop, or cotton or rayon tipped swab can be used. The smear should be taken about 0.5–1 cm into the urethra. A plastic loop is less painful than a Dacron or Rayon swab, while based on sensitivities of microscopy for detection of *Chlamydia*, blunt spatula is better than swab.
- When there is no frank discharge, *milking* of the urethra may provide some exudate. Microscopy has poor sensitivity (≤55%) in asymptomatic men and in identifying rectal infection (≤40%). Microscopy is not recommended for identification of pharyngeal infection due to poor specificity as well as low sensitivity.
- **Methylene blue (MB) or gentian violet (GV) stain** microscopy can also be used instead of Gram stain—purple intracellular diplococci on urethral smear.

3. **Culture**

- Specific, sensitive and cheap diagnostic test at genital sites.
- Culture is appropriate for endocervical, urethral, rectal, pharyngeal, and conjunctival specimens but not for urine samples.
- Culture is the 'gold standard' in the diagnosis of gonococcal urethritis, though newer methods like nucleic acid amplification tests (NAATs) are rapidly becoming popular and the most favored methods. It remains a useful tool to determine antibiotic sensitivity. *N. gonorrhoeae* requires enriched media for growth, such as modified Thayer-Martin, Martin-Lewis, New York City, and GC-Lect **(Table 33.25)**.

  Ideal conditions: 35–36.5°C in a CO_2-enriched atmosphere. Plates are examined every 18–24 hours until 48–72 hrs.

Transport media—**Amies or Stuart medium. Isolation rate 100% within 6 hours** between specimen collection and inoculation, 90% within 12 hours, acceptable result within 2 days.

TABLE 33.25: Anti-microbial agents used in selective media for isolation of *N. gonorrhoeae*

Selective agent	Concentrations used	Organisms inhibited
Vancomycin	2–4 mg/L	Gram-positive bacteria
Lincomycin	1 mg/L	Gram-positive bacteria
Colistin	7.5 mg/L	Gram-negative bacteria (other than *Neisseria*)
Trimethoprim	5 mg/L	Gram-negative bacteria (other than *Neisseria*)
Nystatin	12,500 IU/L	*Candida* spp.
Amphotericin	1–1.5 mg/L	*Candida* spp.

Presumptive identification:

- Gram-negative, oxidase and superoxidase positive diplococci.
- Gonococci form small, round, translucent, soft, emulsifiable, and convex colonies with a fine granular surface. The sensitivity of culture is 80–95%.
- Oxidase is detected either by placing a drop of oxidase reagent (tetramethyl-paraphenylene-diamine-dihydrochloride) on a few representative colonies or by rubbing representative colonies on filter paper moistened with oxidase reagent with a platinum or plastic loop.
- The aim of identification tests is to distinguish between *N. gonorrhoeae* and other species of *Neisseria*, particularly *N. meningitidis* and *N. lactamica*.
- *N. gonorrhoeae* ferments glucose but not maltose, sucrose and lactose.
- There are three available methods for the epidemiologic identification of *N. gonorrhoeae*: Auxotyping, serotyping, and genotyping methods.

Anti-microbial sensitivity: The aim of susceptibility testing is to enable a correlation with treatment outcome **(Table 33.26)**.

- Several tests for β-lactamase are available commercially; these include chromogenic cephalosporin, acidometric, and iodometric tests. The chromogenic cephalosporin (nitrocefin) tests are preferred because the substrate is stable and the reactions are specific and highly sensitive for β-lactamase.

An anti-microbial susceptibility result determined in the laboratory is only a measure of the *in vitro* susceptibility of an isolate. A patient may have a 'positive test-of-cure culture' for a variety of reasons:

1. Failure of therapy because of infection with a resistant isolate.
2. Failure of therapy even when the patient is infected with a strain that is susceptible by *in vitro* measurements because of noncompliance with treatment.
3. Reinfection

Thus, anti-microbial susceptibilities must be used as an *adjunct* to, but cannot be substituted for, clinical findings.

TABLE 33.26: Results of correlation of disk-diffusion susceptibity with clinical outcome

Susceptible	Less than 5% likelihood of treatment failure
Intermediate	Predictable failure rates of 5 to 15% if the patient is treated with the tested antibiotic in the standard dosage (in most cases of intermediate susceptibility, a higher dose or prolonged therapy results in greater than 95% cure rates)
Resistant	May be associated with treatment failure rates of greater than 15%

4. **Nucleic acid amplification tests (NAATs):** There are two types of nucleic acid detection tests—non-amplified tests and amplified tests:
   - *Amplified tests*: The nucleic acid amplification tests (NAATs) include polymerase chain reaction (PCR) (Roche Amplicor; Cepheid GeneXpert CT/NG), transcription-mediated amplification (TMA) (Gen-Probe Aptima), and strand displacement amplification (SDA) (Becton-Dickinson BDProbeTec ET).
     - Amplified tests are FDA-cleared for endocervical specimens from women, urethral specimens from men, and urine specimens from men and women.
     - Multiple studies have shown NAATs are the most sensitive test to detect *N. gonorrhoeae* infections.
   - *Non-amplified tests*: Several non-amplified tests used for *N. gonorrhoeae*, include the DNA probe tests (e.g. Gen-Probe PACE 2 and Digene Hybrid Capture II).
     - A non-amplified test is less likely to be affected by transport conditions than culture, and has the potential for more timely results.
     - These tests are FDA-cleared for endocervical specimens from women and urethral specimens from men.

Pros:
- Among the fastest POCTs
- Generally, more sensitive than culture
- Some specimens can be *non-invasive*, e.g. first pass urine can be used in men and self-taken vaginal swabs in women (NB: Urine is not optimal in women).
- Can also detect *Chlamydia* on the same specimen.

Cons:
- Antibiotic susceptibility testing cannot be carried out.
- Because they are so sensitive, may get false +ve from contamination or non-gonococcal *Neisseria* species.
- Lower sensitivity in female urine (thus, it is not an optimal specimen in women; vaginal or endocervical swabs are better).

5. **Fluorescent antibody methods:** The reagent used for these tests is the globulin fraction of a high titred antiserum against gonococci prepared in rabbits and conjugated with fluorescein isothiocyanate. This unites with gonococci which fluoresce an apple green color when viewed under ultraviolet light.
6. **Other diagnostic tests**
   - DNA hybridization
   - ELISA
   - Complement fixation
   - Latex agglutination, immunofluorescence and anti-surface pili assays
   - Radioimmunoassay
   - Immunoblotting
   - Hemagglutination
7. **For complications: USG, urethroscopy**—to be done by a urologist
8. **HIV, VDRL**

Treatment of Gonorrhea

The treatment of gonorrhea has been updated by CDC 2021:

Regimen for uncomplicated gonococcal infections of the cervix, urethra, or rectum:

- Ceftriaxone **500 mg** IM as a single dose for persons weighing **<150 kg** (since a 250 mg ceftriaxone dose does not reliably achieve levels higher than an MIC ≥0.125 µg/mL for an extended duration. Also, at 500 mg dose, adequate pharyngeal levels are achieved).
- For persons weighing **≥150 kg** (300 lb), **1 g** of IM ceftriaxone should be administered.
- The rationale for eliminating the routine use of azithromycin as dual therapy for the treatment of gonorrhea includes concern for the potential impact of azithromycin on commensal organisms and concurrent pathogens, as well as the trend of increasing *N. gonorrhoeae* resistance to azithromycin (Wind CM).
- If chlamydial infection has not been excluded, providers should treat for *Chlamydia* with doxycycline 100 mg orally twice daily for 7 days.

  (This new recommendation is based on emerging data suggesting lower *Chlamydia* treatment efficacy with azithromycin compared with doxycycline, especially with rectal *Chlamydia*).

Alternative regimens for uncomplicated gonococcal infections of the cervix, urethra, or rectum if ceftriaxone is not available:

- Gentamicin 240 mg IM as a single dose plus azithromycin 2 g orally as a single dose.

  OR
- Cefixime 800 mg orally as a single dose.
- If treating with cefixime, and chlamydial infection has not been excluded, providers should treat for *Chlamydia* with doxycycline 100 mg orally twice daily for 7 days. During pregnancy, azithromycin 1 g as a single dose is recommended to treat *Chlamydia*.

Treatment Failure

This is suspected when there is a recurrence of symptoms or a positive culture after a documented, appropriate treatment (Workowski KA, et al., 2015). The majority of cases of suspected treatment failure are reinfection rather than true treatment failure.

A true treatment failure should be considered in:

1. a person whose symptoms do not resolve within 3–5 days after appropriate treatment, and they report no sexual contact during the post-treatment follow-up period.
2. a person with a failed test-of-cure (i.e. positive culture at least 72 hours or positive NAAT at least 7 days after receiving recommended treatment) when no sexual contact is reported during the post-treatment follow-up period.

Risk factors for treatment failure due to resistant organisms include multiple prior treatment courses for gonorrhea, international travel, or pharyngeal disease.

The steps that should be done next in such a case include:

1. Perform culture and susceptibility testing of all relevant clinical specimens
2. Send samples to the regional reference laboratory
3. Isolate and notify partners of persons with *N. gonorrhoeae* infection suspected for cephalosporin treatment failure or persons whose isolates demonstrate decreased susceptibility to cephalosporins.

4. A test-of-cure at relevant clinical sites should be obtained 7–14 days after retreatment; culture is the recommended test, preferably with simultaneous NAAT and susceptibility testing of *N. gonorrhoeae* if isolated.

2015 STD Treatment Guidelines (CDC)

1. Single dose oral therapy with gemifloxacin 320 mg plus azithromycin 2 grams,
2. Single dose oral therapy with azithromycin 2 grams plus a single intramuscular injection of a 240 mg dose of gentamicin.

Follow-up

- Follow-up should take place to confirm compliance with advice, resolution of symptoms and partner notification issues.

  A follow-up protocol is given in **Table 33.27**. This should be followed at 3 months by a VDRL/HIV test.

TABLE 33.27: Suggested follow-up of a patient of gonococcal urethritis

Day	Glass test	Smear	Culture	Comment
3	+	GC+, PMN+	Negative	Resistance if culture positive
10	+	PMN+	Negative	–
>14	If +	If PMN+	Negative	PGU (post-gonococcal urethritis)
28	Usually (–)	Usually (–)	Usually (–)	Prostate massage

Source: King, Nicol

- Men or women who have been treated for gonorrhea should be **retested 3 months after treatment (due to high rates of reinfection)** regardless of whether they believe their sex partners were treated (CDC, 2021).

Management of Sex Partners

- Recent sex partners (contact within the 60 days preceding onset of symptoms) should be referred for evaluation, testing, and presumptive dual treatment.
- For heterosexual men and women with gonorrhea for whom health department partner—management strategies are impractical or unavailable, **expedited partner therapy (EPT)** is preferred. Cefixime is to be given in a dose of 800 mg, routine dual therapy with azithromycin is not recommended; if concurrent *Chlamydia* was not excluded in the source individual (who was diagnosed with gonorrhea), then the expedited partner therapy should include oral doxycycline 100 mg twice daily for 7 days (for nonpregnant persons).

Test of Cure

Essential in:

- Persisting symptoms or signs.
- Pharyngeal infection (all treatments are less effective at eradicating pharyngeal infection).
- Treatment with anything other than the first-line recommendations.
- Test of cure is ideally needed in all patients:
  - If using NAATs, test 2 weeks after Rx. If +ve → send culture.
  - If using culture, test ≥72 hours after Rx. Note that infection identified after treatment may well be due to reinfection.

Special Considerations

1. *Allergy, Intolerance, and Adverse Reactions*

Use of ceftriaxone or cefixime is contraindicated in persons with a history of penicillin allergy.
- Intramuscular gentamicin 240 mg plus a single dose of oral azithromycin 2 grams.

2. *Pregnancy*

Single intramuscular dose of ceftriaxone 500 mg, with the addition of azithromycin if *Chlamydia* infection was not ruled out.

3. *HIV Infection*

Persons who have gonorrhea and HIV infection should receive the same treatment regimen as those who are HIV negative.

4. *Gonococcal Conjunctivitis*

Ceftriaxone 1 g IM single dose **plus** azithromycin 1 g orally in a single dose.

5. *Treatment of Arthritis and Arthritis-Dermatitis Syndrome* (CDC)

- Ceftriaxone 1 g IM or IV every 24 hours **plus** azithromycin 1 g orally in a single dose.
- After 24–48 hours after clinical improvement, can switch to oral agent for a total treatment course of at least 7 days.

6. *Treatment of Gonococcal Meningitis and Endocarditis* (CDC)

- Ceftriaxone 1–2 g IV every 12–24 hours **plus** azithromycin 1 g orally in a single dose.
- Therapy for meningitis should be continued with recommended parenteral therapy for 10–14 days.
- Parenteral anti-microbial therapy for endocarditis should be administered for at least 4 weeks.

7. *Investigational Therapy for N. Gonorrhoeae*

Single dose oral gepotidacin and single dose oral zoliflodacin. These two agents are now under study in phase 3 trials and both may have a future role in treating drug-resistant gonorrhea, and for treatment of gonorrhea in persons with serious penicillin or cephalosporin allergy. The oral agents solithromycin and delafloxacin showed promising early results, but phase 3 studies have been disappointing and these agents not likely to have a clinical role in the treatment of gonorrhea.

NONGONOCOCCAL URETHRITIS

Etiology

- NGU is the most common treatable STD in men (Moi et al).
- *Chlamydia trachomatis* (commonest)—15–40% of NGU
- *Mycoplasma genitalium*—second most common (15–25% of cases, with a double infection with *C. trachomatis* in 5 to 15%)
- Neither *C. trachomatis* nor *M. genitalium* is detected in 30–60%.
- Pathogen negative NGU is more likely with increasing age, the absence of discharge or clinical symptoms, and engagement in low-risk practices.

Clinical Features

The type of clinical infection caused by *C. trachomatis* is determined by the outer membrane protein A (OmpA—also known as MOMP), which can be determined based on culture (OmpA serovar) or molecular methods (OmpA genotype).

Although the majority of *C. trachomatis* infections caused by OmpA types D through K in women and men are asymptomatic, symptoms and clinical syndromes can develop at any site of infection.

Males

- Urethral discharge—mucoid/watery and sparse (cf copious purulent discharge in GU). This may not have been noticed by the patient or may only be present on urethral massage.
- Dysuria
- Balanoposthitis
- Normal examination otherwise.

Complications

- Epididymo-orchitis
- Prostatitis
- Sexually acquired reactive arthritis/Reiter syndrome. These are infrequent, occurring in fewer than 1% of cases though incomplete forms may be more common.

Females

The majority of women with chlamydial infection initially have no signs or symptoms, but may present later with uncomplicated infection (cervicitis or urethritis); some women develop complicated infections, including pelvic inflammatory disease, perihepatitis, endometritis, salpingitis, or reactive arthritis.

Cervicitis

Is involved in 75–80% of women and is asymptomatic in most cases where it is difficult to distinguish them from uninfected women, due to the infrequency of finding cervicitis (cervical findings of mucopurulent endocervical discharge and/or spontaneous or easily induced endocervical bleeding). The symptoms are non-specific, such as vague discomfort or spotting.

Urethritis

Urethral infection with *Chlamydia* in women is usually asymptomatic, but it can cause 'dysuria-pyuria' syndrome, or an 'acute urethral syndrome', mimicking acute cystitis.

Diagnosis of *Chlamydia trachomatis*

1. **Cell culture (gold standard)**—McCoy, HeLa cells. Sample of columnar cells from the cervix or urethra is necessary. Specimen composed of PMNL or mucopurulent discharge is inadequate (for *Chlamydia*).
2. **Antigen detection**—Direct fluorescent antibody (DFA) and enzyme-linked immunosorbent assay (EIA)
3. **Nucleic acid hybridization**—PAGE 2 assay by Genprobe.
   (NAAT is the preferred method to diagnose chlamydial infection, primarily because of improved sensitivity; this test is FDA approved for use on urine specimens from men and women, urethral swabs in men, and endocervical swabs in women).
4. **DNA amplification tests**—polymerase chain reaction **(PCR)** and ligase chain reaction **(LCR)**, **TMA**.
5. **Serology**—complement fixation test or microimmunofluorescence test.

Treatment of Chlamydial Urethritis

Most studies show comparable efficacy between azithromycin and doxycycline and rectal chlamydial infections are treated similarly to urogenital infection, with the caveat that data from observational trials suggest doxycycline may have greater efficacy than azithromycin for the treatment of rectal *C. trachomatis* infection.

Abstinence from sexual intercourse for 7 days after a single dose of azithromycin or until completion of a 7-day regimen of doxycycline is advised; also they should not resume sexual activity until all symptoms related to the chlamydial infection have resolved and their sex partners have received treatment for *Chlamydia*.

Recommended regimen (CDC 2021)

Doxycycline 100 mg BD for 7 days*

Alternate treatment:

Azithromycin 1 g orally single dose

OR

Azithromycin 500 single dose, then 250 mg OD × 4 days

*Azithromycin no longer recommended as first line drug due to increasing reports of resistance among *Chlamydia* and *M. genitalium*.

Treatment of *M. Genitalium*

Thus, if there is treatment failure, there is a likelihood that resistance has developed on treatment. The need for moxifloxacin is in case of treatment failure, which is defined as persistent symptoms following treatment, or a positive test of cure taken 5 weeks post-treatment. A treatment algorithm is depicted in **Fig. 33.34** and the overview of the treatment is given below, the important consideration is that there is now a rising incidence of macrolide resistance which can undermine the efficacy of azithromycin.

- Doxycycline 100 mg BD × 7 days followed by azithromycin 1 g orally as a single dose then 500 mg orally once daily for 2 days
  (if the organism is known to be macrolide-sensitive or where resisance status is unknown).
- Moxifloxacin 400 mg orally × 10 days
  (if organism is known to be macrolide resistant or where treatment with azithromycin has failed).

PERSISTENT AND RECURRENT NGU

- Persistent urethritis is defined as urethritis that fails to resolve or substantially improve within 1 week of initiating therapy.
- Recurrent urethritis is defined as the return of symptomatic urethritis within 6 weeks following an initial response to therapy of acute NGU.
- It has been estimated that even after successful treatment, 10–20% of patients have persistent or recurrent urethritis. In nonchlamydial NGU, the failure rates may be even beyond 50% and these are the cases that need a careful analysis.
- The basic steps of diagnosis are ***documentation*** of urethritis, confirmation of ***adherence*** with previous therapy and ruling out ***reinfection***.
- As a thumb rule, the longer the duration between episodes of urethritis in a sexually active man, the greater the likelihood that reinfection is the cause.

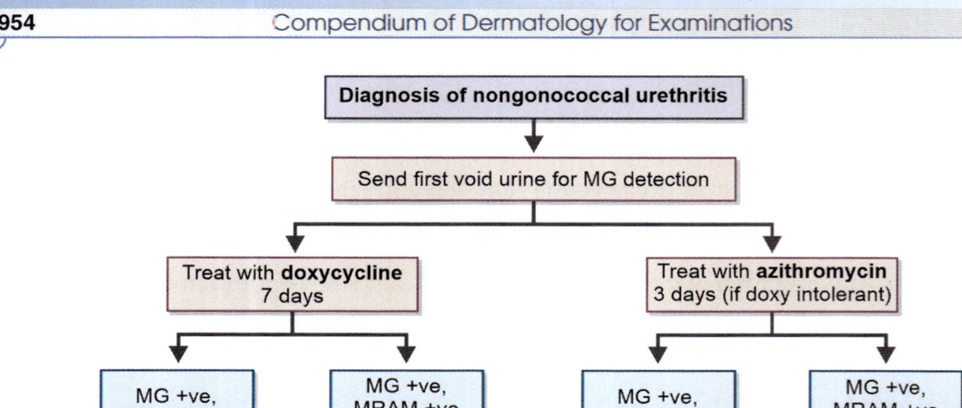

Fig. 33.34: Suggested treatment pathway for men presenting with nongonococcal urethritis who subsequently test positive for *M. genitalium*

Etiology

- First rule out reinfection and poor adherence to treatment.
- *Mycoplasma genitalium (MC, especially following doxycycline therapy)*, *Chlamydia trachomatis*, *Ureaplasma urealyticum*, HSV, *Trichomonas* vaginalis (serovars 2, 5, 8, 9)
- 20–50%—no cause can be identified

A summary of the varied etiologies is given below in **Box 33.9**.

Steps to Investigate

- **Step 1**—R/o reinfection or lack of compliance
- **Step 2**—Gram smear, wet mount, NAAT
- **Step 3**—Four-glass test (prostatitis) ≥5 WBCs per high-power field in expressed prostatic secretions.
- **Step 4**—pain for >3 months within a 6 months period, refer to urologist.

BOX 33.9: Etiology of PRNGU

Infectious causes	*M. genitalium*, *T. vaginalis*, HSV type 1 and 2, anti-microbial resistant *Chlamydia trachomatis*
Noninfectious causes	Immunological reaction to chlamydial heat-shock protein, Reiter syndrome, Kawasaki syndrome, urethral strictures, foreign bodies and periurethral fistulae
Prostatitis	

Treatment Principles

1. Urethritis should be *documented* in all patients presenting with persistent or recurrent symptoms. If no objective evidence of NGU is found, the patients should be reassured and re-examined at a later date if symptoms persist.
2. If there is objective evidence of NGU, and there is *noncompliance* or *reinfection*, then retreatment is advisable.
3. If there is a history of *sexual contact* before resolution of symptoms, the patient should be retreated with the original regimen.
4. Treatment of persistent urethritis should cover *M. genitalium*, *T. vaginalis* and anaerobes.

Recommended regimens

Any treatment of persistent NGU should cover *M. genitalium* (most common cause) and *T. vaginalis* and/or bacterial vaginosis-associated bacteria. An approach to treatment is given in **Fig. 33.35**.

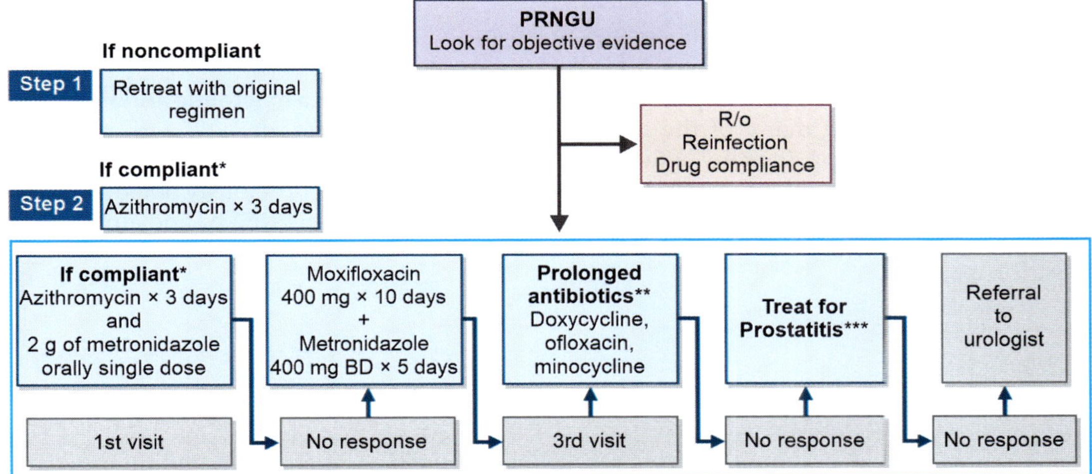

* In this case treatment of *Mycoplasma genitalium* is advised—azithromycin 1 g orally as a single dose then 500 mg orally once daily for 2 days, if non-responsive treat as MRM. For trichomoniasis, metronidazole 400–500 mg BD × 5–7 days can also be given.

** If the patient returns with PRNGU and no new exposure is identified, we do not recommend further evaluation for gonorrhea and *Chlamydia*; antibiotics: Doxycycline 100 mg orally twice daily for 3 weeks; ofloxacin 300 mg orally twice daily for 1 week (levofloxacin, 500 mg/day orally, should be as effective).

*** 4- to 6-week course of fluoroquinolones

Fig. 33.35: An approach to treatment of PRNGU

Treatment (CDC 2021)

Recommended regimen if *M. genitalium* resistance testing is available:

- Macrolide sensitive: Doxycydine 100 mg BD × 7 days followed by Azithromycin 1 g single dose and then 500 mg OD × 3 days
- Macrolide resistant: Doxycycline 100 mg BD × 7 days followed by Moxifloxacin 400 mg OD × 7 days

Recommended regimen if *M. genitalium* resistance testing is not available:

Doxycycline 100 mg BD × 7 days followed by
Moxifloxacin 400 mg OD × 7 days

Trichomonas vaginalis (common cause in heterosexual men)
Metronidazole 2 g single dose

Continuing symptoms

- Rule out chronic abacterial prostatitis, chronic pelvic pain syndrome and psychosexual causes. Chronic pelvic pain syndrome (CPPS)—a complex condition which overlaps with chronic urethritis.
- Recurrent HSV—dysuria and monocytes in smear.
- Female partner may have TV or BV. Treat with doxycycline/metronidazole.
- Most patients with PRNGU improve following retreatment with a macrolide antibiotic and metronidazole, and many of the remaining cases resolve after an extended course of erythromycin therapy. In many of those whose disease recurs or does not improve following those treatments, symptoms resolve spontaneously over time. As previously noted, patients can be reassured that there is no documented association between PRNGU and any serious sequelae **(Fig. 33.35)**.

VAGINAL DISCHARGE, CERVICITIS, AND PID

- **Healthy vagina:** Vagina is a dynamic ecosystem that normally contains approximately 10^9 bacterial colony-forming units per gram of vaginal fluid. Due to lactobacilli the vaginal pH is between 3.8 and 4.5 and this is due to the conversion of glycogen → lactic acid and H_2O_2 production. However, absence of lactobacilli does not inevitably lead to illness. Other lactic acid producing bacteria may maintain healthy vaginal milieu—*Atopobium vaginae*, *Megasphaera*, *Leptotrichia*, etc.
- We will discuss the salient aspects of the important causes of vaginal discharge, while the treatment is given in **Table 33.28**.

1. Bacterial Vaginosis

Most common cause of vaginal discharge/malodor; but a majority of females may be asymptomatic.

Causes

Facultative anaerobic bacteria—*Gardnerella vaginalis*, *Mycoplasma*
Anaerobic GN-rods—*Prevotella*, *Bacteroides*
Anaerobic GP (Gram variable)-rods—*Mobiluncus* spp.
Anaerobic GP-cocci—*Peptostreptococcus*

Risk Factors

- Younger sexual debut
- Douching
- Black race
- Smoking
- Chronic stress
- New or higher number of male sex partners
- IUD use
- Hormonal contraceptives
- Menses

TABLE 33.28: Treatment options for vaginal discharge (CDC 2021)

Drug options for BV*	Drug options for TV*	Drug options for VVC*
Metronidazole 500 mg BID for 7 days OR Metronidazole 0.75% gel 5 g daily intravaginally for 5 days OR Clindamycin 2% vaginal cream, 5 g at bedtime intravaginally for 7 days <u>Alternatives regimen</u> Clindamycin 300 mg BID for 7 days OR Tinidazole 2 g OD for 2 days OR Tinidazole 1 g OD for 5 days OR Secnidazole 2 g oral granules single dose	Metronidazole 500 mg BID for 7 days <u>Alternative regimen</u> Tinidazole 2 g single dose	Miconazole 4% or clotrimazole 2% (5 g) intravaginally for 3 consecutive days OR Fluconazole 150 mg as a single dose

*BV, bacterial vaginosis; TV, trichomoniasis; VVC, vulvovaginal candidiasis.

Symptoms

- Malodorous thin gray homogeneous vaginal discharge (malodor may be intermittent—only after intercourse/during menstruation—as semen/blood increases pH leading to fishy odor).
- Recurrences—30% within 3 months and 50% within 1 year (due to biofilm on vaginal wall).

Complications

- Higher risk of acquiring STDs—HPG, *Chlamydia*, gonorrhea, HIV, trichomoniasis, esp. with higher (>8) Nugent scores.
- Ascending infection (PID)
- Post-operative complications—vaginal stump infections, uterine infections
- Pregnancy—PROM, early and late miscarriage, habitual miscarriage, preterm labor, sepsis after miscarriage, chorioamnionitis, postpartum endometritis.

Diagnosis

- **Amsel criteria (clinical criteria)**—3 out of 4 **(Box 33.10)** to be present to diagnose—almost as effective as Nugent score.
- **Nugent score**—microbiological evaluation of normal and pathogenic flora on Gram stain. Considered gold standard in diagnosis of BV **(Box 33.11)**. This is based on the relative concentration of lactobacillus, *Bacteroides*, *Gardnerella*, and *Mobiluncus* species.

BOX 33.10: Amsel criteria for diagnosis of BV (3 out of 4 should be present for diagnosis)

1. Homogeneous, non-viscous, milky-white discharge adherent to the vaginal walls.
2. Amine (fishy) odor when potassium hydroxide solution is added to vaginal secretions (commonly called the 'whiff test').
3. Presence of clue cells (greater than 20%) in wet mount on microscopy.
4. Vaginal pH greater than 4.5—most sensitive but least specific sign.

BOX 33.11: Nugent score

Organism/morpho type	Number/oil immersion field	Score
Lactobacillus-like (parallel sided, gram-positive rods)	>30	0
	5–30	1
	1–4	2
	<1	3
	0	4
Mobiluncus-like (Curved, Gram positive/Gram variable rods)	>5	2
	1–5	1
	0	0
Gardnerella/Bacteroides-like (tiny, gram variable coccobacilli and pleomorphic rods with vacuoles)	>30	4
	5–30	3
	1–4	2
	<1	1

Total score: 0–3 = Normal; 4–6 = Intermediate, repeat test later; 7–10 = Bacterial vaginosis.

- Hay-Ison criteria: These are also based on the findings on a Gram-stained smear but are easier and quicker to use in clinical practice and do include non-BV-associated bacteria.
- Clue cells: Squamous vaginal epithelial cells covered with vaginal bacteria *Gardnerella, Mobiluncus* amongst others covering the epithelial borders giving a stippled appearance **(Fig. 33.36)**.

Treatment

While the treatment is summarized in **Table 33.28**, a 5–7 days of topical or oral metronidazole or 7 days of intravaginal clindamycin can be considered first line for uncomplicated BV in women. In pregnancy metronidazole is safe and partner treatment is not needed in BV.

2. Vulvovaginal Candidiasis (VVC)

The second most common cause of vaginal discharge. While vulvovaginal candidiasis is not a sexually transmitted disease, it frequently causes clinical manifestations that overlap with several other common sexually transmitted diseases.

Causes

- *Candida albicans*—90%
- *Candida glabrata*—9–10%
- Others— *C. krusei, C. tropicalis, C. parapsilosis*, etc.

Risk Factors

- Low immunity
- Uncontrolled diabetes mellitus
- Antibiotic therapy
- Gene polymorphisms
- Pregnancy
- Estrogens (not low-dose combined OCPs)

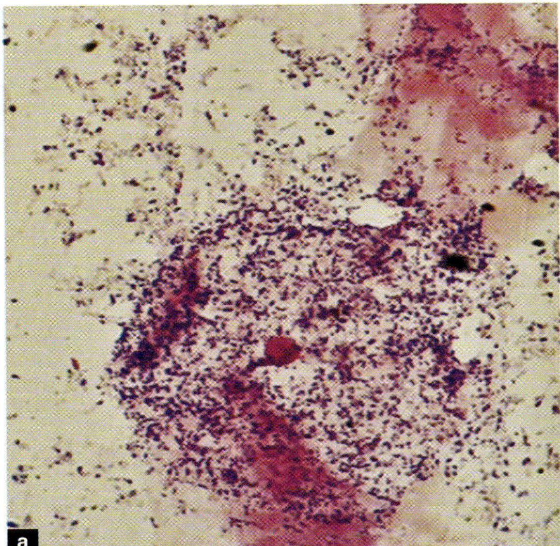

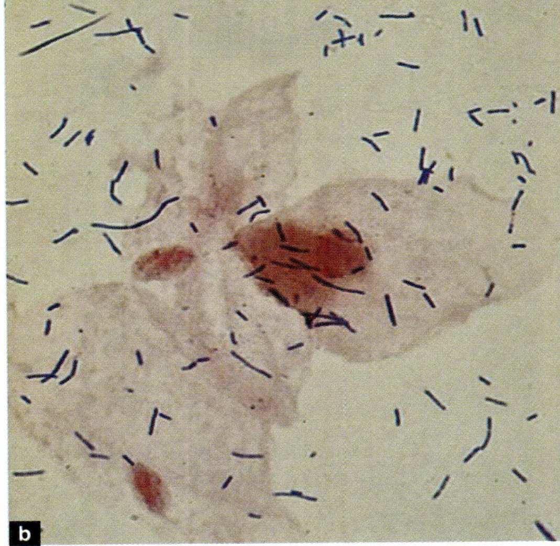

Fig. 33.36: A clue cell studded with bacilli (a) and a normal smear with lactobacilli predominating with vaginal epithelial cells (b). The clue cells should constitute at least 20% of vaginal epithelial cells viewed on saline microscopy (an occasional clue cell does not fulfill this criterion) for diagnosis of BV

Pathogenesis

Disruption of the host vaginal environment can cause *Candida* organisms to transition from a commensurate to pathologic role (Gonçalves B, et al., 2016). Yeast blastospores are typically responsible for asymptomatic colonization, whereas mycelia (pseudohyphae or hyphae forms) cause symptomatic vaginitis through overgrowth and adherence to vaginal epithelial cells (Sobel JD, 2007).

Destruction of host tissue by *Candida* species is mediated by the activity of several hydrolytic enzymes, which promote adhesion and host tissue penetration, as well as other virulence factors, such as biofilm formation and phenotypic switching.

While there are no risk factors for uncomplicated VVC, certain factors suggest complicated VVC and are listed in **Fig. 33.37**.

Clinical Features

Symptoms

- Itching
- Burning, pain, dysuria, dyspareunia
- Tend to flare prior to the onset of menses
- White thick curdy odorless discharge but may be minimal.

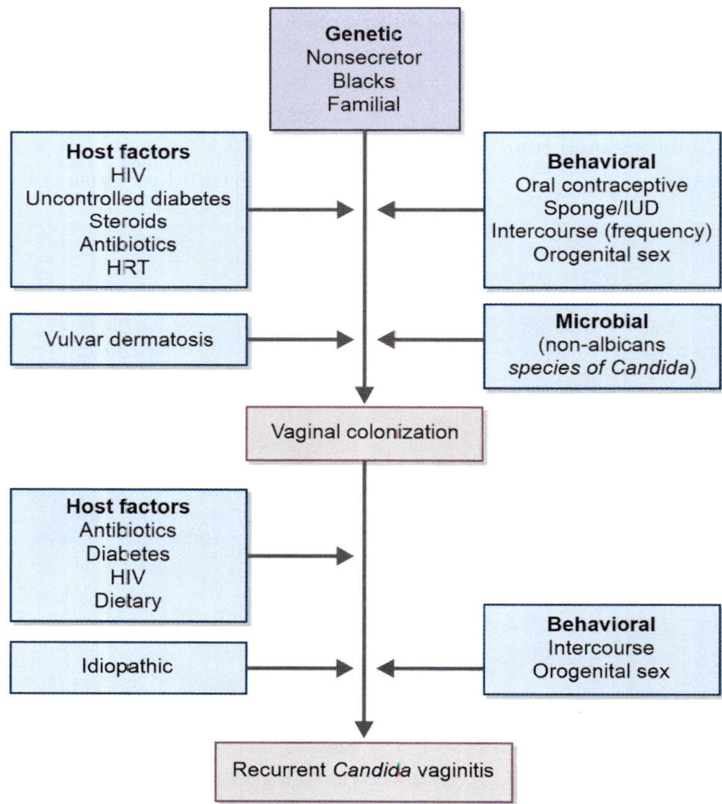

Fig. 33.37: Overview of factors that cause candidal vaginitis

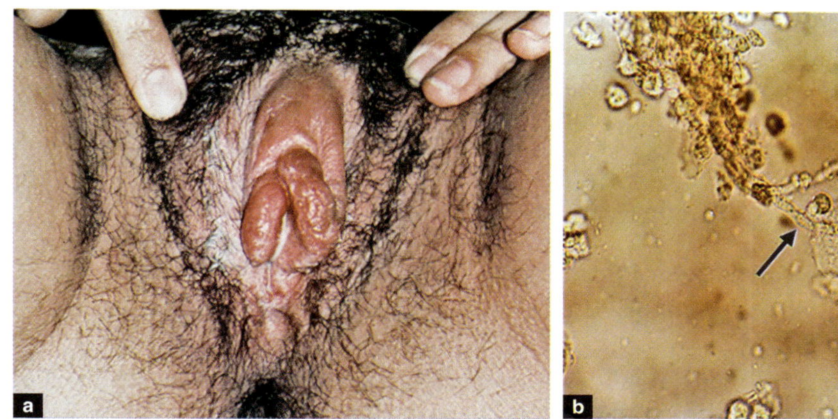
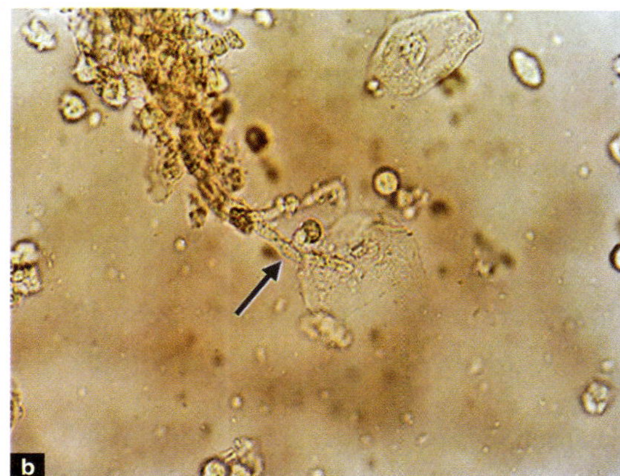

Fig. 33.38: Candidiasis: (a) Lumpy white discharge with the consistency of a pasty, wet talc; (b) KOH smear showing pseudohyphae

- Red edematous vagina
- Vulval candidiasis may be associated—eczematous, vesicular, follicular **(Fig. 33.38)**.

Classification (*Workowski KA*) (Box 33.12)

Uncomplicated vulvovaginal candidiasis is defined as sporadic or infrequent infection in an immunocompetent, non-pregnant woman that is mild-to-moderate in severity, recurs ≤2 times per year, and involves *Candida albicans* strains that respond to all forms of antifungal therapy.

Complicated vulvovaginal candidiasis, by contrast, is defined as infection that is (1) moderate to severe, (2) associated with pregnancy or other concomitant conditions (i.e. immunosuppression, diabetes mellitus), or (3) recurs ≥3 times per year, or (4) is caused by non-*albicans* species of *Candida*.

Diagnosis

- pH: Normal pH (4.0–4.5)—if the pH is abnormally high (>4.5), it suggests an alternative diagnosis of bacterial vaginosis or trichomoniasis, or a mixed infection.
- 10% KOH mount: Sensitivity in identifying germinating yeast is 65–85%. Most patients with vulvovaginal candidiasis do not have abundant white blood cells visualized on microscopy. Large number of white blood cells indicates a diagnosis other than vulvovaginal candidiasis, or a mixed infection.

BOX 33.12: Difference between complicated VCC and uncomplicated VCC

	Complicated VVC	Uncomplicated VVC
Severity	Moderate-to-severe Recurrent VVC	Sporadic/infrequent VVC
Frequency	≥3 episodes/year	≤2 episodes/year
Species	Non-albicans species (*C. glabrata*)	*C. albicans*
Microscopy	Blastospores	Pseudohyphae
Host	Pregnancy/DM/immunocompromised	Healthy/nongravid
Treatment	Intensive regimens	Short course treatment

- Saline wet mount: Yeast cells and mycelia may be seen.
- Culture—fungal cultures are not useful for the routine diagnosis of vulvovaginal candidiasis since positive cultures may detect colonization rather than clinically significant infections. In some circumstances, however, fungal culture may be useful to detect non-albicans species (since *C. glabrata* only forms blastospores and is easily missed on microscopy) or resistant organisms in women with recurrent disease, and is recommended before initiating suppressive therapy for vulvovaginal candidiasis.

Treatment of Recurrent Valvovaginal Candidiasis (RVVC)

The treatment of VVC is listed in **Box 33.13**.

RVVC is best treated by a 3-day induction course of an azole followed by long-term maintenance suppressive regimen for at least 6 months. The salient principles of treatment of recurrent VVC is that intensive initial therapy achieves mycologic remission before using maintenance therapy which has been demonstrated to reduce episodes of vulvovaginal candidiasis, but symptoms recur in about 30–50% of women once maintenance therapy is stopped.

Notably treatment of sexual partners is not needed as it is not a STD. In pregnancy fluconazole should not be given and topical azoles are preferred, even though a large cohort found that the drug even in first trimester is largely safe with a small risk of tetralogy of Fallot (Mølgaard-Nielsen D, et al., 2013).

3. Trichomonas Vaginitis (TV)

Trichomoniasis is almost always sexually transmitted; fomite transmission is extremely rare. *Trichomonas vaginalis* may persist for months to years in epithelial crypts and periglandular areas of the genital tract. Distinguishing persistent, subclinical infection from remote sexual acquisition is not always possible.

(Males—more commonly affected and symptomatic than females).

BOX 33.13: Overview of treatment of VVC

1. **Uncomplicated VVC**
   Fluconazole 150 mg single dose
2. **Recurrent VVC treatment (CDC 2021)**
   Initiation therapy: Longer duration of initial therapy (7–14 days of topical therapy)
   OR
   100 mg, 150 mg, or 200 mg oral fluconazole on Day-1, Day-4, Day-7
   Maintenance: Oral fluconazole (100 mg, 150 mg, or 200 mg) weekly for 6 months
3. **Severe VVC (skin fissuring, edema)**
   Fluconazole 150 mg two doses at 72 hour intervals or 7–14 days of topical therapy
4. **Non-albicans VVC:**
   First-line therapy: Longer duration of therapy (7–14 days) with a non-fluconazole azole regimen (oral or topical)
   Recurrence: 600 mg of boric acid in a gelatin capsule administered vaginally once daily for 3 weeks
   - *C. krusei*: Fluconazole resistant. Treat with topical clotrimazole/ciclopirox olamine × 6–14 days.
   - *C. glabrata*: Fluconazole resistant. But very rarely symptomatic. Fluconazole 800 mg once daily for 2–3 weeks or flucytosine vaginal cream 5 g at night for 14 days or micafungin IV for 15 days.

Symptoms and Signs in Females

- Malodorous greenish—yellow frothy discharge with pruritus but also can be asymptomatic
- Dysuria
- Dyspareunia
- Burning
- Post-coital bleeding (occasionally)
- Vulval edema
- Colpitis macularis
- **'Strawberry cervix'**—due to punctate hemorrhages. Seen in 5% of cases.

Complications

- Cervical dysplasia and cervical neoplasia
- Infertility
- Preterm labor, PROM, low birth weight-if in pregnancy
- HIV acquisition—increased risk
  (BV may coexist with TV)

Diagnosis

- Direct microscopic examination: From vaginal discharge
- Wet mount has sensitivity of 50–70% in females, lesser in males **(Fig. 33.39)**
- Staining methods
  1. Gram
  2. Giemsa
  3. Papanicolaou
  4. PAS acridine orange
  5. Fluoroscein
  6. Neutral red

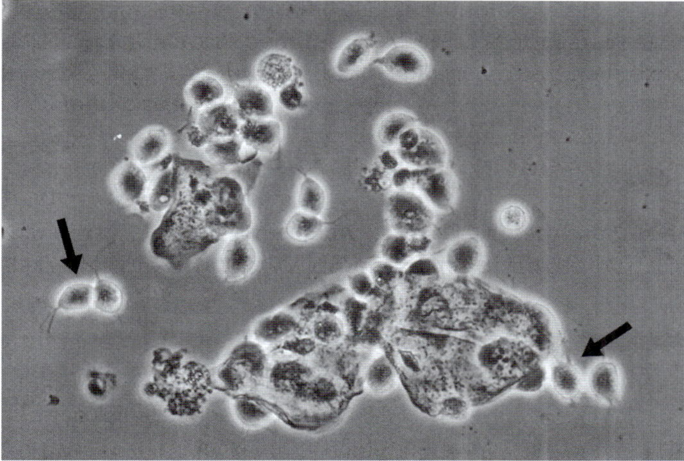

Fig. 33.39: *Trichomonas vaginalis* on a saline mount which should be examined immediately (always within 10 minutes), since the trichomonads will become increasingly sluggish on the wet mount

Treatment

First choice

Metronidazole 500 mg orally twice daily for 7 days or metronidazole 2 g orally in a single dose or tinidazole 2 g orally in a single dose.

Persistent TV

Persistent or recurrent TV is due to inadequate therapy, reinfection, or resistance. Check for compliance and exclude vomiting of metronidazole and exclude the possibility of reinfection from new or untreated partners. Usually, a retreatment or a higher dose is successful (Das S, et al., 2005).

- Metronidazole 400–500 mg twice daily for 7 days
- Metronidazole or tinidazole 2 g daily for 5–7 days
- Metronidazole 800 mg three times daily for 7 days.

4. Cervicitis

Definition

a. Purulent/mucopurulent endocervical exudate (mucopurulent cervicitis), and/or
b. Sustained endocervical bleeding easily induced by gentle passage of a cotton swab through the cervical os.

Leukorrhoea (>10 WBCs/HPF of vaginal fluid) has a high negative predictive value (i.e. cervicitis is unlikely in the absence of leukorrhoea).

Causes

- *C. trachomatis*] most common
- *N. gonorrhoeae*]
- Trichomoniasis
- Genital herpes (esp. HSV2)
- *M. genitalium*
- Often, no organism is isolated

Treatment of cervicitis (CDC 2021)

Recommended regimen
Doxycycline 100 mg BD × 7 days
+/–
Ceftriaxone 500 mg IM single dose (if at risk for gonorrhoea)

Alternative regimen
Azithromycin 1 g single dose

5. Aerobic Vaginitis (AV) and Desquamative Inflammatory Vaginitis

Desquamative inflammatory vaginitis (DIV) occurs more frequently in perimenopausal or post-menopausal women than in women of reproductive age. This chronic syndrome has been documented much more frequently in Caucasians (Mason MJ).

It is not known whether this has an infectious origin or whether it is an inflammatory process followed by a dysbiosis.

Causes

Aerobic microorganisms, like *Escherichia coli*, group B streptococci, and *Staphylococcus aureus* predominate.

Symptoms and Signs

Present with:

- Complaints of vaginal irritation and secondary dyspareunia lasting months or even years.
- Examination shows vaginal erythema with the appearance of a spotted or linear rash or erosions and vestibulitis.
- Changes often resemble 'strawberry' rash.
- A purulent yellow-green discharge may be present.

Laboratory

- Vaginal pH >4.5 (usually >6)
- Amine test—negative (indicates lack of anerobic organism)
- 3–4 Vaginal PMNs
- ↑ parabasal cells + Naked nuclei
- Lack of lactobacilli
- Gram-positive cocci

Treatment

- 2% clindamycin cream 5 g intravaginally for 7–21 days
- Combination use of intravaginal clindamycin and intravaginal steroids,
- In cases with a significant atrophy component, local oestrogens can be added.

Clindamycin is active against staphylococci and streptococci as well as anaerobes. Other anti-microbials which are used with success in AV include kanamycin ovules or moxifloxacin.

6. Pelvic Inflammatory Disease

Pelvic inflammatory disease (PID) is a clinical syndrome comprising a spectrum of infectious and inflammatory diseases of the upper female genital tract. The diagnosis of PID can include any combination of endometritis, salpingitis, tubo-ovarian abscess, or pelvic peritonitis. Each of these disease processes is characterized by ascending spread of organisms from the vagina or cervix to the structures of the upper female genital tract.

The clinical classification is given in **Box 33.14**, though the most common pathogens identified are *N. gonorrhoeae* or *C. trachomatis* (or both); recent data suggest that the proportion of PID cases attributable to these pathogens is decreasing due to widespread screening and treatment of *N. gonorrhoeae* and *C. trachomatis*.

Risk Factors

- <25 years old
- Young age at first intercourse
- Recent new sexual partner/frequent change of sexual partner
- No use of barrier contraceptives
- Intercourse during menstruation
- New placement of IUD within 3–6 weeks
- Prior history of PID

Clinical Features

There are a wide spectrum of features that may be virtually asymptomatic to severe with debilitating symptoms. Women with acute PID may experience subtle, nonspecific symptoms

BOX 33.14: Classification of PID (Brunham RC, et al., 2015)

Acute pelvic inflammatory disease (≤30 days' duration)	Cervical pathogens (*Neisseria gonorrhoeae, Chlamydia trachomatis*, and *Mycoplasma genitalium*) Bacterial vaginosis pathogens (*Peptostreptococcus* species, *Bacteroides* species, *Atopobium* species, *Leptotrichia* species, *M. hominis, Ureaplasma urealyticum*, and *Clostridia* species) Respiratory pathogens (*Haemophilus influenzae, Streptococcus pneumoniae*, group A streptococci, and *Staphylococcus aureus*) Enteric pathogens (*Escherichia coli, Bacteroides fragilis*, group B streptococci, and *Campylobacter* species)
Subclinical pelvic inflammatory disease	*C. trachomatis* and *N. gonorrhoeae*
Chronic pelvic inflammatory disease (>30 days' duration)	*Mycobacterium tuberculosis* and *Actinomyces* species

such as dyspareunia, dysuria, or gastrointestinal symptoms, which they may not attribute to pelvic infection.

Two kinds of complications

Acute: These include local tissue damage, fallopian tube swelling, tubal occlusion, and development of adhesions.

Chronic: These include ectopic pregnancy, infertility, or chronic pelvic pain and may occur after a single episode of symptomatic PID. A recent retrospective cohort study of women admitted with PID or tubo-ovarian abscess (TOA) found that, in follow-up, 25.5% of women met the criteria of infertility, 16.0% had recurrent PID, and 13.8% reported chronic pelvic pain (Chayachinda C, et al., 2016).

The diagnosis is based on clinical suspicion and less precise diagnostic techniques and is given below (Workowski KA, et al., 2015).

Criteria for initiating presumptive treatment for PID—presumptive treatment for PID in sexually active young women and other women at risk for STDs, if they are experiencing pelvic or lower abdominal pain, if no cause for the illness other than PID can be identified, and if one or more of the following minimum clinical criteria are present on pelvic examination:

Cervical motion tenderness OR Uterine tenderness OR Adnexal tenderness

Additional criteria—one or more of the following additional criteria can be used to enhance the specificity of the minimum clinical criteria and support a diagnosis of PID:

- Oral temperature >101°F (>38.3°C);
- Abnormal cervical mucopurulent discharge or cervical friability;
- Presence of abundant numbers of WBC on saline microscopy of vaginal fluid;
- Elevated erythrocyte sedimentation rate;
- Elevated C-reactive protein;
- Laboratory documentation of cervical infection with *N. gonorrhoeae* or *C. trachomatis*.

Most specific criteria for the diagnosis of PID—a diagnostic evaluation that includes one or more of the following more extensive procedures might be warranted in some cases:

Endometrial biopsy with histopathologic evidence of endometritis; OR Transvaginal sonography or magnetic resonance imaging techniques showing thickened, fluid-filled tubes with or without free pelvic fluid or tuboovarian complex, or Doppler studies suggesting pelvic infection (e.g. tubal hyperemia); OR Laparoscopic findings consistent with PID.

Treatment

Treatment regimens must provide empiric, broad-spectrum coverage of likely pathogens (*N. gonorrhoeae*, *C. trachomatis*, anaerobes, gram-negative facultative bacteria, and streptococci).

The treatment is given in **Box 33.15**.

BOX 33.15: CDC 2021 guidelines for treatment of PID

- **Ceftriaxone** 1 g IV every 24 hours + **Doxycycline** 100 mg orally or IV every 12 hours + **Metronidazole** 500 mg orally or IV every 12 hours
  (Oral therapy with doxycycline 100 mg twice daily can be used 24–48 hours after clinical improvement to complete the 14 days of therapy.
- Cefotetan 2 g IV every 12 hours + **Doxycycline** 100 mg orally or IV every 12 hours

Notably, in the parenteral regimen, third generation cephalosprins do not cover anaerobic infections and thus ampicillin-sulbactam 3 g IV every 6 hours can be offered.

Intramuscular/oral therapy can be considered for women with mild-to-moderately severe acute PID, because the clinical outcomes among women treated with these regimens are similar to those treated with intravenous therapy. All the oral regimen components should be continued for a total of 14 days. Patients on oral therapy should be followed up within 72 hours, at which time they should show substantial clinical improvement. If no improvement occurs by 72 hours, the patient should be re-evaluated to confirm the diagnosis and should be switched to parenteral therapy, either in an outpatient or inpatient setting.

ANOGENITAL WARTS

Epidemiology

- **Most common STD worldwide.**
- HPV types 6 and 11—low-risk subtypes (do not integrate in host genome)-90% anogenital warts.
- HPV types 16 and 18—**high risk**, (incorporate into host genome), strongly associated with cervical dysplasia (70% of cervix SCC) → uncontrolled activation of E6 and E7 genes → inactivate tumor suppressor genes (p53 and Rb) → oncongenicity.

Cause: HPV-epitheliotropic DNA virus

- **Genomes**—the early (E) region (E1–E7) are necessary for viral replication and late (L) region that encodes the structural proteins (L1–L2) are required for virion assembly.
- **Immunology:** HPV infections are mostly cleared by cell-mediated immunity (CMI), in which dendritic cells (DC), CD4+ T helper cells and CD8+ T cells play predominant roles.
- **Risk factors:**
  - Higher number of sex partners
  - Abraded genital epithelium
  - HIV seropositive
  - Organ transplant recipients
  - Male partner's—lifetime number of partners (for female patients)
  - Recent partner <8 months
  - Uncircumcised males (circumcision—protective for genital warts)
  - Hormones—estrogen increases, progesterone, controversial role.
- **Most common sites:**
  - Males—penis, scrotum, urethral meatus, perianal.
  - Females—introitus, vulva, perineum, perianal.

Clinical Types (Fig. 33.40)

1. **Condyloma acuminata**—cauliflower-like, on moist partially keratinized epithelium.
2. **Papular warts**—dome-shaped papules, on fully keratinized epithelium.
3. **Keratotic warts/verruca vulgaris**—thick crust-like layer similar to common cutaneous warts on dry fully keratinized epithelium.
4. **Flat macular warts**—macular to slightly raised on partially/fully keratinized epithelium.

Clinical Variants

- **Pigmented genital warts**
- **Leukoplakic genital warts**
- **Bowenoid papulosis**—differential diagnosis of papular warts. Hyperpigmented papules with HSIL (high grade squamous intraepithelial lesion) on histology, **appears at 25–35 years, HPV-16.**
- **Oral florid papillomatosis**—HPV-16, -18
- **Buschke–Lowenstein tumor/giant condyloma**—very large locally invasive and destructive but non-metastasizing growth. Mostly in immunosuppressed. HPV-6.

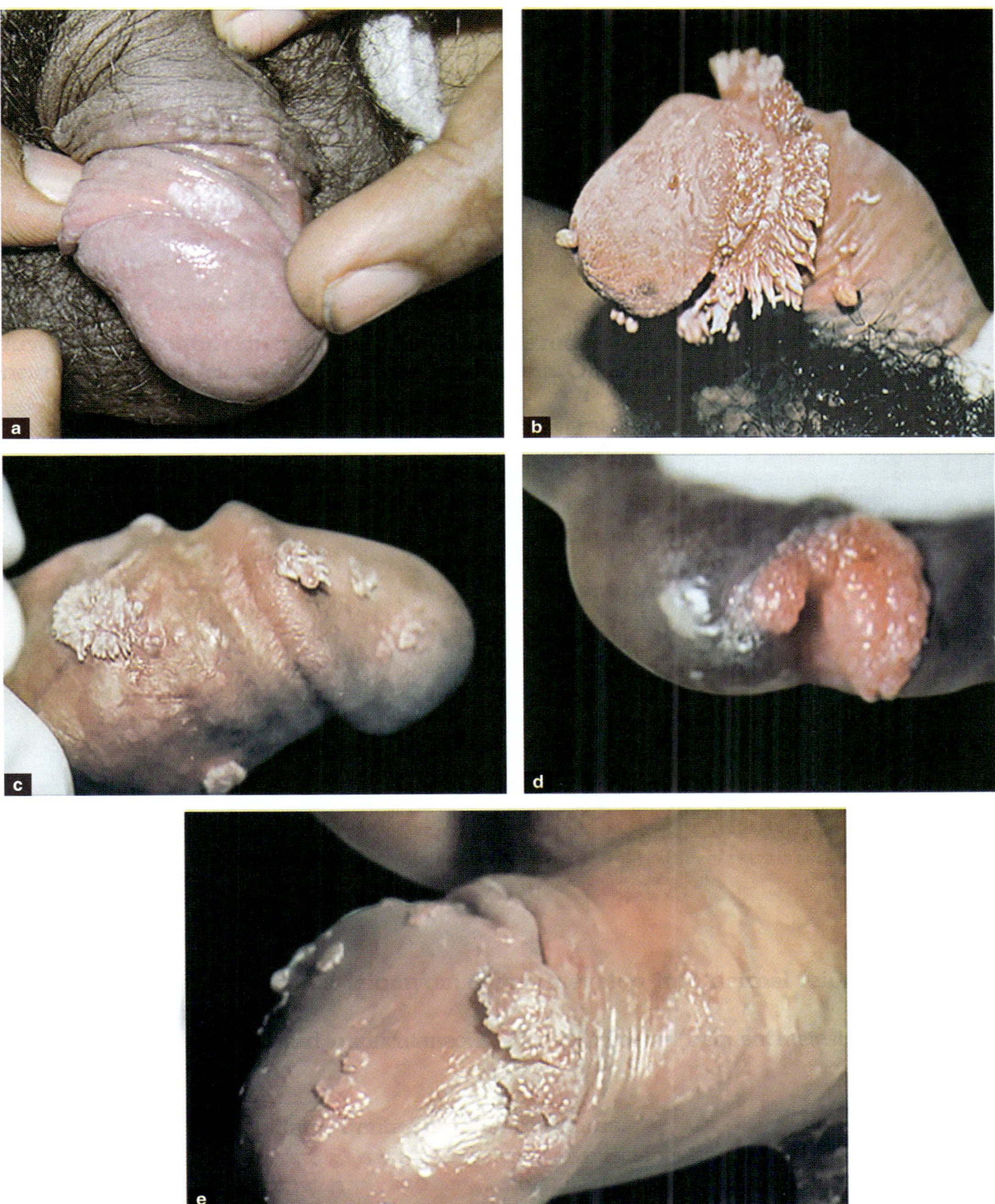

Fig. 33.40: Anogenital warts. Various variants of gental warts are depicted on the genitalia. The severity and extent varies depending on the duration of the disease and previous therapy prescribed to the patient

The transmission characteristics are detailed in **Table 33.29**.

TABLE 33.29: Transmission characteristics of genital HPV infection

- Infection is virtually always sexually transmitted and occurs as a result of microtrauma to skin/mucous membranes.
- Sexual contact with an HPV-infected individual → 75% chance of transmission (1.6 sexual contacts enough to get the infection.)
- Infection is most commonly acquired from persons with asymptomatic and subclinical infection.
- Role of fomite transmission unclear, probably rare.
- Incubation period variable, probably 3–28 months for genital warts and 4–36 months for cervical lesions.
- Vertical transmission may very rarely result in recurrent respiratory papillomatosis in infants and children.
- Genital HPV infection in children as a consequence of sexual abuse, viral inoculation at birth, incidental spread from cutaneous warts (DNA PCR to distinguish HPV types helps to identify nature of transmission—sexual abuse/auto-inoculation).

The complications are listed in **Table 33.30**.

TABLE 33.30: Complications of genital warts

- Most common—psychosocial (anger, guilt, anxiety)
- Occasionally urethral obstruction
- Rarely local invasion (giant condyloma)
- In pregnancy:
  - enlargement of warts causing birth canal obstruction
  - perinatal transmission leading to neonatal respiratory papillomatosis (NRP)
- In immunodeficiency:
  - enlargement, rarely malignant transformation

Differential Diagnosis (Table 33.31)

TABLE 33.31: Differential diagnosis of Condyloma acuminata

Condyloma acuminata	Papular	Keratotic	Flat macular
Acrochordons	Lichen planus	Seborrheic keratosis	Psoriasis
Pearly penile papules	Lichen nitidus		Circinata balanitis in Reiter syndrome
Sebaceous glands (Tyson's)	Bowenoid papulosis		Seborrheic dermatitis
Melanocytic nevi	Molluscum contagiosum	Bowen disease	
Condyloma lata	Pearly penile papules		Erythroplasia of Queyrat
Parafrenular glands			HPV-associated SCC

Diagnosis

Mainly clinical

- Speculum examination/ colposcopy—to look for cervical/vaginal warts in females with external genital warts.
- Anoscopy—if recurrent perianal warts and history of anoreceptive intercourse.
- Urethroscopy—male with warts at urethral meatus + terminal hematuria/abnormal urinary stream.
- **Acetowhite test (3–5% acetic acid)**—no longer recommended due to lack of standardization.

- **HPE:**
  - Parakeratosis, acanthosis, elongated dermal papillae, marked rounded papillomatosis, effacement of granular layer.
  - **Koilocytes**—mature keratinocytes with large hyperchromatic nuclei with large clear perinuclear zone scattered in outer epidermal layers.
  - Dermis—increased vascularization with thrombosed capillaries.

Treatment (Table 33.32 and 33.33)

- Patient—applied therapies are generally more efficacious for warts on moist skin surfaces than for warts on drier, more keratinized skin.
- Fewer and safer options are available for the treatment of genital warts at internal sites.
- Trichloroacetic acid (TCA) or bichloroacetic acid (BCA) is acceptable in vaginal, cervical, and intra-anal warts. The use of TCA, BCA, or podophyllin is contraindicated for urethral meatus warts.
- **Cytodestructive agents**, such as podophyllin and podophyllotoxin, are highly efficacious in rapidly clearing lesions, but they have safety concerns and side effects. For clearing warts, sinecatechins were seen to be significantly less efficacious than podophyllotoxin 0.5% or imiquimod 5%. (Jung, et al., 2020)
- **Immune-modifying or immune-enhancing agents**, such as imiquimod and sinecatechins, take longer time to achieve clearance.
- Imiquimod 1% cream, sinecatechins 15% ointment, imiquimod 5% cream and sinecatechins 10% ointment are the most efficacious for lowering recurrence.
- A recent paper used a combination of 5-fluorouracil 0.5%/salicylic acid 10% solution (5FU/SAsol) in difficult to treat warts which is a novel option (Ciccarese G, et al., 2022).
- Change treatment if no complete resolution after 6 weeks.
- Follow-up after 12 weeks for recurrence.

Summary of Common Treatment Modalities

- Small warts of duration <1 year—respond better to treatment.
- **Podophyllin toxin and podophyllin resin:** Act by disrupting spindle formation, causes metaphase arrest. More effective on mucosal warts than those on keratinized epithelium.
  - Contraindicated in bleeding warts, exceptionally large areas, pregnancy (abortifacient and mutagenic, but not teratogenic in animal studies) **(Table 33.34)**.
  - Podophyllin toxin—contraindicated in intra-anal, rectal, urethral, vaginal, cervical warts. (As these sites have a transitional epithelium and it may be potentially mutagenic here.)
- **Imiquimod**—contraindicated in perianal, rectal, urethral, vaginal, cervical warts. Apply with fingers alternate night (3/week) for 16 weeks. Wash with soap and water after 6–10 hours.
- **TCA/BCA**—for small moist warts only. 80–90%/week for 6 weeks. May apply baking soda to surrounding skin to remove unreacted acid.
- **Cryotherapy**—for small warts only. 1–6 freeze-thaw cycles/wart/session, 1–2/week for 4–6 weeks.
- **Electrosurgery**—contraindicated in patients with pacemakers and in lesions proximal to anal verge.

TABLE 33.32: Patient applied treatment modalities used for genital warts

Technique	Treatment	Mechanism of action	Schedule/procedure	Clearance rate (%)	Recurrence rate (%)
Topical	Podophyllotoxin (Podofilox) 0.5% solution or 0.15% cream	Act by disrupting spindle formation, metaphase arrest	BD × 3 days, followed by 4 rest days, for up to 4 or 5 weeks	36–83	6–100
Immunotherapy*	Imiquimod 5%/3.75%	Immunomodulator: Stimulates interferon and cytokine production	3.75%, once daily up to 8 weeks or 5%, 3 times per week for 6–10 hours at bedtime up to 16 weeks (safer in children)	35–75 after 16 weeks	6–26
	Sinecatechins 15% ointment	Inflammatory Response modulator	3 times daily up to 16 weeks	47–59	7–11% (low)

*Slower to act but with low recurrence rates

TABLE 33.33: Provider administered treatment modalities used for genital warts

Technique	Treatment	Mechanism of action	Schedule/procedure	Clearance rate (%)	Recurrence rate (%)
Topical	Podophyllin resin** (weekly)	Act by disrupting spindle formation, metaphase arrest	Apply with cotton swab, 1–2/week, for up to 6 weeks, ≤0.5 mL/≤10 cm^2 per treatment session	41–77	17–70
Ablative* **	Cryotherapy	Liquid nitrogen freezes and destroys lesions	Applied directly to lesions; repeat 2–3 cycles	46–96	18–39
	CO_2 and Nd:YAG laser	Laser vaporizes lesions	Under local anesthesia, protocol depends on type of laser	23–95	2.5–77
	Electrocautery	High-frequency electrical currents cause thermal damage to infected tissue	Under local anesthesia, base of lesion excised; repeat as required	35–94	20–25
	Surgery	Scissor or scalpel excision	Under local anesthetic using scissors, scalpel or curettage	89–93	18–65
	TCA* (33–50%)	Acid induces a chemical burn	Applied weekly with a wooden/ cotton tipped applicator	70–100	18–36

*TCA, trichloroacetic acid; BCA, bichloroacetic acid. **All treatment modalities given in **Tables 33.32** and **33.33** have level of evidence IA except podophyllin (not generally recommended).*** High recurrence rates in most cases, maximum in laser ablation and in some cases even before healing of laser treatment.

TABLE 33.34: Podophyllotoxin versus podophyllin resin

Podophyllotoxin	Podophyllin resin
Purified from toxin	Crude resin from dried roots of *Podophyllum peltatum P. emodi* (may apply)
Patient applied	Provider administered
0.5% solution in ethanol/0.15% gel	10–25% solution in tincture of benzoin
Stable, long shelf life	Unstable
Apply twice daily with cotton swab (3 days on 4 days off) for up to 4 weeks, should not exceed 10 cm^2/total volume 0.5 mL/day	Apply with cotton swab, 1–2/week, for up to 6 weeks, <0.5 mL/<10 cm^2 per treatment session
No need to wash off	Wash off after 4 hours
No systemic toxicity	Bone marrow depression possible

Site-specific and Management of Anogenital Warts in Special Situations

1. **Extragenital and perianal (penis, groin, scrotum, vulva, perineum, external anus)**
   Patient-applied:
   - Imiquimod—3.75% or 5% cream (1A)
   - Podophyllotoxin—0.5% solution (1B)
   - Sinecatechins—15% ointment (1A)
   - Cidofovir (3)
   - 5–FU (1A)
   - Interferon (1A)

   Provider-administered
   - Cryotherapy (1B)
   - Trichloracetic acid (80–90% solution)
   - Excision (1A)
   - Electrosurgery and electrocautery (2C)
   - Laser (2B)
   - Podophyllin resin (10–25%) (1B)
   - Immunotherapy (1B)
   - Photodynamic therapy (1A)
2. **Cervical warts (podophyllin/podophyllotoxin contraindicated)**
   - Cryotherapy with liquid nitrogen
   - Surgical removal
   - TCA or BCA (80–90% solution)

   Management of cervical warts should include consultation with a gynecologist. For women who have exophytic cervical warts, a biopsy evaluation to exclude high-grade SIL must be performed before treatment is initiated.
3. **Vaginal warts**
   - Cryotherapy with liquid nitrogen. Cryoprobe <u>not recommended</u> due to the risk of vaginal perforation
   - Surgical removal
   - TCA or BCA (80–90% solution)

4. **Urethral meatal warts (<u>TCA not used</u>)**
    - Surgery (including excision, electrosurgery or laser ablation)
    - Podophyllotoxin, imiquimod or cryotherapy are acceptable alternatives if the base of the lesion is clearly visible.
5. **Intra-anal warts (podophyllin/podophyllotoxin <u>contraindicated</u>)**
    - Cryotherapy with liquid nitrogen
    - Surgical removal
    - TCA or BCA (80–90% solution)
6. **Oral warts**
    - Cryotherapy with liquid nitrogen
    - Surgical removal

(Figures in brackets refer to levels of evidence) (Sindhiya, et al., 2022).

Anogenital Warts and Pregnancy

- Genital warts in pregnant women should be treated with <u>TCA/BCA or surgical removal/cryotherapy</u>, both to ameliorate symptoms as well as to prevent their growth and occasional problems with birth canal obstruction.
- Cesarean delivery indicated only if vulvar/vaginal warts obstructing the birth canal as the lesions may avulse and hemorrhage or cause dystocia during an attempted vaginal delivery.

Anogenital Warts and HIV

- More prone to develop anogenital warts
- Bulky, extensive warts
- Require repetitive treatment–greater risk of treatment resistance
- May have more than 1 HPV type
- Higher HPV viral load
- Higher chances of intraepithelial neoplasia and carcinoma

Prevention of Warts

- <u>ABC (**A**bstain/**B**e faithful/use **C**ondoms)</u>
- Male circumcision–conflicting evidence exists.
- HPV prophylactic vaccines (CDC MMWR 16, Dec 2016)

Quadrivalent (4vHPV)—HPV-6, -11, -16, -18. Licensed in males and females (9–26 years)

9-valent (9vHPV)—in routine use in US now. HPV-6, -11, -16, -18, -31, -33, -45, -52, -58. Licensed in males and females, (the 9vHPV vaccine was FDA-approved in 2014 for males and females 9–26 years of age and this was recently expanded by the FDA to include women and men 27–45 years of age.)

Bivalent (2vHPV)—HPV-16, -18. Licensed in females only (9–25 years).

- Routine vaccination for 2vHPV, 4vHPV and 9vHPV: **11–12 years** (9 years onwards)—0.5 mL IM.
- **Dose:** Age <u>≤</u>15 years—**<u>two doses</u> (0, 6–12 months)**, Age >15 years—**<u>three doses</u> (0, 2, 6 months)** **(0, 6 months** for bivalent 2vHPV).
    - Immunosuppressed patients—three doses.
    - HPV vaccines are not recommended for use in pregnant women.

- HPV vaccines can be administered regardless of history of anogenital warts, abnormal Pap/HPV tests, or anogenital precancer.
- A recent meta-analysis showed that prophylactic, quadrivalent HPV vaccination can prevent GW in healthy women and men (Lukacs et al., 2020)
- Women who have received HPV vaccine should continue routine cervical cancer screening if they are aged ≥21 years.

Conclusion

The primary goal of treatment is the removal of visible warts. Currently available therapies may reduce infectivity, but probably not completely. There is no evidence that presence of genital warts is associated with development of cervical or anal cancer, and there are no data that suggest treatment of genital warts impacts the subsequent risk of anogenital HPV-related cancer.

Treatment of warts should be guided by several factors, including preference of the patient, available resources, experience of the healthcare provider, location of the lesion(s), and pregnancy status. As there is no evidence that any treatment is superior to others, and no specific treatment is ideal for all patients or for all warts.

As an important aspect that determines therapeutic results is the size of the lesion, an algorithm is given below that combines the use of immunotherapy and surgical intervention **(Fig. 33.41)**.

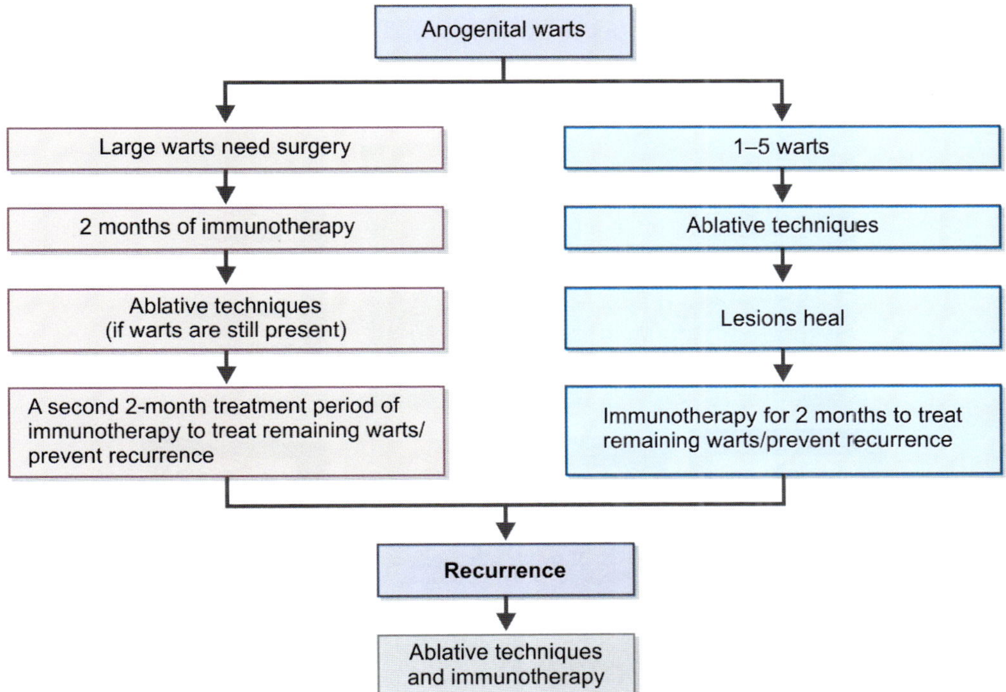

Fig. 33.41: Suggested treatment algorithm for anogenital warts

SYNDROMIC APPROACH

Syndromic management performs well for men presenting with a symptomatic urethral discharge (UD) and for men and women with bacterial genital ulcer disease (GUD). It has high to very acceptable cure rates, thus guaranteeing client satisfaction, prevention of sequelae and complications, as well as further transmission of STIs as well as HIV infection.

The syndromic approach probably performs well in the management of women with vaginitis, although validation of the causes of vaginal discharge may be necessary for different geographical settings. The syndromic algorithms currently used for the management of cervical infection are, however, far from ideal.

The pros and cons of the syndromic approach to STIs are listed in the **Table 33.35**.

TABLE 33.35: Advantages and disadvantages of syndromic management of STIs

Advantages	Disadvantages
• Simple, rapid • No laboratory support required • Treatment given at first visit, preventing complications and further transmission • Simplifies reporting and supervision	• Only applies to patients with <u>symptoms</u> • Leads to <u>over-treatment</u>, especially in women • May lead to problems with partner notification, especially in women who are told they have an STI when they do not

STI Syndromes

There are **9 major STI syndromes**. The STD kits are depicted in **Fig. 33.42** and a salient overview is given below.

- **Urethral** discharge in men (suspected urethritis). This is commonly due to *Neisseria gonorrhoeae* and/or *Chlamydia trachomatis* and/or nongonococcal/nonchlamydial pathogens, e.g. *Mycoplasma genitalium* and *Trichomonas vaginalis*.

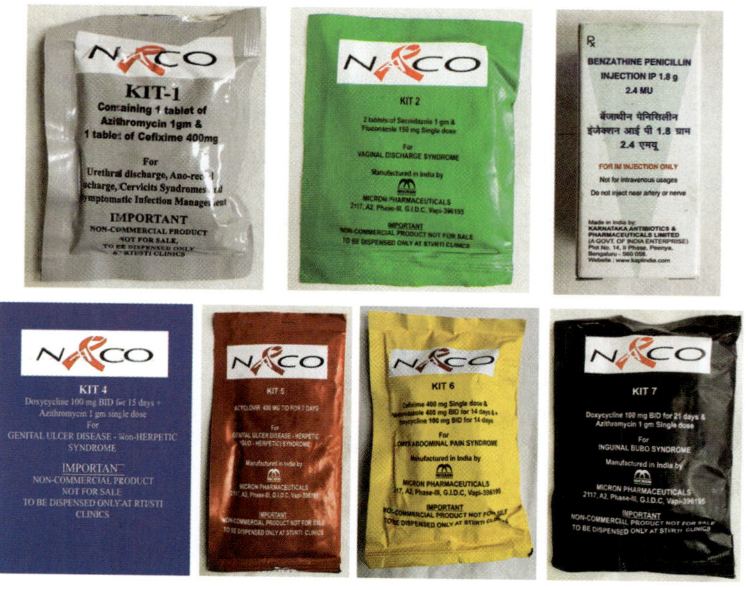

Fig. 33.42: Color coded NACO STI treatment kits

The syndromic approach is depicted in the **Fig. 33.43** and while the treatment given is at variance with the section on urethritis, it is the prevalent NACO protocol.

- **Testicular pain** and swelling (suspected epididymo-orchitis). This is commonly due to *N. gonorrhoeae* and/or *C. trachomatis* **(Fig. 33.44)**.
  Differential diagnosis-non-STI causes include tuberculosis, filariasis, coliforms, Pseudomonas, and mumps. STI causes include trauma, hernia, hydrocele, testicular torsion, testicular tumors.
- Abnormal **vaginal discharge** (vaginitis and/or cervicitis). 'Abnormal' discharge refers to a change in abundance, color, odor, or consistency of genital secretions as perceived by the patient and confirmed by a trained healthcare provider. This syndrome is caused predominantly by organisms causing vaginal infection, such as *T. vaginalis*, *Candida albicans* or bacterial vaginosis, but *N. gonorrhoeae* and *C. trachomatis* (which are of greater public health importance for their complications) can cause a cervical discharge and consequently manifest as a vaginal discharge **(Fig. 33.45)**.
- **Genital ulcers:** The genital ulcer syndrome can be caused by a number of pathogens including *Haemophilus ducreyi* (chancroid), *Treponema pallidum* (syphilis), herpes simplex virus (HSV) type 2, (sometimes, also HSV type 1).

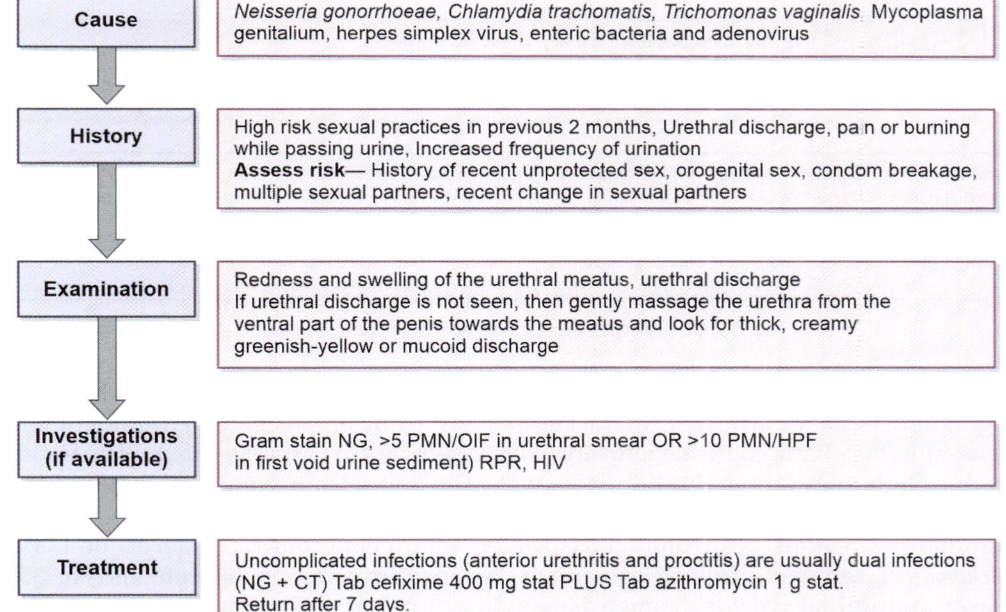

Syndrome-specific guidelines for partner management

- Sexual partners whose last sexual contact within 60 days should be evaluated and treated for UD syndrome
- Advise sexual abstinence during the course of treatment

Follow-up — after 7 days

- To document symptomatic cure and of tests done for HIV and syphilis
- If symptoms/signs persist, assess for TV, if possible treat with tab. secnidazole 2 g orally
- If symptoms/signs persist assess for treatment failure or reinfection and advise prompt referral

Recurrent and persistent urethritis (TV)

Metronidazole 2 g stat **OR**
Tinidazole 2 gm stat **PLUS**
Azithromycin 1 g stat (if not used for initial episode)

Fig. 33.43: Syndromic approach to urethral discharge/burning micturition in males (NACO)

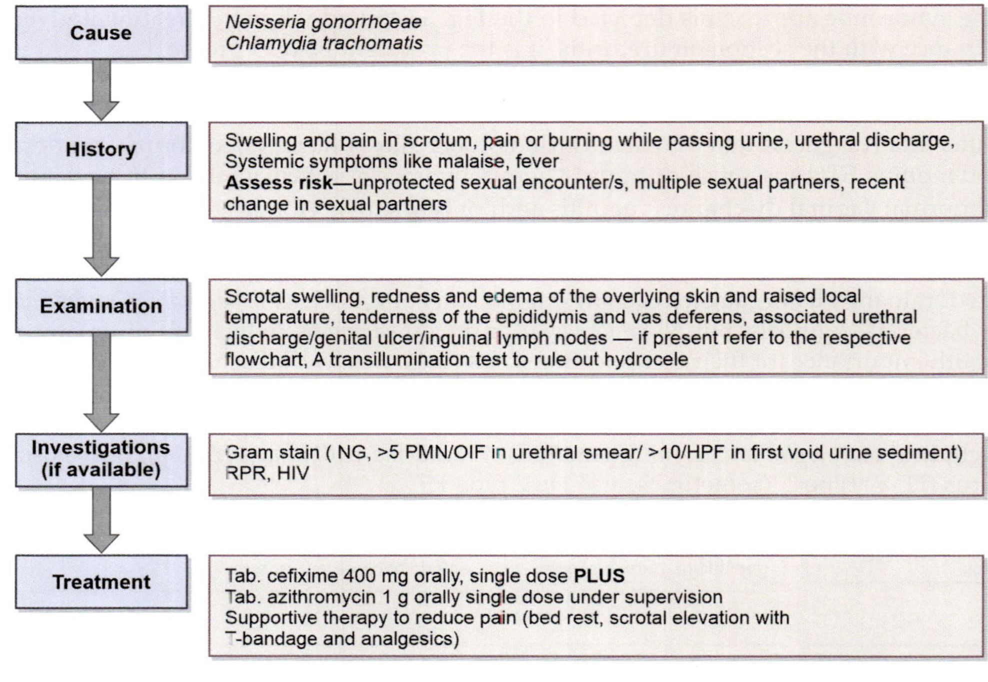

Syndrome-specific guidelines for partner management
- Sexual partners whose last sexual contact within 60 days should be evaluated and treated for UD syndrome
- Advise sexual abstinence during the course of treatment

Follow-up — after 7 days
- To document symptomatic cure, results of tests done for HIV and syphilis
- If symptoms/signs persist assess whether it is due to lack of treatment compliance or treatment failure or recurrence and advise prompt referral to prevent scarring

Fig. 33.44: Syndromic approach to scrotal swelling

Donovanosis (caused by the agent *Klebsiella granulomatis*) may be important in some settings (e.g. South India, South Africa, and Papua New Guinea), as can be lymphogranuloma venereum (LGV) caused by the more invasive L-serovars of *C. trachomatis*, which, however, produce only transient and mild ulcerations. The approach is conveniently divided into two charts **(Fig. 33.46)**.

- Inguinal bubo—this syndrome is associated with chancroid (*H. ducreyi*) or LGV (*C. trachomatis* L-serovars). TB, filariasis and malignancy are common differentials **(Fig. 33.47)**.
- Lower abdominal pain in women [suspicion of pelvic inflammatory disease (PID)]. This condition is due to *N. gonorrhoeae* and/or *C. trachomatis* and/or anaerobic pathogens. **(Fig. 33.48)**.
- Ano-rectal infections—these infections can be divided into **(Fig 33.49)**:
  - *Anal infections* of the external anus and anal canal, involving the stratified squamous epithelium, e.g. human papillomavirus (HPV), herpes simplex virus (HSV), syphilis.
  - *Proctitis infections* from the dentate line to the recto-sigmoid junction, e.g. gonorrhea, *Chlamydia*, HSV.
  - *Proctocolitis* (*infections* of the rectum and colon), e.g. LGV, *Shigella*, *Campylobacter*, *Salmonella*, cytomegalovirus, amoebiasis.

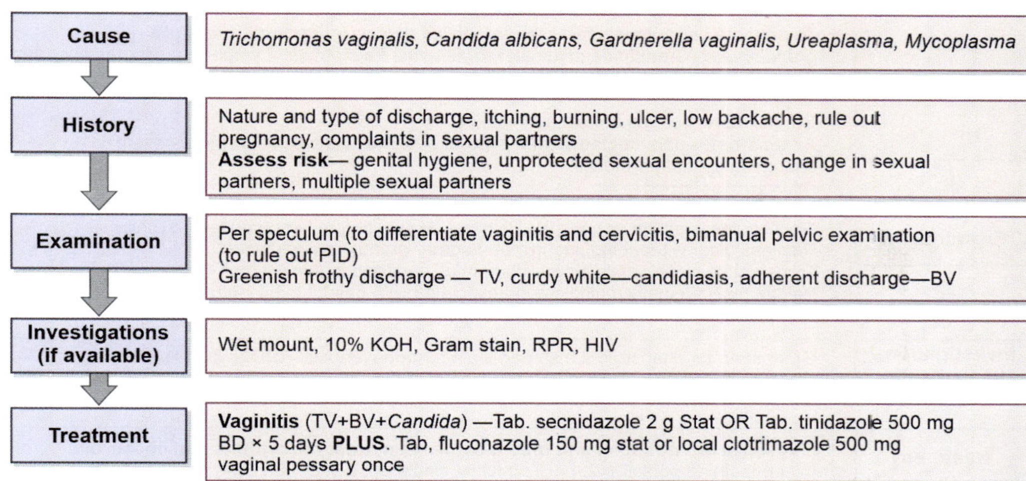

Syndrome-specific guidelines for partner management
- BV and *Candida:* Not required
- *Trichomonas* infection: Treat all sexual partners in the last 30 days with the above protocol
- Advise sexual abstinence during the course of treatment

Follow-up — After 7 days
- Document symptomatic cure, results of tests done for HIV and syphilis
- If symptoms/signs persist assess whether it is due to lack of treatment compliance or treatment failure or re-infection and advise prompt referral

Fig. 33.45a: Approach to vaginal discharge (vaginitis)

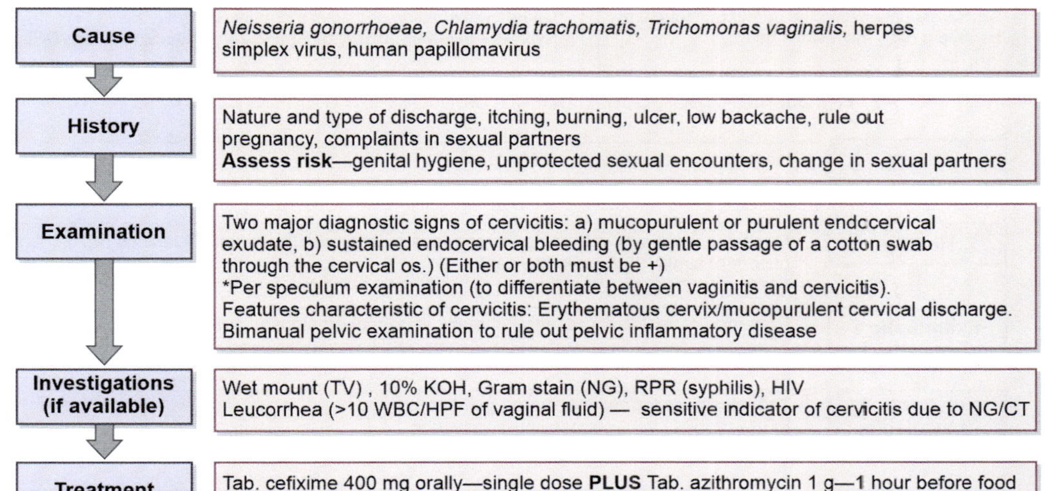

Syndrome-specific guidelines for partner management
- For cervicitis and *Trichomonas* infection: Treat all sexual partners in the last 30 days with the above protocol
- Advise sexual abstinence during the course of treatment

Follow-up — After 7 days
- To document symptomatic cure, results of tests done for HIV and syphilis
- If symptoms/signs persist assess whether it is due to lack of treatment compliance or treatment failure or re-infection and advise prompt referral

**If speculum examination is not possible or client is hesitant, treat both for vaginitis and cervicitis, NG—N. gonorrhoese, CT—C. trachomatis*

Fig. 33.45b: Approach to cervical discharge (cervicitis)

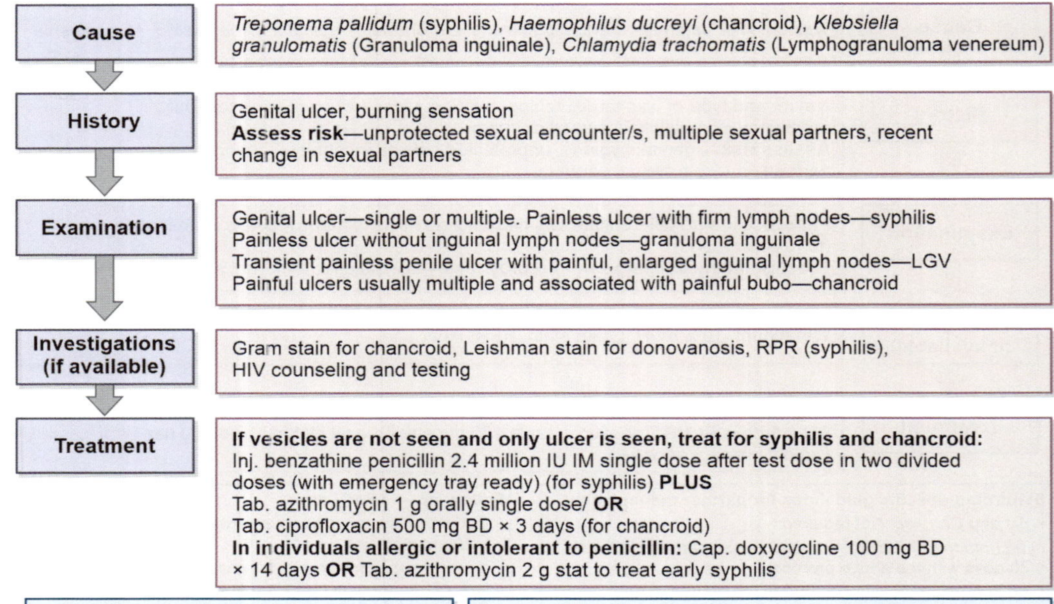

Fig. 33.46a: Approach to genital ulcer disease (non-herpetic)

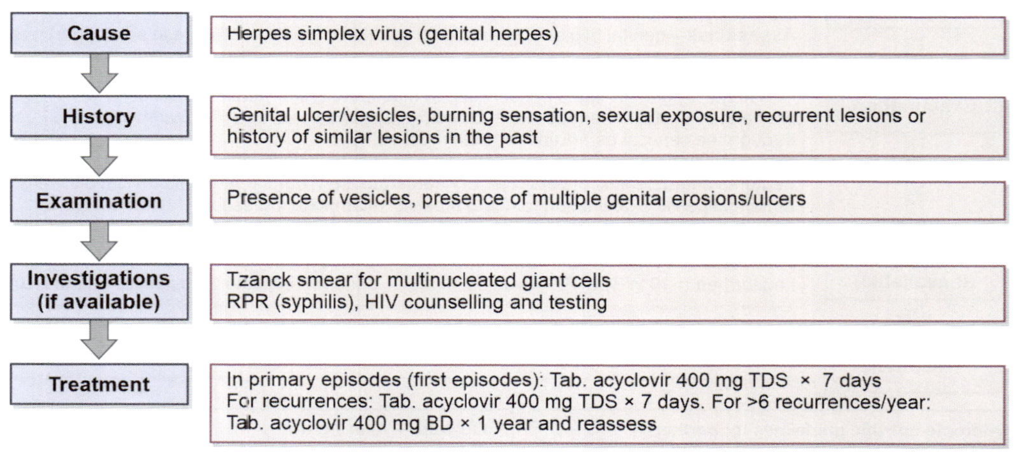

Fig. 33.46b: Approach to genital ulcer disease (herpetic)

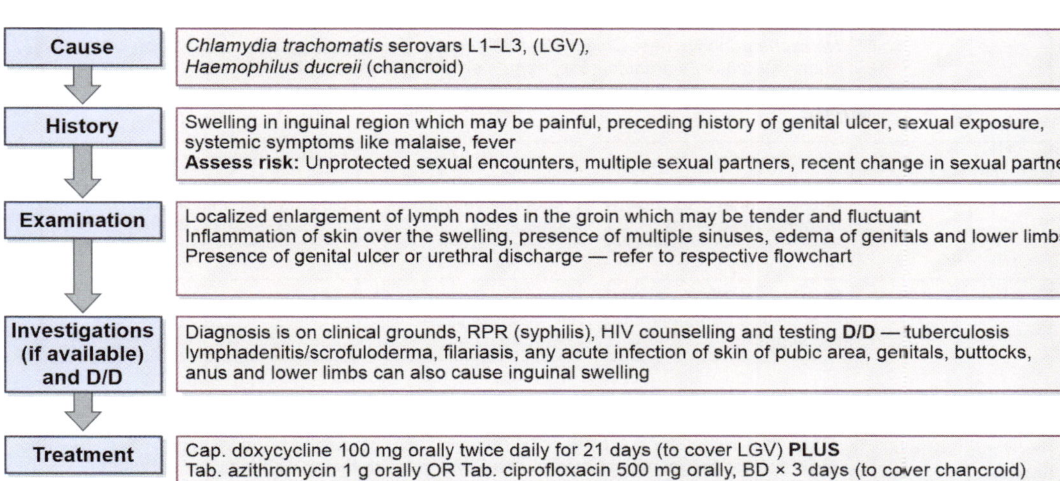

Syndrome-specific guidelines for partner management
- Treat all partners who are in contact with client in last 3 months
- Cap. doxycycline 100 mg BD × 21 days to cover LGV **PLUS**
- Tab. azithromycin 1 g orally stat (to cover chancroid)

Follow-up — After 7 and 21 days
- To document symptomatic cure, results of tests done for HIV and syphilis

** Never incise and drain a bubo, even if fluctuant, as it may lead to a fistula. If fluctuant, always aspirate from non-dependent site.*

Fig. 33.47: Approach to inguinal bubo

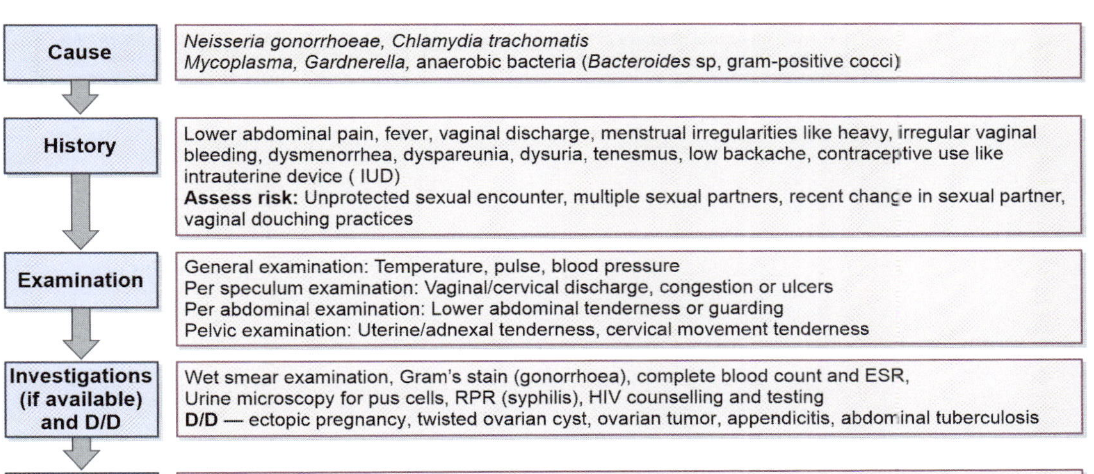

Treatment

Tab. cefixime 400 mg STAT (NG) **PLUS** Tab. metronidazole 400 mg BD × 14 days (anaerobic infection) **PLUS** Cap. doxycyline, 100 mg BD × 14 days (chlamydial infection)
Tab. ibuprofen 400 mg TDS for 3–5 days
Tab. ranitidine 150 mg BD to prevent gastritis
Remove intrauterine device, if present, under antibiotic cover of 24–48 hours (maximal risk in first 3 weeks after insertion)

Syndrome-specific guidelines for partner management
- Those who had sexual contact with the patient during the 60 days preceding the patient's onset of symptoms
- Abstain from sexual intercourse until therapy is completed and until they and their sexual partners no longer have symptoms

Follow-up — After 3, 7 and 14 days
- If not improve within this period usually require hospitalization, additional diagnostic tests, and surgical intervention

Fig. 33.48: Approach to lower abdominal pain in females

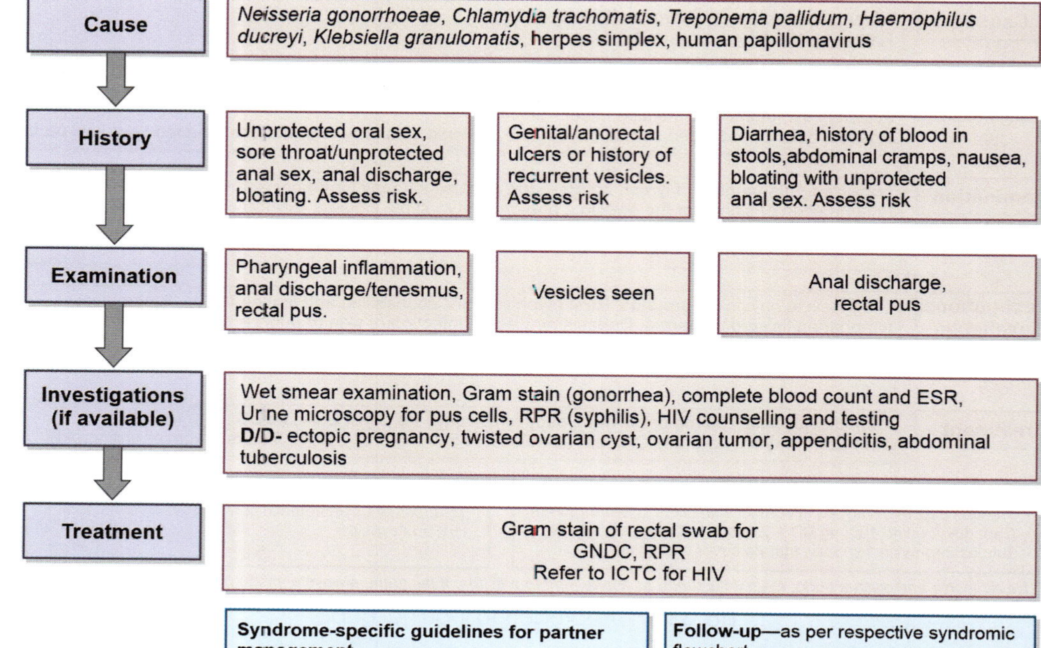

Fig. 33.49: Management of oral and anal STI

SEXUAL ASSAULT AND ABUSE AND STIs

Most guidelines on sexual assault/violence are primarily directed towards the identification, prophylaxis, and treatment of STIs and conditions among female sexual assault survivors. However, some points might apply to male sexual assault survivors as well.

Trichomoniasis, BV, gonorrhea, and chlamydia are the most frequently diagnosed infections among women who have been sexually assaulted. Such conditions are prevalent among the population, and detection of these infections after an assault does not necessarily imply acquisition during the assault. However, a post-assault examination presents an important opportunity for identifying or preventing an STI.

Examination should be conducted by an experienced clinician in a way that minimizes further trauma to the person and should be performed only after written informed consent. The following services should be available in the STI clinic for survivors of sexual assault:

1. Visual Inspection

After obtaining consent and counselling the survivor, a thorough examination of clothes, injuries and genital must be carried out. Look for injury, erosions, scratch marks, bleeding, discharge, odour, irritation, warts, and ulcerative lesions.

2. Collection of Medicolegal Evidence

Medicolegal examination should be available to document evidence if the person chooses to take legal action. Staff should be trained in taking forensic specimens. Forensic examination must include physical and genital examination.

3. Collection of Samples for Detecting STI/RTI

If facilities permit, swabs must be collected from various sites:

- NAATs for *C. trachomatis* and *N. gonorrhoeae* at the sites of penetration or attempted penetration should be performed.
- Females should be offered NAAT testing for *T. vaginalis* from a urine or vaginal specimen.
- POC or wet mount with measurement of vaginal pH and KOH application for the whiff test from vaginal secretions should be performed for evidence of BV and candidiasis, especially if vaginal discharge, malodor, or itching is present.
- MSM should be offered screening for *C. trachomatis* and *N. gonorrhoeae* if they report receptive oral or anal sex during the preceding year, regardless of whether sexual contact occurred at these anatomic sites during the assault. Anoscopy should be considered in instances of reported anal penetration.
- A serum sample should be performed for HIV, HBV, and syphilis infection.

4. Essential Medical Care for Injuries and Health Problems

Medical management of sexual assault includes:

- Care of physical injuries and psychosocial counseling
- Prevention of pregnancy by offering emergency contraception (NACO)
  Levonorgestrel-only pills (0.75 mg levonorgestrel per pill)–2 doses with first dose within 72 hours and second after 12 hours of first dose.

- STI prophylaxis (CDC 2021)
  i. **Recommended regimen for adolescent and adult female sexual assault survivors (against CT, NG, TV)**

Ceftriaxone 500 mg* IM in a single dose
PLUS
Doxycycline 100 mg 2 times/day orally for 7 days
PLUS
Metronidazole 500 mg orally 2 times/day orally for 7 days
*For persons weighing ≥150 kg, 1 g of ceftriaxone should be administered.

  ii. **Recommended regimen for adolescent and adult male sexual assault survivors (against CT, NG)**

Ceftriaxone 500 mg* IM in a single dose
PLUS
Doxycycline 100 mg 2 times/day orally for 7 days
*For persons weighing ≥150 kg, 1 g of ceftriaxone should be administered.

  iii. **Postexposure hepatitis B vaccination** (without HBIG) if the hepatitis status of the assailant is unknown and the survivor has not been previously vaccinated. If the assailant is known to be HBsAg positive, unvaccinated survivors should receive both hepatitis B vaccine and HBIG. Follow-up doses of vaccine should be administered 1–2 and 4–6 months after the first dose.
  iv. **HPV vaccination for female and male survivors aged** 9–26 years who have not been vaccinated or are incompletely vaccinated. The vaccine should be administered to sexual assault survivors at the time of the initial examination and follow-up doses should be administered at 1–2 months and 6 months after the first dose.
  v. **Recommendations for HIV PEP** are made on a case-by-case basis according to risk **(*see* Fig. 33.50)** HIV seroconversion has occurred among persons whose only known risk factor was sexual assault or sexual abuse; however, the frequency of this occurrence likely is low. In consensual sex, the per-act risk for HIV transmission from vaginal intercourse is 0.08%, and for receptive anal intercourse, 1.38%. The per-act risk for HIV transmission from oral sex is substantially lower. Specific circumstances of an assault (e.g. trauma, bleeding) might increase risk for HIV transmission in cases involving vaginal, anal, or oral penetration. Site of exposure to ejaculate, viral load in ejaculate, and the presence of an STI or genital lesions in the assailant or survivor also might increase risk for HIV acquisition.

nPEP (non-occupational post-exposure HIV prevention) guidelines (CDC 2016):

- Tenofovir disoproxil fumarate (TDF)/emtricitabine (FTC) (Truvada) 300/200 mg + dolutegravir 50 mg 1 tablet of each PO daily × 28 days.
- If client is in the first trimester of pregnancy OR may become pregnant within the next 28 days: TDF/FTC (Truvada) 300/200 mg 1 tab PO daily + EITHER dolutegravir 50 mg 1 PO daily OR raltegravir 400 mg 1 tab PO twice a day.
- Possible nPEP drug side effects: Nausea, GI upset, headache, myalgias.
- Possible nPEP drug interactions: Antacids, calcium, iron supplements.

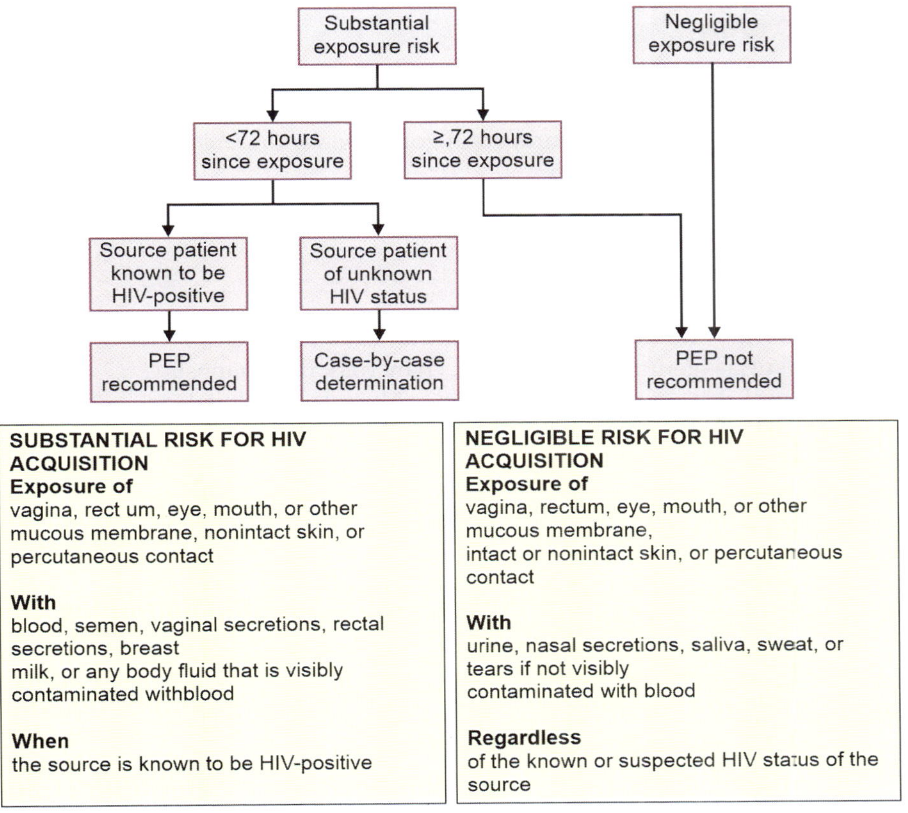

Fig. 33.50: Risk assessment for HIC acquisition (*Source*: Updated Guidelines for Antiretroviral Postexposure Prophylaxis after Sexual, Injection-Drug Use, or Other Nonoccupational Exposure to HIV-United States, 2016. MMWR Morb Mortal Wkly Rep, 2016. 65(17): p. 458)

- Stress the importance of adherence to the nPEP regimen for 28 days, without interruption.
- For those with ongoing risk of HIV infection, offer PrEP initiation immediately after completion of the 28 day course of nPEP follow-up.
- Follow-up should be scheduled at 72 hours and 4–6 weeks after initiating nPEP.
- HIV Ag/Ab test after initial non-reactive test.
- Syphilis test at 4–6 weeks and 3–6 months after exposure.
- HBV and HCV serology tests at 6 months after initial nonreactive test if susceptible at baseline.

HIGH-YIELD STD DATA

Remember while treating STDs

- Treat all recent partners (**EPT:** Expedited partner therapy) (**PDPT:** Patient delivered partner therapy) which is now being encouraged in gonorrhea and *Chlamydia*.
- Condom promotion and education.
- Sexual abstinence during treatment.
- Follow-up after 3 (or 7/14) days.
- Refer to ICTC.

1. STD causes of **dysuria**
   - Internal dysuria—intrameatal chancre, intrameatal HPG, GU, NGU
   - External dysuria—genital ulcers—HPG, chancroid, donovanosis
   - Recurrent urethritis—*Trichomonas vaginalis, Mycoplasma genitalium*
   - Persistent urethritis—*Mycoplasma genitalium*
2. STD causes of **phimosis**
   - Primary HPG
   - Chancroid
   - Phagedenic chancre
3. Causes of **epididymo-orchitis** in sexually active male
   - <35 yrs—GU, NGU
   - >35 yrs—Gram-negative enteric bacilli, e.g. *E. coli, Klebsiella* spp., etc.
4. **Condoms**—↓Risk of HIV, GU, NGU, trichomoniasis, syphilis, chancroid, HPG, HPV-related diseases.
5. **Circumcision**—has a protective role against some STDs.
   - Strong evidence for protective effect in heterosexual men and women (Matoga M et al):
     - HIV
     - HSV-2
     - HPV
     - Syphilis
     - Bacterial vaginosis and trichomoniasis (women)

   Emerging evidence:
   - Hepatitis B and *Mycoplasma genitalium* (heterosexual men)
   - HSV-2, HPV, and syphilis (MSM)
6. HSV urethritis versus *Chlamydia* urethritis
   - Meatitis more in HSV
   - Dysuria disproportionate to the signs of urethritis
7. Inguinal lymphadenopathy more in HSV and almost absent in *Chalmydia* urethritis.

BIBLIOGRAPHY

Genital Herpes

Books

1. ACOG Committee on Practice Bulletins. ACOG Practice Bulletin. Clinical management guidelines for obstetrician-gynecologists. No. 82 June 2007. Management of herpes in pregnancy. Obstet Gynecol 2007; 109:1489. Reaffirmed 2018.
2. Sexually Transmitted Diseases 4th edn. Holmes KK, eds, Tata McGraw, Copyright ©2008.

Journals

1. Hensleigh PA, Andrews WW, Brown Z, et al. Genital herpes during pregnancy: Inability to distinguish primary and recurrent infections clinically. ObstetGynecol 1997;89:891.
2. Management of Genital Herpes in Pregnancy. (2020). Obstetrics & Gynecology, 135(5), e193-e202. doi:10.1097/aog.0000000000003840. N EnglJ Med 2016; 374:2504–06.
3. Patwardhan V, Bhalla P. Role of type-specific herpes simplex virus-1 and 2 serology as a diagnostic modality in patients with clinically suspected genital herpes: A comparative study in Indian population from a tertiary care hospital. Indian J Pathol Microbiol. 2016 Jul-Sep;59(3): 318–21.
4. Shivaswamy KN, Thappa DM, Jaisankar TJ, Sujatha S. High seroprevalence of HSV-1 and HSV-2 in STD clinic attendees and non-high risk controls: A case control study at a referral hospital in South India. Indian J Dermatol Venereol Leprol. 2005 Jan-Feb;71(1):26–30.
5. Taylor, et al. N EnglJ Med 2018; 379:1835–45.
6. van Rooijen MS, Roest W, Hansen G, Kwa D, de Vries HJ. False-negative type-specific glycoprotein G antibody responses in STI clinic patients with recurrent HSV-1 or HSV-2 DNA positive genital herpes, The Netherlands. Sex Transm Infect. 2016 Jun; 92(4):257–60.
7. Vauloup-Fellous C. [Genital herpes and pregnancy: Serological and molecular diagnostic tools. Guidelines for clinical practice from the French College of Gynecologists and Obstetricians (CNGOF)]. Gynecol Obstet Fertil Senol. 2017 Dec; 45(12):655–63.
8. Watts DH, Brown ZA, Money D, et al. A double-blind, randomized, placebo-controlled trial of acyclovir in late pregnancy for the reduction of herpes simplex virus shedding and cesare and elivery. Am J Obstet Gynecol 2003;188:836.
9. Workowski KA, Bolan GA, Centers for Disease Control and Prevention. Sexually transmitted diseases treatment guidelines, 2015. MMWR Recomm Rep 2015;64:1.

Syphilis

1. Castro R, Prieto ES, Santol, et al. Evaluation of an enzyme immunoassay technique for detection of antibodies against *Treponema pallidum*. J Clin Microbiol 2003; 41:250.41.
2. Centers for Disease Control and Prevention (CDC). Discordant results from reverse sequence syphilis screening-five laboratories, United States, 2006–2010. MMWR Morb Mortal Wkly Rep. 2011;60:133–7.
3. Centers for Disease Control and Prevention (CDC). Syphilis testing algorithms using treponemal tests for initial screening-four laboratories, New York City, 2005–2006. MMWR Morb Mortal Wkly Rep 2008; 57:872.32.
4. Chahine LM, Khoriaty RN, Tomford WJ, Hussain MS. The changing face of neurosyphilis. Int J Stroke. 2011;6:136–43.
5. French P. Syphilis. BMJ 2007'334(7585):143–147.
6. Huber TW, Storms S, Young P, et al. Reactivity of microhemagglutination, fluorescent treponemal antibody absorption, Venereal Disease Research Laboratory, and rapid plasma reagin tests in primary syphilis. J Clin Microbiol 1983;17:405.40.
7. Larsen SA. Syphilis. Clin Lab Med 1989;9:545.
8. Lefevre JC, Bertrand MA, Bauriaud R. Evaluation of the Captia enzyme immunoassays for detection of immunoglobulins G and M to *Treponema pallidum* in syphilis. J Clin Microbiol 1990; 28:1704.
9. Liu LL, Lin LR, Tong ML, et al. Incidence and risk factors for the prozone phenomenon inserologic testing for syphilis in a large cohort. Clin Infect Dis 2014;59:384.
10. Lukehart SA, Hook EW 3rd, Baker-Zander SA, Collier AC, Critchlow CW, Handsfield HH. Invasion of the central nervous system by Treponema pallidum: Implications for diagnosis and treatment. Ann Intern Med. 1988;109:855–62.
11. Ratnam S. The laboratory diagnosis of syphilis. Can J Infect Dis Med Microbiol 2005;16:45.
12. Sardana K and Sehgal VN. Tropical medical rounds genital ulcer disease and human immuno-deficiency virus: A focus. Int J dermatol 2005; 44:391–405.
13. Sena AC, white BL, sparling PF. Novel *Treponema pallidum* serologic tests: a paradigm shift in syphilis screening for the 21st century. Clin Infect Dis 2010, 51:700–8.
14. Workowski KA, Bolan GA; Centers for Disease Control and Prevention. Sexually transmitted diseases treatment guidelines, 2015. Syphilis. MMWR Recomm Rep. 2015;64(No. RR-3):1–137.

Donovanosis

1. Sardana K, Garg VK, Arora P, Khurana N. Malignant transformation of donovanosis (granuloma inguinale) in a HIV-positive patient. Dermatol Online J 2008;14:8.

Urethritis

Books

1. PRNGU.STD. Sardana K. Diagnosis & Management of Skin Disorders: An Evidence Based Approach Paperback. LWW. January 2012.
2. Sexually Transmitted Diseases, 4th edn. King K. Holmes, Tata McGraw-Hill, Copyright ©2008.
3. Venereal Diseases by King and Nicol.

Journals

1. Bignell C, Fitzgerald M; Guideline Development Group; British Association for Sexual Health and HIV UK. UK national guideline for the management of gonorrhoea in adults, 2011. IntJ STD AIDS. 2011 Oct;22(10): 541–7.4849.
2. Centers for Disease Control and Prevention. Recommendations for the laboratory-based detection of *Chlamydia trachomatis* and *Neisseria gonorrhoeae*-2014. MMWR Recomm Rep. 2014;63:1–19.
3. Chisholm S, Mouton J, Lewis D, et al. Cephalo-sporin MIC creep among gonococci: Time for a pharmacodynamics rethink? J Antimicrob Chemother 2010;65:2141–18.
4. Crofts M, Mead K, Persad R, et al. Anevaluation of a dedicated chronic pelvic pain syndrome clinic in genitourinary medicine. Sex Transm Infect 2014; 90:373.
5. Furuya R, Nakayama H, Kanayama A, et al. *In vitro* synergistic effects of double combinations of B lactams and azithromycin against clinical isolates of *Neisseria gonorrhoeae*. J Infect Chemother 2006; 12:172–76.
6. Horner P, Blee K, O'Mahony C, MuirP, Evans C, Radcliffe K; Clinical Effectiveness Group of the British Association for Sexual Health and HIV. 2015 UK National Guideline on the management of non-gonococcal urethritis. Int J STD AIDS. 2016 Feb;27(2):85–96.
7. Hooper RR, Reynolds GH, Jones OG, et al. Cohort study of venereal disease. I: The risk of gonorrhea transmission from infected women to men. Am J Epidemiol. 1978;108:136–44.
8. Kenyon S, Crofts M and Horner P. An extended evaluation of a dedicated male chronic pelvic pain clinic within a sexual health service. Sex Transm Infect 2014; 90:572.
9. Komolafe AJ, Sugunendran H, Corkill JE. Gonorrhoea: Test of cure for sensitive bacteria? Use of genotyping to disprove treatment failure. Int J STD AIDS 2004;15:212.
10. Lin JS, Donegan SP, Heeren TC, et al. Transmission of *Chlamydia trachomatis* and *Neisseria gonorrhoeae* among men with urethritis and their female sex partners. J Infect Dis. 1998;178:1707–12.
11. Moi H, Blee K, Horner PJ. Management of non-gonococcal urethritis. BMC Infect Dis 2015;15:294.
12. St. Cyr S, Barbee L, Workowski KA, et al. Update to CDC's Treatment Guidelines for Gonococcal Infection, 2020. MMWR Morb Mortal Wkly Rep 2020;69:1911–1916. DOI: http://dx.doi.org/10.15585/mmwr.mm6950a6external icon.
13. St Cyr S, Barbee L, Workowski KA, et al. Update to CDC's Treatment Guidelines for Gonococcal Infection, 2020. MMWR Morb Mortal Wkly Rep. 2020;69:1911–6.
14. Wind CM, de Vries E, Schim van der Loeff MF, et al. Decreased Azithromycin Susceptibility of *Neisseria gonorrhoeae* Isolates in Patients Recently Treated with Azithromycin. Clin Infect Dis 2017;65:37–45.
15. Wong ES, Hooton TM, HillCC, et al. Clinical and microbiological features of persistent or recurrent non-gonococcal urethritis in men. J Infect Dis 1988; 158:1098–101.
16. Workowski KA, Bolan GA; Centers for Disease Control and Prevention. Sexually transmitted diseases treatment guidelines, 2015. Gonococcal infections. MMWR Recomm Rep 2015;64(No. RR-3):1–137.

Vaginitis

1. Brunham RC, Gottlieb SL, Paavonen J. Pelvic inflammatory disease. N Engl J Med. 2015;372:2039–48.
2. Cartwright CP et al. Comparison of NAA tests with BD Affirm VP III for diagnosis of vaginitis in symptomatic women. J Clin Microbiol 2013;51:3694–9.
3. Chayachinda C, Rekhawasin T. Reproductive outcomes of patients being hospitalised with pelvic inflammatory disease. J Obstet Gynaecol. 2016;1–5.
4. Dan Metal. Performance of a rapidy east test in detecting Candida spp. in the vagina. Diagn Microbiol Infect Dis 2010;67:52–5.
5. Das S, Huengsberg M and Shahmanesh M. Treatment failure of vaginal trichomoniasis in clinical practice. Int J STD AIDS 2005; 16: 284–86.
6. Donders et al. Individualising decreasing-dose maintenance regimen for recurrent vulvo-vaginal candidiasis (ReCiDiFtrial) Am K Obstet Gynecol2008;199:6130–6.
7. Frobenius, et al. Diagnostic value of vaginal discharge, wet mount and vaginal pH—An update on the basis of gynaecologic infectiology. Geburt-shilfe Frauenheilkd 2015;75:355–66.
8. Gonçalves B, Ferreira C, Vulvovaginal candidiasis: Epidemiology, microbiology and risk factors. Crit Rev Microbiol. 2016;42:905–27.
9. Madhivanan Petal. Performance of BV Blue Rapid test in detecting BV among females in Mysore, India. Infect Dis Obstet Gynecol 2014;2014:908313.
10. Mason MJ and Winter AJ. How to diagnose and treat aerobic and desquamative inflammatory vaginitis. Sex Transm Infect 2017; 93: 8–10.
11. Mølgaard-Nielsen D, Pasternak B, Hviid A. Use of oral fluconazole during pregnancy and the risk of birth defects. N Engl J Med. 2013;369:830–9.
12. Rao et al. Diagnosis of bacterial vaginosis: Amsel's criteria versus Nugent's scoring. SchJ App Med Sci 2016;4:2027–31.
13. Sobel JD. Vulvovaginal candidosis. Lancet. 2007;369:1961–71.
14. Workowski KA, Bolan GA; Centers for Disease Control and Prevention. Sexually transmitted diseases treatment guidelines, 2015. Pelvic inflammatory disease (PID). MMWR Recomm Rep. 2015;64 (No. RR-3): 1–137.
15. Workowski KA, Bolan GA; Centers for Disease Control and Prevention. Sexually transmitted diseases treatment guidelines, 2015. Diseases characterized by vaginal discharge: Vulvovaginal candidiasis. MMWR Recomm Rep. 2015;64 (No. RR-3):1–137.

Genital Warts

1. Ciccarese G, Parodi A, Drago F. 5-Fluorouracil 0.5%/salicylic acid 10% solution in the treatment of ano-genital warts. Dermatol Ther. 2022 May;35(5):e15370.
2. Gilson R, Nugent D, Werner RN, Ballesteros J, Ross J. 2019. IUSTI Europe guideline for the management of anogenital warts. Journal of the European Academy of Dermatology and Venereology. 2020 Aug;34(8): 1644–53.
3. Jung JM, Jung CL, Lee WJ, et al. Topically applied treatments for EGWs in non-immuno-compromised patients: A systematic review and network meta-analysis. BJD 2020;183(1):24–36.
4. Lukács A, Máté Z, Farkas N, et al. The quadrivalent HPV vaccine is protective against genital warts: A meta-analysis. BMC Public Health 2020 May 28;20(1):691.
5. Matoga M, Hosseinipour M, Jewett S, et al. Effects of HIV voluntary medical male circumcision programs on sexually transmitted infections, Curr Opin Infect Dis 2021;34:50–55.

Chapter

34

Tumors: Benign Appendageal, Malignant and Premalignant Tumors

Seema Rani, Kabir Sardana, Surabhi Sinha

APPENDAGEAL TUMORS

INTRODUCTION

This section has a daunting list, but not all of these are important for the examination (only the ones in bold are important). But these tumors are important as some of them are seen very commonly and a basic working knowledge will help in the long run. An interesting fact is that these tumors can be predicted by the sites of location as follows:

- The tumors of the pilosebaceous apparatus are concentrated in the **head and neck area**.
- The pilar tumors are seen on the **scalp**.
- The sebaceous elements are seen on the face, chest, and upper back.
- The eccrine tumors are seen all over the body.
- There is an overlap between the apocrine and eccrine tumors as the excretory (ductal) portions of the eccrine and apocrine glands are identical and cannot be differentiated on morphological grounds. Also there are no histochemical or immunohistochemical stains that allow distinction between eccrine and apocrine tumors. Thus, tumors of the eccrine and apocrine glands cannot be clearly delineated.
- Some appendageal tumors are relatively rare, and a brief overview of their clinical features are given in **Table 34.1** while the important cases are discussed in detail.

TABLE 34.1: An overview of appendageal tumors*

Tumors of the hair	Hair follicle tumors	• Inverted follicular keratosis • Dilated pore • Tumor of the follicular infundibulum • Pilar sheath acanthoma • Trichoadenoma • **Comedo nevus**
	External root sheath tumors	• Trichilemmal cyst • Proliferating trichilemmal tumor • **Trichilemmoma** • Trichilemmal carcinoma

(Contd.)

TABLE 34.1: An overview of appendageal tumors* (Contd.)		
	Hamartomas and hair germ tumors and cysts	• Hair follicle nevus • Eruptive vellus hair cyst • Trichofolliculoma • **Trichoepithelioma** • Desmoplastic trichoepithelioma • Solitary giant trichoepithelioma • Trichoblastoma • Cutaneous lymphadenoma • Basaloid follicular hamartoma
	Hair matrix tumors	**Pilomatricoma,** pilomatricarcinoma
	Lesions of hair follicle mesenchyme	Trichodiscoma, perifollicular fibroma, fibrofolliculoma
Sebaceous gland	Sebaceous gland tumor	• **Sebaceous adenomas** and sebaceomas • Superficial epithelioma with sebaceous differentiation • Sebaceous carcinoma
Apocrine gland	Apocrine gland tumors	• Apocrine hidrocystoma • Syringocystadenoma papilliferum • Hidradenoma papilliferum • Erosive adenomatosis of the nipple • Apocrine tubular adenoma • Apocrine carcinoma
Eccrine gland	Eccrine gland hamartomas and tumors	• Eccrine angiomatous nevus • Eccrine hidrocystoma • Hidroacanthoma simplex • Eccrine dermal duct tumor • Eccrine poroma • Eccrine syringofibroadenoma • **Syringoma** • Tubular papillary adenoma
	Eccrine or apocrine/follicular tumors	• Hidradenoma • **Cylindroma** • Spiradenoma • Mixed tumor of the skin • Cutaneous myoepithelioma
Miscellaneous		Paget's disease

*Tumors in bold font are commonly seen.

Though the focus is to cover the commonly seen tumors in this chapter, a list of the other uncommon appendageal skin tumors is given in **Table 34.2**.

TABLE 34.2: A summary of the uncommonly seen appendageal tumors			
Name	**Lesion morphology**	**Site**	**Special features**
Inverted follicular keratoses	Solitary papule or nodule	Head and neck	Usually arises over a nevus sebaceus
Tumor of follicular infundibulum	Nodules	Face	
Pilar sheath acanthoma	Nodule with a central pore	Upper lip, lower lip, and cheeks	
Trichoadenoma	Nodule	Face	
Trichilemmal tumor	Nodule	Head and neck	Rapid growth
Trichilemmoma*	Solitary or multiple papules or nodules, flesh-or yellowish-colored, flat-topped or hyper-keratotic (verrucous) papules or nodules	Face	• Solitary lesions occur sporodically as slow-growing lesions • Multiple papules are seen in Cowden syndrome
Trichilemmal carcinoma	Solitary ulcerated nodule	Face	Looks like a BCC
Hair follicle nevus*	Plaques with a tuft of hair		
Eruptive vellus hair cysts*	Red-brown-blue papules	Chest	Lesions are relatively smaller than cysts of steatocystoma multiplex and are softer than milia
Trichofolliculoma	Raised nodule with 2–3 tufts of hair	Face, scalp, or neck	
Trichoblastoma	Deep dermal nodule, skin-colored or gray	Head and neck	MC neoplasm arising on nevus sebaceous, nonulcerated nodular basal cell carcinoma is a close DD
Basaloid follicular hamartoma	Multiple papules, coalescing to form a palque		
Trichodiscoma (perifollicular fibroma, brofolliculoma)	Flat topped papules on the face		
Sebaceous adenoma*	Raised, rounded, sessile or pedunclated		Muir-Torre syndrome is characterized by solitary or multiple, benign and malignant skin tumors of the sebaceous glands and visceral malignancies
Apocrine* hidrocytoma	Solitary, well defined, dome-shaped, translucent	Eye	Do not show a difference in size during hot weather
Syringocystadenoma papilliferum	Solitary papule, nodule, or plaque, whereas in some cases multiple lesions in groups may be observed		Lesions may be pedunculated, umbilicated or eroded

(*Contd.*)

TABLE 34.2: A summary of the uncommonly seen appendageal tumors *(Contd.)*

Name	Lesion morphology	Site	Special features
Hidradenoma papilliferum	Rounded, mobile, elevated	Vulva	MC tumor of the vulva
Erosive adenomatosis of the nipple	• Nodule → serous, bloody or serosanguineous discharge • Unilateral • Clinically, it may appear as an eczematous lesion	Nipples	Premenstrual flare
Eccrine angiomatous hamartoma	Nodule or plaque, bluish or angiomatous	Palm and sole	Painful
Eccrine hidrocytoma*	Cystic blue lesions	Face	Increases with sweating and heat
Hidroacanthoma simplex	Single nodule	Limbs	Verrucous hyperkeratotic surface
Eccrine poroma	Solitary, soft, sessile, pink or reddish papule, nodule, or plaque that extrudes from a shallow depression	Palms, soles, and sides of the feet	• Bleeding is a sign of carcinoma • Easiest tumor to diagnose
Cylindroma*	• Solitary or multiple lesions, asymptomatic, slow-growing tumor • Pinkish, dome-shaped, smooth nodule with prominent telangiectases • The tumor is firm or rubber-like on palpation	Scalp, face and trunk	Multiple cylindromas are usually familial. They can be seen in familial cylindromatosis and Brooke–Spiegler syndrome
Eccrine spiroadenoma	Solitary, erythematous, blue or gray nodule	Trunk and limbs	Painful
Microcystic adnexal carcinoma	Nodule or an indurated plaque with indistinct border	Nasolabial folds, periorbital areas and the lips	Perineural and intraneural invasion is typical and causes pain
Warty dyskeratoma	Solitary with central plug, foul smellimg discharge with bleeding	Head and neck	Cup-like epidermal invagination with acantholytic dyskeratosis and corp ronds/grains 'cup-shape' and solitary nature distinguishes from Darier disease
Clear cell acanthoma	Red brown, dome-shaped, solitary	Palm and sole	Collarette of scales and vascular puncta

*Important for examination/viva.

SYRINGOMA

- Hidradénomes eruptifs
- Syringocystadenoma
- Syringocystoma—common benign tumor mostly in female adolescence, rarely familial.

Clinical Features

Multiple skin colored, yellowish or mauve sometimes translucent cystic, rounded papules with *angular outline*, tend to have a bilateral symmetrical distribution, size varies from 1 to 5 mm, most common on face, especially over cheeks and eyelids **(Fig. 34.1a)**.

1. Eruptive syringoma—"hyperpigmented" small papules on anterior trunk/neck; most commonly in Africans/Asians and in Down syndrome. Eruptive syringoma have predilection to neck and chest, abdomen and pubic areas.
2. Clear cell syringoma (histologic variant): Associated with diabetes mellitus.
   - Important differential diagnoses are: Trichoepithelioma and milia.
3. Other variants: Linear syringoma (lesions distributed in a linear fashion, either unilateral or bilateral), solitary syringoma, giant syringomas, plaque-type syringoma (focal confluence of individual papules to form a plaque), and lesions with a 'bathing trunk' distribution.

Histology

- Syringomas are derived from intraepidermal eccrine ducts.
- Syringomas are well circumscribed and composed of epithelial cells arranged in cords, nests and small ductal structures within a sclerotic stroma in the upper dermis. Ductal structures have a characteristic feature of '**tadpole or comma'**, i.e. tail-like strands of cells projecting from one side of the duct into the stroma **(Fig. 34.1b)**.
- Eosinophilic cuticle within sweat ducts + amorphous sweat within lumen; surrounding sclerotic stroma; confined to upper half of dermis.

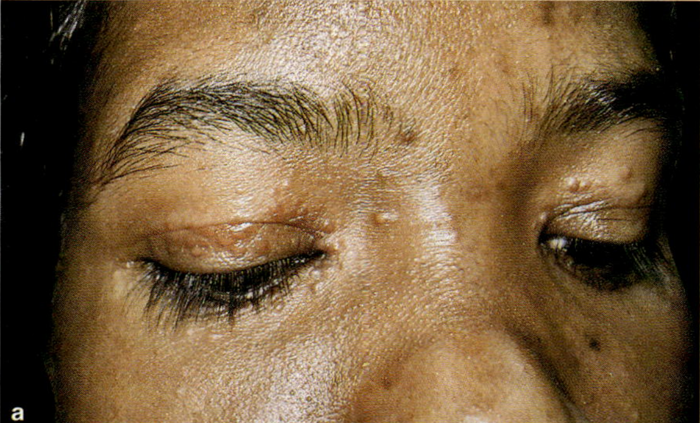

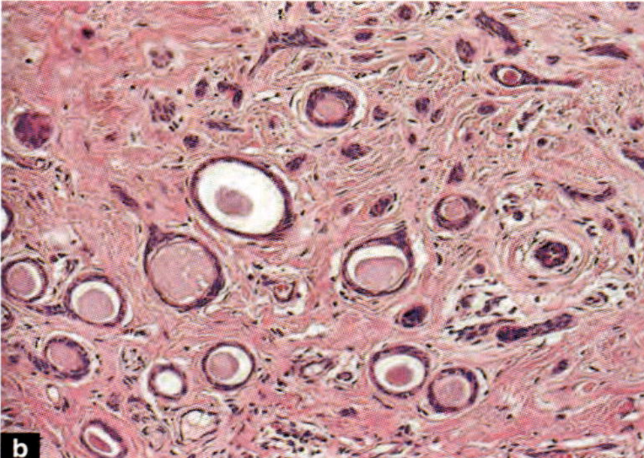

Fig. 34.1: (a) Syringomas presenting as multiple asymptomatic skin colored angular papules over the periorbital area; (b) The pathological changes of syringomas include enmeshed as well as circumscribed tumors in a sclerotic collagenous stroma with 'Comma-like' or 'tadpole-like' elements with epithelial extension

Differential Diagnosis (Box 34.1)

BOX 34.1: Differential diagnosis of syringomas

- Xanthelasma
- Milia
- Angiofibroma

Treatment

For cosmetic reasons. Diathermy has good results compared to carbon dioxide laser ablation. Other T/T options include topical retinoids, chemical peels and surgical excision.

TRICHOEPITHELIOMA

- Epithelioma adenoides cysticum
- Brooke tumor

  A hamartoma of the hair germ cell, mostly in females occurs in young adults.

Gene: Multiple trichoepitheliomas, which are inherited by autosomal dominant transmission, associated with mutations in *CYLD* gene on chromosome 16q12-q13, and *PTCH1* gene on chromosome 9p21.

Clinical Features

- May be solitary or multiple.
- Solitary lesion presents as a smooth nodule, usually on the face, measuring approx. 2–5 mm in size, whereas multiple lesions are small, pearly, mainly on centrofacial skin, often involving the nasolabial folds, may be yellow, pink or sometimes bluish with dilated blood vessels over the surface **(Fig. 34.2a)**. The center of the lesions can be slightly depressed or umbilicated.
- Lesions of trichoepithelioma are asymptomatic with no pruritus or ulceration.
- Syndromes
  - The **Brooke–Spiegler syndrome** inherited by autosomal dominant transmission consists of multiple trichoepitheliomas, cylindromas, and spiradenomas and the gene for this syndrome has been mapped to chromosome 16q12–13.
  - **Rombo syndrome** (atrophoderma vermiculatum, hypotrichosis, acrofacial vasodilation and cyanosis, milia, and multiple BCCs).

Histology

Classical appearance: "Basaloid islands in dermis with finger-like projections and cribriform nodules" **(Fig. 34.2b)**

- Composed of immature islands of basaloid cells with focal primitive follicular differentiation and a cellular stroma, seen around the cellular lobules.
- Reticulated strands and cribriform nodules ('*Swiss cheese*' appearance).
- Numerous horn cysts (much more than BCC), characterized by fully keratinized center surrounded by basophilic cells.
- Peripheral palisading; papillary mesenchymal bodies; highly cellular fibrotic pink stroma (fibroblasts account for 50% of tumors overall cellularity); almost entirely intradermal with minimal to no epidermal connection.

***IHC*:** Scattered CK20+ Merkel cells within tumor; PHLDA1+; stroma CD34+ and CD10+

***Imp*:** BCL-2 only stains periphery of trichoepithelioma (*vs* diffuse in BCC); androgen receptor negative (*vs* AR+ in most BCC).

Histological D/D

***1-BCC*:** The main histological differential diagnosis of trichoepithelioma is BCC. The main differentiating features are mentioned in **Table 34.3**.

Disease course and prognosis: The lesion is benign although it can recur. Number of lesions increase with time. Malignant transformation is extremely rare, although there are reports of its transformation to trichoblastic carcinoma or basal cell carcinoma.

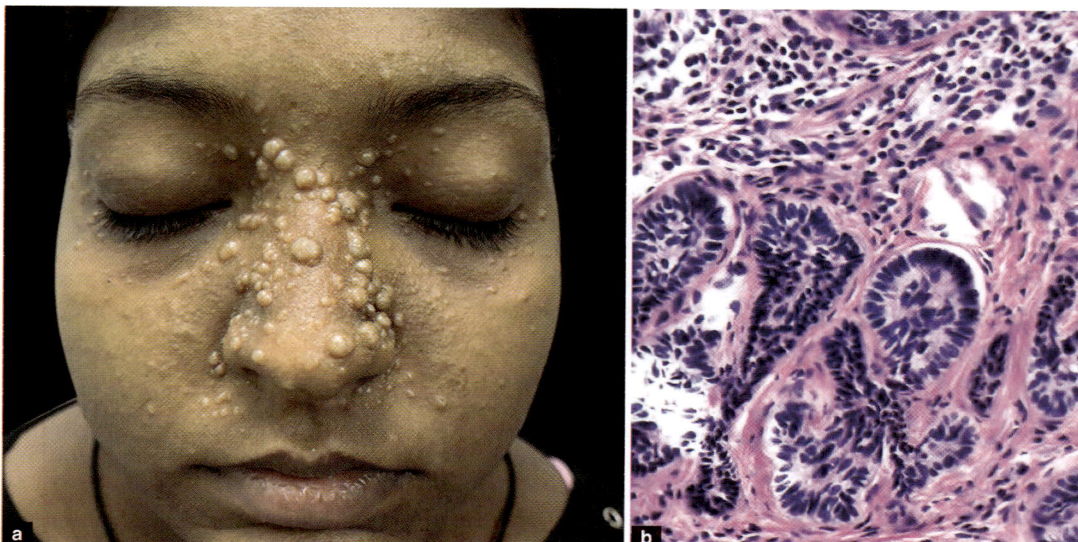

Fig. 34.2: (a) Multiple familial trichoepithelioma presenting as multiple yellowish soft papules in a centrofacial distribution; (b) Collection of "Grape-like" basaloid cells with peripheral palisading surrounded by a fibrotic stroma that may show clefting

TABLE 34.3: Difference between trichoepithelioma and BCC

Criteria	Trichoepithelioma	BCC
Growth	Symmetric growth	Asymmetric growth
Cellular atypia	±	–
Invasion in surrounding tissue	Does not invade	Invades
Stroma	Collagenous stroma	Myxoid stroma
Cribriform architecture	+	–
Retraction from surrounding tissue	–	+
Papillary mesenchymal bodies	+	–
BCL2+	Stains periphery only	Diffuse
CK20	+	–
PHLDAI	+	–
CD 34	+ (stromal cells)	–
Androgen receptor	–	+

Management (Box 34.2)

BOX 34.2: Management of trichoepithelioma

- Surgical excision
- Dermabrasion
- Curettage
- High pulsed CO_2 laser
- Cryotherapy

If malignant change is suspected, surgical excision should be followed by histopathological examination.

PILOMATRICOMA

- Benign calcifying epithelioma of Malherbe
- Trichomatricoma
- Pilomatrixoma

Definition: A benign tumor considered to be a hamartoma of the *hair matrix* composed of cells resembling those of the hair matrix, cortex and inner root sheath.

- **Most common hair follicle tumor.** A number of familial cases are recorded.
- Mutation in the *CTNNB1* gene (encodes β-catenin, involved in WNT pathway).
- Immunohistochemical studies have also demonstrated overexpression of proto-oncogene bcl-2 in the basophilic cells of pilomatrixoma.
- Association with myotonic dystrophy, Turner syndrome and Rubinstein–Taybi syndrome.
- It may occur at any age and is frequently seen in children. The majority of patients are under 20 years of age.
- Females are affected more often than males.

Clinical Features

The lesion is usually a solitary, deep, dermal or subcutaneous tumor 3–30 mm in diameter situated on the head, neck or upper extremities. The lesion has a firm to stone hard consistency with a lobular shape on palpation **(Fig. 34.3)**.

Histology

- Pilomatricoma is classified into four histological stages: Early, fully developed, early regressive and late regressive.
- Well-defined lobulated intradermal tumor with intermediate sized, nucleated, basophilic, basaloid germinative matrical cells on the periphery transitioning into enucleated, eosinophilic shadow cells in the center. Eosinophilic cells represent dead cells that may undergo dystrophic calcification over time **(Fig. 34.4)**.
- Complex cystic proliferation with internal rolls and scrolls appearance: The nuclear outline persists, but the chromatin is sparse and clumped in dark granules; when all basophilic material disappears, a mummified ghost cell remains, calcification can occur in basophilic areas.

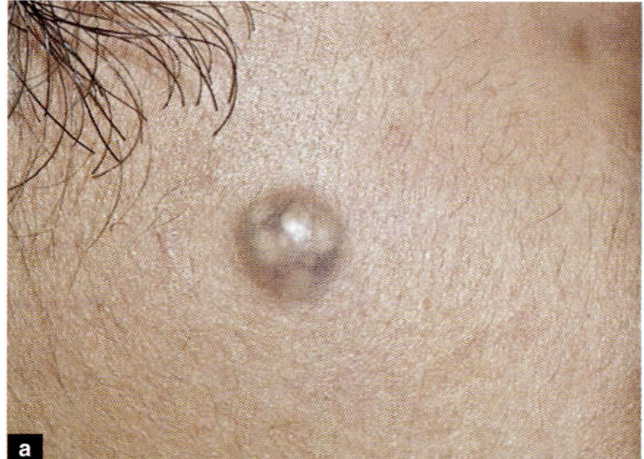

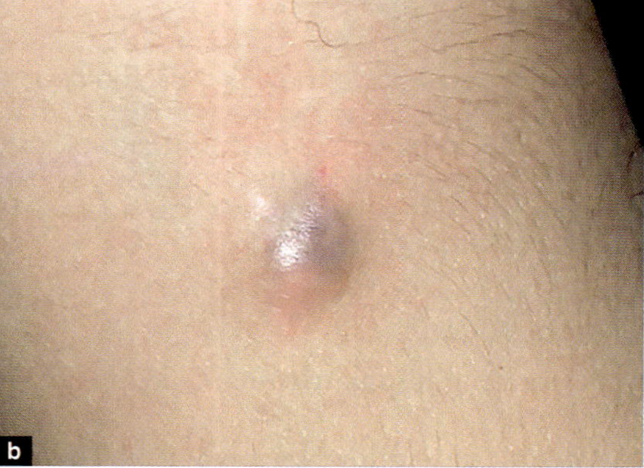

Fig. 34.3: Pilomatricoma (bluish to yellowish nodule)—with a "firm" feel on palpation

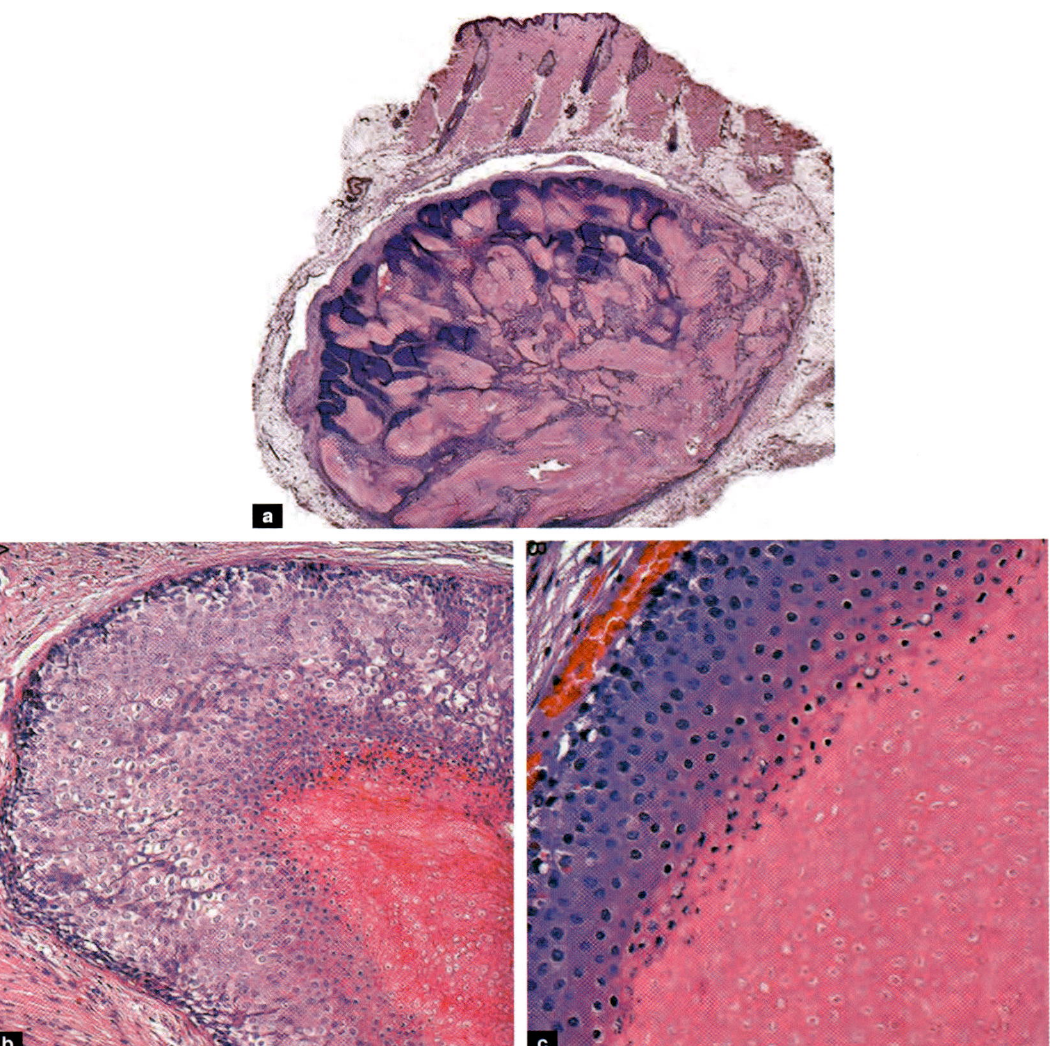

Fig. 34.4: (a) Low power view of a pilomatricoma with basophilic cells transitioning into ghost cells; (b and c) High power shows the transition from the matrical cells which are small, deeply basophilic cells to the supramatrical cells that are large lighter cells which then become pyknotic as they surround the centrally located shadow cell elements (polygonal eosinophilic anucleated cells). Shadow, or ghost cells are often the easiest sign to recognize in neoplasms with predominantly matrical differentiation

Clinical Variants

- **Perforating pilomatricoma:** Calcification extrudes from dermis without altering epidermal integrity.
- **Anetodermic pilomatricoma:** It has bullous appearance. It is characterized by lymphatic congestion and dilation, disruption of collagen fibrils and absence of elastic fibers.

- **Proliferating pilomatricoma:** It is rare, characterized by a lobular proliferation composed mainly of basaloid cells with mitotic figures (4–15 mitoses per HPF).
- **Pigmented pilomatricoma:** Pigmented due to proliferation of dendritic melanocytes within basaloid cell nest with associated shadow cells.

Differential Diagnosis—Cyst

Histological D/D

- Proliferating pilar tumor
- Pilomatrical carcinoma

Treatment

- The lesion is benign, but there is a tendency for local recurrence.
- Malignant change can occur in large pilomatricomas that have been present for many years.
- Wide local surgical excision is required for benign lesions.

CUTANEOUS LEIOMYOMAS

Cutaneous leiomyomas present as solitary or multiple papule(s) or nodule(s) and represent benign smooth muscle tumors in the skin.

Pathogenesis and Associations

Leiomyomas may arise from:

- Arrector pili muscle–piloleiomyoma
- Dartoic/vulvar/mammary smooth muscle–genital leiomyoma
- Muscles enveloping dermal blood vessels–angioleiomyoma.

Multiple piloleiomyomas may occur sporadically or in AD manner as part of the **Reed syndrome** (hereditary leiomyomatosis and renal cell cancer-HLRCC). The gene for Reed syndrome encodes fumarate hydratase but the exact pathogenesis is not yet known.

Multifocal subcutaneous leiomyomas may occur in immunosuppressed and PLHA with EBV infection.

Clinical Features

Piloleimyomas–solitary/multiple firm red-brown or skin-colored papules and nodules with solitary lesions favoring the limbs and multiple lesions mostly occurring on the trunk. They may often be associated with pain, either spontaneous or induced by cold exposure **(Fig. 34.5)**.

Genital leiomyomas–usually a solitary and painless nodule on the scrotum, vulva, areolae or nipple. May be pedunculated.

Angioleiomyomas–usually a solitary firm subcutaneous nodule on the lower limb in middle aged women and almost half of them are painful.

Women are advised a gynecologic review to exclude possible uterine involvement ('fibroids'). Menorrhagia may necessitate hysterectomy, and leiomyosarcoma, although rare, should be excluded.

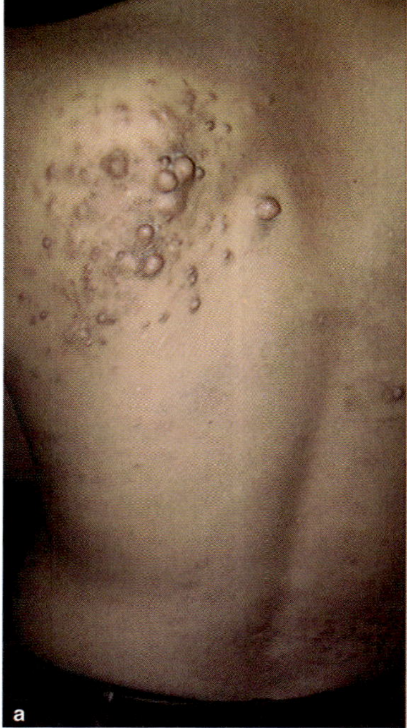

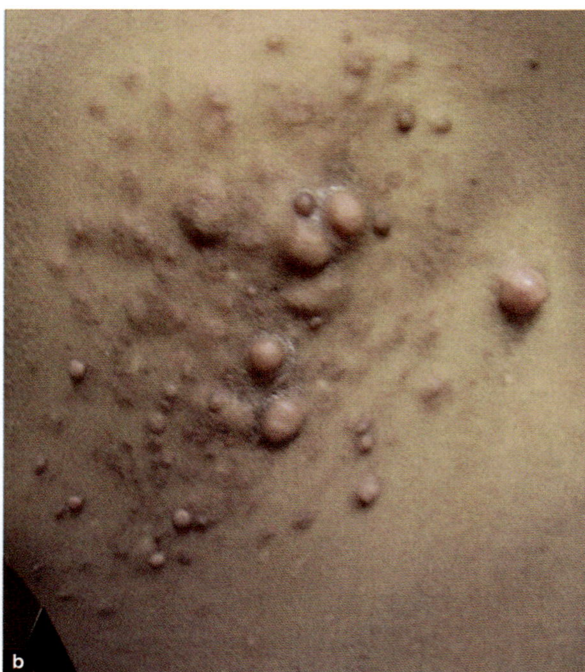

Fig. 34.5: Segmental Painful papules and nodules in a case of Leiomyoma

Histology

Piloleiomyomas are usually within the reticular dermis, with occasional extension into the subcutaneous fat, and closely related to hair follicles. They are composed of interlacing fascicles of relatively bland myocytes which peripherally tend to ramify between surrounding collagen bundles.smooth muscle cells have abundant brightly eosinophilic cytoplasm and blunt-ended, cigar-shaped nuclei.

Special stain for smooth muscle cells include smooth muscle actin (SMA) and desmin.

Differential Diagnosis

Conditions Causing Painless Dermal Nodules

- Dermatofibroma/fibrous histiocytoma
- Neurofibroma
- Eccrine Spiradenoma
- Glomangioma
- Schwannoma
- Leiomyosarcoma
- Kaposi sarcoma
- Agminated Spitz nevus
- Angiolipoma
- Adnexal tumors—trichoepithelioma, cylindroma
- Dermal nevi

- Neuroma
- Giant cell tumor
- Hamartoma
- Keloids
- Fibrosed epidermoid inclusion cyst
- Breast carcinoma (differential diagnosis of genital leiomyoma involving areola or nipple)
- Lipoma
- Poroma

Conditions Causing Painful Dermal Nodules

Acronym for painful skin tumours: BANGLE: Blue rubber bleb nevus syndrome, angiolipoma, neuroma, glioma, leiomyoma, eccrine spiradenoma. Other differentials are given below:

- Adipose
  - Angiolipoma
  - Dercum's disease
  - Piezogenic pedal papule
- Cartilage
  - Chondrodermatitis nodularis helicis
- Deposition
  - Calcinosis cutis
  - Osteoma cutis
- Eccrine
  - Eccrine angiomatous hamartoma
  - Eccrine spiradenoma
  - Hidradenoma
- Fibrous
  - Dermatofibroma
  - Fibromyxoma (digital or superficial acral)
  - Keloid
  - Scar (hypertrophic)
- Infiltration
  - Endometriosis
  - Metastases (cutaneous)
- Muscle
  - Glomus tumor
  - Leiomyoma
  - Leiomyosarcoma
- Neural
  - Granular cell tumor
  - Neurilemmoma
  - Neuroma
- Vascular
  - Angioendotheliomatosis (reactive)
  - Angioma (tufted)
  - Blue rubber bleb nevus
  - Thrombus (organizing)

Complications

- Piloleiomyomas or genital leiomyomas may develop into dermal leiomyosarcomas (metastasis rare).
- Angioleiomyomas may lead to subcutaneous leiomyosarcomas (frequent metastasis—25–40%).

Treatment

- Simple excision for solitary/limited number of tumors.
- For multiple tumors, medications that reduce smooth muscle contraction by blocking mediators (e.g. norepinephrine, epinephrine, and acetylcholine) are used. While not consistent, the agents tried include oral doxazosin (a selective α1-blocker) 1–4 mg daily, oral nifedipine (calcium channel blocker) 10 mg three times daily, amlodipine (calcium channel blocker) 5 mg twice daily, phenoxybenzamine (non-selective α-blocker) 10 mg twice daily, topical 9% hyoscine hydrobromide (anticholinergic), and oral glyceryl trinitrate (nitroglycerin) 0.8–1.6 mg.

Also analgesics that target neuropathic pain (e.g. oral gabapentin 300 mg three times daily and duloxetine) have been tried. Intralesional injection of botulinum toxin A (5 units per sq cm), cryotherapy, and lidocaine patches have shown some benefit.

CUTANEOUS CYSTS

A summary of the common cutaneous cysts is given in **Table 34.4**.

TABLE 34.4: Common cysts and their features

Name	Features
Epidermoid cyst **(Fig. 34.6a)**	• Firm dermal nodule with central punctum; any site, but most commonly head/neck/upper trunk • Derived from follicular infundibular epithelium; lined by stratified squamous epithelium with intact granular layer and no adnexal structures in the wall (*vs* vellus hair cyst and dermoid cyst); laminated/flaky keratin centrally
Proliferating trichilemmal cyst **(Fig. 34.6c)**	• Slow-growing dermal nodule; scalp (90%); usually elderly women • Resembles trichilemmal cyst but more proliferative centrally with areas of multicystic architecture
Dermoid cyst	• Infants; occur along embryonic fusion lines (most commonly lateral eyebrow) • Derived from entrapment of epidermis during embryogenesis; lined by stratified squamous epithelium with granular layer and adnexal structures (hair follicles and sebaceous glands) in cyst wall
Vellus hair cyst **(Fig. 34.6d)**	• Multiple ('eruptive') domed and flesh-colored or hyperpigmented papules; trunk; subset AD inheritance • Same histology as epidermoid cyst, but has multiple vellus hairs in cyst cavit
Steatocystoma **(Fig. 34.6b)**	• Single or multiple (multiplex—AD inheritance) lesions; chest/axilla/groin; drain oily fluid if punctured • Lined by thin stratified squamous epithelium with no granular layer and thin bright pink corrugated ('shark-tooth') cuticle; sebaceous glands in wall-KRT17 mutations; a/w pachyonychia congenita type 2
Hidrocystoma	• Translucent bluish cysts; face • Unilocular or multilocular cyst with low cuboidal lining +/– decapitation secretion (if apocrine); lumen appears empty • Associated with Schöpf-Schulz-Passarge (multiple hidrocystomas, syringofibroadenomas, PPK, hypodontia, and hypotrichosis)
Other cysts	1. Bronchogenic cyst: Solitary; present at birth; suprasternal notch/anterior neck 2. Thyroglossal duct cyst: Children/young adults; midline anterior neck; moves with swallowing 3. Median raphe cyst: Men; ventral penis between urethral meatus and anus 4. Branchial cleft cyst: Second or third decades; lateral neck (anterior SCM, preauricular, and mandibular) 5. Pseudocyst of the auricle: Middle-aged men; scaphoid fossa 6. Omphalomesenteric duct cyst: Umbilical polyp in children

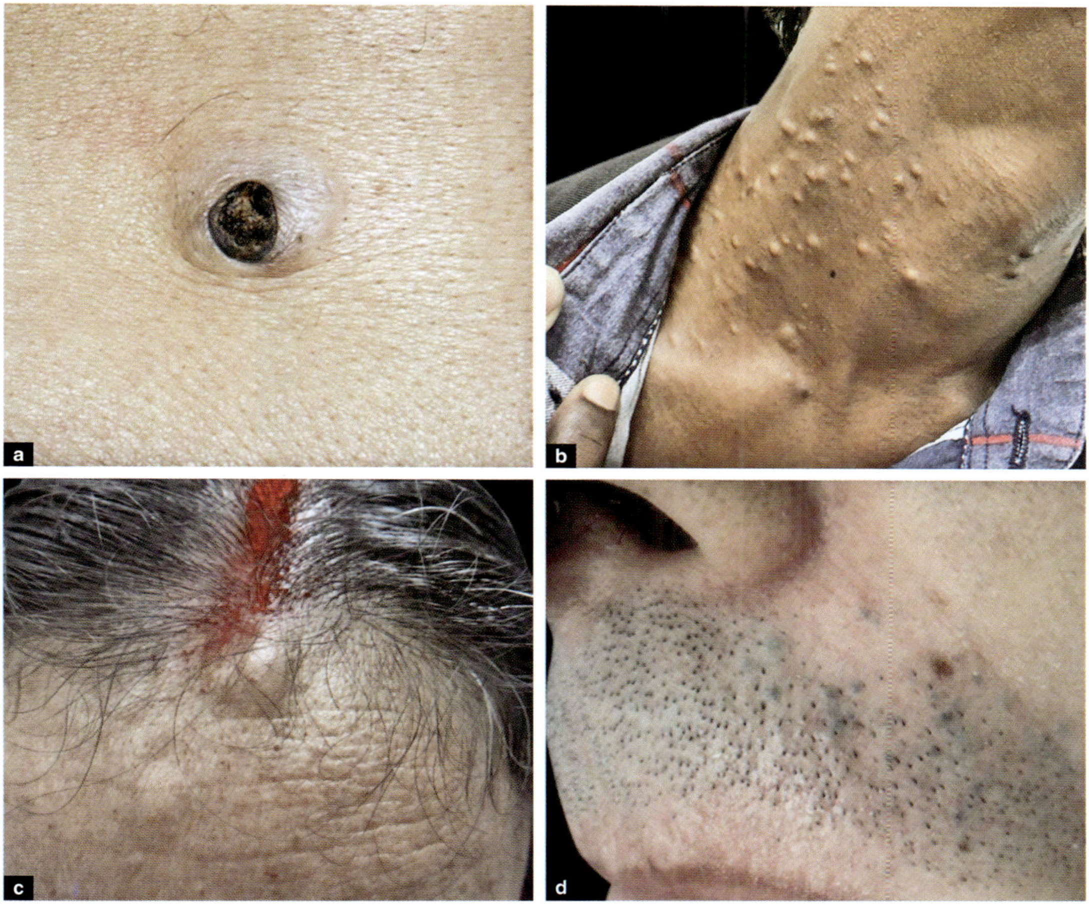

Fig. 34.6a to d: (a) Epidermoid cysts with a central punctum; (b) Steatocytoma; (c) Trichilemmal cysts; (d) Eruptive vellus hair cyst

SEBACEOUS HYPERPLASIA

Sebaceous hyperplasia is a benign condition characterized by hypertrophy of sebaceous glands affecting middle to older aged adults and increases with UV exposure and ageing.

Clinical Features (Fig. 34.6e)

- It presents with multiple yellow papules with central dell on face and upper trunk.
- May assume a linear configuration on clavicle/neck → 'juxtaclavicular beaded lines'.

Clinical D/D

- Sebaceus nevus
- Sebaceous adenoma
- Sebaceous epithelioma

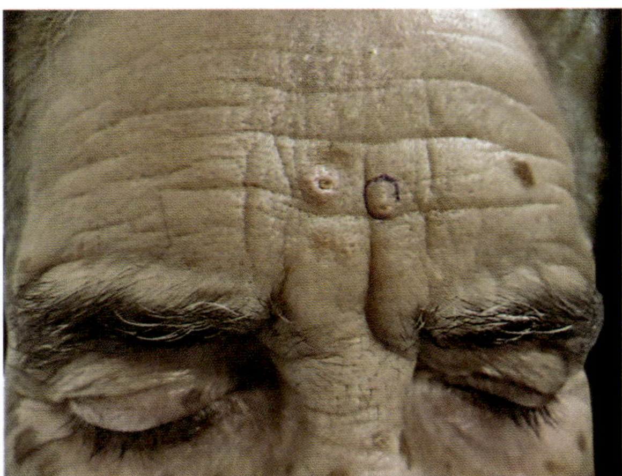

Fig. 34.6e: Sebaceous hyperplasia presenting as yellow papules with a central "dell" on the face

- Basal cell carcinoma
- Molluscum contagiosum
- Xanthoma

Histopathology

Enlarged sebaceous glands with normal internal architecture (peripheral thin layer of immature basaloid seboblasts surrounding central, mature, white sebocytes); enlarged sebaceous lobules circumferentially surround a central infundibulum.

Histological D/D

Sebaceous adenoma.

Treatment

- Oral isotretinoin
- Topical photodynamic therapy
- Cryosurgery
- Electrodessication
- Curettage
- Shave excision
- Topical trichloroacetic acid (TCA)
- CO_2 laser.

PAGET'S DISEASE OF THE NIPPLE

A progressive, marginated, scaling or crusting of the nipple and areola due to invasion of the epidermis by malignant cells, which usually but not always originate from an intraductal carcinoma of the breast.

It occurs chiefly in women, although rare cases have been recorded in men and is most frequent in the fifth and sixth decades.

Pathophysiology

Genetics: NYBY1 expression or loss of pRb expression has been described. Over-expression of ras p21 has been demonstrated in mammary and extramammary Paget's disease.

Clinical Presentation

- The early changes may be minimal, with a small, crusted and intermittently moist area on the nipple producing itching, pricking or burning sensations. The surface changes persist and gradually spread to produce an eczematous appearance **(Fig. 34.7a)**.
- The nipple, areola and, at a later stage, skin of the breast are erythematous and moist or crusted.
- The plaque is sharply marginated and may spare a segment of the areola. The edge is slightly raised and irregular in outline. Itching may be a prominent symptom.
- Retraction of the nipple and areola seen in advanced disease.
- The regional lymph nodes are enlarged in more than half the cases.

Pathology

- The epidermis is thickened, with papillomatosis, characteristic Paget cells are dispersed between the prickle cells.
- The Paget cells have a clear abundant cytoplasm and do not establish intercellular bridges with the adjacent normal keratinocytes, nuclei are rounded, vesicular or hyperchromatic with a high nuclear/cytoplasmic ratio **(Fig. 34.7b)**.
- Paget disease cells are CEA positive, EMA positive and (anticytokeratin) CAM52 positive.

Differential Diagnosis

- Nipple dermatitis
- Erosive adenomatosis
- Dermatophyte infection
- Bowen's disease.

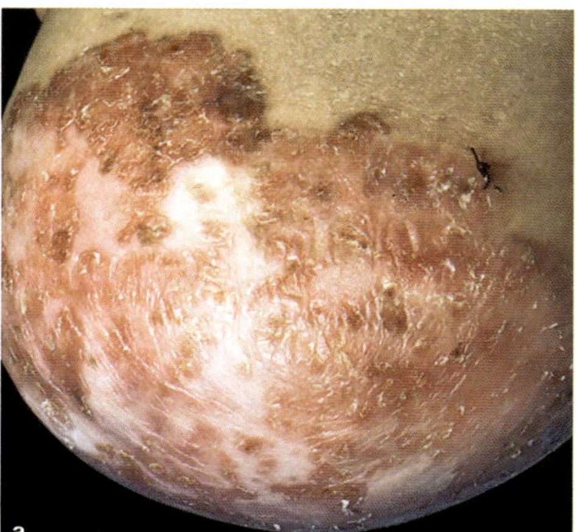

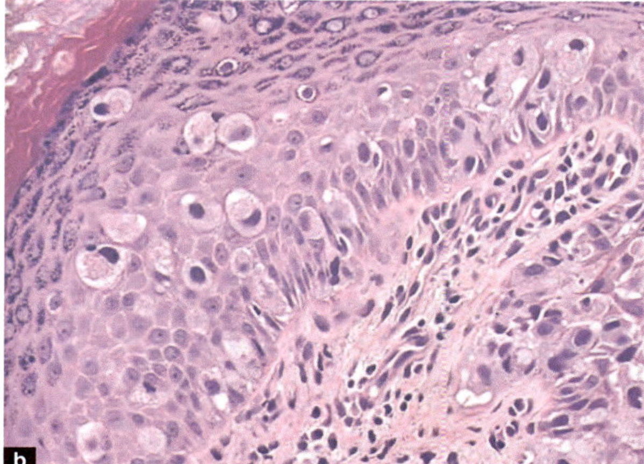

Fig. 34.7: (a) Paget's disease of the nipple; (b) Epidermis shows scattered singly lying large cells and in nests which have expanded cytoplasm and nuclei at periphery

Required Investigations

- Histopathology
- Special stains
- Mammogram
- Ultrasound/MRI.

Treatment

- Mastectomy
- Breast conserving therapy (BCT) plus lymph node evaluation
- Radiotherapy
- Chemotherapy
- Hormonal therapy.

EXTRAMAMMARY PAGET'S DISEASE

- A marginated plaque resembling Paget's disease clinically and histologically, but occurring in sites rich in apocrine glands, such as the vulva, anogenital region and axilla.
- It starts usually in the fifth decade or after and more frequently in women.

Pathophysiology

Genetics: Most common change is amplification at chromosomes Xcentq21 and 19, and losses at chromosome 10q24qter.

Pathology

- The changes in the epidermis are essentially similar to Paget disease.
- Immunohistochemistry shows cells positive for CEA, CAM5.2.

Clinical Features

- The lesion has many features in common with Paget's disease of the nipple.
- The margin is sharp, rounded and slightly raised. Itching is a prominent feature and there may be excoriations or lichenification.
- The commonest area is the vulva, perianal area, the scrotum, penis and axilla.
- Lymph node or distant metastases can occur.

Differential Diagnosis

- Eczema, intertrigo and pruritus vulvae (steady spread, lack of response to topical anti-inflammatory agents and the sharp and extending margin).
- Bowen's disease
- Superficial basal cell carcinoma

Disease Course and Prognosis

Local recurrence is common, even in cases with a wider excision. Poor prognosis is associated with depth of invasion and with elevated serum levels of CEA.

Management

- Adequate tissue sampling and other investigations are essential to establish whether or not there is an associated underlying malignancy requiring surgical excision.
- Photodynamic therapy
- Imiquimod
- Radiotherapy.

MALIGNANT TUMORS

BASAL CELL CARCINOMA (BCC)

Most common non-melanoma skin cancer (NMSC).

Pathophysiology

- 80% cases occurs in people ≥60 years, incidence is higher in male (M:F = 2:1)
- Development risk is associated with genotypic, phenotypic and environmental factors.
- Risk is higher in UV susceptibility such as fair skin color, red hair and inability to tan.
- Other factors, include:
  - actinic keratoses, solar elastosis, solar lentigines and telangiectasia
  - immunosuppression, human papilloma virus infection, acquired immunodeficiency syndrome, non-Hodgkins lymphoma
  - advancing age, male sex, previous BCCs
  - chronic arsenic exposure
  - photosensitizer drugs, PUVA, UVB phototherapy
- Disruption of the hedgehog-patched signalling pathway is closely linked to development of BCC.
- Mutations are seen in following hedgehog pathway genes: *PTCH1* (73%), *SMO* (20%) and *SUFU* (8%).
- **Somatic *PTCH1*** a segment polarity gene (9q22.3) with tumor suppressor functions, mutations have a high frequency in familial BCC.
- 50% of BCC carry a p53 mutation.

Clinical Features

- Runs a slow progressive course of peripheral extension, which produces the thread-like margin, the nodule with a central depression or the expanding rodent ulcer.
- Approximately, 80% of all BCC occur on the head and neck.
- Early lesions are usually small, translucent or pearly, with raised telangiectatic edges.
- However, the presentation can be lichenoid or keratotic, excoriated or ulcerated.
- More advanced lesions can present as classical rodent ulcer with an indurated edge and an ulcerated center.
- Other common subtypes of BCC are nodular or cystic, superficial, morphoeic, pigmented and fibroepithelial BCC.

- Pigment, when present, is usually unevenly distributed throughout the tumor, observed in darker skin type.

Clinical types of BCC:

1. **Nodular basal cell carcinoma, commonest** clinical variant usually present over head and neck, with irregular telangiectatic surface, rolled borders, translucent papule or nodule which may be red or pink with cystic lesion which subsequently ulcerates **(Fig. 34.8a** and **b).**
   Most common differential is melanoma. Other differential include, intradermal nevus and irritated seborrheic keratosis.
2. **Pigmented basal cell carcinoma:** It is a subtype of nodular BCC that exhibits increased melanization. Lesion appears as a hyperpigmented, translucent papule or nodule with hyperpigmented, thready margins **(Fig. 34.8c)**.
3. **Superficial basal cell carcinoma, less common,** commonly present over trunk, well demarcated erythematous patch with thread-like margin with atrophic epidermis may be scaly and pigmented. Mean age at diagnosis is 57 years, that is more common in younger age groups. This type has common differentials like psoriasis, Bowen's disease, discoid eczema and Paget disease of nipple.
4. **Morphoeic basal cell carcinoma, seen in 5% of BCC,** can be difficult to diagnose clinically and often present late. It is an aggressive growth variant of BCC.
   Also known as sclerodermiform, because dense fibrosis of the stroma produces a thickened plaque rather than a tumor have ill-defined borders.
   Morphea form BCC has an ivory white appearance and ill-defined borders. It may resemble a scar or a small lesion of morphea.
5. **Ulcerated basal cell carcinomas,** start as a small macule or papule but with expansion of the thread-like margins, surface may ulcerates **(Fig. 34.8d)**. The edge is usually indurated. The floor of the ulcer is depressed below the skin surface, fleshy in appearance and not very vascular.
   - Nodular lesion is crusted or eroded from an early stage of its evolution.
   - If left, the tumor and its following ulcer may spread deeply and cause great destruction, especially around the eye, nose or ear, periorbital tissues, the bones of the face; the skull; and even the meninges may be invaded.
   - Between 10% and 40% of BCCs contain a mixed pattern of two or more of these subtypes.
6. **Fibroepithelial basal cell carcinoma (premalignant fibroepithelial tumor)** is now classified as a BCC variant. It presents as a pink papule, usually on the lower back.
   Clinical differential diagnosis include intradermal melanocytic nevus or large fibroepithelial polyp.
7. **Advanced and metastatic basal cell carcinomas** (encountered at a rate of 1–2%).
   - Mutilation of the face or scalp, with destruction of the nose or eye and exposure of the paranasal sinuses or the skull, dura or brain may eventually result in death.
   - Progression of advanced BCC to a metastatic form is extremely rare (0.0028–0.55% of BCC).
   - Metastatic BCC usually have a baso-squamous (metatypical) histological subtype.

Genetic Syndromes Associated with BCC

- **Nevoid BCC syndrome (Gorlin syndrome)** is an autosomal dominant disorder with distinct clinical features including palmoplantar pits, odontogenic cysts, calcification of the falx cerebri, skeletal abnormalities, medulloblastomas and multiple BCC.

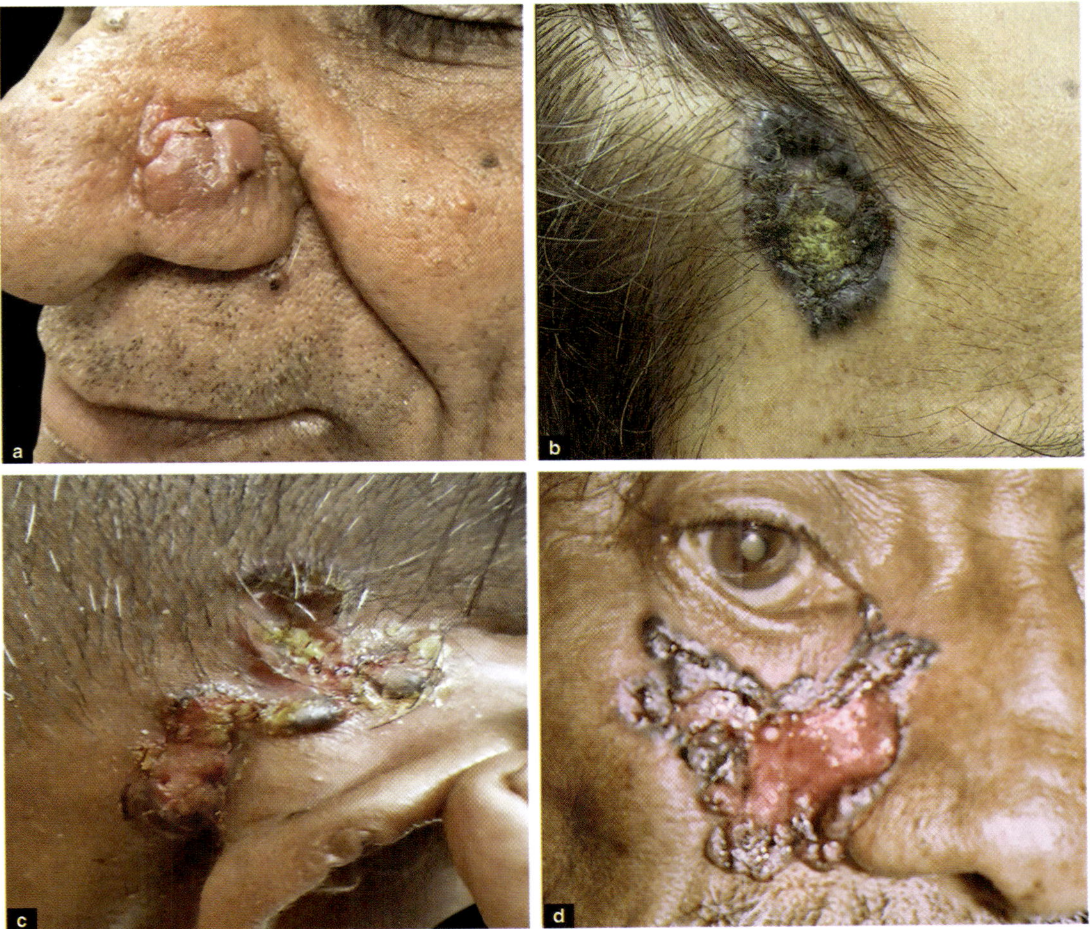

Fig. 34.8: (a) Nodular BCC presented as pink nodule on the nose; (b) Pigmented BCC; (c and d) Ulcerated BCC

- **Bazex-Dupre-Christol syndrome** is X-linked disorder with flexural hyperpigmentation, follicular atrophoderma, hypohidrosis, hypotrichosis, milia and trichoepithelioma.
- **Rombo syndrome** is autosomal dominant with atrophoderma vermiculatum, erythematous lesions, hypotrichosis, milia, telangiectasias and trichoepithelioma.
- **Xeroderma pigmentosum** is autosomal recessive with actinic keratosis/cheilitis, lentigines, atrophy, photosensitivity, telangiectasias, mottled hypo/hyperpigmentation, development delay/mental retardation, eye anomalies, movement disorder, peripheral neuropathy, photophobia, melanomas, squamous cell carcinomas, brain and visceral neoplasms.
- **Generalized follicular basaloid hamartoma** syndrome is autosomal dominant disorder with comedones, hypohidrosis, hypotrichosis, milia.
- **Happle–Tinschert syndrome is sporadic with** lesions over Blaschko's lines, atrophy, hyperpigmentation, teeth abnormalities, body asymmetry, development delay/mental retardation, spine and limb malformations and brain tumors.

Histopathology

- The tumor cells resemble those of the basal layer of the epidermis and the matrix cells of the appendages **(Fig. 34.9)**.
- Their nuclei are compact, rather darkly staining and closely set, cytoplasm stains poorly and the cell margins are rather indistinct.
- Mitotic figures may be frequent.
- In early lesions, the tumor buds can be seen arising from the epidermis as the tumor progresses, the masses extend into the dermis.
- The melanin they produce causes the tumor to be pigmented.

Histological Types of BCC

- **Superficial basal cell carcinoma:**
  - Bud of malignant cells descend from the epidermis which are peripherally lined by palisading basal cells.
  - Palisading basal cells which form slit-like spaces containing alcian blue positive mesenchymal mucoid material.
  - The atypical basaloid cells rarely show mitoses or apoptotic cells but may colonize the hair follicles and rarely the eccrine adnexal structures.
- **Nodular basal cell carcinoma:**
  - Nodular BCCs are composed of islands of cells with peripheral palisading and a haphazard arrangement of the more central cells. Stromal retraction also seen.
  - Basaloid cells in either the papillary or reticular dermis where solar elastosis may be evident.

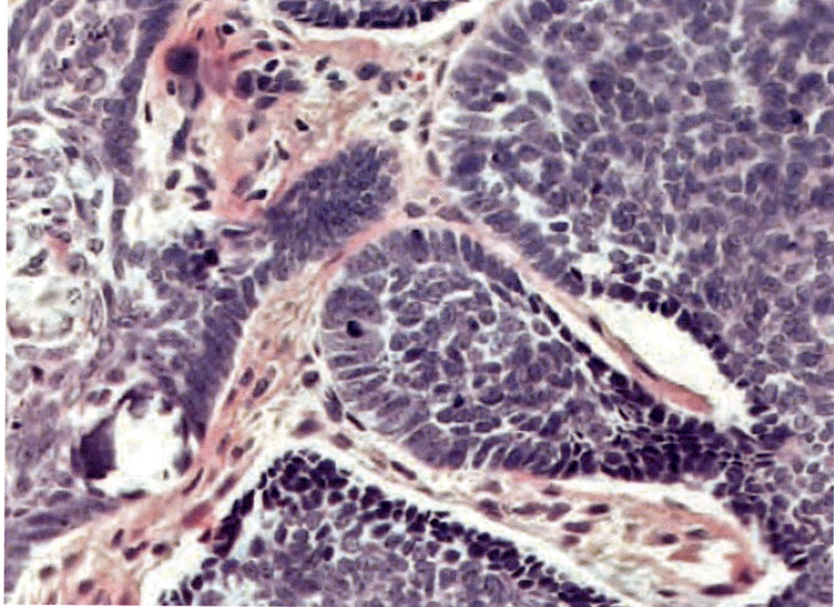

Fig. 34.9: Peripheral palisading of cells with retraction of stroma around individual islands

- **Micronodular basal cell carcinoma:**
  - The tumor nests are smaller than those in nodular BCC, smaller than 15 µm.
  - They are widely and asymmetrically dispersed in the dermis.
  - Surrounding stroma shows either amyxoid or collagenized morphology.
- **Morpheaform basal cell carcinoma:**
  - Sclerosing BCC display one to two cells thick columns of basaloid cells that invade the dermis and are enmeshed in a dense collagenous stroma.
  - Marked cell necrosis and mitotic activity.
- **Infiltrative basal cell carcinoma:** Poorly circumscribed nests of tumor cells which may show invasion of the subcutis and adjacent muscular and other structures.
- **Basosquamous or metatypical basal cell carcinoma:** Appears to have features of both BCC and SCC. The biological significance is that this pathological pattern is associated with a significantly higher incidence of metastatic spread (>5%).

  The cells are larger with a larger paler nucleus than in the classic BCC and have a more eosinophilic cytoplasm.

Differential Diagnosis (Box 34.3)

BOX 34.3: Differential diagnosis of BCC

- Nodular BCC—melanocytic nevi, sebaceous hyperplasia, molluscum contagiosum, keratoacanthoma
- Darkly pigmented ulcerated tumor—malignant melanoma
- Superficial BCC—eczema, psoriasis, Bowen's disease
- Morphoeic BCC—morphea
- Chondrodermatitis nodularis helicis

Disease Course and Prognosis (Box 34.4)

If it does metastasize, it often involves regional lymph nodes, bone, lungs, and skin.

Box 34.4: Disease course and prognosis

- BCC is a slow growing tumor with rare metastases.
- Advanced BCC includes locally advanced BCC (laBCC), with direct tumor spread (0.8% of all BCCs) and occasionally extensive tissue destruction, and metastatic BCC (mBCC)
- Rates of laBCC and mBCC increase after 65 years.

Investigations

- Skin biopsy
- **Dermoscopy**—helps in the diagnosis of non-pigmented and pigmented BCCs
  - White and gray brown structureless areas, blue gray ovoid nests, blue gray globules, maple leaf-like areas, spoke wheel areas, concentric structures, ulcerations and blue gray dots
- High frequency ultrasound
- Optical coherence tomography using infrared light and *in vivo* confocal microscopy.

Management

From treatment point of view BCC is classified into two groups—**easy-to-treat** BCC **(low risk)** and **difficult-to-treat** BCC **(high risk)**.

Difficult-to-treat BCCs include 'all locally advanced BCCs and also common BCCs which, for any reason, pose specific management problems. These reasons may be

1. the technical difficulty of maintaining function and aesthetics due to the size or location (eyes, nose, lips and ears) of the tumor;
2. the poorly defined borders often associated with morphoeic subtype or prior recurrence;
3. multiple prior recurrences on the face (often requiring much larger excision);
4. prior radiotherapy;
5. patient's reluctance to accept the consequences of surgery
6. patient's comorbidities interfering with surgery.

Some apparently easy-to-treat BCCs may still be at risk of **recurrences** such as

a. those located on the H area of the face affecting the invasion of the tumor,
b. those with aggressive histological characteristics (perineural and/or perivascular involvement) and
c. those in immunosuppressed patients

Treatment depends upon the clinical, histological, size and site of tumor and patient factors. It is outlined in **Flowcharts 34.1** to **34.3**.

Prognosis

- With appropriate treatment, the prognosis of BCC is excellent.
- The risk for development of a second primary BCC ranges from 36 to 50% (within 5 years).

Flowchart 34.1: Algorithm for management of BCC (primary *vs* recurrent)

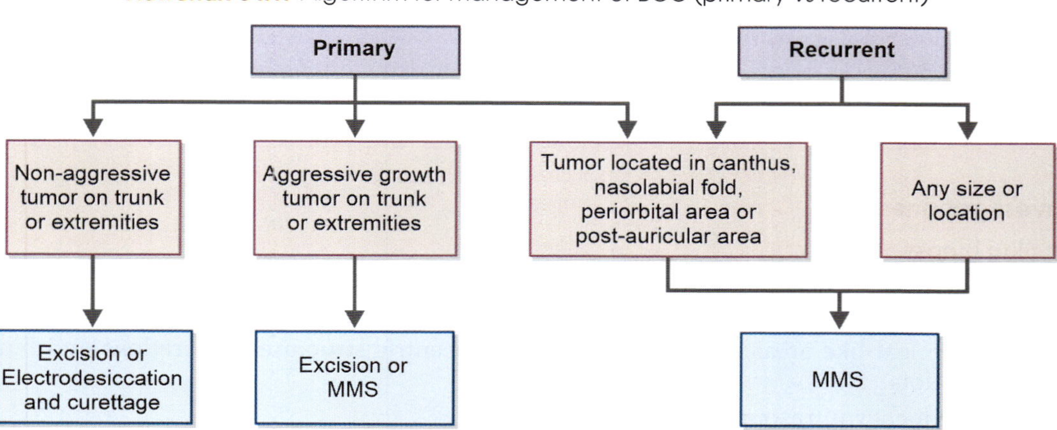

*MMS, Mohs micrographic surgery

Flowchart 34.2: Algorithm for management of BCC (easy-to-treat)

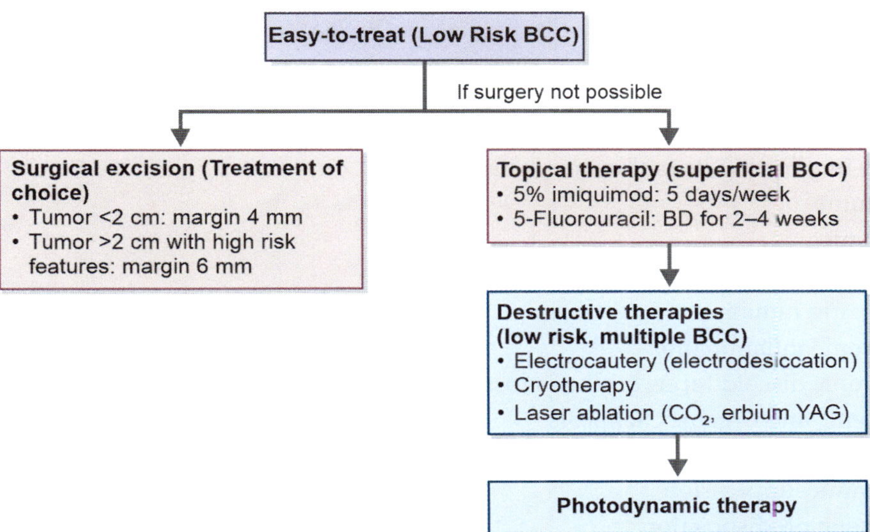

Flowchart 34.3: Algorithm for management of BCC (difficult-to-treat)

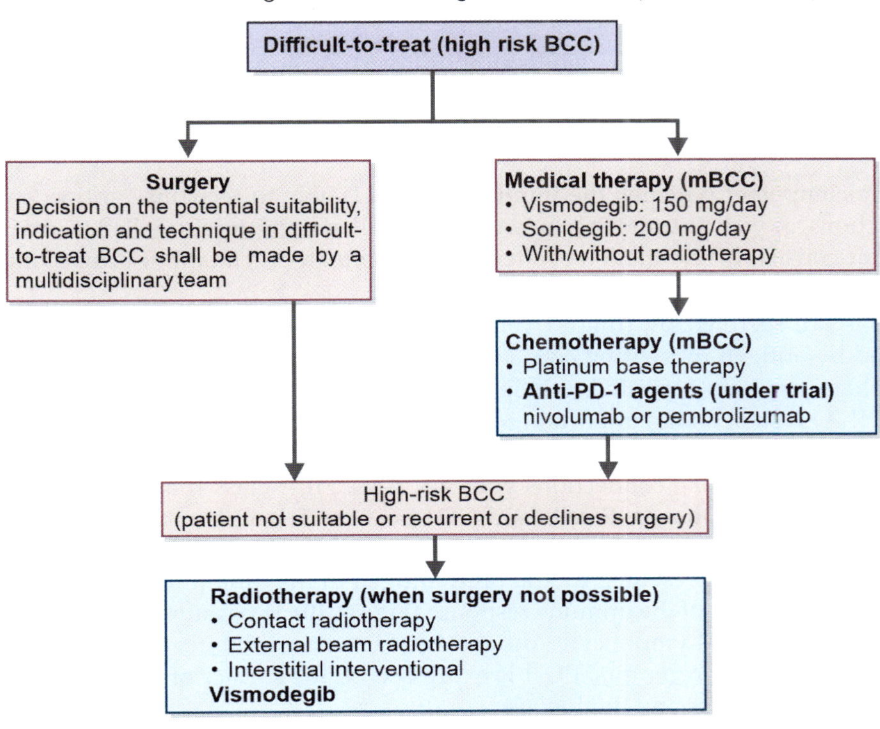

SQUAMOUS CELL CARCINOMA (SCC)

Epidemiology

- Second commonest skin cancer arising from epidermal keratinocytes or its appendages.
- Incidence of SCC increases with age, highest in males and females >85 years of age group.
- Factors implicating its pathogenesis include:
  - Trauma
  - Albinism
  - Burn scar
  - Ionizing radiation
  - Chronic inflammation
  - Chronic discoid lupus erythematosus
  - Arsenic and organic chemicals
  - Human papilloma virus
  - Immunosuppression
  - Genetic predisposition
  - Drugs: Use of hydrochlorothiazide has been associated with an increased risk of cSCC with evidence of a duration-and dose-response relationship.

Precursor lesions—actinic keratoses, Bowen's disease, other non-invasive, precancerous conditions that may evolve into SCC include bowenoid papulosis and erythroplasia of Queyrat.

Associated diseases like, hidradenitis suppurativa, morphea, lymphoedema, Hailey-Hailey disease and dystrophic epidermolysis bullosa.

Pathogenesis

In immunocompetent patients, the immune system is able to recognise antigens related to viral infections, as well as tumour antigens. This is called immune surveillance. An important defence line consists of elimination of altered cells by innate and adaptive arms of the immune system.

Antigens are secreted by tumour cells, and are expressed on the cell membrane and recognized by antigen presenting cells (APC). T lymphocytes and natural killer (NK) cells, among others, are then activated to help eliminate the tumour cells. The human leukocyte antigen (HLA) system has an important role in the recognition of antigens. HLA class I can be found on all cells in the human body. Its function is to present antigens to the CD8 positive T lymphocytes and to make connections with NK cells. HLA class II are expressed on APCs (dendritic cells, macrophages, B cells and CD4 positive T lymphocytes). HLA class III has involvements within the complement system and cytokine formation. When a T lymphocyte recognises the peptide presented by the HLA antigen in the tumour cell, co-receptors act as activators and inhibtors of the immune response **(Fig. 34.10)**. Programmed cell death 1 protein (PD-1) and Cytotoxic T-Lymphocyte Antigen 4 (CTLA4) are inhibitory receptors and known as immune check-point receptors. PD-1 is expressed on the surface of T cells, B cells, natural killer cells, dendritic cells and monocytes.

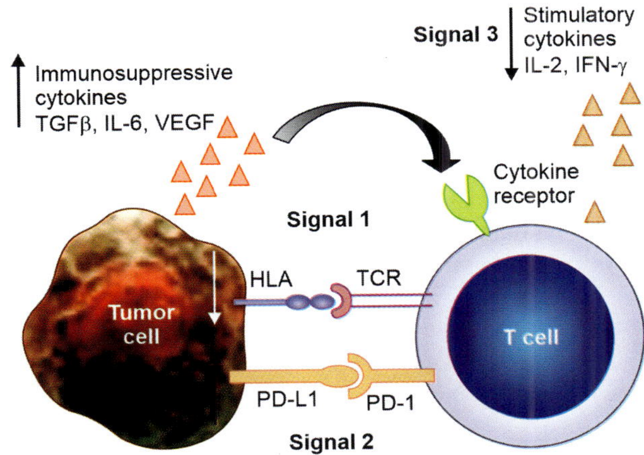

Fig. 34.10: T-cell activation requires three simultaneous signals in order to carry out its anti-tumour effects including signal 1, signal 2 and signal 3. Programmed cell death 1 protein (PD-1) is an inhibitory receptor. Immune evasion can occur at any of these signals impairing the immune system from effectively eradicating malignant cells.

Pathology

- Mutations of tumor protein TP53 caused by UVR leading to pyrimidine dimers, are seen approximately 90% of SCCs.
- Mutation of p16, a tumor suppressor protein involved in the arrest of the cell cycle at G1, suppressing the entry into the S phase, caused by UVR leads to continuous cell cycling.
- Inactivated p16 advances actinic keratoses (AK) to SCC.
- Mutation or activation in pathways including HRAS, Wnt/β-catenin/TCF, mitogen activated protein kinase (MAPK) and STAT3, epidermal growth factor receptor (EGFR) and mammalian target of rapamycin (mTOR) resulting in SCC formation.
- In invasive SCC, atypical keratinocytes breach the epidermal basement membrane and invade the dermis.
- **Histological variants of SCC:**
  - Classic/no special type
  - Acantholytic
  - Spindle cell
  - Desmoplastic
  - Basaloid
  - Verrucous
  - Pseudovascular and follicular
- **Classic SCC**—comprises well-differentiated lesions (large, polygonal cells with vesicular nuclei, prominent nucleoli and abundant cytoplasm) to poorly differentiated lesions (pleomorphic cells).
- Histological grading, identification of *in situ* tumor and expression of cytokerátin markers by the tumor cells on immuno-histochemistry are required as it guides the pathological staging, prognosis and treatment options.

Clinical Features

- **Most common sites are sun-exposed areas,** backs of the hands and forearms, the upper part of the face and, especially in males, on the lower lip and pinna **(Figs 34.11 and 34.12)**.
- **First clinical sign is induration may present as** plaque-like, verrucous, tumid or ulcerated lesion with inflammed edge.
- **Well-differentiated tumors** are usually papillomatous and are capped by a keratotic crust in the earlier stages which shed later to reveal an ulcer or eroded tumor with an indurated margin and a purulent exuding surface that bleeds rather easily **(Fig. 34.13)**.

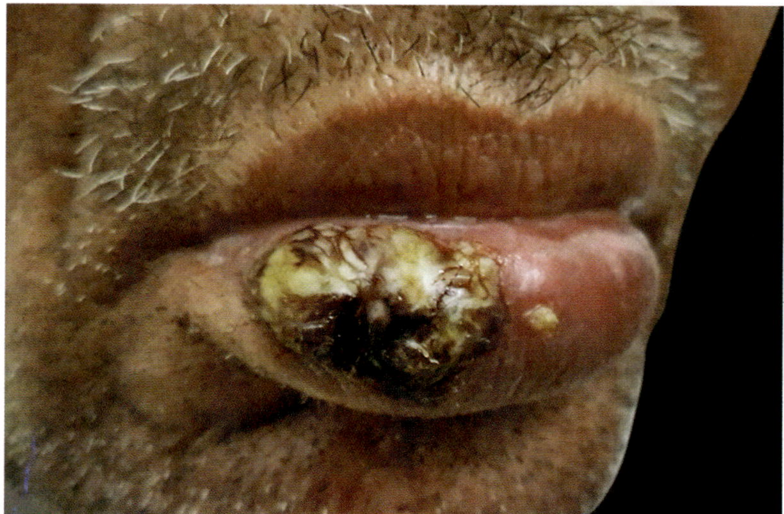

Fig. 34.11: SCC over lower lip with ulcerated, purulent exuding surface

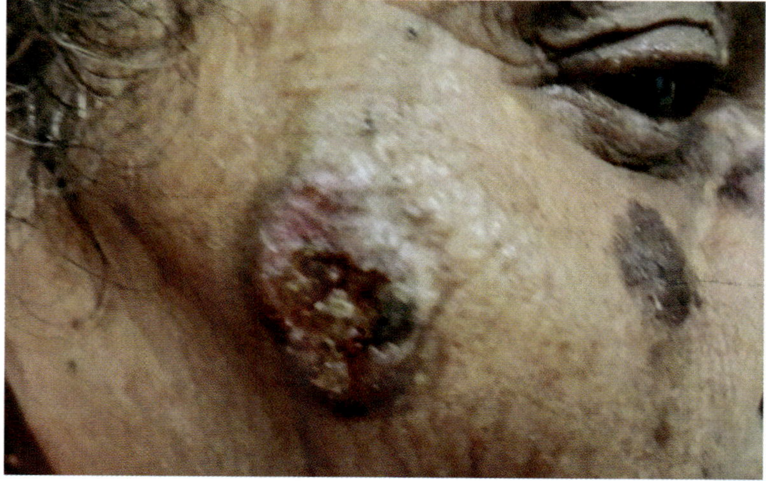

Fig. 34.12: SCC over cheek presenting as hyperkeratotic, ulcerated plaque that developed over a long standing actinic keratosis

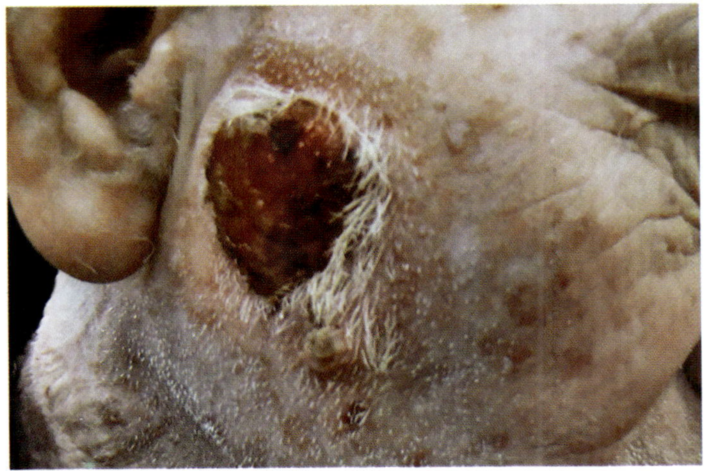

Fig. 34.13: An eroded ulcerative SCC in an albino

Clinical Variants

- Verrucous carcinoma known as epithelioma cuniculatum, slow growing rarely metastasizes immunosuppression
- Recurrent SCC
  - An exophytic verruciform appearance may exhibit hyperkeratosis, ulceration, or a malodorous discharge
  - Unknown etiology, may arise from areas of chronic inflammation
  - Association of HPV-11 and-16

Differential Diagnosis

- **Keratoacanthoma**—a faster rate of growth and involute to leave a scar
- **Actinic keratosis**—tend to be multiple and lack a dermal component on palpation
- **BCC**
- **Amelanotic melanoma**
- **Seborrheic keratosis**—frequently multiple and non-indurated
- **Warts**

Classification of Severity

- SCC has a low rate of metastasis of 5%. For patients with Cut SCC, the risk of local recurrence (LR) is 2% and the risk of nodal metastasis (NM) is 5%. Disease-specific death is estimated to be 1.5–2.1%.

  A subset of cSCC, namely the high-risk cSCCs are associated with worse prognosis and up to 37% of high-risk cSCCs may progress to advanced cSCC.
- **High risk** features of primary cutaneous SCC as below.
  i. **Clinical features**
    - Tumor diameter >20 mm
    - SCC on ear

- Immunosuppression
- Recurrent SCC

ii. **Pathological features**
- Tumor thickness >4 mm
- Tumor extension beyond dermis to subcutaneous
- Perineural invasion
- Poorly differentiated
- Desmoplastic subtype

- **Risk factors** for recurrence or metastasis of cutaneous squamous cell carcinoma are listed below
  - Breslow thickness >2 mm
  - Invasion beyond subcutaneous fat
  - Perineural invasion
  - Diameter >20 mm
  - Poor differentiation
  - Immunosuppression
  - Location on the lip, ear or temple.

Complications and Comorbidity

Do not involute spontaneously, so if left untreated will metastasize by local invasion

Stages: Risk of local recurrence, nodal metastases or disease-specific death based on the number of high-risk features (%).

T1 No high-risk features (tumors smaller than 2 cm in diameter) 4/134 (3%)

T2A 1 high-risk feature (>2 mm thickness) 9/67 (13%)

T2B 2–3 high-risk features 37/49 (76%)

T3 4 of 4 high-risk features (tumors that invade muscle, bone, or cartilage of maxilla, mandible or orbit) 8/8 (100%).

Disease Course and Prognosis

- Excellent prognosis with low risk SCC following definite treatment.
- High risk have greater potential for local invasion and for metastasis.
- Risk of metastasis—5-year metastatic rate of 5%, and 85% of metastatic cases are nodal disease.

Investigations

- **Skin biopsy**
- Reflectance confocal microscopy
- High resolution optical coherence tomography
- MRI for PNI (peripheral nerve invasion)
- High resolution micro oil MRI
- PET, CT scan
- FNAC and ultrasound

Management

First line

- **Squamous cell carcinomas:**
  - **Surgical excision**—completely excise the tumor taking a peripheral and deep margin of normal skin.
  - A clinical peripheral margin of 6 mm is recommended during excision.
  - Required long follow-up of the patients.
- **Low risk SCC**
  - Curettage and cautery
  - Cryotherapy
  - PDT
  - 5% FU
  - 5% Imiquimod
  - Interferon-α

Second line

Radiotherapy (contraindicated in cases of previously irradiated sites and for genodermatoses predisposing to skin cancer).

Secondary prevention

- Retinoids—acitretin 25 mg daily
- Sirolimus
- Cyclosporin

High Risk SCC

The management of High risk SCC is depicted in the **Flowchart 34.4**.

Until recently treatment of advanced CSCC represented a high unmet need since there were no approved systemic therapy and no standard of care. The different medical option include.

1. *Chemotherapy*

Cytotoxic agents as cisplatin or carboplatin, 5-fluorouracil, bleomycin, methotrexate, Adriamycin, taxanes and gemcitabine have been used off-label in patients with advanced CSCC.

2. *Targeted Therapies–EGFR inhibitors*

Among EGFR inhibitors, only cetuximab is approved for the treatment of head and neck SCC but not for cSCC.

3. *Immunotherapy: Immune Checkpoint Inhibitors*

Immune checkpoint inhibitors have represented a major breakthrough for the treatment of advanced cSCC, addressing a large unmet need. Cemiplimab and pembrolizumab are two anti-PD1 agents approved by FDA (while pembrolizumab is not yet approved by EMA), Cemiplimab, a humanized IgG4 PD-1 blocker,binds to the extracellular domain of the PD-1 receptor limiting the interaction of PD-1 with its ligands (PD-L1 and PD-L2), thus restoring the activation of the T cells and the anti-tumour response.

Flowchart 34.4: Management of high-risk and advanced cutaneous squamous cell carcinoma (cSCC)

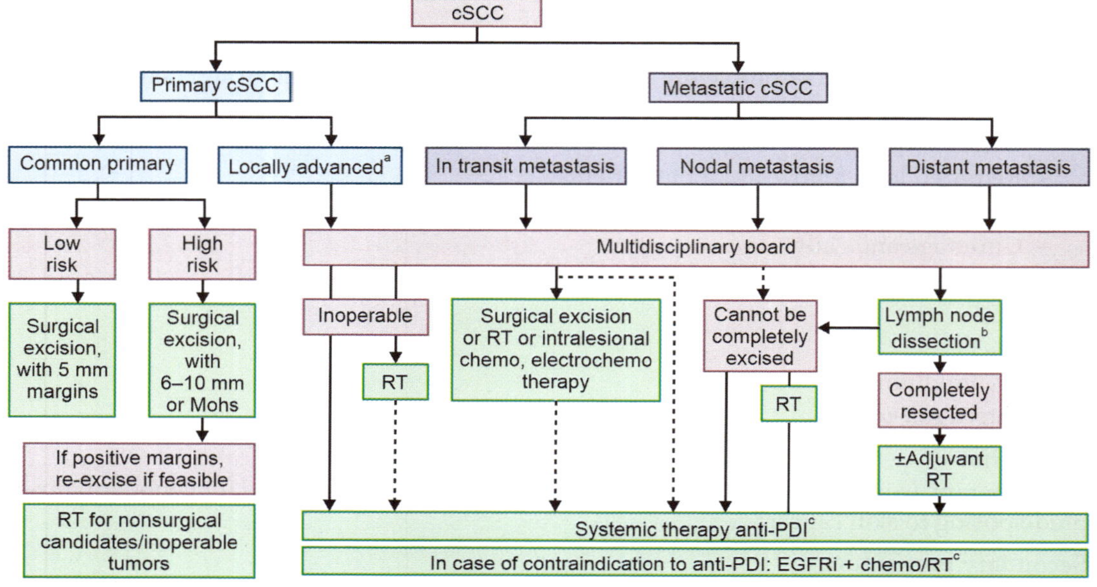

EGFRi, EGFR inhibitors; La, locally advanced; RT, radiotherapy.
[a]Locally advanced by definition not amenable to curative surgery or curative RT. [b]Lymph node dissection as indicated. [c]All systemic treatments are off-label, except for anti-PD-1 agent cemiplimab that is approved by FDA/EMA for patients with locally advanced or metastatic cSCC who are not candidates for curative surgery or curative radiation. Anti-PD-1 agent pembrolizumab has been approved by US FDA for patients with recurrent or metastatic cSCC that is not curable by surgery or radiation.
(C. Dessiniot. JEADV 2021, 36 (Suppl. 1), 11–18)

MALIGNANT MELANOMA

Malignant tumor that arises from melanocytes, due to its metastatic potential, leads to death of >75% of skin cancer death.

Etiopathogenesis

- Most commonly has cutaneous origin, can also arise on mucosal surfaces (e.g. oral, conjunctival, vaginal) and within the uveal tract of the eye as well as the leptomeninges.
- Increased annual incidence (3–7%).
- Several factors like genetic predisposition, mutagenic environmental events and anti-tumor host response play a role in tumor progression.
- Genetic aberrations in melanoma affect signaling pathways, discovery of specific sites within these pathways has led to the era of targeted therapies.

Predisposing Factors

- **Melanoma precursors:** 70–80% of melanoma arises from normal skin, hence 20–25% of melanoma are thought to arise from cutaneous melanocytic nevi.
- **Congenital melanocytic nevi (CMN):** Increase risk of melanoma with size of CMN.

- Risk of 5–15% in CMN of size >20 cm, whereas the risk is between 2.6 and 4.9% in CMN <4.5 cm in diameter.
- **Common nevi:** The estimated lifetime risks of transformation of any given mole is about 1/3000 for males and 1/10000 for females.
- **Atypical/dysplastic nevi (AN/DN):** Number of AN/DN is a risk factor for melanoma (risk increases with the number of DN).
- **Family history of melanoma was overall associated with a 2-fold increased risk of melanoma.**
- **Phenotypic traits:** Increased risk have been found in skin type 1, fair skin, blue color eyes, red color hair and 2-fold for high density freckles.
- **Nevus phenotype:** Depends upon number, size and the features of melanocytic nevi which depends upon genetic and amount of sun exposure since birth.
- **Risk increases with numbers and clinical atypia of nevi,** high nevus count (100–120 common nevi) is associated with an approximately 7-fold increased risk of melanoma as compared to less than 15 nevi.
- **Risk increases in familial AN/DN syndrome, 49% in 10–50 years of age group and 82% in >72 years.**
- **Gene susceptibility:**
  i. The cyclin-dependent kinase (CDK) inhibitor 2A gene (CDKN2A), 40% of individuals with familial melanoma.
  ii. Melanocortin 1 receptor **(*MC1R*)** gene, carries a moderate risk.
  iii. Microphthalmia-associated transcription factor **(*MITF*)** is a master regulator gene of melanocyte development and differentiation, missing link between melanoma and renal cancer.
  iv. ***BAP1*** hereditary cancer predisposition syndrome includes uveal melanoma, mesothelioma, CM, renal cell carcinoma and atypical melanocytic tumors/nevi.
- **Environment factors:** UV and sunlight exposure—low risk factor.
- Presence or history of premalignant skin conditions like actinic keratosis, SCC, BCC carries a risk of 4.28 and presence of actinic damage such as solar lentigines and elastosis, a risk of 2.02.

Pathology

Classification of melanoma (given by McGovern in 1973 based upon the hypothesis of pattern of tumor growth—radial growth or vertical growth).

Four main types

- **Nodular melanoma (NM)**—poor prognosis as it grows vertical directly and no radial growth.
- **Superficial spreading melanoma (SSM)**
- **Lentigo maligna melanoma (LMM)**
- **Acral lentiginous melanoma (ALM)**

Clinical Features

Four general principles of examination

1. Analytical examination
2. Pattern recognition

3. Comparative analysis
4. Dynamic analysis

- **Analytical examination**
  - Most commonly described diagnostic clue known as ABCDE algorithm **(Box 34.5)**.

BOX 34.5: ABCDE algorithm

Asymmetry	**B**order irregularity	**C**olor variegation
Diameter >6 mm	**E**volution	

- **Pattern recognition:** More important than the application of a combination of criteria such as ABCDE
- **Comparative analysis (ugly duckling sign)—major sign for melanoma suspicion**
- **Dynamic analysis**
  - Melanoma grow and change faster, as compared to nevi
  - Dynamic assessment is an important criteria for suspecting a melanoma
  - Includes changes, in the size, color or shape of pre-existing pigmented lesions
  - Or development of any new growing skin lesion.

Diagnostic Tool

- **Dermoscopy**
  - Sensitivity increases by 10–27%
  - Atypical pigment network, irregular brown, black dots/globules, streaks, and pigmentation with multiple colors asymmetrically distributed.
  - Limitation—based mainly on an analysis of color distribution, which are not a perfect reflection of malignancy.
- **Computed dermoscopy devices**
- **Reflectance confocal microscopy**
- **Computer-aided diagnostic system:** Uses dermoscopic images for pigmented lesions.

Clinical Presentations

Cutaneous melanoma is classified as melanoma *in situ* (confined to epidermis) and invasive melanoma (atypical melanocytes progressively invade into the dermis) which are of the following syptypes.

1. **An atypical nevus (superficial spreading melanoma)**
   - 60–70% cases of melanoma correspond to SSM histoclinical subtype
   - Flat pigmented macule, which progressively become irregular in size, with changing color shades like brown, black, gray, red or depigmented over several months to years.
2. **'A pigmented or red nodule' (nodular melanoma) (Fig. 34.14a)**
   - 10–20% of melanoma correspond to NM histoclinical subtype.
   - Fast growing subgroup of melanoma with predominant aggressive vertical growth phase.
   - Present regular, symmetrical, elevated, dome-shaped or rarely polypoid or sometimes pedunculated lesions, with color ranges from black, dark brown to red.
   - Ulceration and bleeding are common.
   - Important differential are BCC, angioma, histiocytoma and dermatofibroma.

3. **'A lentigo of the face in the elderly' (lentigo maligna melanoma) (Fig. 34.14b)**
   - Corresponds to LMM histoclinical subtype.
   - Slow growing subgroup of melanoma.
   - Presents as a flat, brown or black, irregularly-shaped lesion on chronically sunexposed areas of the skin (face, neck, forearms) in the elderly
   - Important differentials are solar lentigo, a pigmented actinic keratosis or a flat seborrhoeic keratosis.
4. **'A pigmented stain on the soles' (acral lentiginous melanoma) (Fig. 34.14c)**
   - Corresponds to ALM histoclinical subtype and c-kit mutated group.
   - Different racial occurrence, ranging from 2 to 10% of melanoma in white to 60–72% in black populations.
   - Presented as discrete light brown or black macule, often described as a 'dirty-like stain', within distinct borders on the soles in elderly.

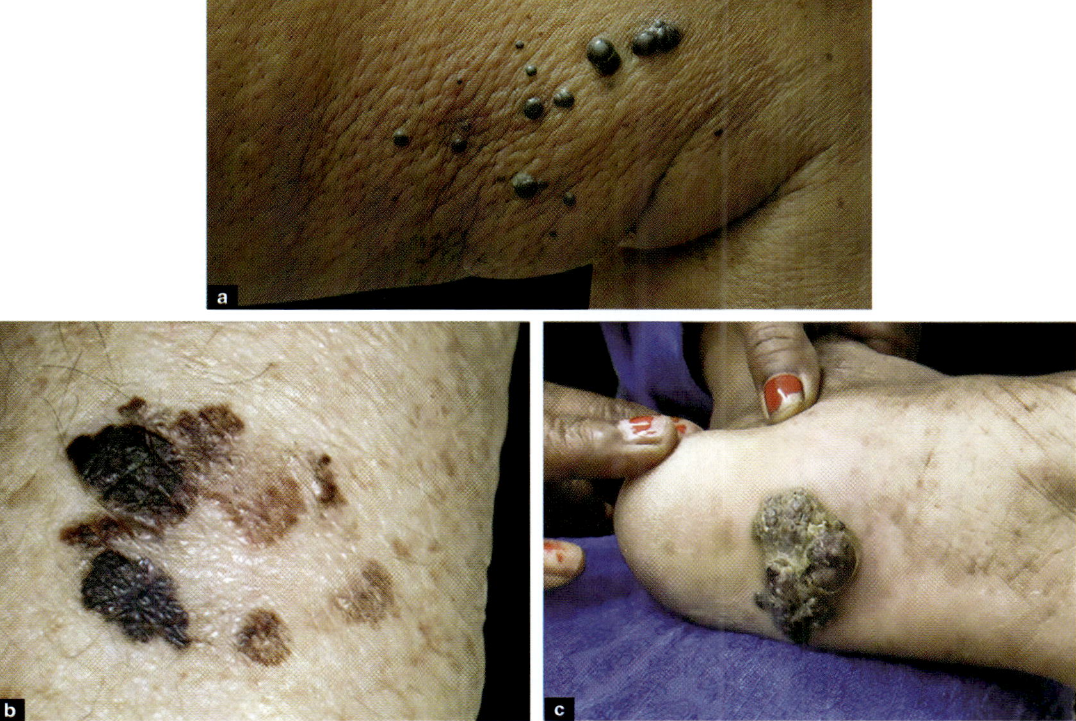

Fig. 34.14: (a) Nodular melanoma; (b) Malignant melanoma—lentigo maligna; (c) Acral melanoma

5. **'Pigmentation in the nail area' (subungual melanoma)**
   - Presents mainly in dark population and only 2–3% in white skinned.
   - The first sign is a brown to black linear discoloration in the nail bed hard resembling benign melanonychia.
   - Changes in color, width of nail band may raises the suspicious.
   - Hutchinson's sign (pigmentation in the adjacent skin) and inflammatory or pigmented paronychia developed later on.
   - Dermoscopy may be helpful.
   - Important differentials are onychomycosis, paronychia, nevus and pyogenic granuloma.
6. **Other clinical variants:**
   - **Pigmented lesions on the vulva or mouth (<5%).**
     - Present as an irregular macular pigmentation, ulceration and bleeding are common.
     - **Poor prognosis as diagnosis is delayed.**
   - **Melanoma arising within congenital nevi.**
7. **Misleading clinical situations: Melanomas are present either in hidden areas or have nonsuspicious clinical appearance**
   i. **Amelanotic melanoma**
      - Mimic inflammatory lesions, angiomas, sarcoma, squamous cell carcinoma, basal cell carcinoma
      - May present on sole as warty or nodular growth.

   ii. **Regressive melanoma**

   iii. **Malignant blue nevus**

   iv. **Sinonasal melanoma**.

Ocular Melanoma

- Second most common melanoma after cutaneous melanoma.
- Arising from melanocytes situated in the conjunctival membrane and uveal tract of the eye.
- Choroidal melanoma is predominant (86.3%), whilst iris and ciliary body melanomas are far less frequent and conjunctival melanoma is very rare.
- Presentation can vary from asymptomatic to visual disturbances or visual loss depending upon the size and location of melanoma.

Strategies for Early Detection

- Early detection
- Screening in high risk population
- Dermatological periodic monitoring
- Education on self-examination or examination
- Public health education

Metastasis

Melanomas can metastasize via lymphatic or haematogenous route. Two-thirds of metastases are confined to regional lymph nodes. Regional metastases can appear as follows.

- Satellite metastases (up to 2 cm from primary tumor)
- In-transit metastases

- Micrometastases
- Clinically or radiologically recognizable regional lymph node metastases.

Investigations

1. *Histopathological Examination*

Most important tool, malignancy criteria depends upon

- Architectural
- Pagetoid spread
- **Cytology:** Nuclear pleomorphism, enlargement and hyperchromatism, prominent nucleoli and mitotic activity are important diagnostic features.
- **Brisk and asymmetrical host-inflammatory response:** Features of regression like, focal disappearance of melanocytes replaced by pigment, dermal fibrosis.
  Verticalization of the blood vessels and lymphocytic inflammation are commonly observed.
- Breslow thickness should also be evaluated (tumor thickness in mm).

2. *Immunohistochemistry*

- S100 protein is expressed by 99% of all melanomas and melanocytic nevi
- HMB45 is most specific, but lacks some sensitivity.

Melan A (MART1) and MITF are more sensitive.

3. *Novel Techniques*

a. **Fluorescence *in situ* hybridization (FISH)**—detects copy number changes as well as chromosomal translocations.
   Sensitive and molecular tool for the diagnosis of non-ambiguous melanocytic lesions.
b. **Comparative genomic hybridization (CGH)**

Prognostic Markers (Box 34.6)

BOX 34.6: Main prognostic factors for primary melanoma

- Thickness (Breslow index)***
- Sentinel node status***
- Ulceration**
- Mitotic rate** (negative value especially in thin tumors)
- Regression* (under estimation of Breslow)
- Age* (negative for older age)
- Sex* (negative for males)
- Location* (negative for head and neck)

(Predictive value from *** high to *low, **between higher and low)

A list of prognostic factors incorporated into diagnostic tools worldwide is given in **Table 34.5**.

Management

Staging Primary Melanoma

- TNM staging categories for cutaneous melanoma **(Tables 34.6** to **34.8)**.

Table 34.5: A list of prognostic factors incorporated into diagnostic tools for melanoma available in different countrires

Test types	Test	Key features	Regions/Countries
Blood tests	LDH	• Tested for initial staging and during follow-up. • Independent predictive factor for poor prognosis. • Part of the staging system for melanoma.	USA, Canada, Europe, Australia and New Zealand
	S100B	• Tested in high-risk melanoma patients during follow-ups. • To facilitate early detection of relapse	Germany, Switzerland
	MIA	• Tested for initial staging and during follow-up. • High serum concentraion correlates with an elevated risk of recurrence	Germany
Molecular test	BRAF, KIT, and NRAS gene mutations	• Next-generation sequencing, single-gene assays, small multigene panels, and immunohistochemistry. • Prediction of risk for recurrence and overall survival.	USA
Molecular test	31-GEP test	• Risk stratification of melanoma • Prediction of metastatic risk	USA
Molecular test	8-GEP test	• Risk stratification of melanoma	Germany
Molecular test	CP-GEP (Merlin Assay)	• Prediction of sentinel lymph node metastasis. • To reduce unnecessary sentinel lymph node biopsy (invasive procedures)	USA, Sweden, Netherlands

GEP, gene expression profiling; LDH, lactate dehydrogenase; MIA, melanoma inhibitory activity; S100B, S100 calcium-binding protein B.

TABLE 34.6: T classification of primary tumor for melanoma

T category	Tumor thickness	Additional prognostic parameters
Tis		Melanoma *in situ*, no tumor invasion
Tx	No information	Tumor thickness cannot be determined[a]
T1	≤1.0 mm	a. <0.8 mm, no ulceration b. <0.8 mm, with ulceration or 0.8e1.0 mm with or without
T2	>1.0–2.0 mm	a. No ulceration b. Ulceration
T3	>2.0–4.0 mm	a. No ulceration b. Ulceration
T4	>4.0 mm	a. No ulceration b. Ulceration

[a]Tumor thickness or information on ulceration not available or unknown primary tumor.

TABLE 34.7: N classification of the regional lymph nodes for melanoma

N category	Number of involved lymph nodes (LN)	Presence of in-transit, satellite, and/or microsatellite metastases
NX	Not assessed (not required for T1 melanoma)	No
N0	0	No
N1	1 LN+ or any in-transit, satellite, and/or microsatellite metastasis	
N1a	1 LN+, clinically occult	No
N1b	1 LN+, clinically detected	No
N1c	0 LN+	Yes
N2	2,3 LN+ or any in-transit, satellite, and/or microsatellite metastasis with 1 LN+	
N2a	2,3 LN+, clinically occult	No
N2b	2,3 LN+, clinically detected	No
N2c	1 LN+, clinically detected or not	Yes
N3	≥4 LN+, or any in-transit, satellite, and/or microsatellite metastasis with 2,3 LN+	
N3a	≥4 LN+, clinically occult	No
N3b	≥4 LN+, of which ≥1 clinically detected	No
N3c	≥2 LN+, clinically detected or not	Yes

LN+ denotes lymph node with melanoma deposit.

TABLE 34.8: M classification of distant metastases for melanoma

M category	Anatomic site of metastasis	LDH level
M0	No evidence of distant metastasis	Not applicable
M1a	Skin, subcutaneous tissue and/or non-regional lymph node	Not recorded or unspecified
M1a(0)	*idem*	Not elevated
M1a(1)	*idem*	Elevated
M1b	Lung, with or without M1a sites of metastasis	Not recorded or unspecified
M1b(0)	*idem*	Not elevated
M1b(1)	*idem*	Elevated
M1c	Distant metastasis to non-CNS sites, with or without M1a or M1b sites of disease	Not recorded or unspecified
M1c(0)	*idem*	Not elevated
M1c(1)	*idem*	Elevated
M1d	Distant metastasis to CNS, with or without M1a, M1b, or M1c sites of disease	Not recorded or unspecified
M1d(0)	*idem*	Not elevated
M1d(1)	*idem*	Elevated

idem (L)—same as above.

Clinicopathological Staging (Table 34.9)

- Primary T1A melanoma with normal physical examination—no further imaging or sentinel lymph node biopsy is required. Sentinel lymph node biopsy is the most important prognostic factor in primary tumor with Breslow >1 mm.
- USG of the local regional lymph nodes is advised in patients with stage IB and higher. Presence of LN metastasis is confirmed by FNAC or USG guided needle biopsy.
- Distant metastasis in stage III and higher, is detected by CT thorax, abdomen, and PET-CT scan. Brain metastasis is better detected on MRI brain.
- No routine blood tests are recommended except for stage IV patients in whom plasma LDH should be assessed.
- In patients with localized melanoma (stage I and II), 5-year and 10-year survival rate estimates ranging from 97% and 93%
- 5-year survival rates are 78%, 59% and 40% for patients with stage IIIA, IIIB and IIIC melanoma, respectively.
- Prognosis depends upon:
  - **Tumor thickness,**
  - **Mitotic rate (histologically defined as mitoses/mm^2) and**
  - **Ulceration.**

TABLE 34.9: AJCC pathological (pTNM) prognostic stage groups

T	N	M	Pathological stage
Tis	N0	M0	0
T1a	N0	M0	IA
T1b	N0	M0	IA
T2a	N0	M0	IB
T2b	N0	M0	IIA
T3a	N0	M0	IIa
T3b	N0	M0	IIB
T4a	N0	M0	IIB
T4b	N0	M0	IIC
T0	N1b, N1c	M0	IIIB
T0	N2b, N2c, N3b, or N3c	M0	IIIC
T1a/b–T2a	N1a or N2a	M0	IIIA
T1a/b–T2a	N1b/c or N2b	M0	IIIB
T2b/T3a	N1a–N2b	M0	IIIB
T1a–T3a	N2c or N3a/b/c	M0	IIIC
T3b/T4a	Any N ≥ N1	M0	IIIC
T4b	N1a–N2c	M0	IIIC

CUTANEOUS LYMPHOMAS

Cutaneous lymphomas are predominantly of the T cell type (Cutaneous T cell lymphomas or CTCL) and only a minority of all primary cutaneous lymphomas are cutaneous B cell lymphomas. 75% of primary cutaneous lymphomas are T-cell derived, two-thirds of which may be classified as mycosis fungoides (MF) or Sézary syndrome (SS). **Mycosis fungoides** (MF) is the most common primary CTCL and has an indolent clinical behavior (88% 5-year survival) while **Sezary syndrome** (SS) is a well-described CTCL believed to have an aggressive clinical behavior (only 11% 5-year survival and a median survival of 32 months from diagnosis). We shall discuss mainly MF and SS in this section. The 2018 revised WHO-EORTC classification of primary cutaneous lymphomas is given in **Table 34.10**.

It is important to note that the site of origin of extranodal lymphomas determines the clinical behavior and prognosis, rather than just the tumor morphology. For example, nodal CD30+ anaplastic large-cell lymphomas usually have a poor prognosis, while primary cutaneous CD30+ anaplastic large-cell lymphomas have a good prognosis.

TABLE 34.10: Primary cutaneous lymphomas included in the 2018 update of the WHO-EORTC classification
With primary cutaneous manifestations
Cutaneous T-cell and NK-cell lymphomas
Mycosis fungoides
MF variants and subtypes
Folliculotrophic MF
Pagetoid reticulosis
Granulomatous slack skin
Sézary syndrome
Adult T-cell leukemia/lymphoma
Primary cutaneous CD30+ lymphoproliferative disorders
Primary cutaneous anaplastic large cell lymphoma
Lymphomatoid papulosis
Subcutaneous panniculitis-like T-cell lymphoma*
Extranodal NK/T-cell lymphoma, nasal type
Primary cutaneous peripheral T-cell lymphoma, unspecified
Primary cutaneous aggressive epidermotropic CD8+ T-cell lymphoma (provisional)
Cutaneous γ/δ T-cell lymphoma (provisional)
Primary cutaneous CD4+ small/medium-sized pleomorphic T-cell lymphoma (provisional)
Cutaneous B-cell lymphomas
Primary cutaneous marginal zone B-cell lymphoma
Primary cutaneous follicle center lymphoma
Primary cutaneous diffuse large B-cell lymphoma, leg type
Primary cutaneous diffuse large B-cell lymphoma, other
Intravascular large B-cell lymphoma
Precursor hematologic neoplasm
CD4+/CD56+ hematodermic neoplasm (blastic NK-cell lymphomat)†

Cells of Origin in MF and SS

Some T cells expressing the cutaneous lymphocyte antigen (HECA 452) have been identified that bind to E-selectin on dermal endothelial cells, thus supporting the concept that there is a subset of T cells with a special affinity for the skin. These T cells comprise the skin associated lymphoid tissue SALT). In MF, there is CCR4 and CCR10 expression, responsible for the epidermotropism, while there is expression of the lymph node chemokine receptor CCR7 in SS, leading to tumor dissemination. MF is derived from skin-resident effector memory T cells, whereas SS is derived from central memory T cells.

MYCOSIS FUNGOIDES

MF is a primary CTCL, characterized by clonal proliferation of skin-resident epidermotropic T cells and accounts for more than half of all cutaneous lymphomas. The staging system for MF/SS is given in **Table 34.11**.

Predisposing Factors

No specific etiological factor has been confirmed in the causation of MF. HTLV-1 virus, occupational exposure, atopic eczema, have all been investigated but no role has been proven. UV radiation has a protective role probably because the incidence of CTCL increases with increasing distance from the equator. TNFi along with thiopurines (but not alone) have been associated with increased risk of CTCL.

Histopathology

HPE Varies According to the Clinical Stage

- **Earliest change (Patch Stage)**–moderate lymphocytic infiltrate in the papillary dermis-small lymphoid cells that may be hyperchromatic and show tendency to "line up" at the DEJ **(Fig. 34.15)**. Spongiosis typically absent. Since MF lesions are chronic, papillary dermal fibrosis must be present and is often composed of thin, wiry collagen fibers. MF tends to have frequent intraepidermal lymphocytes and relatively scant spongiosis **(disproportionate exocytosis)**, while the opposite proportion of lymphocytes versus spongiosis is seen in spongiotic/eczematous dermatitis.
- **Thicker plaque stage**–prominent epidermotropism develops–selective colonization of epidermis by atypical T cells–either as single cell colonization along basal layer or as clusters in the epidermis (Pautrier microabscesses) **(Fig. 34.16)**. Malignant T cells–strikingly cerebriform (Cell of Lutzner) large cells (larger than surrounding keratinocytes) **(Fig. 34.17)** with a very irregular nuclear outline and heavily stained nucleus and a halo appearance of the cells. Since MF lesions are chronic, dermal fibrosis must be present. There may be some extension of the infiltrate into the reticular dermis.
- **Advanced stages (Tumor stage)**–epidermotropic infiltrate may be lost. Scattered larger tumor cells with marked cellular atypia. Large cell transformation [defined as presence of more than 25–50% large cells (which may be CD30 +ve or-ve) within the dermal infiltrate or the development of microscopic dermal nodules consisting of larger cells with pleomorphic and occasionally anaplastic morphology] is a poor prognostic indicator-increased risk of disease progression **(Fig. 34.18)**.
- Large cell transformation should be differentiated from the primary cutaneous CD30+ disorders which have excellent prognosis. Development of large tumors in a patient with

TABLE 34.11: ISCL/EORTC staging classification for MF/SS

TNMB stages	
Skin	
T_1	Limited patches, papules, and/or plaques covering <10% of the skin surface. May further stratify into T_{1a} (patch only) *vs* T_{1b} (plaque ± patch).
T_2	Patches, papules or plaques covering ≥10% of the skin surface. May further stratify into T_{2a} (patch only) *vs* T_{2b} (plaque = patch).
T_3	One or more tumors (≥1 cm diameter)
T_4	Confluence of erythema covering ≥80% body surface area.
Node	
N_0	No clinically abnormal peripheral lymph nodes; biopsy not required
N_1	Clinically abnormal peripheral lymph nodes; histopathology Dutch grade 1 or NCI LN_{0-2}
N_{1a}	Clone negative
N_{1b}	Clone positive
N_2	Clinically abnormal peripheral lymph nodes; histopathology Dutch grade 2 or NCI LN_3
N_{2a}	Clone negative
N_{2b}	Clone positive
N_3	Clinically abnormal peripheral lymph nodes; histopathology Dutch grades 3–4 or NCI LN_4; clone positive or negative
N_x	Clinically abnormal peripheral lymph nodes; no histologic confirmation
Visceral	
M_0	No visceral organ involvement
M_1	Visceral involvement (must have pathology confirmation and organ involved should be specified
Blood	
B_0	Absence of significant blood involvement: ≤5% of peripheral blood lymphocytes are atypical (Sézary) cells
B_{0a}	Clone negative
B_{0b}	Clone positive
B_1	Low blood tumore burden: >5% of peripheral blood lymphocytes are atypical (Sézary) cells but does not meet the criteria of B_2
B_{1a}	Clone negative
B_{1b}	Clone positive
B_2	High blood tumore burden: ≥1000/μL Sézary cells with positive clone

typical patches and plaques of MF would suggest large cell transformation if HPE criteria are fulfilled. In contrast, very large numbers (>75%) of CD30+ large cells in one or a few isolated tumors developing in a patient with no evidence of MF suggests a primary cutaneous CD30+ lymphoproliferative disorder.

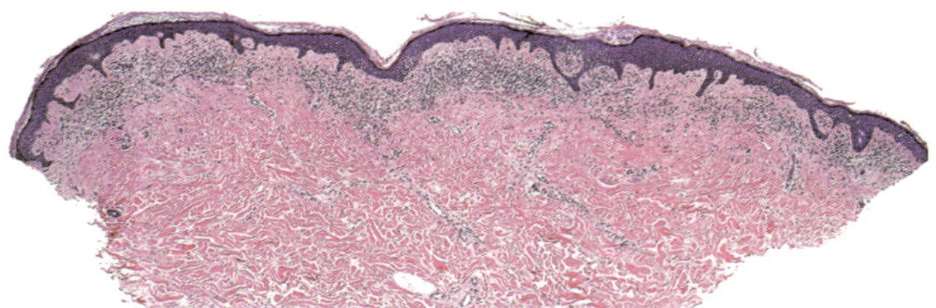

Fig. 34.15: Histopathologic features of early mycosis fungoides. Band-like lymphocytic infiltrate with focal, scant spongiosis

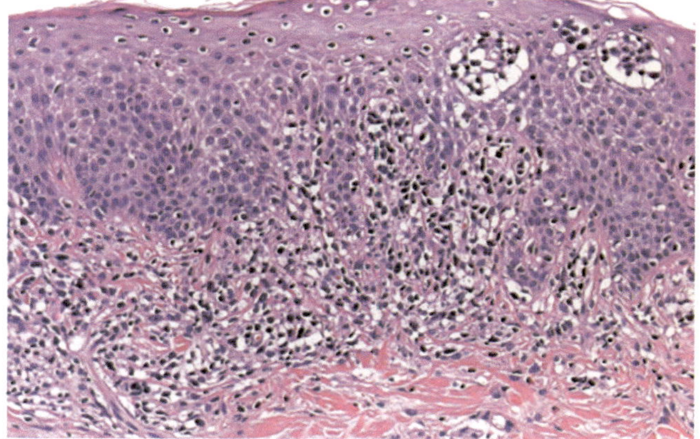

Fig. 34.16: Epidermotropism with Darier's nests (Pautrier's microabscesses) with interspersed eosinophils

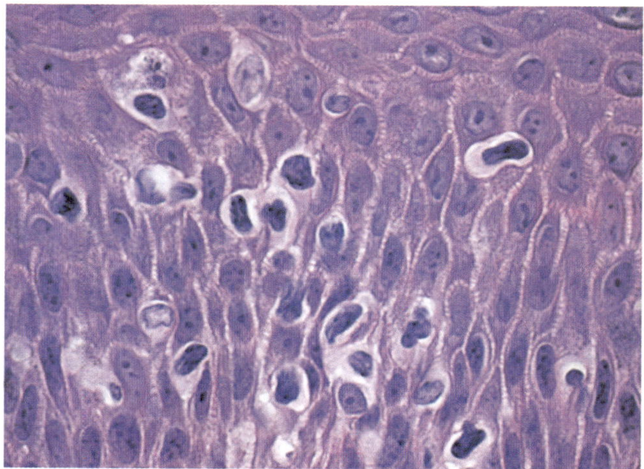

Fig. 34.17: Mycosis fungoides. Intraepidermal lymphocytes with predominance of medium-sized pleomorphic ("cerebriform") lymphocytes

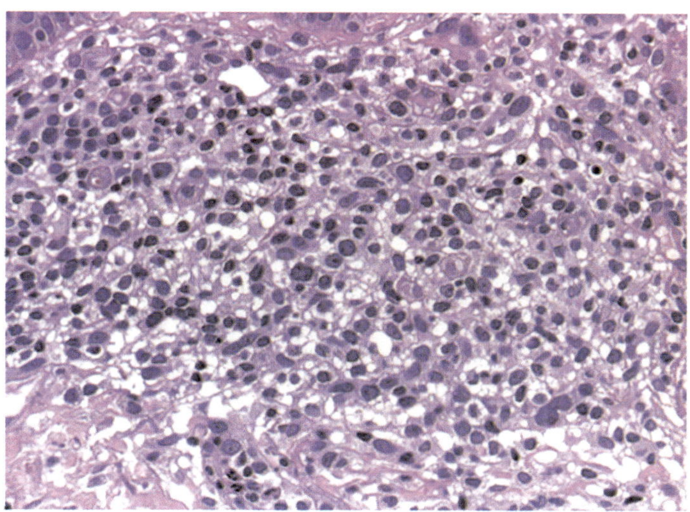

Fig. 34.18: Many mid-sized and large pleomorphic lymphocytes. Large cell transformation is diagnosed when there are at least 25% of large atypical cells

Immunopathology

- **Tumor phenotype:** CD4+ CD45RO+ CD7-(CD8+ more likely in childhood and hypopigmented MF)
- **Skin homing:** CLA+, CCR4+, CCR10+
- Tregs CTLA4+ CD25 FoxP3–protective probably–good prognostic factor.

Table 34.12 lists the ISCL diagnostic criteria for early diagnosis of MF. **Box 34.7** list histopathologic clues for an early diagnosis while for increasing the yield in skin biopsies.

TABLE 34.12: International Society for Cutaneous Lymphomas (ISCL)diagnostic criteria for early MF (>=4 points required for diagnosis of MF)

Criteria	Major (2 points each)	Minor (1 point each)
Clinical • Persistent and/or progressive patches and plaques PLUS 1. Non-sun-exposed/sanctuary location 2. Size/ shape variation 3. Poikiloderma	Any 2	Any 1
Histopathological • Superficial lymphoid infiltrate PLUS 1. Epidermotropism 2. Atypia	Both	Either
Molecular/Biological • Clonal TCR rearrangement		Present
Immunopathological 1. CD2, 3, 5 <50% 2. CD7 < 10% 3. Epidermal discordance		Any 1

BOX 34.7: Histopathologic and immunopathologic checklist for diagnosis of MF (Hodak E, 2023)

Histopathologic features suggestive of early MF	Pitfalls
Epidermis	
Pautrier micro-abscesses	Spongiotic Langerhans' cell vesicles
Lymphocytic epidermotropism generally without spongiosis	Spongiosis
Epidermal lymphocytes larger than dermal lymphocytes	
Tagging (lining up) of lymphocytes at the dermoepidermal junction	Interface or lichenoid dermatitis
High nuclear variability, hyperchromatic and/or folded nuclei, pericellular halo	Nuclear irregularities seen with interface/ lichenoid dermatitis
Dermis	
Superficial dermal band-like lymphoid infiltrate	Lichenoid dermatitis, PPD
Fibrosis of papillary dermis (sign of chronicity)	Chronic/lichenified dermatitis
Variant folliculotropic MF: perifollicular lymphocytic infiltrate with folliculotropism with/without follicular mucinosis	Perifollicular infiltrates may be sparse
Immunopathologic features suggestive of early MF	
Increased CD4:CD8 ratio ($CD4^-$, $CD8^+$ or $CD4^-$ $CD8^-$)	$CD4^-$ $CD8^-$ can also be observed after skin-directed (e.g. topical steroid) therapy
Loss of T-cell-marker expression on CD4+ lymphocytes	BID (drug- and contact-related) associated with loss of pan T-cell markers, particularly CD7

Clinical Features

- Polymorphic patches and plaques on limb/girdle sites-especially buttock and breast ("bathing suit" distribution) **(Fig. 34.19)**.
- Only 1/3rd patients progress to extensive plaque/tumor/erythroderma
  - Patches-subtle fine scaly slightly atrophic erythematous patches on limb/girdles, mild pruritus +/–, usually asymptomatic **(Fig. 34.20a)**.
  - Plaques-more visible, persistent, polymorphic erythematous plaques on limb/girdles **(Fig. 34.20b and c)**. May regress to form arcuate plaques, may have psoriasiform scaling, may become eroded or ulcerated. Overall thickness has prognostic relevance.
  - Tumors-nodules form **(Fig. 34.20d)** (tumor d'emblee form of MF is now believed to be due to other CTCL variants).
  - Erythrodermic-needs to be differentiated from SS and other dermatitic causes of erythroderma.
- Histological involvement of lymph nodes-very poor prognostic marker.
- Most common visceral organs involved-lung, bones, nasopharynx and CNS.

Box 34.8 Lists the clinical clues to the diagnosis of MF.

Clinical Variants

- **Follicular mucinosis/folliculotropic MF/pilotropic MF**–has a poor prognosis and poor response to treatment.

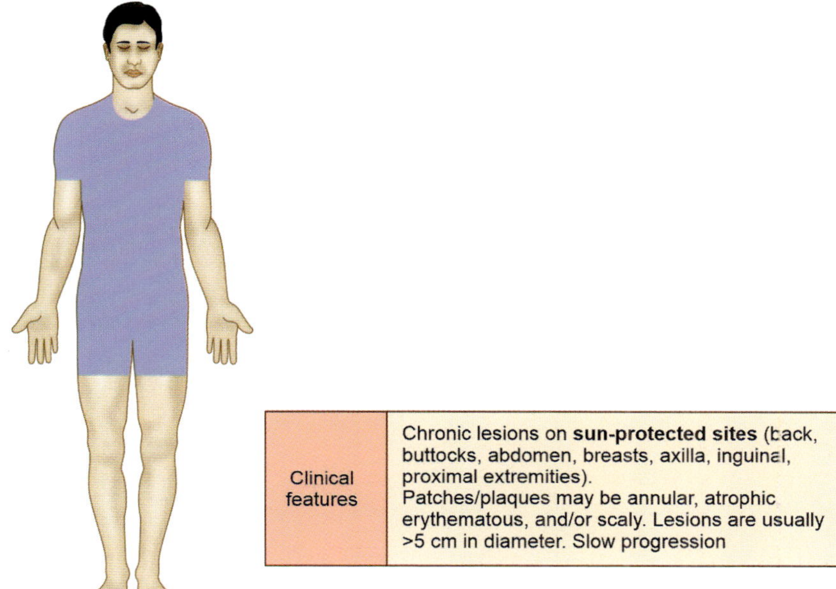

Fig. 34.19: Classical sites affected by MF (sunprotected sites)

- **Pagetoid reticulosis**–rare, younger adults. Isolated persistent scaly plaque usually on an acral site-may be psoriasiform or Bowenoid. Has marked epidermotropism on HPE. Has very slow extension and excellent prognosis.
- **Granulomatous slack skin disease**–rare, middle aged adults. Slow development of pendulous folds of lax erythematous skin with dermal granulomas and elastolysis on HPE. May have HL/NHL associated. Excellent prognosis.
- **Other MF variants**
  - Poikiloderma-atrophy, reticulate hyperpigmentation and telangiectasia on trunk and breast and pelvic girdle.
  - Hypopigmented-younger patients, skin of color, scaly hypopigmented patches especially on the pelvic girdle and trunk. Marked epidermotropism and loss of melanocytes on HPE due to direct cytotoxicity by CD8+ (instead of the more usual CD4+) tumor cells.
  - Capillaritis-like
  - Verrucous/hyperkeratotic
  - Psoriasiform
  - Icthyosiform
  - Bullous.

Differential Diagnosis

- Allergic contact dermatitis
- Atopic eczema
- Pityriasis rosea
- Psoriasis
- Dermatophytoses.

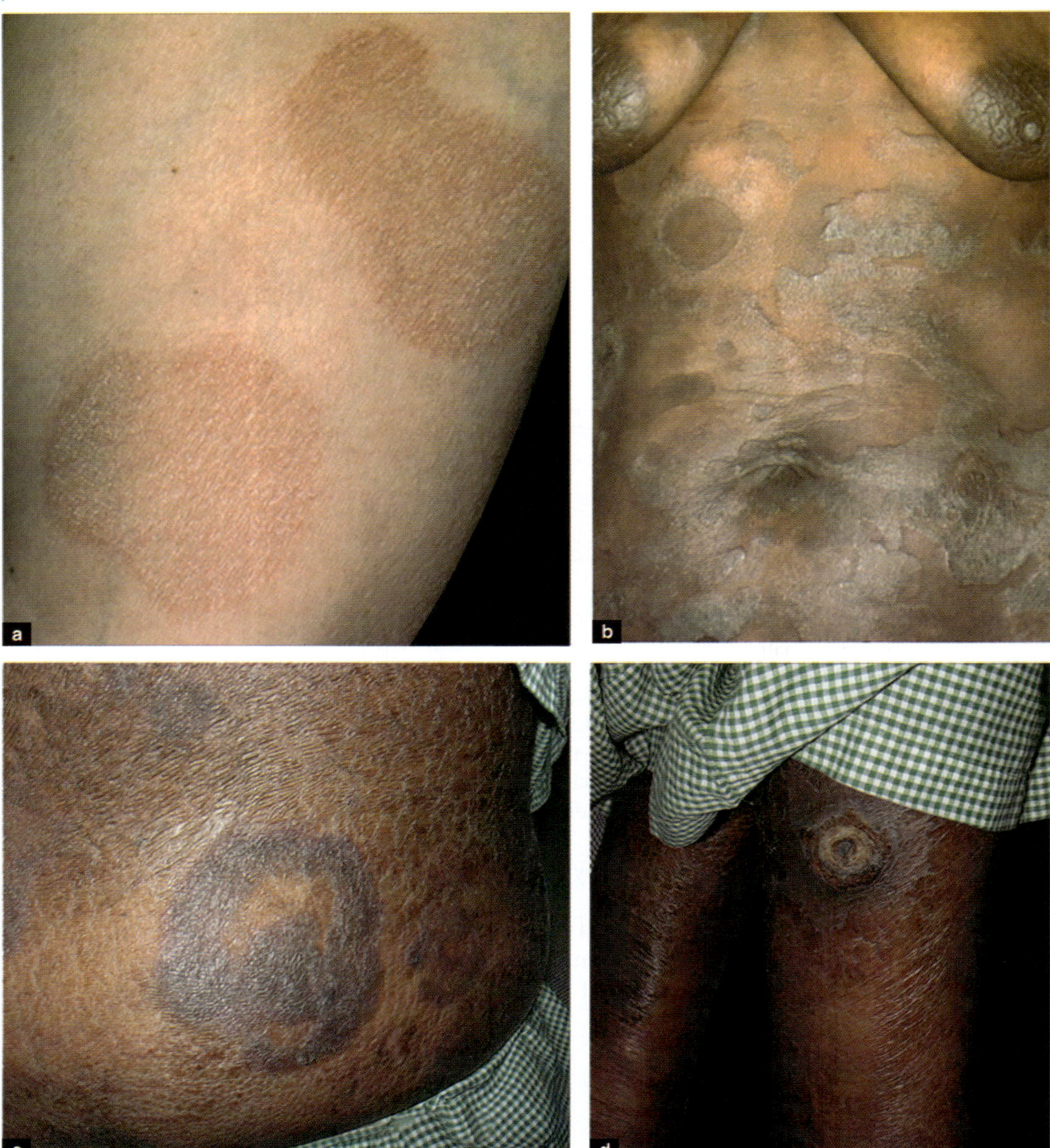

Fig. 34.20: (a) Patch stage of MF (Note the wrinkled appearance); (b and c) Plaque stage of MF; (d) Tumor stage

Investigations

Any patient with persistent polymorphic plaques, particularly on pelvic girdle, should have a skin biopsy. **Box 34.9** gives a few pointers to a appropriate biopsy.

Box 34.10 lists the important investigations for MF/SS.

BOX 34.8: Main clinical clues for early MF or MF variant

- Persistent and/or progressive erythematous patches/plaques, sometimes with skin atrophy, especially in sanctuary areas.
- Persistent and/or progressive hypopigmented or hyperpigmented patches/plaques, sometimes with skin atrophy, especially in sanctuary areas.
- Elongated patches/plaques, especially that follow the cleavage lines, or kidney-shaped lesions located along the sides of the trunk and/or inner aspects of the extremities.
- 'Non-specific dermatitis' on non-sanctuary areas that may be associated with pruritus, especially if progressive.
- Any unusual atopic dermatitis:
  - Presumed 'late-onset atopic dermatitis', especially in the absence of a family/personal history of atopic dermatitis or atopic diathesis during childhood
  - Absence of pruritus
  - Prominent infiltration/induration of lesions on palpation
  - Worsening of an eruption diagnosed as atopic dermatitis during treatment with appropriate therapies: topical agents and systemic treatment.
- Any unusual psoriasis vulgaris:
  - Psoriasiform lesions with erosions/ulceration and/or impetiginization
  - Worsening of an eruption diagnosed as psoriasis during treatment with appropriate therapies: topical agents and systemic treatment
  - 'Psoriatic lesions' with erosions/ulceration and/or impetiginization.
- Any unusual keratoderma palmaris and/or plantaris after excluding the most common causes:
  - Psoriasis, contact dermatitis/atopic dermatitis, and/or tinea
- Any unusual follicular-based rash:
  - Erythematous, hypopigmented and/or hyperpigmented patches/plaques with follicular accentuation
  - Lesions resembling keratosis pilaris but in an unusual distribution and/or in clusters sometimes on faint base.
  - Acneiform eruptions in the absence of any relevant drug or known relevant associated condition; comedones in locations not characteristic of acne or hidradenitis suppurativa; acneiform and concomitant eczematous or psoriasiform lesions in the same areas.
  - Localized hair loss on what seems to be 'dermatitis' or in areas without lesions but only with scales (also look for focal eyebrow loss).
- Any unusual chronic pigmented purpuric dermatosis:
  - Patches/plaques in an extensive distribution (beyond the lower legs, occasionally with the buttocks-the usual locations in most cases)
  - Coexisting with 'nonspecific dermatitis'.

BOX 34.9: Recommendations to increase biopsy yield for early diagnosis of MF (Hodak E, 2023)

1. Topical corticosteroids and other skin-directed therapies should be discontinued ≥2 weeks before biopsy; sunbathing should be avoided.
2. Perform two or more punch biopsies of the most representative lesions. If lesions are variable, multiple biopsies should be taken from several lesions.
3. Punch size: 6 mm diameter is preferable. Deeper-punch biopsies are preferred in cases of clinical suspicion of adnexotropic/folliculotropic involvement. In case hair follicles are not observed, additional deeper sections should be ordered.
4. Of note, if the biopsy is inconclusive, lesions should be monitored for changes or progression. Confirmation of an uncertain diagnosis may require multiple biopsies taken over several years, which can be distressing for patients.

BOX 34.10: Investigations for MF/SS

- Skin biopsies from representative patches/plaques/tumors (multiple may be required)
- Hematology, peripheral smear examination, Sézary cell count, lymphocyte subsets, CD4:CD8 ratio, (flow cytometry)
- LDH, beta 2 microglobulin
- HTLV-1 serology
- TCR gene analysis of skin, peripheral blood lymphocytes and any node
- PET/CT scans for stages IIB-IV
- Lymph node excision for histopathology/LN core biopsies (FNAC is inadequate) for peripheral nodes >1.5 cm in short axis or peripheral palpable nodes or central lymph nodes >1 cm.
- Bone marrow trephine biopsy if unexplained hematological findings.

Staging

Refer to **Table 34.11** depicts the ISCL/EORTC staging system for MF/SS.

Course and Prognosis

TNMB (tumor, node, metastasis, blood) staging remains the most important prognostic factor in MF/SS. Age at onset, male gender, skin stage, nodal (IVA) or visceral (IVB) disease, large cell transformation (LCT), and increased LDH are independent prognostic factors in MF. The disease-specific survival (DSS) rates are 81–89% and 75% at 5 and 10 years, respectively. **Box 34.11** lists independent prognostic factors used in the cutaneous lymphoma prognostic index (CLIPi) for MF/SS.

Patients with MF have a high incidence of second malignancies-NMSC (and a small increase in melanoma) and small cell lung cancer while lymphomas and leukemia are increased in the relatives of patients.

BOX 34.11: Independent prognostic factors for MF/SS

Stage IA-IIA

- Male
- >60 years
- Plaques
- Folliculotropic
- N1/Nx

Late stage IIB- IVB

- Male
- >60 years
- B1/B2
- N2/N3
- Visceral (M1)

Based on the number of factors, the risk categories are low risk (0–1 factors), intermediate risk (2) and high risk (3–5) that are seen to correlate with the 10-year overall survival.

Treatment (Hristov AC, 2023)

1. *Treatment of Limited Stage MF*

As the majority of CTCL patients present with patch/plaque stage MF and have an excellent prognosis, the initial goal of therapy is to improve symptoms and quality of life while avoiding treatment-related toxicity. For many patients, this may involve either expectant management (i.e. "watch and wait") or skin-directed therapies.

Patients with limited-stage disease who require therapy are best approached with skin-directed therapies, usually under the direction of a dermatologist and/or radiation oncologist.

- Topical therapies
  - Topical steroids–clobetasol propionate 0.05%
  - Topical chemotherapy–mechlorethamine 0.02% gel (nitrogen mustard) and carmustine (BCNU)
  - Topical retinoids–bexarotene 1% gel
  - TLR agonists–imiquimod 5%, resiquimod
- Phototherapy
  - Used alone or in combination with topical therapies
  - narrowband UVB (NBUVB, 311 nm)
  - 8-methoxypsoralen plus ultraviolet A (PUVA)
- Radiation
  - MF/SS are radiosensitive, thus radiation therapy, with curative intent, may be considered in patients with localized, unilesional MF.
  - For those with more widespread disease, palliative local radiation or low-dose total skin electron beam therapy (TSEBT) are effective.

2. *Treatment of Advanced Stage MF/SS*

Patients with advanced-stage MF/SS require a multidisciplinary approach, as various combinations of skin-directed therapies, biologic-response modifiers (e.g. bexarotene and interferon-alpha), histone deacetylase inhibitors (e.g. romidepsin), or monoclonal antibodies or antibody-drug conjugates (e.g. mogamulizumab, brentuximab vedotin) and ultimately the sequential use of systemic chemotherapeutic agents are frequently employed. Allogeneic stem cell transplantation may represent a curative option.

SÉZARY SYNDROME

It is a leukemic form of CTCL and consists of a clinical triad of erythroderma, peripheral lymphadenopathy and atypical mononuclear cells (Sézary cells) comprising >20% of total lymphocyte count or a total Sezary cell count of $>1000 \times 10^9/L$ (peripheral blood stage B2). The following three conditions are now required for confirmation of clonality/malignant disease:

- presence of a peripheral blood T-cell clone as indicated by a CD4:CD8 ratio >10,
- aberrant expression of pan T-cell antigens
- TCR gene analysis.

It is important to remember that the total lymphocyte count (TLC) does not have to be raised in SS. Also, even in the presence of a normal TLC, careful examination of the "tail" of a blood smear or of a buffy coat preparation is required.

Most patients are elderly males and develop the disease either *de novo* or rarely as progression from MF.

Histopathology

Many atypical mononuclear cells in dermis with epidermotropism are seen usually. Atypical cerebriform mononuclear cells resembling Sezary cells have been reported in inflammatory conditions including actinic reticuloid, erythrodermic eczema, psoriasis and severe drug reactions, though the percentage would be lower than in SS. T cells with similar morphological features can even be seen in peripheral blood of normal individuals.

Immunopathology

Sezary cells are usually CD3+, CD4+, CD7-AND CD26-. Absolute CD4 and CD4:CD8 ratios are invariably elevated.

Clinical Features

- Generalized erythroderma
- Complications of erythroderma-high output cardiac failure, temperature dysregulation
- Peripheral lymphadenopathy
- Ectropion
- Scalp alopecia
- Palmoplantar keratoderma and fissuring
- Gross subungual hyperkeratosis.

Differential Diagnosis

The most important D/D is erythrodermic MF (T4, N0-3, M0/stage IIIa-IVA1). It can be differentiated on the degree of peripheral blood involvement.

Course and Prognosis

Poor prognosis with 11% 5-year overall survival. Lymph node disease is an independent prognostic factor, and peripheral blood involvement may be important. Age and gender are also key factors. Most patients die of opportunistic infections.

Management

Allogeneic stem cell transplantation may represent a curative option.

Extracorporeal photopheresis, interferon-α, retinoids (alone or in combination), denileukin diftitox, methotrexate, combination treatments. Several other options, including PUVA associated with other modalities, chlorambucil combined with prednisone (Winkelmann scheme), and multi-agent or single-agent chemotherapy. Allogeneic stem cell transplantation may provide a chance for cure.

PREMALIGNANT TUMORS

ACTINIC KERATOSES (AK)

- Hyperkeratotic lesions occurring on chronically light exposed adult skin which are focal areas of abnormal proliferation and differentiation.
- Carry a low risk of progression to invasive squamous cell carcinoma (SC) (5–10%).
- The prevalence is influenced by the amount of ambient UV radiation (UVR).
- More common in elderly and in male sex and in white population (Fitzpatrick skin type I and II).

- Immunosuppressed patients developing AKs earlier in life and with a more rapid malignant transformation,
- Mutations of *tumor protein 53* (TP53) are frequently seen in AK prevents apoptosis of tumorigenic cells

Clinical Features (Fig. 34.21)

- Actinic keratoses are commonly present on light exposed areas such as the face, scalp and dorsa of the hands (80%),
- Asymptomatic, multiple lesions comprise either macules or papules with a rough scaly surface resulting from disorganized keratinization and a variable degree of inflammation, size may vary from 1 mm to 2 cm.

Flat, atrophic or lichenoid variants are seen over face and pigmented AK can be on any sun-exposed area.

Clinical Classification (Olsen et al.)

- Grade 1 (mild)
  - Slight palpability
  - AK better felt than seen
- Grade 2 (moderate)
  - Moderately thick AK
  - Easily seen and felt
- Grade 3 (severe)
  - Very thick or obvious AK.

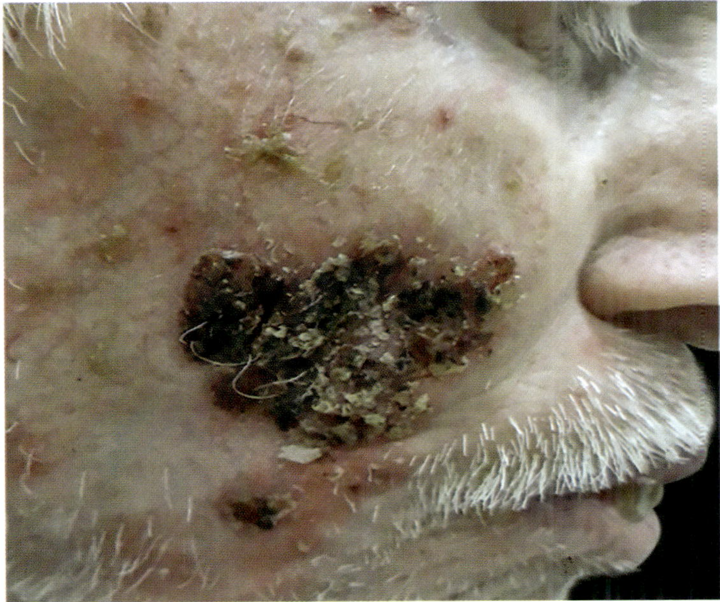

Fig. 34.21: Actinic keratosis with development of BCC in a patient of albinism

Differential Diagnosis (Box 34.12)

BOX 34.12: Differential diagnosis

Seborreic keratoses	Mimic pigmented AK, usually larger, darker, and multiple with raised greasy, warty surface.
Squamous cell carcinoma	Indurating, enlarging lesion, raised shoulder or nodule and tenderness.
Bowen disease	Usually larger, solitary with irregular erythematous base mainly seen in female over lower legs.
Keratoacanthoma	Larger, solitary, and more hyperkeratotic lesion.
BCC	Usually solitary irregular erythematous base, less hyperkeratotic than AK.

Risk of SCC: Increases with the number of thick AKs, previous nonmelanoma skin cancer (NMSC) and immunosuppression, extensive actinic damage and tender enlarging lesion. Patients with AK are at a higher risk of concurrent SCC, BCC, *in situ* and invasive melanoma.

- Average risk of malignant transformation (invasive SCC) is 5–10%.
- Induration, pain, inflammation and ulceration are the signs of transition of AK to SCC.

Histology

- Basal layer atypia (lower one-third epidermis) with budding/finger-like projections into dermis.
- **'Flag sign':** Overlying parakeratosis (pink) alternating with orthohyperkeratosis (blue); atypia and parakeratosis often spares follicles; solar elastosis in dermis.

Dermoscopy

Actinic keratosis are characterized by a 'strawberry pattern' and include an erythematous vessel pseudonetwork, prominent follicular openings and a surrounding white halo.

Disease Course and Prognosis

Regression can occur in 15–63% in solitary lesions, recurrence rate of 15–53%.

Investigation

- Skin biopsy
- Non-invasive techniques such as reflectance confocal microscopy and high definition optical coherence tomography.

Management (Box 34.13)

BOX 34.13: Management of actinic keratosis

- Cryotherapy
- 0.5% 5-FU with salicylic acid
- Ingenol
- 3% diclofenac
- Curettage
- 5% imiquimod
- PDT
- Retinoids

DISSEMINATED SUPERFICIAL ACTINIC POROKERATOSIS (DSAP)

- Most common clinical type of porokeratosis
- Middle age with female preponderance
- Risk factors for developing DSAP include genetic factors, UVR exposure and immuno-suppression.

Clinical Features (Fig. 34.22a to c)

- Usually affects light exposed sites appearing mainly on the distal extremities, with mild pruritus.
- Begins as follicular papules which expand with development of raised sharp keratotic ring.
- The skin within the ring is somewhat atrophic and mildly reddened or hyperpigmented.

The classic description is of oval or gyrate plaques with an atrophic center and a thin, elevated, guttered, keratotic rim that may show peripheral expansion.

It is important that the biopsy is taken across the edge of the peripheral rim to show the typical cornoid lamella.

Pathology

- Cornoid lamella at the margin, is a narrow column of altered or parakeratotic keratin, seated in a slight depression in the epidermis and directed obliquely inwards in some cases there is classically absent or decreased underlying granular zone and vacuolated or dyskeratotic cells in the spinous layer. It may involve the ostia of follicles and sweat ducts **(Fig. 34.22d)**.
- The granular layer may be absent.
- There is a marked inflammatory changes seen in DSAP with a superficial band-like infiltrate with a lichenoid (interface) resemblance but the cornoid lamellae differentiates it form LP like lesions The infiltrate is usually present inside the porokeratotic rim.

Dermoscopic Features (Fig. 34.22e)

- A white border circumscribing the lesion
- Homogenous central white scar like area
- Brownish globules or dots
- Vascular structures: Pinpoint vessels or irregular linear vessels crossing the lesion.

Clinical Variants

- Porokeratosis of Mibelli
- Linear porokeratosis
- Disseminated superficial porokeratosis

  Two types: DSAP1 linked to the 12q24.1 region, and DSAP2 on chromosome 15q25.1–26.
- Porokeratosis palmaris and plantaris diffuse
- Punctuate porokeratosis
- *Porokeratosis ptychotropica*, an unusual variant in which pruritic, red to brown papules and plaques develop in the intergluteal cleft and on the buttocks.

Differential Diagnosis

- Actinic keratoses
- Granuloma annulare
- BCC
- Bowen's disease.

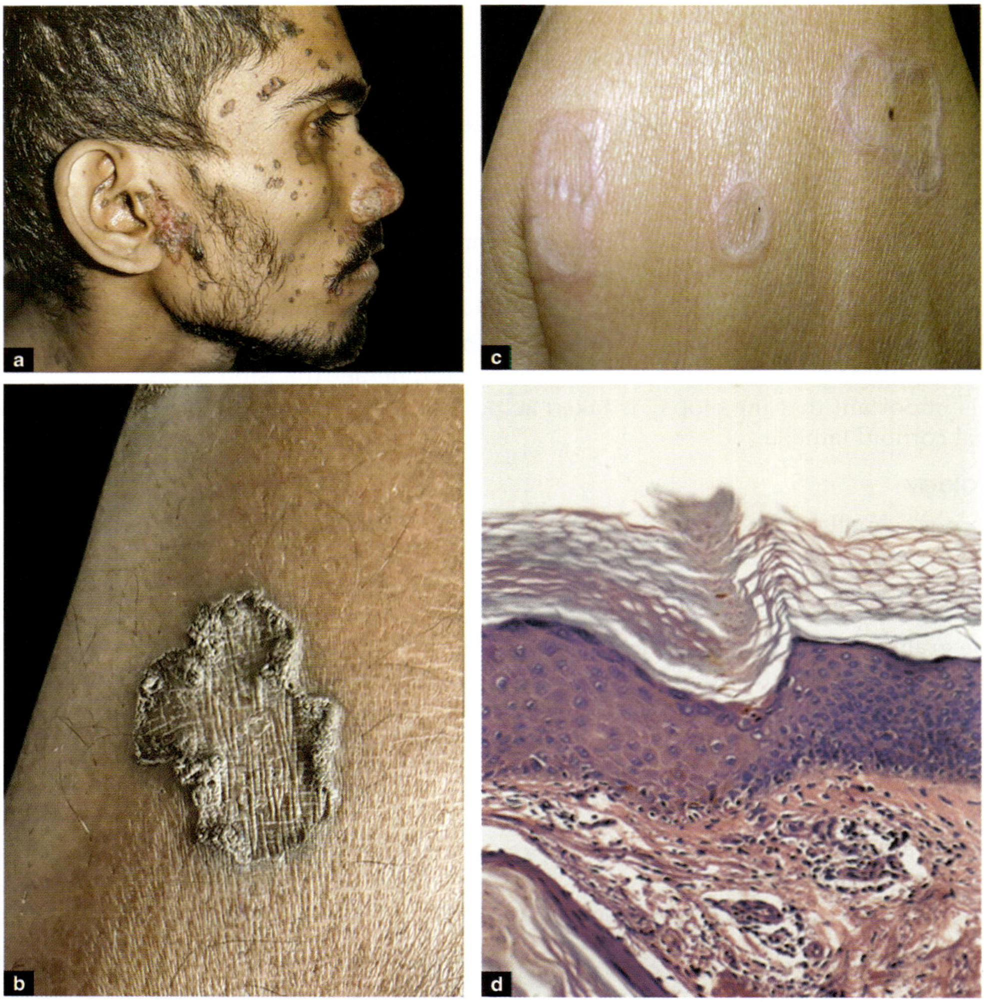

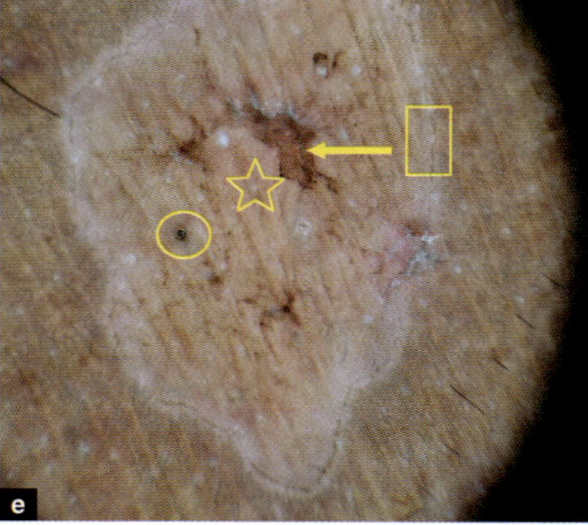

Fig. 34.22: (a) Disseminated superficial actinic porokeratosis; (b) Closer view of Porokeratosis, note the raised peripheral edge with a furrow; (c) Close-up of Porokeratosis showing central atrophy and a thin, elevated, guttered, keratotic rim; (d) Histology is characterized by a parakeratotic column of cells (cornoid lamella) that overlies a past of epiderms wherein the granular layer is absent. (e) Dermoscopy of porokeratosis demonstrates peripheral double track (box), brown structureless area (star) with red areas (arrow) in the centre. Comedo-like openings (circle) are well appreciated (*Courtesy*: Ankad Balachandra)

Disease Course and Prognosis

Tends to increase in numbers with time with low risk of malignancy.

Lesions in older patients, those of long standing duration, and linear variants all have higher rates of malignant degeneration.

DSAP has the lowest risk of malignant change.

Investigation

Skin biopsy.

Management

While the management is depcited in **Box 34.14**, there has been increasing focus on treatment with topical combination of cholesterol and simvastatin. The treatment was based on the fact that this disorder is caused by mevalonate pathway gene variants associated with a buildup of metabolites that impair keratinocyte maturation. Cholesterol is an end product of this pathway and a key component of the extracellular lipid matrix of the stratum corneum.

A recent RCT has confirmed that lovastatin cream is a useful as monotherapy (Santa Lucia G, 2023).

BOX 34.14: Management of Erythroplasia of Queyrat

- Topical sunscreen
- Diclofenac gel
- Imiquimod 5%
- Laser—CO_2, ND:YAG, QSRL
- Cryotherapy
- Vitamin D_3 analogues
- 5-FU

ERYTHROPLASIA OF QUEYRAT

- Carcinoma *in situ*.

Aetiopathogenesis

- Carcinogenic influences in uncircumcized man like, poor hygiene, smegma, trauma, friction, heat, maceration, inflammation, phimosis, dermatoses such as lichen sclerosus and smoking (tar metabolites in urine)
- Associated with co-infection with the rare epidermodysplasia verruciformis-associated HPV-8 and the genital high risk HPV-16.
- Immunosuppression—50% of HIV patients with anogenital warts
- Risk of progression to SCC is 10–30%.

Pathology

- The histology is of an intraepithelial carcinoma, shows prominent epithelial hypoplasia and plasma cells in the dermal infiltrate.

Clinical Features

- Seen in older men. Red shiny patches or plaques of the 'mucosal' penis (glans and prepuce of the uncircumcized) **(Fig. 34.23)**.

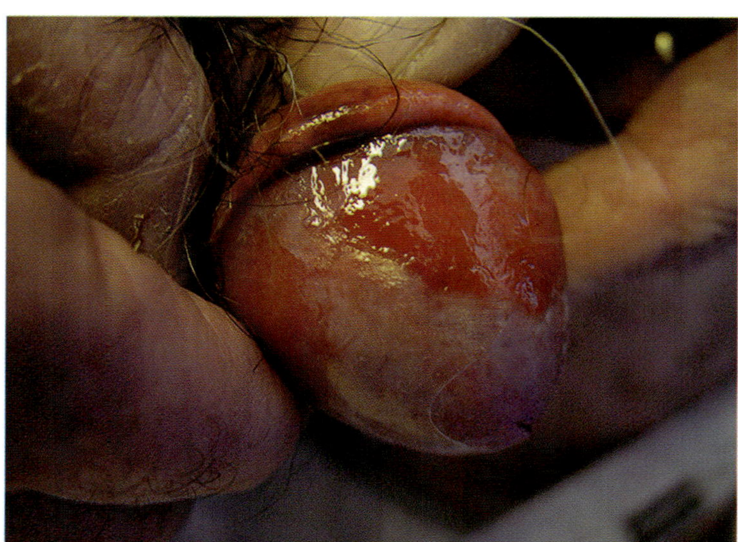

Fig. 34.23: A sharply circumscribed, asymptomatic, bright red shiny plaque seen in erythroplasia. It can resemble closely Zoon's plasmacellular Balanitis and the differene lies in the histology as Zoon's balanitis has characteristic diamond, or "lozenge-shaped," keratinocytes and a lack of significant epithelial atypia. Both may have plasma cell-rich dermal infiltrates.

Differential Diagnosis

- Lichen planus, zoon balanitis and extramammary Paget's disease.

Treatment

- Local excision,
- Cryosurgery,
- Ablative lasers (CO_2-laser),
- Imiquimod, 5-FU, topical cidofovir
- Preventive measures comprise circumcision, proper hygiene, stopping smoking, and avoiding genital UV exposure.

BOWEN'S DISEASE (BD)

Bowen's disease is a form of intraepidermal (*in situ*) SCC.

Etiopathogenesis

- More common in person >60 years
- Commonly seen in females (70–85%)
- Associated disease—other UVR-induced cancer, BCC (30–50%).

Predisposing Factors

- Ingestion of arsenic
- Immunosuppression—solid organ transplant, HIV
- Chronic lymphocytic leukemia,

- HPV—up to 30% of extragenital BD lesions have been found to harbour HPV DNA.
- Radiations—UV, PUVA
- Chronic lupus erythematosus, lupus vulgaris.

Pathology

- Full thickness epidermal dysplasia with loss of epithelial polarity (windblown).
- Keratinocytes show variable pleomorphism, nuclear hyperchromasia and nuclear enlargement.
- Multinucleate cells may be seen and mitotic figures can be frequent.
- The dermal–epidermal junction remains distinct.
- HPV-associated viral cytopathic changes are frequently seen, particularly in lesions from genital skin.
- The dermal inflammatory cell infiltrate may have a band-like distribution mimicking lichenoid dermatoses.

Clinical Variants

Psoriasiform, atrophic, verrucous, papillated, pigmented and irregular, periungual, and subungual BD.

Clinical Features

- Usually solitary plaque, multiple in 10–20% of cases **(Fig. 34.24)**.
- Bowen disease is more common on light-exposed sites such as the lower legs, head and neck can occur on the perianal skin, subungual region, palms and soles.
- Characterized by a persistent, non-elevated, red, scaly or crusted plaque, margin is well demarcated, lesions slightly raised, surface is flat may become hyperkeratotic or crusted
- Ulceration may occur late, sign of invasive carcinoma.

Differential Diagnosis (Box 34.15)

BOX 34.15: Clinical differential diagnosis of Bowen disease

Erythematous Bowen's disease
- Superficial basal cell carcinoma
- Dermatitis, eczema
- Psoriasis
- Seborrheic dermatitis
- Lichen planus
- Benign lichenoid keratosis
- Irritated or inflammed seborrheic keratosis
- Actinic keratosis

Hyperkeratotic Bowen's disease
- Verruca vulgaris
- Seborrheic keratosis
- Discoid lupus erythematosus
- Hypertrophic lichen planus

Pigmented Bowen's disease
- Melanoma
- Bowenoid papulosis

Intertriginous Bowen's disease
- Inverse psoriasis
- Seborrheic dermatitis
- Candidiasis
- Paget's disease
- Hailey–Hailey disease

Subungual or periungual Bowen's disease
- Nail dystrophy
- Onychomycosis
- SCC

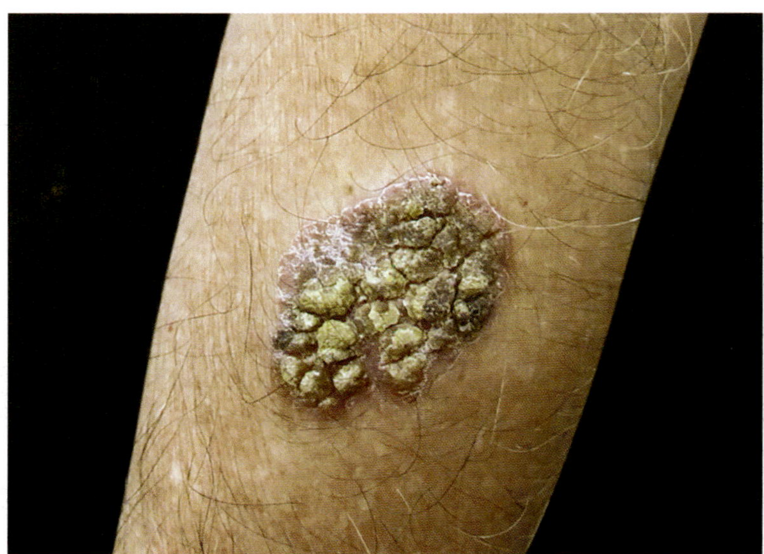

Fig. 34.24: Bowen's disease

Complications and Comorbidities

Risk of malignant transformation: 3–5% (invasive SCC).

Disease Course and Prognosis

- Runs a chronic course
- With development of single or multiple lesions.

Investigations

Skin biopsy.

Management (Sharma A, 2022)

Topical

- Offer topical 5-fluorouracil (5%) monotherapy to people with SCC in situ, for small lesions (e.g. < 2?cm) in low-risk sites, immunosuppressed individuals with multiple recurrent lesions and in those who will not or cannot undergo alternative treatments. OD-BD for 3–4 weeks.
- Consider topical imiquimod (5%) in people with SCC in situ at low-risk sites, when there is no suitable alternative. OD thrice weekly for 4 weeks, up to 12 weeks.

Cryotherapy

- Offer cryotherapy as a first-line treatment option to people with small (< 2?cm) SCC *in situ* lesions.

Curettage with Cautery

- Offer curettage with cautery as a first-line treatment option to people with small SCC *in situ* lesions, especially if a histological diagnosis is desirable.

Surgical Excision

- Offer* standard surgical excision to people with SCC in situ if there is diagnostic uncertainty regarding invasive disease. Depending on the anatomical location and clinical assessment, a 3–5-mm margin may be preferable.

Mohs Micrographic Surgery

- Consider Mohs micrographic surgery in people with SCC in situ when tissue conservation is important, such as around the eyes and the nail unit.

Laser

- Consider laser treatment in people with SCC *in situ* where other treatments have failed or are not suitable. Ablative CO2 laser may be more effective than nonablative neodymium: YAG.

BIBLIOGRAPHY

Books

1. Grob JJ, Marqueste GC, Melanoma. In: Rook's Textbook of Dermatology (ninth edition) UK. Blackwell publishers. Part 4, Chapter141:p143.1–143.35.
2. Gupta G, Madan V, John T. Lear. Squamous Cell Carcinoma. In: Rook's Textbook of Dermatology (ninth edition) UK. Blackwell publishers. Part 4, Chapter 142:p142.1–141.20.
3. Hodak E, Geskin L, Guenova E, et al. Real-Life Barriers to Diagnosis of Early Mycosis Fungoides: An International Expert Panel Discussion. Am J Clin Dermatol. 2023;24(1):5-14. doi:10.1007/s40257-022-00732-w.
4. Hristov AC, Tejasvi T, Wilcox RA. Cutaneous T-cell lymphomas: 2023 update on diagnosis, risk-stratification, and management. Am J Hematol 2023 Jan;98(1):193-209. doi: 10.1002/ajh.26760. Epub 2022 Oct 20.
5. Madan V, John T Lear. Basal Cell Carcinoma. In: Rook's Textbook of Dermatology (ninth edition) UK. Blackwell publishers. Part 4, Chapter141:p141.1–141.21.
6. Part 20, Neoplasia, Chapter 109–112,114, Fitzpatrick's Dermatology 9th edition.
7. Peris K, Fargnoli MC, Garbe C, European Dermatology Forum (EDF), the European Association of Dermato-Oncology (EADO) and the European Organization for Research and Treatment of Cancer (EORTC). Diagnosis and treatment of basal cell carcinoma: European consensus-based interdisciplinary guidelines. Eur J Cancer. 2019 Sep;118:10–34.
8. Rook's textbook of dermatology 9th edition.
9. Sethi T, Montanari F, Foss F, Reddy N. How we treat advanced stage cutaneous T-cell lymphoma-mycosis fungoides and Se?zary syndrome. Br J Haematol 2021;195: 352-364. https://doi.org/10.1111/bjh.17458.
10. Soyer HP, Rigel DS, McMeniman E. Actinic keratosis, Basal cell carcinoma and Squamous cell carcinoma. Bolognia JL, Schaffer JV, Cerroni L (Editors). In: Dermatology (fourth edition). Elsevier, 2018. Section 18, Chapter 108:p1872–1892.

Journals

1. Cohen PR, Erickson CP, Calame A. Painful tumors of the skin: "CALM HOG FLED PEN AND GETS BACK". Clin Cosmet Investig Dermatol. 2019 Feb 13;12:123-132. doi: 10.2147/CCID.S193359.
2. Ding L, Gosh A, Lee DJ, Emri G, Huss WJ, Bogner PN, Paragh G. Prognostic biomarkers of cutaneous melanoma. Photodermatol Photoimmunol Photomed. 2022 Sep;38(5):418–434.
3. Garbe C et. al.; European consensus-based interdisciplinary guideline for melanoma. Part 1: Diagnostics Update 2019, European Journal of Cancer, https://doi.org/10.1016/j.ejca.2019.11.014.
4. Jones CD, et al. Pilomatrixoma: A comprehensive review of the literature. Am J Dermatopathol 2018: 40(9): 631–38.
5. Karimzadeh I, Namazi MR, Karimzadeh A. Trichoepithelioma: A Comprehensive Review. Acta dermatovenerologic a Croatica 2018:26(2):162–65.
6. Santa Lucia G, Safety and Efficacy of Topical Lovastatin Plus Cholesterol Cream vs Topical Lovastatin Cream Alone for the Treatment of Disseminated Superficial Actinic Porokeratosis: A Randomized Clinical Trial. JAMA Dermatol. 2023 Mar 22:e230205.

Chapter

35

Xanthomas and Hyperlipoproteinemia

Kabir Sardana, Surabhi Sinha, Sweta Singh

Hyperlipoproteinemias are clinically characterized by subcutaneous lipid deposits (xanthomas).

OVERVIEW OF LIPOPROTEIN TRANSPORT

- Lipoprotein transport plasma lipids to peripheral cells. **Figure 35.1** depicts the transport and metabolism of triglycerides (TG).

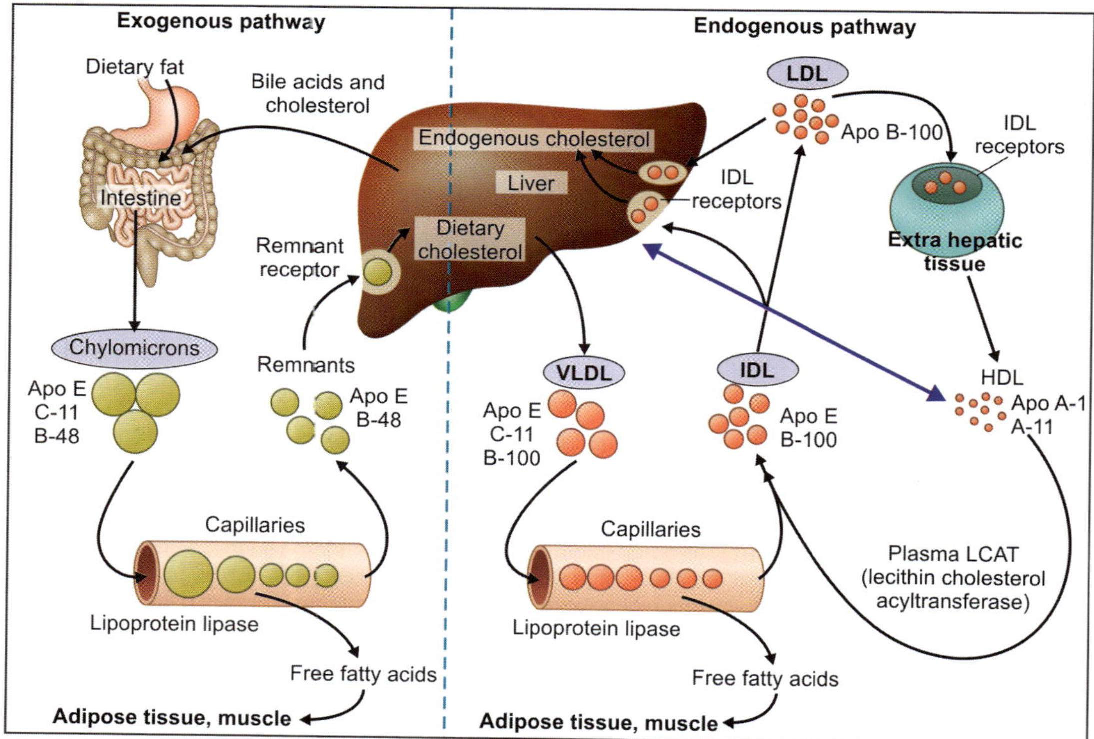

Fig. 35.1: Overview of lipoprotein metabolism and transport

- Types of lipoproteins:
  i. **Chylomicrons:** Mainly *exogenous production*
  Central core of mainly triglycerides; outer shell contains various apoproteins (B-48, E, A-I, A-II, and C-II).
  Becomes *chylomicron remnant* after most of the triglyceride content is hydrolyzed.
  ii. **VLDL:** Mainly *endogenous production* in liver.
  Central core of mainly triglycerides; outer shell contains B-100, E and C-II. C-II needed for lipoprotein lipase activation.
  iii. **IDL:** Remnant of VLDL after hydrolysis of most of the triglycerides by lipoprotein lipase
  iv. **LDL:** Product of further triglyceride hydrolysis of IDL (now mainly cholesterol ester core and B-100 on surface).
  Uptake into *hepatocytes* by apo B-100/E.
  v. **HDL:** *Removes cholesterol* from tissues. Free cholesterol esterified by lecithin: Cholesterol acyltransferase. Requires apoprotein A-I on HDL **(Fig. 35.1)**.

CLINICAL TYPES, PATHOGENESIS AND TREATMENT OF HYPERLIPOPROTEINEMIAS

An overview of the **hyperlipoproteinemias** is listed in **Table 35.1**.

Clinical Features

The clinical features can be localized to the skin or systemic and are listed in **Table 35.1**. As xanthomas are an obvious clinical marker, a detailed overview and the possible disorders are depicted in **Figs 35.2** and **35.3** and listed in **Table 35.2**.

Investigations

I—**plasma chylomicrons, triglycerides markedly** ↑; cholesterol normal; very low-density lipoprotein (VLDL), high-density lipoprotein (HDL), low-density lipoprotein (LDL) normal or decreased; enzyme assay for lipoprotein lipase/apo C-II activity; **creamy top layer** on standing at 4°C for 18 hours.

II—plasma **LDL, cholesterol** markedly ↑; LDL receptor assay; **turbid plasma**.

III—plasma **cholesterol, triglycerides** ↑; presence of beta-VLDL on lipoprotein electrophoresis; apoE phenotyping; **turbid plasma**.

IV—plasma **VLDL, triglycerides** markedly ↑; turbid plasma.

V—plasma **chylomicrons, triglycerides, VLDL** markedly ↑; cholesterol increased; **creamy top layer**.

Treatment

1. Close routine care by primary physician-screen children with family history of early infarcts, hyperlipoproteinemia
2. Nutritional management:
   I, V—restriction of fat intake/medium-chain triglyceride diet
   II—low-fat, low-cholesterol diet with reduction of saturated fats, increase in polyunsaturated and monounsaturated fats
   III—low-calorie/cholesterol/saturated-fat diet
   IV—low-calorie, low-carbohydrate diet
3. Plasmapheresis, liver transplantation (II)
4. Medical therapy: Lipid lowering agents including HMG-CoA reductase inhibitors, nicotinic acid, gemfibrozil, cholestyramine (II, III, IV, V).
5. Treatment of diabetes, hypothyroidism, obesity (III, IV, V).

TABLE 35.1: Fredrickson classification of hyperlipoproteinemias

Type	Pathogenesis	Laboratory findings	Clinical findings	Systemic features	Treatment	Age at presentation, incidence and prognosis
Type I (primary hyperlipoproteinemia, familial hyperchylomicronemia)	• Deficient or abnormal LPL • Apo C-11 deficiency • Deficient glycosyl phosphatidylinositol HDL binding protein	Elevated chylomicrons and TG	Skin: Eruptive xanthoma lipemia retinalis Systemic: Associated with hepatomegaly, pancreatitis, abdominal pain **('horrible, screaming pain')**	No increased risk of coronary artery disease	Diet control only	Childhood onset very rare, may succumb prematurely to pancreatitis; otherwise normal lifespan
Type IIa (familial hypercholesterolemia)	• **LDL receptor defect** • Reduced affinity of LDL for LDL receptor due to dysfunction of apo B-100 (ligand)	Elevated LDL and cholesterol, normal TG	Skin: Tendinous, tuberoeruptive, tuberous, plane (xanthelasma, intertriginous areas, interdigital web spaces) Systemic: Associated with hepatoma, obstructive biliary disease, porphyria, hypothyroidism, anorexia, nephrotic syndrome, Cushing syndrome	Atherosclerosis of peripheral and coronary arteries	Bile acid sequestrants, statins, niacin	Less common, premature myocardial infarction or death secondary to atherosclerotic event in first few decades of life; may improve with early intervention (medication, diet modification, plasmapheresis, transplantation)

(Contd.)

TABLE 35.1: Fredrickson classification of hyperlipoproteinemias *(Contd.)*

Type	Pathogenesis	Laboratory findings	Clinical findings	Systemic features	Treatment	Age at presentation, incidence and prognosis
Type IIb (familial combined hyper-lipidemia)	• Decreased LDL receptor and increased Apo B	Elevated LDL, VLDL, cholesterol, TG	Skin: Tendinous, tuberoeruptive, tuberous, plane (xanthelasma, intertriginous areas, interdigital web spaces) Systemic: Nephrotic syndrome and Cushing syndrome **(see Fig. 35.3)**	Atherosclerosis of peripheral and coronary arteries	Statins, niacin, fibrates	Commonest, premature myocardial infarction or death secondary to atherosclerotic event in first few decades of life; may improve with early intervention (medication, diet modification, plasmapheresis, transplantation)
Type III (familial dysbetalipo-proteinemia, remnant particle disease, broad beta disease)	Hepatic remnant clearance impaired due to apo E abnormality; only apo E2 isoform expressed—poorly binds to apo E receptor	• Elevated chylomicron remnants and IDLs • Elevated TG, cholesterol	Skin: **Plane (palmar creases)**—most characteristic, tuberoeruptive, tuberous, tendinous Systemic: Diabetes, gout, and obesity	Atherosclerosis of peripheral and coronary arteries	Fibrates, niacin, statins	Fourth–fifth decade: Rare, lipid changes very responsive to diet modification/caloric restriction and medication; treatment may decrease cardiovascular events
Type IV (familial hypertri-glyceridemia)	Elevated production of VLDL associated with glucose intolerance and hyperinsulinemia	• Highly elevated VLDL • Elevated TG	Eruptive xanthoma	Frequently associated with type 2 non-insulin dependent diabetes mellitus, obesity, alcoholism	Fibrate, niacin, statins	Early adulthood: Common, lipid changes respond to weight loss, caloric restriction, medication; unknown decrease in cardiovascular events with treatment
Type V (familial combined hyper-triglyceridemia)	Elevated chylomicrons and VLDLs; subset related to apo A-V defect	• Highly elevated VLDL, chylomicrons • Elevated TG, cholesterol	Eruptive xanthoma	Diabetes mellitus	Niacin, fibrates	Adulthood: Less common, may succumb prematurely to pancreatitis; otherwise normal lifespan

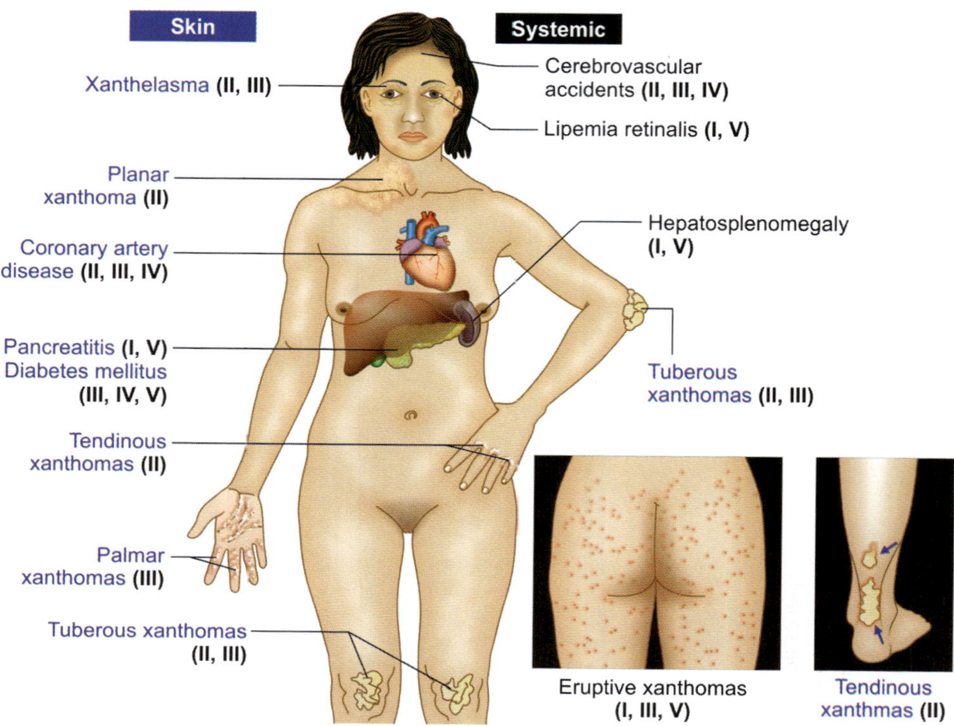

Fig. 35.2: A depiction of the various forms of xanthomas, the salient systemic associations and the associated types of hyperlipoproteinemia

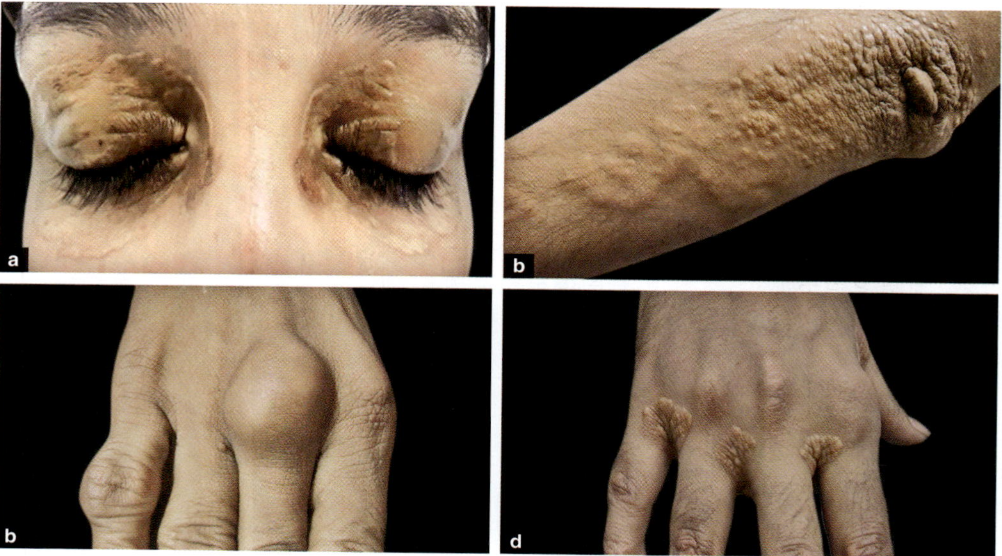

Fig. 35.3: Xanthoma variants—xanthelasma, eruptive xanthomas, tuberous xanthoma and xanthomas on interdigital web spaces

TABLE 35.2: Xanthomas due to hyperlipidemia

Types of xanthomas	Subtypes	Site	Associated disease	Clinical features	Differential diagnosis	Investigations	Management
Tendon xanthomas		Extensor tendons—knuckles, Achilles tendon	• Familial hypercholesterolemia • Secondary hypercholesterolemia	As cholesterol is deep within tendons so skin not yellow, contains collagen + cholesterol, so feels hard	• Rheumatoid nodules • Gouty tophi • Subcutaneous granuloma annulare • Erythema elevatum diutinum	• LDL • LFT	Treatment of hypercholesterolemia
Tuberous xanthomas		Sites of pressure—elbows, knees, sometimes heel and soles	• Type II and III hyperlipoproteinemia • Monoclonal gammopathies	Firm yellow-red nodules	• Rheumatoid nodules • Gouty tophi • Subcutaneous granuloma annulare • Erythema elevatum diutinum	Extended lipid profile—apo E, apo E genotyping, lipid electrophoresis/ultracentrifugation	Treatment of dyslipidemia
Eruptive xanthomas		Extensors—buttocks, back, legs, arms	• Primary: Type I, IV, and V hyperlipidemias • Secondary: Obesity, diabetes, alcohol abuse, medication-induced (oral/retinoids, protease inhibitors, olanzapine and estrogen replacement)	Multiple small yellow 2–5 mm papules on erythematous base, pruritus +/–, 'lipemia retinalis'—yellow discoloration of retinal vessels, lipemic blood/serum samples	• Generalized granuloma annulare • Molluscum contagiosum • Subepidermal calcified nodules • Xanthoma disseminatum • Sarcoidosis	Triglycerides usually >3000 (mg/dL)	Treatment of hypertriglyceridemia

(Contd.)

TABLE 35.2: Xanthomas due to hyperlipidemia *(Contd.)*

Types of xanthomas	Subtypes	Site	Associated disease	Clinical features	Differential diagnosis	Investigations	Management
Dyslipidemic plane xanthomas	**Xanthelasma**	**Around the eyes**	• Types IIa and III hyperlipoproteinemia • Chronic cholestasis (primary biliary cirrhosis)	Upper eyelids, area around medial canthus, soft pale yellow plane plaques	• Sebaceous hyperplasia • Juvenile xanthogranuloma, Syringoma • Nodular basal cell carcinoma	Lipid profile, LFT	Surgical excision, electrocautery, topical TCA, CO_2 lasers, drugs lowering LDL
	Plane xanthomas	Anywhere on the body, 2nd interdigital web space in homozygous familial hypercholesterolemia only	• Type II and III hyperlipoproteinemias • Palmar/finger creases (xanthoma striatum palmare) nearly pathognomonic for dysbetalipoproteinemia • May occur in monoclonal gammopathy (plasma cell dyscrasia usually) with no lipid abnormalitites	Wide-based flat macules	• Necrobiotic xanthogranuloma • Syringeal palmar keratoderma • Digital fibromatosis	Lipid profile, serum electrophoresis, autoimmune screen	Treatment of dyslipidemia
	Palmar xanthomas	Palmar creases, occasionally flexor creases of wrists	Type III hyperlipoproteinemia	Orange—yellow lipid deposition	• Necrobiotic xanthogranuloma, • Syringeal palmar keratoderma • Digital fibromatosis	Lipid profile, LFT, TFT, apo E genotyping, lipid electrophoresis/ ultracentrifugation	Treatment of type III hyperlipoproteinemia

LFT = Liver function test; TFT = Thyroid function test.

BIBLIOGRAPHY

Book

Rook's Textbook of Dermatology, 9th edition.

Journals

1. Cuchel M, et al. Eur Heart J 2014; 35:2146–57.
2. Laftah Z, et al. J Cutan Aesthet Surg 2018;11:1–6.

Chapter

36

Dermatopathology

Kabir Sardana, Geeti Khullar, Surabhi Sinha, Purnima Paliwal

INTRODUCTION

Dermatopathology is a minor yet important component of postgraduate curriculum and examination. A sound knowledge of dermatopathology is a prerequisite to make a correct diagnosis, often by means of clinicopathological correlation. It is, therefore, essential that the postgraduates visualize glass slides under microscope and attempt to make diagnoses to develop a good understanding of the subject.

There is a list of common slides that are usually kept for assessment by the examiners. Each slide should be viewed in steps, starting from the lowest magnification (scanner view) and then going to medium and higher magnifications. The lowest power is to get an idea of where the pathology lies—epidermis and/or dermis and/or subcutis, and also to identify the major reaction patterns. Medium and higher magnifications are helpful to further confirm the initial findings and delineate the composition of inflammatory infiltrate. It is also important to view all the sections in a given slide so as not to miss any findings. Finally, the histopathologic description should include standard terminologies that are used in dermatopathology, accompanied with the likely diagnosis.

We are listing images of common cases asked in MD/DVD/National Board Examinations but many other images are given in the book.

The list of images given in this chapter includes psoriasis, lichen planus, lichen nitidus, DLE, morphea, pemphigus vulgaris, pemphigus foliaceus, bullous pemphigoid, dermatitis herpetiformis, molluscum contagiosum, verruca vulgaris, lupus vulgaris, leprosy, and BCC.

HISTOLOGICAL FEATURES

The histological features relevant to dermatologists and postgraduates can be divided into:

- **Epidermal changes**

- Acantholysis
- Atrophy
- Dyskeratosis
- Follicular plugging
- Hypergranulosis
- Hyperplasia of epidermis
- Hypogranulosis
- Liquefaction degeneration of basal layer
- Necrotic keratinocytes
- Papillomatosis
- Parakeratosis
- Transepidermal elimination
- Vacuolization of keratinocytes

- **Dermal changes**
- **Cells**
- **Patterns**

Epidermal Changes

- **Epidermal atrophy:** Thinning of the entire epidermis to just 2–4 cell layers thick. It mainly affects the spinous layer
- **Acanthosis**

  Acanthosis is a thickened Malpighian (spinous) layer **(Fig. 36.1)**, secondary to—
  a. An increase in number of cells.
  b. Occasionally, to an increase in size of cells or both number and size concurrently.

- Increase in number of spinous cells is seen in **psoriasis.**[Q]
- Increase in size of spinous cells in seen in **lichen planus.**[Q]
- Increase in number and size of spinous cells is seen in some cases of **lichen simplex chronicus.**

[Q], commonly asked questions in postgraduate examinations.

- **Hyperkeratosis:** Thickened stratum corneum. It is of two types:
  a. Orthokeratosis, in which no nuclei are visible in cornified cells, thus this is hyperkeratosis without parakeratosis, it is of two types—basket weave and compact.
  b. Parakeratosis, in which nuclei are retained in cornified cells.

  It results either from acceleration in epidermopoiesis (e.g. in psoriasis) or from faulty maturation of keratocytes (e.g. in Bowen's disease).

  While hyperkeratosis and acanthosis often occur together (papillomatosis), there are some exceptions, like lichen sclerosus. True hyperkeratosis and acanthosis are often accompanied by parakeratosis **(Fig. 36.2)**.

Cornoid Lamella

Cornoid lamella is a localized area of faulty keratinization with a thin column of parakeratotic cells with an absent or decreased underlying granular layer and vacuolated or dyskeratotic cells in the spinous layer. Although cornoid lamellation is a characteristic feature of porokeratosis and its clinical variants, it can be found as an incidental phenomenon in a range of inflammatory, hyperplastic, and neoplastic conditions of the skin.

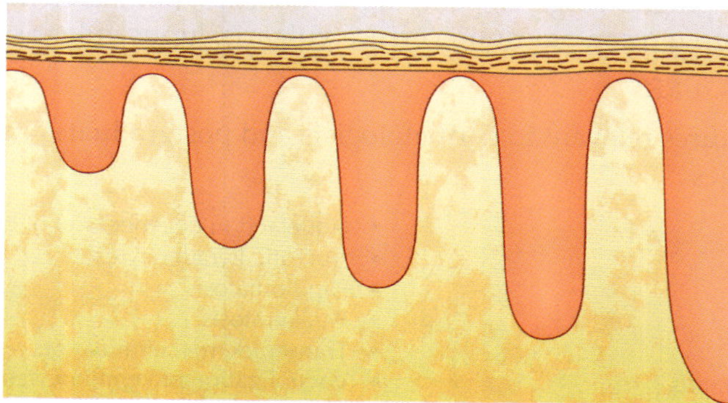

Fig. 36.1: Acanthosis: Thickening of Malphigian layer

Fig. 36.2: Normal epidermis (left) and hyperkeratosis (right)

Abscess

Clinically, a circumscribed collection of pus which histopathologically correlates with a localized collection of neutrophils. There can be collection of other cells on histology.

Examples:

- Abscesses of non-infectious nature are seen histopathologically in eruptive lesions of psoriasis-'pustular' psoriasis-an exaggerated histological response of a neutrophilic collection which is named depending on the site of collection: **Munro's microabscess** (stratum corneum) and **spongiform pustule of Kogoj** (stratum spinulosum).
- Abscesses in eccrine units, designated **neutrophilic eccrine hidradenitis**, are seen in various conditions including insect 'bite' reaction and in response to treatment for cancer by chemotherapeutic agents, such as cytarabine.
- Eosinophilic abscess—pemphigus vegetans.
- Lymphocytic abscess—Pautrier's abscess seen in mycosis fungoides.

Hypergranulosis

The stratum granulosum is thickened (e.g. lichen planus) **(Fig. 36.3)**.

As any hyperkeratosis is accompanied by hypergranulosis, it has limited value in diagnosis.

Hypogranulosis (Fig. 36.3)

A thinned granular zone as a consequence of a decreased number of cells containing keratohyaline granules. As it may occur in any condition where there is parakeratosis (sometimes indicating a faster epidermal turnover time with less time to develop a granular layer), the finding of hypogranulosis has limited diagnostic importance except in ichthyosis vulgaris. It may occur across the entire front of a lesion, such as in ichthyosis vulgaris, or in foci of diseases like psoriasis, inflammatory linear verrucous epidermal nevus, and solar keratosis.

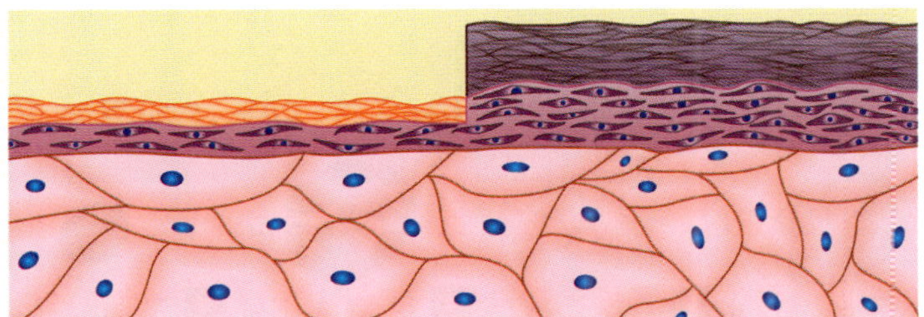

Fig. 36.3: Hypogranulosis (left) and hypergranulosis (right)

Dyskeratosis

Dyskeratotic cells are abnormally or prematurely cornified individual keratinocytes in the epidermis that stain intensely pink with the H&E stain. A small remnant of a basophilic nucleus may be present. Dyskeratotic cells have dark pyknotic nuclei and eosinophilic cytoplasm **(Fig. 36.4c)**, the latter is consequent to the keratin filaments which aggregate in a perinuclear location.

Notably the terms **colloid bodies**, **cytoid bodies**, **hyaline bodies**, **Kamino bodies**, or **Civatte bodies** essentially represent the same process.

- **Colloid bodies** are seen in conditions with basal cell degeneration and represent collagen or basement membrane, fibrin, and immunoglobulin, as well as degenerated keratinocytes.
- **Caterpillar bodies** are seen in PCT (porphyria cutanea tarda) in the roof of the blister and are linear in shape.
- **Corps ronds and grains** are acantholytic dyskeratotic cells seen in Darier disease. Corps ronds have a round nucleus, often with a perinuclear halo, while grains have a more oval, grain-like nucleus.
- The distinction between dyskeratotic, apoptotic, and necrotic keratinocytes is hazy and all appear intensely pink with the H&E stain. They may be impossible to distinguish with routine staining, or they may all represent the same thing.
- Grover's disease, Verrucous stage of incontinentia pigmenti, Neoplastic diseases, such as Bowen's disease and subungual keratoacanthoma, genodermatoses such as Darier disease and cystic conditions such as warty dyskeratoma show dyskeratotic cells on histopathology.

Karyolysis

Karyolysis (ghosts of nuclei), karyorrhexis (fragmentation of nuclei), and pyknosis (shrinkage and darkening of nuclei) are three cardinal signs of necrosis **(Fig. 36.5)**. Karyolysis may be observed in herpes virus infection and pilomatricoma.

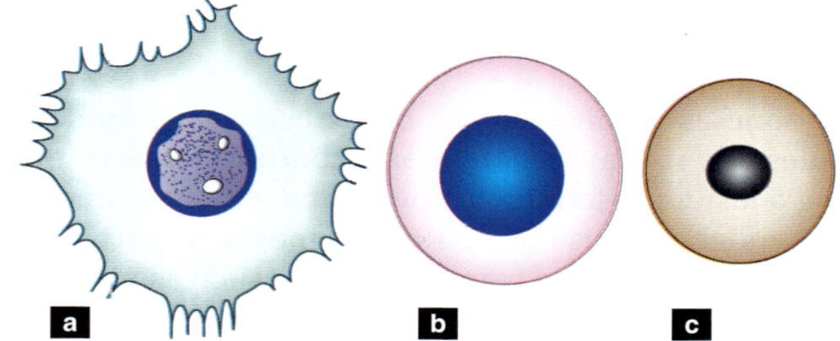

Fig. 36.4: (a) Normal cell; (b) Acantholytic cell; (c) Dyskeratotic cell

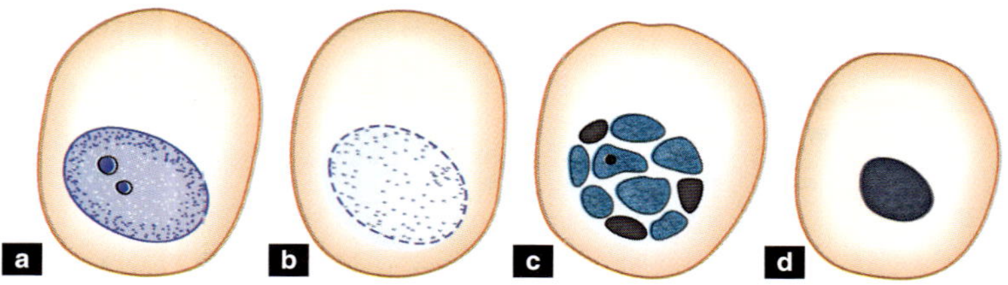

Fig. 36.5: (a) Normal nucleus; (b) Karyolysis; (c) Karyorrhexis; (d) Pyknosis

Acantholysis

Loss of cohesion between keratinocytes causing individual cells to become rounded and resulting in clefts and vesicles **(Figs 36.4b** and **36.6)**. Here the term is derived from the old name of keratinocyte, "acanthocyte", which referred to the "prickle cells" (name derived from the desmosomal spines that connect the cells). Dyscohesive melanocytes in melanoma may also resemble acantholysis, but here the term used is "dyscohesion".

This can be either primary or secondary.

a. *Primary*: Damage occurs to the intercellular adhesion mechanism (pemphigus, Hailey-Hailey disease).
b. *Secondary*: Damage occurs to the cell directly (SCC, herpes infections, warty dyskeratoma, solitary keratosis).

Acantholytic Dyskeratosis

When acantholysis occurs rapidly in an inflammatory disease, such as in pemphigus vulgaris, the cells affected die rapidly, becoming necrotic. When, however, acantholysis develops more slowly in an inflammatory disorder, such as in Hailey–Hailey disease, the cells separated from their neighbours die slowly, permitting time for cornification to occur and the result is acantholytic dyskeratotic cells, which tend to be polygonal rather than round.

Hence here there is acantholysis with:

a. Corps ronds: Rounded basophilic cells, large nuclei, perinuclear halo (epidermal cells maturing toward granular layer in an unusual fashion, instead of "dyskeratosis").
b. Grains: Resemble rice grains, flattened nuclei, eosinophilic cytoplasm (the parakeratotic remnants of the dyskeratotic cells).

It may be a generalized process (Darier disease), a systematized process (a variant of epidermal nevus), transient (Grover's disease), palmar–plantar (a very rare form of keratoderma), solitary (warty dyskeratoma), an incidental finding, or a feature of solar keratosis (acantholytic solar keratosis).

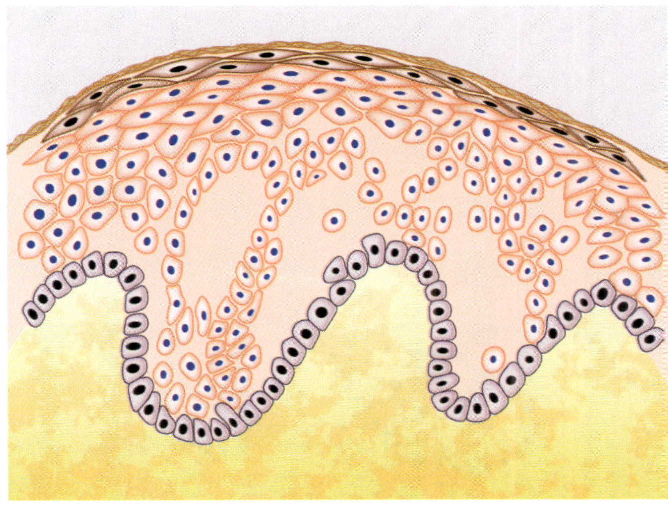

Fig. 36.6: Separation of cells with acantholysis

Ballooning Degeneration (Fig. 36.7)

'Intracellular edema' of epidermis and epithelial structures of adnexa, recognizable morphologically as swollen pale cytoplasm of affected spinous cells. Rupture of the ballooned keratocytes leads to formation of a pattern of epidermis that resembles a net and, therefore, is termed "reticular alteration".

Examples: Herpes, chickenpox, and coxsackie viruses infection; also in non-infectious conditions like erythema multiforme, fixed drug eruption, and Mucha–Habermann disease.

Spongiosis (Fig. 36.8)

Epidermal intercellular edema with exocytosis of inflammatory cells into the epidermis.

Epidermal Proliferation or Epidermal Hyperplasia (Fig. 36.9)

Hyperplasia means an increase in the thickness of a tissue, usually through an increase in the number of cells. It differs from neoplasia by its theoretical capability of a return to a normal condition, whereas neoplasia implies uncontrolled, progressive growth that usually does not regress. A "collarette" of epithelium is defined as epithelium at the edge of a lesion, which tend to bow inwardly and clutch alterations of the dermis. Examples of lesions that often have collarettes include lichen nitidus, verruca vulgaris, Spitz nevus, angiokeratoma circumscriptum, pyogenic granuloma, and lymphangioma circumscriptum.

A proliferation of epithelial cells in skin may be divided into those that are epidermal and those that are adnexal.

i. A proliferation of epidermal keratocytes may be regular **psoriasiform** **(Fig. 36.9a)**, i.e. elongated rete ridges of about equal length, those alternating with dermal papillae of about equal length, as in psoriasis.

   Other disorders–PRP, syphilis, MF, nutritional deficiency disorders.

ii. Irregular psoriasiform **(Fig. 36.9b)**, i.e. elongated rete ridges that are not of uniform length, jagged, i.e. serrations at the base of a thickened epidermis, as in lichen planus, lichen simplex chronicus.

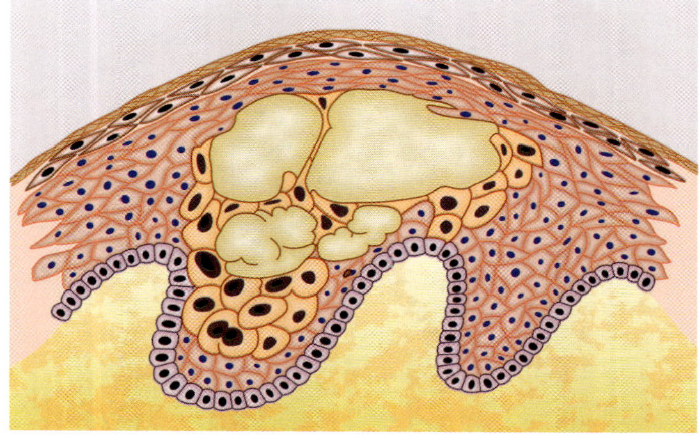

Fig. 36.7: Ballooning degeneration

Fig. 36.8: Spongiosis with separation of cells seen in eczema

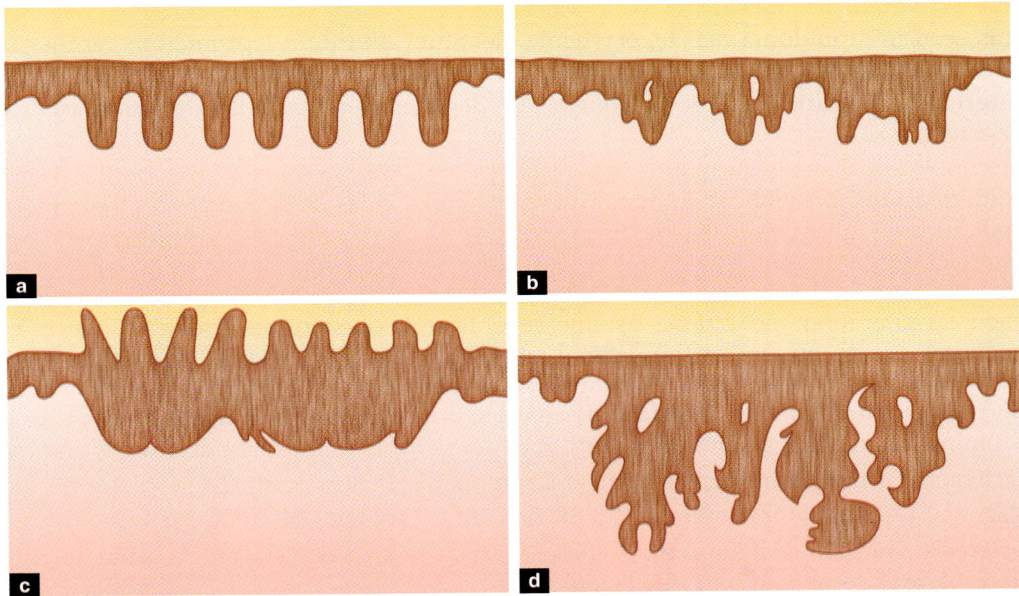

Fig. 36.9: Epidermal hyperplasia: (a) Psoriasiform—regular; (b) Psoriasiform—irregular; (c) Papillomatous; (d) Pseudocarcinomatous

iii. Papillomatosis **(Fig. 36.9c)** refers to the presence of undulations or projections of the epidermal surface. This may vary from tall "steeple-like" projections to quite small, somewhat broader elevations of the epidermal surface. The term church-spiring is sometimes used to refer to this change.

iv. Proliferation of cells of epithelial structures of adnexa, i.e. the upper part of eccrine ducts (and of infundibular epidermis) may be slight or marked, the latter sometimes simulating squamous carcinoma (pseudocarcinomatous) **(Fig. 36.9d)**, as seen in some examples of halogenodermas, infections by deep fungi and atypical mycobacteria, and the verrucous stage of incontinentia pigmenti.

Epidermolytic Hyperkeratosis

Compact hyperkeratosis accompanied by granular and vacuolar degeneration of the cells of the spinous and granular layers.

Seen in diseases or lesions that are

- generalized (bullous ichthyosiform erythroderma)
- systematized (epidermal nevus variant)
- palmar–plantar (a variant of palmoplantar keratoderma)
- solitary (epidermolytic acanthoma)
- follicular (nevoid follicular hyperkeratosis).

Dermal Changes

- **Grenz zone:** Uninvolved and largely cell-free area of dermis beneath the epidermis or adjacent to a hair follicle (term derived from the German word for boundary)

  It is seen in granuloma faciale, erythema elevatum diutinum lepromatous leprosy and pseudolymphoma.
- **Interface dermatitis** (basal layer liquefaction degeneration/vacuolar alteration/hydropic degeneration)

  Interface dermatitis is dermatitis in which there is a degenerative change at the dermal–epidermal junction, with inflammation (mostly lymphocytes) at the junction of the epidermis and dermis. Liquefaction degeneration and vacuolar or hydropic degeneration are types of interface dermatitis and used synonymously and, while the term liquefaction degeneration was the preferred term until Ackerman and his trainees started popularizing the term vacuolar alteration, most books use the latter term because of his strong influence. Tiny vacuolar spaces appear at the dermal-epidermal junction, often leaving the junction indistinct. This may result in formation of a subepidermal blister. The term lichenoid dermatitis overlaps with interface dermatitis, but "lichenoid" is used when there is a prominent band-like inflammatory infiltrate. The 2 types of interface dermatitis are:

  Lichenoid (usually lymphocyte rich)—Lichen planus, lichen striatus.

  Vacuolar (Fewer Lymphocytes)—LE, PLC, PLEVA, GVHD, FDE, EM.
- **Sclerosis:** Thickening of the dermis with increased numbers of collagen fibers but decreased fibroblasts as compared to normal skin.

  Example: Morphea **(Fig. 36.10a)**, scleroderma, lichen sclerosus, sclerodermoid graft-versus-host disease (GVHD)

  Collagen bundles thicker than normal and oriented perpendicular to the epidermis **(Fig. 36.10b)** are seen in conditions where there is constant rubbing or itching and is seen in persistent forceful rubbing of skin, as occurs in lichen simplex chronicus and its variant, prurigo nodularis.
- **Fibrosis:** Increased collagen with relative increase in fibroblasts from normal skin.

  e.g. hypertrophic scar, keloid, scleromyxedema, reactive perforating collagenosis, chondrodermatitis nodularis helicis.
- Granuloma (*see* under "Patterns").

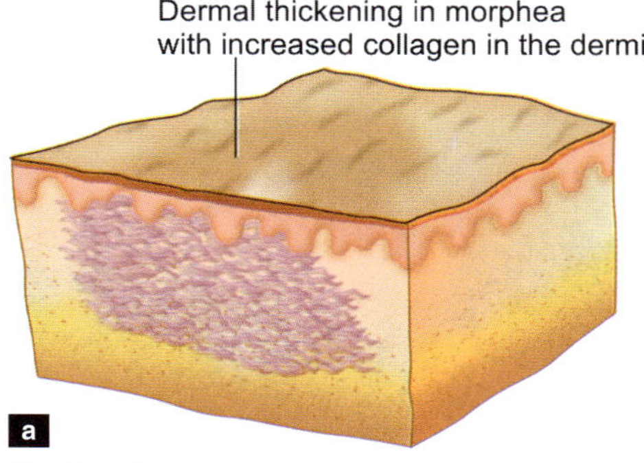

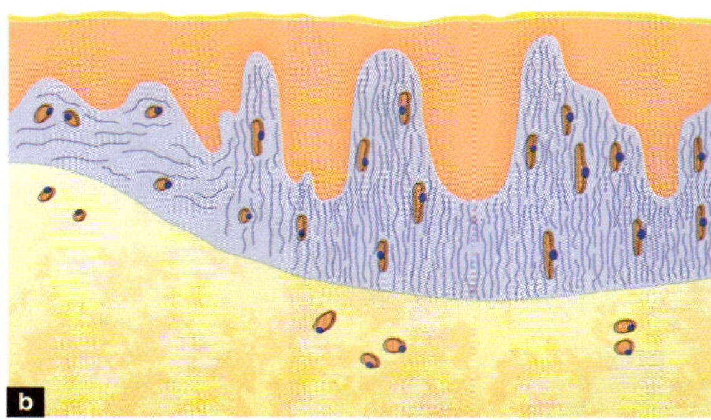

Fig. 36.10: (a) Depiction of dermal thickening causing bound down skin; (b) Vertical bands of collagen in pruritic disorders

INFLAMMATORY PATTERNS

The most common inflammatory dermatopathology patterns observed on low power microscopy are:

1. **Spongiotic (Fig. 36.11)**
   a. Conditions grouped under the term "eczema"-display epidermal spongiosis (edema between keratinocytes), e.g. allergic contact dermatitis.
   b. Can be acute, subacute or chronic spongiotic dermatitis.
2. **Psoriasiform (Fig. 36.12)**
   a. Regular psoriasiform hyperplasia-elongation of epidermal rete ridges in an even pattern. e.g. psoriasism PRP
   b. Irregular psoriasiform hyperplasia-elongation of rete in an uneven pattern, e.g. lichen simplex chronicus (LSC)
3. **Interface dermatitis**
   a. "Interface" means the presence of inflammation at the dermal–epidermal junction.
   b. Usually, the infiltrate is lymphocytic

   The specific diagnosis of a disease within the lichenoid tissue reaction requires an assessment of several other morphological features:

   i. Type of basal damage—vacuolar change is sometimes more prominent than cell death in lupus erythematosus, dermatomyositis, the poikilodermas, and drug reactions.
   ii. Distribution of the accompanying inflammatory cell infiltrate
   iii. Prominent pigment incontinence
   iv. Satellite cell necrosis (lymphocyte-associated apoptosis)-defined as two or more lymphocytes in close proximity to a Civatte body.
4. **Bullous**
   a. Subcorneal-split just below the stratum corneumm, e.g. bullous impetigo, SSSS, pemphigus foliaceus.
   b. Suprabasal-split due to acanthloysis suprabasally, e.g. pemphigus vulgaris, Hailey–Hailey disease.
   c. Subepidermal **(Fig. 36.13)** split is subepidermal, e.g. bullous pemphigoid.

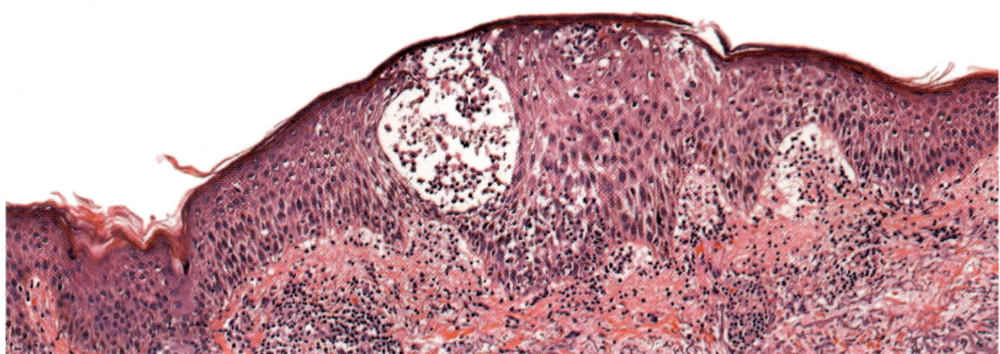

Fig. 36.11: Spongiotic pattern

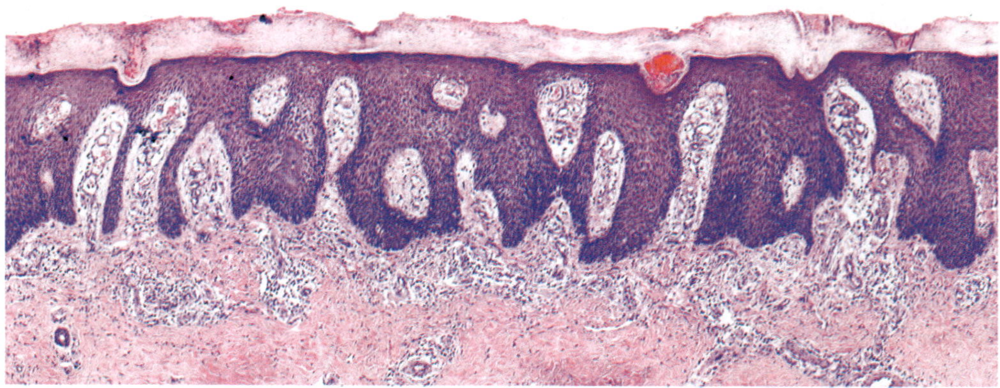

Fig. 36.12: Psoriasiform pattern

5. **Cutaneous vasculitis (Fig. 36.14)**
   a. Inflammation of vessels in the skin
      i. Small vessel
      ii. Medium vessel
      iii. Large vessel
6. **Panniculitis**
   a. Septal, e.g. erythema nodosum **(Fig. 36.15)**
   b. Lobular, e.g. lupus panniculitis **(Fig. 36.16)**
7. **Granulomatous:** A granuloma is an aggregate of monocyte-derived histiocytes, sometimes mixed with other inflammatory cells. Large histiocytes in a granuloma are often called epithelioid cells. These epithelioid cells may fuse to form multinucleated giant cells. It is important to stress that such multinucleated giant cells do not have to be present to meet the criteria for a granuloma.

Fig. 36.13: Subepidermal bulla in bullous pemphigoid

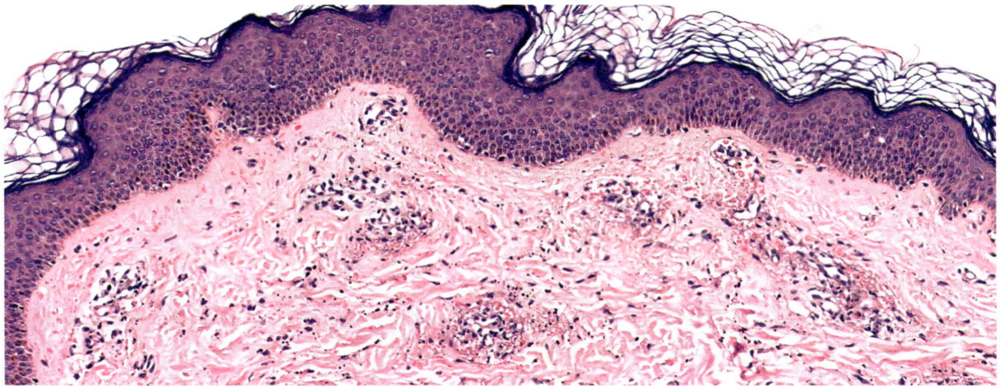

Fig. 36.14: Leukocytoclastic vasculitis

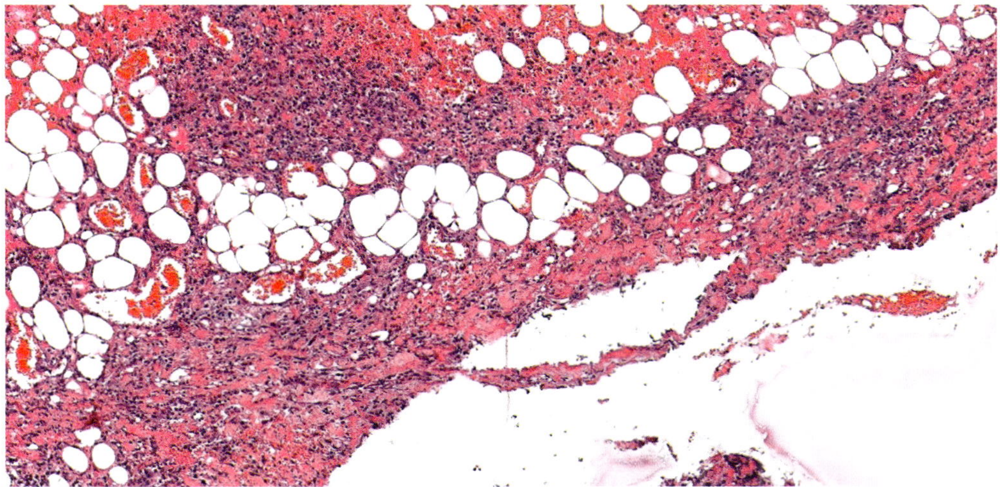

Fig. 36.15: Septal panniculitis

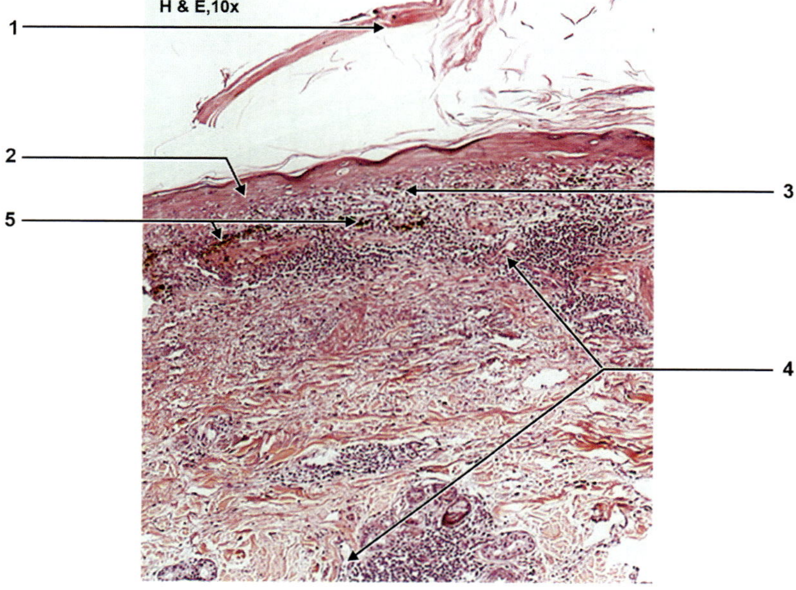

Fig. 36.25

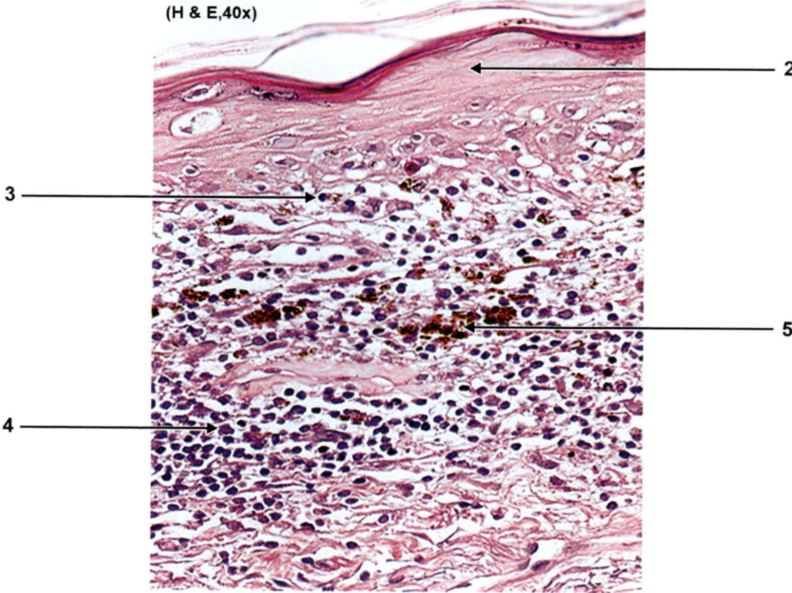

Fig. 36.26

Figs 36.25 and 36.26: Discoid lupus erythematosus (DLE) showing hyperkeratosis (1), thinning of stratum malpighii (2) and vacuolar degeneration of basal cells (3). There is superficial and deep perivascular and periappendageal lymphohistiocytic infiltrate (4) and pigment incontinence (5) in the dermis

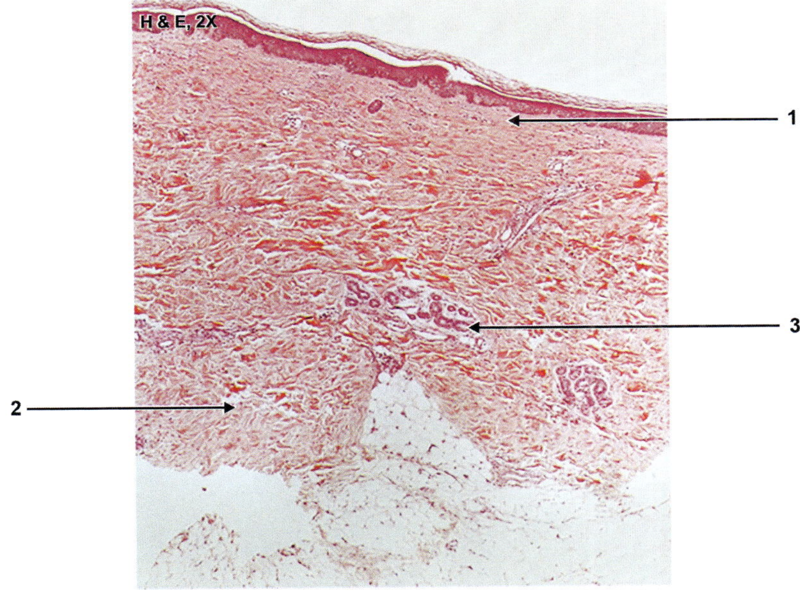

Fig. 36.27

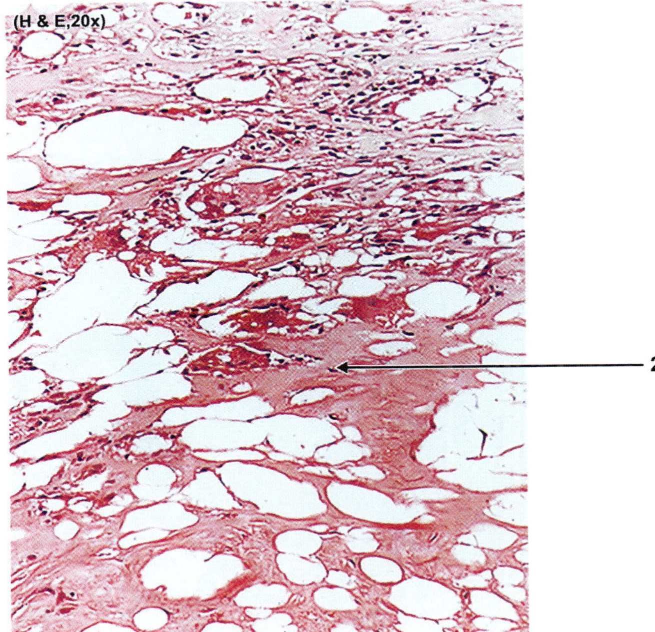

Fig. 36.28

Figs 36.27 and 36.28: Morphea showing atrophic epidermis (1). Collagen bundles in reticular dermis appear thickened, closely packed and hypocellular (2). Eccrine glands are atrophic and appear higher in the dermis (3) as a result of replacement of subcutaneous fat by newly formed collagen

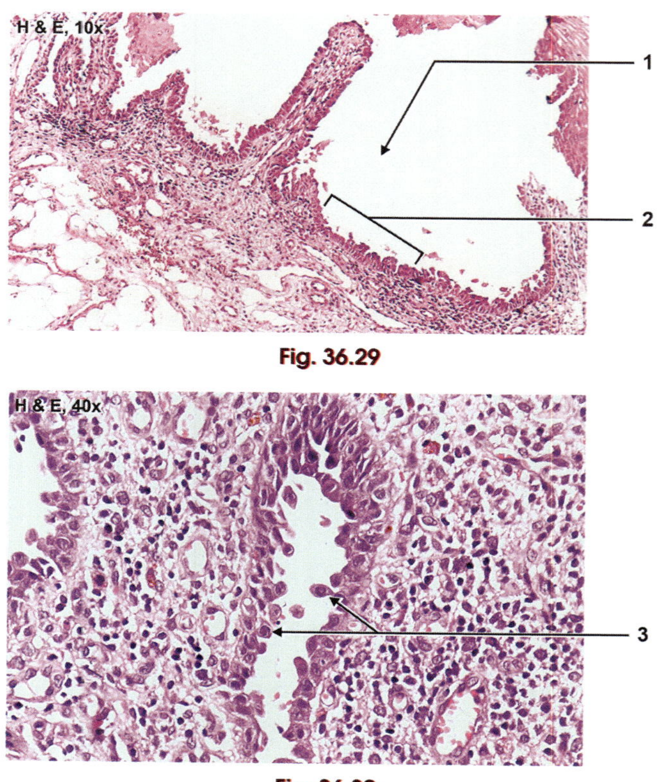

Fig. 36.29

Fig. 36.30

Figs 36.29 and 36.30: Pemphigus vulgaris showing a suprabasal split in the epidermis (1). The basal keratinocytes, although separated from each other, are attached to the basement membrane, giving a "row of tombstone" appearance (2). Within the blister cavity, the acantholytic keratinocytes are round in shape with hypertrophic nuclei, increased nuclear to cytoplasmic ratio, and peripheral condensation of cytoplasm with a perinuclear halo (3)

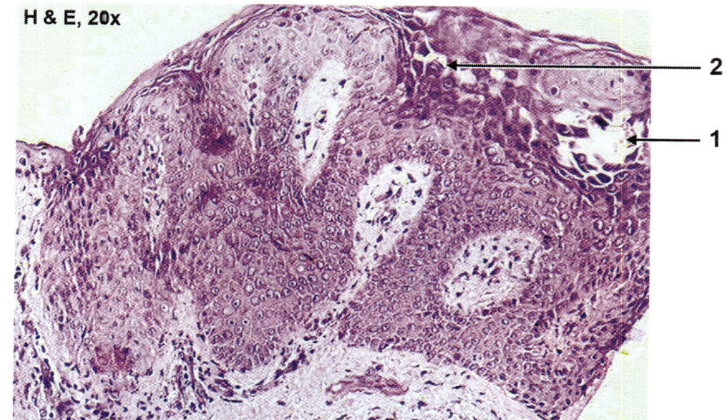

Fig. 36.31: Pemphigus foliaceus showing a subcorneal split in the granular layer (1) containing dyskeratotic keratinocytes and acantholytic cells (2)

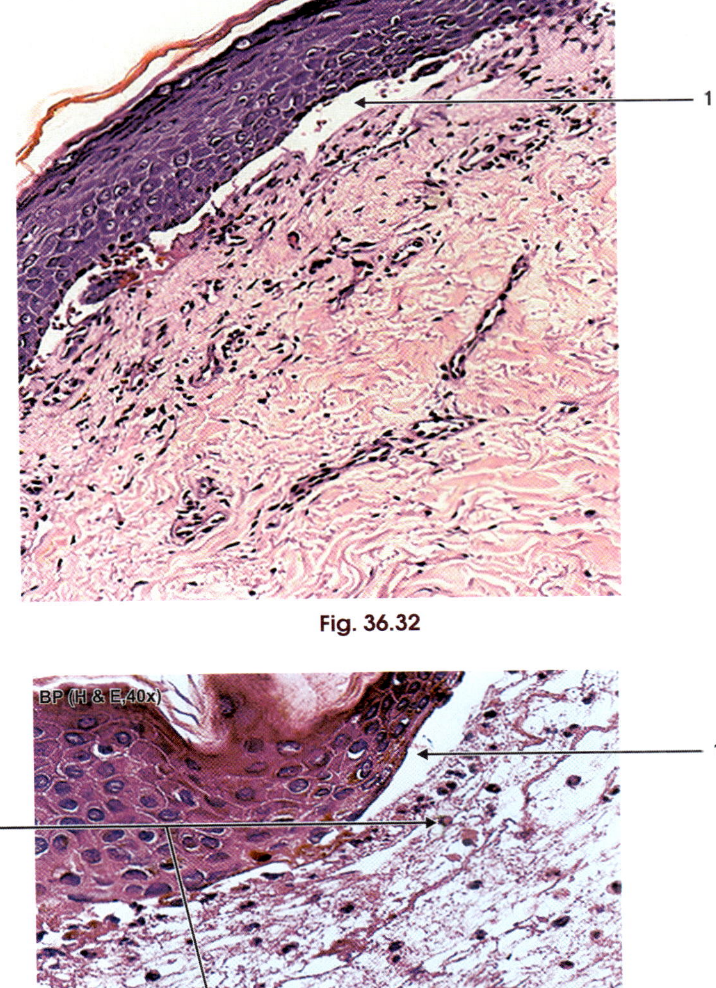

Fig. 36.32

Fig. 36.33

Figs 36.32 and 36.33: Bullous pemphigoid showing an unremarkable epidermis. There is a subepidermal split (1) with blister cavity containing predominantly eosinophils (2) and occasional neutrophils (3)

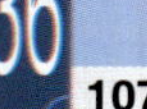

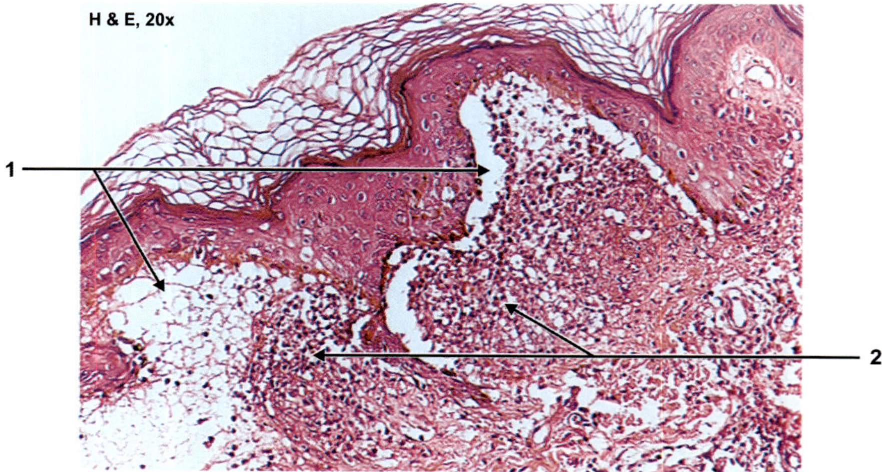

Fig. 36.34: Dermatitis herpetiformis showing an essentially normal epidermis. There is subepidermal multilocular blister (1) with cavity rich in neutrophils and some lymphocytes (2)

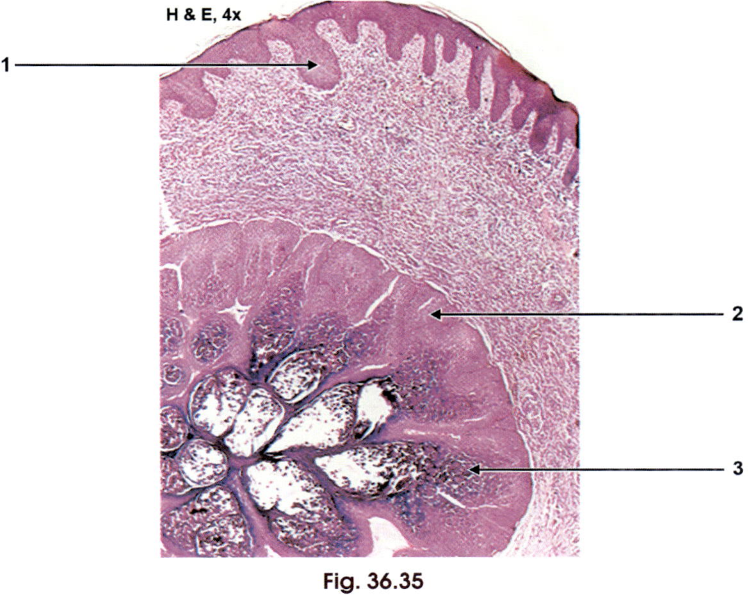

Fig. 36.35

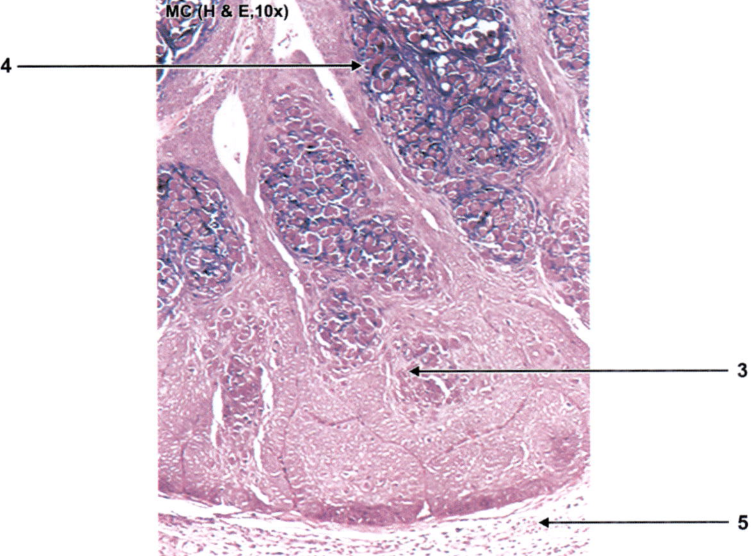

Fig. 36.36

Figs 36.35 and 36.36: Molluscum contagiosum showing an acanthotic epidermis (1). There are lobules of hyperplastic squamous epithelium expanding into the dermis (2), which are separated by fine septae. The keratinocytes contain large intracytoplasmic inclusion bodies called molluscum bodies, which appear as ovoid eosinophilic structures in the lower layers of stratum malpighii above the basal layer (3). These bodies increase in size as infected cells move towards the surface. At the level of granular layer, the molluscum bodies appear basophilic (4). The underlying dermis shows inflammatory reaction (5)

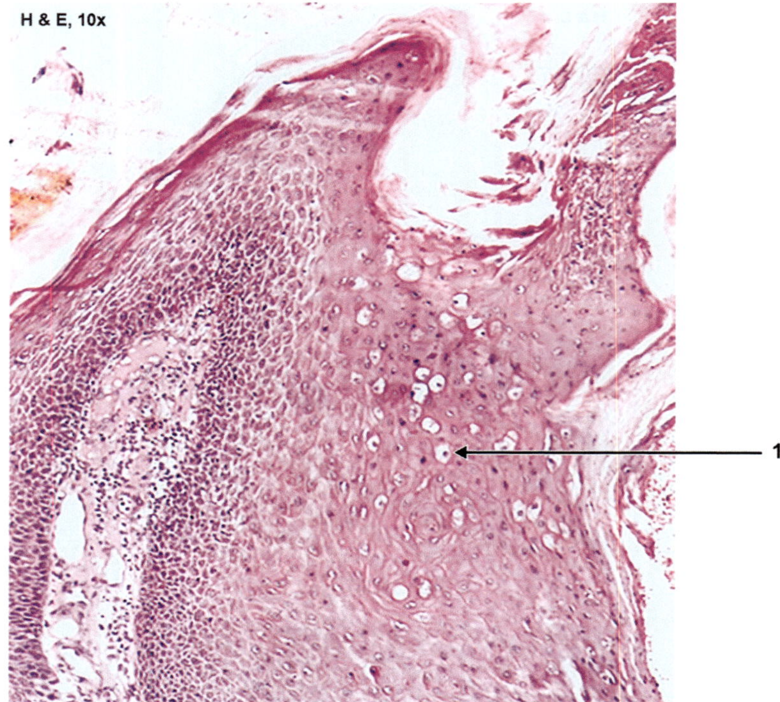

Fig. 36.37: Verruca vulgaris with the epidermis showing hyperkeratosis, acanthosis and papillomatosis. The rete ridges are elongated and bent inward at both the margins and thus appear to point radially toward the centre (arborization). Characteristic features include foci of koilocytic cells (1), vertical tiers of parakeratotic cells, and foci of clumped keratohyaline granules

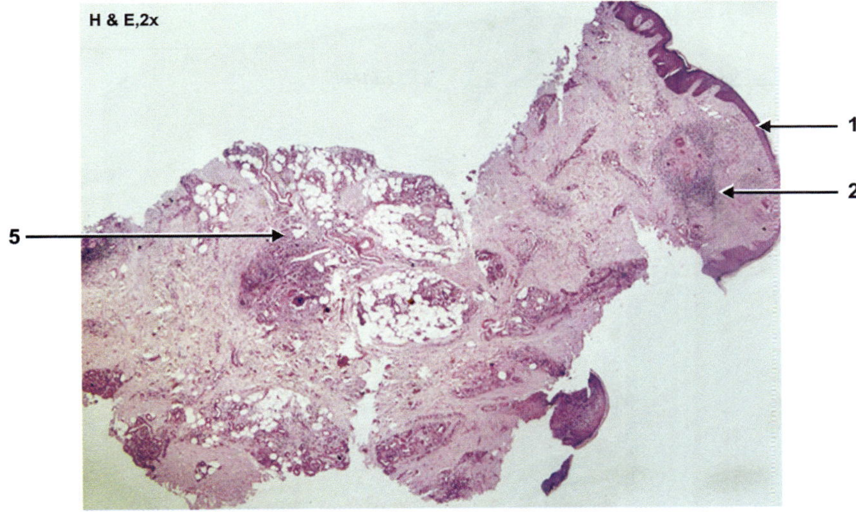

Fig. 36.38

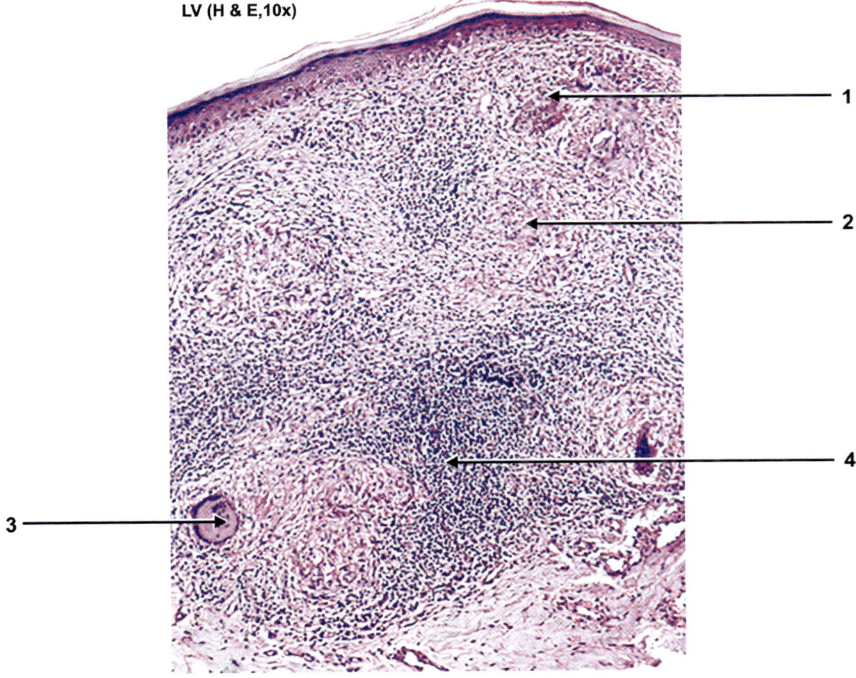

Fig. 36.39

Figs 36.38 and 36.39: Lupus vulgaris with an atrophic epidermis overlying the infiltrate. (1) The upper dermis shows confluent lichenoid granulomatous infiltrate comprising of epithelioid cells (2) Langhans' giant cells (3), with dense cuffing of lymphocytes (4). Lower dermis and subcutis also show discrete granulomas (5)

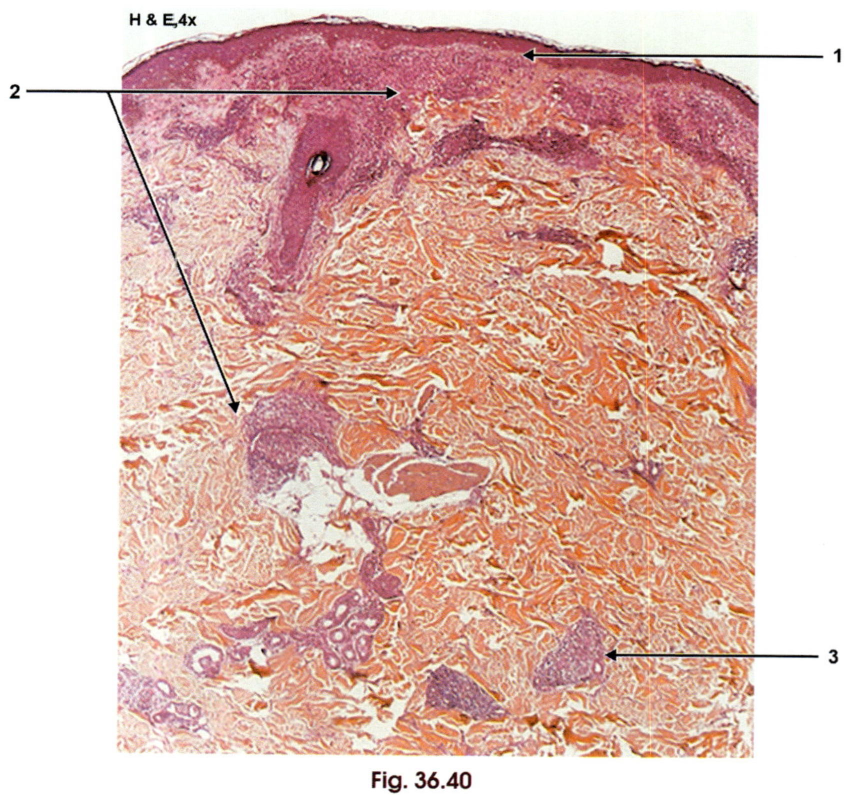

Fig. 36.40

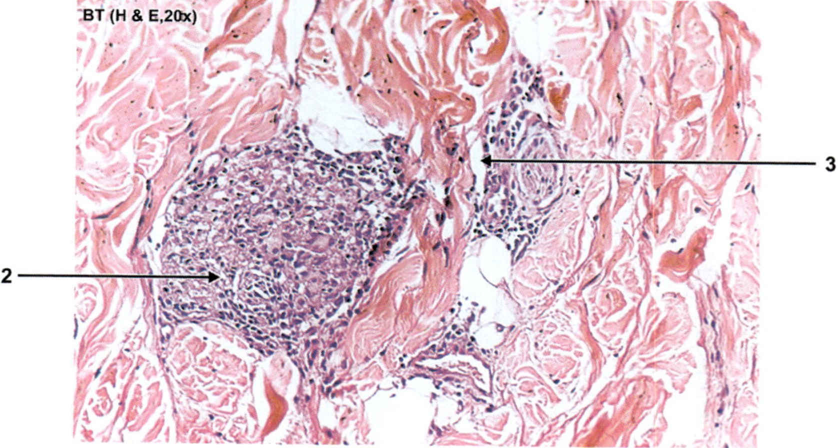

Fig. 36.41

Figs 36.40 and 36.41: Borderline tuberculoid leprosy showing an atrophic epidermis (1). Dermis shows superficial and deep, oblong, sharply demarcated granulomas (2) composed of epithelioid cells, Langhans' giant cells and dense cuff of peripheral lymphocytes in perivascular, periadnexal and perineural (3) distributions

BL (10x)

Fig. 36.42

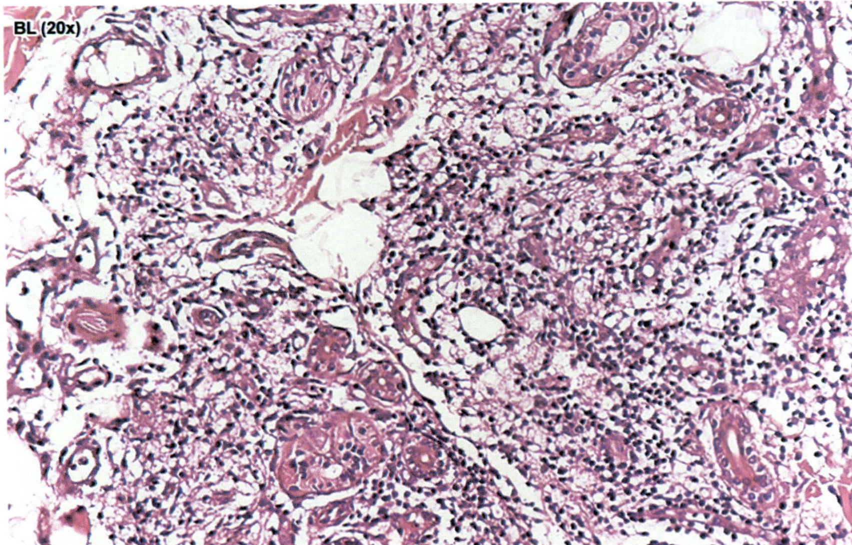

Fig. 36.43

Figs 36.42 and 36.43: Borderline lepromatous leprosy. The lymphocytes are prominent and accumulate around neurovascular bundles, the superficial and deep dermal vessels, sweat gland and erector pili muscles. There is tendency for activation of macrophages to form poorly to moderately defined granulomas. Perineural fibroblast proliferation, forming an "onion skin" in crcss section, is typical. BI ranges from 4 to 5

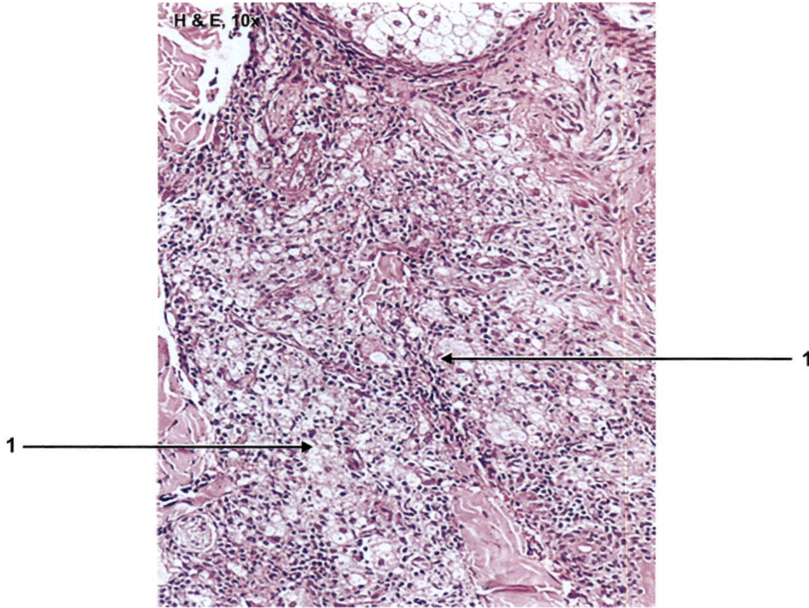

Fig. 36.44

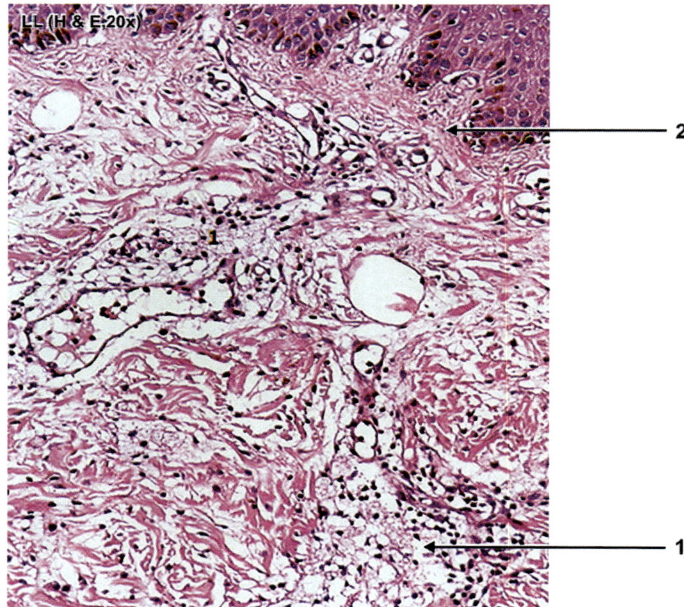

Fig. 36.45

Figs 36.44 and 36.45: Lepromatous leprosy shows an extensive cellular infiltrate separated (1) from the flattened epidermis by a narrow grenz label zone of normal collagen (2). There is diffuse infiltrate of foamy histiocytes (1)

Fig. 36.46

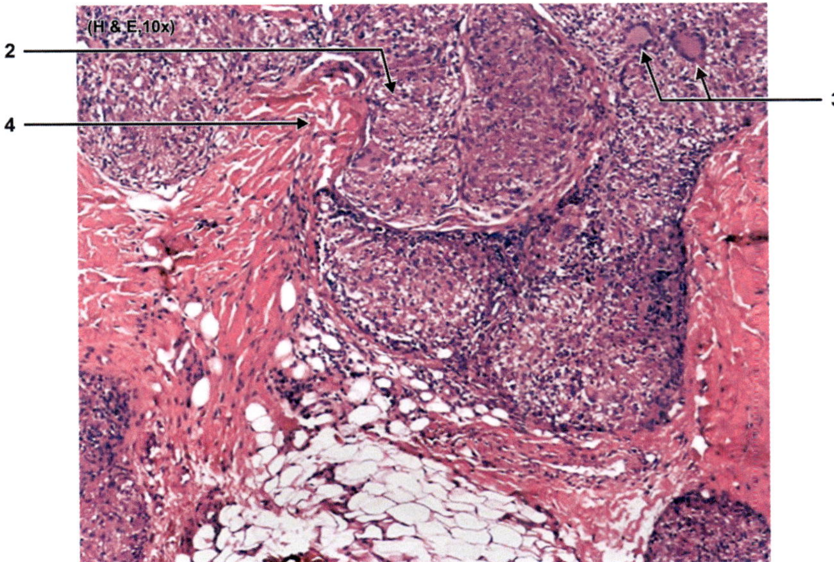

Fig. 36.47

Figs 36.46 and 36.47: Sarcoidosis showing an atrophic epidermis (1). There are compact non-necrotizing granulomas (2) composed of epithelioid cells, Langhans' giant cells (3) and sparse lymphocytes (naked granulomas) throughout the dermis and extending to the subcutis. Perigranulomatous fibrosis is present (4)

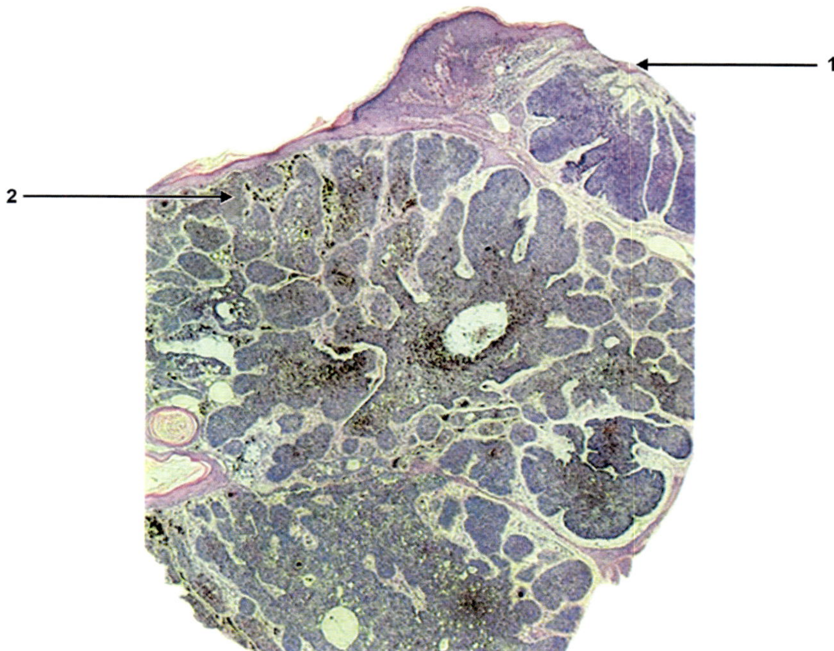

Fig. 36.48

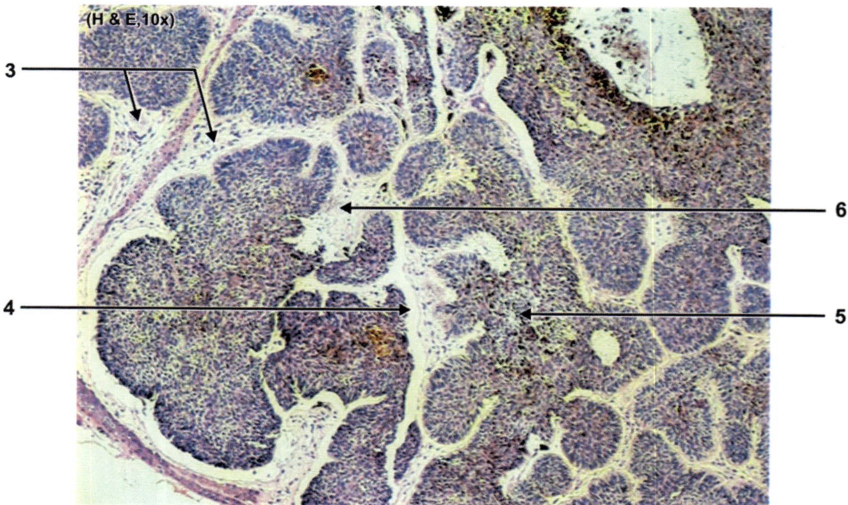

Fig. 36.49

Figs 36.48 and 36.49: Basal cell carcinoma with focally ulcerated epidermis (1). Entire dermis shows nests of basaloid cells arising from the epidermis (2), with palisading of cells in the periphery (3). The tumor cells demonstrate hyperchromatic nuclei and little cytoplasm. Between the tumor islands and surrounding stroma, retraction spaces are present (4). Melanin pigment is prominent within tumor nests (5). The stroma appears myxoid (6)

Bibliography

1. **Dermatology**
    - **Rook's** Textbook of Dermatology 9th edn
    - **Fitzpatrick's** Dermatology 9th Edition
    - **Bolognia**. Dermatology, 4th ed, 2018.
    - Diagnosis and Management of Skin Disorders: An Evidence Based Approach. Paperback-1, January 2012. 1st Edn LWW. Delhi.
2. **Immunology**
    - **Clinical Immunology** Principles and Practice Fourth Edition © 2013, Elsevier Limited All rights reserved.
    - **Immunology**, 8th edn, https://www.inkling.com/read/immunology-male-brostoff-roth-roitt-8th/chapter-11/t-cell-regulation-of-the-immune-system.
3. **Eczema**
    - **Contact Dermatitis**, DOI: 10.1007/978-3-642-03827-3_19,© Springer-Verlag Berlin Heidelberg 2011.
    - **Handbook of Eczema for Dermatologists**. Sardana K, Khurana A, Rani S. CBS Publishers, New Delhi,2018.
    - Pigmented Contact Dermatitis and Chemical Depigmentation. JD Johansen, et al. (eds.): Contact Dermatitis,DOI: 10.1007/978-3-642-03827-3_19,© Springer-Verlag Berlin Heidelberg 2011.
4. **Infectious Diseases**
    - Infectious Diseases Mandell, **Douglas, and Bennett's** Principles and Practice of Infectious Diseases,8th Edition.
5. **Rheumatology**
    - **Kelly** Textbook of Rheumatology, 10th edition, 2017.
    - Rheumatology—**Hochbergs** https://expertconsult.inkling.com/read/hochberg-rheumatology-2-vol-set-7e. [Hochberg Rheumatology]
6. **Leprosy**
    - Handbook of Leprosy, 5E (Pb-2015). WH Jopling AC McDougall CBS, 2015.
    - Leprosy, 2nd ed, Hastings Churchill Livingstone, Edinburgh; New York.
    - Jopling's Handbook of Leprosy, 7th edition, CBS Publishers, 2020, New Delhi.
7. **Dermatopathology**

    McKee's Pathology of the Skin, 4th edn, 2011.
8. **Nail Disorders**

    Nails: Scher and Daniel's Nails, accessed on 2 January 2019.
9. **STD**
    - Sexually Transmitted Diseases, 4th edn. Holmes KK (eds). Tata McGraw, Copyright ©2008.
    - Venereal Diseases by King and Nicol.

10. **Specialized Books**
    - Dermoscopy in Darker Skin. Chatterjee M, Neema S, Malakar S., Eds. Jaypee Bros. New Delhi, India, 2017.
    - Genodermatoses: A Clinical Guide to Genetic Skin Disorders, Second Edition, 2005.
    - Hair Loss Disorders, Restoration and Management, 2nd ed. 2018 CBS.
    - Handbook of Pigmentary Disorders for Practitioners. CBS Publishers, 2018.
    - Lasers and Energy Devices in Aesthetic Dermatology, Practice 1st edn. 2018. Jaypee.
    - **Clinical Approach to Acne Vulgaris** (Hb-2015) 1st edn. CBS.
    - **Diagnosis and Management of Skin Disorders: An Evidence Based Approach**. Paperback-1, January 2012. 1st Edn LWW. Delhi.

Index

C

D

E

F

G

M

N

O

P

R

S